Minidictionary for Nurses

Eighth Edition

SEE WEB LINKS

For recommended web links for this title, visit www.oxfordreference.com/page/nursing when you see this sign.

Minidictionary for **Nurses**

Eighth Edition

CONSULTANT

Tanya A. McFerran MA, SRN, RSCN, Cert. Ed.
Senior Lecturer, Department of Midwifery, Child and Community Nursing, Faculty of Health, Social Care and Education, Anglia Ruskin University, Essex

EDITOR

Elizabeth A. Martin MA
Market House Books Ltd

OXFORD
UNIVERSITY PRESS

OXFORD
UNIVERSITY PRESS

Oxford University Press is a department of the University of Oxford. It furthers the University's objective of excellence in research, scholarship, and education by publishing worldwide. Oxford is a registered trademark of Oxford University Press in the UK and in certain other countries

Published in India by
Oxford University Press
2/11 Ground floor, Ansari Road, Daryaganj, New Delhi 110002, India

First edition, published as *Pocket Dictionary for Nurses*, 1984
Second edition 1991
Third edition 1995
Fourth edition 1998
Fifth edition 2003
Sixth edition 2008
Seventh edition 2014
Eighth edition 2017

ISBN: 978-0-19-881717-8

Reprinted 2017

Printed in India by Replika Press Pvt. Ltd,

Preface

This new edition of the *Minidictionary for Nurses* provides, in almost 10,500 entries, explanations of the terms and concepts likely to be encountered by student and practising nurses and allied health professionals during the course of their work and training. In addition to terms relating specifically to the nursing profession and the nursing process, there are many entries in the fields of medicine, surgery, anatomy and physiology, ethics, statistics, endocrinology, psychiatry, and pharmacology. For this edition, many new terms have been added, increasing the coverage of such fields as lymphology, medical research, and critical care nursing. Drug names reflect the use of recommended International Non-proprietary Names (rINNs).

Each entry contains a pronunciation guide, the part of speech, and a concisely written definition without the use of unnecessary technical jargon. The pronunciation guide follows that used in the *Oxford Paperback Dictionary* and provides an easy and accessible guide to correct pronunciation without the use of special symbols. Most definitions comprise a single sentence, but, where necessary, further explanation is given. Many terms in medicine are used in combination (for example, **acute abscess**, **apical abscess**, etc.) and each of these phrases is treated as a separate definition within the main entry (**abscess** in this example). Derived terms (for example, adjectives derived from nouns) are not normally included as separate entries except where their meanings cannot be deduced from the words from which they are derived. Instead they are listed at the end of the definition of the parent word together with the part of speech and, where necessary, a pronunciation guide.

The Appendices include a comprehensive selection of tables of reference values for biochemical data, obtained from the *Oxford Textbook of Medicine* (fifth edition, 2005), together with tables of SI units, conversion tables to and from other systems of units, formulae for calculating drug dosages, and immunization schedules. For this edition we have also included the most recent version of the NMC Code of professional conduct.

In the preparation of this dictionary a range of entries has been adapted from the *Concise Medical Dictionary*, first published by the Oxford University Press in 1980 (ninth edition published 2015).

J. L.
T. McF
2016

Credits

Editors (Market House Books Ltd)

Elizabeth Martin MA
Jonathan Law BA

Contributors and Advisers

Dr Sandeep Bajwa MRCP
Dr Deborah Bowman MA, PhD
Dr Mark Donnelly FRCP
P. J. T. Drew MD, FRCP
Peter Glennon MD, FRCP
Pamela A. Hall BM, DPH, MFPHM
T. Q. Howes MA, MB, BS, MD, MRCP(I)
Dr J. Craig Jobling MA, MB, BChir, FRCS, FRCR
Nikhil Kaushik FRCOphth
Matthew Kurien MRCP
Dr Peter Lepping MD, MRCPsych, MSc
H. Manji MA, MD, FRCP
D. J. McFerran MA, FRCS
Tanya McFerran MA, SRN, RSCH, Cert. ed.
Dr Alpa Patel MB, BS, MRCGP, DRCOG
Amin Rahemtulla PhD, FRCP
Dr Alexandra Taylor MRCP, FRCR, MD
Jonathan White BSc (Hons), MRCP (UK)
Clare Willocks MBChB, BSc (Hons), MRCOG

Contents

Pronunciation guide

A pronunciation guide is given in brackets after the entry word and before the part of speech. Words of two or more syllables are broken up into small units, usually of one syllable, separated by hyphens. The stressed syllable in a word of two or more syllables is shown in bold type.

The sounds represented are as follows:

a *as in* back (bak), active (**ak**-tiv)
ă *as in* abduct (ăb-**dukt**), gamma (**gam**-ă)
ah *as in* after (**ahf**-ter), palm (pahm)
air *as in* aerosol (**air**-ŏ-sol), care (kair)
ar *as in* tar (tar), heart (hart)
aw *as in* jaw (jaw), gall (gawl)
ay *as in* mania (**may**-nia), grey (gray)
b *as in* bed (bed)
ch *as in* chin (chin)
d *as in* day (day)
e *as in* red (red)
ĕ *as in* bowel (**bow**-ĕl)
ee *as in* see (see), haem (heem), caffeine (**kaf**-een)
eer *as in* fear (feer), serum (**seer**-ŭm)
er *as in* dermal (**der**-măl), labour (**lay**-ber)
ew *as in* dew (dew), nucleus (**new**-kli-ŭs)
ewr *as in* pure (pewr), dura (**dewr**-ă)
f *as in* fat (fat), phobia (**foh**-biă), cough (kof)
g *as in* gag (gag)
h *as in* hip (hip)
i *as in* fit (fit), acne (**ak**-ni), reduction (ri-**duk**-shŏn)
I *as in* eye (I), angiitis (an-ji-**I**-tis)
j *as in* jaw (jaw), gene (jeen), ridge (rij)
k *as in* kidney (**kid**-ni), chlorine (**klor**-een)
ks *as in* toxic (**toks**-ik)
kw *as in* quadrate (**kwod**-rayt)
l *as in* liver (**liv**-er)
m *as in* milk (milk)

n *as in* nit (nit)
ng *as in* sing (sing)
nk *as in* rank (rank), bronchus (**bronk**-ŭs)
o *as in* pot (pot)
ŏ *as in* buttock (**but**-ŏk)
oh *as in* home (hohm), post (pohst)
oi *as in* boil (boil)
oo *as in* food (food), croup (kroop), fluke (flook)
oor *as in* pruritus (proor-**I**-tŭs)
or *as in* organ (**or**-găn), wart (wort)
ow *as in* powder (**pow**-der), pouch (powch)
p *as in* pill (pil)
r *as in* rib (rib)
s *as in* skin (skin), cell (sel)
sh *as in* shock (shok), action (**ak**-shŏn)
t *as in* tone (tohn)
th *as in* bath (bahth)
th as in then (*th*en)
u *as in* pulp (pulp), blood (blud)
ŭ *as in* typhus (**ty**-fŭs)
uu *as in* hook (huuk)
v *as in* vein (vayn)
w *as in* wind (wind)
y *as in* yeast (yeest) or, when preceded by a consonant, *as in* bite (byt)
yoo *as in* unit (**yoo**-nit), formula (**form**-yoo-lă)
yoor *as in* ureter (yoor-**ee**-ter)
yr *as in* fire (fyr)
z *as in* zinc (zink), glucose (**gloo**-kohz)
zh as in vision (**vi*zh***-ŏn)

A consonant is sometimes doubled to prevent accidental mispronunciation of a syllable resembling a familiar word; for example **ass**-id (acid), rather than **as**-id; ultră-**sonn**-iks (ultrasonics), rather than ultră-**son**-iks.

An apostrophe is used (i) between two consonants forming a syllable, as in **den**-t'l (dental), and (ii) between two letters when the syllable might otherwise be mispronounced through resembling a familiar word, as in **th'e**-ră-pi (therapy), th'y (thigh), and tal'k (talc).

Aa

a- (an-) *prefix denoting* absence of; lacking; not.

AA *n.* *see* Alcoholics Anonymous.

AAA *n.* *see* (abdominal aortic) aneurysm.

A & E medicine *n.* accident and emergency medicine: an important specialty dealing with the immediate problems of the acutely ill and injured. *See also* ED.

ab- *prefix denoting* away from.

abarticulation (ab-ar-tik-yoo-lay-shŏn) *n.* **1.** the dislocation of a joint. **2.** a synovial joint (*see* diarthrosis).

abasia (ă-bay-ziă) *n.* inability to walk normally for which there is no identifiable physical cause. The patient displays normal motor ability when sitting or lying down, suggesting that a psychogenic reaction may be involved (*see* conversion disorder). **Astasia-abasia** (also known as **Blocq's disease**) is abasia with the inability to stand.

abbreviated injury scale (a-**bree**-vi-ay-tid) *n.* a quick method for determining the severity of a case of serious trauma. It can be used for purposes of triage and clinical audit.

abdomen (**ab**-dŏm-ĕn) *n.* the part of the body cavity below the chest (*see* thorax), from which it is separated by the diaphragm. The abdomen contains the organs of digestion (stomach, liver, intestines, etc.), excretion (kidneys, bladder, etc.), and in women reproduction (ovaries and

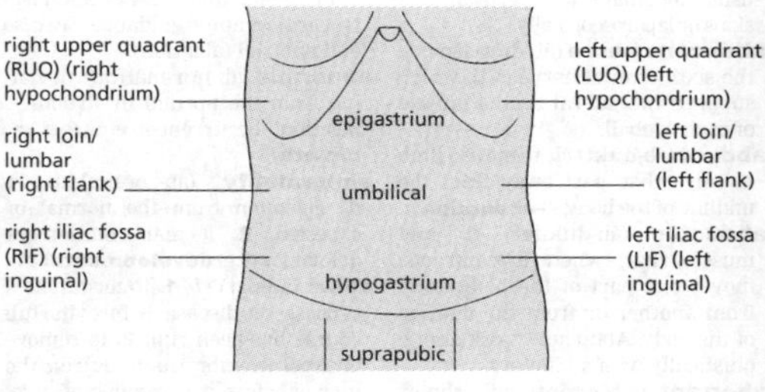

Regions and quadrants of the abdomen

uterus). It is lined by a membrane, the peritoneum. See illustration. **—abdominal** (ăb-**dom**-i-năl) *adj.*

abdominal dehiscence (di-**hiss**-ĕns) *n. see* burst abdomen.

abdominal thrusts (Heimlich manoeuvre) *pl. n.* a manoeuvre for the treatment of choking in which the patient is held firmly around the midriff just under the ribcage. The hands of the rescuer are held as a fist and short sharp thrusts into the patient's upper abdomen are made in order to dislodge the obstructing article from the airway. This procedure should not be performed on children under the age of one year.

abdominoperineal resection (ăb-dom-in-oh-pe-ri-**nee**-ăl) *n.* surgical excision of the anal sphincter, rectum, and part of the sigmoid colon due to cancer. The remaining length of sigmoid colon is brought through the abdominal wall (*see* colostomy). This procedure may be performed using abdominal and perineal incisions or laparoscopically.

abducens nerve (ăb-**dew**-sĕnz) *n.* the sixth cranial nerve (VI), which supplies the lateral rectus muscle of each eyeball.

abduct (ăb-**dukt**) *vb.* to move a limb or any other part away from the midline of the body. **—abduction** *n.*

abductor (ăb-**duk**-ter) *n.* any muscle that, when it contracts, moves one part of the body away from another or from the midline of the body. Abductors work antagonistically with adductors.

aberrant (ă-**b'e**-rănt) *adj.* abnormal: usually applied to a blood vessel or nerve that does not follow its normal course.

aberration (ab-er-**ay**-shŏn) *n.* **1.** deviation from the normal. **2.** a defect in the image formed by an optical device (e.g. a lens). **chromatic a.** a defect in which the image has coloured fringes as a result of the different extent to which light of different colours is refracted. **spherical a.** a defect in which the image is blurred because curvature of the lens causes light rays from the object to come to a focus in slightly different positions.

ABGs *pl. n. see* arterial blood gases.

ablation (ăb-**lay**-shŏn) *n.* the removal or destruction of tissue or an abnormal growth by surgery, heat, hormones, or other drugs. **radiofrequency a.** the destruction of abnormal conducting tissue in the heart in patients with supraventricular tachycardia by the use of radiofrequency energy delivered via catheter under X-ray and electrocardiographic guidance. *See also* endometrial (ablation).

abnormal (ab-**nor**-măl) *adj.* deviating from the normal in structure, position, occurrence, etc. (e.g. **a. growth**).

abnormality (ab-nor-**mal**-iti) *n.* **1.** deviation from the normal or expected. **2.** a malformation or deformity (e.g. **developmental a.**).

abort (ă-**bort**) *vb.* **1.** to terminate a process or disease before its full course has been run. **2.** to remove or expel an embryo or fetus from the uterus before it is capable of independent existence. *See* abortion.

abortifacient (ă-bor-ti-fay-shĕnt) *n.* a drug that induces abortion or miscarriage.

abortion (ă-bor-shŏn) *n.* **1. (induced abortion, termination of pregnancy)** the removal of an embryo or fetus from the uterus at a stage of pregnancy when it is deemed incapable of independent survival (i.e. at any time between conception and the 24th week of pregnancy). In the UK the procedure must be carried out within the terms of the Abortion Act 1967 as amended by the Human Fertilization and Embryology Act 1990. **2. (spontaneous abortion)** *see* miscarriage. **—abortive** *adj.*

SEE WEB LINKS

- Information on induced abortion from Marie Stopes International UK

abortus (ă-bor-tŭs) *n.* a fetus, weighing less than 500 g, that is expelled from the uterus either dead or incapable of surviving.

ABO system *n. see* blood group.

ABPI *n. see* ankle–brachial pressure index.

abrasion (ă-bray-zhŏn) *n.* a minor wound in which the surface of the skin or a mucous membrane is worn away by rubbing or scraping.

abreaction (ab-ree-**ak**-shŏn) *n.* the therapeutic release of strong emotion commonly associated with the retrieval of a buried memory. This intervention is now largely obsolete in psychiatric practice.

abruptio placentae (placental abruption) (ă-brup-ti-oh plă-sent-i) *n.* bleeding from the placenta causing its complete or partial detachment from the uterine wall after the 24th week of gestation. Abruptio placentae is often associated with hypertension and pre-eclampsia. It is often an unanticipated emergency, as a small bleed (antepartum haemorrhage) can suddenly evolve into a major abruption and disseminated intravascular coagulation.

abscess (**ab**-sis) *n.* a collection of pus and necrotic tissue enclosed by damaged and inflamed tissues. **acute a.** an abscess associated with pain, inflammation, and some fever. **apical a.** an abscess in the bone around the tip of the root of a tooth. **Brodie's a.** a chronic abscess of bone that develops from acute bacterial osteomyelitis. **cerebral a.** an abscess resulting from infection of the brain or its meninges. **cold** or **chronic a.** an abscess, usually due to tuberculosis bacilli, in which there is little pain or inflammation. **psoas a.** a cold abscess in the psoas muscle (in the groin), which has spread from diseased vertebrae in the lower part of the spine. **subphrenic a.** an abscess below the diaphragm, usually resulting from a spread of infection from the abdomen. **tropical** (or **amoebic**) **a.** an abscess of the liver caused by infection with *Entamoeba histolytica*. *See also* ischiorectal abscess.

absence (**ab**-sĕns) *n.* (in neurology) *see* epilepsy.

absorption (ăb-**sorp**-shŏn) *n.* the uptake of digested food from the intestine into the blood and lymphatic systems. *See also* assimilation, digestion.

a.c. (ante cibum) Latin: before food, used as a direction in prescriptions.

acanthosis (ak-ăn-**thoh**-sis) *n.* an increase in the number of prickle cells in the innermost layer of the epidermis, leading to thickening of the epidermis. **a. nigricans** acanthosis associated with insulin resistance and overweight, characterized by papillomatous growths, mainly in the armpits, neck, and groin, which give the skin a pigmented appearance and a velvety texture. It may be benign or malignant.

acapnia (hypocapnia) (ă-**kap**-niă) *n.* a condition in which there is an abnormally low concentration of carbon dioxide in the blood.

acarbose (ass-ar-bohz) *n.* an oral hypoglycaemic drug that reduces the breakdown and absorption of carbohydrates in the intestine by blocking the action of an important enzyme (α-glucosidase) in this process. Trade name: **Glucobay**.

acardia (ay-**kar**-diă) *n.* congenital absence of the heart. The condition may occur in conjoined twins; the twin with the heart controls the circulation for both.

acariasis (akă-**ry**-ă-sis) *n.* an infestation of mites and ticks.

acaricide (ă-**ka**-ri-syd) *n.* any chemical agent used for destroying mites and ticks.

acatalasia (ă-kat-ă-**lay**-ziă) *n.* a rare inborn lack of the enzyme catalase, leading to recurrent infections of the gums (gingivitis) and mouth.

accessory muscles (ăk-**sess**-er-i) *pl. n.* muscles of the shoulder girdle and chest wall that (in addition to the intercostal muscles and the diaphragm) are utilized during respiratory distress to help the flow of air in and out of the lungs.

accessory nerve (spinal accessory nerve) *n.* the eleventh cranial nerve (XI), which arises from two roots, cranial and spinal. Fibres from the cranial root form the recurrent laryngeal nerve, which supplies the internal laryngeal muscles; fibres from the spinal root supply the sternomastoid and trapezius muscles, in the neck region.

accident (**ak**-sid-ĕnt) *n.* a traumatic incident involving any part of the body. **Accident and emergency** (**A & E**) **medicine** is a specialized area of patient care dealing with acute illness.

accommodation (ă-kom-ŏ-**day**-shŏn) *n.* adjustment of the shape of the lens to change the focus of the eye. When the ciliary muscle (*see* ciliary body) is relaxed, the lens is flattened and the eye is then able to focus on distant objects. To focus the eye on near objects the ciliary muscles contract and the lens becomes more spherical. Adjustments in convergence also contribute to accommodation. **a. reflex** the change in shape of the lens (which becomes more convex), constriction of the pupils, and inward turning of the eyes that occur when an individual focuses on a near object.

accouchement (ă-**koosh**-mahnt) *n.* delivery of a baby.

accountability (ă-kownt-ă-**bil**-iti) *n.* (in nursing) the obligation of being answerable for one's own judgments and actions to an appropriate person or authority recognized as having the right to demand information and explanation, according to the terms of reference of the NMC Code of Professional Conduct (see Appendix 17). A registered practitioner (nurse, midwife, health visitor) is accountable for her or his actions as a professional at all times, on or off duty, whether engaged in current practice or not. *See also* responsibility.

accreditation (ă-kred-i-**tay**-shŏn) *n.* **1.** formal recognition by an organization of an individual as an approved and acknowledged representative, e.g. of a union or staff organization. **2.** (in the USA, Australasia, and some European countries) the licensing of a hospital by government agencies, subject to its meeting certain prerequisite conditions.

Accreditation of Prior (Experiential) Learning *n. see* APEL.

accretion (ă-**kree**-shŏn) *n.* the accumulation of deposits in an organ or cavity. Calculi may be formed by accretion.

acebutolol (ass-i-**bew**-toh-lol) *n.* a beta blocker drug used to treat high blood pressure, angina pectoris, and irregular heart rhythms. It is administered by mouth. Trade name: **Sectral**.

ACE inhibitor (ayss) *n.* angiotensin-converting enzyme inhibitor: any one of a group of drugs used in the treatment of raised blood pressure and heart failure. ACE inhibitors act by interfering with the action of the enzyme that converts the inactive angiotensin I to the powerful artery constrictor angiotensin II. ACE inhibitors are administered by mouth; they include **perindopril arginine** (Coversyl Arginine) and **ramipril** (Tritace). *See also* captopril, enalapril.

acephalus (ă-**sef**-ă-lŭs) *n.* a fetus without a head. —**acephalous** *adj.*

acetabuloplasty (ass-i-**tab**-yoo-loh-plas-ti) *n.* an operation in which the shape of the acetabulum is modified to correct congenital dislocation of the hip or to treat osteoarthritis.

acetabulum (cotyloid cavity) (ass-i-**tab**-yoo-lŭm) *n.* (*pl.* **acetabula**) either of the two deep sockets, one on each side of the hip bone, into which the head of the thigh bone (femur) fits at the hip joint.

acetaminophen (ass-ee-tă-**min**-ŏ-fen) *n. see* paracetamol.

acetate (ass-it-ayt) *n.* any salt or ester of acetic acid.

acetazolamide (ass-ee-tă-**zol**-ă-myd) *n.* a carbonic anhydrase inhibitor used mainly in the treatment of glaucoma to reduce the pressure inside the eyeball and also as a preventative for epileptic seizures and altitude sickness. Trade name: **Diamox**.

acetic acid (ă-**see**-tik) *n.* the acid that is present in vinegar. It is used in the preparation of astringent and antiseptic medicines and in urine testing. Formula: CH_3COOH.

acetoacetic acid (ass-i-toh-ă-**see**-tik) *n.* an organic acid produced in large amounts by the liver in such conditions as starvation. Formula: CH_3COCH_2COOH. *See also* ketone.

acetonaemia (ass-i-toh-**nee**-miă) *n.* the presence of ketone bodies in the blood. *See* ketone.

acetone (**ass**-i-tohn) *n.* an organic compound that is produced by the liver in such conditions as starvation. Acetone is of great value as a solvent. Formula: CH_3COCH_3. **a. body** *see* ketone.

acetonuria (ass-i-toh-**newr**-iă) *n. see* ketonuria.

acetylcholine (ass-i-tyl-**koh**-leen) *n.* the acetic acid ester of the organic base choline: the neurotransmitter released at the synapses of parasympathetic nerves and at neuromuscular junctions. Acetylcholine (Miochol-E, Miphtel) is instilled into the anterior chamber of the eye as a miotic during intraocular surgery.

acetylcholinesterase inhibitor (ass-i-tyl-koh-lin-**est**-er-ayz) *n.* a drug that blocks the action of acetylcholinesterase (*see* cholinesterase). Acetylcholinsterase inhibitors are used to slow down the rate of cognitive decline in mild to moderate Alzheimer's disease, which is associated with a reduction in acetylcholine levels. The group includes **donepezil** (Aricept), **galantamine** (Reminyl), and **rivastigmine** (Exelon).

acetylcoenzyme A (ass-i-tyl-koh-**en**-zym) *n.* a compound formed by the combination of an acetate molecule with coenzyme A. Acetylcoenzyme A has an important role in the Krebs cycle.

acetylcysteine (ass-i-tyl-**sis**-ti-een) *n.* a drug that is administered as eye drops for the treatment of dry eyes, as in Sjögren's syndrome; as an intravenous infusion, it is used to prevent liver damage in paracetamol overdosage. Trade name: **Ilube**.

acetylsalicylic acid (ass-i-tyl-sa-li-**sil**-ik) *n. see* aspirin.

achalasia (ak-ă-**lay**-ziă) *n.* a disorder of the oesophagus (gullet) characterized by uncoordinated or absent contraction of oesophageal smooth muscle and incomplete relaxation of the lower oesophageal sphincter (LOS), leading to disturbances of swallowing (*see* dysphagia).

Achilles tendon (ă-**kil**-eez) *n.* the tendon of the muscles of the calf of the leg (the gastrocnemius and soleus muscles), situated at the back of the ankle and attached to the calcaneus (heel bone).

achillorrhaphy (ak-i-**lo**-răfi) *n.* surgical repair of the Achilles tendon.

achillotomy (ak-i-**lot**-ŏmi) *n.* surgical division of the Achilles tendon.

achlorhydria (ay-klor-**hy**-driă) *n.* absence of hydrochloric acid in the stomach. It is associated with many conditions, including autoimmune diseases (such as pernicious anaemia), Helicobacter infection, and previous gastric surgery.

acholia (ă-**koh**-liă) *n.* absence or deficiency of bile secretion or failure of the bile to enter the alimentary canal.

acholuria (ak-oh-**lewr**-iă) *n.* absence of the bile pigments from the urine, which occurs in some forms of jaundice (**acholuric jaundice**). —**acholuric** *adj.*

achondroplasia (ă-kon-droh-**play**-ziă) *n.* a disorder, inherited as a dominant characteristic, in which the bones of the arms and legs fail to grow to normal size. It results in a type of dwarfism characterized by short limbs, a normal-sized head and body, and normal intelligence. —**achondroplastic** (ă-kon-droh-**plas**-tik) *adj.*

achromatic (ak-roh-**mat**-ik) *adj.* without colour. —**achromasia** (ak-roh-**may**-ziă) *n.*

achromatopsia (ă-kroh-mă-**top**-siă) *n.* the inability to differentiate different shades of colour. Such complete colour blindness is very rare and is usually determined by hereditary factors.

aciclovir (acyclovir) *n.* (ay-**sy**-klŏ-veer) an antiviral drug that inhibits DNA synthesis in cells infected by herpesviruses. Administered topically, by mouth, or intravenously, it is used in the treatment of herpes simplex, herpes zoster, and herpes encephalitis. Trade name: **Zovirax**.

acid (ass-id) *n.* a substance that releases hydrogen ions when dissolved in water, has a pH below 7 and turns litmus paper red, and reacts with a base to form a salt and water only. *Compare* base.

acidaemia (asid-**ee**-miă) *n.* a condition of abnormally high blood acidity. *See also* acidosis. *Compare* alkalaemia.

acid-base balance *n.* the balance between the amount of carbonic acid and bicarbonate in the blood, which must be maintained at a constant ratio of 1:20 in order to keep the hydrogen ion concentration of the plasma at a constant value (pH 7.4).

acid-fast *adj.* **1.** describing bacteria that have been stained and continue to hold the stain after treatment with an acidic solution (**a.-f. bacilli**, **AFB**). **2.** describing a stain that is not removed from a specimen by washing with an acidic solution.

acidity (ă-**sid**-iti) *n.* the state of being acid. The degree of acidity of a solution is measured on the pH scale (*see* pH).

acidosis (asid-**oh**-sis) *n.* a condition in which the acidity of body fluids and tissues is abnormally high. This arises because of a failure of the mechanisms responsible for maintaining a balance between acids and alkalis in the blood (*see* acid-base balance). *See also* ketoacidosis, lactic acidosis. —**acidotic** (asid-**ot**-ik) *adj.*

acid phosphatase *n.* an enzyme secreted in the seminal fluid by the prostate gland.

acinus (ass-in-ŭs) *n.* (*pl.* **acini**) **1.** a small sac or cavity surrounded by the secretory cells of a gland. **2.** (in the lung) the tissue supplied with air by one terminal bronchiole. —**acinous** *adj.*

acne (acne vulgaris) (ak-ni vul-**gar**-iss) *n.* a common inflammatory disorder of the sebaceous glands. It involves the face, back, and chest and is characterized by the presence of blackheads with papules, pustules, and – in more severe cases – cysts and scars. Mild cases respond to topical therapy with benzoyl peroxide; treatment for more refractory conditions includes long-term antibiotics and oral isotretinoin. Exogenous or occupational factors, such as occlusion from tight or impermeable clothes, make-up, or chemicals, may trigger or exacerbate acne.

acoustic (ă-**koo**-stik) *adj.* of or relating to sound or the sense of hearing. **a. nerve** *see* cochlear nerve. **a. neuroma** *see* (vestibular) schwannoma.

acquired (ă-**kwyrd**) *adj.* describing a condition or disorder contracted after birth and not attributable to hereditary causes. *Compare* congenital.

acquired immune deficiency syndrome *n. see* AIDS.

acro- *combining form denoting* **1.** extremity; tip. **2.** height; promontory. **3.** extreme; intense.

acrocentric (ak-roh-**sen**-trik) *n.* a chromosome in which the centromere is situated at or very near one end. **—acrocentric** *adj.*

acrocyanosis (ak-roh-sy-ă-**noh**-sis) *n.* bluish-purple discoloration of the hands and feet due to slow circulation of the blood through the small vessels in the skin.

acrodermatitis enteropathica (ak-roh-der-mă-**ty**-tis en-ter-oh-**path**-ikă) *n.* an inherited inability to absorb sufficient zinc, which causes patchy sparse hair, patches of dry scaly skin on the hands, feet, scalp, and around the mouth and anogenital region, and chronic diarrhoea.

acrodynia (ak-roh-**din**-iă) *n. see* pink disease.

acromegaly (ak-roh-**meg**-ăli) *n.* overgrowth of soft tissues and bones due to excessive secretion of growth hormone, usually by a benign tumour of the anterior pituitary gland.

acromion (ă-**kroh**-mi-ŏn) *n.* an oblong process at the top of the spine of the scapula, part of which articulates with the clavicle (collar bone) to form the **acromioclavicular joint**. **—acromial** *adj.*

acronyx (**ak**-rŏ-niks) *n.* an ingrowing toenail or fingernail. *See* ingrowing toenail.

acroparaesthesia (ak-roh-paris-**theez**-i-ă) *n.* a tingling sensation in the hands and feet.

acrophobia (ak-rŏ-**foh**-biă) *n.* a morbid dread of heights.

acrosclerosis (ak-roh-skleer-**oh**-sis) *n.* a skin disease thought to be a type of generalized scleroderma, causing stiffness of the skin mainly affecting the hands, face, and feet.

acrosome (**ak**-rŏ-sohm) *n.* the cap-like structure on the front end of a spermatozoon.

ACTH (adrenocorticotrophic hormone, adrenocorticotrophin, corticotrophin) *n.* a hormone synthesized and stored in the anterior pituitary gland, controlling the secretion of corticosteroid hormones from the adrenal gland. Its release is stimulated by corticotrophin-releasing hormone.

actin (**ak**-tin) *n.* a protein, found in muscle, that plays an important role in the process of contraction. *See* striated muscle.

Actinomyces (ak-ti-noh-**my**-seez) *n.* a genus of Gram-positive nonmotile fungus-like bacteria that cause disease in animals and humans. **A. israelii** the causative organism of human actinomycosis.

actinomycin D (ak-ti-noh-**my**-sin) *n. see* dactinomycin.

actinomycosis (ak-ti-noh-my-**koh**-sis) *n.* a noncontagious disease caused by the bacterium *Actinomyces israelii* and resulting in the formation of multiple sinus tracts that open onto the skin. Actinomycosis most commonly affects the jaw but may also affect the lungs, brain, or intestines.

actinotherapy (ak-ti-noh-**th'**e-ră-pi) *n.* the treatment of disorders with infrared or ultraviolet radiation.

action potential (**ak**-shŏn) *n.* the change in voltage that occurs across the membrane of a nerve or muscle cell when a nerve impulse is triggered.

activator (**ak**-ti-vay-ter) *n.* a substance that stimulates a chemical change or reaction.

active movement (**ak**-tiv) *n.* movement brought about by a patient's own efforts. *Compare* passive movement.

active principle *n.* an ingredient of a drug that is actively involved in its therapeutic effect.

activin (**ak**-ti-vin) *n.* a protein complex that enhances the biosynthesis and secretion of follicle-stimulating hormone and helps to regulate the menstrual cycle. **Inhibin** is closely related and exerts an opposite effect.

activities of daily living (activities of living, ADLs, ALs) (ak-**tiv**-it-iz) *pl. n.* the routine activities that an individual does for himself or herself during the course of the day, such as eating, drinking, and washing. *See* Roper, Logan, and Tierney model.

actomyosin (ak-toh-**my**-oh-sin) *n.* a protein complex formed in muscle between actin and myosin during the process of contraction. *See* striated muscle.

acuity (ă-**kew**-iti) *n. see* visual acuity.

acupuncture (**ak**-yoo-punk-cher) *n.* a complementary therapy, developed by Eastern physicians, in which thin metal needles are inserted into selected points beneath the skin. It is used to relieve the symptoms of a wide range of physical and psychological conditions.

SEE WEB LINKS

- Website of the British Acupuncture Council, the UK's main regulatory body for the practice of acupuncture

acute (ă-**kewt**) *adj.* **1.** describing a disease of rapid onset, severe symptoms, and brief duration. *Compare* chronic. **2.** describing any intense symptom, such as severe pain.

acute abdomen *n.* the sudden uncontrolled development of severe abdominal symptoms secondary to disease or injury. Failure to establish a prompt diagnosis may lead to rapid clinical decline.

acute kidney injury (AKI, acute renal failure) *n.* kidney failure of rapid onset, usually diagnosed by changes in the serum creatinine concentration or the presence of oliguria. Dehydration often leads to AKI.

acute renal failure *n.* *see* acute kidney injury.

acute respiratory distress syndrome *n.* *see* adult respiratory distress syndrome.

acute rheumatism *n.* *see* rheumatic fever.

acyclovir *n.* *see* aciclovir.

acystia (ă-sis-tiă) *n.* congenital absence of the bladder.

ad- *prefix denoting* towards or near.

ADA deficiency *n.* *see* adenosine deaminase deficiency.

Adam's apple (laryngeal prominence) (ad-ămz) *n.* a projection, lying just under the skin, of the thyroid cartilage of the larynx.

adaptation (ad-ăp-tay-shŏn) *n.* **1.** the phenomenon in which a sense organ shows a gradually diminishing response to continuous or repetitive stimulation. **2.** a process of change to enable adjustment to a condition or an environment.

addiction (ă-dik-shŏn) *n.* a state of dependence produced either by the habitual taking of drugs or by regularly engaging in certain behaviours (e.g. gambling). *See also* alcoholism, tolerance.

Addisonian crisis (ad-i-soh-niăn) *n.* an acute medical emergency due to a lack of corticosteroid production by the body, caused by disease of the adrenal glands or long-term suppression of production by steroid medication. It manifests as low blood pressure and collapse, biochemical abnormalities, hypoglycaemia, and (if untreated) coma and death. [T. Addison (1793–1860), British physician]

Addison's disease (ad-i-sŏnz) *n.* a syndrome due to inadequate secretion of corticosteroid hormones by the adrenal glands. Symptoms include progressive deterioration, low blood pressure, and dark pigmentation of the skin. [T. Addison]

adduct (ă-dukt) *vb.* to move a limb or any other part towards the midline of the body. **—adduction** *n.*

adductor (ă-duk-ter) *n.* any muscle that moves one part of the body towards another or towards the midline of the body.

Adelaide Coma Scale (Paediatric Coma Scale) (ad-ĕ-layd) *n.* the Glasgow Coma Scale (GCS) adapted for use in children. Like the GCS, it assesses eye opening, verbal response, and motor response, giving a score out of 15, but takes account of the child's age and neurological development when evaluating responses.

aden- (adeno-) *combining form denoting* a gland or glands.

adenine (ad-ĕ-neen) *n.* one of the nitrogen-containing bases (*see* purine) that occurs in the nucleic acids DNA and RNA. *See also* ATP.

adenitis (ad-ĕ-ny-tis) *n.* inflammation of one or more glands or lymph nodes.

adenocarcinoma (ad-in-oh-kar-si-noh-mă) *n.* (*pl.* **adenocarcinomata**) a malignant epithelial tumour arising from glandular tissue. The term is also applied to tumours showing a glandular growth pattern.

adenohypophysis (ad-in-oh-hy-pof-i-sis) *n. see* pituitary gland.

adenoidectomy (ad-in-oid-**ek**-tŏmi) *n.* surgical removal of the adenoids.

adenoids (nasopharyngeal tonsil) (ad-in-oidz) *n.* a collection of lymphatic tissue in the nasopharynx. Enlargement of the adenoids can cause obstruction to breathing through the nose and can block the Eustachian tubes, causing glue ear.

adenolymphoma (ad-in-oh-lim-**foh**-mă) *n. see* Warthin's tumour.

adenoma (ad-in-**oh**-mă) *n.* (*pl.* **adenomata**) a benign tumour of epithelial origin that is derived from glandular tissue or exhibits clearly defined glandular structures. Adenomas may become malignant (*see* adenocarcinoma). **—adenomatous** *adj.*

adenomyoma (ad-in-oh-my-**oh**-mă) *n.* a benign tumour derived from glandular and muscular tissue. Adenomyomas frequently occur in the uterus.

adenomyosis (ad-in-oh-my-**oh**-sis) *n.* the infiltration of tissue resembling endometrium into the wall of the uterus. *See* endometriosis.

adenopathy (ad-in-**op**-ăthi) *n.* disease of a gland or glandlike structure, especially a lymph node.

adenosclerosis (ad-in-oh-skleer-**oh**-sis) *n.* hardening of a gland, usually due to calcification.

adenosine (ă-**den**-ŏ-seen) *n.* a compound containing adenine and the sugar ribose: it occurs in ATP (*see also* nucleoside). It is also injected or infused as an anti-arrhythmic drug to stop supraventricular tachycardias and restore a normal heart rhythm.

adenosine deaminase deficiency (ADA deficiency) (dee-am-in-ayz) *n.* a genetic disorder characterized by a defect in the enzyme **adenosine deaminase (ADA)**, which is involved in purine metabolism. Deficiency of this enzyme results in damage to the antibody-producing lymphocytes, which leads to severe combined immune deficiency (SCID).

adenosine diphosphate *n. see* ADP.

adenosine monophosphate *n. see* AMP.

adenosine triphosphate *n. see* ATP.

adenosis (ad-in-**oh**-sis) *n.* (*pl.* **adenoses**) **1.** excessive growth or development of glands. **2.** any disease of a gland or gland-like structure, especially of a lymph node.

adenovirus (ad-in-oh-**vy**-rŭs) *n.* one of a group of DNA-containing viruses causing infections of the upper respiratory tract that produce symptoms resembling those of the common cold.

ADH *n.* antidiuretic hormone (*see* vasopressin).

ADHD *n. see* attention-deficit/hyperactivity disorder.

adherence (ăd-**heer**-ĕnss) *n.* the degree to which a patient follows medical advice, as in attending appointments for courses of therapy. **medicines a. (compliance)**

taking medication in accordance with instructions. *Compare* nonadherence.

adhesion (ăd-**hee**-zhŏn) *n.* **1.** a fibrous band of connective tissue that develops in response to inflammation, trauma, or surgery, resulting in the union of two adjacent structures. Adhesions between loops of intestine often occur following abdominal surgery and may predispose to symptoms of abdominal pain or intestinal obstruction. **2.** a healing process in which the edges of a wound fit together.

adiaphoresis (ă-dy-ă-fŏ-**ree**-sis) *n.* deficient or reduced secretion of sweat. **—adiaphoretic** (ă-dy-ă-fŏ-**ret**-ik) *adj.*

Adie's pupil (ay-diz) *n. see* tonic (pupil). [W. J. Adie (1886–1935), British physician]

adipose tissue (ad-i-pohs) *n.* fibrous connective tissue packed with masses of fat cells. In adults it consists mostly of **white fat** (accounting for 20–25% body weight), which stores energy. Adipose tissue forms a thick layer under the skin and occurs around the kidneys and in the buttocks.

adiposis (liposis) (ad-i-**poh**-sis) *n.* the presence of abnormally large accumulations of fat in the body. The condition may arise from overeating, hormone irregularities, or a metabolic disorder. *See also* obesity.

adiposuria (ad-i-poh-**sewr**-iă) *n. see* lipuria.

aditus (ad-i-tŭs) *n.* an anatomical opening or passage; for example, the opening of the tympanic cavity (middle ear) to the air spaces of the mastoid process.

adjunct (aj-unkt) *n.* a subsidiary drug used in treating a disorder, which is administered in conjunction with, and provides additional benefits to, the main drug used in treatment. **—adjunctive** (ă-**junk**-tiv) *adj.*

adjuvant (aj-oo-vănt) *n.* any substance used in conjunction with another to enhance its activity.

adjuvant therapy *n.* treatment given to cancer patients after the primary therapy, which is usually surgical removal of the tumour, when there is known to be a high risk of future recurrence. *Compare* neoadjuvant chemotherapy.

ADLs *pl. n. see* activities of daily living.

admission rate (ăd-**mish**-ŏn) *n.* the number of people from a specified population with a specified disease or condition admitted to hospitals in a given geographical area over a specified time period.

adnexa (ad-**neks**-ă) *pl. n.* adjoining parts. **uterine a.** the Fallopian tubes and ovaries.

adolescence (ad-ŏ-**less**-ĕns) *n.* the period of development between childhood and adulthood. It begins with the start of puberty and usually lasts until 19 years of age. **—adolescent** *n., adj.*

ADP (adenosine diphosphate) *n.* a compound containing adenine, ribose, and two phosphate groups. ADP occurs in cells and is involved in processes requiring the transfer of energy (*see* ATP).

adrenalectomy (ă-dree-năl-**ek**-tŏmi) *n.* surgical removal of an adrenal gland, usually performed because of cancer.

adrenal glands (suprarenal glands) (ă-**dree**-năl) *pl. n.* two triangular endocrine glands, each of which covers the superior surface of a kidney. The **medulla** forms the grey core of the gland and produces adrenaline and noradrenaline. The **cortex** is a yellowish tissue surrounding the medulla; it produces corticosteroid hormones.

adrenaline (epinephrine) (ă-**dren**-ă-lin) *n.* an important hormone secreted by the medulla of the adrenal gland. It has widespread effects on circulation, the muscles, and sugar metabolism. The action of the heart is increased, the rate and depth of breathing are increased, and the metabolic rate is raised; the force of muscular contraction improves and the onset of muscular fatigue is delayed. At the same time the blood supply to the bladder and intestines is reduced, their muscular walls relax, and the sphincters contract. Adrenaline is administered by injection for the emergency treatment of anaphylaxis and cardiac arrest. It is also included in some local anaesthetic solutions, particularly those used in dentistry, to prolong anaesthesia, and is used as eye drops in treating glaucoma.

adrenarche (**ad**-ren-ar-ki) *n.* the start of secretion of androgens by the adrenal glands, occurring at around 6–7 years of age in girls and 7–8 in boys. Adrenal androgens are dehydroepiandrosterone (DHEA), DHEA sulphate, and androstenedione. *Compare* gonadarche.

adrenergic (ad-rĕ-**ner**-jik) *adj.* describing or relating to nerve fibres that release noradrenaline as a neurotransmitter. **a. receptor** (**adrenoceptor**) any of the receptors that are stimulated by noradrenaline and/or adrenaline, of which there are two types, alpha (α) and beta (β), each with subtypes (α_1, α_2, β_1, and β_2). *Compare* cholinergic.

adrenoceptor (ă-**dree**-noh-sep-ter) *n. see* adrenergic (receptor).

adrenocorticotrophic hormone (adrenocorticotrophin) (ă-dree-noh-kor-ti-koh-**trof**-ik) *n. see* ACTH.

adrenogenital syndrome (ă-dree-noh-**jen**-it-ăl) *n.* a hormonal disorder resulting from abnormal steroid production by the adrenal cortex, due to a genetic fault. It may cause masculinization in girls, precocious puberty in boys, and adrenocortical failure (*see* Addison's disease) in both sexes. Treatment is by lifelong steroid replacement.

adrenoleukodystrophy (ALD) (ă-dree-noh-loo-koh-**dis**-trŏ-fi) *n.* a genetically determined condition of neurological degeneration with childhood and adult forms. Inherited as an X-linked (*see* sex-linked) trait resulting in demyelination, it is characterized by progressive spastic paralysis of the legs, sensory loss, and cognitive impairment, associated with adrenal gland insufficiency and small gonads.

adrenolytic (ă-dree-noh-**lit**-ik) *adj.* inhibiting the activity of adrenergic nerves. Adrenolytic activity is opposite to that of noradrenaline.

ADRs *pl. n.* adverse drug reactions. *See* side-effect.

adsorbent (ăd-**sor**-bĕnt) *n.* a substance that attracts other substances to its surface to form a film. Charcoal and kaolin are adsorbents.

adsorption (ăd-**sorp**-shŏn) *n.* the formation of a layer of atoms or molecules of one substance on the surface of a solid or liquid of different substance. *See* adsorbent.

adult respiratory distress syndrome (acute respiratory distress syndrome, ARDS) (**ad**-ult) *n.* a form of acute respiratory failure that occurs after a precipitating event, such as trauma, aspiration, or inhalation of a toxic substance; it is particularly associated with septic shock.

advance decision, directive, or statement (ăd-**vahns**) *n.* under the Mental Capacity Act 2005, a legally recognized decision or statement made by an adult with capacity that identifies any specific or general treatments the patient does not want in the event that he or she loses capacity. An **advance directive** or **decision** (formerly often called a living will) should be informed, made voluntarily, and must be shown to be valid and applicable to the medical situation that arises. An **advance statement** is a more general and less legally binding expression of the person's values and views on the sort of treatment he or she may or may not wish to undergo.

advanced life support (ALS) (ăd-**vahnst**) *n.* a structured and algorithm-driven method of life support for use in the severest of medical emergencies, especially cardiac arrest. Personnel involved in ALS receive special training in the use of equipment (e.g. defibrillators and appropriate drugs). *Compare* basic life support.

advanced paediatric life support paediatric resuscitation with the incorporation of critical illness identification and stabilization techniques.

advanced trauma life support *n. see* ATLS.

advancement (ăd-**vahns**-mĕnt) *n.* the detachment by surgery of a muscle, musculocutaneous flap, or tendon and its reattachment at a more advanced (anterior) point while preserving its previous nerve and blood supply. The technique is used, for example, in the treatment of squint, and extensively in plastic surgery.

adventitia (tunica adventitia) (ad-ven-**ti**-shă) *n.* **1.** the outer coat of the wall of a vein or artery. **2.** the outer covering of various other organs or parts.

adventitious (ad-ven-**ti**-shŭs) *adj.* **1.** occurring in a place other than the usual one. **2.** relating to the adventitia.

advocate (**ad**-vŏ-kăt) *n.* **1.** (in health care) a practitioner, usually a nurse, who utilizes this role to promote and safeguard the well-being and interests of his or her patients or clients by ensuring they are aware of their rights and have access to information to make informed decisions. Advocacy in health care is an integral part of professional practice. **2.** a person who acts as a proxy for or speaks on behalf of a patient who lacks capacity. **—advocacy** (ad-vŏ-kă-si) *n.*

SEE WEB LINKS

- Explanation of an advocate's role in mental health care from the National Archives

Aëdes (ay-ee-deez) *n.* a genus of widely distributed mosquitoes occurring throughout the tropics and subtropics. **A. aegypti** the principal vector of dengue and yellow fever.

aegophony (e-gof-ŏni) *n. see* vocal resonance.

-aemia *combining form denoting* a specified condition of the blood.

aer- (aero-) *combining form denoting* air or gas.

aerobe (air-ohb) *n.* any organism, especially a microbe, that requires the presence of free oxygen for life and growth. *Compare* anaerobe. **—aerobic** (air-oh-bik) *adj.*

aerobic exercise *n. see* exercise.

aerobic respiration *n.* a type of cellular respiration in which foodstuffs (carbohydrates) are completely oxidized by atmospheric oxygen, with the production of maximum chemical energy from the foodstuffs.

aerogenous (air-oj-in-ŭs) *adj.* producing gas. The term is applied to bacteria such as *Clostridium perfringens*, which causes gas gangrene.

aerophagia (aerophagy) (air-o-fay-jiă) *n.* the swallowing of air. Voluntary aerophagia is used to permit oesophageal speech after surgical removal of the larynx (usually for cancer).

aerosol (air-ŏ-sol) *n.* a suspension of extremely small liquid or solid particles in a gas. Drugs for inhalation are in aerosol form.

aetiology (etiology) (ee-ti-ol-ŏji) *n.* **1.** the study or science of the causes of disease. **2.** the cause of a specific disease.

AF *n. see* (atrial) fibrillation.

AFB *pl. n. see* acid-fast (bacilli).

afebrile (ay-feb-ryl) *adj.* without, or not showing any signs of, a fever.

affect (af-ekt) *n.* (in psychiatry) **1.** the predominant emotion in a person's mental state at a particular moment. **2.** the emotion associated with a particular idea. **blunted a.** diminished intensity of emotional response, which is a feature of some forms of schizophrenia and depression. **incongruent a.** an inappropriate emotional response to a situation, which may be seen in psychotic illnesses. **—affective** (ă-fek-tiv) *adj.*

affective disorder (mood disorder) (dis-or-der) *n.* any psychiatric disorder featuring abnormalities of mood or emotion (affect). The most serious of these are depression and mania. Other affective disorders include SAD (seasonal affective disorder).

afferent (af-er-ĕnt) *adj.* **1.** designating nerves or neurons that convey impulses to the brain or spinal cord. **2.** designating blood vessels that feed a capillary network in an organ or part. **3.** designating lymphatic vessels that enter a lymph node. *Compare* efferent.

affinity (ă-**fin**-iti) *n.* the chemical attraction of one substance to another or others.

aflatoxin (af-lă-**toks**-in) *n.* a poisonous substance produced in the spores of the fungus *Aspergillus flavus*, which infects peanuts. It is known to produce cancer in certain animals.

AFP *n. see* alpha-fetoprotein.

afterbirth (**ahf**-ter-berth) *n.* the placenta, umbilical cord, and ruptured membranes associated with the fetus, which normally become detached from the uterus and expelled within a few hours of birth.

aftercare (**ahf**-ter-kair) *n.* **1.** long-term surveillance or rehabilitation as an adjunct or supplement to formal medical treatment of those who are chronically sick or disabled. Aftercare includes the provision of equipment and the adaptation of homes to aid activities of daily living. **2.** surveillance of convalescents.

after-image (**ahf**-ter-im-ij) *n.* an impression of an image that is registered by the brain for a brief moment after an object is removed from in front of the eye, or after the eye is closed.

afterpains (**ahf**-ter-paynz) *pl. n.* pains caused by uterine contractions after childbirth, especially during breast feeding, due to release of the hormone oxytocin.

AGA *adj.* appropriate for gestational age.

agammaglobulinaemia (ă-gam-ă-glob-yoo-lin-**ee**-miă) *n.* a total deficiency of the plasma protein gammaglobulin. *Compare* hypogammaglobulinaemia.

agar (**ay**-ger) *n.* an extract of certain seaweeds that forms a gel suitable for the solidification of liquid bacteriological culture media. Agar may also be used as a laxative.

agenesis (ă-**jen**-ĕsis) *n.* absence of an organ, usually due to total failure of its development in the embryo.

age-related macular degeneration (ayj-ri-lay-tid) *n. see* macular degeneration.

agglutination (clumping) (ă-gloo-tin-**ay**-shŏn) *n.* the sticking together of such microscopic antigenic particles as red blood cells or bacteria so that they form visible clumps. **—agglutinative** *adj.*

agglutinin (ă-**gloo**-tin-in) *n.* an antibody that brings about the agglutination of bacteria, blood cells, or other antigenic particles.

agglutinogen (ă-**gloo**-tin-oh-jĕn) *n.* any antigen that provokes formation of an agglutinin in the serum and is therefore likely to be involved in agglutination.

aglossia (ă-**gloss**-iă) *n.* congenital absence of the tongue.

aglutition (a-gloo-**ti**-shŏn) *n.* inability to swallow. *See also* dysphagia.

agnosia (ag-**noh**-ziă) *n.* a disorder of the brain whereby the patient cannot interpret sensations correctly although the sense organs and nerves conducting sensation to the brain are functioning normally.

agonist (**ag**-ŏ-nist) *n.* **1. (prime mover)** a muscle whose active contraction causes movement of a part of the body. Contraction of an agonist is associated with relaxation of its antagonist. **2.** a drug or other substance that acts at a cell-receptor site to produce an effect that is the same as, or similar to, that of the body's normal chemical messenger. Sympathomimetic drugs (alpha agonists and beta agonists) are examples.

agoraphobia (ag-er-ă-**foh**-biă) *n.* a morbid fear of public places and/or of open spaces. *See also* phobia.

agranulocytosis (ă-gran-yoo-loh-sy-**toh**-sis) *n.* a disorder in which there is a severe acute deficiency of certain blood cells (neutrophils) as a result of damage to the bone marrow by toxic drugs or chemicals. It is characterized by fever, with ulceration of the mouth and throat, and may lead rapidly to prostration and death.

agraphia (dysgraphia) (ă-graf-iă) *n.* an acquired inability to write, although the strength and coordination of the hand remain normal.

ague (ay-gew) *n. see* malaria.

AHF *n.* antihaemophilic factor (*see* Factor VIII).

AIDS (acquired immune deficiency syndrome) (aydz) *n.* a syndrome caused by the human immunodeficiency virus (HIV), which destroys a subgroup of lymphocytes, resulting in suppression of the body's immune response (*see* (helper) T cell). AIDS is largely a sexually transmitted disease, either homosexually or heterosexually, but it can also be spread via infected blood or blood products and from an infected mother to her child in the uterus, during parturition, or in breast milk.

Acute (primary) infection following exposure to the virus results in the production of antibodies (seroconversion). Symptoms, lasting about 14 days, include fever, fatigue, enlarged lymph nodes, and headache. The chronic stage, lasting an average of ten years, may be asymptomatic; it is followed by the development of AIDS. This is characterized by recurrent pneumonia (especially pneumonia caused by *Pneumocystis jiroveci*), Kaposi's sarcoma, any of various lymphomas, and/or any of certain cytomegalovirus-related diseases.

Ordinary social contact with HIV-positive subjects involves no risk of infection. However, high standards of clinical practice are required by all health workers in order to avoid inadvertent infection via blood, blood products, or body fluids from HIV-positive people. Staff who become HIV-positive are expected to declare their status and will be counselled.

AIH *n. see* artificial insemination (by husband).

air bed (air) *n.* a bed with a mattress whose upper surface is perforated with thousands of holes through which air is forced under pressure, so that the patient is supported on a cushion of air. Air beds are invaluable for the treatment of patients with large areas of burns.

air embolism *n.* an air bubble that suddenly obstructs the bloodflow down a blood vessel. Air may gain access to the circulation as a result of surgery, injury, intravenous infusions, or intravascular catheters.

air hunger *n.* difficulty in breathing characterized by sighing and gasping. It is caused by anoxia.

air sickness *n.* *see* motion sickness.

airway (air-way) *n.* **1.** any of the passages of the respiratory system. **2.** any device that enables the flow of air into and out of the lungs. *See* nasopharyngeal airway, oropharyngeal airway.

akathisia (ak-ă-**thiz**-iă) *n.* a pattern of involuntary movements induced by antipsychotic drugs or, more rarely, antidepressants. An affected person is driven to restless overactivity, which is most commonly experienced as restless legs syndrome.

AKI *n. see* acute kidney injury.

akinesia (ak-in-**ee**-ziă) *n.* a loss of normal muscular tonicity or responsiveness. **akinetic epilepsy** a form of epilepsy in which there is a sudden loss of muscular tonicity, making the patient fall with momentary loss of consciousness. **akinetic mutism** a state of complete physical unresponsiveness although the patient's eyes remain open and appear to follow movements. It is a consequence of damage to the brainstem. **akinetic rigid syndrome** a condition, such as parkinsonism or progressive supranuclear palsy, characterized by akinesia. **—akinetic** (a-kin-**et**-ik) *adj.*

ala (al-ă) *n.* (*pl.* **alae**) (in anatomy) a winglike structure.

alanine (al-ă-neen) *n.* *see* amino acid.

alanine aminotransferase (ALT) (ă-mee-noh-**trans**-fer-ayz) *n.* an enzyme involved in the transamination of amino acids. Measurement of ALT in the serum is of use in the diagnosis and study of acute liver disease. It was formerly called **serum glutamic pyruvic transaminase (SGPT)**.

alastrim (ă-**las**-trim) *n.* a mild form of smallpox, causing only a sparse rash and low-grade fever. Medical name: **variola minor**.

Albee's operation (awl-beez) *n.* **1.** an operation to produce ankylosis of the hip. The upper surface of the femur and the corresponding part of the acetabulum are removed and the two exposed surfaces allowed to remain in contact. **2.** an operation to immobilize part of the spinal column, using a bone graft from the tibia.[F. H. Albee (1876–1945), US surgeon]

albendazole (al-**ben**-dă-zohl) *n.* an anthelmintic drug used for treating hydatid disease, hookworm disease, strongyloidiasis, and creeping eruption. It is administered by mouth.

Albers-Schönberg disease (al-bers **shern**-berg) *n.* *see* osteopetrosis. [H. E. Albers-Schönberg (1865–1921), German radiologist]

Alberti regime (GIK regime) (al-**ber**-ti ray-*zh*eem) *n.* a method for controlling blood-sugar levels in diabetic patients who are being fasted. It involves infusing a solution of glucose (G), insulin (I), and potassium (K) chloride intravenously over a standard period using a sliding scale. [K. G. M. M. Alberti (1937–), British physician]

albinism (al-bin-izm) *n.* the inherited absence of pigmentation in the skin, hair, and eyes (*see* albino).

albino (al-bee-noh) *n.* an individual lacking the normal body pigment (melanin). Albinos have white hair and pink skin and eyes, reduced visual acuity, and sensitivity to light (*see* photophobia).

Albright's hereditary osteodystrophy (awl-bryts) *n.* the skeletal abnormalities, collectively, of pseudohypoparathyroidism. These include short stature, abnormally short fingers and toes (particularly involving the fourth and fifth metacarpals and metatarsals), and soft-tissue calcification. [F. Albright (1900–69), US physician]

albumin (al-bew-min) *n.* a protein that is soluble in water and coagulated by heat. **serum a.** a protein found in blood plasma that is important for the maintenance of plasma volume.

albuminuria (proteinuria) (al-bew-min-**yoor**-iă) *n.* the presence of serum albumin, serum globulin, or other serum proteins in the urine, which may be associated with kidney or heart disease. **orthostatic a.** albuminuria not associated with disease, occurring after strenuous exercise or after a long period of standing.

albumose (al-bew-mohz) *n.* a substance, intermediate between albumin and peptones, produced during the digestion of proteins by pepsin and other endopeptidases (*see* peptidase).

alcaptonuria (alkaptonuria) (al-kap-tŏn-**yoor**-iă) *n.* accumulation in the tissues and excretion in the urine of homogentisic acid due to congenital absence of homogentisic acid oxidase, an enzyme essential for the normal breakdown of the amino acids tyrosine and phenylalanine.

alclometasone (al-kloh-**met**-ă-zohn) *n.* a corticosteroid drug applied as a cream to treat inflammatory skin disorders. Trade name: **Modrasone**.

alcohol (al-kŏ-hol) *n.* any of a class of organic compounds formed when a hydroxyl group (–OH) is substituted for a hydrogen atom in a hydrocarbon. **ethyl a. (ethanol)** the alcohol in alcoholic drinks, produced by the fermentation of sugar by yeast. Formula: C_2H_5OH. 'Pure' alcohol contains not less than 94.9% by volume of ethyl alcohol. A solution of 70% alcohol can be used as a preservative or antiseptic. *See also* alcoholism. **—alcoholic** (al-kŏ-**hol**-ik) *adj., n.*

alcohol-fast *adj.* describing bacteria that have been stained and continue to hold the stain after treatment with alcohol.

Alcoholics Anonymous (AA) *n.* an international voluntary agency of mutual support that is organized and operated locally among those with alcoholic dependency.

SEE WEB LINKS

• The AA website

alcoholism (al-kŏ-hol-izm) *n.* the syndrome due to physical dependence on alcohol, such that sudden deprivation may cause withdrawal symptoms – tremor, anxiety, hallucinations, and delusions (*see* delirium (tremens)). Alcoholism impairs intellectual function, physical skills, memory, and judgment. Heavy consumption of alcohol also causes cardiomyopathy, peripheral neuropathy, cirrhosis of the liver, and enteritis.

alcoholuria (al-kŏ-hol-**yoor**-iă) *n.* the presence of alcohol in the urine.

ALD *n. see* adrenoleukodystrophy.

aldesleukin (al-des-**loo**-kin) *n. see* interleukin.

Aldomet (al-dŏ-met) *n. see* methyldopa.

aldosterone (al-**dos**-ter-ohn) *n.* a steroid hormone (*see* corticosteroid) that is synthesized and released by the adrenal cortex and acts on the kidney to regulate salt (potassium and sodium) and water balance.

aldosteronism (hyperaldosteronism) (al-**dos**-tĕ-rŏ-nizm) *n.* overproduction of aldosterone, causing electrolyte imbalance and raised blood pressure (hypertension). *See also* Conn's syndrome.

alendronic acid (sodium alendronate) (al-en-**dron**-ik, ă-**len**-drŏ-nayt) *n. see* bisphosphonates.

Aleppo boil (ă-**lep**-oh) *n. see* oriental sore.

alerting device (ă-**lert**-ing) *n.* a device for helping people with hearing difficulties that indicates the occurrence of an event by other than an auditory signal, such as a doorbell with a visible (as well as an audible) alarm.

alexia (ă-**leks**-iă) *n.* an acquired inability to read due to disease in the left (dominant) hemisphere of the brain in a right-handed person. **agnostic a.** (**word blindness**) inability to identify letters and words not affecting the patient's ability to write. *See also* dyslexia.

alexithymia (ă-lex-i-**thim**-iă) *n.* inability to express or describe one's emotions in words, commonly accompanied by a lack of empathy for the feelings of others. Most often seen in males, it is associated with autistic spectrum disorders (*see* autism) and also with certain eating disorders.

alfacalcidol (al-fă-**kal**-sid-ol) *n.* 1α-hydroxycholecalciferol: a derivative of vitamin D used to raise blood-calcium levels for the prevention and treatment of rickets and osteomalacia in patients with severe kidney disease. It is administered by mouth or by intravenous injection. Trade name: **One-Alpha**.

alfentanil (al-**fen**-tă-nil) *n.* an opioid analgesic used mainly for pain relief during surgery. It is administered by intravenous injection or infusion. Trade name: **Rapifen**.

alfuzosin (al-few-zoh-sin) *n.* an alpha blocker commonly used in the treatment of men with lower urinary tract symptoms thought to be due to benign prostatic hyperplasia (*see* prostate gland). It is administered orally. Trade names: **Besavar XL**, **Vasran XL**, **Xatral**.

ALG *n.* antilymphocyte globulin. *See* antilymphocyte serum.

algesimeter (al-jĕ-**sim**-it-er) *n.* a piece of equipment for determining the sensitivity of the skin to various touch stimuli, especially those causing pain.

-algia *combining form denoting* pain.

algid (**al**-jid) *adj.* cold: usually describing the cold clammy skin associated with certain forms of malaria.

alginates (**al**-jin-ayts) *pl. n.* complex carbohydrates, derived from certain seaweeds, that readily absorb water to form a gel. They are included in many antacid preparations (e.g. **Gaviscon**) for the relief of heartburn caused by gastro-oesophageal reflux and are also used in dressings for exuding wounds.

algorithm (**al**-gŏ-rith-ĕm) *n.* a sequential set of instructions used in calculations or problem solving, such as a stepwise series of instructions with branching pathways to be followed to assist a physician in coming to a diagnosis (**diagnostic a.**) or deciding on a management strategy (**therapeutic a.**).

alienation (ay-li-ĕn-**ay**-shŏn) *n.* (in psychiatry) **1.** *see* thought alienation. **2.** insanity.

alien limb syndrome *n.* a rare neurological condition in which upper limb movements occur without an individual's awareness or volition. It is caused by damage to connections between the cerebral hemispheres or the frontal or occipital brain areas and can occur following stroke or in dementia.

alimemazine (ali-**mem**-ă-zeen) *n.* an antihistamine drug (a phenothiazine derivative) that also possesses sedative properties. Given by mouth, it is mainly used in the treatment of pruritus and urticaria (nettle rash) but also for premedication.

alimentary canal (ali-**ment**-er-i) *n.* the long passage, extending from the mouth to the anus, through which food passes to be digested and absorbed. See illustration.

aliquot (**al**-i-kwot) *n.* one of a known number of equal parts of a compound or solution.

alkalaemia (al-kă-**lee**-miă) *n.* abnormally high blood alkalinity. *See also* alkalosis. *Compare* acidaemia.

alkali (**al**-kă-ly) *n.* a base that is soluble in water. Alkaline solutions turn litmus paper blue. *See* base.

alkaloid (**al**-kă-loid) *n.* one of a diverse group of nitrogen-containing substances that are produced by plants and have potent effects on body function. Many alkaloids are important drugs, including morphine, quinine, atropine, and codeine.

alkalosis (al-kă-**loh**-sis) *n.* a condition in which the alkalinity of body fluids and tissues is abnormally high. This arises because of a failure of the mechanisms that usually maintain a balance between alkalis and acids in the arterial blood (*see* acid-base balance).

alkaptonuria *n. see* alcaptonuria.

alkylating agent (**al**-ki-lay-ting) *n.* a drug, such as cyclophosphamide, that disrupts the growth of a malignant tumour by damaging the DNA in the tumour cell nuclei. Side-effects are those of other cytotoxic drugs; these agents may also cause sterility in men.

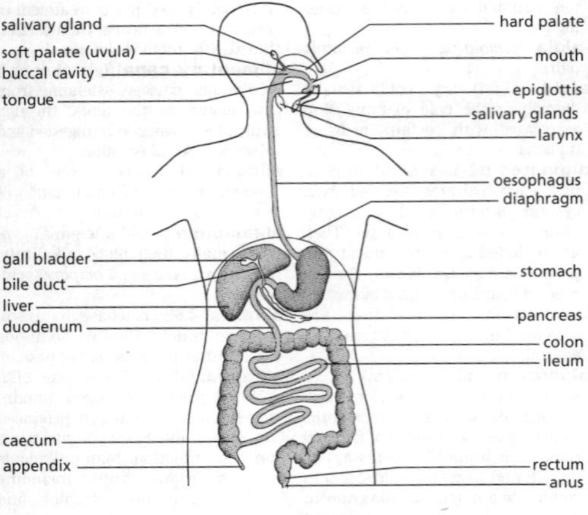

The alimentary canal

ALL *n.* acute lymphoblastic leukaemia. *See* leukaemia, lymphoblast.

allantois (al-ăn-**toh**-iss) *n.* the membranous sac that develops as an outgrowth of the embryonic hindgut. Its outer (mesodermal) layer carries blood vessels to the placenta and so forms part of the umbilical cord. **—allantoic** *adj.*

allele (allelomorph) (ă-leel) *n.* one of two or more alternative forms of a gene, only one of which can be present in a chromosome. *See also* dominant, recessive. **—allelic** *adj.*

allelomorph (ă-leel-oh-morf) *n.* *see* allele.

allergen (al-er-jĕn) *n.* any antigen that causes allergy in a hypersensitive person. **—allergenic** *adj.*

allergy (al-er-ji) *n.* a disorder in which the body becomes hypersensitive to particular antigens (called allergens), which provoke characteristic symptoms whenever they are subsequently encountered. Different allergies afflict different tissues and may have either local or general effects, varying from asthma and hay fever to severe dermatitis or gastroenteritis or extremely serious shock (*see* anaphylaxis). **—allergic** *adj.*

SEE WEB LINKS

- Overview of allergies from the NHS Choices website

allied health professional (al-yd) *n.* a health-care professional with expert knowledge and experience in certain fields but without medical or nursing qualifications. Allied health professionals include speech and language therapists, radiographers, physiotherapists, occupational therapists, and dietitians.

alloantibody (a-loh-**an**-ti-bo-di) *n.* *see* isoantibody.

alloantigen (a-loh-**an**-ti-jĕn) *n.* *see* isoantigen.

allocheiria (al-oh-**keer**-iă) *n.* a condition in which the sensation aroused by a stimulus applied to one side of the body is referred to the opposite side.

allodynia (a-loh-**din**-iă) *n.* pain due to a stimulus that would not normally cause pain, such as a light touch. It occurs acutely after injury but also in many chronically painful conditions, including peripheral neuropathy.

allogeneic (al-oh-jĕ-**nay**-ik) *adj.* describing grafted tissue derived from a donor of the same species as the recipient but with different histocompatibility.

allograft (**al**-oh-grahft) *n.* a living tissue or organ graft between two members of the same species. Unless the graft is from an identical twin, it will not survive unless the recipient is treated to suppress the body's immune response to the foreign tissue.

allopathy (ă-**lop**-ă-thi) *n.* (in homeopathic medicine) the orthodox system of medicine, in which the use of drugs is directed to producing effects in the body that will directly oppose and so alleviate the symptoms of a disease. *Compare* homeopathy.

allopurinol (al-oh-**pewr**-i-nol) *n.* a drug administered by mouth for the prevention of acute attacks of gout and of kidney stones. It acts by reducing the level of uric acid in tissues and blood. Trade name: **Zyloric**.

all-or-none law *n.* the principle that tissue, such as nerve fibres, can produce only one of two reactions to a stimulus. Regardless of the intensity of the stimulus, such tissue will show either a total response or no response at all.

almotriptan (al-moh-**trip**-tan) *n.* *see* $5HT_1$ agonist.

alopecia (baldness) (al-ŏ-**pee**-shiă) *n.* absence of hair from areas where it normally grows. **a. areata** a condition characterized by bald patches that may regrow; it is an example of an organ-specific autoimmune disease. **a. totalis** total scalp hair loss, due to an autoimmune condition. **a. universalis** loss of all body hair. **androgenetic a.** hair loss in women, which is associated with increasing age. **scarring** (or **cicatricial**) **a.** alopecia in which the hair does not regrow, as occurs in lichen planus and discoid lupus erythematosus.

alpha agonist (al-fă) *n.* *see* sympathomimetic.

alpha blocker (alpha-adrenergic blocker) *n.* a drug that prevents the stimulation of alpha-adrenergic receptors at the nerve endings of the sympathetic nervous system by noradrenaline and adrenaline: it therefore relaxes smooth muscle, causing (among other effects) widening of arteries (vasodilatation) and a drop in blood pressure. Alpha blockers include alfuzosin, doxazosin, phentolamine, phenoxybenzamine, indoramin, prazosin, and tamsulosin.

alpha cells *pl. n.* the cells in the islets of Langerhans that produce glucagon. *Compare* beta cells, D cells.

alpha-fetoprotein (AFP) (al-fă-fee-toh-**proh**-teen) *n.* a protein that is formed in the liver and yolk sac of the fetus and is present in the fetal serum and secondarily in maternal blood. Maternal AFP is used as a marker in prenatal screening tests, performed between the 15th and 20th weeks of pregnancy. Levels are elevated in spina bifida, multiple pregnancies, and certain other conditions and decreased in Down's syndrome.

Alport's syndrome (awl-ports) *n.* a hereditary disease that causes nephritis accompanied by deafness. Affected males usually develop end-stage renal failure and, unless treated with a kidney transplant, die before the age of 40. Females have a better prognosis. [A. C. Alport (1880–1959), South African physician]

alprazolam *n.* a benzodiazepine used for the short-term relief of anxiety. It is administered by mouth. Trade name: **Xanax**.

alprostadil (al-pros-tă-dil) *n.* a prostaglandin drug administered by infusion to improve lung blood flow in newborn babies with congenital heart defects who are awaiting surgery and by injection into the corpora cavernosa of the penis or by application into the urethra to treat erectile dysfunction in men. Trade names: **Caverject**, **MUSE**, **Prostin VR**, **Viridal Duo**.

ALS *n.* **1.** *see* advanced life support. **2.** *see* antilymphocyte serum. **3.** *see* (amyotrophic lateral) sclerosis.

ALT *n.* *see* alanine aminotransferase.

alteplase (al-tĕ-playz) *n.* a tissue-type plasminogen activator made by genetic engineering. Administered by intravenous injection and infusion, it is used to dissolve blood clots (*see* fibrinolytic) in the treatment of myocardial infarction, ischaemic stroke, and pulmonary embolism. Trade names: **Actilyse**, **Actilyse Cathflo**.

alternative medicine (awl-ter-nă-tiv) *n.* *see* complementary medicine.

altitude sickness (mountain sickness) (al-ti-tewd) *n.* the condition that results from unaccustomed exposure to a high altitude (4500 m or more above sea level). Reduced atmospheric pressure and shortage of oxygen cause deep rapid breathing, which lowers the concentration of carbon dioxide in the blood.

altruistic donation (al-troo-is-tik) *n.* organ donation where the donor offers an organ (often a kidney) for transplantation into a stranger. This may form a chain of donation to allow a suitable match for the donor's relative or partner if the pair are incompatible.

aluminium chloride hexahydrate (al-yoo-**min**-iŭm) *n.* a powerful antiperspirant used in the treatment of conditions associated with excessive sweating (*see* hyperhidrosis). It is applied to the skin in the form of a solution. Trade names: **Anhydrol Forte**, **Driclor**.

aluminium hydroxide *n.* a safe slow-acting antacid. It is administered by mouth, alone, or in combination with magnesium hydroxide (as **co-magaldrox**; Maalox, Mucogel) in the treatment of indigestion, gastric and duodenal ulcers, and reflux oesophagitis. Trade name: **Alu-Cap**.

alveolitis (al-vee-oh-**ly**-tis) *n.* inflammation of an alveolus or alveoli. Chronic inflammation of the walls of the alveoli of the lungs is usually caused by inhaled organic dusts (**extrinsic allergic a.**; *see* bird-fancier's lung, farmer's lung) but may occur spontaneously (**cryptogenic fibrosing a.** or **idiopathic pulmonary fibrosis, IPF**).

alveolus (al-vee-**oh**-lŭs) *n.* (*pl.* **alveoli**) **1.** (in the lung) a blind-ended air sac of microscopic size. **2.** the part of the upper or lower jawbone that supports the roots of the teeth (*see also* mandible, maxilla). **3.** the sac of a racemose gland (*see also* acinus). **4.** any other small cavity, depression, or sac. **—alveolar** *adj.*

alverine citrate (al-vě-reen) *n.* a bulking agent and antispasmodic drug used to treat irritable bowel syndrome and diverticular disease. It is administered by mouth. Trade names: **Audmonal**, **Spasmonal**.

Alzheimer's disease (alts-hy-merz) *n.* the most common form of dementia, occurring in middle age or later. It is characterized by memory impairment and, as the disease progresses, language difficulties, apraxia, and visuospatial problems, leading to a loss of judgment and the inability to carry out even basic functions. At post-mortem there are excess deposits of amyloid protein and neurofibrillary tangles (twisted filaments of abnormal tau protein) in the brain. [A. Alzheimer (1864–1915), German physician]

SEE WEB LINKS

- Website of the Alzheimer's Society

amalgam (ă-**mal**-găm) *n.* any of a group of alloys containing mercury. In dentistry amalgam fillings are made by mixing a silver–tin alloy with mercury in a machine known as an **amalgamator**.

amantadine (ă-**man**-tă-deen) *n.* an antiviral drug that also increases the action of dopamine in the brain and is used mainly to treat Parkinson's disease.

amaurosis (am-aw-**roh**-sis) *n.* partial or complete blindness. **a. fugax** a condition in which loss of vision is transient. **—amaurotic** (am-aw-**rot**-ik) *adj.*

ambivalence (am-**biv**-ălĕns) *n.* (in psychology) the condition of holding opposite feelings (such as love and hate) for the same person or object.

amblyopia (am-blee-**oh**-piă) *n.* poor sight, not due to any detectable disease of the eyeball or visual system, known colloquially as **lazy eye**. **a. ex anopsia** a condition in which factors such as squint (*see* strabismus), cataract, and other abnormalities of the optics of the eye (*see* refraction) impair its normal use in early childhood by preventing the formation of a clear image on the retina.

amblyoscope (orthoptoscope, synoptophore) (am-blee-ŏ-skohp) *n.* an instrument for measuring the angle of a squint and assessing the degree to which a person uses both eyes together.

ambulant (**am**-bew-lănt) *adj.* able to walk.

ambulatory (am-bew-**layt**-er-i) *adj.* relating to walking. **a. treatment** treatment that enables or encourages a patient to remain on his or her feet.

AMD *n.* *see* (age-related) macular degeneration.

amelia (ă-**mee**-liă) *n.* congenital total absence of the arms or legs due to a developmental defect. It is one of the fetal abnormalities induced by the drug thalidomide taken early in pregnancy. *See also* phocomelia.

amelioration (ă-mee-li-er-**ay**-shŏn) *n.* general improvement in the condition of a patient; reduction in severity of the symptoms of a disease.

ameloblastoma (ă-mee-loh-blas-**toh**-mă) *n.* a locally invasive tumour of the jaw that develops from enamel-forming cells (**ameloblasts**) but does not contain enamel.

amenorrhoea (am-en-ŏ-**ree**-ă) *n.* the absence or stopping of the menstrual periods. **primary a.** the nonappearance of menstrual periods at puberty. This may be due to absence of the uterus or ovaries, a genetic disorder, or hormonal imbalance. **secondary a.** the stopping of menstrual periods after establishment at puberty, for reasons such as pituitary or thyroid hormone deficiency or anorexia nervosa.

amethocaine (ă-**meth**-ŏ-kayn) *n.* *see* tetracaine.

ametropia (am-ĕ-**troh**-piă) *n.* any abnormality of refraction of the eye, resulting in blurring of the image formed on the retina. *See* (errors of) refraction.

amiloride (ă-**mil**-ŏ-ryd) *n.* a potassium-sparing diuretic that causes the increased excretion of sodium and chloride; it is often combined with a thiazide or loop diuretic to reduce the potassium loss that occurs with these drugs.

amino acid (ă-**mee**-noh) *n.* an organic compound that contains an amino group ($-NH_2$) and a carboxyl group ($-COOH$). Amino acids are fundamental constituents of all proteins (see table). They are classified as essential amino acids, i.e. those that cannot be synthesized by the body and must be obtained from protein in the diet; and

The amino acids occurring in proteins

Amino acid	*Abbreviation*	*Amino acid*	*Abbreviation*
alanine	ala	*leucine	leu
arginine	arg	*lysine	lys
asparagine	asn	*methionine	met
aspartic acid	asp	*phenylalanine	phe
cysteine	cys	proline	pro
glutamic acid	glu	serine	ser
glutamine	gln	*threonine	thr
glycine	gly	*tryptophan	trp
histidine	his	tyrosine	tyr
*isoleucine	ile	*valine	val

*an essential amino acid

nonessential amino acids, which can be synthesized by the body.

aminoacidopathy (ă-mee-noh-asid-**op**-ă-thi) *n. see* maple syrup urine disease.

aminoglycosides (ă-mee-noh-**gly**-koh-sydz) *pl. n.* a group of antibiotics active against a wide range of bacteria. Included in the group are gentamicin, neomycin, and streptomycin. Because of their toxicity, they are used only when less toxic antibacterials are ineffective or contraindicated. They are usually administered by injection.

aminopeptidase (ă-mee-noh-**pep**-ti-dayz) *n.* any one of several enzymes in the intestine that cause the breakdown of a peptide, removing an amino acid.

aminophylline (ami-**nof**-il-een) *n.* a drug that relaxes smooth muscle and stimulates respiration. Administered by mouth, intravenous injection, or infusion, it is used in the treatment of severe asthma and chronic obstructive pulmonary disease. *See also* theophylline. Trade name: **Phyllocontin Continus**.

amiodarone (ami-**oh**-dă-rohn) *n.* an anti-arrhythmic drug used to control a variety of abnormal heart rhythms, including atrial fibrillation and abnormally rapid heartbeat. It is administered by mouth or intravenous infusion. Trade name: **Cordarone X**.

amitosis (ami-**toh**-sis) *n.* division of the nucleus of a cell by a process, not involving mitosis, in which the nucleus is constricted into two.

amitriptyline (ami-**trip**-til-een) *n.* a tricyclic antidepressant drug that has a mild tranquillizing action.

Because it may cause abnormal heart rhythms, amitriptyline is now rarely used to treat depression, but it can be used in the treatment of chronic pain.

AML *n.* acute myeloid leukaemia. *See* myeloid (leukaemia).

amlodipine (am-loh-**dy**-peen) *n.* a calcium-channel blocker used to treat hypertension and prevent angina pectoris. It is administered by mouth. Trade name: **Istin**.

ammonia (ă-**moh**-niă) *n.* a colourless gas with a pungent odour that can be cooled and compressed to form a liquid (formula: NH_3). **Ammonium chloride** is occasionally used to acidify urine.

amnesia (am-**nee**-ziă) *n.* total or partial loss of memory following physical injury, disease, drugs, or psychological trauma. **anterograde a.** loss of memory for events following the trauma. **retrograde a.** loss of memory for events preceding the trauma.

amnestic MCI (am-**nes**-tik) *n. see* mild cognitive impairment.

amnihook (**am**-ni-huuk) *n.* a small plastic hooked instrument introduced through the cervix for performing amniotomy.

amniocentesis (am-ni-oh-sen-**tee**-sis) *n.* withdrawal of a sample of amniotic fluid surrounding a fetus in the uterus, by means of a syringe inserted through the abdominal wall under direct ultrasound guidance, to enable chromosome analysis of fetal cells in the fluid and hence prenatal diagnosis of chromosomal abnormalities (such as Down's syndrome) and metabolic and other congenital disorders (such as spina bifida). The procedure is usually performed after the 15th completed week of gestation and carries a 1–2% risk of miscarriage.

amnion (**am**-ni-ŏn) *n.* the membrane that forms initially over the dorsal part of the embryo but soon expands to enclose it completely within the amniotic cavity. **—amniotic** (am-ni-**ot**-ik) *adj.*

amniotic cavity *n.* the fluid-filled cavity between the embryo and the amnion. *See also* amniotic fluid.

amniotic fluid *n.* the fluid contained within the amniotic cavity. It surrounds the growing fetus, protecting it from external pressure. **a. f. embolism** a rare condition in which amniotic fluid enters the maternal circulation causing features similar to anaphylactic and septic shock, including cardiopulmonary collapse and disseminated intravascular coagulation. *See also* amniocentesis.

amniotomy (artificial rupture of membranes, ARM) (am-ni-**ot**-ŏmi) *n.* a method of surgically inducing labour by puncturing the amnion surrounding the baby in the uterus using an amnihook or similar instrument.

amobarbital (amylobarbitone) (am-oh-**bar**-bi-tal) *n.* an intermediate-acting barbiturate used to treat severe insomnia in patients already taking barbiturates. Trade name: **Sodium Amytal**.

amoeba (ă-**mee**-bă) *n.* (*pl.* **amoebae**) any protozoan of irregular and constantly changing shape. Some amoebae cause disease in humans (*see* entamoeba). **—amoebic** *adj.* **—amoeboid** *adj.*

amoebiasis (ami-**by**-ă-sis) *n. see* dysentery.

amoebicide (ă-**mee**-bi-syd) *n.* an agent that kills amoebae.

amorolfine (am-oh-**rol**-feen) *n.* an antifungal drug used to treat fungal infections of the skin and nails. It is applied externally as a nail lacquer. Trade name: **Loceryl**.

amoxicillin (ă-mok-si-**sil**-in) *n.* a semisynthetic penicillin used to treat infections caused by a wide range of bacteria and other micro-organisms. It is administered by mouth or injection. Trade name: **Amoxil**.

AMP (adenosine monophosphate) *n.* a compound containing adenine, ribose, and one phosphate group. AMP occurs in cells and is involved in processes requiring the transfer of energy (*see* ATP).

ampere (**am**-pair) *n.* the basic SI unit of electric current. It is equal to the current flowing through a conductor of resistance 1 ohm when a potential difference of 1 volt is applied between its ends. Symbol: A.

amphetamines (am-**fet**-ăminz) *pl. n.* a group of sympathomimetic drugs that have a marked stimulant action on the central nervous system. **Dexamfetamine** (**dexamphetamine**), administered by mouth, is used in the treatment of narcolepsy and attention-deficit/hyperactivity disorder. Tolerance to amphetamines develops rapidly, and prolonged use may lead to dependence.

amphiarthrosis (am-fi-arth-**roh**-sis) *n.* a slightly movable joint in which the bony surfaces are separated by fibrocartilage (*see* symphysis) or hyaline cartilage (*see* synchondrosis).

amphoric breath sounds (am-**fo**-rik) *pl. n. see* cavernous breath sounds.

amphotericin (am-foh-**te**-ri-sin) *n.* an antifungal drug used to treat deep-seated fungal infections. It can be administered by mouth, but is usually given by intravenous infusion. Trade names: **Abelcet**, **AmBisome**, **Fungizone**.

ampicillin (am-pi-**sil**-in) *n.* a semisynthetic penicillin administered by mouth, injection, or infusion in the treatment of a variety of infections, including those of the urinary, respiratory, biliary, and intestinal tracts. Trade names: **Penbritin**, **Rimacillin**.

ampoule (ampule) (**am**-pool) *n.* a sealed glass or plastic capsule containing one dose of a drug in the form of a sterile solution for injection.

ampulla (am-**puul**-ă) *n.* (*pl.* **ampullae**) an enlarged or dilated ending of a tube or canal. **a. of Vater** the dilated part of the common bile duct where it is joined by the pancreatic duct. (A. Vater (1684–1751), German anatomist)

amputation (am-pew-**tay**-shŏn) *n.* the removal of a limb, part of a limb, or any other portion of the body (such as a breast).

amylase (**am**-i-layz) *n.* an enzyme that occurs in saliva and pancreatic juice and aids the digestion of starch, which it breaks down into glucose, maltose, and dextrins.

amylobarbitone (ami-loh-**bar**-bi-tohn) *n. see* amobarbital.

amyloid (**am**-i-loid) *n.* a glycoprotein, resembling starch, that is deposited in the internal organs in amyloidosis. β-amyloid protein has been found in the brains of Alzheimer's patients.

amyloidosis (ami-loid-**oh**-sis) *n.* infiltration of the liver, kidneys, spleen, and other tissues with amyloid. **primary a.** amyloidosis without any apparent cause. **secondary a.** a late complication of such chronic infections as tuberculosis or leprosy.

amylopectin (ami-loh-**pek**-tin) *n. see* starch.

amylopsin (ami-**lop**-sin) *n.* an amylase found in the pancreatic juice.

amylose (**am**-i-lohz) *n. see* starch.

amyotonia congenita (floppy baby syndrome) (ay-my-ŏ-**toh**-niă kon-**jen**-ită) *n.* a former diagnosis for various conditions, present at birth, in which the baby's muscles are weak and floppy (i.e. hypotonic). The term is becoming obsolete as more specific diagnoses are discovered to explain the cause of floppiness in babies.

amyotrophy (ami-**ot**-rŏfi) *n.* a progressive loss of muscle bulk (wasting) associated with weakness, caused by disease of the motor nerve that supplies the affected muscle. **diabetic a.** wasting of the quadriceps muscle and loss of the knee jerk due to disease of the femoral nerve, associated with poor diabetic control.

an- *prefix. see* a-.

anabolic (ană-**bol**-ik) *adj.* promoting tissue growth by increasing the metabolic processes that are involved in protein synthesis. Anabolic steroids are synthetic forms of male sex hormones. *See* nandrolone.

anabolism (ă-**nab**-ŏl-izm) *n.* the synthesis of complex molecules, such as proteins and fats, from simpler ones by living organisms. *See also* anabolic, metabolism.

anacidity (ană-**sid**-iti) *n.* a deficiency or abnormal absence of acid in the body fluids.

anacrotism (ăn-**ak**-rŏt-izm) *n.* the condition in which there is an abnormal curve in the ascending line of a pulse tracing. It may be seen in cases of aortic stenosis. **—anacrotic** *adj.*

anaemia (ă-**nee**-miă) *n.* a reduction in the quantity of the oxygen-carrying pigment haemoglobin in the blood. The main symptoms are excessive tiredness and fatigability, breathlessness on exertion, pallor, and poor resistance to infection. The many causes of anaemia include loss of blood (**haemorrhagic a.**); lack of iron (**iron-deficiency a.**); the increased destruction of red blood cells (**haemolytic a.**); and the impaired production of red blood cells (*see* aplastic anaemia, leukaemia, pernicious (anaemia)). Anaemias can be classified on the basis of the size of the red cells, which may be large (**macrocytic a.**), small (**microcytic a.**), or normal-sized (**normocytic a.**). **—anaemic** *adj.*

anaerobe (**an**-air-rohb) *n.* any organism, especially a microbe, that is able to live and grow in the absence of free oxygen. *Compare* aerobe. **—anaerobic** (an-air-**roh**-bik) *adj.*

anaerobic respiration *n.* a type of cellular respiration in which foodstuffs (usually carbohydrates) are never completely oxidized because molecular oxygen is not used.

anaesthesia (anis-**theez**-iă) *n.* loss of feeling or sensation in a part or all of the body, especially when induced by drugs. **general a.** total unconsciousness, usually achieved by administering a combination of injections and gases. **local a.** loss of feeling in a limited area of the body, induced for minor operations, particularly many dental procedures. It may be achieved by injections of substances such as lidocaine close to a local nerve, which deadens the tissues supplied by that nerve. **regional a.** anaesthesia (usually of a limb) achieved by encircling local anaesthetic solutions or by direct application of anaesthetic to one or more peripheral nerves. *See also* epidural, spinal anaesthesia.

anaesthetic (anis-**thet**-ik) **1.** *n.* an agent that reduces or abolishes sensation. **general a.** an anaesthetic, such as halothane, that affects the whole body. **local a.** an anaesthetic, such as lidocaine, that affects a particular area or region of the body. **2.** *adj.* reducing or abolishing sensation.

anaesthetist (ăn-**ees**-thĕt-ist) *n.* a medically qualified doctor who administers an anaesthetic to induce unconsciousness in a patient before a surgical operation.

anagen (**an**-ă-jĕn) *n.* the growth phase of a hair follicle, lasting two to three years. It is followed by a transitional stage, called **catagen**, which lasts for about two weeks, and then a resting phase, **telogen**. On average about 85% of hairs are in anagen and hence growing actively.

anal (**ay**-năl) *adj.* of, relating to, or affecting the anus. **a. canal** the terminal portion of the large intestine, which is surrounded by the muscles of defecation (**a. sphincters**). The canal ends on the surface at the anal orifice (*see* anus). **a. fissure** *see* fissure.

analeptic (respiratory stimulant) (ană-**lep**-tik) *n.* a drug that acts on the central nervous system to stimulate the muscles involved in breathing. An example is doxapram.

analgesia (an-ăl-**jeez**-iă) *n.* reduced sensibility to pain, without loss of consciousness and without the sense of touch necessarily being affected.

analgesic (an-ăl-**jee**-sik) **1.** *n.* a drug that relieves pain. Aspirin and paracetamol are **nonopioid analgesics**; morphine and pethidine (**opioid analgesics**) are more potent. *See* opiate. **2.** *adj.* relieving pain.

analogous (ă-**nal**-ŏ-gŭs) *adj.* describing organs or parts that have similar functions in different organisms although they do not have the same evolutionary origin or development. *Compare* homologous.

analogue (an-ă-log) **1.** *n.* a drug that differs in minor ways in molecular structure from its parent compound. Useful analogues of existing drugs are either more potent or cause fewer side-effects. Carboplatin and oxaliplatin, for example, are less toxic analogues of cisplatin. *See also* gonadorelin analogue, insulin. **2.** *adj.* relating to or designating information that can be represented by a continuously varying quantity. **a. hearing aid** *see* hearing aid. **a. image** a traditional X-ray image on film in shades ranging smoothly from black to white. It can be converted to digital format. *Compare* digital.

analysis (ă-**nal**-i-sis) *n.* (in psychology) any means of understanding complex mental processes or experiences. *See also* psychoanalysis.

analyst (**an**-ă-list) *n.* a person who performs analysis.

anaphase (**an**-ă-fayz) *n.* the third stage of mitosis and of each division of meiosis.

anaphylaxis (ană-fil-**aks**-iss) *n.* an emergency condition resulting from an abnormal and immediate allergic response to a substance to which the body has become intensely sensitized. It results in flushing, itching, nausea and vomiting, swelling of the mouth and tongue and airway enough to often cause obstruction, wheezing, a sudden drop in blood pressure, and even sudden death. In this extreme form it is called **anaphylactic shock**. Treatment, which must be given immediately, consists of adrenaline (epinephrine) injection, oxygen with possible advanced support of the airway, intravenous fluids, intravenous corticosteroids, and antihistamines. **—anaphylactic** *adj.*

anaplasia (ană-**play**-ziă) *n.* a loss of normal cell characteristics or differentiation. Anaplasia is typical of rapidly growing malignant tumours (called **anaplastic tumours**).

anasarca (ană-**sar**-kă) *n.* massive swelling of the legs, trunk, and genitalia due to retention of fluid (oedema): found in congestive heart failure and some forms of renal failure.

anastomosis (ă-nass-tŏ-**moh**-sis) *n.* **1.** (in anatomy) a communication between two blood vessels without any intervening capillary network. **arteriovenous a.** a thick-walled blood vessel that connects an arteriole directly with a venule, found in the skin of the lips, nose, ears, hands, and feet. **2.** (in surgery) an artificial connection between two tubular organs or parts, especially between two normally separate parts of the intestine or two blood vessels. *See also* shunt.

anastrazole (an-**ass**-tră-zohl) *n.* *see* aromatase inhibitor.

anatomy (ă-**nat**-ŏmi) *n.* the study of the structure of living organisms. In medicine it refers to the study of the form and gross structure of the various parts of the human body. *See also* cytology, histology, physiology. **—anatomical** (ană-**tom**-i-k'l) *adj.* **—anatomist** *n.*

anconeus (an-**koh**-niŭs) *n.* a muscle behind the elbow that assists in extending the forearm.

Ancylostoma (Ankylostoma) (an-si-loh-**stoh**-mă) *n.* a genus of small parasitic nematodes that inhabit the small intestine (*see* hookworm). **A. duodenale** the species that most commonly infests humans.

ancylostomiasis (an-si-loh-stoh-**my**-ăsis) *n.* an infestation of the small intestine by the parasitic hookworm *Ancylostoma duodenale*. *See* hookworm (disease).

ANDI (**an**-di) *n.* an acronym for *ab*normal *d*evelopment and *i*nvolution, used to tabulate benign disorders of the breast.

andr- (andro-) *combining form denoting* men or the male sex.

androgen (**an**-drŏ-jĕn) *n.* one of a group of steroid hormones, including testosterone and dihydrotestosterone, that stimulate the development of male sex organs and male secondary sexual characteristics. The principal source of these hormones is the testis but they are also secreted by the adrenal cortex (*see* dehydroepiandrosterone) and ovaries in small amounts. In women excessive production of androgens gives rise to masculinization. Naturally occurring and synthetic androgens are used in replacement therapy and as anabolic agents. **—androgenic** *adj.*

androgen insensitivity syndrome (AIS) *n.* an X-linked (*see* sex-linked) disorder in which the body does not react to androgens because of structural abnormalities in androgen receptors. **complete AIS** (formerly known as **testicular feminization syndrome**) the most extreme form of AIS, in which there is a fully female body appearance with breast development and a short vagina (but no uterus; testes are present internally). Psychosexuality is female orientated. **partial AIS** a form of AIS that becomes most obvious at puberty, with poor development of male genitalia and breast development.

androgenization (an-droj-ĕn-I-**zay**-shŏn) *n.* the final effects of the exposure of sensitive tissues to androgens, i.e. the development of secondary male sexual characteristics. Androgenization can also occur abnormally in females, who may develop excessive body hair, male pattern baldness, and clitoromegaly.

andrology (an-**drol**-ŏji) *n.* **1.** the study of male infertility and erectile dysfunction. It includes seminal analysis and other investigation procedures to determine the causes of infertility, which determine the treatment undertaken. **2.** the study of androgen production and the relationship of plasma androgen to androgen action. **—andrologist** *n.*

androstenedione (an-drŏ-steen-**dy**-ohn) *n. see* adrenarche, dehydroepiandrosterone, testosterone.

androsterone (an-**drost**-er-ohn) *n.* a steroid that is formed in the liver as a metabolite of testosterone.

anencephaly (an-en-**sef**-ăli) *n.* partial or complete absence of the bones of the rear of the skull, the meninges, and the cerebral hemispheres of the brain. It occurs as a developmental defect and most affected infants are stillborn; if born live they do not survive for more than a few hours. *See also* alpha-fetoprotein. **—anencephalic** *adj.*

anergy (an-er-ji) *n.* **1.** lack of response to a specific antigen or allergen. **2.** lack of energy. **—anergic** *adj.*

aneurine (vitamin B_1) (an-yoor-in) *n. see* vitamin B.

aneurysm (an-yoor-izm) *n.* an abnormal balloon-like swelling in the wall of an artery, due to disease or congenital deficiency. **aortic a.** an aneurysm that most frequently occurs in the abdominal aorta, below the level of the renal arteries (**abdominal aortic a.**, **AAA**). Beyond a certain size it is prone to rupture: an acute surgical emergency. **arteriovenous a.** a direct communication between an artery and vein, without an intervening capillary bed. **berry a.** a small saccular aneurysm commonly affecting branches of the circle of Willis in the brain. Usually associated with congenital weakness of the vessels, they are a cause of cerebral haemorrhage in young adults. **Charcot-Bouchard a.** a small aneurysm found within the brain of elderly and hypertensive subjects. Such aneurysms may rupture, causing cerebral haemorrhage. **dissecting a.** a condition in which a tear occurs in the lining of (usually) the first part of the aorta, which allows blood to enter the wall and track along (dissect) the muscular coat. A dissecting aneurysm may rupture or it may compress the blood vessels arising from the aorta and produce infarction (localized necrosis) in the organs they supply. **ventricular a.** a condition that may develop in the wall of the left ventricle after myocardial infarction. Heart failure may result or thrombosis within the aneurysm may act as a source of embolism. **—aneurysmal** *adj.*

Angelman syndrome (happy puppet syndrome) (ayn-jĕl-măn) *n.* a disorder characterized by severe developmental delay, absence of speech, seizures, a jerky puppet-like gait, and paroxysmal laughter. It is usually caused by an abnormality of maternal chromosome 15. [H. Angelman (1915–96), British paediatrician]

angi- (angio-) *combining form denoting* blood or lymph vessels.

angiectasis (an-ji-**ek**-tă-sis) *n.* abnormal dilation of blood vessels.

angiitis (an-ji-**I**-tis) *n. see* vasculitis.

angina (an-**jy**-nă) *n.* a sense of suffocation or suffocating pain. **a. pectoris** pain in the centre of the chest, which is induced by exercise and relieved by rest and may spread to the jaws and arms. Angina pectoris occurs when the demand for blood by the heart exceeds the supply of the coronary arteries and it usually results from coronary artery atheroma. It may be prevented or relieved by such drugs as glyceryl trinitrate and beta blockers or by surgery (*see* angioplasty, coronary artery bypass graft). *See also* Ludwig's angina.

angiodysplasia (an-ji-oh-dis-**play**-ziă) *n.* an abnormal collection of small blood vessels found in the lining of the gastrointestinal tract, which can bleed.

angiogenesis (an-ji-oh-**jen**-i-sis) *n.* the formation of new blood vessels. This process occurs during wound healing and the development of malignant tumours and is promoted by growth factors. **a. inhibitor** an agent that interferes with angiogenesis, used in treating certain cancers. *See* bevacizumab.

angiography (an-ji-**og**-răfi) *n.* X-ray imaging of blood vessels after injection of radiopaque X-ray dye (contrast medium). **computerized tomographic a.** angiography in which a contrast agent, usually injected into a vein, increases the visibility of the blood vessels, which can then be seen on two- or three-dimensional images, with surrounding tissues hidden by the computer. **coronary a.** an X-ray technique for examining the coronary arteries and chambers of the heart in which video images are recorded during contrast-medium injection. *See* arteriography. **fluorescein a.** a technique for visualizing blood flow in the retina, in which the dye fluorescein sodium, injected into the bloodstream, causes the retinal blood vessels to fluoresce. **indocyanine green a.** a technique for visualizing blood flow in the choroid layer of the eye after the injection of the dye indocyanine green. **magnetic resonance a.** magnetic resonance imaging of blood vessels, either with (contrast-enhanced) or without (noncontrast) injection of magnetic resonance contrast agent. Contrast-enhanced MRA will show the blood vessels better.

angiology (an-ji-**ol**-ŏji) *n.* the branch of medicine concerned with the structure, function, and diseases of blood vessels.

angioma (an-ji-**oh**-mă) *n.* (*pl.* **angiomata**) a benign tumour composed of blood vessels or lymph vessels. **arteriovenous a.** (**arteriovenous malformation**, **AVM**) a knot of distended blood vessels that may occur in many parts of the body. When overlying and compressing the surface of the brain, it may cause epilepsy or subdural haematoma. **cherry a.** (**Campbell de Morgan spot**) a small red spot, consisting of a minor vascular malformation, occurring on the trunk in middle-aged and elderly people. *See also* haemangioma, lymphangioma.

angio-oedema (angioneurotic oedema) (an-ji-oh-ee-**dee**-mă) *n.* *see* urticaria.

angioplasty (**an**-ji-oh-plasti) *n.* repair or reconstruction of narrowed or completely obstructed blood vessels. **balloon a.** (**percutaneous transluminal a.**, **PTA**) enlargement of the lumen of a blood vessel by means of an inflatable balloon, mounted on the tip of a flexible catheter, under X-ray screening control. **coronary a.** balloon angioplasty of a section of coronary artery narrowed by atheroma.

angiosarcoma (an-ji-oh-sar-**koh**-mă) *n.* a sarcoma arising in the blood vessels.

angiospasm (an-ji-oh-spazm) *n.* *see* Raynaud's disease.

angiotensin (an-ji-oh-**ten**-sin) *n.* either of two peptides. **a. I** a peptide derived, by the action of renin, from a protein secreted by the liver into the bloodstream. **a. II** a peptide, formed from angiotensin I by enzyme action, that causes constriction of blood vessels and stimulates the release of vasopressin and aldosterone, which increase blood pressure. *See also* ACE inhibitor.

angiotensin II antagonist *n.* a drug that blocks the action of the hormone angiotensin II, which constricts blood vessels, and is therefore useful in treating hypertension. Such drugs include **candesartan** (Amias), **irbesartan** (Aprovel), **losartan** (Cozaar), **telmisartan** (Micardis), and **valsartan** (Diovan). They are taken by mouth.

angstrom (**ang**-strŏm) *n.* a unit of length equal to one ten millionth of a millimetre (10^{-10} m), sometimes used to express wavelengths and interatomic distances. Symbol Å.

anhedonia (an-hee-**doh**-niă) *n.* a reduction in or total loss of the feeling of pleasure in acts that normally give pleasure.

anhidrosis (an-hy-**droh**-sis) *n.* the absence of sweating in the presence of an appropriate stimulus for sweating, such as heat, which may accompany disease or occur as a congenital defect. *See also* hypohidrosis.

anhidrotic (an-hy-**drot**-ik) **1.** *n.* any drug that inhibits the secretion of sweat, such as an antimuscarinic drug. **2.** *adj.* inhibiting sweating.

anhydraemia (an-hy-**dree**-miă) *n.* a decrease in the proportion of water, and therefore plasma, in the blood.

anhydrous (an-**hy**-drŭs) *adj.* containing no water.

aniline (**an**-il-een) *n.* an oily compound obtained from coal tar and widely used in the preparation of dyes.

anion (**an**-I-ŏn) *n.* a negatively charged ion, which moves towards the anode (positive electrode) when an electric current is passed through the solution containing it. *Compare* cation. **a. gap** the difference between the concentrations of cations (positively charged ions) and anions, calculated from the formula $(Na^+ + K^+) - (HCO_3^- + Cl^-)$: it is used to estimate the unaccounted-for anions in the blood in cases of metabolic disturbance.

aniridia (ani-**rid**-iă) *n.* congenital absence of the iris (of the eye).

anisocytosis (an-I-soh-sy-**toh**-sis) *n.* an excessive variation in size between individual red blood cells.

anisomelia (an-I-soh-**mee**-liă) *n.* a difference in size or shape between the arms or the legs.

anisometropia (an-I-soh-mĕ-**troh**-piă) *n.* the condition in which the power of refraction in one eye differs markedly from that in the other.

ankle (**an**-k'l) *n.* **1.** the hinge joint between the leg and the foot. It consists of the talus (ankle bone), which projects into a socket formed by the lower ends of the tibia and fibula. **2.** the whole region of the ankle joint, including the tarsus and the lower parts of the tibia and fibula.

ankle–brachial pressure index (ABPI) *n.* the ratio of systolic blood pressure at the ankle (measured by a Doppler ultrasound probe placed over the dorsalis pedis artery; *see* pulse) to that measured at the brachial artery: used to quantify the severity of arterial occlusion in the leg. Peripheral arterial disease is present if the ABPI is less than 0.95.

ankyloblepharon (anki-loh-**blef**-er-on) *n.* abnormal fusion (partial or complete) of the upper and lower eyelid margins.

ankylosing spondylitis (anki-**loh**-zing) *n. see* spondylitis.

ankylosis (anki-**loh**-sis) *n.* pathological fusion of two bones across a joint space resulting from prolonged joint inflammation or infection, either by bony tissue (**bony a.**) or by shortening of connecting fibrous tissue (**fibrous a.**).

Ankylostoma (anki-loh-**stoh**-mă) *n. see* Ancylostoma.

annulus (**an**-yoo-lŭs) *n.* (in anatomy) a circular opening or ring-shaped structure. —**annular** *adj.*

ano- *combining form denoting* the anus.

anodyne (**an**-ŏ-dyn) *n.* any treatment or drug that soothes and eases pain.

anomaly (ă-**nom**-ăli) *n.* any deviation from the normal, especially a congenital or developmental defect. —**anomalous** *adj.*

anomia (ă-**noh**-miă) *n.* a form of aphasia in which the patient is unable to give the names of objects, but retains the ability to put words together into speech.

anomie (**an**-oh-mi) *n.* a condition in which a person is no longer able to identify with or relate to others, resulting in apathy, loneliness, and distress.

anonychia (anŏ-**nik**-iă) *n.* congenital absence of one or more nails.

Anopheles (ă-**nof**-i-leez) *n.* a genus of widely distributed mosquitoes. The malarial parasite (*see* plasmodium) is transmitted to humans solely through the bite of female *Anopheles* mosquitoes.

anophthalmos (an-off-**thal**-mŏs) *n.* congenital absence of the eye.

anoplasty (**ay**-noh-plasti) *n.* a surgical technique used to repair a weak or injured anal sphincter.

anorchism (an-**or**-kizm) *n.* congenital absence of one or both testes.

anorexia (an-er-**eks**-iă) *n.* loss of appetite. **a. nervosa** a psychiatric illness, most common in female adolescents, in which the patients starve themselves or use other techniques, such as vomiting or taking laxatives, to induce weight loss. The result is severe loss of weight with amenorrhoea. The causes of the illness are not clearly understood. Patients must be persuaded to eat enough to maintain a normal body weight and their emotional disturbance is usually treated with psychotherapy supported by a dietitian. *See also* bulimia.

SEE WEB LINKS

- Overview of anorexia from the NHS Choices website

anosmia (an-**oz**-miă) *n.* absence of the sense of smell. Permanent anosmia may follow certain viral infections, head injuries, and tumours affecting the olfactory nerve.

anovular (anovulatory) (an-**ov**-yoo-ler) *adj.* not associated with the development and release of a female germ cell (ovum) in the ovary, as in **anovular menstruation**.

anoxaemia (an-oks-**ee**-miă) *n.* a condition in which there is less than the normal concentration of oxygen in the blood. *See also* hypoxaemia.

anoxia (an-**oks**-iă) *n.* a condition in which the tissues of the body receive inadequate amounts of oxygen. *See also* hypoxia. **—anoxic** *adj.*

ant- (anti-) *prefix denoting* opposed to; counteracting; relieving.

Antabuse (**ant**-ă-bews) *n.* *see* disulfiram.

antacid (ant-**ass**-id) *n.* a drug, such as aluminium or magnesium hydroxide, that neutralizes the hydrochloric acid secreted in the digestive juices of the stomach. Antacids are used to relieve discomfort in disorders of the digestive system.

antagonist (an-**tag**-ŏn-ist) *n.* **1.** a muscle whose action (contraction) opposes that of another muscle (*see* agonist). **2.** a drug or other substance with opposite action to that of another drug or natural body chemical. **—antagonism** *n.*

ante- *prefix denoting* before.

anteflexion (anti-**flek**-shŏn) *n.* the bending forward of an organ. A mild degree of anteflexion of the uterus is considered to be normal. *Compare* retroflexion.

ante mortem (**an**-ti **mor**-tĕm) *adj.* before death. *Compare* post mortem.

antenatal (anti-**nay**-t'l) *adj.* of or relating to the period of pregnancy; before birth. **a. diagnosis** *see* prenatal diagnosis.

antepartum (anti-**par**-tŭm) *adj.* occurring before the onset of labour. **a. haemorrhage (APH)** bleeding from the genital tract after the 20th week of pregnancy until the birth of the baby.

anterior (an-**teer**-i-er) *adj.* **1.** describing or relating to the front (ventral) portion of the body or limbs. **2.** describing the front part of any organ. **a. chamber** the part of the eye between the cornea and lens, which is filled with aqueous humour.

anteversion (anti-**ver**-shŏn) *n.* the forward inclination of an organ, especially the normal forward inclination of the uterus. *Compare* retroversion.

anthelmintic (an-thel-**min**-tik) **1.** *n.* any drug, such as piperazine, or chemical agent used to destroy parasitic worms (helminths) and/or remove them from the body. **2.** *adj.* having the power to destroy or eliminate helminths.

anthracosis (an-thră-**koh**-sis) *n.* *see* coal-worker's pneumoconiosis.

anthracycline (an-thră-**sy**-kleen) *n.* any of numerous antibiotics synthesized or isolated from species of *Streptomyces*. Doxorubicin is the most important member of this group of compounds, which have wide activity against tumours, particularly breast cancer and lymphoma. *See* cytotoxic drug.

anthrax (**an**-thraks) *n.* an acute infectious disease of farm animals caused by the bacterium *Bacillus anthracis*. In humans the disease attacks either the lungs, causing pneumonia, or the skin, producing severe ulceration (**malignant pustule**). **Woolsorter's disease** is a serious infection of the skin or lungs by *B. anthracis*, affecting those handling wool or pelts (*see* occupational disease). Anthrax can be treated with penicillin or tetracycline.

anthrop- (anthropo-) *combining form denoting* the human race.

anti-androgen (anti-**an**-drŏ-jĕn) *n.* any one of a group of drugs that inhibit the action of testosterone on the prostate gland and are therefore used in the treatment of prostate cancer, which is an androgen-dependent tumour. An example is **abiraterone acetate** (Zytiga). *See also* bicalutamide, cyproterone, finasteride, flutamide.

anti-arrhythmic (anti-ă-**ri***th*-mik) *n.* any of a group of drugs used to correct irregularities in the heartbeat (*see* arrhythmia). They include adenosine, amiodarone, verapamil, disopyramide, and lidocaine.

antibacterial (anti-bak-**teer**-iăl) *adj.* describing an antibiotic that is active against bacteria.

antibiotic (anti-by-**ot**-ik) *n.* a substance, produced by or derived from a microorganism, that destroys or inhibits the growth of other microorganisms. Antibiotics are used to treat infections caused by organisms that are sensitive to them, usually bacteria or fungi. *See also* aminoglycosides, antifungal, antiviral drug, cephalosporin, penicillin, quinolone, tetracyclines.

antibody (**an**-ti-bodi) *n.* a special kind of blood protein that is synthesized in lymphoid tissue in response to the presence of a particular antigen and circulates in the plasma to attack the antigen and render it harmless. Antibody formation is the basis of both immunity and allergy.

anticholinergic (anti-koli-**ner**-jik) *adj. see* antimuscarinic.

anticholinesterase (anti-koli-**nes**-ter-ayz) *n.* any drug or other substance that inhibits the action of cholinesterase and therefore allows acetylcholine to continue transmitting nerve impulses.

anticoagulant (anti-koh-**ag**-yoo-lănt) *n.* an agent, such as heparin or warfarin, that prevents the clotting of blood and is used in the treatment of such conditions as thrombosis and embolism. Incorrect dosage may result in haemorrhage.

anticonvulsant (anti-kŏn-**vul**-sănt) *n.* a drug, such as sodium valproate, carbamazepine, lamotrigine, or levetiracetam (Keppra), that prevents or reduces the severity of seizures in various types of epilepsy. Anticonvulsants are also known as **antiepileptic drugs**.

anti D *n.* the rhesus-factor antibody, formed by rhesus-negative individuals following exposure to rhesus-positive blood. **Anti-D immunoglobulin** (**anti-D Ig**) is administered to Rh-negative women within 72 hours of giving birth to a Rh-positive child (or following miscarriage or abortion) to prevent the risk of haemolytic disease of the newborn in a subsequent child.

antidepressant (anti-di-**press**-ănt) *n.* a drug designed to alleviate the symptoms of depression. A widely prescribed group are the **tricyclic antidepressants** (**TCAs**), such as doxepin and imipramine. Side-effects include dry mouth, blurred vision, and difficulty in urination. *See also* MAO inhibitor, SNRI, SSRI.

antidiabetic drugs (anti-dy-ă-**bet**-ik) *pl. n.* drugs used to control diabetes mellitus. Type 1 diabetes is treated with the wide range of formulations of insulin. Type 2 diabetes is treated mainly with oral hypoglycaemic drugs but in some cases insulin may be required.

antidiuretic hormone (ADH) (anti-dy-yoor-**et**-ik) *n.* *see* vasopressin.

antidote (**an**-ti-doht) *n.* a drug that counteracts the effects of a poison.

antiemetic (anti-i-**met**-ik) *n.* a drug that prevents vomiting, used to treat such conditions as motion sickness and vertigo and to counteract nausea and vomiting caused by other drugs.

antiepileptic drug (anti-epi-**lep**-tik) *n.* *see* anticonvulsant.

antifibrinolytic (anti-fib-rin-ŏ-**lit**-ik) *adj.* describing an agent that inhibits the dissolution of blood clots (*see* fibrinolysis). Antifibrinolytic drugs include tranexamic acid.

antifungal (antimycotic) (anti-**fung**-ăl) *adj.* describing a drug that kills or inactivates fungi and is used to treat fungal (including yeast) infections. Antifungal drugs include amphotericin, griseofulvin, the imidazoles, nystatin, and terbinafine.

antigen (**an**-ti-jĕn) *n.* any substance that may be specifically bound by an antibody molecule. —**antigenic** *adj.*

antihaemophilic factor (anti-heem-ŏ-**fil**-ik) *n.* *see* Factor VIII.

anti HBc *n.* antibody against hepatitis B core antigen.

anti HBs *n.* antibody against hepatitis B surface antigen.

antihistamine (anti-**hist**-ă-meen) *n.* a drug that inhibits the action of histamine by blocking specific histamine receptors. Four such receptors have been identified (H_1 to H_4). **H_1-receptor antagonists** are used to relieve the symptoms of allergic conditions, such as hay fever, pruritus (itching), and urticaria (nettle rash). Many H_1-receptor antagonists (e.g. cyclizine, promethazine) have a strong anti-emetic activity and are used to prevent motion sickness. The most common side-effect of these drugs, especially the older ones (e.g. alimemazine, promethazine), is drowsiness and because of this they are sometimes used to promote sleep. Newer antihistamines (e.g. cetirizine, loratidine, mizolastine) are less sedating. H_2 receptors are found mainly in the stomach, where stimulation by histamine causes secretion of acid gastric juice. **H_2-receptor antagonists** (e.g. cimetidine, famotidine, nizatidine, ranitidine) block these receptors and so reduce gastric acid secretion; they are used in the treatment of dyspepsia, peptic ulcers, and gastro-oesophageal reflux disease. H_3- and H_4-receptor antagonists have yet to find a clinical role.

antihypertensive (anti-hy-per-**ten**-siv) *adj.* describing drugs or other agents used in treating high blood pressure.

anti-inflammatory (anti-in-**flam**-ă-tŏ-ri) **1.** *adj.* describing a drug that reduces inflammation. The various groups of anti-inflammatory drugs act against one or more of the mediators that initiate or maintain inflammation. They include antihistamines, the glucocorticoids (*see* corticosteroid), and the nonsteroidal anti-inflammatory drugs (*see* NSAID). **2.** *n.* an anti-inflammatory drug.

antilymphocyte serum (antilymphocyte globulin, ALS, ALG) (anti-**lim**-foh-syt) *n.* an antiserum containing antibodies that suppress lymphocytic activity. ALS may be given to prevent the immune reaction that causes tissue rejection following transplantation of organs (e.g. kidneys) or bone marrow.

antimetabolite (anti-mi-**tab**-ŏ-lyt) *n.* a drug that interferes with the normal metabolic processes within cells by combining with the enzymes responsible for them. Some drugs used in the treatment of cancer, e.g. fluorouracil, methotrexate, and mercaptopurine, are antimetabolites. Side-effects can include blood cell disorders and digestive disturbances. *See also* cytotoxic drug.

antimitotic (anti-my-**tot**-ik) *n.* a drug that inhibits cell division and growth. The drugs used to treat cancer are mainly antimitotics. *See also* antimetabolite, cytotoxic drug.

antimuscarinic (anticholinergic) (anti-musk-er-**in**-ik) *adj.* inhibiting the action of acetylcholine, a neurotransmitter in the parasympathetic nervous system. Antimuscarinic drugs relax smooth muscle, decrease the secretion of saliva, sweat, and digestive juice, and dilate the pupil of the eye.

antimycotic (anti-my-**kot**-ik) *adj. see* antifungal.

anti-oestrogen (oestrogen-receptor antagonist) (anti-**ees**-trŏ-jĕn) *n.* one of a group of drugs that oppose the action of oestrogen by binding to oestrogen receptors in the body's tissues. It includes tamoxifen, which is used in the treatment of breast cancers dependent on oestrogen. Because they stimulate the production of pituitary gonadotrophins, some anti-oestrogens (e.g. clomifene) are used to induce or stimulate ovulation in infertility treatment (*see* superovulation). Side-effects of anti-oestrogens include hot flushes, itching of the vulva, nausea, vomiting, and fluid retention.

antioxidant (anti-**oks**-i-dănt) *n.* a substance capable of neutralizing oxygen free radicals, the highly active and damaging atoms and chemical groups produced by various disease processes and by poisons, radiation, smoking, and other agencies. Antioxidants include vitamin C (ascorbic acid), vitamin E (tocopherols), and beta carotene.

antiphospholipid antibody syndrome (Hughes syndrome) (anti-fos-foh-**lip**-id) *n.* an autoimmune disease in which the presence of antibodies against phospholipid is associated with a tendency to arterial or venous thrombosis and – in women of childbearing age – recurrent (three or more) miscarriages. Treatment is by low-dose aspirin or heparin.

antiplatelet drug (anti-**playt**-lit) *n.* a drug, such as aspirin or clopidogrel, that reduces platelet aggregation and therefore the formation of clot (*see* thrombosis).

antipruritic (anti-proor-**it**-ik) *n.* an agent, such as doxepin or crotamiton, that relieves itching (pruritus).

antipsychotic (anti-sy-**kot**-ik) *n.* any one of a group of drugs used to treat severe mental disorders (psychoses), including schizophrenia and mania; some are administered in small doses to relieve anxiety and tic disorders. They were formerly known as **major tranquillizers**. **first generation** (or **typical**) **a.** any one of a group of antipsychotic drugs including the phenothiazines (e.g. chlorpromazine), butyrophenones (e.g. haloperidol), and thioxanthenes (e.g. flupentixol). Side-effects include abnormal involuntary movements (extrapyramidal effects), sedation, dry mouth, blurred vision, and weight gain. **second generation** (or **atypical**) **a.** any one of a group of antipsychotics, including clozapine, risperidone, **olanzapine** (Zyprexa), and **quetiapine** (Seroquel), that are used in treating patients unresponsive to first-generation antipsychotics. Extrapyramidal side-effects are less troublesome.

antipyretic (anti-py-**ret**-ik) *n.* a drug that reduces fever by lowering the body temperature.

antiretroviral (ARV) (anti-ret-roh-vy-răl) *adj.* describing a drug or therapy that inhibits or slows the growth of retroviruses, specifically HIV, and is used in the treatment of HIV infection and AIDS. Antiretroviral drugs include didanosine, zidovudine, and the protease inhibitors. **highly active a. therapy** (**HAART**) treatment with a combination of antiretroviral drugs.

antisecretory drug (anti-si-**kree**-tŏri) *n.* any drug that reduces the normal rate of secretion of a body fluid, usually one that reduces acid secretion into the stomach. Such drugs include antimuscarinic drugs, H_2-receptor antagonists (*see* antihistamine), and proton-pump inhibitors.

antisepsis (anti-**sep**-sis) *n.* the elimination of bacteria, fungi, viruses, and other microorganisms that cause disease by the use of chemical or physical methods.

antiseptic (anti-**sep**-tik) *n.* a chemical, such as chlorhexidine or cetrimide, that destroys or inhibits the growth of disease-causing bacteria and other microorganisms. Antiseptics are used externally to cleanse wounds and internally to treat infections of the intestine and bladder.

antiserum (anti-**seer**-ŭm) *n.* (*pl.* **antisera**) a serum that contains antibodies against antigens of a particular kind; it may be injected to treat, or give temporary protection against, specific diseases. Antisera are prepared in large quantities in such animals as horses.

antisocial (anti-**soh**-shăl) *adj.* contrary to the accepted standards of behaviour in society.

antisocial personality disorder *n.* a personality disorder characterized by callous unconcern for others, irresponsibility, violence, disregard for social rules, and an incapacity for maintaining enduring relationships. It is also known as **dyssocial personality**, **psychopathy**, or **sociopathy**.

antispasmodic (anti-spaz-**mod**-ik) *n.* a drug, such as alverine citrate or dicycloverine, that relieves spasm of smooth muscle in the gut.

antispastic (anti-**spas**-tik) *n.* a drug that relieves spasm of skeletal muscle. *See also* muscle relaxant.

antistatic (anti-**stat**-ik) *adj.* preventing the accumulation of static electricity.

antithrombin (anti-**throm**-bin) *n.* a substance or effect that inhibits the action of thrombin in the circulation, preventing unwanted clotting.

antithyroid drug (anti-**th'y**-roid) *n.* a drug, such as carbimazole, that is used to counteract the excessive production and release of thyroid hormones in thyrotoxic states.

antitoxin (anti-**toks**-in) *n.* an antibody produced by the body to counteract a toxin formed by invading bacteria or from any other source.

antitragus (anti-**tray**-gŭs) *n.* a small projection of cartilage above the lobe of the ear, opposite the tragus. *See* pinna.

antitussive (cough suppressant) (anti-**tuss**-iv) *n.* a drug, such as pholcodine, that suppresses coughing.

antivenene (antivenin) (anti-**ven**-een) *n.* an antiserum containing antibodies against specific poisons in the venom of such an animal as a snake, spider, or scorpion.

antiviral drug (anti-**vy**-răl) *n.* a drug effective against viruses that cause disease. Antiviral drugs include aciclovir, ganciclovir, foscarnet, oseltamivir, and ribavirin, used for treating herpes, cytomegalovirus, influenza, and respiratory syncytial virus infections; and antiretroviral drugs, used for treating HIV infections and AIDS.

antrectomy (an-**trek**-tŏmi) *n.* **1.** surgical removal of the bony walls of an antrum. *See* antrostomy. **2.** (**distal gastrectomy**) a surgical operation in which a part of the stomach (the antrum) is removed. Indications for antrectomy include peptic ulcer disease resistant to medical treatment, tumours, perforation, and gastric outlet obstruction.

antroscopy (an-**tros**-kŏpi) *n.* inspection of the inside of the maxillary sinus (*see* paranasal sinuses) using an endoscope (called an **antroscope**).

antrostomy (an-trost-ŏmi) *n.* a surgical operation to produce an artificial opening to an antrum in a bone, so providing drainage for any fluid. The operation is sometimes carried out to treat infection or inflammation of the paranasal sinuses.

antrum (an-trŭm) *n.* **1.** a cavity, especially a cavity in a bone. **a. of Highmore** the maxillary sinus (*see* paranasal sinuses). [N. Highmore (1613–85), English physician] **mastoid** (or **tympanic**) **a.** the space connecting the air cells of the mastoid process with the chamber of the inner ear. **2. (gastric antrum)** the distal third of the stomach.

anuria (ă-newr-iă) *n.* failure of urine production.

anus (ay-nŭs) *n.* the opening at the lower end of the alimentary canal, through which the faeces are discharged. It opens out from the anal canal and is guarded by two sphincters. **—anal** *adj.*

anvil (an-vil) *n.* (in anatomy) *see* incus.

anxiety (ang-zy-iti) *n.* generalized pervasive fear. **a. disorder** any one of a group of mental or behavioural disorders in which anxiety dominates the patient's life or is experienced in particular situations. *See* generalized anxiety disorder, neurosis, panic disorder, post-traumatic stress disorder. **a. management** a behaviour therapy designed to allow patients who suffer from anxiety disorders to reduce their symptoms by learning how to relax and avoid excessive rumination.

anxiolytic (angk-si-oh-**lit**-ik) *adj.* describing a group of drugs used to treat anxiety of various causes. Formerly known as **minor tranquillizers**, they include the benzodiazepines and buspirone. Prolonged use may result in dependence.

aorta (ay-or-tă) *n.* (*pl.* **aortae** or **aortas**) the main artery of the body, from which all others derive. **abdominal a.** the part of the descending aorta below the diaphragm. **arch of the a.** the part of the aorta that arches over the heart. **ascending a.** the part of the aorta that arises from the left ventricle. **descending a.** the part of the aorta that descends in front of the backbone. **thoracic a.** the part of the descending aorta from the arch of the aorta to the diaphragm. **—aortic** (ay-or-tik) *adj.*

aortic aneurysm *n. see* aneurysm.

aortic regurgitation *n.* a leak of the aortic valve resulting in reflux of blood from the aorta into the left ventricle during diastole. Aortic regurgitation is most commonly due to degenerative wear and tear of the aortic valve.

aortic replacement *n.* a surgical technique used to replace a diseased length of aorta, most often the abdominal aorta. It usually involves inserting into the aorta a flexible tube of artificial material, which functions as a substitute for the diseased section.

aortic stenosis *n.* narrowing of the opening of the aortic valve due to fusion of the cusps that comprise the valve. It may result from previous rheumatic fever, or from calcification and scarring in a valve that has two cusps instead of the normal three, or it may be congenital.

aortic valve *n.* a semilunar valve in the heart, lying between the left ventricle and the aorta, that prevents the backflow of blood from the aorta to the left ventricle.

aortitis (ay-or-**ty**-tis) *n.* inflammation of the aorta, which is often associated with a variety of poorly understood autoimmune conditions, such as Behçet's syndrome and Takayasu's disease.

aortography (ay-or-**tog**-răfi) *n.* X-ray examination of the aorta in which a series of images is taken during the injection of X-ray dye (see angiography) into the aorta via a catheter inserted in the groin. It has now largely been replaced by other cross-sectional imaging techniques.

APACHE scoring system *n.* *a*cute *p*hysiological *a*nd *c*hronic *h*ealth *e*valuation: a tool used to assess the severity of illness in a critically ill patient and to estimate mortality. The assessment uses information from twelve physiological measurements, including temperature, blood pressure, arterial pH, and certain blood results.

apareunia (ap-ă-**roo**-niă) *n.* inability to have penetrative intercourse due to physical discomfort, vaginismus, or an underlying psychological problem. *See* dyspareunia.

apathetic hyperthyroidism (apă-**thet**-ik) *n. see* hyperthyroidism.

apathy (**a**-pă-thi) *n.* an individual's lack of interest in or concern for issues that may affect him or her significantly. A sign of impaired motivation, it is associated with depression.

APD *n.* **1.** *see* auditory processing disorder. **2.** automated peritoneal dialysis: a method of treating renal failure in which fluid is delivered through a soft silastic catheter that is tunnelled out of the peritoneal cavity and is designed to stay in place for years.

APEL (APL) *n.* Accreditation of Prior (Experiential) Learning: a system for the award of credit, based on previous experience and learning, that enables students to avoid repetition of assessment and to maximize their learning potential. Evidence for the learning and experience must be provided for scrutiny. The level at which learning and experience are valued is measured using education-based tariffs. *See also* CATS.

aperient (ă-**peer**-iĕnt) *n.* a mild laxative.

aperistalsis (ay-pe-ri-**stal**-sis) *n.* the absence of peristaltic movement in the intestines.

apex (**ay**-peks) *n.* the tip or summit of an organ; for example the heart or lung. The apex of a tooth is the tip of the root. *See also* apical.

apex beat *n.* the impact of the heart against the chest wall during systole. It can be felt to the left of the breastbone, in the space between the fifth and sixth ribs.

Apgar score (**ap**-gar) *n.* a method of rapidly assessing the general

Apgar score

Apgar score	0	1	2
Appearance	Blue	Acrocyanotic	Pink
Pulse rate (bpm)	Absent	<100	>100
Reflex irritability	No response	Grimace	Vigorous cough/sneeze
Muscle tone	Limp	Some flexion of extremities	Active movement
Respiratory effort	Absent	Slow/irregular breaths	Good respiratory effort and cry

state of a baby immediately after birth. A score of 0, 1, or 2 points is given for each sign, usually measured at one minute and five minutes after delivery (see table). [V. Apgar (1909–74), US anaesthetist]

aphagia (ă-fay-jiă) *n.* loss of the ability to swallow.

aphakia (ă-fay-kiă) *n.* absence of the lens of the eye: the state of the eye after a cataract has been removed and no intraocular lens has been inserted. **—aphakic** *adj.*

aphasia (dysphasia) (ă-fay-ziă) *n.* a disorder of language affecting the generation and content of speech and its understanding. It is caused by damage to the language-dominant half of the brain, usually the left hemisphere in a right-handed person. **expressive a.** difficulty in producing language. **receptive a.** difficulty with comprehension of the spoken word. **—aphasic** *adj.*

aphonia (ă-foh-niă) *n.* absence or loss of the voice caused by disease of the larynx or mouth or disease of the nerves and muscles involved in the generation and articulation of speech.

aphrodisiac (afrŏ-diz-iak) *n.* an agent that stimulates sexual excitement.

aphthous ulcer (af-thŭs) *n.* a small ulcer, occurring singly or in groups in the mouth as white or red spots.

apical (ay-pi-k'l) *adj.* of or relating to the apex of an organ or tooth. **a. abscess** *see* abscess.

apicectomy (ay-pi-sek-tŏmi) *n.* (in dentistry) surgical removal of the apex of the root of a tooth, now often called **root end resection**.

APL *n. see* APEL.

aplasia (ă-play-ziă) *n.* total or partial failure of development of an organ or tissue. *See also* agenesis. **—aplastic** (ay-plas-tik) *adj.*

aplastic anaemia *n.* a severe form of anaemia, resistant to therapy, in which the bone marrow fails to produce new blood cells (*see* pancytopenia). There are several causes, including a reaction to toxic drugs.

apnoea (ap-**nee**-ă) *n.* temporary cessation of breathing from any cause, formally defined as a reduction in nasal air flow to less than 30% of normal for more than 10 seconds. **a. index** the number of apnoea episodes per hour of sleep. **a. monitor** an electronic alarm, responding to a baby's breathing movements, that can monitor babies at risk from sudden infant death syndrome. *See also* sleep apnoea. **—apnoeic** *adj.*

apocrine (ap-ŏ-kryn) *adj.* **1.** describing sweat glands that occur only in hairy parts of the body, especially the armpit and groin. These glands develop in the hair follicles and appear after puberty has been reached. *Compare* eccrine. **2.** describing a type of gland that loses part of its protoplasm when secreting. *See* secretion.

apolipoprotein (Apo) (apŏ-lip-oh-**proh**-teen) *n.* the protein component of a lipoprotein. Apolipoproteins have a variety of functions, which include acting as ligands for the binding of enzymes (ApoB) and as cofactors for the action of other enzymes (ApoA and ApoC).

apomorphine (apŏ-**mor**-feen) *n.* a drug used mainly in the treatment of Parkinson's disease that is poorly controlled by levodopa. It is administered by subcutaneous injection or infusion. Trade name: **APO-go**.

aponeurosis (apŏ-newr-**oh**-sis) *n.* a thin but strong fibrous sheet of tissue that replaces a tendon in muscles that are flat and sheetlike and have a wide area of attachment (e.g. to bones). **—aponeurotic** (apŏ-newr-**ot**-ik) *adj.*

apophysis (ă-**pof**-i-sis) *n.* a protuberance of bone to which a tendon is attached. **a. cerebri** the pineal gland. **—apophyseal** *adj.*

apophysitis (ă-pof-i-**sy**-tis) *n.* inflammation of an unfused apophysis caused by excessive pull of an attached tendon. *See* Osgood-Schlatter disease, Sever's disease.

apoplexy (ap-ŏ-plek-si) *n. see* stroke.

apoptosis (ă-**pop**-tŏ-sis) *n.* programmed cell death, which results in the ordered removal of cells and occurs naturally as part of the normal development, maintenance, and renewal of cells, tissues, and organs. Defects in apoptosis have been implicated in the uncontrolled division of cells that occurs in cancer.

appendectomy (ap-ĕn-**dek**-tŏmi) *n. US* appendicectomy.

appendicectomy (ă-pen-di-**sek**-tŏmi) *n.* surgical removal of the vermiform appendix. *See also* appendicitis.

appendicitis (ă-pen-di-**sy**-tis) *n.* inflammation of the vermiform appendix. The typical presentation of **acute a.** is abdominal pain, first central and later in the right lower abdomen, over the appendix. If not treated by surgical removal (appendicectomy) the condition may progress to cause abscess formation, perforation, peritonitis, life-threatening sepsis, and circulatory shock.

appendicular (ap-ĕn-**dik**-yoo-ler) *adj.* **1.** relating to or affecting the vermiform appendix. **2.** relating to the limbs.

appendix (vermiform appendix) (ă-**pen**-diks) *n.* the short thin blind-ended tube, 7–10 cm long, that is attached to the end of the caecum. It has no known function in humans and is liable to become infected and inflamed (*see* appendicitis).

apperception (ap-er-**sep**-shŏn) *n.* (in psychology) the process by which the qualities of an object, situation, etc., perceived by an individual are correlated with his/her preexisting knowledge.

appestat (**ap**-ĕs-tat) *n.* a region in the brain that controls the amount of food intake. Appetite suppressants probably decrease hunger by changing the chemical characteristics of this centre.

applanation (ap-lă-**nay**-shŏn) *n.* flattening of the cornea. It is used to determine intraocular pressure (**a. tonometry**). *See* tonometer.

applicator (**ap**-li-kay-ter) *n.* any device used to apply medication or treatment to a particular part of the body.

apposition (apŏ-**zish**-ŏn) *n.* the state of two structures, such as parts of the body, being in close contact. For example, the fingers are brought into apposition when the fist is clenched.

appraisal (ă-**pray**-z'l) *n.* the evaluation of an individual's performance, usually by an immediate line manager. Appraisals are performed on a regular basis for National Health Service employees.

apraclonidine (ap-ră-**kloh**-ni-deen) *n.* a sympathomimetic drug administered in the form of eye drops to reduce or prevent raised intraocular pressure, mostly used after laser surgery. Trade name: **Iopidine**.

apraxia (ă-**praks**-iă) *n.* an inability to make skilled movements with accuracy. This is a disorder of the cerebral cortex most often caused by disease of the parietal lobes of the brain. *Compare* dyspraxia. **gait a.** difficulty in walking, caused by disease of the frontal lobes.

APT *n.* alum precipitated toxoid: a preparation used for immunization against diphtheria. *See also* DtaP/IPV, DTaP/IPV/Hib.

APTT *n.* activated partial thromboplastin time (*see* PTTK).

APUD cells *pl. n.* cells that share the metabolic property of *a*mine-*p*recursor *u*ptake and *d*ecarboxylation. They are widely distributed, especially in the mucosa of the gastrointestinal tract and pancreas, and their function is to synthesize and release polypeptides that serve as regulator peptides and neurotransmitters.

apudoma (apuud-**oh**-mă) *n.* a tumour that contains APUD cells and may give rise to symptoms caused by excessive production of the hormones and other peptides that these cells produce. Carcinoids are examples.

apyrexia (ap-I-**reks**-iă) *n.* the absence of fever.

aqua (**ak**-wă) *n.* water. **a. destillata** distilled water. **a. fortis** nitric acid.

aqueduct (ak-wi-dukt) *n.* (in anatomy) a canal containing fluid. **cerebral a.** (**a. of Sylvius**) a canal connecting the third and fourth ventricles. [F. Sylvius de la Boe (1614–72), French anatomist]

aqueous humour (ay-kwi-ŭs) *n.* the watery fluid that fills the chamber of the eye immediately behind the cornea and in front of the lens.

arachidonic acid (ă-rak-i-**don**-ik) *n.* *see* essential fatty acid.

arachnodactyly (ă-rak-noh-**dak**-tili) *n.* *see* Marfan's syndrome.

arachnoid (arachnoid mater) (ă-**rak**-noid) *n.* the middle of the three membranes covering the brain and spinal cord (*see* meninges), which has a fine, almost cobweb-like, texture. **a. villi** thin-walled projections of the arachnoid into the blood-filled sinuses of the dura, through which cerebrospinal fluid flows from the subarachnoid space into the bloodstream. Large villi (**Pacchionian bodies**) are found in the region of the superior sagittal sinus.

arachnoiditis (ă-rak-noid-I-tis) *n.* an inflammatory process causing thickening and scarring (fibrosis) of the membranous linings (meninges) of the spinal canal. The resulting entrapment of nerve roots may result in weakness, pain, and numbness in the affected area. Arachnoiditis may result from infection of the meninges, surgery, or as a response to the oil-based dyes formerly used in myelography.

arbor (ar-ber) *n.* (in anatomy) a treelike structure. **a. vitae 1.** the treelike outline of white matter seen in sections of the cerebellum. **2.** the treelike appearance of the inner folds of the cervix (neck) of the uterus.

arborization (ar-ber-I-zay-shŏn) *n.* the branching termination of certain neurone processes.

arbovirus (ar-boh-vy-rŭs) *n.* one of a group of RNA-containing viruses that are transmitted by arthropods (hence *ar*thropod-*bo*rne viruses) and cause diseases resulting in encephalitis or serious fever, such as dengue and yellow fever.

ARC *n.* AIDS-related complex: *see* AIDS.

arch- (arche-, archi-, archo-) *combining form denoting* first; beginning; primitive; ancestral.

arcus (ar-kŭs) *n.* (in anatomy) an arch. **a. senilis** (**corneal a.**) a white or greyish line in the periphery of the cornea, common in the elderly. In a younger person (**a. juvenilis**) it may indicate hyperlipidaemia.

ARDS *n.* *see* adult respiratory distress syndrome.

areola (ă-ree-ŏlă) *n.* **1.** the brownish or pink ring of tissue surrounding the nipple of the breast. **2.** the part of the iris that surrounds the pupil of the eye. **3.** a small space in a tissue. **—areolar** (ă-ree-ŏler) *adj.*

areolar tissue *n.* loose connective tissue consisting of a meshwork of collagen, elastic tissue, and reticular fibres interspersed with numerous connective tissue cells.

ARF *n.* **1.** acute renal failure. **2.** acute respiratory failure.

argentaffin cells (ar-jen-tă-fin) *pl. n.* cells that stain readily with silver salts. Such cells occur, for example, in the crypts of Lieberkühn in the intestine.

arginine (ar-ji-neen) *n.* an amino acid that plays an important role in the formation of urea by the liver.

argon laser (ar-gŏn) *n. see* laser.

Argyll Robertson pupil (ar-gyl **rob**-ert-sŏn) *n.* a disorder of the eyes, which may result from syphilis or diabetes, in which the pupillary (light) reflex is absent. Although the pupils contract normally for near vision, they fail to contract in bright light. [D. Argyll Robertson (1837–1909), Scottish ophthalmologist]

ariboflavinosis (ă-ry-boh-flay-vin-**oh**-sis) *n.* the group of symptoms caused by deficiency of riboflavin (vitamin B_2). These symptoms include inflammation of the tongue and lips and sores in the corners of the mouth.

ARM *n.* artificial rupture of membranes: *see* amniotomy.

ARMD *n. see* (age-related) macular degeneration.

Arnold–Chiari malformation (**ar**-n'ld ki-**ar**-i) *n.* a congenital disorder in which there is distortion of the base of the skull with protrusion of the lower brainstem and parts of the cerebellum. [J. Arnold (1835–1915) and H. Chiari (1851–1916), German pathologists]

Aromasin (ă-**roh**-mă-sin) *n. see* aromatase inhibitor.

aromatase inhibitor (ă-**roh**-mă-tayz) *n.* any of a class of drugs used in the treatment of oestrogen-dependent breast cancer in postmenopausal women. By inhibiting the action of aromatase, an enzyme that promotes the conversion of testosterone to oestradiol, they reduce oestrogen levels. Aromatase inhibitors include **anastrazole** (Arimidex), **exemestane** (Aromasin), and **letrozole** (Femara).

aromatherapy (ă-roh-mă-**th'e**-ră-pi) *n.* the therapeutic use of fragrances derived from essential oils. These can be inhaled through an infusion of the essential oils that produce them, or the oils can be combined with a base oil and massaged into the skin.

arrector pili (ă-**rek**-tor **py**-ly) *n.* (*pl.* **arrectores pilorum**) a small erector muscle attached to the hair follicle. Contraction of the arrectores pilorum causes goose flesh.

arrhythmia (ă-**ri*th***-miă) *n.* any deviation from the normal rhythm (sinus rhythm) of the heart. Arrhythmias include ectopic beats, ectopic tachycardias, atrial and ventricular fibrillation, and heart block. **sinus a.** (**SA**) a normal variation in the heart rate, which accelerates slightly on inspiration and slows on expiration.

arsenic (**ar**-sĕn-ik) *n.* a poisonous greyish metallic element producing the symptoms of nausea, vomiting, diarrhoea, cramps, convulsions, and coma when ingested in large doses. Arsenic was formerly used in medicine, the most important arsenical drugs being **arsphenamine** (Salvarsan) and **neoarsphenamine**, used in the treatment of syphilis and dangerous parasitic diseases. Symbol: As.

arter- (arteri-, arterio-) *combining form denoting* an artery.

arterial blood gases (ABGs) (ar-**teer**-iăl) *pl. n.* gases present in arterial blood, normally including oxygen, carbon dioxide, and nitrogen. Measurements of the partial pressures of oxygen and carbon dioxide, together with the blood's pH, give information on the oxygen saturation of the haemoglobin and the acid-base state of the blood, which is relevant in critical care situations and for those requiring respiratory support.

arterial line *n.* a narrow catheter inserted into an artery for the purposes of continuous monitoring or blood gas analysis. It is used during phases of acute or critical illness for short periods and should be clearly labelled to prevent inadvertent use as a medication conduit. The femoral, axillary, or posterior tibial arteries can be used as insertion sites.

arterial ulcer *n. see* ulcer.

arteriectomy (ar-teer-i-**ek**-tŏmi) *n.* surgical excision of an artery or part of an artery.

arteriography (ar-teer-i-**og**-răfi) *n.* imaging of arteries (*see* angiography). The major roles of arteriography are to demonstrate the site and extent of atherosclerotic narrowing or occlusion, especially in the coronary arteries (*see* coronary angiography) and leg arteries (**peripheral a.**), and to demonstrate the anatomy of aneurysms within the skull (**carotid** and **vertebral a.**). The technique is also used to image a bleeding vessel prior to blocking it.

arteriole (ar-**teer**-i-ohl) *n.* a small branch of an artery, leading into many smaller vessels – the capillaries. By their constriction and dilation, under the regulation of the sympathetic nervous system, arterioles are the principal controllers of blood flow and pressure.

arteriolosclerosis (ar-teer-i-oh-loh-skleer-**oh**-sis) *n.* replacement of smooth muscle cells in the middle layer of the wall of an arteriole by connective tissue.

arteriopathy (ar-teer-i-**op**-ăthi) *n.* disease of an artery.

arterioplasty (ar-**teer**-i-oh-plas-ti) *n.* surgical reconstruction of an artery; for example, in the treatment of aneurysms.

arteriorrhaphy (ar-teer-i-**o**-răfi) *n.* suture of an artery.

arteriosclerosis (ar-teer-i-oh-skleer-**oh**-sis) *n.* any of several conditions affecting the arteries, especially atherosclerosis.

arteriotomy (ar-teer-i-**ot**-ŏmi) *n.* an incision into, or a needle puncture of, the wall of an artery.

arteriovenous (ar-teer-i-oh-**vee**-nŭs) *adj.* relating to or affecting an artery and a vein. **a. anastomosis** *see* anastomosis. **a. fistula** *see* fistula. **a. malformation** *see* angioma.

arteritis (ar-ter-**I**-tis) *n.* an inflammatory disease affecting the muscular walls of the arteries. The affected vessels are swollen and tender and may become blocked. **temporal** (or **giant-cell**) **a.** a condition that occurs in the elderly. It most commonly affects the arteries of the scalp and blindness may

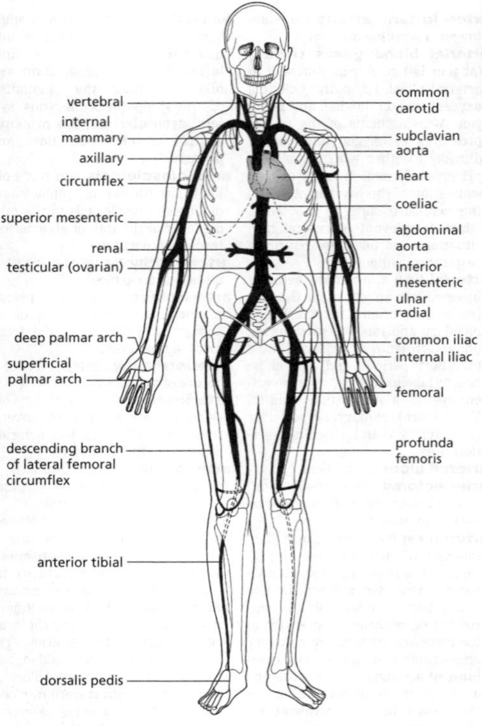

The principal arteries of the body

result from thrombosis of the arteries to the eyes.

artery (ar-ter-i) *n.* a blood vessel carrying blood away from the heart. The walls of arteries contain smooth muscle fibres, which contract or relax under the control of the sympathetic nervous system. See illustration. *See also* aorta, arteriole. **—arterial** *adj.*

arthr- (arthro-) *combining form denoting* a joint.

arthralgia (arthrodynia) (arth-**ral**-jă) *n.* severe ache or pain in a joint, without swelling or other signs of arthritis. *Compare* arthritis.

arthrectomy (arth-**rek**-tŏmi) *n.* surgical excision of a joint.

arthritis (arth-**ry**-tis) *n.* inflammation of one or more joints, characterized by pain, swelling, warmth, redness of the overlying skin, and restriction of motion. Any disease involving the synovial membranes or resulting in the degeneration of cartilage may cause arthritis. Treatment of arthritis depends on the cause, but NSAIDs are often used to suppress inflammation, and hence reduce pain and swelling. *See also* juvenile chronic arthritis, osteoarthritis, psoriasis, rheumatoid arthritis, septic (arthritis), haemarthrosis, pyarthrosis, hydrarthrosis. **—arthritic** (arth-**rit**-ik) *adj.*

arthrocentesis (arth-roh-sen-**tee**-sis) *n.* aspiration (removal) of fluid from a joint through a puncture needle into a syringe.

arthroclasia (arth-roh-**klay**-ziă) *n.* the surgical breaking down of ankylosis in a joint to permit freer movement.

arthrodesis (arth-roh-**dee**-sis) *n.* artificial ankylosis: the fusion of bones across a joint space by surgical means, in order to eliminate movement.

arthrodynia (arth-roh-**din**-iă) *n.* *see* arthralgia.

arthrography (arth-**rog**-răfi) *n.* an imaging technique for examining joints. A contrast medium (either radiolucent gas or radiopaque material) is injected into the joint space, outlining its contents and extent accurately. Conventional arthrography has now largely been replaced by magnetic resonance arthrography (*see* magnetic resonance imaging).

arthropathy (arth-**rop**-ăthi) *n.* any disease or disorder involving a joint.

arthroplasty (**arth**-roh-plasti) *n.* surgical refashioning of a diseased joint to relieve pain and to maintain or regain movement. **excision** (or **resection**) **a.** arthroplasty involving the excision of enough bone to create a gap at which movement can occur. **interposition a.** arthroplasty in which a biological or artificial barrier is placed between the two bony surfaces. **total a.** arthroplasty in which both joint surfaces are replaced by prostheses. *See also* hemiarthroplasty.

arthroscope (**arth**-roh-skohp) *n.* a rigid telescope fitted with fibreoptic illumination that is inserted into a joint through a small incision and generates a magnified image of the joint interior on a television monitor (*see* arthroscopy).

arthroscopy (ar-**thros**-kŏpi) *n.* inspection of a joint cavity with an arthroscope, enabling percutaneous surgery (such as meniscectomy) and biopsy to be performed.

arthrostomy (ar-**thros**-tŏmi) *n.* a procedure to enable a temporary opening to be made into a joint cavity.

arthrotomy (arth-**rot**-ŏmi) *n.* the surgical opening of a joint in order to inspect the interior or carry out any of various procedures.

articular (ar-**tik**-yoo-ler) *adj.* relating to a joint. **a. cartilage** the layer of cartilage at the ends of adjoining bones at a joint.

articulation (ar-tik-yoo-**lay**-shŏn) *n.* (in anatomy) the point or type of contact between two bones. *See* joint.

artificial heart (ar-ti-**fish**-ăl) *n.* a titanium pump that is implanted into the body to take over the function of a failing left ventricle in patients with heart disease. This allows the diseased ventricle time to recover its function. The pump is powered by an external battery, strapped to the patient's body, to which it is connected by wires passed through the patient's skin. The most recent devices are small enough to fit into the heart itself.

artificial insemination *n.* instrumental introduction of semen into the vagina in order that a woman may conceive. The semen specimen may be provided by the husband (**AIH** – **artificial insemination by husband**) in cases of erectile dysfunction or by an anonymous donor (**DI** – **donor insemination**), usually in cases where the husband is sterile.

artificial respiration (artificial ventilation) *n.* an emergency procedure for maintaining a flow of air into and out of a patient's lungs when the natural breathing reflexes are absent or insufficient. The simplest and most efficient method is mouth-to-mouth resuscitation.

artificial rupture of membranes (ARM) *n. see* amniotomy.

artificial sphincter *n.* an apparatus designed to replace or support a sphincter that is either absent or ineffective. *See also* neosphincter.

ARV *adj. see* antiretroviral.

arytenoid cartilage (a-ri-**tee**-noid) *n.* either of the two pyramid-shaped cartilages that lie at the back of the larynx next to the upper edges of the cricoid cartilage.

arytenoidectomy (a-ri-tee-noid-**ek**-tŏmi) *n.* surgical excision of the arytenoid cartilage of the larynx in the treatment of paralysis of the vocal folds.

ASA classification *n.* a widely used classification for grading patients' fitness for surgery prior to the operation. It was developed by the American Society of Anesthesia (ASA), but is now used worldwide. Patients are assigned grades between 1 and 6.

asbestos (ass-**best**-os) *n.* a fibrous mineral that is incombustible and does not conduct heat. It is used in the form of fabric or boards for its heat-resistant properties.

asbestosis (ass-best-**oh**-sis) *n.* a lung disease – a form of pneumoconiosis – caused by fibres of asbestos inhaled by those who are exposed to the mineral. *See also* mesothelioma.

ascariasis (askă-ry-ăsis) *n.* a disease caused by an infestation with the parasitic worm *Ascaris lumbricoides*. Adult worms in the intestine can cause abdominal pain, vomiting, constipation, diarrhoea, appendicitis, and peritonitis; migrating larvae in the lungs can provoke pneumonia.

Ascaris (ass-kă-ris) *n.* a genus of parasitic nematode worms. **A. lumbricoides** the largest of the human intestinal nematodes. Larvae hatch out in the intestine and then migrate via the hepatic portal vein, liver, heart, lungs, windpipe, and pharynx, before returning to the intestine where they later develop into adult worms (*see also* ascariasis).

Aschoff nodules (ash-off) *pl. n.* nodules that occur in the muscular and connective tissue of the heart in rheumatic myocarditis. [K. A. L. Aschoff (1866–1942), German pathologist]

ascites (hydroperitoneum) (ă-sy-teez) *n.* the accumulation of fluid in the peritoneal cavity, causing abdominal swelling. Causes include heart failure, cirrhosis, and various cancers (particularly of the liver and ovary). **chylous a.** ascites that occurs when the drainage of lymph from the abdomen is obstructed. **pancreatic a.** ascites due to direct communication between the pancreatic duct and peritoneal cavity. *See also* oedema.

ascorbic acid (ă-skor-bik) *n. see* vitamin C.

ASD *n. see* (atrial) septal defect.

-ase *suffix denoting* an enzyme.

asepsis (ay-sep-sis) *n.* the complete absence of bacteria, fungi, viruses, or other microorganisms that could cause disease. Asepsis is the ideal state for the performance of surgical operations and is achieved by using sterilization techniques. **—aseptic** *adj.*

Asherman syndrome (ash-er-măn) *n.* a condition in which amenorrhoea and infertility follow a major haemorrhage in pregnancy. It may result from overvigorous curettage of the uterus in an attempt to control the bleeding. This removes the lining, the walls adhere, and the cavity is obliterated to a greater or lesser degree. *Compare* Sheehan's syndrome. [J. G. Asherman (20th century), Czechoslovakian gynaecologist]

asparaginase (ă-spa-ră-jin-ayz) *n.* an enzyme that inhibits the growth of certain tumours and is used (in the form of **crisantaspase**) in the treatment of acute lymphoblastic leukaemia. Trade name: **Erwinase**.

asparagine (ă-spa-ră-jeen) *n. see* amino acid.

aspartame (as-pă-taym) *n.* an artificial sweetener 200 times sweeter than sugar. Aspartame is metabolized by the body into its constituents – aspartic acid, phenylalanine, and methanol – and is therefore not suitable for people with phenylketonuria. It can be used in diabetic foods.

aspartate aminotransferase (AST) (ass-par-tayt] *n.* an enzyme involved in the transamination of amino acids. Measurement of AST in the serum may be used in the diagnosis of acute myocardial infarction and acute liver disease. It was formerly called serum glutamic oxaloacetic transaminase (SGOT).

aspartic acid (aspartate) (ă-**spar**-tik) *n. see* amino acid.

Asperger's syndrome (ass-per-gerz) *n.* a mild form of autism characterized by social aloofness, stilted and pedantic styles of speech, a limited range of interests, and an excessive preoccupation with a very specialized interest (such as timetables). [H. Asperger (1906–80), Austrian paediatrician]

aspergillosis (ass-per-jil-**oh**-sis) *n.* a group of conditions caused by fungi of the genus *Aspergillus*, usually *Aspergillus fumigatus*. These conditions nearly always arise in patients with pre-existing lung disease and fall into three categories. The allergic form most commonly affects asthmatic patients and may cause collapse of segments or lobes of a lung. The colonizing form leads to formation of a fungus ball (**aspergilloma**), usually within a pre-existing cavity in the lung. In the third form the fungus spreads throughout the lungs and may even disseminate throughout the body; this form is rare but potentially fatal.

Aspergillus (ass-per-**jil**-ŭs) *n.* a genus of fungi, including many common moulds, some of which cause infections of the respiratory system in humans. **A. fumigatus** the cause of aspergillosis.

aspermia (ă-**sperm**-iă) *n.* strictly, a lack or failure of formation of semen. More usually, however, the term is used to mean the total absence of sperm from the semen (*see* azoospermia).

asphyxia (ă-**sfiks**-iă) *n.* suffocation: a life-threatening condition in which oxygen is prevented from reaching the tissues by obstruction of or damage to any part of the respiratory system.

aspiration (ass-per-**ay**-shŏn) *n.* the withdrawal of fluid from the body by means of suction. **vacuum a.** the removal by suction of the products of conception, either to terminate a pregnancy or to evacuate the uterus following miscarriage. *See also* (aspiration) cytology, endometrial (aspiration).

aspirator (ass-per-ay-ter) *n.* any of various instruments used for aspiration. Some employ hollow needles for removing fluid from cysts, inflamed joint cavities, etc.; another kind is used to suck debris and water from the patient's mouth during dental treatment.

aspirin (acetylsalicylic acid) (ass-prin) *n.* a drug that relieves pain and also reduces inflammation and fever. Largely superseded by modern anti-inflammatory agents (*see* NSAID), aspirin is now most commonly taken regularly in low doses as an antiplatelet drug, to prevent coronary thrombosis and strokes in those at risk. Aspirin works by inhibiting the production of prostaglandins; it may irritate the lining of the stomach, causing nausea, vomiting, pain, and bleeding. It has been implicated as a cause of Reye's syndrome and should therefore not be given to children below the age of 16 years unless specifically indicated.

assent (ă-**sent**) *n.* agreement to undergo medical treatment sought from an adult or child who lacks capacity to consent.

assertion (ă-**ser**-shŏn) *n.* the skill to communicate positively in order to press one's own claims, rights, or opinions.

assessment (ă-**ses**-mĕnt) *n.* **1.** the first stage of the nursing process, in which data about the patient's health status is collected and from which a nursing care plan may be devised. **2.** an examination set by an examining body to test a candidate's theoretical and practical nursing skills.

assimilation (ă-simi-**lay**-shŏn) *n.* the process by which food substances are taken into the cells of the body after they have been digested and absorbed.

assisted suicide (ă-**sis**-tid) *n. see* suicide.

assistive listening device (ă-**sis**-tiv) *n.* a type of environmental hearing aid that increases the loudness of the desired sound without increasing the level of any background noise.

associate nurse (ă-**soh**-si-ăt) *n.* a nurse who provides care for a patient on the instructions of the patient's primary nurse or in her absence. *See* primary nursing.

associate practitioner (assistant practitioner) *n.* a senior support worker who works as part of the multidisciplinary team in a wide variety of clinical areas undertaking a range of skills under the supervision of a registered healthcare professional.

association area (ă-soh-si-**ay**-shŏn) *n.* an area of cerebral cortex that lies away from the main areas that are concerned with the reception of sensory impulses and the start of motor impulses but is linked to them by many neurons (**association fibres**).

association of ideas *n.* (in psychology) linkage of one idea to another in a regular way according to their meaning. **Loosening of associations** is a form of formal thought disorder in which the linkage of a person's train of thoughts is lost or disrupted. *See also* free association.

AST *n. see* aspartate aminotransferase.

astasia-abasia *see* abasia.

astereognosis (ă-ste-ri-ŏg-**noh**-sis) *n. see* agnosia.

asteroid hyalosis (ass-tĕ-roid hy-ă-**loh**-sis) *n.* **1.** a degenerative condition, formerly known as **asteroid hyalitis**, in which tiny deposits of calcium are suspended in the vitreous humour. Vision is usually not affected. **2.** *see* synchysis (scintillans).

asthenia (ass-**theen**-iă) *n.* weakness or loss of strength.

asthenopia (ass-thi-**noh**-piă) *n. see* eyestrain.

asthenospermia (ass-thi-noh-**sper**-miă) *n.* the presence in the semen of spermatozoa with poor motility, revealed by seminal analysis.

asthma (ass-mă) *n.* the condition of subjects with widespread narrowing of the bronchial airways, which changes in severity over short periods of time and leads to coughing, wheezing, and difficulty in breathing. **bronchial a.** asthma that may be precipitated by exposure to one or more of a wide range of stimuli, including allergens, drugs (such as aspirin), exertion, emotion, infections, and air pollution. Treatment is with bronchodilators, with or without corticosteroids, usually administered via aerosol or dry-powder inhalers, or – if the condition is more severe – via a nebulizer. Severe asthmatic attacks may need large doses or oral corticosteroids (*see* status asthmaticus). **cardiac a.** asthma that occurs in left ventricular heart failure and must be distinguished from bronchial asthma, as the treatment is quite different. **—asthmatic** (ass-**mat**-ik) *adj.*

SEE WEB LINKS

- Website of the charity Asthma

astigmatism (ă-**stig**-mă-tizm) *n.* a defect of vision in which the image of an object is distorted because not all the light rays come to a focus on the retina. This is usually due to irregular curvature of the cornea and/or lens, whose surface resembles part of the surface of an egg (rather than a sphere). **—astigmatic** (ass-tig-**mat**-ik) *adj.*

astragalus (ass-**trag**-ălŭs) *n. see* talus.

astringent (ă-**strin**-jĕnt) *n.* a drug that causes cells to shrink by precipitating proteins from their surfaces. Astringents are used in lotions to harden and protect the skin and to reduce bleeding from minor abrasions.

astrocytoma (ass-troh-sy-**toh**-mă) *n.* any brain tumour derived from non-nervous supporting cells (glia), which may be benign or malignant. In adults astrocytomas are usually found in the cerebral hemispheres but in children they also occur in the cerebellum.

asymmetric tonic neck reflex *n.* a primitive reflex that is present from birth but should disappear by six months of age. If the infant is lying on its back and the head is turned to one side, the arm and leg on the side to which the head is turned should straighten, and the arm and leg on the opposite side should bend (the 'fencer' position). Persistence of the reflex beyond six months is suggestive of cerebral palsy.

asymmetry (ay-**sim**-it-ri) *n.* (in anatomy) the state in which opposite parts of an organ or parts at opposite sides of the body do not correspond with each other. **—asymmetric** (ay-si-**met**-rik) *adj.*

asymptomatic (ay-simp-tŏm-**at**-ik) *adj.* not showing any symptoms of disease, whether disease is present or not.

asynclitism (ă-**sin**-klit-izm) *n.* tilting of the fetal skull towards one or other shoulder causing the top of the skull to be either nearer to the sacrum (**anterior a.** or **Naegele's obliquity**) or nearer to the pubis (**posterior a.** or **Litzmann's**

obliquity). These mechanisms enable the fetal head to pass more easily through the maternal pelvis.

asystole (ă-sis-tŏ-li) *n.* a condition in which the heart no longer beats, accompanied by the absence of complexes in the electrocardiogram. **—asystolic** (a-sis-**tol**-ik) *adj.*

atavism (at-ă-vizm) *n.* the phenomenon in which an individual has a character or disease known to have occurred in a remote ancestor but not in his parents.

ataxia (ă-**taks**-iă) *n.* the shaky movements and unsteady gait that result from the brain's failure to regulate the body's posture and the strength and direction of limb movements. **cerebellar a.** a condition, due to disease of the cerebellum, in which the patient staggers when walking, cannot pronounce words properly, and may have nystagmus. **Friedreich's a.** an inherited disorder appearing first in adolescence. It has the features of cerebellar ataxia, together with spasticity of the limbs. **sensory a.** ataxia caused by disease of the sensory nerves, which is exaggerated when the patient closes his eyes (*see* Romberg's sign). *See also* ataxia telangiectasia, tabes dorsalis (locomotor ataxia). **—ataxic** *adj.*

ataxia telangiectasia (til-an-ji-ek-**tay**-ziă) *n.* an inherited (autosomal recessive) neurological disorder. Ataxia is usually noted early in life. Prominent blood vessels are visible in the sclerae of the eyes, and learning disability, growth retardation, abnormal eye movements, skin lesions, and immune deficiency may be found.

atel- (atelo-) *combining form denoting* imperfect or incomplete development.

atelectasis (at-ĕ-**lek**-tă-sis) *n.* failure of part of the lung to expand. This occurs when the cells lining the alveoli are immature, as in premature babies; it also occurs when the larger bronchial tubes are blocked by retained secretions, inhaled foreign bodies, bronchial cancers, or enlarged lymph nodes.

atenolol *n.* a drug (*see* beta blocker) used to treat angina, high blood pressure, and arrhythmias. It is administered by mouth or by intravenous injection or infusion. Trade name: **Tenormin**.

atherogenic (ath-er-oh-**jen**-ik) *adj.* denoting a factor that may cause atheroma. Such factors include cigarette smoking, excessive consumption of animal fats and refined sugar, obesity, and inactivity.

atheroma (ath-er-**oh**-ma) *n.* degeneration of the walls of the arteries due to the formation in them of fatty plaques and scar tissue. This limits blood circulation and predisposes to thrombosis. **—atheromatous** *adj.*

atherosclerosis (ath-er-oh-skleer-**oh**-sis) *n.* a disease of the arteries in which fatty plaques develop on their inner walls, with eventual obstruction of blood flow. *See* atheroma. **—atherosclerotic** *adj.*

athetosis (ath-ĕ-**toh**-sis) *n.* a writhing involuntary movement especially affecting the hands, face, and tongue. It is usually a form of cerebral palsy but can be caused by drugs used to treat parkinsonism or by phenothiazines. **—athetotic** *adj*.

athlete's foot (ath-leets) *n*. a fungal infection of the skin between the toes: a type of ringworm. Medical name: **tinea pedis**.

atlas (at-lăs) *n*. the first cervical vertebra, by means of which the skull is articulated to the backbone.

ATLS *n*. advanced trauma life support, which comprises the treatment programmes for patients who have been subjected to major trauma (e.g. serious road traffic accidents, missile injuries). Doctors, nurses, and paramedical personnel involved in ATLS receive special training for dealing with such emergencies.

ATN *n. see* (acute) tubular necrosis.

atom (at-ŏm) *n*. the smallest constituent of an element that can take part in a chemical reaction. An atom consists of a positively charged nucleus with negatively charged electrons orbiting around it.

atomizer (at-ŏ-my-zer) *n*. an instrument that reduces liquids to a fine spray of minute droplets.

atony (at-ŏni) *n*. a state in which muscles are floppy, lacking their normal elasticity. **—atonic** (ă-**ton**-ik) *adj*.

atopen (at-oh-pĕn) *n. see* atopy.

atopy (at-oh-pi) *n*. a form of allergy in which there is a hereditary or constitutional tendency to develop hypersensitivity reactions (e.g. hay fever, allergic asthma, atopic eczema) in response to allergens (**atopens**). Individuals with this predisposition – and the conditions provoked in them by contact with allergens – are described as **atopic**.

atorvastatin (at-or-vas-tă-tin) *n*. a drug used to reduce abnormally high levels of cholesterol and other lipids in the blood (*see* statin). It is administered by mouth. Trade name: **Lipitor**.

ATP (adenosine triphosphate) *n*. a compound that contains adenine, ribose, and three phosphate groups and occurs in cells. The chemical bonds of the phosphate groups store energy needed by the cell, for muscle contraction; this energy is released when ATP is split into ADP or AMP. ATP is formed from ADP or AMP using energy produced by the breakdown of carbohydrates or other food substances. *See also* mitochondrion.

atracurium besilate (at-ră-**kewr**-iŭm **bes**-il-ayt) *n*. a muscle relaxant administered by injection and infusion during anaesthesia or intensive care. Trade name: **Tracrium**.

atresia (ă-**tree**-ziă) *n*. **1.** congenital absence or abnormal narrowing of a body opening. **biliary a.** obstruction of bile flow due to destruction or absence of the bile extrahepatic ducts, causing jaundice in affected babies. **duodenal a.** narrowing of the duodenum, causing complete obstruction of its lumen. **tricuspid a.** absence of the tricuspid valve, with resultant lack of communication between the right atrium and right ventricle of the heart. **2.** the degenerative process that affects the majority of ovarian follicles. Usually only one Graafian follicle will ovulate in each menstrual cycle. —**atretic** (ă-tret-ik) *adj.*

atri- (atrio-) *combining form denoting* an atrium, especially the atrium of the heart.

atrial (ay-tri-ăl) *adj.* of or relating to the atrium or atria. **a. fibrillation** *see* fibrillation. **a. septal defect** *see* septal defect.

atrioventricular (AV) (ay-tri-oh-ven-**trik**-yoo-ler) *adj.* relating to the atria and ventricles of the heart.

atrioventricular bundle (AV bundle, bundle of His) *n.* a bundle of modified heart muscle fibres (**Purkinje fibres**) passing from the atrioventricular (AV) node forward to the septum between the ventricles, where it divides into right and left bundles, one for each ventricle. The fibres transmit contraction waves from the atria, via the AV node, to the ventricles.

atrioventricular node (AV node) *n.* a mass of modified heart muscle situated in the lower middle part of the right atrium. It receives the impulse to contract from the sinoatrial node, via the atria, and transmits it through the atrioventricular bundle to the ventricles.

at-risk register *n.* a listing of children and other vulnerable individuals whose social circumstances render them liable to abuse.

atrium (ay-tri-ŭm) *n.* (*pl.* **atria**) **1.** either of the two upper chambers of the heart. The left atrium receives arterial blood from the lungs via the pulmonary artery; the right atrium receives venous blood from the venae cavae. *See also* auricle. **2.** any of various anatomical chambers into which one or more cavities open. —**atrial** *adj.*

atrophy (**at**-rŏ-fi) *n.* the wasting away of a normally developed organ or tissue due to degeneration of cells. Pathological atrophy may occur through starvation, disuse, denervation, or ischaemia. **muscular a.** atrophy of muscular tissue associated with various diseases, such as poliomyelitis. *See also* multiple system atrophy, spinal muscular atrophy, Sudek's atrophy.

atropine (**at**-rŏ-peen) *n.* an antimuscarinic drug extracted from belladonna. Atropine is used as a mydriatic (*see* cycloplegia, mydriasis). It is also used in surgery (as premedication and to reverse the action of muscle relaxants) and sometimes to relieve gut spasms. Trade names: **Minijet Atropine**, **Minims Atropine Sulphate**.

ATT *n.* antitetanus toxoid. *See also* DTaP/IPV, DTaP/IPV/Hib.

attachment (ă-**tach**-mĕnt) *n.* **1.** (in psychology) the process of developing the first close selective relationship of a child's life, most commonly with the mother. **a. disorder** a psychiatric disorder in infants and young children resulting from institutionalization, poor parenting, emotional neglect, or child abuse. Affected children may be withdrawn or aggressive, and fearful or attention-seeking and indiscriminately friendly. **2.** (in the NHS) a working arrangement by which district nurses, social workers, etc., are engaged in association with specific general practitioners, caring for their registered patients rather than working solely on a geographical or district basis. **clinical a.** (in the NHS) an arrangement in which a person shadows a clinical professional, often in order to gain experience in that professional's field.

attention-deficit/hyperactivity disorder (ADHD, hyperkinetic disorder) (ă-ten-shŏn def-i-sit dis-**or**-der) *n.* a developmental disorder, characterized by grossly excessive levels of activity and a marked impairment of the ability to attend and concentrate. The behaviour may be predominantly hyperactive-impulsive, predominantly inattentive, or a combination of these. Learning is impaired and behaviour can be disruptive and may be defiant or aggressive. Treatment can involve drugs (such as methylphenidate) and behaviour therapy.

SEE WEB LINKS

- This US website focuses on people with ADHD

attenuation (ă-ten-yoo-**ay**-shŏn) *n.* reduction of the disease-producing ability (virulence) of a bacterium or virus so that it may be used for immunization.

atticotomy (at-i-**kot**-ŏmi) *n.* a surgical operation to remove cholesteatoma from the ear. It is a form of limited mastoidectomy.

atypical (ay-**tip**-ik-ăl) *adj.* not conforming to type. **a. antipsychotic** *see* antipsychotic. **a. pneumonia** pneumonia, caused by such organisms as *Mycoplasma pneumoniae*, that does not respond to penicillin but does respond to such antibiotics as tetracycline and erythromycin.

audi- (audio-) *combining form denoting* hearing or sound.

audiogram (aw-di-oh-gram) *n.* the graphic record of a test of hearing carried out on an audiometer.

audiology (awdi-**ol**-ŏji) *n.* the study of disorders of hearing.

audiometer (awdi-**om**-it-er) *n.* an apparatus for testing hearing at different sound frequencies, so helping in the diagnosis of deafness. **—audiometry** *n.*

audit (aw-dit) *n.* *see* clinical audit, nursing audit.

AUDIT (Alcohol Use Disorders Identification Tool) (**or**-dit) *n.* an international tool, developed by the WHO, used as an outcome or a screening measure for alcohol problems. It consists of ten questions that review consumption, drinking behaviours, and alcohol-related issues using an interview or a self-report approach. A score of 8 or above suggests hazardous or harmful alcohol consumption; 20 or above suggests alcohol dependence.

auditory (aw-dit-er-i) *adj.* relating to the ear or to the sense of hearing. **a. canal** the canal leading from the pinna to the eardrum. **a. nerve** *see* cochlear nerve.

auditory brainstem response audiometry (brainstem evoked response audiometry, BSER) *n.* an objective test of hearing that measures the electrical activity in the auditory nerve and brainstem following sound stimulation using repeated clicks or brief tones.

auditory processing disorder (APD, central auditory processing disorder, CAPD) *n.* a series of conditions characterized by difficulty in hearing and processing auditory information, especially in poor acoustic environments, despite normal or near-normal ear function.

auditory verbal therapy (AVT) *n.* a technique for teaching deaf children to communicate that focuses on speech and residual hearing rather than sign language.

Auerbach's plexus (myenteric plexus) (ow-er-bahks) *n.* a collection of nerve fibres – fine branches of the vagus nerve – within the walls of the intestine. It supplies the muscle layers and controls the movements of peristalsis. [L. Auerbach (1828–97), German anatomist]

AUR *n. see* (acute urinary) retention.

aura (or-ă) *n.* the forewarning of an attack, as occurs in epilepsy (e.g. as an odd smell or taste) and migraine (e.g. fortification spectra (zigzag lines) or scotomas (black holes in the visual field) or pins and needles).

aural (or-ăl) *adj.* relating to the ear.

auricle (or-i-k'l) *n.* **1.** a small pouch in the wall of each atrium of the heart: the term is also used incorrectly as a synonym for atrium. **2.** *see* pinna.

auriscope (auroscope, otoscope) (or-i-skohp) *n.* an apparatus for examining the eardrum and the ear canal (external meatus). See illustration.

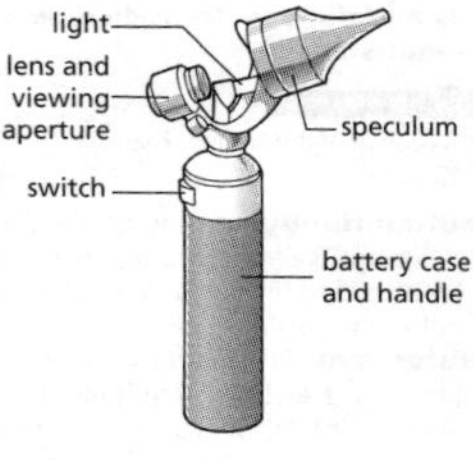

An auriscope

auscultation (aw-skŭl-tay-shŏn) *n.* the process of listening, usually with a stethoscope, to sounds produced by movement of gas or liquid within the body, as an aid to diagnosis. **—auscultatory** *adj.*

Australia antigen (oss-tray-liă) *n.* a former name for the hepatitis B antigen, which was first found in the blood of an Australian aborigine.

aut- (auto-) *combining form denoting* self.

autism (aw-tizm) *n.* a psychiatric disorder of childhood, with an onset before the age of 2½ years, marked by severe difficulties in communicating and forming relationships with other people, in developing language, and in using abstract concepts; repetitive and limited patterns of behaviour; and obsessive resistance to tiny changes in familiar surroundings. About 50% of autistic children have learning disabilities. Autism and similar developmental disorders (including Asperger's syndrome and Rett's syndrome) are known as **autistic spectrum disorders**. —**autistic** *adj*.

SEE WEB LINKS

- Website of the National Autistic Society

autoantibody (aw-toh-**an**-ti-bodi) *n.* an antibody formed against one of the body's own components in an autoimmune disease.

autoclave (aw-tŏ-klayv) **1.** *n.* a piece of sterilizing equipment in which surgical instruments, dressings, etc., are treated with steam at high pressure. **2.** *vb.* to sterilize in an autoclave.

autogenous (aw-**toj**-in-ŭs) *adj.* originating within the body of the patient. **a. vein graft** a graft to bypass a blocked artery, made from material derived from the body of the patient receiving the graft.

autograft (aw-tŏ-grahft) *n.* a tissue graft taken from one part of the body and transferred to another part of the same individual. Unlike allografts, autografts are not rejected by the body's immunity defences. *See also* skin (graft).

autoimmune disease (aw-toh-i-**mewn**) *n.* one of a group of otherwise unrelated disorders caused by inflammation and destruction of tissues by the body's own immune response. These disorders include pernicious anaemia, rheumatic fever, rheumatoid arthritis, glomerulonephritis, myasthenia gravis, and Hashimoto's disease.

autoimmunity (aw-toh-i-**mewn**-iti) *n.* a disorder of the body's defence mechanisms in which an immune response is generated against components or products of its own tissues, treating them as foreign material and attacking them. *See* autoimmune disease, immunity.

autoinfection (aw-toh-in-**fek**-shŏn) *n.* **1.** infection by an organism that is already present in the body. **2.** infection transferred from one part of the body to another via the fingers, towels, etc.

autointoxication (aw-toh-in-toks-i-**kay**-shŏn) *n.* poisoning by a toxin formed within the body.

autologous (aw-**tol**-ŏ-gŭs) *adj.* denoting a graft that is derived from the recipient of the graft.

autolysis (aw-**tol**-i-sis) *n.* the destruction of tissues or cells brought about by the actions of their own enzymes. *See* lysosome.

automatism (aw-**tom**-ă-tizm) *n.* behaviour that may be associated with epilepsy, in which the patient performs well-organized movements or tasks while unaware of doing so.

autonomic nervous system (aw-tŏ-**nom**-ik) *n.* the part of the peripheral nervous system responsible for the control of involuntary muscles (e.g. heart, bladder, bowels) and hence bodily functions that are not consciously directed. *See* parasympathetic nervous system, sympathetic nervous system.

autonomy (aw-**ton**-ŏmi) *n.* literally 'self-rule', the capacity for reasoned self-determination. Respect for the autonomy of all persons with capacity, particularly patients, is a fundamental principle of medical ethics. In law it is formally safeguarded by the need for valid consent to any proposed treatment or research. **professional a.** reflection and attempting to follow one's own principles consistently and confidently.

autopsy (necropsy, post mortem) (aw-top-si) *n.* a review of the clinical history of a deceased person followed by external examination and dissection of the body and ancillary investigations (e.g. toxicology) in order to determine the cause of death.

autoradiography (radioautography) (aw-toh-ray-di-og-răfi) *n.* a technique for examining the distribution of a radioactive tracer in the tissues of an experimental animal.

autoscopy (aw-tos-kŏpi) *n.* the experience of seeing one's whole body as though from a vantage point some distance away. It can be a symptom in epilepsy. *See also* out-of-body experience.

autosomal (aw-tŏ-soh-măl) *adj.* relating to an autosome. **a. dominant** denoting hereditary diseases in which the defective gene is dominant and will therefore tend to be inherited by (and be expressed in) 50% of the offspring (of either sex) of the person with the disease. **a. recessive** denoting inherited diseases in which the defective gene is recessive but not sex-linked. *See also* recessive.

autosome (aw-tŏ-sohm) *n.* any chromosome that is not a sex chromosome and that occurs in pairs in diploid cells.

autotransfusion (aw-toh-trans-few-*zhŏn*) *n.* reintroduction into a patient of his or her own blood, which has either been previously drawn and stored in a blood bank or lost and then collected from the patient's circulation during surgical operation.

aux- (auxo-) *combining form denoting* increase; growth.

AV *adj. see* atrioventricular.

avascular (ă-vas-kew-ler) *adj.* lacking blood vessels or having a poor blood supply.

Avastin (ă-vas-tin) *n. see* bevacizumab.

aversion therapy (ă-ver-shŏn) *n.* a form of behaviour therapy that is used (now rarely) to reduce the occurrence of undesirable behaviour. The patient is conditioned by repeated pairing of some unpleasant stimulus with a stimulus related to the undesirable behaviour. *See also* sensitization.

avian influenza (ay-vi-ăn) *n. see* H5N1, influenza.

AVM *n.* arteriovenous malformation (*see* angioma).

avoidant (ă-void-ănt) *adj.* describing a personality disorder characterized by self-consciousness, hypersensitivity to rejection and criticism from others, avoidance of normal situations because of their potential risk, high levels of tension and anxiety, and consequently a restricted life.

AVPU *n.* a system for assessing the depth of unconsciousness: A = alert; V = voice responses present; P = pain responses present; U = unresponsive. It is useful for judging the severity of head injury and the need for specialized neurosurgical assistance before formal evaluation using the Glasgow Coma Scale.

AVT *n. see* auditory verbal therapy.

avulsion (ă-vul-shŏn) *n.* the tearing or forcible separation of part of a structure.

axilla (ak-sil-ă) *n.* (*pl.* **axillae**) the armpit. **—axillary** *adj.*

axis (aks-is) *n.* **1.** a real or imaginary line through the centre of the body or one of its parts or a line about which the body or a part rotates. **2.** the second cervical vertebra, which articulates with the atlas vertebra above and allows rotational movement of the head.

axon (aks-on) *n.* a nerve fibre: a single process extending from the cell body of a neuron and carrying nerve impulses away from it.

axonotmesis (aks-on-ŏt-mee-sis) *n.* rupture of nerve fibres (axons) within an intact nerve sheath. This may result from prolonged pressure or crushing and it is followed by peripheral degeneration of the nerve beyond the point of rupture. The prognosis for nerve regeneration is good.

azathioprine (ază-th'y-ŏ-preen) *n.* a drug (*see* immunosuppressant) administered by mouth mainly to aid the survival of organ or tissue transplants. It may also be used in the treatment of severe Crohn's disease, rheumatoid arthritis, myasthenia gravis, and severe eczema. Trade name: **Imuran**.

azelaic acid (az-ĕ-lay-ik) *n.* an antibacterial drug applied externally as a cream or gel in the treatment of acne. Trade names: **Finacea**, **Skinoren**.

azelastine (ay-zel-ă-steen) *n.* an antihistamine drug that is administered in a metered-dose nasal spray for the treatment of hay fever and as eye drops to treat allergic conjunctivitis. Trade names: **Optilast**, **Rhinolast**.

azithromycin (ă-zith-roh-my-sin) *n.* an antibiotic used to treat respiratory, skin, eye, soft-tissue, and other infections, including genital infections caused by *Chlamydia trachomatis*. It is administered by mouth or as eye drops. Trade names: **Azyter**, **Zithromax**.

azo- (azoto-) *combining form denoting* a nitrogenous compound, such as urea.

azoospermia (aspermia) (ay-zoh-ŏ-sperm-iă) *n.* the complete absence of sperm from the seminal fluid.

azotaemia (azŏ-tee-miă) *n.* a former name for uraemia.

azoturia (azŏ-tewr-iă) *n.* the presence in the urine of an abnormally high concentration of nitrogen-containing compounds, especially urea.

aztreonam (az-tree-ŏ-nam) *n.* an antibiotic administered by injection or inhalation that is used to treat infections caused by Gram-negative organisms (*see* gram's stain). It is especially useful for treating lung infections in children with cystic fibrosis. Trade names: **Azactam**, **Cayston**.

azygos vein (az-i-gos) *n.* an unpaired vein that arises from the inferior vena cava and drains into the superior vena cava, returning blood from the thorax and abdominal cavities.

Bb

Babinski reflex (extensor response) (ba-**bin**-ski) *n.* an upward movement of the big toe that is an abnormal plantar reflex indicating damage to the pyramidal system in the brain or spinal cord in those over the age of 18 months. [J. F. F. Babinski (1857–1932), French neurologist]

baby blues (**bay**-bi) *n. see* postpartum (blues).

baby-friendly hospital initiative (BFHI) *n.* an international programme, supported by the World Health Organization and UNICEF, that was established in 1992 to encourage maternity hospitals to support and enhance breastfeeding. It aims to ensure a high standard of care in relation to infant feeding through a range of teaching resources and individual support. There are ten criteria that must be met to have BFHI accreditation.

bacillaemia (ba-si-**lee**-miă) *n.* the presence of bacilli in the blood, resulting from infection.

bacille Calmette-Guérin (ba-**seel** kal-**met** gay-**ran**) *n. see* BCG. [A. L. C. Calmette (1863–1933) and C. Guérin (1872–1961), French bacteriologists]

bacilluria (ba-sil-**yoor**-iă) *n.* the presence of bacilli in the urine, resulting from a bladder or kidney infection. *See* cystitis.

bacillus (bă-**sil**-ŭs) *n.* (*pl.* **bacilli**) any rod-shaped bacterium. *See also* Lactobacillus, Streptobacillus.

Bacillus *n.* a large genus of Gram-positive spore-bearing rodlike bacteria. They are widely distributed in soil and air (usually as spores). **B. anthracis** a nonmotile species that causes anthrax. **B. polymyxa** the source of the polymyxin group of antibiotics. **B. subtilis** a species that may cause conjunctivitis; it also produces the antibiotic bacitracin zinc.

bacitracin zinc (ba-si-**tray**-sin) *n.* an antibiotic effective against a number of microorganisms. Combined with polymyxin B, it is applied externally to treat infections of the skin and eyes.

backbone (spinal column, spine, vertebral column) (**bak**-bohn) *n.* the flexible bony column, extending from the base of the skull to the small of the back, that encloses and protects the spinal cord. It is made up of individual bones (*see* vertebra) connected by discs of fibrocartilage (*see* intervertebral disc). The backbone of a newborn baby contains 33 vertebrae: seven cervical, 12 thoracic, five lumbar, five sacral, and four coccygeal. In the adult the sacral and coccygeal vertebrae become fused into two single bones (sacrum and coccyx, respectively). See illustration. Anatomical name: **rachis**.

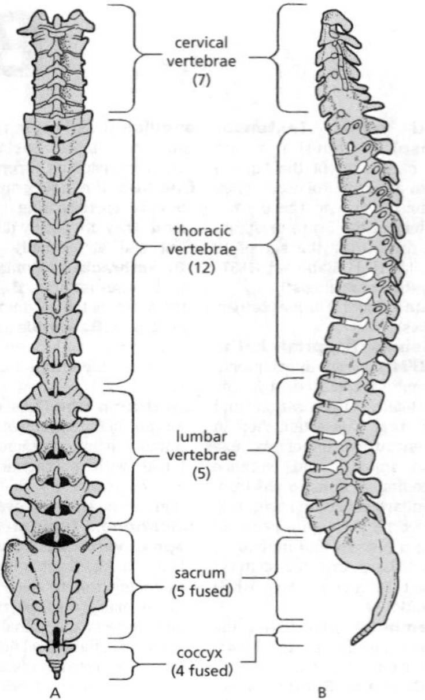

The backbone, seen from the back (A) and left side (B)

back slaps (bak) *pl. n.* a manoeuvre for the treatment of a choking patient. Firm slaps are given to the patient's back in an attempt to dislodge the obstructing article from the upper airway.

baclofen (bak-lŏ-fen) *n.* a skeletal muscle relaxant administered orally or by intrathecal injection to relieve spasm resulting from injury or disease of the brain or spinal cord, including cerebral palsy and multiple sclerosis. Trade name: **Lioresal**.

bacteraemia (bak-ter-**ee**-miă) *n.* the presence of bacteria in the blood: a sign of infection. —**bacteraemic** *adj.*

bacteri- (bacterio-) *combining form denoting* bacteria.

bacteria (bak-**teer**-iă) *pl. n.* (*sing.* **bacterium**) a group of microorganisms all of which lack a distinct nuclear membrane and most of which have a cell wall of unique composition. Most bacteria are unicellular; the cells may be spherical (*see* coccus), rodlike (*see* bacillus), spiral (*see* Spirillum), comma-shaped (*see* Vibrio), or corkscrew-shaped (*see* spirochaete). Generally, they range in size between 0.5 and 5 μm. Motile species bear one or more fine hairs (flagella) arising from their surface. Bacteria reproduce asexually by simple division of cells. They live in soil, water, or air or as parasites of humans, animals, and plants. Some parasitic bacteria cause diseases by producing poisons (*see* endotoxin, exotoxin). —**bacterial** *adj.*

bacterial vaginosis *n. see* vaginosis.

bactericidal (bak-teer-i-**sy**-dăl) *adj.* capable of killing bacteria. Substances with this property include antibiotics, antiseptics, and disinfectants. *Compare* bacteriostatic. —**bactericide** *n.*

bacteriology (bak-teer-i-**ol**-ŏji) *n.* the science concerned with the study of bacteria. *See also* microbiology. —**bacteriological** *adj.* —**bacteriologist** *n.*

bacteriolysin (bak-teer-i-**ol**-i-sin) *n. see* lysin.

bacteriolysis (bak-teer-i-**ol**-i-sis) *n.* the destruction of bacteria by lysis. —**bacteriolytic** *adj.*

bacteriophage (phage) (bak-**teer**-i-oh-fayj) *n.* a virus that attacks bacteria. The phage grows and replicates in the bacterial cell, which is eventually destroyed with the release of new phages. Each phage acts specifically against a particular species of bacterium. This is utilized in **phage typing**, a technique of identifying bacteria by the action of known phages on them.

bacteriostatic (bak-teer-i-oh-**stat**-ik) *adj.* capable of inhibiting or retarding the growth and multiplication of bacteria. *Compare* bactericidal.

bacterium (bak-**teer**-iŭm) *n. see* bacteria.

bacteriuria (bak-teer-i-**yoor**-iă) *n.* the presence of bacteria in the urine, with or without symptoms of urinary tract infection.

bagassosis (bag-ă-**soh**-sis) *n.* a form of external allergic alveolitis caused by exposure to the dust of mouldy bagasse, the residue of sugar cane after the sugar has been extracted. Symptoms include fever, malaise, irritant cough, and respiratory distress.

Baghdad boil (bag-**dad**) *n. see* oriental sore.

BAHA *n. see* (bone-anchored) hearing aid.

BAI *n.* *see* Beck Anxiety Inventory.

Baker's cyst (popliteal cyst) (**bay**-kerz) *n.* a cyst behind the knee resulting from rupture or herniation of the synovial membrane from a knee joint affected by osteoarthritis or rheumatoid arthritis. [W. M. Baker (1839–96), British surgeon]

BAL *n.* **1.** *see* bronchoalveolar lavage. **2.** British Anti-Lewisite.

balanced salt solution (BSS) (**bal**-ănst) *n.* a solution containing physiological concentrations of sodium chloride, acetate, and citrate, potassium chloride, calcium chloride, and magnesium chloride. Such fluids are used during intraocular surgery and to replace intraocular fluids.

balanitis (bal-ă-**ny**-tis) *n.* inflammation of the glans penis, usually associated with tightness of the foreskin (phimosis). **b. xerotica obliterans** (**BXO**) an autoimmune condition characterized by ivory-white patches on the glans.

balanoposthitis (bal-ă-noh-pos-**th'y**-tis) *n.* inflammation of the foreskin and the surface of the underlying glans penis. It usually occurs as a consequence of phimosis and represents a more extensive local reaction than simple balanitis.

balantidiasis (bal-ăn-ti-**dy**-ă-sis) *n.* an infestation of the large intestine of humans with the parasitic protozoan *Balantidium coli*. The parasite invades and destroys the intestinal wall, causing ulceration and necrosis, and the patient may experience diarrhoea and dysentery.

baldness (**bawld**-nis) *n.* *see* alopecia.

Balkan beam (Balkan frame) (**bawl**-kăn) *n.* a rectangular frame attached over a bed, used for the support of splints, pulleys, or slings for an immobilized limb.

ball-and-socket joint (bawl-ănd-**sok**-it) *n.* *see* enarthrosis.

balloon (bă-**loon**) *n.* an inflatable plastic cylinder of variable size that is mounted on a thin tube and used for dilating narrow areas in blood vessels or in the alimentary or urinary tracts. **b. angioplasty** *see* angioplasty.

ballottement (bă-**lot**-mĕnt) *n.* the technique of examining a fluid-filled part of the body to detect a floating object. During pregnancy, a sharp tap with the fingers, applied to the uterus through the abdominal wall or the vagina, causes the fetus to move away and then return, with an answering tap, to its original position.

balneotherapy (bal-ni-oh-**th'e**-ră-pi) *n.* the treatment of disease by bathing, originally in the mineral-containing waters of hot springs. Today, specialized remedial treatment in baths is used to alleviate pain and improve blood circulation and limb mobility in conditions such as arthritis.

balsam (**bawl**-săm) *n.* an aromatic resinous substance of plant origin. **b. of Peru** a South American balsam used in skin preparations as a mild antiseptic. *See* friar's balsam.

bandage (**band**-ij) *n.* a piece of material, in the form of a pad or strip, applied to a wound or bound around an injured or diseased part of the body. **b. lens** *see* contact lenses.

Bandl's ring (ban-d'lz) *n.* an abnormal retraction ring (*see* retraction) that occurs in obstructed labour. It is a sign of impending rupture of the lower segment of the uterus, which becomes progressively thinner as Bandl's ring rises upwards. Immediate action to relieve the obstruction is then necessary, usually in the form of Caesarean section. [L. Bandl (1842–92), German obstetrician]

Bankart's operation (**bank**-arts) *n.* an operation to repair a defect in the glenoid cavity in cases of recurrent dislocation of the shoulder. [A. S. B. Bankart (1879–1951), British orthopaedic surgeon]

Banti's syndrome (ban-teez) *n.* a disorder in which enlargement and overactivity of the spleen occurs as a result of increased pressure within the splenic vein. This arises primarily in children and also occurs with cirrhosis of the liver. [G. Banti (1852–1925), Italian pathologist]

barbiturate (bar-**bit**-yoor-ăt) *n.* any of a group of drugs, derived from barbituric acid, that depress activity of the central nervous system. Because barbiturates produce psychological and physical dependence and have serious toxic side-effects (*see* barbiturism), their use has declined. *See* amobarbital, butobarbital, phenobarbital, thiopental.

barbiturism (bar-**bit**-yoor-izm) *n.* addiction to drugs of the barbiturate group. Signs of intoxication include slurring of speech, sleepiness, and loss of balance. Withdrawal of the drugs must be undertaken slowly.

barbotage (bar-bŏ-**tahzh**) *n.* a method of spinal anaesthesia in which a small amount of anaesthetic is injected into the subarachnoid space followed by withdrawal of cerebrospinal fluid into the syringe. This process is repeated until all the anaesthetic has been injected.

bariatric surgery (ba-ri-**at**-rik) *n.* surgery performed for the purposes of weight loss in obese patients. Most procedures are restrictive, being designed to promote feelings of fullness and satiety after meals (*see* gastric (banding), stomach stapling).

barium enema (**bair**-iŭm) *n. see* enema.

barium follow-through *n. see* small bowel (meal).

barium sulphate *n.* a barium salt, insoluble in water, that is opaque to X-rays and is used as a contrast medium in radiography of the gastrointestinal tract. *See* (barium) enema, barium swallow and meal, small bowel (meal).

barium swallow and meal *n.* a radiological technique used to assess the anatomy and function of the upper gastrointestinal tract. The patient swallows radiopaque contrast (barium sulphate), which coats the mucosal surfaces of the oesophagus, stomach, and duodenum. The descent of the barium is charted by a series of radiographs. Gas-forming agents (such as sodium bicarbonate) may be given to distend the stomach and improve the quality of the images.

Barlow's disease (**bar**-lohz) *n.* infantile scurvy: scurvy occurring in young children due to dietary deficiency of vitamin C. [Sir T. Barlow (1845–1945), British physician]

Barlow's manoeuvre (mă-noo-ver) *n.* a test for congenital dislocation of the hip. A clunk felt and sometimes heard when the hip is gently adducted and backward pressure is applied to the head of the femur indicates instability of the joint. [Sir T. Barlow]

baroreceptor (baroceptor) (ba-roh-ri-**sep**-ter) *n.* a collection of sensory nerve endings specialized to monitor changes in blood pressure. The main receptors lie in the carotid sinuses and the aortic arch.

Barr body (bar) *n. see* sex chromatin. [M. L. Barr (1908–95), Canadian anatomist]

Barrett's oesophagus (ba-rĕts) *n.* a condition in which the squamous epithelium lining the oesophagus is replaced by columnar epithelium of the type normally lining the intestine. Barrett's oesophagus is caused by chronic inflammation and damage resulting from gastro-oesophageal reflux or (less frequently) by corrosive oesophagitis. [N. R. Barrett (1903–79), British surgeon]

barrier cream (**ba**-ri-er) *n.* a preparation used to protect the skin against water-soluble irritants (e.g. detergents, breakdown products of urine). Usually applied in the form of a cream or ointment and often containing a silicone (e.g. dimeticone), barrier creams are useful in the alleviation of various skin disorders, including napkin rash and pressure sores.

barrier nursing *n.* the nursing care of an infectious patient in isolation from other patients, to prevent the spread of infection.

Barthel index (Barthel scale) (bar-**thel**) *n.* a scale used to assess a person's functioning in relation to activities of daily living and mobility. Each of ten items is allocated a score: the person receives a score based on whether or not they need help to do the task. The higher the aggregated score, the more independent the person is. This tool can be used in a variety of settings to monitor improvement in independence over a period of time.

bartholinitis (vulvovaginitis) (bar-thŏ-li-**ny**-tis) *n.* inflammation of Bartholin's glands. **acute b.** bartholinitis in which abscess formation may occur (**Bartholin's abscess**). **chronic b.** bartholinitis in which cysts may form in the glands as a result of blockage of their ducts.

Bartholin's glands (greater vestibular glands) (bar-thŏ-linz) *pl. n.* a pair of glands that open at the junction of the vagina and the vulva. Their secretions lubricate the vulva and so assist penetration by the penis during coitus. [C. Bartholin (1655–1738), Danish anatomist]

Bartter syndrome (bar-tĕr) *n.* an inherited condition of the kidney, which causes abnormalities in the excretion and reabsorption of salts from the blood. This results in lowered levels of potassium and chloride and an increased level of calcium. The baby fails to grow properly and becomes progressively weaker and dehydrated.

[F. C. Bartter (1914–83), US physician]

basal cell carcinoma (BCC) (bay-săl) *n.* the commonest form of skin cancer: a slow-growing tumour that usually occurs on the central area of the face, especially in fair-skinned people. The prevalence increases greatly with episodes of sunburn. Treatment involves topical chemotherapy (e.g. with 5-fluorouracil), curettage and cautery, surgical excision, cryotherapy, or radiotherapy. If neglected for decades, a BCC eventually becomes a **rodent ulcer** and destroys the surrounding tissue. The term 'rodent ulcer' is sometimes used to mean any basal cell carcinoma.

basal ganglia *pl. n.* several large masses of grey matter embedded deep within the white matter of the cerebrum. They include the **caudate** and **lenticular nuclei** (together known as the **corpus striatum**) and the **amygdaloid nucleus**. The lenticular nucleus consists of the **putamen** and **globus pallidus**. The basal ganglia are involved with the regulation of voluntary movements at a subconscious level.

basal metabolism *n.* the minimum amount of energy expended by the body to maintain vital processes, e.g. respiration, circulation, and digestion. It is expressed in terms of heat production per unit of body surface area per day (**basal metabolic rate – BMR**). BMR is normally determined indirectly, by measuring the respiratory quotient. Measurements are best taken during a period of least activity, i.e. during sleep and 12–18 hours after a meal, under controlled temperature conditions.

basal narcosis *n.* preliminary unconsciousness induced in a patient by administration of an opioid drug prior to administration of a general anaesthetic by inhalation.

base (bayss) *n.* **1.** the main ingredient of an ointment or other medicinal preparation. **2.** a substance that releases hydroxyl ions when dissolved in water, has a pH greater than 7 and turns litmus paper blue, and reacts with an acid to form a salt and water only. *Compare* acid.

basement membrane (bayss-mĕnt) *n.* the thin delicate membrane that lies at the base of an epithelium.

basic life support (BLS) (bay-sik) *n.* the provision of treatment designed to maintain adequate circulation and ventilation to a patient in cardiac arrest, without the use of drugs or specialist equipment. *See also* cardiopulmonary resuscitation. *Compare* advanced life support.

basilar artery (ba-si-ler) *n.* an artery in the base of the brain, formed by the union of the two vertebral arteries.

basilic vein (bă-zil-ik) *n.* a large vein in the arm, extending from the hand along the back of the forearm, then passing forward to the inner side of the arm at the elbow.

basophil (bay-sŏ-fil) **1.** *n.* a variety of white blood cell (*see* polymorph) distinguished by the presence in its cytoplasm of coarse granules that stain purple-black with Romanowsky stains. Basophils are capable of ingesting foreign particles and contain histamine and heparin. **2.** *adj.* **(basophilic)** describing any cell that stains well with basic dyes.

basophilia (bay-sŏ-fil-iă) *n.* **1.** a property of a microscopic structure whereby it shows an affinity for basic dyes. **2.** an increase in the number of basophils in the blood.

Batchelor plaster (ba-chĕ-ler) *n.* a type of plaster that keeps both legs abducted and medially rotated, used to correct congenital dislocation of the hip. [J. S. Batchelor (20th century), British orthopaedic surgeon]

bat ears (bat) *pl. n.* protuberent external ears as a result of the absence of the antihelical fold in the pinna. It can be surgically corrected using an otoplasty operation.

Batten's disease (bat-t'nz) *n.* a rare hereditary disorder of lipid metabolism. Fatty substances accumulate in the cells of the nervous system, causing progressive dementia, epilepsy, spasticity, and visual failure. The condition starts in late infancy or childhood. [F. E. Batten (1865–1918), British neurologist]

battered baby syndrome (bat-erd) *n. see* nonaccidental injury.

battery (bat-er-i) *n.* (in law) the criminal or wrongful touching of another person (the latter is also known as **trespass against the person**). Any intentional touching of another is a potential battery unless it occurs with the consent of the person involved. Consent therefore provides a defence against a charge of battery brought in relation to medical treatment.

battledore placenta (bat-t'l-dor) *n.* a placenta to which the umbilical cord is attached at the margin (rather than at the centre).

Battle's sign (ba-t'lz) *n.* an area of extreme tenderness and bruising behind the ear in the region of the mastoid process of the skull. It is an acute sign of basal skull fracture with local bleeding and is indicative of recent head trauma. [W. H. Battle (1855–1936), British surgeon]

Bazin's disease (ba-zanz) *n.* a rare disease of young women in which tender nodules develop under the skin in the calves; it is a tuberculide. The nodules may break down and ulcerate though they may clear up spontaneously. Medical name: **erythema induratum**. [A. P. E. Bazin (1807–78), French dermatologist]

BBB *n.* **1.** *see* bundle branch block. **2.** *see* blood-brain barrier.

BBV *n.* blood-borne virus.

BCC *n. see* basal cell carcinoma.

B cell *n. see* lymphocyte.

BCG (bacille Calmette-Guérin) *n.* a strain of tubercle bacillus that has lost the power to cause tuberculosis but retains its antigenic activity; it is therefore used to prepare a vaccine against the disease.

b.d. (bis die) Latin: twice daily, used as a direction in prescriptions.

BDI *n. see* Beck Depression Inventory.

bearing down (bair-ing down) *n.* **1.** the expulsive uterine contractions of a woman in the second stage of labour. **2.** a sensation of heaviness and descent in the pelvis associated with pelvic tumours and certain other disorders.

Beck Anxiety Inventory (BAI) (bek) *n.* a questionnaire that assesses levels of anxiety experienced by patients. It consists of an evaluation of the cognitive and physical manifestations of anxiety, which are rated on a scale from 0 to 3. [A. T. Beck (1921–), US psychiatrist]

Beck Depression Inventory (BDI) *n.* a screening tool or self-rating scale consisting of 21 questions reflecting attitudes often displayed by depressed people. Each question is rated on a scale from 0 (normality) to 3 (severe disturbance). The BDI can act as a measure of effective therapy if completed before and after treatment. (A. T. Beck)

Becker muscular dystrophy (**bek**-er) *n.* a sex-linked (X-linked) disorder in which affected males develop an increase in muscle size followed by weakness and wasting. It usually starts between the ages of 5 and 15, and 25 years after onset most patients are wheelchair-bound. Although most men become severely disabled, life expectancy is close to normal. The disorder is similar to Duchenne muscular dystrophy but less severe. [P. E. Becker (1908–2000), German geneticist]

Beck Scale for Suicide Ideation (BSS) *n.* an assessment tool designed to identify vulnerability to and risk of suicide in patients. (A. T. Beck)

Beck's triad *n.* **1.** the classical diagnostic features of cardiac tamponade: dilated neck veins, a fall in blood pressure, and muffled heart sounds. [C. S. Beck (1894–1971), US surgeon] **2.** pessimistic views of oneself, the future, and the present: a triad of symptoms characteristic of clinical depression. [A. T. Beck]

beclometasone (bek-loh-**met**-a-zohn) *n.* a corticosteroid drug that is administered by mouth to treat ulcerative colitis, by nasal spray to treat hay fever, as a cream or ointment to treat severe skin infections, and by inhaler for the prevention of asthma (for which it may be combined with formoterol as **Fostair**). It is applied externally in the treatment of severe inflammatory skin disorders. Trade names: **Beconase**, **Clenil Modulite**, **Clipper**, **Qvar**.

becquerel (bek-er-**el**) *n.* the SI unit of activity of a radioactive source, being the activity of a radionuclide decaying at a rate of one spontaneous nuclear transition per second. It has replaced the curie. Symbol: Bq.

bed bug (**bed** bug) *n.* a bloodsucking insect of the genus *Cimex*, especially *C. lectularius*. They live and lay their eggs in the crevices of walls and furniture and emerge at night to suck blood; their bites leave a route for bacterial infection.

bed occupancy *n.* the number of hospital beds occupied by patients expressed as a percentage of the total beds available in the ward, specialty, hospital, area, or region. It is used to assess the demands for hospital beds and hence to gauge an appropriate balance between demands for health care and number of beds.

bedsore (**bed**-sor) *n. see* pressure sore.

bedwetting (**bed**-wet-ing) *n. see* enuresis.

behavioural objective (bi-**hayv**-yer-ăl) *n.* the goal of a particular nursing intervention or a specific lesson, in terms of what a person is expected to be able to do as a result of it.

behaviourism (bi-**hayv**-yer-izm) *n.* an approach to psychology postulating that only observable behaviour need be studied, thus denying any importance to unconscious processes. **—behaviourist** *n.*

behaviour therapy (bi-**hayv**-yer) *n.* treatment based on the belief that certain psychological problems are the products of faulty learning. *See also* aversion therapy, conditioning, desensitization, exposure.

Behçet's syndrome (**bay**-setz) *n.* a disease of the immune system characterized by oral and genital ulceration, inflammation of the uveal tract, and skin lesions. It may also involve the joints and nervous system and cause inflammation of the veins. The condition occurs more often in men. [H. Behçet (1889–1948), Turkish dermatologist]

bejel (endemic syphilis) (**bej**-ĕl) *n.* a long-lasting nonvenereal form of syphilis, particularly prevalent where standards of personal hygiene are low. The disease is spread among children and adults by direct body contact.

belladonna (bel-ă-**don**-ă) *n.* **1.** deadly nightshade (*Atropa belladonna*). **2.** the alkaloid derived from deadly nightshade, from which atropine is extracted. Preparations containing belladonna are used for treating diarrhoea. Trade names: **Alophen**, **Bellocarb**.

belle indifférence (bel an-di-fay-**rahns**) *n.* a symptom of conversion disorder in which an apparently grave physical affliction or disability (which has no physical cause) is accepted in a calm and smiling fashion. It can also be a sign of dementia or psychosis.

Bellocq's cannula (Bellocq's sound) (bel-**oks**) *n.* a curved hollow tube used for inserting a plug into the nose to arrest nosebleeding. [J. J. Bellocq (1732–1807), French surgeon]

Bell's palsy (belz) *n.* paralysis of the facial nerve causing weakness of the muscles of one side of the face and an inability to close the eye. The cause is usually a viral infection. [Sir C. Bell (1774–1842), Scottish physiologist]

Bell's phenomenon *n.* the normal outward and upward rotation of the eyes that occurs when the lids are closed. [Sir C. Bell]

belly (**bel**-i) *n.* **1.** the abdomen or abdominal cavity. **2.** the central fleshy portion of a muscle.

Bence-Jones protein (benss-**joh'nz**) *n.* a protein of low molecular weight found in the urine of patients with multiple myeloma and rarely in patients with lymphoma, leukaemia, and Hodgkin's disease. [H. Bence-Jones (1814–73), British physician]

benchmarking (**bench**-mark-ing) *n.* a process by which best practice is identified and continuous improvement is generated through the sharing of evidence and the comparison of practice.

SEE WEB LINKS

- Pamphlets setting out basic health-care benchmarks from the Department of Health

bendroflumethiazide (bendrofluazide) (ben-droh-floo-mi-**th'**y-ă-zyd) *n.* a potent thiazide diuretic used in the treatment of conditions involving retention of fluid, such as hypertension and oedema. Trade names: **Aprinox**, **Neo-NaClex**.

bends (bendz) *n.* *see* compressed air illness.

Benedict's test (**ben**-i-dikts) *n.* a test for the presence of sugar in urine or other liquids, using a solution of sodium or potassium citrate, sodium carbonate, and copper sulphate (**Benedict's solution**). [S. R. Benedict (1884–1936), US chemist]

beneficence (bi-**nef**-i-sĕns) *n.* (in ethics) doing good: the obligation to act in the patient's best interests at all times, which should be what the patient considers to be doing good.

benign (bi-**nyn**) *adj.* **1.** describing a tumour that is not cancerous. **2.** describing any disorder or condition that does not produce harmful effects. *Compare* malignant.

benign paroxysmal positional vertigo (BPPV) *n.* brief episodes of rotatory vertigo precipitated by sudden head movements: a common cause of vertigo. It is thought to be due to microscopic debris in one of the semicircular canals (usually the posterior canal) and is treated by a predetermined set of head movements to move the debris.

benign prostatic hyperplasia (BPH) *n.* *see* prostate gland.

benperidol (ben-**pe**-ri-dol) *n.* a butyrophenone antipsychotic drug used mainly to treat deviant and antisocial sexual behaviour. It is administered by mouth. Trade name: **Anquil**.

benserazide (ben-**ser**-ă-zyd) *n.* *see* levodopa.

benzalkonium (ben-zăl-**koh**-niŭm) *n.* an antiseptic used in preparations for treating mouth and throat infections and skin conditions.

benzene (**ben**-zeen) *n.* a toxic liquid hydrocarbon. Continued inhalation of benzene vapour may result in aplastic anaemia or a form of leukaemia. Formula: C_6H_6.

benzhexol (benz-**heks**-ol) *n.* *see* trihexyphenidyl.

benzodiazepines (ben-zoh-dy-**az**-ĕ-peenz) *pl. n.* a group of anxiolytics and hypnotics, including diazepam, oxazepam, and temazepam.

benzoic acid (ben-**zoh**-ik) *n.* an antiseptic used as a preservative and (combined with salicylic acid) in an ointment (Whitfield's ointment) to treat ringworm.

benzoin (**ben**-zoh-in) *n.* a fragrant gum resin used as a constituent of friar's balsam.

benzoyl peroxide (ben-zoh-il pĕ-**rok**-syd) *n.* a preparation administered as a cream or gel in the treatment of acne. It removes the surface layers of the epidermis, unblocks skin pores, and has an antiseptic effect. Trade names: **Acnecide**, **Brevoxyl**, **PanOxyl**.

benzydamine hydrochloride (ben-zy-dă-meen hy-droh-**klor**-ryd) *n.* an anti-inflammatory drug (*see* NSAID) administered as a mouthwash or throat spray. Trade name: **Difflam**.

benzyl benzoate (**ben**-zyl **ben**-zoh-ayt) *n.* an oily aromatic liquid that is applied externally for the treatment of scabies.

benzylpenicillin (ben-zyl-pen-i-sil-in) *n. see* penicillin.

bereavement (bi-reev-mĕnt) *n.* the state or feeling of having lost a loved one, especially through death. It is usually manifest as mental anguish (**grief**), and bereaved people may lose weight, cry without ceasing, withdraw and wish themselves dead, or suffer from abnormal perceptions (e.g. they hear or see the departed). As in other forms of loss, acceptance will usually come with time.

beriberi (b'e-ri-**b'e**-ri) *n.* a nutritional disorder due to deficiency of vitamin B_1 (thiamine). It is widespread in communities in which the diet is based on polished rice. **dry b.** a form of beriberi in which there is extreme emaciation. **wet b.** a form of beriberi in which there is an accumulation of tissue fluid (oedema). There is nervous degeneration in both forms of the disease and death from heart failure is often the outcome.

berry aneurysm (b'e-ri) *n. see* aneurysm.

berylliosis (b'e-ri-li-**oh**-sis) *n.* poisoning by beryllium or its compounds, either by inhalation or by skin contamination. Inhalation of fumes from molten beryllium causes an acute alveolitis and is usually fatal. Subacute and chronic forms can result from exposure to the powder and can produce granulomata in the skin or lungs. In the lungs, these can lead to fibrosis unless prevented by prompt use of oral corticosteroids.

Best's disease (bests) *n. see* vitelliform degeneration. [F. Best (1878–1920), German physician]

beta agonist (bee-tă) *n. see* sympathomimetic.

beta blocker *n.* a drug that prevents stimulation of the beta-adrenergic receptors at the nerve endings of the sympathetic nervous system. Beta blockers decrease the activity of the heart and some reduce the production of aqueous humour (and therefore pressure) inside the eye. They include propranolol, oxprenolol, sotalol, levobunolol, and timolol.

beta cells *pl. n.* the cells of the islets of Langerhans that produce insulin. *Compare* alpha cells, D cells.

betahistine (bee-tă-**hist**-een) *n.* a drug that is an analogue of histamine and increases blood flow through the inner ear. It is administered by mouth to treat Ménière's disease. Trade name: **Serc**.

betamethasone (bee-tă-**meth**-ă-sohn) *n.* a synthetic corticosteroid drug used to treat a wide range of inflammatory and allergic conditions. The side-effects are those of cortisone. Trade names: **Betnesol**, **Betnovate**, **Vista-methasone**, etc.

betaxolol (bet-**aks**-oh-lol) *n.* a beta blocker administered as eye drops to treat chronic simple glaucoma. Trade name: **Betoptic**.

bevacizumab (bee-vă-**siz**-oo-mab) *n.* a monoclonal antibody that interferes with the growth of new blood vessels (*see* angiogenesis). Administered by intravenous infusion, it is used in the treatment of metastatic colorectal cancer, breast cancer, ovarian cancer, and non-small-cell lung cancer. Trade name: **Avastin**.

bezafibrate (bee-ză-**fy**-brayt) *n.* a drug used to treat hyperlipidaemia that fails to respond to diet (*see* fibrate). It is administered by mouth. Trade name: **Bezalip**.

bezoar (**bee**-zor) *n.* a mass of swallowed indigestible material within the stomach.

bi- *combining form denoting* two; double.

bias (**bi**-ăs) *n.* systematic deviation of results from the truth. The different types include **selection bias** (failing to select a sample that is representative of the wider population), **nonresponse bias** (respondents differing from nonrespondents in statistical surveys), and **social desirability bias** (respondents giving false answers they believe to be more socially acceptable than the truth).

bicalutamide (bik-ă-**loot**-ă-myd) *n.* a nonsteroidal anti-androgen commonly used to treat locally advanced and metastatic prostate cancer. It binds to and blocks the androgen receptor but does not reduce levels of testosterone in the blood, thus preserving libido and general energy levels. It is administered by mouth. Trade name: **Casodex**.

bicarbonate (by-**kar**-bŏ-nit) *n.* a salt containing the ion HCO_3^-. **b. of soda** *see* sodium bicarbonate.

biceps (**by**-seps) *n.* a muscle with two heads. **b. brachii** a muscle that extends from the shoulder to the elbow and is responsible for flexing the arm and forearm (see illustration). **b. femoris** a muscle at the back of the thigh, responsible for flexing the knee.

biconcave (by-**kon**-kayv) *adj.* having a hollowed surface on both

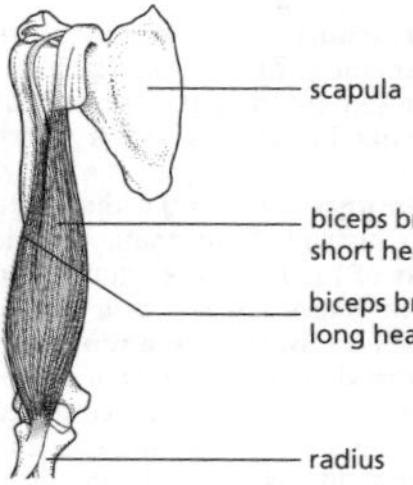

The biceps muscle of the arm

sides. Biconcave lenses are used to correct short-sightedness. *Compare* biconvex.

biconvex (by-**kon**-veks) *adj.* having a surface on each side that curves outwards. Biconvex lenses are used to correct long-sightedness. *Compare* biconcave.

bicornuate (by-**kor**-new-it) *adj.* having two hornlike processes or projections. The term is applied to an abnormal uterus that is divided into two separate halves at the upper end.

bicuspid (by-**kus**-pid) *adj.* having two cusps, as in the premolar teeth and the mitral valve of the heart. **b. valve** *see* mitral valve.

bifid (**by**-fid) *adj.* split or cleft into two parts.

bifocal lens (by-**foh**-kăl) *n.* a lens with two principal focal lengths: usually the upper part of the lens gives a sharp image of distant objects and the lower part is for near vision, such as reading. *See also* multifocal lens.

bifurcation (by-fer-**kay**-shŏn) *n.* (in anatomy) the point at which division into two branches occurs; for example in blood vessels or in the trachea.

bigeminy (by-**jem**-ini) *n.* the condition in which alternate ectopic beats of the heart are transmitted to the pulse and felt as a double pulse beat (**pulsus bigeminus**).

biguanide (by-**gwah**-nyd) *n.* any of a class of drugs that increase glucose uptake by the muscles and reduce glucose release by the liver. These drugs, which include metformin, are taken by mouth in the treatment of type 2 diabetes mellitus.

bilateral (by-**lat**-er-ăl) *adj.* (in anatomy) relating to or affecting both sides of the body or of a tissue or organ or both of a pair of organs.

bile (byl) *n.* a thick alkaline fluid that is secreted by the liver and stored in the gall bladder. It is ejected intermittently into the duodenum, where it helps to emulsify fats so that they can be more easily digested. Bile may be yellow, green, or brown; its constituents include bile pigments and salts, lecithin, and cholesterol.

bile acids *pl. n.* the organic acids in bile; mostly occurring as bile salts. They are cholic acid, deoxycholic acid, glycocholic acid, and taurocholic acid.

bile-acid sequestrant (si-**kwes**-trănt) *n.* a drug that binds to bile acids, forming a complex that is excreted in the faeces. The reduction in bile acids causes cholesterol to be oxidized to bile acids, decreases low-density lipoprotein serum levels, and decreases serum cholesterol levels. *See* colestipol, colestyramine.

bile duct *n.* any of the ducts that convey bile from the liver. Many small ducts drain into the right and left hepatic ducts, which unite to form the main bile duct, the **common hepatic duct**. This joins the **cystic duct**, which leads from the gall bladder, to form the **common bile duct**, which drains into the duodenum.

bile pigments *pl. n.* coloured compounds – breakdown products of the blood pigment haemoglobin – that are excreted in bile. The two most important bile pigments are **bilirubin**, which is orange or yellow, and its oxidized form **biliverdin**, which is green. Mixed with the intestinal contents, they give the brown colour to the faeces (*see* urobilinogen).

bile salts *pl. n.* sodium glycocholate and sodium taurocholate – the alkaline salts of bile – necessary for the emulsification of fats.

bi-level positive airways pressure (by-lev-ĕl) *n. see* BiPAP.

Bilharzia (bil-harts-iă) *n. see* Schistosoma.

bilharziasis (bil-harts-I-ă-sis) *n. see* schistosomiasis.

bili- *combining form denoting* bile.

biliary (bil-yer-i) *adj.* relating to or affecting the bile duct or bile. **b. atresia** *see* atresia. **b. colic** severe steady pain in the upper abdomen (in the mid-line or to the right) resulting from obstruction of the gall bladder or common bile duct, most commonly by a gallstone. Vomiting often occurs. **b. fistula** *see* fistula.

bilious (bil-yŭs) *adj.* **1.** containing bile. **2.** a lay term used to describe attacks of nausea or vomiting.

bilirubin (bili-roo-bin) *n. see* bile pigments.

biliuria (choluria) (bili-yoor-iă) *n.* the presence of bile in the urine: a feature of certain forms of jaundice.

biliverdin (bili-ver-din) *n. see* bile pigments.

Billings method (bil-ingz) *n.* a method of planning pregnancy involving the daily examination of cervical mucus, which varies in consistency and colour throughout the menstrual cycle. [J. and E. Billings (20th century), Australian physicians]

Billroth's operation (bil-rohts) *n.* an operation in which the lower part of the stomach is removed and the remaining portion joined to the duodenum (**B. o. I**) or the lower stomach and duodenum are removed, with attachment of the remaining stomach to the jejunum (**B. o. II**). *See* gastrectomy. [C. A. T. Billroth (1829–94), Austrian surgeon]

bimanual (by-man-yoo-ăl) *adj.* using two hands to perform an activity, such as a gynaecological examination.

binaural (byn-or-ăl) *adj.* relating to or involving the use of both ears.

binder (byn-der) *n.* a bandage that is wound around a part of the body, usually the abdomen, to apply pressure or to give support or protection.

binge–purge syndrome (binj-perj) *n. see* bulimia.

binocular (bin-ok-yoo-ler) *adj.* relating to or involving the use of both eyes. **b. vision** the acquired ability to focus both eyes on an object at the same time, so that only one image is seen.

binovular (bin-ov-yoo-ler) *adj.* derived from two separate ova, as are fraternal twins. *Compare* uniovular.

bio- *combining form denoting* life or living organisms.

bioassay (by-oh-ass-ay) *n.* estimation of the activity or potency of a drug or other substance by comparing its effects on living organisms with effects of a preparation of known strength.

bioavailability (by-oh-ă-vayl-ă-**bil**-iti) *n.* the proportion of a drug that is delivered to its site of action in the body. This is usually the amount entering the circulation and may be low when the drugs are given by mouth.

biochemistry (by-oh-**kem**-istri) *n.* the study of the chemical processes and substances occurring in living things. —**biochemical** *adj.* —**biochemist** *n.*

bioengineering (by-oh-en-ji-**neer**-ing) *n.* the application of biological and engineering principles to the development and manufacture of equipment and devices for use in biological systems. Examples of such products include orthopaedic prostheses and heart pacemakers.

bioethics (by-oh-**eth**-iks) *n.* an area of applied ethics relating to the life sciences generally. Medical ethics is commonly considered to be a subspecialty of bioethics (**biomedical ethics**).

biofeedback (by-oh-**feed**-bak) *n.* a treatment method in which patients are guided to improve their health by using physiological signals or symptoms (e.g. heart rate) from their own bodies, often detected by means of monitoring devices. Physiotherapists and psychologists can identify or elicit a response to a particular condition (e.g. stress) and then promote ways of learning how to deal with it. This heightened sensitivity and awareness enables effective personal or professional supervision of the condition.

biofilm (**by**-oh-film) *n.* an organized layer of microorganisms that forms on a surface. Biofilm may be implicated in several disease processes, including dental infections, endocarditis, infections of surgical implants, lung infections in people with cystic fibrosis, and glue ear.

biogenesis (by-oh-**jen**-i-sis) *n.* the theory that living organisms can arise only from other living organisms and not from nonliving matter.

biological response modifier (BRM) *n.* a therapeutic agent that stimulates the body's defence mechanisms against infection and disease. In small amounts, they are produced naturally by the body; larger doses have been genetically developed for use against cancer, rheumatoid arthritis, and hepatitis. *See* immunotherapy.

biological therapy *n.* any treatment that facilitates the ability of the immune system to fight disease, as opposed to acting directly against the disease. Such treatments, most commonly used for cancer and rheumatic disease, include biological response modifiers, immunotherapy, and monoclonal antibodies.

biology (by-**ol**-ŏji) *n.* the study of living organisms including their structure and function and their relationships with one another and with the inanimate world. —**biological** (by-ŏ-**loj**-ik-ăl) *adj.* —**biologist** *n.*

bionics (by-**on**-iks) *n.* the science of mechanical or electronic systems that function in the same way as, or have characteristics of, living systems. *Compare* cybernetics. —**bionic** *adj.*

bionomics (by-ŏ-**nom**-iks) *n. see* ecology.

biophysical profile (by-oh-**fiz**-ikăl **proh**-fyl) *n.* a physiological assessment of fetal wellbeing, based on scores for fetal movement, breathing, tone, and heart rate and amniotic fluid volume.

biopsy (**by**-op-si) *n.* the removal of a small piece of living tissue from an organ or part of the body for microscopic examination.

biostatistics (by-oh-stă-**tist**-iks) *n.* statistical information and techniques used with special reference to studies of health and social problems. *See also* demography, vital statistics.

biotin (**by**-ŏ-tin) *n.* a vitamin of the B complex that is an essential coenzyme for several enzymes involved in fatty acid synthesis, gluconeogenesis, and the metabolism of branched-chain amino acids. Rich sources of the vitamin are egg yolk, yeast, and liver.

BiPAP (bi-level positive airways pressure) *n.* trade name (now widely used generically) for a device that provides ventilation for patients by delivering air to the lungs at two levels of pressure, either cyclically in an anaesthetized patient or triggered by the patient's attempts at breathing when awake.

bipolar (by-**poh**-ler) *adj.* (in neurology) describing a neuron (nerve cell) that has two processes extending in different directions from its cell body.

bipolar affective disorder (BPAD) *n.* a severe mental illness causing repeated episodes of depression and mania (**Type I BPAD**) or depressive episodes with occasional phases of hypomania (**Type II BPAD**). Antidepressants and antipsychotics are used to treat depressive episodes together with mood stabilizers (e.g. lithium) or antiepileptics. Mood stabilizers are also used to prevent or lessen future episodes. Mania is most commonly treated with benzodiazepines, antipsychotics, and mood stabilizers. To prevent future episodes many patients need combinations of mood stabilizers with antidepressants or antipsychotics.

bird-fancier's lung (**berd**-fan-si-erz) *n.* a form of extrinsic allergic alveolitis caused by the inhalation of avian proteins present in the droppings and feathers of certain birds, especially pigeons and caged birds (such as budgerigars). There is an acute and a chronic form. *See also* alveolitis.

birth (berth) *n.* (in obstetrics) *see* labour.

birth asphyxia (hypoxic-ischaemic encephalopathy) *n.* brain damage in a newborn infant as a result of the brain receiving inadequate oxygen. Surviving infants may have developmental delay, cerebral palsy, or learning disability.

birth control *n.* the use of contraception or sterilization (male or female) to prevent unwanted pregnancies.

birthing chair (berth-ing) *n.* a chair specially adapted to allow childbirth to take place in a sitting position. Its introduction in the Western world followed the increasing demand by women for greater mobility during labour. The chair is electronically powered and can be tilted back quickly and easily should the need arise.

birthmark (berth-mark) *n.* a skin blemish or mark present at birth.

birth rate (live birth rate) *n.* the number of live births occurring in a year per 1000 total population. *See also* fertility rate.

bisacodyl (bis-ak-oh-dil) *n.* a stimulant laxative that acts on the large intestine to cause reflex movement and bowel evacuation. It is administered by mouth or as a suppository. Trade name: **Dulcolax**.

bisexual (by-seks-yoo-ăl) *adj.* **1.** describing an individual who is sexually attracted to both men and women. **2.** describing an individual who possesses the qualities of both sexes.

bismuth (biz-mŭth) *n.* a white metallic element. Its salts are used in some antacid mixtures and as protective agents in skin powders and pastes. They were formerly widely used in the treatment of syphilis. Symbol: Bi.

bisoprolol (by-soh-proh-lol) *n.* a beta blocker drug used to treat hypertension, angina pectoris, and heart failure. It is administered by mouth. Trade name: **Cardicor**.

bisphosphonates (bis-fos-fŏ-nayts) *pl. n.* a class of drugs that inhibit the resorption of bone by blocking the action of osteoclasts. Bisphosphonates are used in the treatment of Paget's disease and hypercalcaemia due to cancer and in the treatment and prevention of postmenopausal osteoporosis. They include **disodium etidronate** (Didronel), **pamidronate disodium**, **alendronic acid**, **risedronate** (Actonel), **sodium clodronate** (Bonefos, Clasteon, Loron), and **zoledronic acid**.

bistoury (bis-ter-i) *n.* a narrow surgical knife, with a straight or curved blade.

bite-wing (byt-wing) *n.* a dental X-ray film that provides a view of the crowns of the teeth in part of both upper and lower jaws.

Bitot's spots (bee-tohz) *pl. n.* cheesy foamy greyish spots that form on the surface of dry patches of conjunctiva at the sides of the eyes. They consist of fragments of keratinized epithelium. A common cause is vitamin A deficiency. [P. A. Bitot (1822–88), French physician]

bivalve (by-valv) *adj.* consisting of or possessing two valves or sections. **b. cast** a plaster cast that is cut into anterior and posterior sections to monitor pressure beneath the cast. **b. speculum** a vaginal speculum that has two blades.

black eye (blak) *n.* bruising of the eyelids.

blackhead (blak-hed) *n.* a plug formed of fatty material (sebum and keratin) in the outlet of a sebaceous gland in the skin. *See also* acne. Medical name: **comedo**.

black heel *n.* a black area resulting from the rupture of capillaries in the skin in those who play basketball, squash, etc. It may be mistaken for malignant melanoma.

blackwater fever (blak-waw-ter) *n.* a rare and serious complication of malignant (falciparum) malaria in which there is massive destruction of the red blood cells, leading to the presence of the blood pigment haemoglobin in the urine.

bladder (blad-er) *n.* **1. (urinary bladder)** a sac-shaped organ that has a wall of smooth muscle and stores the urine produced by the kidneys. **b. neck incision** *see* incision. **b. outflow obstruction** *see* BOO. **2.** any of several other hollow organs containing fluid, such as the gall bladder.

bladder pressure study *n.* a combined X-ray and manometry examination of the bladder to look for abnormal function. The bladder is filled slowly with contrast medium using a small urinary catheter and the pressure is monitored during filling and voiding (micturition).

bladderworm (blad-er-werm) *n.* *see* cysticercus.

Blalock-Taussig operation (blay-lok taw-sig) *n.* an operation in which the pulmonary artery is anastomosed to the subclavian artery, performed on patients with tetralogy of Fallot. [A. Blalock (1899–1964), US surgeon; H. B. Taussig (20th century), US paediatrician]

bland (bland) *adj.* nonirritating; mild; soothing: applied to foods and diets.

blast (blahst) *n.* an important cause of serious soft-tissue injury that is associated with explosions or high-velocity missiles. The eardrums, lungs, and gastrointestinal tract are especially vulnerable to the indirect effects of the blast wave.

-blast *combining form denoting* a formative cell.

blasto- *combining form denoting* a germ cell or embryo.

blastocyst (blast-oh-sist) *n.* an early stage of embryonic development that consists of a hollow ball of cells with a localized thickening (the **inner cell mass**) that will develop into the actual embryo. *See also* implantation.

blastomycosis (blast-oh-my-koh-sis) *n.* any disease caused by parasitic fungi of the genus *Blastomyces*, which may affect the skin (forming wartlike ulcers and tumours) or involve various internal tissues.

blastula (blast-yoo-lă) *n.* an early stage of the embryonic development of many animals. The equivalent stage in mammals (including humans) is the blastocyst.

bleb (bleb) *n.* a blister or large vesicle. **filtering b.** a blister-like cyst underneath the conjunctiva resulting from a surgical procedure such as trabeculectomy, used in the treatment of glaucoma.

bleeding (bleed-ing) *n.* *see* haemorrhage.

bleeding time *n.* the time taken for bleeding to cease from a small wound, such as a puncture in a finger or ear lobe. It is used as a test of platelet function.

SEE WEB LINKS
- Explanation of blood clotting tests from a comprehensive health information website

blenn- (blenno-) *combining form denoting* mucus.

blennorrhagia (blen-ŏ-**ray**-jiă) *n.* a copious discharge of mucus, particularly from the urethra.

blennorrhoea (blen-ŏ-**ree**-ă) *n.* a profuse watery discharge from the urethra.

bleomycin (bli-oh-**my**-sin) *n.* an antibiotic with action against cancer cells (*see* cytotoxic drug), administered intravenously or intramuscularly in the treatment of germ-cell cancer, non-Hodgkin's lymphoma, and squamous cell carcinoma.

blephar- (blepharo-) *combining form denoting* the eyelid.

blepharitis (blef-ă-**ry**-tis) *n.* inflammation of the eyelids.

blepharochalasis (blef-er-oh-kă-**lay**-sis) *n.* excessive eyelid skin resulting from recurrent episodes of oedema and inflammation of the eyelid. It occurs in young people, causing drooping of the lid. *Compare* dermatochalasis.

blepharoconjunctivitis (blef-er-oh-kŏn-junk-ti-**vy**-tis) *n.* inflammation involving the eyelid margins and conjunctiva.

blepharon (**blef**-er-ŏn) *n. see* eyelid.

blepharoptosis (blef-er-**op**-tŏ-sis) *n. see* ptosis.

blepharospasm (**blef**-er-oh-spazm) *n.* involuntary tight contraction of the eyelids, either in response to painful conditions of the eye or as a form of dystonia.

blind and partially sighted register (blynd) *n.* (in Britain) a list of persons who are technically blind or partially sighted due to reduced visual acuity or who have severely restricted fields of vision. The list is maintained by local authorities (England and Wales), regional or island councils (Scotland), or the Health and Social Services Board (Northern Ireland). Registration is voluntary, but it is a precondition for the receipt of some financial benefits.

blind loop syndrome (stagnant loop syndrome) *n.* a condition of stasis of the small intestine that alters the normal bacterial flora of the gut, leading to malabsorption, nutrient deficiency, and the passage of fatty stools (*see* steatorrhoea). It is usually a result of chronic obstruction, surgical bypass operations producing a stagnant length of bowel, or conditions in which a segment of intestine is out of continuity with the rest.

blindness (**blynd**-nis) *n.* the inability to see. For administrative purposes, the term covers both total blindness and certain degrees of visual impairment (*see* blind register). The commonest causes of blindness worldwide are trachoma, onchocerciasis, and vitamin

A deficiency, and in Great Britain age-related macular degeneration, glaucoma, cataract, myopic retinal degeneration, and diabetic retinopathy. *See also* colour blindness, day blindness, night blindness, snow blindness.

blind spot *n.* the small area of the retina of the eye where the nerve fibres from the light-sensitive cells lead into the optic nerve. There are no rods or cones in this area and hence it does not register light. Anatomical name: **punctum caecum**.

blind trial *n.* a controlled trial in which the participants are not aware of which group they are assigned to.

blister (blis-ter) *n.* a swelling containing watery fluid (serum) and sometimes also blood (**blood b.**) or pus, within or just beneath the skin.

bloating (bloh-ting) *n.* the subjective experience of abdominal fullness, often (but not always) accompanied by distension. Causes include air swallowing (*see* aerophagia), abnormal intestinal gas handling or abdominal wall reflexes, increased gas production, and organ hypersensitivity. Bloating may be associated with changes in bowel habit, particularly constipation. It tends to be aggravated by meals and fluctuates in severity throughout the day. Treatment includes changes in diet and reassurance; antispasmodics, laxatives, and tricyclic antidepressants (to reduce hypersensitivity) may be tried.

block (blok) *n.* any interruption of physiological or mental function, brought about intentionally (as part of a therapeutic procedure) or by disease. *See also* heart block, nerve block.

Blocq's disease *see* abasia.

blood (blud) *n.* a fluid that circulates throughout the body, via the arteries and veins, providing a vehicle by which an immense variety of different substances are transported between the various organs and tissues. It is composed of cells (*see* blood cell), which are suspended in a liquid medium (*see* plasma).

blood bank *n.* a department within a hospital or blood transfusion centre in which blood collected from donors is stored prior to transfusion.

blood-brain barrier (BBB) *n.* the mechanism that controls the passage of molecules from the blood into the cerebrospinal fluid and the tissue spaces surrounding the cells of the brain and thus protects the brain from the effects of substances harmful to it. The endothelial cells lining the walls of the brain capillaries are more tightly joined together at their edges than those lining capillaries supplying other parts of the body, which allows the passage of solutions and fat-soluble compounds but excludes particles and large molecules.

blood casts *pl. n.* fragments of cellular material (*see* cast) to which blood cells are attached, which are derived from the kidney tubules and are excreted in the urine in certain kidney diseases.

blood cell (blood corpuscle) *n.* any of the cells that are present in the blood in health or disease. The cells may be subclassified into three major categories: red cells (*see* erythrocyte), white cells (*see* leucocyte), and platelets. See illustration.

blood clot *n.* a solid or semisolid mass formed as the result of blood coagulation, either within the blood vessels and heart or elsewhere. *See also* thrombosis.

blood clotting *n.* *see* blood coagulation.

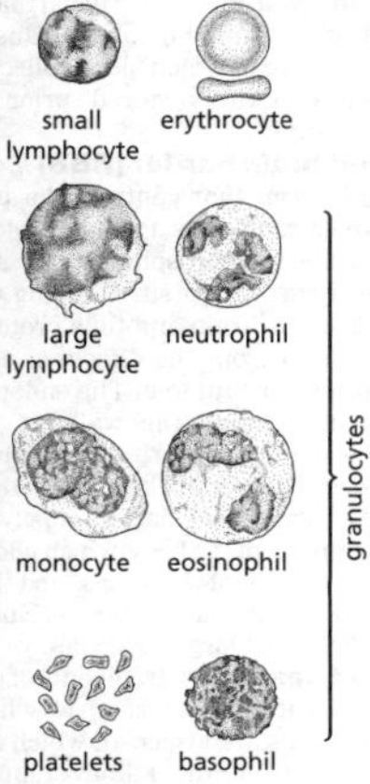

Types of blood cells

blood coagulation (blood clotting) *n.* the process whereby blood is converted from a liquid to a solid state. The process involves the interaction of a variety of substances (*see* coagulation factors) and leads to the production of the enzyme thrombin, which converts the soluble blood protein fibrinogen to the insoluble protein fibrin, forming the blood clot. Blood coagulation is an essential mechanism for the arrest of bleeding (haemostasis).

blood corpuscle *n.* *see* blood cell.

blood count *n.* the numbers of different blood cells in a known volume of blood, usually expressed as the number of cells per litre. **full b. c. (FBC)** a blood count that includes measures of the amount of haemoglobin and size of red cells, as well as counts of red cells, white cells, and platelets. *See also* differential leucocyte count.

blood donor *n.* a person who gives blood for storage in a blood bank.

blood group *n.* any one of the many types into which a person's blood may be classified, based on the presence or absence of certain inherited antigens on the surface of the red blood cells. Blood of one group contains antibodies in the serum that react against the cells of other groups. One of the most important blood group systems is the **ABO system**. It is based on the presence or absence of antigens A and B: blood of groups A and B contains antigens A and B, respectively; group AB contains both antigens and group O neither. Blood of group A contains antibodies to

Blood groups of the ABO system

Donor's blood group	*Blood group of people donor can receive blood from*	*Blood group of people donor can give blood to*
A	A, O	A, AB
B	B, O	B, AB
AB	A, B, AB, O	AB
O	O	A, B, AB, O

antigen B; group B blood contains anti-A antibodies or isoagglutinins; group AB has neither antibody and group O has both. The table below illustrates which blood groups can be used in transfusion for each of the four groups. *See also* rhesus factor.

blood plasma *n. see* plasma.

blood poisoning *n.* the presence of either bacterial toxins or large numbers of bacteria in the bloodstream causing serious illness. *See* pyaemia, septicaemia, toxaemia.

blood pressure (BP) *n.* the pressure of blood against the walls of the main arteries. Pressure is highest during systole, when the ventricles are contracting (**systolic pressure**), and lowest during diastole, when the ventricles are relaxing and refilling (**diastolic pressure**). Blood pressure is measured – in millimetres of mercury (mmHg) – by means of a sphygmomanometer at the brachial artery of the arm. A young adult would be expected to have a systolic pressure of around 120 mmHg and a diastolic pressure of 80 mmHg. These are recorded as 120/80 mmHg. *See also* hypertension, hypotension.

blood serum *n. see* serum.

blood sugar *n.* the concentration of glucose in the blood, normally expressed in millimoles per litre. The normal range is 3.5–5.5 mmol/l. Blood-sugar estimation is an important investigation in a variety of diseases, most notably in diabetes mellitus. fasting b. s. (**FBS**) the concentration of glucose in the blood after an overnight fast. *See also* hyperglycaemia, hypoglycaemia.

blood test *n.* any test designed to discover abnormalities in a sample of a person's blood or to determine the blood group.

blood transfusion *n. see* transfusion.

SEE WEB LINKS

- Website of the National Blood Service

blood vessel *n.* a tube carrying blood away from or towards the heart. *See* artery, arteriole, vein, venule, capillary.

Bloom's syndrome (bloomz) *n.* a specific abnormality of chromosome

15 in which the individual suffers from recurrent infections, blisters on the hands and lips, and poor growth. Such children have a much higher than normal risk of developing cancer. [D. Bloom (20th century), US dermatologist]

Blount disease (blownt) *n.* a condition causing bow-legs as a result of abnormal growth at the epiphysis at the top of the tibia. It is more common in Africans and is most noticeable in childhood. [W. P. Blount (1900–92), US orthopaedic surgeon]

BLS *n. see* basic life support.

blue baby (bloo) *n.* an infant suffering from congenital heart disease in which the circulation is misdirected. This results in the presence of partially deoxygenated blood (which is blue in colour) in the peripheral circulation, which gives the skin and lips a characteristic purple colour (*see* cyanosis).

B lymphocyte *n. see* lymphocyte.

BMI *n. see* body mass index.

BMR *n.* basal metabolic rate (*see* basal metabolism).

BMT *n.* bone-marrow transplant. *See* transplantation.

BNF *n. see* British National Formulary.

BNP *n.* brain natriuretic peptide (*see* natriuretic peptide). **BNP test** measurement of the level of BNP in the blood, which is increased (>99 ng/l) in cases of congestive heart failure. The test is used to assess the degree of heart failure and monitor response to treatment.

Boari flap (boh-ah-ri) *n.* a tube of bladder tissue constructed to replace the lower third of the ureter when this has been injured or surgically excised because of the presence of a tumour or stricture. *See also* ureteroplasty. [A. Boari (19th century), Italian surgeon]

body (bod-i) *n.* **1.** an entire animal organism. **2.** the trunk of an individual, excluding the limbs. **3.** the main or largest part of an organ. **4.** a solid discrete mass of tissue; e.g. the carotid body. *See also* corpus.

body image (body schema) *n.* the individual's concept of the disposition of his limbs and the identity of the different parts of his body.

body mass index (BMI) *n.* the weight of a person (in kilograms) divided by the square of the height of that person (in metres): used as an indicator of whether or not a person is over- or underweight. A BMI of between 20 and 25 is considered normal, between 25 and 30 is overweight, and greater than 30 indicates clinical obesity. See Appendix 5: Body mass index (BMI).

body temperature *n.* the temperature of the body, as measured by a thermometer. In most normal individuals body temperature is maintained at about 37°C (98.4°F). A rise in body temperature occurs in fever.

Boeck's disease (beeks) *n. see* sarcoidosis. [C. P. M. Boeck (1845–1913), Norwegian dermatologist]

boil (boil) *n.* a tender inflamed area of the skin containing pus. The infection is usually caused by the bacterium *Staphylococcus aureus*, which enters through a hair follicle or a break in the skin. Boils usually heal when the pus is released or with antibiotic treatment, though occasionally they may cause more widespread infection. Medical name: **furuncle**.

Bolam and Bolitho tests (boh-lăm bŏ-**leeth**-oh) *n.* where negligence involving medical treatment is claimed, tests used to determine the standard of care owed to patients by doctors or other health professionals. The 1957 case of *Bolam v Friern Hospital Management Committee* established that if a doctor acts in accordance with a responsible body of medical opinion, he or she will not be negligent. In 1997 this standard of care test was amended by the case of *Bolitho v City and Hackney Health Authority*, which requires the doctor's behaviour to satisfy the judgment not only of responsible medical opinion but also of a court's own independent logical analysis.

bolus (**boh**-lŭs) *n.* **1.** a soft mass of chewed food. **2.** a large dose of a drug administered by rapid injection, as opposed to infusion.

bonding (**bond**-ing) *n.* **1.** (in psychology) the development of a close and selective relationship, such as that of attachment. **2.** (in dentistry) the attachment of dental restorations, sealants, and orthodontic brackets to teeth.

bone (bohn) *n.* the hard extremely dense connective tissue that forms the skeleton of the body. It is composed of a matrix of collagen fibres impregnated with bone salts, chiefly calcium carbonate and calcium phosphate (hydroxyapatite), in which bone cells (osteocytes) are embedded. **compact** (or **cortical**) **b.** the outer shell of bones, consisting of a hard virtually solid mass made up of bony tissue arranged in concentric layers (**Haversian systems**). **spongy** (or **cancellous**) **b.** bone found beneath the outer shell; it consists of a meshwork of bony bars (**trabeculae**) with many interconnecting spaces containing marrow. See illustration.

bone graft *n. see* graft.

bone marrow (marrow) *n.* the tissue contained within the internal cavities of the bones. At birth, these cavities are filled entirely with blood-forming **myeloid tissue** (**red marrow**) but in later life the marrow in the limb bones is replaced by fat (**yellow marrow**).

Bonney's blue (**bon**-iz) *n.* a dye consisting of a mixture of crystal violet and brilliant green. It is used as a skin disinfectant and to demonstrate the presence of a fistula, by instilling it via a cannula and tracing its path. [W. F. V. Bonney (1872–1953), British gynaecologist]

bony labyrinth (**boh**-ni) *n. see* labyrinth.

BOO (bladder outlet obstruction) *n.* a condition in which urine flow from the bladder through the urethra is impeded. It is usually caused by an enlarged prostate gland but sometimes also by a high bladder neck or uncoordinated contraction of the urinary sphincter and detrusor muscle of the bladder.

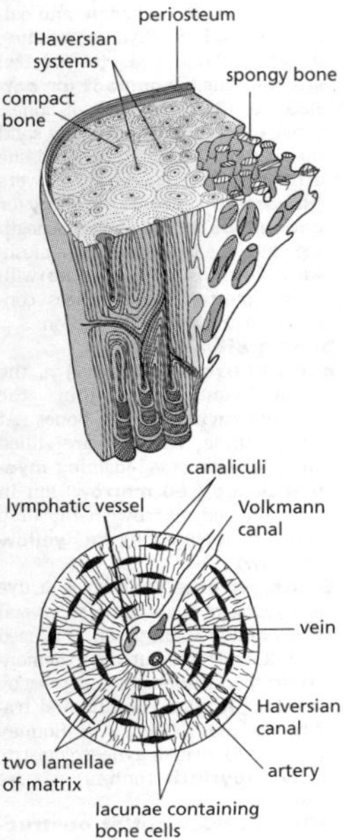

Section of the shaft of a long bone (above) with detail of a single Haversian system (below)

BOOP *n. see* bronchiolitis (obliterans organizing pneumonia).

borborygmus (bor-ber-**ig**-mŭs) *n.* (*pl.* **borborygmi**] an abdominal gurgling sound due to movement of fluid and gas in the intestine.

borderline (**bor**-der-lyn) *adj. see* emotionally unstable personality disorder.

Bordetella (bor-dĕ-**tel**-ă) *n.* a genus of tiny Gram-negative aerobic bacteria. **B. pertussis** the cause of whooping cough.

borneol (**bor**-nee-ol) *n.* an essential oil used, in preparations with other essential oils, such as camphene, cineole, and pinene, to disperse gallstones and kidney stones. It is administered by mouth. Trade names: **Rowachol**, **Rowatinex**.

Bornholm disease (devil's grip, epidemic myalgia, epidemic pleurodynia) (**born**-holm) *n.* a disease caused by Coxsackie viruses. It is spread by contact; symptoms include fever, headache, and attacks of severe pain in the lower chest. The illness lasts about a week and is rarely fatal.

bortezomib (bor-**tez**-ŏ-mib) *n.* a cytotoxic drug that is administered intravenously or subcutaneously in the treatment of relapsed myeloma and, in combination with other agents, for the first-line treatment of myeloma. Side-effects include peripheral neuropathy, thrombocytopenia, and nausea. Trade name: **Velcade**.

Bosniak classification (**boz**-ni-ak) *n.* a system for classifying renal cysts seen on CT imaging to aid in determining their degree of malignancy. Cysts are classified according to smoothness or irregularity of margins, degree of calcification, number and thickness of septa, and whether or not they enhance with contrast material.

bottom shuffling (bot-ŏm shuf-ling) *n.* a normal variant of crawling in which babies sit upright and move on their bottoms, usually by pulling forward on their heels. Babies who bottom-shuffle tend to walk slightly later. There is often a family history of bottom shuffling.

botulinum toxin (bot-yoo-ly-nŭm) *n.* a powerful nerve toxin (types A and B), produced by the bacterium Clostridium botulinum, that is injected, in minute dosage, for the treatment of various conditions of muscle dysfunction, such as dystonia (including blepharospasm and torticollis) and spastic paralysis associated with cerebral palsy and stroke. It is also used to treat severe hyperhidrosis and wrinkles between the eyebrows and to prevent chronic migraine. Trade names: **Botox**, **Dysport**, **NeuroBloc**, **Vistabel**, **Xeomin**.

botulism (bot-yoo-lizm) *n.* a rare and potentially life-threatening form of food poisoning due to ingestion of foods contaminated with toxins produced by the bacterium *Clostridium botulinum*, which thrives in improperly preserved foods. Botulinum toxin selectively targets motor nerve fibres of the central nervous system, causing flaccid paralysis.

Bouchard's node (boo-shahdz) *n.* a bony thickening arising at the proximal interphalangeal joint of a finger in osteoarthritis. It is often found together with Heberden's nodes. [J. C. Bouchard (1837–1915), French physician]

bougie (boo-*zhee*) *n.* a hollow or solid cylindrical instrument, usually flexible, that is inserted into tubular passages, such as the oesophagus (gullet), rectum, or urethra. Bougies are used in diagnosis and treatment, particularly by enlarging strictures.

Bourneville's disease (born-ĕ-veez) *n. see* tuberous (sclerosis). [D.-M. Bourneville (1840–1909), French neurologist]

bowel (bow-ĕl) *n. see* intestine.

Bowen's disease (boh-ĕnz) *n.* a type of in situ carcinoma of the squamous epidermal cells of the skin that does not spread to the basal layers. It can mimic psoriasis clinically. [J. T. Bowen (1857–1941), US dermatologist]

bow-legs (boh-legz) *pl. n.* abnormal out-curving of the legs at the knees, resulting in a gap between the knees on standing. Medical name: **genu varum**.

Bowman's capsule (boh-mănz) *n. see* glomerulus. [Sir W. P Bowman (1816–92), British physician]

BP *n. see* blood pressure.

BPAD *n. see* bipolar affective disorder.

BPD *n. see* bronchopulmonary (dysplasia).

BPH *n.* benign prostatic hyperplasia. *See* prostate gland.

BPPV *n. see* benign paroxysmal positional vertigo.

BPRS *n. see* Brief Psychiatric Rating Scale.

brachi- (brachio-) *combining form denoting* the arm.

brachial (**brayk**-iăl) *adj.* relating to or affecting the arm.

brachial artery *n.* an artery that extends from the axillary artery at the armpit, down the side and inner surface of the upper arm to the elbow, where it divides into the radial and ulnar arteries.

brachial plexus *n.* a network of nerves, arising from the spine at the base of the neck, from which arise the nerves supplying the arm, forearm and hand, and parts of the shoulder girdle. *See also* radial (nerve).

brachiocephalic artery (bray-ki-oh-si-**fal**-ik) *n.* *see* innominate artery.

brachium (**brayk**-iŭm) *n.* (*pl.* **brachia**) the arm, especially the part of the arm between the shoulder and the elbow.

brachy- *combining form denoting* shortness.

brachycephaly (brak-i-**sef**-ăli) *n.* shortness of the skull, with a cephalic index of about 80. —**brachycephalic** *adj.*

brachytherapy (brak-i-**th'**e-răpi) *n.* radiotherapy administered by implanting a radioactive source into or close to a tumour. This technique is used in the treatment of many accessible tumours (e.g. gynaecological cancers and localized prostate cancer).

Braden Q scale *n.* an assessment scale for the care of children (in hospital or the community) under the age of 8 who are at risk of developing pressure ulcers. It was modified in 1996 from the adult tool (*see* Braden scale), to which was added tissue perfusion to reflect a developmentally appropriate focus.

Braden scale (**bray**-dĕn) *n.* a predictive risk assessment tool, developed in the USA in 1987, that uses six factors to identify patients at risk of developing pressure ulcers. It includes an assessment of skin integrity, sensory perception, nutrition, mobility, activity level, and whether assistance is required when changing position. Each factor is accorded a score, the total score ranging from 6 to 23: the lower the score, the greater the risk of developing ulcers. [B. J. Braden]

Bradford's frame (**brad**-ferdz) *n.* a rectangular metal frame with canvas slings attached, used to support and immobilize a patient in a prone or supine position. [E. H. Bradford (1848–1926), US orthopaedic surgeon]

brady- *combining form denoting* slowness.

bradyarrhythmia (brad-i-ă-**ri*th***-miă) *n.* any deviation from the normal sinus rhythm of the heart that involves a decrease in heart rate.

bradycardia (brad-i-**kar**-diă) *n.* slowing of the heart rate to less than 50 beats per minute.

bradykinin (brad-i-**ky**-nin) *n.* a naturally occurring polypeptide consisting of nine amino acids; it is a very powerful vasodilator and causes contraction of smooth muscle.

brain (brayn) *n.* the enlarged and highly developed mass of nervous tissue that forms the upper end of the central nervous system. It is invested by three connective tissue

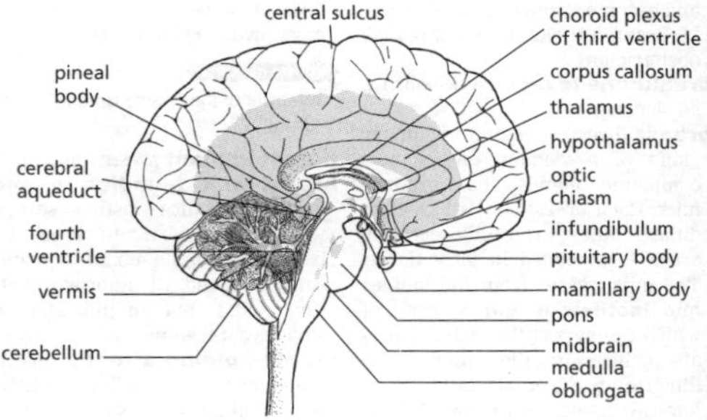

The brain (midsagittal section)

membranes (*see* meninges) and floats in cerebrospinal fluid within the rigid casing formed by the bones of the skull. See illustration. *See also* forebrain, hindbrain, midbrain. Anatomical name: **encephalon**.

brain death *n.* *see* death.

brain natriuretic peptide *n.* *see* BNP, natriuretic peptide.

brainstem (**brayn**-stem) *n.* the enlarged extension upwards within the skull of the spinal cord, consisting of the medulla oblongata, the pons, and the midbrain.

brainstem evoked response audiometry (BSER) *n.* *see* auditory brainstem response audiometry.

branchial cyst (**brank**-iăl) *n.* a cyst that arises at the site of an embryonic pharyngeal pouch due to a developmental anomaly.

branchial pouch *n.* *see* pharyngeal (pouch).

Brandt Andrews method (brant **an**-drooz) *n.* a technique for expelling the placenta from the uterus. Upward pressure is applied to the uterus through the abdominal wall while holding the umbilical cord taut. When the uterus is elevated in this way, the placenta will be in the cervix or upper vagina and is then expelled by applying pressure below the base of the uterus. [T. Brandt (1819–95), Swedish obstetrician; H. R. Andrews (1872–1942), British gynaecologist]

Braun's splint (brawnz) *n.* a metal splint with attachments for pulleys, used to support or apply traction to a fractured lower limb. See illustration. [H. F. W. Braun (1862–1934), German surgeon]

Braxton Hicks contractions (**braks**-tŏn hiks) *pl. n.* painless contractions of the uterus that occur intermittently during pregnancy and become stronger towards term. [J. Braxton Hicks (1825–97), British obstetrician]

breakbone fever (brayk-bohn) *n.* *see* dengue.

breast (brest) *n.* **1.** the mammary gland of a woman: one of two compound glands that produce milk. Each breast consists of glandular lobules – the milk-secreting areas – embedded in fatty tissue. The milk passes from the lobules into **lactiferous ducts**, each of which discharges through a separate orifice in the nipple. See illustration. *See also* lactation. Anatomical name: **mamma**. **2.** the front part of the chest (thorax).

breastbone (brest-bohn) *n.* *see* sternum.

breast cancer *n.* a malignant tumour of the breast, usually a carcinoma, rarely a sarcoma. It is unusual in men but is the commonest form of cancer in women, in some cases involving both breasts.

SEE WEB LINKS

- Website of the charity Breast Cancer Care

breast implant *n.* *see* implant.

breast-milk jaundice *n.* prolonged jaundice lasting several weeks after birth in breast-fed babies for which no other cause can be found. It improves with time and is not an indication to stop breast-feeding.

breath-holding attacks (breth-hohld-ing) *pl. n.* episodes in which a young child cries, holds its breath, and goes blue, which may result in loss of consciousness. The attacks cease spontaneously.

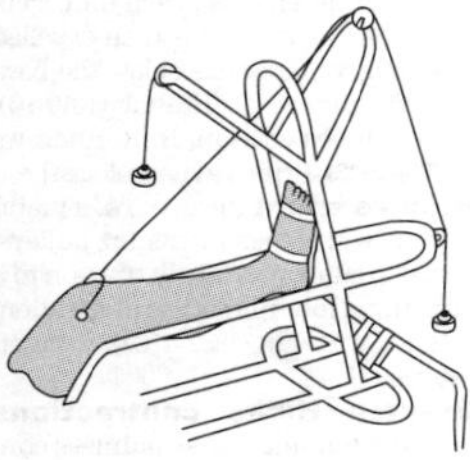

Braun's splint

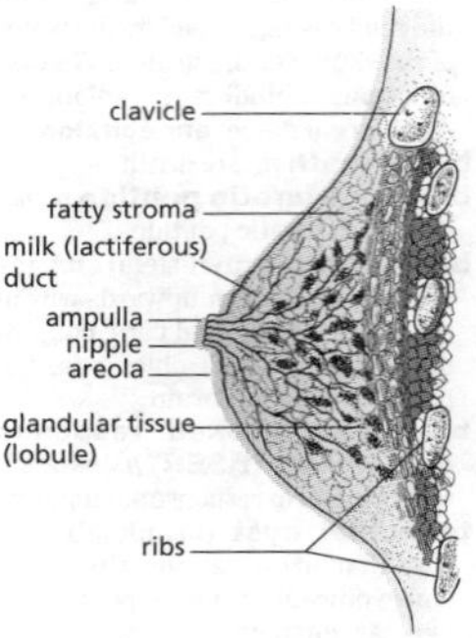

Longitudinal section through a breast

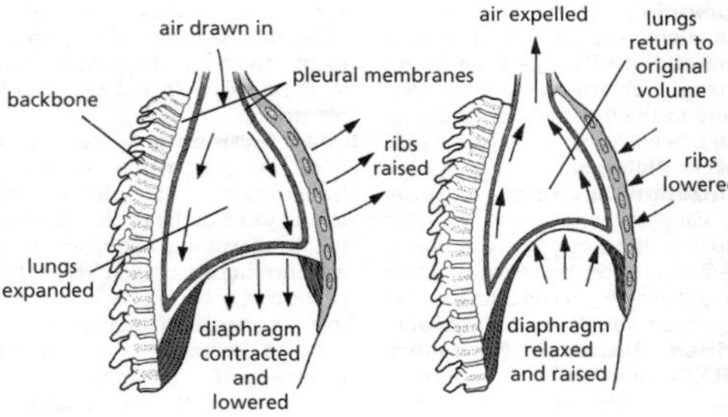

Position of the diaphragm (from the side) during breathing

breathing (bree*th*-ing) *n.* the alternation of active inhalation of air into the lungs through the mouth or nose with the passive exhalation of the air. Breathing is part of respiration and is sometimes called **external respiration**. See illustration.

breathlessness (**breth**-lis-nis) *n.* *see* dyspnoea.

breath sounds (breth) *pl. n.* the sounds heard through a stethoscope placed over the lungs during breathing. *See* bronchial breath sounds, cavernous breath sounds, vesicular breath sounds.

breech presentation (breech) *n.* the position of a baby in the uterus such that it would be delivered buttocks first (instead of the normal head-first delivery).

bregma (**breg**-mă) *n.* the point on the top of the skull at which the coronal and sagittal sutures meet. In a young infant this is an opening, the anterior fontanelle.

Breslow's thickness (brez-lohz) *n.* the distance (in millimetres) between the surface and the deepest extent of a malignant melanoma. The measurement is the best prognostic indicator in melanoma; tumours that are less than 0.76 mm thick have a five-year survival in well over 90% of patients. [A. Breslow (1928–80), US pathologist]

Brief Psychiatric Rating Scale (BPRS) *n.* a measure of general psychiatric symptoms based on patients' verbal responses and observation of patients at the time of interview.

Bright's disease (bryts) *n.* *see* nephritis. [R. Bright (1789–1858), British physician]

brilliant green (**bril**-yănt) *n.* an aniline dye used as an antiseptic.

brimonidine (bri-**mon**-i-deen) *n.* an alpha agonist (*see* sympathomimetic) used in the form of eye drops to reduce intraocular pressure in the treatment of glaucoma and ocular hypertension. Trade name: **Alphagan**.

brinzolamide (brin-**zol**-ă-myd) *n.* a carbonic anhydrase inhibitor used in the form of eye drops to reduce intraocular pressure in the treatment of glaucoma and ocular hypertension. Trade name: **Azopt**.

British National Formulary (BNF) (**brit**-ish) *n.* a reference source published by the Royal Pharmaceutical Society of Great Britain and the *British Medical Journal (BMJ)* Group twice a year (in March and September). It contains comprehensive information on medications from various sources, including the manufacturer as well as regulatory and professional bodies, resulting in information that is relevant to practice and takes into account national guidelines.

British Sign Language (BSL) *n.* the form of sign language most commonly used in Great Britain.

SEE WEB LINKS

- This interactive website explains British Sign Language

brittle diabetes (**brit**'l) *n.* type 1 diabetes mellitus that constantly causes disruption of lifestyle due to recurrent attacks of hypo- or hyperglycaemia.

BRM *see* biological response modifier.

Broadbent's sign (**brawd**-bents) *n.* retraction of the left side and back near the 11th and 12th ribs with every heartbeat, indicating adhesions between the pericardium and the diaphragm. [Sir W. H. Broadbent (1835–1907), British physician]

broad ligaments (brawd) *pl. n.* folds of peritoneum extending from each side of the uterus to the lateral walls of the pelvis, supporting the uterus and Fallopian tubes, and forming a partition across the pelvic cavity.

Broca's area (**broh**-kăz) *n.* the area of cerebral motor cortex responsible for the initiation and control of speech. It is situated in the left frontal lobe in most (but not all) right-handed people. [P. P. Broca (1824–80), French surgeon]

Brodie's abscess (**broh**-diz) *n.* *see* abscess. [Sir B. C. Brodie (1783–1862), British surgeon]

bromism (**broh**-mizm) *n.* a group of symptoms, including drowsiness, loss of sensation, and slurred speech, caused by excessive intake of bromides.

bromocriptine (broh-moh-**krip**-teen) *n.* a drug, derived from ergot, that is administered by mouth in the treatment of galactorrhoea, acromegaly, tumours associated with excessive secretion of prolactin, and (rarely) parkinsonism. Trade name: **Parlodel**.

Brompton cocktail (**bromp**-tŏn **kok**-tayl) *n.* a mixture of alcohol, morphine, and cocaine sometimes given to control severe pain in terminally ill people, especially those dying of cancer. The mixture was first tried at the Brompton Hospital, London.

bromsulphthalein (brom-**sulf**-thă-lin) *n.* a blue dye used in tests of liver function.

bronch- (broncho-) *combining form denoting* the bronchial tree.

bronchial breath sounds (**bronk**-iăl) *pl. n.* breath sounds transmitted through consolidated lungs in pneumonia; they are similar to the sounds heard normally over the larger bronchi and are louder and harsher than vesicular breath sounds.

bronchial carcinoma *n.* cancer of the bronchus, one of the commonest causes of death in smokers. *See also* lung cancer, small-cell lung cancer.

bronchial tree *n.* a branching system of tubes conducting air from the trachea to the lungs: includes the bronchi and their subdivisions and the bronchioles.

bronchiectasis (bronk-i-**ek**-tă-sis) *n.* widening of the bronchi or their branches. It may be congenital or it may result from infection or obstruction. Pus may form in the widened bronchus so that the patient coughs up purulent sputum, which may contain blood. Treatment consists of antibiotic drugs to control the infection and physiotherapy to drain the sputum. Surgery may be used if only a few segments of the bronchi are affected.

bronchiole (**bronk**-i-ohl) *n.* a subdivision of the bronchial tree that does not contain cartilage or mucous glands in its wall. The smallest bronchioles open into the alveoli. —**bronchiolar** *adj.*

bronchiolitis (bronk-i-oh-**ly**-tis) *n.* inflammation of the small airways in the lungs (*see* bronchiole) due to infection by viruses, usually the respiratory syncytial virus, and occurring most commonly in infants of less than one year. **b. obliterans organizing pneumonia** (**BOOP**) a flulike illness with cough, fever, and shortness of breath; there are patchy infiltrates on X-ray. It may result from a viral infection, be caused by certain drugs, or be associated with connective tissue disease.

bronchitis (brong-**ky**-tis) *n.* inflammation of the bronchi. **acute b.** bronchitis caused by viruses or bacteria. It is characterized by coughing, the production of mucopurulent sputum, and bronchospasm. **chronic b.** bronchitis in which the patient coughs up excessive mucus secreted by enlarged bronchial mucous glands on most days for at least three consecutive days in at least two consecutive years; the bronchospasm cannot be relieved by bronchodilator drugs. The disease is particularly prevalent in Britain in association with cigarette smoking, air pollution, and emphysema.

bronchoalveolar lavage (BAL) (brong-koh-al-vee-**oh**-ler) *n.* a method of obtaining cellular material from the lungs that is used particularly in the investigation and monitoring of interstitial lung disease and in the investigation of pulmonary infiltrates in immunosuppressed patients.

bronchoconstrictor (brong-koh-kŏn-**strik**-ter) *n.* a drug that causes narrowing of the air passages by producing spasm of bronchial smooth muscle.

bronchodilator (brong-koh-dy-**lay**-ter) *n.* an agent, such as formoterol, terbutaline, salbutamol, ipratropium, or theophylline, that causes widening of the air passages by relaxing bronchial smooth muscle.

bronchography (brong-**kog**-răfi) *n.* X-ray examination of the bronchial tree after it has been made visible by the injection of radiopaque dye or contrast medium. It has been largely superseded by CT scanning.

bronchomycosis (brong-koh-my-**koh**-sis) *n.* any of various fungal infections of the bronchi, such as candidiasis of the lungs.

bronchophony (brong-**kof**-ŏni) *n.* *see* vocal resonance.

bronchopleural (brong-koh-**ploor**-ăl) *adj.* relating to a bronchus and the pleura. **b. fistula** an abnormal communication (*see* fistula) between a bronchus and the pleural cavity.

bronchopneumonia (brong-koh-new-**moh**-niă) *n.* *see* pneumonia.

bronchopulmonary (brong-koh-**pul**-mŏn-er-i) *adj.* relating to the lungs and the bronchial tree. **b. dysplasia** (**BPD**) a condition seen usually in premature babies as a result of respiratory distress syndrome, requiring prolonged treatment with oxygen beyond the age of 28 days.

bronchoscope (**bronk**-ŏ-skohp) *n.* an instrument used to look into the trachea and bronchi. With the aid of a bronchoscope the bronchial tree can be washed out (*see* bronchoalveolar lavage) and samples of tissue and foreign bodies can be removed with long forceps. —**bronchoscopy** (brong-**kos**-kŏ-pi) *n.*

bronchospasm (**brong**-koh-spazm) *n.* narrowing of bronchi by muscular contraction in response to some stimulus, as in asthma and bronchitis. Some types of bronchospasm can usually be relieved by bronchodilator drugs; others, such as chronic bronchitis, usually cannot.

bronchus (**bronk**-ŭs) *n.* (*pl.* **bronchi**) any of the air passages beyond the trachea that has cartilage and mucous glands in its wall. *See also* bronchiole. —**bronchial** *adj.*

bronze diabetes (bronz) *n.* *see* haemochromatosis.

brown fat (brown) *n.* a form of fat in adipose tissue that is a rich source of energy and can be converted rapidly to heat. It accounts for 5% of body weight in infants; adults have little or no brown fat. Some forms of obesity may be linked to lack of – or inability to synthesize – brown fat.

Brown-Séquard syndrome (brown say-**kar**) *n.* the neurological condition resulting when the spinal cord has been damaged. Below the lesion there is a spastic paralysis on the same side and a loss of pain and temperature sensation on the opposite side. [C. E. Brown-Séquard (1818–94), French physiologist]

Brucella (broo-**sel**-ă) *n.* a genus of Gram-negative aerobic spherical or rodlike parasitic bacteria resp[illegible] sible for brucellosis (undulant in humans and contagious abortion in cattle, pigs, sheep, and goats. The principal species are *B. abortus* and *B. melitensis*.

brucellosis (Malta fever, Mediterranean fever, undulant fever) (broo-si-**loh**-sis) *n.* a chronic disease of farm animals caused by bacteria of the genus *Brucella*, which can be transmitted to humans either by contact with an infected animal or by drinking nonpasteurized contaminated milk. Symptoms include headache, fever, aches and pains, and sickness; occasionally a chronic form develops with recurrent symptoms.

Bruch's membrane (bruuks) *n.* the transparent innermost layer of the choroid, which is in contact with the retinal pigment epithelium (*see* retina). [K. W. L. Bruch (1819–84), German anatomist]

Brudzinski sign (bruud-**zin**-ski) *n.* a sign present when there is irritation of the meninges (the membranes covering the brain); it is present in meningitis. As the neck is pulled forward, the hips and knees bend involuntarily. [J. von Brudzinski (1874–1917), Polish physician]

Brufen (broo-fĕn) *n. see* ibuprofen.

bruise (contusion) (brooz) *n.* an area of skin discoloration caused by the escape of blood from ruptured underlying vessels following injury. A bruise may be the sign of previous assault.

bruit (broot) *n.* a sharp or harsh systolic sound, heard on auscultation, that is due to turbulent blood flow in a peripheral artery, usually the carotid or iliofemoral artery. Bruits can also be heard over arteriovenous fistulae or malformations.

Brunner's glands (**brun**-erz) *pl. n.* compound glands of the small intestine, found in the duodenum and the upper part of the jejunum. They are embedded in the submucosa and secrete mucus. [J. C. Brunner (1653–1727), Swiss anatomist]

Brushfield spots (**brush**-feeld) *pl. n.* greyish-brown spots seen in the iris of the eye. They can be found in normal individuals but are usually associated with Down's syndrome. [T. Brushfield (1858–1937), British physician]

BSA *n.* body surface area.

BSE *n.* bovine spongiform encephalopathy. *See* Creutzfeldt-Jakob disease, spongiform encephalopathy.

BSER *n.* brainstem evoked response audiometry. *See* auditory brainstem response audiometry.

BSL *n. see* British Sign Language.

BSS *n.* **1.** *see* balanced salt solution. **2.** *see* Beck Scale for Suicide Ideation.

bubo (**bew**-boh) *n.* a swollen inflamed lymph node in the armpit or groin, commonly developing in soft sexually transmitted diseases (e.g. soft sore), bubonic plague, and leishmaniasis.

bubonic plague (bew-**bon**-ik) *n. see* plague.

buccal (**buk**-ăl) *adj.* relating to the mouth or the hollow part of the cheek.

buccinator (**buks**-i-nay-ter) *n.* a muscle of the cheek that has its origin in the maxilla and mandible.

It is responsible for compressing the cheek and is important in mastication.

Budd-Chiari syndrome (bud-ki-**ah**-ri) *n.* a rare condition that follows obstruction of the hepatic veins by a blood clot. It is characterized by abdominal pain, jaundice, ascites, and rapid decline in liver function. [G. Budd (1808–82), British physician; H. Chiari (1851–1916), German pathologist]

budesonide (bew-**dess**-ŏ-nyd) *n.* a corticosteroid drug used in a nasal spray to treat hay fever or as an inhalant for asthma or for asthma and chronic obstructive pulmonary disease (for which it is combined with formoterol in **Symbicort**). It is also administered by mouth or enema for the treatment of Crohn's disease and ulcerative colitis. Trade names: **Budelin Novolizer**, **Budenofalk**, **Entocort**, **Pulmicort**, **Rhinocort Aqua**.

Buerger's disease (**ber**-gerz) *n.* an inflammatory condition affecting the arteries, especially the arteries of the legs. The condition may lead to gangrene of the limbs and venous or coronary thrombosis. Medical name: **thromboangiitis obliterans**. [L. Buerger (1879–1943), US physician]

Buffalo hump (**buf**-ă-loh) *n.* excessive subcutaneous adipose tissue forming a hump on the back over the lower cervical (neck) and upper thoracic regions of the spine. It is seen classically in Cushing's syndrome but also in patients who are obese. *Compare* dowager's hump.

buffer (**buf**-er) *n.* a solution whose hydrogen ion concentration (pH) remains virtually unchanged by dilution or by the addition of acid or alkali. *See also* acid-base balance.

bulb (bulb) *n.* (in anatomy) any rounded structure or a rounded expansion at the end of an organ or part.

bulbar (**bul**-ber) *adj.* **1.** relating to or affecting the medulla oblongata. **2.** relating to a bulb. **3.** relating to the eyeball.

bulbourethral glands (bul-bo-yoor-**ee**-thrăl) *n. see* Cowper's glands.

bulimia (bew-**lim**-iă) *n.* insatiable overeating. This symptom may be psychogenic, as in anorexia nervosa (**b. nervosa** or the **binge–purge syndrome**); or it may be due to neurological causes, such as a lesion of the hypothalamus.

bulla (**buul**-ă) *n.* (*pl.* **bullae**) **1.** a large blister, containing serous fluid. **2.** (in anatomy) a rounded bony prominence. **3.** a thin-walled air-filled space within the lung, arising congenitally or in emphysema. **—bullous** *adj.*

Buller's shield (**buul**-erz) *n.* a protective shield placed over one eye when the other is infected. It consists of a watch glass fixed in position with adhesive tape. [F. Buller (1844–1905), Canadian ophthalmologist]

bullous pemphigoid (**buul**-ŭs) *n. see* pemphigoid.

bumetanide (bew-**met**-ă-nyd) *n.* a quick-acting loop diuretic used to relieve the fluid retention (oedema) occurring in heart failure, kidney disease, or cirrhosis of the liver. It is administered by mouth, injection, or infusion.

bundle (bun-d'l) *n.* a group of muscles or nerve fibres situated close together and running in the same direction.

bundle branch block (BBB) *n.* a defect in the specialized conducting tissue of the heart that is identified on an electrocardiogram.

bundle of His (hiss) *n. see* atrioventricular bundle. [W. His (1863–1934), Swiss anatomist]

bunion (bun-yŏn) *n.* an area of thickened tissue overlying the joint at the base of the big toe. It arises when a bursa develops around the joint in response to friction and pressure from ill-fitting footwear and is commonly associated with hallux valgus.

buphthalmos (hydrophthalmos) (buf-thal-mŏs) *n.* infantile or congenital glaucoma: increased pressure within the eye due to a defect in the development of the tissues through which fluid drains from the eye.

bupivacaine (bew-piv-ă-kayn) *n.* a potent local anaesthetic used for regional nerve block, including epidural anaesthesia during labour and to relieve postoperative pain. Trade name: **Marcain**.

buprenorphine (bew-prĕn-or-feen) *n.* a powerful opioid analgesic used for the relief of moderate to severe pain and to treat opioid dependence (*see* opiate). It acts for 6–8 hours and is administered by mouth, injection, or skin patches. Trade names: **BuTrans**, **Subutex**, **Temgesic**, **Transtec**.

bur (ber) *n.* **1.** a cutting instrument that fits in a dental handpiece (*see* drill). Burs are mainly used for cutting cavities in teeth, removing old restorations, and preparing teeth to receive crowns. **2. (burr)** a surgical drill for cutting through bone or other tissue. **b. hole** a circular hole drilled through the skull to release pressure inside the skull or to facilitate biopsies and other procedures.

buried bumper syndrome *n.* a condition in which feeding via a PEG tube (*see* gastrostomy) is blocked. It occurs when the internal retention disc (bumper) of the tube, which holds it in place inside the stomach, is overgrown by mucous membranes and becomes embedded in the stomach wall. This serious complication requires surgical removal of the tube.

Burkitt's lymphoma (Burkitt's tumour) (ber-kits) *n.* a malignant tumour of the lymphatic system, most commonly affecting children and largely confined to tropical Africa. It is the most rapidly growing malignancy, with a tumour doubling time of about five days. It can arise at various sites, most commonly the facial structures, such as the jaw, and in the abdomen. [D. P. Burkitt (1911–93), Irish surgeon]

burn (bern) *n.* tissue damage caused by such agents as heat, cold, chemicals, electricity, ultraviolet light, or nuclear radiation. Burns cause swelling and blistering; loss of plasma from damaged blood vessels may lead to severe shock. There is also a risk of bacterial infection. **first-degree b.** a burn affecting only the outer layer (epidermis) of the skin. **second-degree b.** a burn in which both the epidermis and the underlying dermis are damaged. **third-degree b.** a burn that involves damage or destruction of the skin to its full depth and damage to the tissues beneath.

burr (ber) *n. see* bur.

bursa (ber-să) *n.* (*pl.* **bursae**) a small sac of fibrous tissue that is lined with synovial membrane and filled with fluid. Bursae help to reduce friction; they are normally formed round joints and in places where ligaments and tendons pass over bones. —**bursal** *adj.*

bursa of Fabricius (fă-**brish**-ŭs) *n.* a mass of lymphoid tissue occurring as an outgrowth of the cloaca of young birds. It is an important source of B-lymphocytes. [H. Fabricius (1537–1619), Italian anatomist]

bursitis (bursal synovitis) (ber-**sy**-tis) *n.* inflammation of a bursa, resulting from repetitive slight injury, pressure, friction, infection, or inflammatory conditions. It produces pain and sometimes restricts joint movement. *See also* housemaid's knee.

burst abdomen (abdominal dehiscence) (berst) *n.* spontaneous opening of a surgical wound after an abdominal operation.

buserelin (bew-sĕ-**rel**-in) *n.* a gonadorelin analogue that is administered as a nasal spray or by subcutaneous injection for the treatment of endometriosis and infertility and to help in the management of advanced prostate cancer. Trade names: **Suprecur**, **Suprefact**.

buspirone (bew-**spy**-rohn) *n.* a drug used for the short-term relief of symptoms of anxiety (*see* anxiolytic).

busulfan (busulphan) (bew-**sul**-fan) *n.* an alkylating agent that destroys cancer cells by acting on the bone marrow. It is administered mainly by mouth in the treatment of chronic myeloid leukaemia. Trade name: **Myleran**.

butobarbital (butobarbitone) (bew-toh-**bar**-bi-tal) *n.* an intermediate-acting barbiturate taken by mouth for the treatment of severe insomnia.

buttock (**but**-ŏk) *n.* either of the two fleshy protuberances at the lower posterior section of the trunk, consisting of muscles (*see* gluteus) and fat. Anatomical name: **natis**.

butyrophenone (bew-ti-roh-**fee**-nohn) *n.* one of a group of chemically related antipsychotic drugs that includes haloperidol, benperidol, and droperidol.

bypass (**by**-pahs) *n.* diversion of a flow from its normal channels, usually by means of surgery. *See* anastomosis, cardiopulmonary bypass, coronary artery bypass graft, shunt.

byssinosis (bis-i-**noh**-sis) *n.* an industrial disease of the lungs caused by inhalation of dusts of cotton, flax, hemp, or sisal.

Cc

C 1. *symbol for* carbon. **2.** *symbol for* Celsius *or* centigrade.

Ca *symbol for* calcium.

cabergoline (kă-**ber**-gŏ-leen) *n.* a drug used as an adjunct to levodopa for the treatment of Parkinson's disease and to treat disorders caused by excessive secretion of prolactin. It is administered by mouth. Trade names: **Cabaser**, **Dostinex**.

CABG *n. see* coronary artery bypass graft.

cac- (caco-) *combining form denoting* disease or deformity.

cachet (**kash**-ay) *n.* a flat capsule containing a drug that has an unpleasant taste. The cachet is swallowed intact by the patient.

cachexia (kă-**keks**-iă) *n.* a condition of abnormally low weight, weakness, and general bodily decline associated with chronic disease, such as cancer.

cadaver (kă-**dav**-er) *n.* a dead body, especially one preserved and used for dissection and anatomical study.

caecosigmoidostomy (see-koh-sig-moid-**ost**-ŏmi) *n.* an operation in which the caecum is joined to the sigmoid colon.

caecostomy (see-**kost**-ŏmi) *n.* the creation of an artificial stoma that serves as a bridge between the caecum and the anterior abdominal wall. Its purpose is to facilitate lavage in patients with refractory constipation or decompress the intestine.

caecum (see-kŭm) *n.* a blind-ended pouch at the junction of the small and large intestines, to which the vermiform appendix is attached. **—caecal** *adj.*

Caesarean section (siz-**air**-iăn) *n.* a surgical operation for delivering a baby through the abdominal wall, usually by a transverse incision in the lower portion of the uterus (**lower uterine segment C. s.**). It is carried out when there are risks to the baby or to the mother from normal childbirth and may be performed, if necessary, as soon as the child is viable.

caesium-137 (seez-iŭm) *n.* an artificial radioactive isotope of the metallic element caesium, used rarely in radiotherapy. Symbol: ^{137}Cs.

CAF *n. see* common assessment framework.

café au lait spots (kaf-ay-oh-**lay**) *pl. n.* well-defined pale-brown patches on the skin. The presence of six or more in an individual is strongly suggestive of neurofibromatosis type I.

caffeine (**kaf**-een) *n.* an alkaloid drug, present in coffee and tea, that has a stimulant action on the central nervous system and is a weak diuretic. It is included in some analgesic preparations.

Caffey's disease (**kaf**-iz) *n. see* hyperostosis. [J. Caffey (1895–1966), US paediatrician]

CAGE questionnaire *n.* a screening tool for alcoholism, widely used in hospitals, primary care, and psychiatric services. The name derives from an acronym of its four questions: (1) Have you ever felt you needed to *c*ut down on your drinking? (2) Have people *a*nnoyed you by criticizing your drinking? (3) Have you ever felt *g*uilty about drinking? (4) Have you ever felt you needed a drink first thing in the morning (*e*ye-opener)? Two or more yes answers indicate a reasonably high likelihood of alcohol problems.

CAH *n. see* congenital adrenal hyperplasia.

caisson disease (**kay**-sŏn) *n. see* compressed air illness.

calamine (**kal**-ă-myn) *n.* a preparation of zinc carbonate used as a mild astringent on the skin in the form of a lotion, cream, or ointment.

calc- (calci-, calco-) *combining form denoting* calcium or calcium salts.

calcaneus (heel bone) (kal-**kay**-niŭs) *n.* the large bone in the tarsus of the foot that forms the projection of the heel behind the foot.

calcareous (kal-**kair**-iŭs) *adj.* containing calcium, especially calcium carbonate; chalky.

calciferol (kal-**sif**-er-ol) *n. see* vitamin D.

calcification (kal-si-fi-**kay**-shŏn) *n.* the deposition of calcium salts in tissue. This occurs as part of the normal process of bone formation (*see* ossification).

calcinosis (kal-si-**noh**-sis) *n.* the abnormal deposition of calcium salts in the tissues.

calcipotriol (kal-si-**pot**-ri-ol) *n.* a vitamin D analogue administered as an ointment, or scalp solution for the treatment of psoriasis. Trade name: **Dovonex**.

calcitonin (thyrocalcitonin) (kal-si-**toh**-nin) *n.* a hormone, produced by the C cells of the thyroid gland, that lowers the levels of calcium and phosphate in the blood. A recombinant form of salmon calcitonin, **salcatonin** (Miacalcic), is given by injection or nasal spray to treat malignant hypercalcaemia and Paget's disease of the bone. It is also used as a tumour marker in cases of medullary thyroid cancer. *Compare* parathyroid hormone.

calcium (**kal**-siŭm) *n.* a metallic element that is an important constituent of bones, teeth, and blood. It is also essential for many metabolic processes, including nerve function, muscle contraction, and blood clotting. The best sources are dairy products (milk and cheese). Symbol: Ca.

calcium carbonate (**kar**-bŏ-nayt) *n.* a salt of calcium that neutralizes acids and is used in many antacid preparations. It is also used as a calcium supplement and to reduce high blood levels of phosphates (which it binds) in patients with renal failure. Formula: $CaCO_3$.

calcium-channel blocker (calcium antagonist) *n.* a drug that inhibits the influx of calcium ions into cardiac and smooth-muscle cells; it therefore reduces the strength of heart-muscle contraction, reduces conduction of impulses in the heart, and causes vasodilatation. Calcium-channel blockers, which include amlodipine, diltiazem, nicardepine, nifedipine, and verapamil, are used to treat angina and high blood pressure.

calcium gluconate and lactate (gloo-kŏ-nayt, **lak**-tayt) *n.* salts of calcium that are used to treat and prevent disorders caused by calcium deficiency, such as tetany and rickets, and to prevent osteoporosis. Formulae: $(CH_2OH(CHOH)_4COO)_2Ca.H_2O$; $(CH_3CHOHCOO)_2Ca.5H_2O$.

calculosis (kal-kew-**loh**-sis) *n.* the presence of multiple calculi in the body.

calculus (**kal**-kew-lŭs) *n.* (*pl.* **calculi**) **1.** a stone: a hard pebble-like mass formed within the body, particularly in the gall bladder (*see* gallstone) or anywhere in the urinary tract. Calculi may also occur in the ducts of the salivary glands. **2.** a calcified deposit that forms on the surface of a tooth as it is covered with plaque.

Caldwell-Luc operation (kawld-wel look) *n.* an operation in which the maxillary sinus is drained through an incision above the upper canine tooth. [G. W. Caldwell (1834–1918), US otolaryngologist; H. Luc (1855–1925), French laryngologist]

Calgary Depression Scale (CDS) (**kal**-gă-ri) *n.* a structured interview tool that enables the assessment of depression in people suffering from schizophrenia.

calibrator (**kal**-i-bray-ter) *n.* **1.** an instrument used for measuring the size of a tube or opening. **2.** an instrument used for dilating a tubular part, such as the gullet.

caliectasis (hydrocalycosis) (kal-i-**ek**-tă-sis) *n.* dilatation or distension of the calyces of the kidney, mainly associated with hydronephrosis and usually demonstrated by ultrasound, intravenous urography, or computerized tomography (CT).

calliper (caliper) (**kal**-i-per) *n.* **1.** an instrument with two prongs or jaws, used for measuring diameters, particularly of the pelvis in obstetrics. **2. (calliper splint)** a surgical appliance (*see* orthosis) that is used to correct or control deformity of a joint in the leg. It consists of a metal bar that is fixed to the shoe and held to the leg by means of straps.

callosity (callus) (kă-**los**-iti) *n.* a hard thick area of skin occurring in parts of the body subject to pressure or friction, particularly the soles of the feet and palms of the hands.

callus (**kal**-ŭs) *n.* **1.** the composite mass of tissue that forms between bone ends when a fracture is healing. It initially consists of blood clot and granulation tissue, which develops into cartilage and eventually new bone, which unites the fracture. **2.** *see* callosity.

calor (**kal**-er) *n.* heat: one of the four classical signs of inflammation in a tissue. *See also* dolor, rubor, tumor.

calorie (**kal**-er-i) *n.* a unit commonly defined as the approximate amount of energy required to raise the temperature of 1 gram of water by 1°C at atmospheric pressure. One **kilocalorie** is equal to 1000 calories; this unit is used to indicate the energy value of foods. The SI unit is the joule (1 calorie = 4.1855 joules). The average adult requires 1994 kcal (women) or 2250 kcal (men) per day.

calorific (kal-er-**if**-ik) *adj.* producing heat.

calorimeter (kal-er-**im**-it-er) *n.* any apparatus used to measure the heat lost or gained during various chemical and physical changes. Calorimeters are used to determine the energy value of different foods. **—calorimetry** *n.*

calvaria (kal-**vair**-iă) *n.* the vault of the skull.

calyx (**kay**-liks) *n.* (*pl.* **calyces**) a cup-shaped part, especially any of the divisions of the pelvis of the kidney.

camphor (**kam**-fer) *n.* a crystalline aromatic substance obtained from the tree *Cinnamomum camphora*. It is used in liniments, creams, and sprays as a counterirritant and antipruritic.

Campylobacter (kam-pi-loh-**bak**-ter) *n.* a genus of motile Gram-negative bacteria that have a characteristic spiral appearance when viewed under an electron microsope. They are a common cause of food poisoning, producing headache, nausea, diarrhoea, and vomiting. **C. pylori** *see* Helicobacter.

canal (kă-**nal**) *n.* a tubular channel or passage; e.g. the alimentary canal.

canaliculitis (ka-nă-lik-yoo-**ly**-tis) *n.* inflammation of a canaliculus, especially a lacrimal canaliculus (*see* lacrimal (apparatus)).

canaliculus (ka-nă-**lik**-yoo-lŭs) *n.* (*pl.* **canaliculi**) a small channel or canal. Canaliculi occur, for example, in compact bone, linking lacunae containing bone cells; in the liver, transporting bile to the bile duct; and as part of the lacrimal apparatus of the eye.

cancellous (**kan**-si-lŭs) *adj.* lattice-like. **c. bone** spongy porous bone tissue, which forms the interior of a bone and has a lower density than the surrounding cortical bone.

cancer (**kan**-ser) *n.* any malignant tumour, including carcinoma and sarcoma. It arises from the abnormal and uncontrolled division of cells that then invade and destroy the surrounding tissues. The cancer cells spread (*see* metastasis), setting up secondary tumours (metastases) at sites distant from the original tumour. There are probably many causative factors, some of which are known; for example, cigarette smoking is associated with lung cancer, radiation with some sarcomas and leukaemia, and several viruses are implicated; genetic factors are involved in the development of many cancers. Treatment of cancer depends on the type of tumour, the site of the primary tumour, and the extent of spread.

SEE WEB LINKS

• Website of Cancer Research UK

cancer phobia *n.* a disorder in which minor symptoms are interpreted as signs of cancer and panic attacks may occur. *See also* phobia.

candesartan (kan-**dess**-ar-tan) *n. see* angiotensin II antagonist.

Candida (**kan**-di-dă) *n.* a genus of yeasts (formerly called *Monilia*) that inhabit the vagina and alimentary tract. **C. albicans** a small oval budding species primarily responsible for candidiasis. **—candidal** *adj.*

candidiasis (candidosis) (kan-di-**dy**-ă-sis) *n.* a common yeast infection of moist areas of the body, usually caused by *Candida albicans*. It is common in the vagina, where it is known as **thrush**, but is also found in the mouth and skin folds. On the skin the lesions are bright red with small satellite pustules, while in the mouth candidiasis appears as white patches on the tongue or inside the cheeks. In the vagina it produces itching and sometimes a thick white discharge. Topical, intravaginal, or oral therapy with imidazoles is effective; nystatin, administered by mouth, helps to reduce candidal infection of the bowel.

canine (**kay**-nyn) *n.* the third tooth from the midline of each jaw. There are thus four canines, two in each jaw. It is known colloquially as the **eye tooth**.

cannabis (**kan**-ă-bis) *n.* a drug prepared from the Indian hemp plant (*Cannabis sativa*), also known as **pot**, **marijuana**, **hashish**, and **bhang**. It produces euphoria and altered perceptions. Cannabis extract (Sativex) is licensed for treating spasticity in patients with multiple sclerosis. The nonmedical use of cannabis is illegal. *See also* dependence.

cannula (**kan**-yoo-lă) *n.* a hollow tube designed for insertion into a body cavity. The tube contains a sharp pointed solid core (**trocar**), which facilitates its insertion and is withdrawn when the cannula is in place.

cantholysis (kan-**thol**-i-sis) *n.* a surgical procedure to divide the attachment of the canthus (corner of the eye) from its underlying bone and tendon. It is performed as part of some eye operations.

canthoplasty (**kan**-thoh-plasti) *n.* a surgical procedure to reconstruct the canthus.

canthus (**kan**-thŭs) *n.* either corner of the eye; the angle at which the upper and lower eyelids meet. **—canthal** *adj.*

cap (kap) *n.* **1.** a covering or a cover-like part. **2.** (in contraception) *see* diaphragm.

CAP *see* community-acquired pneumonia.

capacity (mental capacity) (kă-**pas**-iti) *n.* the ability to learn or retain knowledge and to make a decision about an issue; specifically, to consent to or refuse treatment. For a person to have capacity for a decision, he or she must be able to understand information, make choices, and communicate the decision to others. The patient must understand the nature, purpose, and possible consequences of having and not having treatment. The term competence is often used as a synonym, but since the Mental Capacity Act 2005 came into force, capacity has been the preferred term. *Compare* incompetence.

CAPD *n.* **1.** chronic (or continuous) ambulatory peritoneal dialysis: a method of treating renal failure on an out-patient basis. *See* (peritoneal) dialysis. **2.** *see* (central) auditory processing disorder.

CAPE *n.* *see* Clifton Assessment Procedures for the Elderly.

capecitabine (kap-i-**sit**-ă-been) *n.* a drug that is used in treatment of cancers of the rectum, colon, stomach, or breast that have spread to other sites (*see* cytotoxic drug). It is taken by mouth. Trade name: **Xeloda**.

capillary (kă-**pil**-er-i) *n.* an extremely narrow blood vessel. Capillaries form networks in most tissues; they are supplied with blood by arterioles and drained by venules. The vessel wall is only one cell thick, which enables exchange of oxygen, carbon dioxide, water, salts, etc., between the blood and the tissues.

capillary refill time *n.* a quickly performed test to assess the adequacy of circulation in an individual with poor cardiac output. An area of skin is pressed firmly by (say) a fingertip until it loses its colour; the number of seconds for the area to return to its normal colour indicates capillary refill time. Normal capillary refill takes around 2 seconds.

capitate (**kap**-i-tayt) *adj.* head-shaped; having a rounded extremity. **c. bone** the largest bone of the wrist (*see* carpus). It articulates with the scaphoid and lunate bones behind, with the second, third, and fourth metacarpal bones in front, and with the trapezoid and hamate laterally.

capitellum (kap-i-**tel**-ŭm) *n.* *see* capitulum.

capitulum (kă-**pit**-yoo-lŭm) *n.* the small rounded end of a bone that articulates with another bone. **c. humeri** (or **capitellum**) the round prominence at the elbow end of the humerus that articulates with the radius.

capreomycin (kap-ri-oh-**my**-sin) *n.* an antibiotic drug, derived from the bacterium *Streptomyces capreolus*, that is administered by intramuscular injection in the treatment of tuberculosis.

capsule (**kaps**-yool) *n.* **1.** a membrane, sheath, or other structure that encloses a tissue or organ. **joint c.** the fibrous tissue, including the synovial membrane, that surrounds a freely movable joint. **2.** a soluble case, usually made of gelatin, in which certain drugs are administered. **3.** the slimy substance that forms a protective layer around certain bacteria.

capsulitis (kaps-yoo-**ly**-tis) *n.* inflammation of a joint capsule. **adhesive c.** *see* frozen shoulder.

capsulorrhexis (kaps-yoo-loh-**rek**-sis) *n.* a surgical procedure in which a continuous tear is made in the lens capsule of the eye. **anterior c.** a tear made in the anterior surface of the lens capsule during cataract surgery, which makes the residual capsule much more resilient to being torn during surgery.

capsulotomy (kaps-yoo-**lot**-ŏmi) *n.* an incision into the capsule of the lens. **posterior c.** an incision into the posterior capsule using a YAG laser, to provide a path for light rays to reach the retina.

captopril (**kap**-tŏ-pril) *n.* a drug used in the treatment of heart failure, hypertension, and diabetic nephropathy; it acts by inhibiting the action of angiotensin (*see* ACE inhibitor). Trade name: **Capoten**.

caput succedaneum (**kap**-ŭt suk-si-**day**-niŭm) *n.* a temporary swelling of the soft parts of the head of a newly born infant that occurs during labour, due to compression by the muscles of the cervix (neck) of the uterus, and resolves after delivery.

carbamazepine (kar-bă-**maz**-ĕ-peen) *n.* an anticonvulsant drug used in the treatment of epileptic tonic–clonic seizures, the prophylaxis of bipolar affective disorder, and to relieve the pain of trigeminal neuralgia. It is given by mouth or as rectal suppositories. Trade names: **Carbagen SR**, **Tegretol**, **Tegretol Prolonged Release**.

carbidopa (**kar**-bi-doh-pă) *n. see* levodopa.

carbimazole (kar-**bim**-ă-zohl) *n.* a drug administered by mouth to reduce the production of thyroid hormone in cases of overactivity of the gland (thyrotoxicosis).

carbohydrate (kar-boh-**hy**-drayt) *n.* any one of a large group of compounds, including the sugars and starch, that contain carbon, hydrogen, and oxygen and have the general formula $C_x(H_2O)_y$. Carbohydrates are important as a source of energy: they are manufactured by plants and obtained by animals and humans from the diet, being one of the three main constituents of food. *See also* disaccharide, monosaccharide, polysaccharide.

carbol fuchsin (**kar**-bol **fuuk**-sin) *n.* a red stain for bacteria and fungi, consisting of carbolic acid and fuchsin dissolved in alcohol and water.

carbolic acid (kar-**bol**-ik) *n. see* phenol.

carbon dioxide (**kar**-bŏn dy-**ok**-syd) *n.* a colourless gas formed in the tissues during metabolism and carried in the blood to the lungs, where it is exhaled (an increase in the concentration of this gas in the blood stimulates respiration). It forms a solid (dry ice) at –75°C (at atmospheric pressure) and in this form is used as a refrigerant. Formula: CO_2.

carbonic anhydrase (kar-**bon**-ik an-**hy**-drayz) *n.* an enzyme that catalyses the breakdown of carbonic acid into carbon dioxide and water or the combination of carbon dioxide and water to form carbonic acid. It therefore facilitates the transport of carbon dioxide from the tissues to the lungs.

carbonic anhydrase inhibitor *n.* a drug that blocks the action of carbonic anhydrase, which is present in high concentrations in the eye, kidneys, stomach lining, and pancreas. Carbonic anhydrase inhibitors reduce the production of aqueous humour in the eye and are used mainly in treating glaucoma. *See* acetazolamide, brinzolamide, dorzolamide.

carbon monoxide (mŏn-**ok**-syd) *n.* a colourless almost odourless gas that is very poisonous. When breathed in it combines with haemoglobin in the red blood cells (*see* carboxyhaemoglobin). Carbon monoxide is present in coal gas and motor exhaust fumes. Formula: CO.

carbon tetrachloride (tet-ră-**klor**-ryd) *n.* a pungent volatile fluid used as a dry-cleaner. When inhaled or swallowed it may severely damage the heart, liver, and kidneys. Treatment is by administration of oxygen. Formula: CCl_4.

carboplatin (kar-boh-**plat**-in) *n.* a derivative of platinum that is used in the treatment of advanced ovarian and lung cancers. Given intravenously, it is similar to cisplatin but causes less nausea and kidney damage and more myelosuppression. Trade name: **Paraplatin**.

carboxyhaemoglobin (kar-boks-i-heem-ŏ-**gloh**-bin) *n.* a substance formed when carbon monoxide combines with the pigment haemoglobin in the blood. Carboxyhaemoglobin is incapable of transporting oxygen to the tissues and this is the cause of death in carbon monoxide poisoning.

carboxyhaemoglobinaemia (kar-boks-i-heem-ŏ-gloh-bi-**nee**-miă) *n.* the presence of carboxyhaemoglobin in the blood.

carbuncle (**kar**-bung-kŭl) *n.* a collection of boils with multiple drainage channels. The infection is usually caused by *Staphylococcus aureus* and may result in an extensive slough of skin.

carcin- (carcino-) *combining form denoting* cancer or carcinoma.

carcinogen (kar-**sin**-ŏ-jin) *n.* any substance that, when exposed to living tissue, may cause the production of cancer. **—carcinogenic** (kar-sin-ŏ-**jen**-ik) *adj.*

carcinogenesis (kar-sin-oh-**jen**-ĕ-sis) *n.* the evolution of an invasive cancer cell from a normal cell, a process resulting from successive genetic mutations caused by carcinogens.

carcinoid (argentaffinoma) (**kar**-sin-oid) *n.* a tumour of the argentaffin cells in the glands of the intestine (*see* apudoma). Carcinoids typically occur in the tip of the appendix and are among the commonest tumours of the small intestine. **c. syndrome** the combination of flushing, headache, diarrhoea, and bronchial constriction that occurs when a carcinoid has spread to the liver and is caused by the peptides it releases.

carcinoma (kar-sin-**oh**-mă) *n.* cancer that arises in epithelium, the tissue that lines the skin and internal organs of the body. It may occur in any tissue containing epithelial cells. Organs may exhibit more than one type of carcinoma; for example, an adenocarcinoma and a squamous carcinoma may be found in the cervix (but not usually concurrently). **—carcinomatous** *adj.*

carcinoma in situ (CIS) *n.* the earliest stage of cancer spread, in which the tumour is confined to the epithelium and surgical removal of the growth should lead to cure. ductal c. i. s. (DCIS) the earliest stage of breast cancer, which is confined to the lactiferous (milk) ducts. *See also* cervical (cancer), CIN (cervical intraepithelial neoplasia).

carcinomatosis (kar-sin-oh-mă-**toh**-sis) *n.* carcinoma that has spread widely throughout the body.

carcinosarcoma (kar-sin-oh-sar-**koh**-mă) *n.* a malignant tumour of the cervix, uterus, or vagina containing a mixture of adenocarcinoma and cells with a sarcoma appearance.

cardi- (cardio-) *combining form denoting* the heart.

cardia (**kar**-diă) *n.* **1.** the opening at the upper end of the stomach that connects with the oesophagus (gullet). **2.** the heart.

cardiac (**kar**-di-ak) *adj.* **1.** of, relating to, or affecting the heart. **2.** of or relating to the upper part of the stomach (*see* cardia).

cardiac arrest *n.* the cessation of effective pumping action of the heart, which may be because the heart stops beating altogether (asystole), because there is normal electrical activity without mechanical pumping activity (pulseless electrical activity), or because there is rapid, chaotic, electrical and mechanical activity (ventricular fibrillation). There is abrupt loss of consciousness, absence of the pulse, and breathing stops. Unless treated promptly, irreversible brain damage and death follow within minutes. Some patients may be resuscitated by massage of the heart, artificial ventilation, and defibrillation.

cardiac-arrest team *n.* a designated team of doctors in a hospital who attend cardiac arrests as they occur and administer treatment according to the latest guidelines. *See also* medical emergency team.

cardiac cycle *n.* the sequence of events between one heartbeat and the next, normally occupying less than a second. *See* diastole, systole.

cardiac index *n.* the volume of blood pumped from the left ventricle divided by body surface area, expressed as litres per minute per square metre ($l/min/m^2$). It is determined by heart rate and stroke volume index (the volume of blood pumped by the heart with each beat), and provides a normal range (2.5–4.0 $l/min/m^2$) regardless of the size of the patient.

cardiac muscle *n.* the specialized muscle of which the walls of the heart are composed. It consists of a network of branching elongated cells (fibres).

cardiac output *n.* the amount of blood ejected by the heart in a minute, measured with a pulmonary artery catheter. The range is 4.0–8.0 l/min.

cardiac reflex *n.* reflex control of the heart rate.

cardiac rehabilitation *n.* a programme of staged exercises and lifestyle classes designed for people recovering from a heart attack and run through the local hospital by dedicated health-care professionals, who may include specialist nurses, occupational therapists, and physiotherapists.

cardiac tamponade *n. see* tamponade.

cardinal ligaments (Mackenrodt's ligaments) (kar-din-ăl) *pl. n.* fan-shaped sheets of fascia that extend from the vagina and the cervix of the uterus to the walls of the pelvis.

cardiogenic shock (kar-di-oh-**jen**-ik) *n.* peripheral circulatory failure resulting from an extreme form of heart failure, most commonly caused by myocardial infarction. Features include cool extremities, oliguria, hypotension, and poor cardiac output and cerebral function.

cardiology (kar-di-**ol**-ŏji) *n.* the science concerned with the study of the structure, function, and diseases of the heart. **nuclear c.** the study and diagnosis of heart disease by the intravenous injection of a radionuclide, which emits gamma rays, enabling a gamma camera and computer to form an image of the heart. **—cardiologist** *n.*

cardiomyopathy (kar-di-oh-my-**op**-ă-thi) *n.* any chronic disorder affecting the muscle of the heart. **hypertrophic c.** a familial condition characterized by thickening of the left ventricle. The most severely affected patients may suffer chest pain, arrhythmia causing a fast heart rate, heart failure, and sudden death. **hypertrophic obstructive c.** hypertrophic cardiomyopathy in which thickening of the muscle around the left ventricular outflow tract restricts blood flow to the body.

cardiomyotomy (Heller's operation) (kar-di-oh-my-**ot**-ŏmi) *n.* surgical splitting of the muscular ring at the junction of the stomach and oesophagus to relieve achalasia.

cardiopathy (kar-di-**op**-ă-thi) *n.* any disease of the heart. **—cardiopathic** (kar-di-oh-**path**-ik) *adj.*

cardioplegia (kar-di-oh-**plee**-jiă) *n.* a technique in which the heart is stopped by injecting it with a solution of salts, by hypothermia, or by an electrical stimulus. This has enabled complex cardiac surgery and transplants to be performed safely.

cardiopulmonary bypass (kar-di-oh-**pul**-mŏn-er-i) *n.* a method by which the circulation to the body is maintained while the heart is deliberately stopped during heart surgery. The function of the heart and lungs is carried out by a pump-oxygenator (heart-lung machine) until the natural circulation is restored.

cardiopulmonary resuscitation (CPR) *n.* an emergency procedure for life support, consisting of artificial respiration and manual external cardiac massage. It is used in cases of cardiac arrest or apparent sudden death resulting from electric shock, drowning, respiratory arrest, or other causes, to establish effective circulation and ventilation in order to prevent irreversible brain damage.

cardiotocograph (kar-di-oh-**tok**-oh-graf) *n.* the instrument used in cardiotocography to produce a **cardiotocogram**, the graphic printout of the measurements obtained.

cardiotocography (kar-di-oh-tŏ-**kog**-răfi) *n.* the electronic monitoring of the fetal heart rate (detected by means of an external transducer or a fetal scalp electrode) and the frequency of uterine contractions (using a second transducer).

cardiotomy syndrome (postcardiotomy syndrome) (kar-di-**ot**-ŏmi) *n.* a condition that may develop after heart surgery and is characterized by fever and pericarditis. Pneumonia and pleurisy may form part of the syndrome.

cardiovascular system (circulatory system) (kar-di-oh-**vas**-kew-ler) *n.* the heart together with two networks of blood vessels – the systemic circulation and the pulmonary circulation. The cardiovascular system effects the circulation of blood around the body, which brings about transport of nutrients and oxygen to the tissues and the removal of waste products.

cardioversion (countershock) (**kar**-di-oh-ver-shŏn) *n.* restoration of normal heart rhythm in patients with increased heart rate caused by arrhythmia. It involves the application of a controlled shock through electrodes placed on the chest wall of the anaesthetized patient. The apparatus is called a **cardiovertor**.

care assistant (kair) *n.* a person who helps with the general care of a patient, usually assisting a nurse or social worker with care of the vulnerable elderly in the community.

Caregiver Strain Index (CSI) (**kair**-giv-er) *n.* an assessment tool used by nurses (predominantly mental health nurses) to assess stress in caregivers.

care pathway *n.* *see* integrated care pathway.

care plan *n.* *see* planning.

Care Quality Commission (CQC) *n.* a publicly funded independent organization established in 2009 and responsible for regulation of health and social care in England; it replaced the **Healthcare Commission**, the **Commission for Social Care Inspection**, and the **Mental Health Act Commission**. Its responsibilities include publication of national health-care standards; annual assessment of the performance of NHS and social-care organizations; reviewing other (i.e. private and voluntary) health and social-care organizations; reviewing complaints about the services when it has not been possible to resolve them locally; and investigating serious service failures.

caries (**kair**-eez) *n.* decay and crumbling of the substance of a bone. **dental c.** tooth decay, caused by the metabolism of the bacteria in plaque attached to the surface of the tooth. Acid formed by bacterial breakdown of sugar in the diet gradually etches and decomposes the enamel of the tooth; if left unrepaired, it spreads in and progressively destroys the tooth completely. **—carious** *adj.*

carina (kă-**ree**-nă) *n.* a keel-like structure, such as the keel-shaped cartilage at the bifurcation of the trachea into the two main bronchi.

cariogenic (kair-i-oh-**jen**-ik) *adj.* causing caries, particularly dental caries.

carminative (kar-min-ă-tiv) *n.* a drug that relieves flatulence, used to treat gastric discomfort and colic.

carmustine (kar-**mus**-teen) *n.* an alkylating agent administered intravenously or as implants in the treatment of myeloma, non-Hodgkin's lymphomas, and some brain tumours. Trade name: **Gliadel**.

carneous mole (**kar**-niŭs) *n.* a fleshy mass in the uterus consisting of pieces of placenta and products of conception that have not been expelled after miscarriage or abortion.

Caroli's disease (ka-rŏ-leez) *n.* an inherited condition in which the bile ducts, which drain the liver, are widened, causing an increased risk of infection or cancer in the gall bladder. *Compare* Caroli's syndrome. [J. Caroli (20th century), French physician]

Caroli's syndrome *n.* an inherited condition in which the bile ducts, which drain the liver, are widened and there are fibrous changes in the liver and cysts within the kidneys. *Compare* Caroli's disease. [J. Caroli]

carotenaemia (ka-rŏ-ti-**nee**-miă) *n. see* xanthaemia.

carotene (**ka**-rŏ-teen) *n.* a yellow, orange, red, or brown plant pigment; one of the carotenoids. The most important form, β-carotene, is an antioxidant and can be converted in the body to retinol (vitamin A).

carotenoid (kă-**rot**-in-oid) *n.* any one of a group of about 100 naturally occurring yellow to red pigments found mostly in plants.

carotid artery (kă-**rot**-id) *n.* either of the two main arteries in the neck (**right** or **left common c. a.**) whose branches supply the head and neck. See illustration.

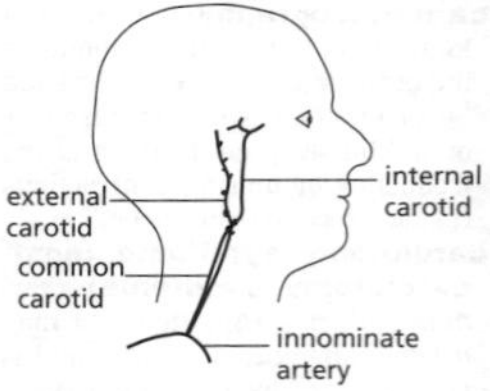

The origin and main branches of the right common carotid artery

carotid-artery stenosis (carotid stenosis) *n.* narrowing of the carotid artery, which reduces the supply of blood to the brain and is a cause of strokes. It is treated by surgical excision or bypass of the narrowed segment, or by inserting a stent into the carotid artery.

carotid body *n.* a small mass of tissue in the carotid sinus containing chemoreceptors that monitor levels of oxygen, carbon dioxide, and hydrogen ions in the blood.

carotid sinus *n.* a pocket in the wall of the carotid artery, at its division in the neck, containing receptors that monitor blood pressure (baroreceptors).

carp- (carpo-) *combining form denoting* the wrist (carpus).

carpal (**kar**-păl) **1.** *adj.* relating to the wrist. **2.** *n.* any of the bones forming the carpus.

carpal tunnel syndrome *n.* tingling, numbness, and pain in the hand affecting the thumb, index, and middle fingers and sometimes extending to the fourth finger; there may be weakness of grip due to wasting of the thenar eminence of the thumb. It is caused by pressure on the median nerve as it passes through the wrist, which may result from any continuous repetitive movements of the hand, such as keyboarding, or any condition causing local swelling.

carphology (kar-**fol**-ŏji) *n. see* floccillation.

carpopedal spasm (kar-poh-**pee**-d'l) *n. see* spasm.

carpus (**kar**-pŭs) *n.* the eight bones of the wrist (see illustration). The carpus articulates with the metacarpals distally and with the ulna and radius proximally.

carrier (**ka**-ri-er) *n.* **1.** a person who harbours the microorganisms causing a particular disease without experiencing signs or symptoms of infection and who can transmit the disease to others. **2.** (in genetics) a person who bears a gene for an abnormal trait without showing signs of the disorder. **3.** an animal, usually an insect, that passively transmits infectious organisms from one animal to another or from an animal to a human being. *See also* vector.

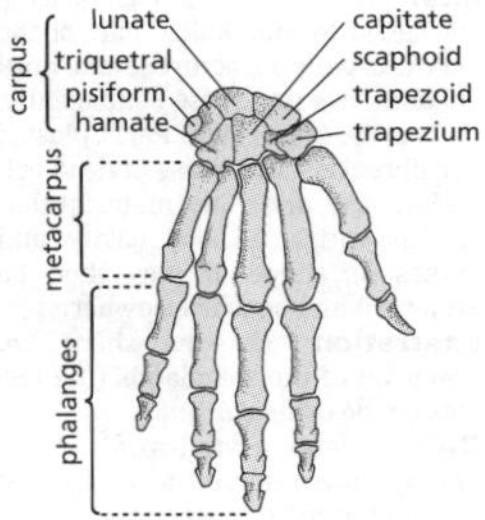

Bones of the left wrist and hand

carteolol (kar-**tee**-ŏ-lol) *n.* a beta blocker used as eye drops in the treatment of glaucoma. Trade name: **Teoptic**.

cartilage (**kar**-til-ij) *n.* a dense connective tissue, consisting chiefly of chondroitin sulphate, that is capable of withstanding considerable pressure. In the fetus and infant cartilage occurs in many parts of the body, but most of this cartilage disappears during development. Cartilage is the precursor of bone following a fracture (*see* callus). **elastic c.** cartilage occurring in the external ear. **fibrocartilage** cartilage occurring in the intervertebral discs and tendons. **hyaline c.** cartilage found in the costal cartilages, larynx, trachea, bronchi, nose, and covering the surface of the bones at joints. See illustration.

caruncle (**ka**-rŭng-kŭl) *n.* a small red fleshy swelling. **hymenal c.** a caruncle occurring around the mucous membrane lining the vaginal opening. **lacrimal c.** the red prominence at the inner angle of the eye.

cascara (cascara sagrada) (kas-**kar**-ă) *n.* the dried bark of an

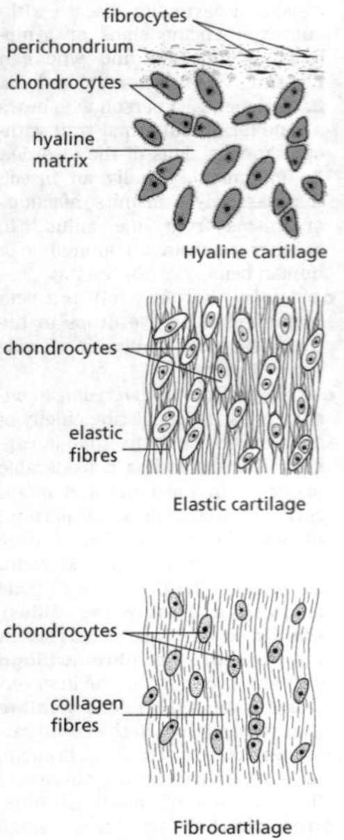

Types of cartilage

American buckthorn, *Rhamnus purshiana*, used as a laxative.

caseation (kay-si-ay-shŏn) *n.* the breakdown of diseased tissue into a dry cheeselike mass: a type of necrosis associated with tubercular lesions.

casein (kay-si-in) *n.* a milk protein. Casein is precipitated out of milk in acid conditions or by the action of rennin. It is very easily prepared and is useful as a protein supplement, particularly in the treatment of malnutrition.

caseinogen (kay-si-in-ŏ-jin) *n.* a protein, present in milk, that is converted into casein by the action of rennin.

Casey's model (kay-siz) *n.* a model of family-centred care for paediatric nursing in which the care of children (well or sick) is regarded as best carried out by their families, with varying degrees of assistance from members of a suitably qualified health-care team as necessary. *See also* nursing models. [A. Casey (1951–), British nurse theorist]

cast (kahst) *n.* **1.** a rigid casing designed to immobilize part of the body, usually a fractured limb, until healing has progressed sufficiently. It is made of plaster of Paris, plastic, or fibreglass. **2.** a mass of dead cellular, fatty, and other material that forms within a body cavity and takes its shape. It may then be released and appear elsewhere.

castration (kas-tray-shŏn) *n.* removal of the sex glands (the testes or the ovaries).

CAT *n.* computerized axial tomography, now referred to as CT (*see* computerized tomography).

cata- *prefix denoting* downward or against.

catabolism (kă-tab-ŏl-izm) *n.* the chemical decomposition of complex substances by the body to form simpler ones, accompanied by the release of energy. *See also* metabolism. —**catabolic** (kat-ă-**bol**-ik) *adj.*

catagen (**kat**-ă-jĕn) *n. see* anagen.

catalase (**kat**-ă-layz) *n.* an enzyme, present in many cells (including red blood cells and liver cells), that catalyses the breakdown of hydrogen peroxide.

catalepsy (**kat**-ă-lep-si) *n.* the abnormal maintenance of postures occurring in catatonia.

catalyst (**kat**-ă-list) *n.* a substance that alters the rate of a chemical reaction but is itself unchanged at the end of the reaction. The catalysts of biochemical reactions are the enzymes.

cataphoresis (kat-ă-fŏ-**ree**-sis) *n.* the introduction into the tissues of positively charged ionized substances (cations) by the use of a direct electric current. *See* iontophoresis.

cataplexy (**kat**-ă-pleks-i) *n.* a sudden onset of muscle weakness that may be precipitated by excitement or emotion. There may be total loss of muscle tone, resulting in collapse, or simply jaw dropping or head nodding. It occurs in 60–90% of patients with narcolepsy.

cataract (**kat**-ă-rakt) *n.* an opacity in the lens of the eye that may result in blurred vision. Cataracts most commonly occur as a result of ageing (**senile c.**), but some are congenital or result from metabolic disease (such as diabetes) or from injury to the lens or exposure of the eye to harmful radiation.

cataract extraction *n.* surgical removal of a cataract from the eye. **extracapsular c. e.** removal of the cataract alone, leaving the lens capsule behind. **intracapsular c. e.** removal of the whole lens, including the capsule that surrounds it.

catarrh (kă-**tar**) *n.* the excessive secretion of thick phlegm or mucus by the mucous membrane of the nose, nasal sinuses, nasopharynx, or air passages.

catatonia (kat-ă-**toh**-niă) *n.* a state in which a person becomes mute or stuporous or adopts bizarre postures (*see also* flexibilitas cerea). Catatonia was once a noted feature of schizophrenia but is now hardly ever seen in developed countries. It remains common in developing countries. —**catatonic** *adj.*

CATCH-22 *n.* *C*ardiac abnormalities, *A*bnormal facies, *T*-cell deficiency (from absent thymus), *C*left palate, *H*ypocalcaemia, chromosome *22* (in which the defect lies): another name for di George syndrome.

catchment area (**kach**-mĕnt) *n.* the geographic area from which a hospital can expect to receive patients and on which (in Britain) the designated population of the hospital is based.

catecholamines (kat-ĕ-**kol**-ă-meenz) *pl. n.* a group of physiologically important substances, including adrenaline, noradrenaline, and dopamine, with different roles (mainly as neurotransmitters) in the functioning of the sympathetic and central nervous systems.

categorical data (kat-ĕ-gor-i-kăl) *pl. n.* data that are assigned to categories, such as gender (i.e. male or female), socioeconomic groups, or illness types.

catgut (**kat**-gut) *n.* a natural fibrous material prepared from the tissues of animals, usually from sheep intestines, formerly widely used to sew up wounds and tie off blood vessels during surgery. The catgut gradually dissolves and is absorbed by the tissues, so that the stitches do not have to be removed later.

catharsis (kă-**thar**-sis) *n.* **1.** purging or cleansing out of the bowels by giving the patient a laxative (cathartic) to stimulate intestinal activity. **2.** the release of strong pent-up emotions. *See* abreaction.

cathartic (kă-**thar**-tik) *n. see* laxative.

catheter (**kath**-it-er) *n.* a flexible tube for insertion into a narrow opening so that fluids may be introduced or removed. **suprapubic c.** a catheter passed through the abdominal wall above the pubis into the bladder, usually when this is very enlarged to relieve urinary retention. **urinary c.** a catheter passed into the bladder through the urethra to allow drainage of urine in certain disorders and to empty the bladder before abdominal operations.

catheterization (kath-it-er-I-**zay**-shŏn) *n.* the introduction of a catheter into a hollow organ. **cardiac c.** the introduction of special catheters into the chambers of the heart, usually via the arteries and veins of the arms or legs. It allows the measurement of pressures in the chambers and pressure gradients across the valves and the introduction of contrast medium for visualization of structures using X-rays (*see* coronary angiography). **urethral c.** the introduction of a catheter into the bladder in order to relieve obstruction to the outflow of urine (*see also* intermittent self-catheterization). **vascular c.** the introduction, via catheters, into the arteries or veins of contrast medium for radiography, drugs to constrict or expand vessels or to dissolve a thrombus, metal coils or other solid materials to block bleeding vessels or to thrombose aneurysms (*see* embolization), devices for monitoring pressures within important vessels, or balloons and stents to relieve obstruction.

cation (**kat**-I-ŏn) *n.* a positively charged ion, which moves towards the cathode (negative electrode) when an electric current is passed through the solution containing it. *Compare* anion.

CATS *n.* Credit Accumulation Transfer Scheme: a system in educational establishments in which credit ratings are awarded at various levels of achievement (certificate, diploma, and first-degree level). *See also* APEL.

cat-scratch disease (**kat**-skrach) *n.* an infectious disease caused by the bacterium *Bartonella henselae*, which infects cats and is transmitted to humans by a cat scratch or bite. Swelling of the lymph nodes (usually those closest to the wound) develops a week to two months after infection.

cauda (kaw-dă) *n.* a tail-like structure. **c. equina** a bundle of nerve roots from the lumbar, sacral, and coccygeal spinal nerves that descend from the spinal cord to their respective openings in the vertebral column.

caudal (kaw-d'l) *adj.* relating to the lower part or tail end of the body.

caul (kawl) *n.* **1.** (in obstetrics) the amnion, a piece of which may cover an infant's head at birth. **2.** (in anatomy) *see* omentum.

causal agent (kaw-zăl) *n.* a factor associated with the definitive onset of an illness (or other response, including an accident). Examples of causal agents are bacteria, trauma, and noxious agents.

causalgia (kaw-zal-jiă) *n.* an intensely unpleasant burning pain felt in a limb where there has been partial damage to the sympathetic and somatic sensory nerves.

caustic (kaw-stik) *n.* an agent, such as silver nitrate, that destroys tissue. Caustic agents may be used to remove dead skin, warts, etc.

cauterize (kaw-tĕ-ryz) *vb.* to destroy tissues by direct application of a heated instrument (known as a **cautery**): used for the removal of small warts or other growths and also to stop bleeding from small vessels. **—cautery** *n.*

cavernosography (kav-er-noh-sog-răfi) *n.* a radiological examination of the erectile tissue of the penis that entails the infusion of radiopaque contrast material into the corpora cavernosa via a small butterfly needle. Radiographs taken during the infusion give information regarding any abnormality of the veins draining the penis. It is chiefly used in the evaluation of erectile dysfunction.

cavernosometry (kav-er-noh-som-itri) *n.* the measurement of pressure within the corpora cavernosa of the penis during infusion. The flow rate required to produce an erection is recorded and also the flow necessary to maintain the induced erection. The examination is important in the investigation of erectile dysfunction.

cavernous breath sounds (amphoric breath sounds) (kav-er-nŭs) *pl. n.* hollow breath sounds heard over cavities in the lung.

cavernous sinus *n.* one of the paired cavities within the sphenoid bone, at the base of the skull behind the eye sockets, into which blood drains from the brain, eye, nose, and upper cheek before leaving the skull through connections with the internal jugular and facial veins.

cavity (kav-iti) *n.* **1.** (in anatomy) a hollow enclosed area; for example, the abdominal cavity or the buccal cavity (mouth). **2.** (in dentistry) the hole in a tooth caused by caries or abrasion or formed by a dentist to retain a filling.

CBF *n.* cerebral blood flow.

CBT *n. see* cognitive behavioural therapy.

C cells *pl. n.* parafollicular cells of the thyroid gland, which produce calcitonin.

CCF *n.* congestive cardiac failure. *See* heart failure.

CCU *n.* *see* coronary care (unit).

CD *n.* controlled drug. *See* Misuse of Drugs Act 1971.

CD4 *n.* a surface antigen on helper T cells that is particularly important for immune resistance to viruses. It is also a receptor for HIV; progressive reduction of CD4-bearing T cells reflects the progression of AIDS.

CDH *n.* **1.** congenital diaphragmatic hernia. **2.** *see* congenital dislocation of the hip.

C. diff. *n. Clostridium difficile. See* Clostridium.

CDS *n.* *see* Calgary Depression Scale.

cefaclor (sef-ă-klor) *n.* *see* cephalosporin.

cefadroxil (sef-ă-**droks**-il) *n.* *see* cephalosporin.

cefalexin (sef-ă-**leks**-in) *n.* *see* cephalosporin.

ceftazidime (sef-taz-i-deem) *n.* *see* cephalosporin.

cefuroxime (sef-yoor-**oks**-eem) *n.* *see* cephalosporin.

-cele (-coele) *combining form denoting* swelling, hernia, or tumour.

celecoxib (sel-i-**koks**-ib) *n.* an anti-inflammatory drug (*see* COX-2 inhibitor) that is taken by mouth in the treatment of osteoarthritis, rheumatoid arthritis, and ankylosing spondylitis. Trade name: **Celebrex**.

cell (sel) *n.* the basic unit of all living organisms, which can reproduce itself exactly (*see* mitosis). Cells contain cytoplasm, in which are suspended a nucleus and other structures (organelles) specialized to carry out particular activities in the cell. Complex organisms are built up of millions of cells that are specially adapted to carry out particular functions. See illustration.

cell division *n.* reproduction of cells by division first of the chromosomes (karyokinesis) and then of the cytoplasm (cytokinesis). Cell division to produce more body (somatic) cells is by mitosis; cell division during the formation of gametes is by meiosis.

cellulitis (sel-yoo-ly-tis) *n.* an infection of the deep layers of the skin and subcutaneous tissue by staphylococci, streptococci, or other bacteria. It is most common on the lower legs and there may be associated lymphangitis and lymphadenitis. It is otherwise similar to erysipelas, but the margins are less clearly defined because the infection is deeper.

cellulose (sel-yoo-lohz) *n.* a carbohydrate consisting of linked glucose units. It is an important constituent of plant cell walls. Cellulose cannot be digested by humans and is a component of dietary fibre (roughage).

Celsius temperature (centigrade temperature) (sel-si-ŭs) *n.* temperature expressed on a scale in which the melting point of ice is assigned a temperature of 0° and the boiling point of water a temperature of 100°. The formula for converting from Celsius (C) to Fahrenheit (F) is: $F = 9/5C + 32$. *See also* Fahrenheit temperature.

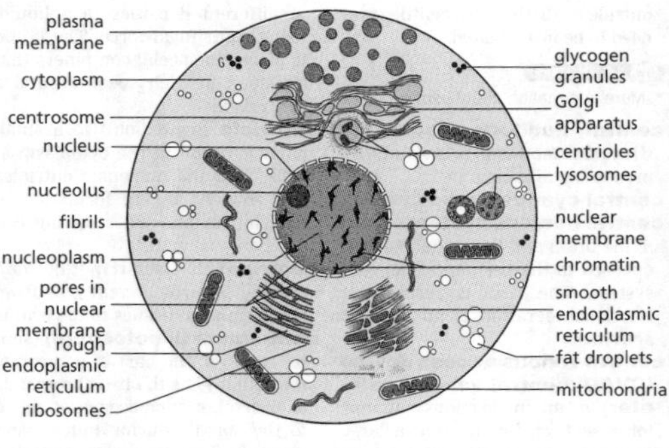

An animal cell (microscopical structure)

[A. Celsius (1701–44), Swedish astronomer]

CEMACH *n.* Confidential Enquiry into Maternal Deaths and Child Health. *See* confidential enquiries.

cement (si-ment) *n.* **1.** any of a group of materials used in dentistry either as fillings or as lutes for crowns. **2.** *see* cementum.

cementum (cement) (si-men-tŭm) *n.* a thin layer of hard tissue on the surface of the root of a tooth. It anchors the fibres of the periodontal membrane to the tooth.

censor (sen-ser) *n.* (in psychology) the mechanism, postulated by Freud, that suppresses or modifies desires that are inappropriate or feared.

-centesis *combining form denoting* puncture or perforation.

centi- *prefix denoting* one hundredth or a hundred.

centigrade temperature (sent-i-grayd) *n. see* Celsius temperature.

centile chart (sen-tyl) *n.* a graph with lines showing average measurements of height, weight, and head circumference compared with age and sex, against which a child's physical development can be assessed. The lines of growth on the graph are called **centiles** (or **percentiles**), and the number of a centile predicts the percentage of children who are below that measurement at a given age; for example, the 10th centile means that 10% of the age- and sex-matched population will be smaller and 90% will be bigger. Children whose growth lies outside the 97th or 3rd centiles may need to be investigated.

SEE WEB LINKS

- More information about centile charts

central auditory processing disorder (sen-trăl) *n. see* auditory processing disorder.

central cyanosis *n. see* cyanosis.

central nervous system (CNS) *n.* the brain and the spinal cord, as opposed to the peripheral nervous system. The CNS is responsible for the integration of all nervous activities.

central venous access device (CVAD, central venous catheter) *n.* an intravenous catheter for insertion directly into a large vein, most commonly the subclavian under the clavicle or the jugular in the neck, or indirectly via a peripheral vein (e.g. the femoral vein in the groin). Its tip lies in the inferior or superior vena cava. The CVAD enables intravenous drugs and fluids to be given and intravenous pressures to be measured during operations or in intensive care.

central venous pressure (CVP) *n.* blood pressure in the right atrium, recorded by means of a catheter inserted into the vena cava and attached to a manometer. It is monitored particularly after heart surgery.

centri- *combining form denoting* centre.

centrifugal (sen-tri-**few**-găl) *adj.* moving away from a centre, as from the brain to the peripheral tissues.

centrifuge (**sen**-tri-fewj) *n.* a device for separating components of different densities in a liquid, using centrifugal force. The liquid is placed in special containers that are spun at high speed around a central axis.

centriole (sen-tri-ohl) *n.* a small particle found in the cytoplasm of cells, near the nucleus. Centrioles are involved in the formation of the spindle and aster during cell division.

centripetal (sen-**trip**-it'l) *adj.* moving towards a centre, as from the peripheral tissues to the brain.

centromere (kinetochore) (sen-trŏ-meer) *n.* the part of a chromosome that joins the two chromatids to each other and becomes attached to the spindle during mitosis and meiosis. When chromosome division takes place the centromeres split longitudinally.

centrosome (centrosphere) (**sen**-trŏ-sohm) *n.* an area of clear cytoplasm, found next to the nucleus in nondividing cells, that contains the centrioles.

centrosphere (sen-trŏ-sfeer) *n.* **1.** an area of clear cytoplasm seen in dividing cells around the poles of the spindle. **2.** *see* centrosome.

cephal- (cephalo-) *combining form denoting* the head.

cephalalgia (sef-ă-**lal**-jiă) *n.* pain in the head; headache.

cephalhaematoma (sef-ăl-heem-ă-**toh**-mă) *n.* a swelling on the head caused by a collection of bloody fluid between one or more of the skull bones and its covering membrane (periosteum). It is most commonly seen in newborn infants delivered with the aid of forceps or subjected to pressures during passage through the birth canal. No treatment is necessary and the swelling disappears in a few months. If it is extensive, the blood in the fluid may break down, releasing bilirubin into the bloodstream and causing jaundice.

cephalic (si-fal-ik) *adj.* of or relating to the head.

cephalic index *n.* a measure of the shape of a skull, commonly used in craniometry.

cephalic version (external cephalic version) *n.* a procedure in which a fetus that is lying in the breech position is turned so that its head will enter the birth canal first.

cephalocele (si-fal-ŏ-seel) *n.* protrusion of the contents of the skull through a defect in the bones of the skull. *See* neural tube defects.

cephalogram (sef-ă-loh-gram) *n.* a special standardized X-ray picture that can be used to measure alterations in the growth of skull bones.

cephalometry (sef-ă-**lom**-itri) *n.* the study of facial growth by examination of standardized lateral radiographs of the head. It is used mainly for diagnosis in orthodontics.

cephalosporin (sef-ă-loh-**spo**-rin) *n.* any one of a group of semisynthetic antibiotics, derived from the mould *Cephalosporium*, which are effective against a wide range of microorganisms and are therefore used to treat a variety of infections. The older (first-generation) cephalosporins include **cefadroxil** and **cefalexin**; more recent (second-generation) drugs include **cefaclor** and **cefuroxime**; **ceftazidime** is a third-generation cephalosporin. Cross-sensitivity with penicillin may occur and the principal side-effects are allergic reactions and irritation of the digestive tract.

cerclage (ser-**klah***zh*) *n. see* cervical (cerclage).

cerebellum (se-ri-**bel**-ŭm) *n.* the largest part of the hindbrain, bulging back behind the pons and the medulla oblongata and overhung by the occipital lobes of the cerebrum. The cerebellum is essential for the maintenance of muscle tone, balance, and the synchronization of activity in groups of muscles under voluntary control, converting muscular contractions into smooth coordinated movement. **—cerebellar** *adj.*

cerebr- (cerebri-, cerebro-) *combining form denoting* the cerebrum or brain.

cerebral abscess (se-ri-brăl) *n. see* abscess.

cerebral aqueduct *n. see* aqueduct.

cerebral cortex *n.* the intricately folded outer layer of the cerebrum, making up some 40% of the brain by weight. It is directly responsible for consciousness, with essential roles in perception, memory, thought, mental ability, and intellect, and it is responsible for initiating voluntary activity.

cerebral haemorrhage *n.* bleeding from a cerebral blood vessel into the tissue of the brain. It is commonly caused by degenerative disease of the arteries and high blood pressure but may result from bleeding from congenital abnormalities of blood vessels. The symptoms vary from a transient weakness or numbness to profound coma and death. *See also* atheroma, hypertension, stroke.

cerebral hemisphere *n.* one of the two paired halves of the cerebrum.

cerebral palsy *n.* a disorder of movement and/or posture as a result of nonprogressive but permanent damage to the developing brain, which may occur before, during, or immediately after delivery. Causes include an inadequate supply of oxygen to the brain, low levels of glucose in the blood, and infection. Cerebral palsy is often associated with other problems, such as learning difficulties, hearing difficulties, poor speech, and epilepsy. There are three main types: **spastic**, in which the limbs are difficult to control; **ataxic hypotonic**, in which the main problem is poor balance and uncoordinated movements; and **dyskinetic**, in which there is involuntary movement of the limbs.

SEE WEB LINKS
- Website of Scope

cerebration (se-ri-**bray**-shŏn) *n.* **1.** the functioning of the brain as a whole. **2.** the unconscious activities of the brain.

cerebrospinal fever (spotted fever) (se-ri-broh-**spy**-năl) *n.* a former name for meningococcal meningitis.

cerebrospinal fluid (CSF) *n.* the clear watery fluid that surrounds and protects the brain and spinal cord. It is contained in the subarachnoid space and circulates in the ventricles of the brain and in the central canal of the spinal cord.

cerebrovascular accident (CVA) (se-ri-broh-**vas**-kew-ler) *n.* the clinical syndrome accompanying a sudden and sometimes severe attack of cerebrovascular disease, which leads to a stroke.

SEE WEB LINKS
- Website of the Stroke Association

cerebrovascular disease *n.* any disorder of the blood vessels of the brain and its covering membranes (meninges). Most cases are due to atheroma and/or hypertension, clinical effects being caused by rupture of diseased blood vessels or inadequacy of the blood supply to the brain, due to cerebral thrombosis or embolism.

cerebrum (telencephalon) (se-ri-brŭm) *n.* the largest and most highly developed part of the brain, composed of the two cerebral hemispheres, separated from each other by the longitudinal fissure in the midline and connected at the base by the corpus callosum. The cerebrum is responsible for the initiation and coordination of all voluntary activity in the body and for governing the functioning of lower parts of the nervous system. See illustration. —**cerebral** *adj.*

cerumen (earwax) (si-**roo**-men) *n.* the waxy material that is secreted by the sebaceous glands in the external auditory meatus of the outer ear.

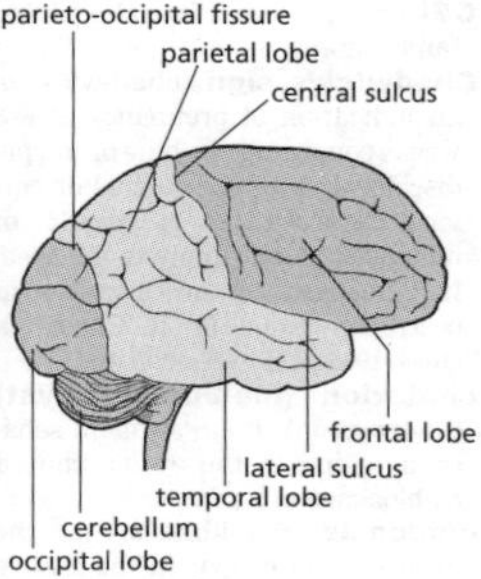

Lobes of the cerebrum (from right side)

cervic- (cervico-) *combining form denoting* **1.** the neck. **2.** the cervix, especially of the uterus.

cervical (ser-vy-kăl) *adj.* **1.** of or relating to the neck. **c. vertebrae** the seven bones making up the neck region of the backbone. *See also* (cervical) fracture, vertebra. **2.** of, relating to, or affecting the cervix of an organ, especially the cervix of the uterus. **c. cancer** cancer of the cervix of the uterus. The growth can be detected at an early stage by cervical screening. **c. cerclage** a procedure to help prevent preterm delivery. It involves placing a stitch around the cervix of the uterus to keep it closed and reduce the possibility of preterm cervical dilatation and rupture of membranes. **c. ectopy** *see* ectropion. **c. incompetence** spontaneous dilatation of the cervix of the uterus during the second trimester of pregnancy. The membranes bulge and subsequently rupture, and the fetus is expelled prematurely in a late miscarriage. **c. intraepithelial neoplasia** *see* CIN. **c. screening** screening tests, using cervical smears, to detect precancerous changes in the cervix of the uterus. Colposcopy is indicated when abnormal cells (*see* dyskaryosis) are found. **c. smear** a specimen of cellular material, scraped from the cervix of the uterus, that is stained and examined under a microscope in order to detect cell abnormalities indicating the presence of precancerous change.

cervicitis (ser-vi-**sy**-tis) *n.* inflammation of the cervix of the uterus.

cervix (ser-viks) *n.* a necklike part. **c. uteri** the neck of the uterus, which at its lower end projects into the vagina and contains the cervical canal.

cestode (ses-tohd) *n. see* tapeworm.

cetirizine (sĕ-**ti**-ri-zeen) *n.* a non-sedating antihistamine used to treat such allergic conditions as hay fever and urticaria. It is administered by mouth.

cetrimide (**set**-ri-myd) *n.* a detergent disinfectant, used for cleansing skin surfaces and wounds, treating minor burns and abrasions, and included as an ingredient in barrier creams.

cetuximab (si-**tuks**-i-mab) *n.* a cytotoxic drug (a monoclonal antibody) administered by intravenous infusion in the treatment of metastatic colorectal cancer and squamous cell carcinoma of the head and neck. It is given by intravenous infusion. Trade name: **Erbitux**.

CEWS *n.* children's early warning score (*see* paediatric early warning score).

CF *n. see* cystic fibrosis.

CFS/ME/PVF *n.* a condition, known variously as **chronic fatigue syndrome**, **myalgic encephalomyelitis** (or **encephalopathy**), and **postviral fatigue syndrome**, characterized by extreme disabling fatigue that has lasted for at least six months, is made worse by physical or mental exertion, does not resolve with bed rest, and cannot be attributed to other disorders. The fatigue is accompanied by at least some of the following: muscle pain or weakness (*see* fibromyalgia), poor coordination, joint pain, recurrent sore throat, slight fever, painful lymph nodes in the neck and armpits, depression, cognitive impairment (especially an inability to concentrate), and general malaise. The cause is unknown, but in some cases certain viral conditions (especially glandular fever) are thought to trigger the disease.

CFTR gene *n.* the gene, lying on chromosome no. 7, that encodes a protein, cystic fibrosis transmembrane regulator (CFTR), enabling the transport of chloride ions across cell membranes. Patients with cystic fibrosis lack CFTR due to a mutation in this gene.

CGI *n. see* Clinical Global Impression.

Chadwick's sign (**chad**-wiks) *n.* an indication of pregnancy at 6–8 weeks consisting of a blue or purple discoloration of the vaginal or cervical mucosa as a result of increased blood supply to the area. It is caused by an increase in oestrogen levels. [J. R. Chadwick (1844–1905), US gynaecologist]

chalazion (meibomian cyst) (kă-lay-zi-ŏn) *n.* a swollen sebaceous gland in the eyelid, caused by blockage of its duct.

chalcosis (kal-**koh**-sis) *n.* the deposition of copper in the tissues of the eye, usually resulting from the presence of a copper foreign body within the eye.

chancre (**shang**-ker) *n.* a painless ulcer that develops at the site where infection enters the body, e.g. on the lips, penis, urethra, or eyelid. It is the primary symptom of such infections as sleeping sickness and syphilis.

chancroid (**shank**-roid) *n. see* soft sore.

charcoal (**char**-kohl) *n.* a fine black powder, a form of carbon that is the residue from the partial burning of wood and other organic materials. **activated c.** charcoal that has been treated to increase its properties as an adsorbent, used as an emergency antidote to various poisons.

Charcot-Bouchard aneurysm (shar-**koh boo**-shard) *n. see* aneurysm. [J. M. Charcot (1825–93), French neurologist; C. J. Bouchard (1837–1915), French physician]

Charcot-Marie-Tooth disease (peroneal muscular atrophy, hereditary sensorimotor neuropathy) (mă-ree tooth) *n.* a group of inherited diseases of the peripheral nerves causing a gradually progressive weakness and wasting of the muscles of the legs and the lower part of the thighs. The hands and arms are eventually affected. [J. M. Charcot; P. Marie (1853–1940), French physician; H. H. Tooth (1856–1925), British physician]

Charcot's joint (neuropathic arthritis) *n.* an extreme form of osteoarthritis resulting from damage to the sensory nerves that supply a joint, which becomes unstable, swollen, and painless. Causes include diabetes mellitus, syringomyelia, tabes dorsalis, and leprosy. [J. M. Charcot]

Charcot's triad *n.* the combination of pain in the right upper quadrant (*see* abdomen), fever, and jaundice that is seen in acute cholangitis. [J. M. Charcot]

Charnley clamps (**charn**-li) *pl. n.* an apparatus used to encourage arthrodesis between the ends of two bones on either side of a joint. Parallel pins driven through the bone ends are connected on each side of the joint by bolts bearing wing nuts; tightening of the screw arrangements forces the surfaces of the bones together. [Sir J. Charnley (1911–82), British orthopaedic surgeon]

CHD *n.* coronary heart disease (*see* ischaemic heart disease).

Chediak-Higashi syndrome (**ched**-i-ak hi-**gash**-i) *n.* a rare fatal hereditary (autosomal recessive) condition causing enlargement of the liver and spleen, albinism, and abnormalities of the eye. It is thought to be due to a disorder of glycolipid metabolism. [A. Chediak (20th century), Cuban physician; O. Higashi (20th century), Japanese paediatrician]

cheil- (cheilo-) *combining form denoting* the lip(s).

cheilitis (ky-**ly**-tis) *n.* inflammation of the lips. **angular c.** cheilitis that affects the angles of the lips and may be caused by a staphylococcal or candidal infection.

cheiloplasty (**ky**-loh-plasti) *n. see* labioplasty.

cheiloschisis (ky-**losk**-i-sis) *n. see* cleft lip.

cheilosis (ky-**loh**-sis) *n.* swollen cracked bright-red lips. This is a common symptom of many nutritional disorders, including ariboflavinosis (vitamin B_2 deficiency).

cheir- (cheiro-) *combining form denoting* the hand(s).

cheiroarthropathy (ky-roh-arth-**rop**-ăthi) *n.* the restricted hand movement seen in long-standing diabetes, due to chronic thickening of the skin limiting joint flexibility. *See* diabetic hand syndrome.

cheiropompholyx (ky-roh-**pom**-fŏ-liks) *n.* a type of blistering eczema affecting the palms and fingers. *See* pompholyx.

chelating agent (kee-layt-ing) *n.* a chemical compound that forms complexes by binding metal ions. Some chelating agents, including desferrioxamine and penicillamine, are drugs used to treat metal poisoning: the metal is bound to the drug and excreted safely.

chem- (chemo-) *combining form denoting* chemical or chemistry.

chemoradiotherapy (kee-moh-ray-di-oh-**th'**e-ră-pi) *n.* the use of concurrent chemotherapy (as a radiosensitizer) and radical irradiation in the treatment of malignant disease.

chemoreceptor (kee-moh-ri-**sep**-ter) *n.* a cell or group of cells that responds to the presence of specific chemical compounds by initiating an impulse in a sensory nerve. Chemoreceptors are found in the taste buds and in the mucous membranes of the nose. *See also* receptor.

chemosis (ki-**moh**-sis) *n.* swelling (oedema) of the conjunctiva.

chemotaxis (kee-moh-**taks**-iss) *n.* movement of a cell or organism in response to the stimulus of a gradient of chemical concentration.

chemotherapy (kee-moh-**th'**e-ră-pi) *n.* the prevention or treatment of disease by the use of chemical substances. The term is increasingly restricted to the treatment of cancer with antimetabolites and similar drugs (in contrast to radiotherapy). *See also* cytotoxic drug.

cherry angioma (**che**-ri) *n. see* angioma.

chest (chest) *n. see* thorax.

Cheyne–Stokes respiration (chayn-**stohks**) *n.* a striking form of breathing in which there is a cyclical variation in the rate, which becomes slower until breathing stops for several seconds before speeding up to a peak and then slowing again. It occurs particularly in states of coma. [J. Cheyne (1777–1836), Scottish physician; W. Stokes (1804–78), Irish physician]

CHF *n. see* (congestive) heart failure.

chiasm (**ky**-az'm) *n. see* optic (chiasm).

chickenpox (**chik**-in-poks) *n.* a highly infectious disease caused by the varicella-zoster virus (a herpesvirus), which is transmitted by airborne droplets. Symptoms are mild fever followed by an itchy rash of red pimples that spread from the trunk to the face, scalp, and limbs. These develop into vesicles and then scabs, which drop off after about 12 days. The patient is infectious from the onset of symptoms until all the spots have gone. Medical name: **varicella**.

Chief Nursing Officer (cheef) *n.* the UK government's chief nursing adviser, who is responsible for providing an expert professional contribution and advice on nursing, midwifery, and health visiting matters to ministers and senior officials. There are separate officers appointed to advise the devolved governments in Scotland, Wales, and Northern Ireland.

SEE WEB LINKS

- Chief Nursing Officer's page on the NHS England website

chilblains (perniosis) (**chil**-blaynz) *pl. n.* dusky red itchy swellings that develop on the extremities in cold weather. They usually settle in two weeks but treatment with nifedipine is helpful in severe cases.

child abuse (chyld) *n.* the maltreatment of children. It may take the form of **sexual abuse**, when a child is involved in sexual activity by an adult; **physical abuse**, when physical injury is caused by cruelty or undue punishment (*see* nonaccidental injury); **neglect**, when basic physical provision for needs is lacking; and **emotional abuse**, when lack of affection and/or hostility from caregivers damage a child's emotional development.

childbirth (**chyld**-berth) *n. see* labour.

child health clinic *n.* (in Britain) a special clinic for the routine care of infants and preschool children. The service provides screening tests for such conditions as congenital dislocation of hips, suppressed squint, and impaired speech and/or hearing, education for mothers (especially those having their first child) in feeding techniques and hygiene, and immunizations against infectious diseases.

child protection register *n.* a confidential list of children whose social circumstances render them at risk of neglect or abuse. Each local authority maintains a child protection register, and children who are subject to a child protection plan will be on the register and will receive extra support and surveillance from health and/or social services.

children's centre (**chil**-drĕnz) *n.* a building housing a range of services to support children up to five years of age and their families, including childcare, early education, parenting advice, and access to health advice.

children's early warning score *see* paediatric early warning score.

chir- (chiro-) *combining form denoting* the hand(s). *See also* cheir-.

chiropody (ki-**rop**-ŏdi) *n. see* podiatry.

chiropractic (ky-rŏ-**prak**-tik) *n.* a system of treating diseases by manipulation, mainly of the vertebrae of the backbone. It is based on the theory that nearly all disorders can be traced to the incorrect alignment of bones, with consequent malfunctioning of nerves and muscle throughout the body. —**chiropractor** (**ky**-rŏ-prak-ter) *n.*

chi-square test (**ky**-skwair) *n.* (in statistics) a test to determine if the difference between two groups of observations is statistically significant (*see* significance), used in controlled trials and other studies. It measures the differences between theoretical and observed frequencies (*see* frequency distribution) and identifies whether or not variables are dependent (*see* variable).

Chlamydia (klă-**mid**-iă) *n.* a genus of Gram-negative bacteria that are obligate intracellular parasites of humans and other animals, in which they cause disease. **C. pneumoniae** a cause of pneumonia. **C. psittaci** the cause of psittacosis. **C. trachomatis** the causative agent of the eye disease trachoma and a common cause of sexually transmitted infections (*see* urethritis). —**chlamydial** *adj.*

chloasma (melasma) (kloh-**az**-mă) *n.* ill-defined symmetrical brown patches on the cheeks or elsewhere on the face. Chloasma is a photosensitivity reaction in women on combined oral contraceptive pills or who are pregnant; very rarely it occurs in men.

chlor- (chloro-) *combining form denoting* **1.** chlorine or chlorides. **2.** green.

chloracne (klor-**ak**-ni) *n.* an occupational acne-like skin disorder that occurs after regular contact with chlorinated hydrocarbons.

chloral hydrate (**klor**-ăl **hy**-drayt) *n.* a sedative and hypnotic drug formerly widely used (as a syrup) to induce sleep, mainly in children and the elderly; its derivative **chloral betaine** (Welldorm) is formulated as an elixir or tablets. Prolonged use may lead to dependence.

chlorambucil (klor-**am**-bew-sil) *n.* an alkylating agent used in chemotherapy, mainly in the treatment of chronic leukaemias and some lymphomas. It is given by mouth; prolonged large doses may cause damage to the bone marrow. Trade name: **Leukeran**.

chloramphenicol (klor-am-**fen**-i-kol) *n.* an antibiotic that is effective against a wide variety of microorganisms. However, due to its serious side-effects, especially damage to the bone marrow, it is usually reserved for serious infections (especially those caused by *Haemophilus influenzae*) when less toxic drugs are ineffective. It is also used, in the form of eye drops and ear drops, to treat superficial eye and outer ear infections. Trade names: **Chloromycetin**, **Kemicetine**, **Minims Chloramphenicol**.

chlordiazepoxide (klor-dy-az-i-**pok**-syd) *n.* a benzodiazepine with muscle relaxant properties, administered by mouth for the short-term relief of anxiety and to lessen the severity of symptoms in alcohol withdrawal. Trade name: **Librium**.

chlorhexidine (klor-**heks**-i-deen) *n.* an antiseptic used in solutions to disinfect and cleanse the skin (before surgery and to treat wounds and burns). It is also used as a mouthwash, gel, or spray for treating mouth ulcers and gingivitis and as a cream for treating dry and itchy skin conditions. Trade names: **Cepton**, **ChloraPrep**, **Chlorohex**, **Corsodyl**, **Hibitane**, **Hibitane Obstetric**, etc.

chlorine (**klor**-een) *n.* an extremely pungent gaseous element with antiseptic and bleaching properties. It is widely used to sterilize drinking water and purify swimming pools. In high concentrations it is toxic. Symbol: Cl.

chlormethiazole (klor-mi-**th'y**-ă-zohl) *n.* *see* clomethiazole.

chloroform (**klo**-rŏ-form) *n.* a volatile liquid formerly widely used as a general anaesthetic. Chloroform is now used only in low concentrations as a flavouring agent and preservative, in the treatment of flatulence, and in liniments as a rubefacient.

chlorophenothane (klo-roh-**feen**-ŏ-thayn) *n.* *see* DDT.

chloroquine (**klo**-roh-kween) *n.* a drug used principally in the treatment and prevention of benign malarias but also used in the treatment of rheumatoid arthritis and lupus erythematosus. It is administered by mouth; a side-effect of prolonged use in large doses is eye damage. Trade names: **Avloclor**, **Malarivon**.

chlorphenamine (chlorpheniramine) (klor-**fen**-ămeen) *n.* a potent antihistamine used to treat such allergies as hay fever and urticaria and in the emergency treatment of anaphylactic shock. It is administered by mouth or, to relieve severe conditions, by injection. Trade name: **Piriton**.

chlorpromazine (klor-**prom**-ă-zeen) *n.* a phenothiazine antipsychotic drug, administered by mouth or injection or as a rectal suppository. It is used in the treatment of schizophrenia and mania and to control nausea and vomiting in terminal illness. Trade name: **Largactil**.

chlortalidone (chlorthalidone) (klor-**tal**-i-dohn) *n.* a thiazide diuretic administered by mouth to treat fluid retention, hypertension, heart failure, and diabetes insipidus. Trade name: **Hygroton**.

choana (**koh**-ă-nă) *n.* (*pl.* **choanae**) a funnel-shaped opening, particularly either of the two openings between the nasal cavity and the pharynx.

chocolate cyst (**chok**-ŏ-lit) *n.* a cyst filled with dark fluid, occurring in the ovary in endometriosis.

chol- (chole-, cholo-) *combining form denoting* bile.

cholaemia (kol-**eem**-iă) *n.* the presence of bile or bile pigments in the blood. *See* jaundice.

cholagogue (**kol**-ă-gog) *n.* a drug that stimulates the flow of bile from the gall bladder and bile ducts into the duodenum.

cholangiocarcinoma (kol-anji-oh-kar-sin-**oh**-mă) *n.* a rare malignant tumour of the bile ducts. A tumour located at the junction of the right and left hepatic ducts within the liver is known as a **Klatskin tumour**.

cholangiography (kol-anji-**og**-răfi) *n.* imaging of the bile ducts in order to demonstrate congenital anatomical abnormalities, biliary diseases, and the presence of gallstones or strictures. It may be combined with imaging of the pancreatic duct (*see* cholangiopancreatography). **operative** (or **on-table**) **c.** cholangiography in which a radi-opaque contrast medium is injected into the bile ducts during cholecystectomy, to make sure there are no remaining gallstones in the ducts. **percutaneous transhepatic c. (PTC)** an invasive fluoroscopic technique in which a catheter is manipulated through the anterior abdominal wall, across the liver, and into a bile duct; contrast solution is injected to outline the bile ducts, and drains or stents can be placed to treat infection or malignant strictures. **T-tube c.** cholangiography that involves the postoperative injection of radi-opaque contrast material via a drain (T-tube) left in the main bile duct after cholecystectomy.

cholangiopancreatography (kol-anji-oh-pank-ri-ă-**tog**-răfi) *n.* imaging of the bile ducts and pancreatic duct. **endoscopic retrograde c.** *see* ERCP. **magnetic resonance c. (MRCP)** magnetic resonance imaging of the bile ducts and pancreatic duct, often used in the diagnosis of obstructive jaundice and pancreatic disease.

cholangitis (kol-an-jy-tis) *n.* inflammation and secondary bacterial infection of the bile ducts, due to biliary obstruction and stasis. Treatment includes antibiotics and decompression of the biliary system.

cholecalciferol (koli-kal-**sif**-er-ol) *n. see* vitamin D.

cholecyst- *combining form denoting* the gall bladder.

cholecystectomy (koli-sis-**tek**-tŏmi) *n.* surgical removal of the gall bladder (usually for cholecystitis), gallstones, or biliary colic.

cholecystenterostomy (koli-sist-en-ter-**ost**-ŏmi) *n.* a surgical procedure in which the gall bladder is joined to the small intestine. It is performed in order to allow bile to pass freely from the liver to the intestine, bypassing an obstructed common bile duct.

cholecystitis (koli-sis-**ty**-tis) *n.* inflammation of the gall bladder.

cholecystoduodenostomy (koli-sis-toh-dew-oh-di-**nost**-ŏmi) *n.* a form of cholecystenterostomy in which the gall bladder is joined to the duodenum.

cholecystography (koli-sis-**tog**-răfi) *n.* X-ray examination of the gall bladder in which a radiopaque contrast agent is administered by mouth and an X-ray image (**cholecystogram**) is taken.

cholecystojejunostomy (koli-sis-toh-jĕ-joo-**nost**-ŏmi) *n.* a form of cholecystenterostomy in which the gall bladder is joined to the jejunum.

cholecystokinin (koli-sis-toh-**ky**-nin) *n.* a hormone secreted by cells of the duodenum in response to the presence of partly digested food in the duodenum. It causes contraction of the gall bladder and expulsion of bile into the intestine and stimulates the production of digestive enzymes by the pancreas.

cholecystolithiasis (koli-sis-toh-lith-**I**-ă-sis) *n. see* cholelithiasis.

cholecystotomy (koli-sis-**tot**-ŏmi) *n.* a surgical operation in which the gall bladder is opened, usually to remove gallstones.

choledoch- (choledocho-) *combining form denoting* the common bile duct.

choledocholithiasis (koli-dok-oh-lith-**I**-ă-sis) *n.* gallstones within the common bile duct. The stones usually form in the gall bladder and pass into the common bile duct, but they may develop within the duct itself, even after cholecystectomy.

choledochotomy (koli-dŏ-**kot**-ŏmi) *n.* a surgical operation in which the common bile duct is opened, to search for or to remove stones within it.

cholelithiasis (cholecystolithiasis) (koli-lith-**I**-ă-sis) *n.* the formation of gallstones in the gall bladder or bile common duct (*see* gallstone).

cholelithotomy (koli-lith-**ot**-ŏmi) *n.* the surgical removal of gallstones by cholecystotomy.

cholera (kol-er-ă) *n.* an acute infection of the small intestine by the bacterium *Vibrio cholerae*, which causes severe vomiting and diarrhoea (known as **ricewater stools**) leading to dehydration. The disease is contracted from contaminated food or drinking water and often occurs in epidemics. Initial treatment is concentrated on replacing the fluid loss by oral rehydration therapy; tetracycline eradicates the bacteria and hastens recovery. The mortality rate in untreated cases is over 50%. Vaccination against cholera is effective for only 6–9 months.

choleresis (kol-er-**ee**-sis) *n.* the production of bile by the liver.

choleretic (kol-er-**et**-ik) *n.* an agent that stimulates the secretion of bile by the liver thereby increasing the flow of bile.

cholestasis (koli-**stay**-sis) *n.* failure of normal amounts of bile to reach the intestine. The chief symptom is itching (pruritus); others include jaundice, dark urine, and pale stools. **obstetric c.** intense itching during pregnancy with abnormal liver function tests and raised bile acids, which may endanger the fetus.

cholesteatoma (koli-sti-ă-**toh**-mă) *n.* a skin-lined sac containing debris from dead skin cells that grows from the eardrum into the mastoid bone. Unless treated (by mastoidectomy), it can carry infection to the brain, causing meningitis or a cerebral abscess.

cholesterol (kŏl-**est**-er-ol) *n.* a fat-like material (a sterol) present in the blood and most tissues, especially nervous tissue. Elevated blood concentration of cholesterol (**hypercholesterolaemia**) is often associated with atheroma, of which cholesterol is a major component. Cholesterol is also a constituent of gallstones.

cholesterosis (kŏl-est-er-**oh**-sis) *n.* an uncommon form of chronic inflammation of the gall bladder in which small crystals of cholesterol are deposited on the internal wall. The crystals may enlarge to become gallstones.

cholestyramine *n. see* colestyramine.

cholic acid (cholalic acid) (**kol**-ik) *n. see* bile acids.

choline (**koh**-leen) *n.* a basic compound important in the synthesis of phosphatidylcholine (lecithin) and other phospholipids and of acetylcholine. It is also involved in the transport of fat in the body. Choline is sometimes classed as a vitamin but, although it is essential for life, it can be synthesized in the body.

cholinergic (koh-lin-**er**-jik) *adj.* **1.** describing or relating to nerve fibres that release acetylcholine as a neurotransmitter. **c. receptor** a receptor at which acetylcholine acts to pass on messages from cholinergic nerve fibres. **c. urticaria** *see* urticaria. **2.** describing drugs that mimic the actions of acetylcholine (*see* parasympathomimetic). *Compare* adrenergic.

cholinesterase (koh-lin-**est**-er-ayz) *n.* an enzyme that breaks down a choline ester into its choline and acid components. The term usually refers to **acetylcholinesterase**, which breaks down the neurotransmitter acetylcholine into choline and acetic acid.

choluria (kol-**yoor**-iă) *n.* the presence of bile in the urine, which lends it a dark brown colour. Choluria is caused by liver disease, usually in cases of obstructive jaundice.

chondr- (chondro-) *combining form denoting* cartilage.

chondritis (kon-**dry**-tis) *n.* any inflammatory condition affecting cartilage.

chondroblast (**kon**-droh-blast) *n.* a cell that produces the matrix of cartilage.

chondroblastoma (kon-droh-blas-**toh**-mă) *n.* a tumour derived from chondroblasts, having the appearance of a mass of well-differentiated cartilage.

chondroclast (**kon**-droh-klast) *n.* a cell that is concerned with the absorption of cartilage.

chondrocyte (**kon**-droh-syt) *n.* a cartilage cell, found embedded in the matrix.

chondroma (kon-**droh**-mă) *n.* a relatively common benign tumour of cartilage-forming cells, which may occur at the growing end of any bone but is found most commonly in the bones of the feet and hands.

chondromalacia (kon-droh-mă-**lay**-shiă) *n.* softening, inflammation, and degeneration of cartilage at a joint. **c. patellae** chondromalacia affecting the undersurface of the kneecap, resulting in pain in the front of the knee and grating, which is made worse by kneeling, squatting, or climbing stairs.

chondrosarcoma (kon-droh-sar-**koh**-ma) *n.* (*pl.* **chondrosarcomata**) an uncommon malignant tumour of cartilage cells occurring in a bone, usually the femur, humerus, pelvis, or a rib.

chord- (chordo-) *combining form denoting* **1.** a cord. **2.** the notochord.

chorda (**kor**-da) *n.* (*pl.* **chordae**) a cord, tendon, or nerve fibre. **chordae tendineae** stringlike processes in the heart that attach the margins of the mitral and tricuspid valve leaflets to projections of the wall of the ventricle (**papillary muscles**).

chordee (**kor**-dee) *n.* abnormal curvature or angulation of the penis. It may occur as a result of Peyronie's disease or, in a child, of hypospadias.

chordotomy (kor-**dot**-ŏmi) *n. see* cordotomy.

chorea (ko-**ree**-ă) *n.* a jerky involuntary movement particularly affecting the head, face, or limbs. The symptoms are most commonly due to disease of the basal ganglia. **Huntington's c.** *see* Huntington's disease. **Sydenham's c.** chorea that mainly affects children and typically occurs after an infection caused by β-haemolytic streptococci (such as rheumatic fever or scarlet fever).

chorioamnionitis (intra-amniotic infection) (kor-i-oh-am-ni-on-**I**-tis) *n.* acute inflammation of the fetal membranes (amnion and chorion), usually due to ascending Gram-negative bacterial infection following membrane rupture, although it can occur in the presence of intact membranes. Maternal fever during labour is the most common sign. It can result in premature labour.

choriocarcinoma (chorionepithelioma) (kor-i-oh-kar-sin-**oh**-mă) *n.* a rare malignant tumour of the placenta originating in the chorion. It is a complication of a hydatidiform mole, although it may follow a miscarriage or even a normal pregnancy.

chorion (**kor**-iŏn) *n.* the embryonic membrane that totally surrounds the embryo from the time of implantation. **—chorionic** *adj.*

chorionic gonadotrophin (kor-i-**on**-ik) *n.* *see* human chorionic gonadotrophin.

chorionic villi *pl. n.* *see* villus.

chorionic villus sampling (CVS) *n.* a procedure for the prenatal diagnosis of chromosomal abnormalities (e.g. Down's syndrome) in which a sample of placental tissue (containing chorionic villi) is aspirated through the cervix or abdomen under ultrasound visualization. The cells so obtained are subjected to chromosomal and biochemical analysis. CVS is usually performed between the 10th and 13th weeks of gestation.

chorioretinopathy (kor-i-oh-ret-in-**op**-ă-thi) *n.* any eye disease involving both the choroid and the retina. **central serous c.** shallow retinal detachment in the area of the macula due to leakage through the retinal pigment epithelium (*see* retina) into the subretinal space. The cause is unknown. It affects young adult males, causing reduced or distorted vision that usually settles in a few months.

choroid (**ko**-roid) *n.* the layer of the eyeball between the retina and the sclera. It contains blood vessels and a pigment that absorbs excess light and so prevents blurring of vision. *See* eye. **—choroidal** (kŏ-**roid**-ăl) *adj.*

choroidal detachment *n.* the separation of the choroid from the sclera of the eye as a result of leakage of fluid from the vessels of the choroid. It occurs when pressure inside the eyeball is very low, usually after trauma or intraocular surgery.

choroiditis (ko-roid-**I**-tis) *n.* inflammation of the choroid layer of the eye. Vision becomes blurred but the eye is usually painless. *See* uveitis.

choroidocyclitis (ko-roid-oh-sy-**kly**-tis) *n.* inflammation of the choroid layer and the ciliary body of the eye.

choroid plexus *n.* a rich network of blood vessels, derived from those of the pia mater, in each of the brain's ventricles. It is responsible for the production of cerebrospinal fluid.

Christmas disease (haemophilia B) (**kris**-măs) *n.* a disorder that is identical in its effects to haemophilia A, but is due to a deficiency of a different blood coagulation factor, Factor IX. [S. Christmas (20th century), in whom the factor was first identified]

Christmas factor *n.* *see* Factor IX.

chrom- (chromo-) *combining form denoting* colour or pigment.

-chromasia *combining form denoting* staining or pigmentation.

chromat- (chromato-) *combining form denoting* colour or pigmentation.

chromatid (**kroh**-mă-tid) *n.* one of the two threadlike strands formed by longitudinal division of a chromosome during mitosis and meiosis. They remain attached at the centromere.

chromatin (**kroh**-mă-tin) *n.* the material of a cell nucleus that stains with basic dyes and consists of DNA and protein: the substance of which the chromosomes are made.

chromatography (kroh-mă-**tog**-răfi) *n.* any of several techniques for separating the components of a mixture by selective absorption. In two such techniques, widely used in medicine, a sample of the mixture is placed at the edge of a sheet of filter paper (**paper c.**) or a column of a powdered absorbent (**column c.**). The components of the mixture are absorbed to different extents and thus move along the paper or column at different rates.

chromatolysis (kroh-mă-**tol**-i-sis) *n.* the dispersal or disintegration of the microscopic structures within the nerve cells that normally produce proteins. It is part of the cell's response to injury.

chromatophore (**kroh**-mă-tŏ-for) *n.* a cell containing pigment. In humans chromatophores containing melanin are found in the skin, hair, and eyes.

chromatosis (kroh-mă-**toh**-sis) *n.* abnormal pigmentation of the skin, as occurs in Addison's disease.

chromic acid (**kroh**-mik) *n.* a compound of chromium used in solution as a caustic for the removal of warts. Formula: CrO_3.

chromosome (**kroh**-mŏ-sohm) *n.* one of the threadlike structures in a cell nucleus that carry the genetic information in the form of genes. It is composed of a long double filament of DNA coiled into a helix together with associated proteins. The nucleus of each human somatic cell contains 46 chromosomes, 23 being of maternal and 23 of paternal origin. *See also* chromatid, centromere, sex chromosome. **—chromosomal** *adj.*

chronic (**kron**-ik) *adj.* describing a disease of long duration involving very slow changes. Such disease is often of gradual onset. *Compare* acute. **—chronicity** (kron-**iss**-iti) *n.*

chronic fatigue syndrome *n. see* CFS/ME/PVF.

chronic obstructive pulmonary disease (COPD, chronic obstructive airways disease, COAD) *n.* a disease of adults, especially those over the age of 45 with a history of smoking or inhalation of airborne pollution. It has features of emphysema and chronic bronchitis and is diagnosed, according to the GOLD guidelines, at different stages (0–4) based on the value of the forced expiratory volume in 1 second (FEV_1). Different treatment regimens are recommended for different stages: inhaled corticosteroids and long-acting beta agonists can improve quality of life and survival in the later stages.

Chronic Sick and Disabled Persons Act 1970 *n.* (in Britain) an Act providing for the identification and care of those suffering from a chronic or degenerative disease for which there is no cure and which can be only partially alleviated by treatment.

Churg-Strauss syndrome (eosinophilic granulomatosis with polyangitis) (cherg-strows) *n.* a systemic autoimmune vasculitis comprising severe asthma, allergic rhinitis, and sinusitis associated with an increased eosinophil count in the peripheral blood and eosinophilic deposits in the small vessels of the lungs. It usually responds to oral corticosteroids. [J. Churg (1910–2005) and L. Strauss (1913–85), US pathologists]

Chvostek's sign (vos-teks) *n.* a spasm of the facial muscles elicited by lightly tapping the facial nerve. It is a sign of tetany. [F. Chvostek (1835–84), Austrian surgeon]

chyle (kyl) *n.* an alkaline milky liquid found within the lacteals after a period of absorption. It consists of lymph with a suspension of minute droplets of digested fats (triglycerides), which have been absorbed from the small intestine.

chyluria (kyl-**yoor**-iă) *n.* the presence of chyle in the urine.

chyme (kym) *n.* the semiliquid acid mass that is the form in which food passes from the stomach to the small intestine. It is produced by the action of gastric juice and the churning of the stomach.

chymotrypsin (ky-moh-**trip**-sin) *n.* a protein-digesting enzyme (*see* peptidase). It is secreted by the pancreas in an inactive form, **chymotrypsinogen**, that is converted into chymotrypsin in the duodenum by the action of trypsin.

chymotrypsinogen (ky-moh-trip-**sin**-ŏ-jin) *n. see* chymotrypsin.

cicatricial (sik-ă-**trish**-ăl) *adj.* associated with scarring. **c. alopecia** *see* alopecia.

ciclosporin (cyclosporin) (sik-loh-**spo**-rin) *n.* an immunosuppressant drug used to prevent and treat rejection of a transplanted organ or bone marrow. It is also used to treat severe rheumatoid arthritis, psoriasis, atopic eczema, and ulcerative colitis. Ciclosporin is administered orally or by intravenous infusion. Trade names: **Capimune**, **Capsorin**, **Deximune**, **Neoral**, **Sandimmun**.

-cide *combining form denoting* killer or killing.

ciliary body (**sil**-i-er-i) *n.* the part of the eye that connects the choroid with the iris. It consists of three zones: the **ciliary ring**, which adjoins the choroid; the **ciliary processes**, a series of about 70 radial ridges behind the iris to which the suspensory ligament of the lens is attached; and the **ciliary muscle**, contraction of which alters the curvature of the lens (*see* accommodation).

cilium (**sil**-iŭm) *n.* (*pl.* **cilia**) **1.** a hairlike process, large numbers of which are found on certain epithelial cells, particularly the epithelium that lines the upper respiratory tract, and on certain protozoa. **2.** an eyelash or eyelid. **—ciliary** *adj.*

cimetidine (si-**met**-i-deen) *n.* an H_2-receptor antagonist (*see* antihistamine) that reduces gastric acidity and is used to treat gastro-oesophageal reflux and peptic ulcers. It is administered by mouth. Trade name: **Tagamet**.

Cimex (sy-meks) *n. see* bed bug.

CIN (cervical intraepithelial neoplasia) *n.* cellular changes in the cervix of the uterus preceding the invasive stages of cervical cancer. The CIN grading system distinguishes three stages: **CIN 1** (mild dysplasia); **CIN 2** (moderate dysplasia); and **CIN 3** (severe dysplasia, carcinoma in situ).

cinchocaine (sink-ŏ-kayn) *n.* a local anaesthetic used in combination with corticosteroids in ointments and suppositories to relieve the pain of haemorrhoids.

cinchona (sing-**koh**-nă) *n.* the dried bark of *Cinchona* trees, formerly used in medicine to stimulate the appetite and to prevent haemorrhage and diarrhoea. Cinchona is the source of quinine.

cinchonism (sink-ŏ-nizm) *n.* poisoning caused by an overdose of cinchona or the alkaloids quinine, quinidine, or cinchonine derived from it. The symptoms include ringing noises in the ears, dizziness, and blurring of vision.

cine- *combining form denoting* any technique of recording a rapid series of X-ray images on cine film for later analysis. Examples: **cineangiography**; **cinefluorography**. Cine film has largely been replaced by electronic storage (digital) media.

cingulectomy (sing-yoo-**lek**-tŏmi) *n.* surgical excision of the cingulum, occasionally carried out as psychosurgery for intractable mental illness.

cingulum (**sing**-yoo-lŭm) *n.* (*pl.* **cingula**) a curved bundle of nerve fibres in each cerebral hemisphere, nearly encircling its connection with the corpus callosum. It is the part of the brain controlling anger and depression. *See* cerebrum.

ciprofibrate (sip-roh-**fy**-brayt) *n.* a drug used for treating hyperlipidaemia (*see* fibrate). It is administered by mouth.

ciprofloxacin (sip-roh-**floks**-ă-sin) *n.* a broad-spectrum quinolone antibiotic that can be given orally or by intravenous infusion and is particularly useful against Gram-negative bacteria, such as *Pseudomonas*, that are resistant to all other oral antibiotics. It is also applied as eye drops or ointment to treat eye infections and corneal ulcers. Trade names: **Ciloxan**, **Ciproxin**.

circadian rhythm (ser-**kay**-diăn) *n.* the periodic rhythm, synchronized approximately to the 24-hour day/night cycle, seen in various metabolic activities of most living organisms (e.g. sleeping, hormone secretion).

circle of Willis (ser-kŭl ŏv wil-iss) *n.* a circle on the undersurface of the brain formed by linked branches of the arteries that supply the brain. [T. Willis (1621–75), English anatomist]

circulation (ser-kew-**lay**-shŏn) *n.* **1.** the movement of a fluid in a circular course, especially the passage of blood through the cardiovascular system. **2.** the system of vessels effecting this passage. **pulmonary c.** circulation of blood between the heart and lungs. Deoxygenated blood passes to the lungs from the right ventricle via the pulmonary artery; oxygenated blood returns to the left atrium via the pulmonary vein. **systemic c.** circulation of blood between the heart and all parts of the body except the lungs. Oxygenated blood leaves the aorta and deoxygenated blood returns into the vena cava. *See also* collateral circulation. **—circulatory** *adj.*

circum- *prefix denoting* around; surrounding.

circumcision (ser-kŭm-**sizh**-ŏn) *n.* surgical removal of the foreskin of the penis. This operation is usually performed for religious and ethnic reasons but may be required for medical conditions, mainly phimosis and paraphimosis. **female c.** *See* female genital mutilation.

circumduction (ser-kŭm-**duk**-shŏn) *n.* a circular movement, such as that made by a limb.

circumflex nerve (ser-kŭm-fleks) *n.* a mixed sensory and motor nerve of the upper arm. It arises from the fifth and sixth cervical segments of the spinal cord and is distributed to the deltoid muscle of the shoulder and the overlying skin.

circumoral (ser-kŭm-**or**-ăl) *adj.* situated around the mouth.

cirrhosis (si-**roh**-sis) *n.* a condition in which the liver responds to injury or death of some of its cells by replacing damaged tissue with interlacing strands of fibrous tissue and nodules of regenerating cells. Causes include chronic alcoholism (**alcoholic c.**), viral hepatitis, nonalcoholic fatty liver disease, chronic obstruction of the common bile duct (**secondary biliary c.**), autoimmune diseases **(primary biliary c., PBC)**, and chronic heart failure (**cardiac c.**). Complications include portal hypertension, ascites, hepatic encephalopathy, and hepatoma. **—cirrhotic** *adj.*

cirs- (cirso-) *combining form denoting* a varicose vein.

cirsoid (ser-soid) *adj.* describing the distended knotted appearance of a varicose vein.

CIS *n. see* carcinoma in situ.

CISC *n. see* (clean) intermittent self-catheterization.

cisplatin (sis-**plat**-in) *n.* a platinum-containing compound: a cytotoxic drug that impedes cell division by damaging DNA. Administered intravenously, it is used in the treatment of testicular tumours and cancers of the lung, bladder, and head and neck; side-effects include nausea and vomiting, kidney damage, hearing loss, and peripheral neuropathy.

cisterna (sis-**ter**-nă) *n.* (*pl.* **cisternae**) **1.** one of the enlarged spaces beneath the arachnoid that act as reservoirs for cerebrospinal fluid. **c. magna** the largest of the cisternae, lying beneath the cerebellum and behind the medulla oblongata. **2.** a dilatation at the lower end of the thoracic duct, into which the great lymph ducts of the lower limbs drain.

citalopram (sit-al-ŏ-pram) *n.* a drug (*see* SSRI) that is taken by mouth for the treatment of depression and panic disorder.

citric acid (sit-rik) *n.* an organic acid found naturally in citrus fruits. Citric acid is formed in the first stage of the Krebs cycle. Formula: $CH_2(COOH)C(OH)(COOH)CH_2COOH$.

citric acid cycle *n.* *see* Krebs cycle.

Citrobacter (sit-roh-bak-ter) *n.* a genus of Gram-negative anaerobic rod-shaped bacteria widely distributed in nature. The organisms cause infections of the intestinal and urinary tracts, gall bladder, and the meninges that are usually secondary, occurring in the elderly, newborn, debilitated, and immunocompromised.

citrulline (sit-rŭ-leen) *n.* an amino acid produced by the liver as a by-product during the conversion of ammonia to urea.

CIWA-Ar (Clinical Institute Withdrawal Assessment for Alcohol, revised scale) *n.* a scale consisting of a series of symptoms rated from 0 (not present) to 7 (most extreme), the cumulative score of which provides the basis for treatment of patients undergoing alcohol withdrawal. Medication is optional for patients with a score of 8–14, a score of over 15 requires treatment with chlordiazepoxide, and a score of over 20 poses a strong risk of delirium tremens.

CJD *n.* *see* Creutzfeldt-Jakob disease.

clamp (klamp) *n.* a surgical instrument designed to compress a structure, such as a blood vessel or a cut end of the intestine. See illustration.

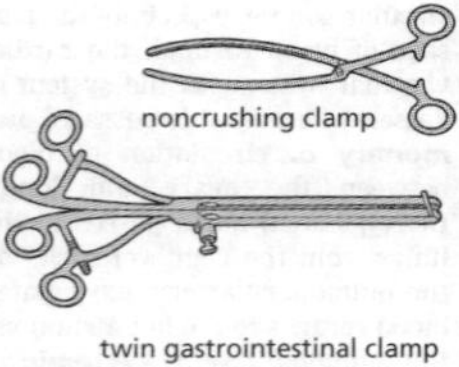

Intestinal clamps

clasp-knife rigidity (klahsp-nyf) *n.* *see* spasticity.

claudication (klaw-di-kay-shŏn) *n.* limping. **intermittent c.** a cramping pain in the calf and leg muscles, induced by exercise and relieved by rest, that is caused by an inadequate supply of blood to the affected muscles.

claustrophobia (klaw-strŏ-foh-biă) *n.* a morbid fear of enclosed places. *See also* phobia.

clavicle (klav-i-kŭl) *n.* the collar bone: a long slender curved bone, a pair of which form the front part of the shoulder girdle. Fracture of the clavicle is a common sports injury: the majority of cases require no treatment other than supporting the weight of the arm in a sling. **—clavicular** (klă-vik-yoo-ler) *adj.*

clavulanic acid (klav-yoo-lan-ik) *n.* a drug that interferes with the enzymes (penicillinases) that inactivate many penicillin-type antibiotics, such as amoxicillin. Combined with the antibiotic, clavulanic acid can overcome drug resistance.

clavus (klay-vŭs) *n.* a sharp pain in the head, as if a nail were being driven in.

claw-foot (klaw-fuut) *n.* an excessively arched foot, giving an unnaturally high instep. In most cases the cause is unknown, but the deformity may sometimes be due to an imbalance between the muscles flexing the toes and the shorter muscles that extend them. Medical name: **pes cavus**.

claw-hand (klaw-hand) *n.* flexion and contraction of the fingers with extension at the joints between the fingers and the hand, giving a claw-like appearance. Causes of claw-hand include injuries, syringomyelia, and leprosy. *See also* Dupuytren's contracture.

clearance (renal clearance) (kleer-ăns) *n.* a quantitative measure of the rate at which waste products are removed from the blood by the kidneys or through the process of dialysis. It is expressed in terms of the volume of blood that could be completely cleared of a particular substance in a specified unit of time.

cleavage (kleev-ij) *n.* (in embryology) the process of repeated cell division of the fertilized egg to form a ball of cells that becomes the blastocyst.

cleft lip (harelip) (kleft) *n.* the congenital deformity of a cleft in the upper lip, on one or both sides of the midline. It is often associated with a cleft palate. Medical name: **cheiloschisis**.

cleft palate *n.* a fissure in the midline of the palate due to failure of the two sides to fuse in embryonic development. Only part of the palate may be affected, or the cleft may extend the full length with bilateral clefts at the front of the maxilla; it may be accompanied by a cleft lip and disturbance of tooth formation.

cleid- (cleido-, clid-, clido-) *combining form denoting* the clavicle (collar bone).

cleidocranial dysostosis (kly-doh-**kray**-niăl dis-os-**toh**-sis) *n.* a congenital defect of bone formation in which the skull bones ossify imperfectly and the collar bones (clavicles) are absent.

clemastine (klem-ă-steen) *n.* an antihistamine used to relieve the symptoms of hay fever and urticaria. It is administered by mouth. Trade name: **Tavegil**.

Clifton Assessment Procedures for the Elderly (CAPE) (klif-tŏn) *n.* an assessment tool designed to assess quality of life and physical and cognitive dependency levels in the elderly, which gives an indication of current met and unmet needs.

climacteric (kly-**mak**-ter-ik) *n. see* menopause. **male c.** declining sexual drive and fertility in men, usually occurring around or after middle age.

clindamycin (klin-dă-**my**-sin) *n.* an antibiotic administered by mouth or injection to treat serious bacterial infections. The most severe side-effect is pseudomembranous colitis caused by overgrowth of *Clostridium difficile*, which limits its use. Trade name: **Dalacin C**.

clinic (klin-ik) *n.* **1.** an establishment or department of a hospital devoted to the treatment of particular diseases or the medical care of out-patients. **2.** a gathering of instructors, students, and patients, usually in a hospital ward, for the examination and treatment of the patients.

clinical audit (klin-i-kăl) *n.* a process by which doctors, nurses, and other health-care professionals systematically review the procedures used for diagnosis, care, and treatment against agreed standards, examining how associated resources are used and investigating the effects care has on the outcome and quality of life for the patient.

clinical commissioning group *n.* (in England) a group of health-care professionals forming a statutory body within the NHS whose decision-making role involves communication across other groups, increased accountability, and strategic planning to reduce inequalities in public health and social care. Commissioning groups were developed from primary care trusts, which were disbanded in 2013; they must have a registered nurse, a hospital doctor, and two lay members on their board. The geographical boundaries of these groups should not normally cross those of local authorities and they must have a clear link to their locality.

Clinical Global Impression (CGI) *n.* rating scales used by clinicians to measure symptom severity and treatment response in patients with psychiatric illnesses. They are considered to be a good measure of the clinical utility of a treatment. The Clinical Global Impression – Severity scale (**CGI-S**) is used to rate the severity of the patient's symptoms relative to other patients with the same diagnosis. The Clinical Global Impression – Improvement scale (**CGI-I**) measures change in the patient's presentation from baseline.

clinical governance (guv-er-năns) *n.* a system for making local health services responsive to patients and aiming to reduce variations in clinical practice, thus improving national standards. It consists of audit, continuing professional development, standard setting, workforce planning, complaints handling, user involvement, risk assessment, and research and development.

clinical medicine *n.* the branch of medicine dealing with the study of actual patients and the diagnosis and treatment of disease at the bedside, as opposed to the study of disease by pathology or other laboratory work.

clinical supervision *n.* a formal process of professional support and learning that enables individual practitioners to develop knowledge and competence, assume responsibility for their own practice, and enhance patient protection and safety of care in a wide range of situations. The Nursing and Midwifery

Council recognizes clinical supervision as an important part of clinical governance and a means of maintaining and improving standards of patient care. Clinical supervision is a statutory requirement for midwives but not for nurses or health visitors.

clinical trial *n.* *see* intervention study.

clinodactyly (klin-oh-**dak**-tili) *n.* congenital deflection of one or more digits from the central axis of the hand or foot. Clinodactyly may affect both hands (or feet) but most commonly affects the fifth finger (which curves towards the fourth); it may be found in association with other congenital malformations or as a part of certain syndromes (e.g. Down's).

clitoridectomy (klit-er-id-**ek**-tŏmi) *n.* surgical removal of the clitoris. *See* female genital mutilation.

clitoris (**klit**-er-iss) *n.* the female counterpart of the penis, which contains erectile tissue (*see* corpus (cavernosum)) but is unconnected with the urethra. It becomes erect under conditions of sexual stimulation.

clitoromegaly (klit-er-oh-**meg**-ăli) *n.* abnormal development of the clitoris due to excessive exposure to androgens, either from abnormal endogenous production or exogenous administration.

cloaca (kloh-**ay**-kă) *n.* the most posterior part of the embryonic hindgut. It becomes divided into the rectum and the urinogenital sinus.

clomethiazole (chlormethiazole) (kloh-mi-**th'y**-ă-zohl) *n.* a sedative and hypnotic drug administered by mouth to treat severe insomnia in the elderly (when associated with confusion, agitation, and restlessness) and alcohol withdrawal symptoms.

clomifene (clomiphene) (**kloh**-mi-feen) *n.* a synthetic nonsteroidal compound (*see* anti-androgen) administered by mouth to induce ovulation and subsequent menstruation in women who fail to ovulate. Trade name: **Clomid**.

clomipramine (kloh-**mip**-ră-meen) *n.* a tricyclic antidepressant administered by mouth to treat depressive illness, phobias, and obsessional states.

clonazepam (kloh-**naz**-ĕ-pam) *n.* a drug with anticonvulsant properties, administered by mouth to treat epileptic seizures. Trade name: **Rivotril**.

clone (klohn) **1.** *n.* a group of cells (usually bacteria) descended from a single cell by asexual reproduction and therefore genetically identical to each other and to the parent cell. **2.** *n.* an organism derived from a single cell of its parent and therefore genetically identical to it. **gene c.** a group of identical genes produced by techniques of genetic engineering. **3.** *vb.* to form a clone.

clonic (**klon**-ik) *adj.* of, relating to, or resembling clonus. The term is most commonly used to describe the rhythmical limb movements seen as part of a generalized tonic-clonic seizure (*see* epilepsy).

clonidine (**kloh**-ni-deen) *n.* a drug, administered by mouth, occasionally used to treat high blood pressure (hypertension). Trade name: **Catapres**.

clonus (kloh-nŭs) *n.* rhythmical contraction of a muscle in response to a suddenly applied and then sustained stretch stimulus. It is most readily obtained at the ankle and is usually a sign of disease in the brain or spinal cord.

clopidogrel (kloh-**pid**-oh-grel) *n.* an antiplatelet drug administered by mouth to prevent strokes or heart attacks in those at risk. Trade name: **Plavix**.

Clostridium (klo-**strid**-iŭm) *n.* a genus of mostly Gram-positive anaerobic spore-forming rodlike bacteria commonly found in soil and in the intestinal tract of humans and animals. **C. botulinum** a species that grows freely in badly preserved canned foods, producing a toxin causing serious food poisoning (*see* botulism). **C. difficile** (**C. diff.**) a species found in the intestine that causes pseudomembranous colitis, an increasingly common hospital-acquired infection. **C. tetani** a species that causes tetanus on contamination of wounds. **C. perfringens** (**Welch's bacillus**) a species that causes blood poisoning, food poisoning, and gas gangrene.

SEE WEB LINKS

- A guide to *Clostridium difficile* from the NHS Choices website, including the ways in which it can cause infection

clotrimazole (kloh-**trim**-ă-zohl) *n.* an antifungal drug used to treat all types of fungal skin infections (including ringworm), outer ear infection, and vaginal thrush. It is applied to the infected part as a cream, spray, or solution or as vaginal pessaries. Trade name: **Canesten**.

clotting factors (**klot**-ing) *pl. n.* *see* coagulation factors.

clotting time *n.* *see* coagulation time.

clozapine (**kloz**-ă-peen) *n.* an atypical antipsychotic drug administered by mouth in the treatment of schizophrenia resistant to conventional antipsychotics. Trade names: **Clozaril**, **Denzapine**, **Zaponex**.

clubbing (**klub**-ing) *n.* thickening of the tissues at the bases of the finger and toe nails so that the normal angle between the nail and the digit is filled in. In extreme cases the digit end becomes bulbous like a club or drumstick. Clubbing is seen in some diseases of the heart and respiratory system, cirrhosis, and as a harmless congenital abnormality.

club-foot (**klub**-fuut) *n.* *see* talipes.

clumping (**klump**-ing) *n.* *see* agglutination.

cluster headache (**klust**-er) *n.* a variant of migraine more common in men than in women. The unilateral pain around one eye is very severe and lasts between 15 minutes and three hours. It is associated with drooping of the eyelid (ptosis), a bloodshot eye, a small pupil, and/or excessive production of tears in the eye.

Clutton's joint (**klu**-t'nz) *n.* a painless joint effusion in a child, usually in the knee, caused by inflammation of the synovial membranes due to congenital syphilis. [H. H. Clutton (1850–1909), British surgeon]

CML *n.* chronic myeloid leukaemia. *See* myeloid (leukaemia).

CMV *n.* *see* cytomegalovirus.

CNS *n.* *see* central nervous system.

COAD *n.* chronic obstructive airways disease (*see* chronic obstructive pulmonary disease).

coagulant (koh-ag-yoo-lănt) *n.* any substance capable of converting blood from a liquid to a solid state. *See* blood coagulation.

coagulase (koh-ag-yoo-layz) *n.* an enzyme, formed by disease-producing varieties of certain bacteria of the genus *Staphylococcus*, that causes blood plasma to coagulate. Staphylococci that are positive when tested for coagulase production are classified as belonging to the species *Staphylococcus aureus*.

coagulation (koh-ag-yoo-lay-shŏn) *n.* the process by which a colloidal liquid changes to a jelly-like mass. *See* blood coagulation.

coagulation factors (clotting factors) *pl. n.* a group of substances present in blood plasma that are responsible for the conversion of blood from a liquid to a solid state (*see* blood coagulation). Although they have specific names, most coagulation factors are referred to by an agreed set of Roman numerals (*see* Factor VIII, Factor IX, Factor XI).

coagulation time (clotting time) *n.* the time taken for blood or blood plasma to coagulate (*see* blood coagulation).

coagulum (koh-ag-yoo-lŭm) *n.* a mass of coagulated matter, such as that formed when blood clots.

coalesce (koh-ă-less) *vb.* to grow together or unite. **—coalescence** *n.*

coal tar (kohl) *n.* *see* tar.

coal-worker's pneumoconiosis (anthracosis) (kohl-werkerz) *n.* a lung disease caused by coal dust. It affects mainly coal miners but also other exposed workers, such as lightermen, if the lungs' capacity to accommodate and remove the particles is exceeded. *See* pneumoconiosis.

coarctation (koh-ark-tay-shŏn) *n.* (of the aorta) a congenital narrowing of a short segment of the aorta, resulting in high blood pressure in the upper part of the body and arms and low blood pressure in the legs. The defect is corrected by surgery or stent implant.

Coats' disease (kohts) *n.* a congenital anomaly of the blood vessels of the retina, which are abnormally dilated and leaking. This results in subretinal haemorrhage and retinal detachment. [G. Coats (1876–1915), British ophthalmologist]

cobalt (koh-bawlt) *n.* a metallic element that forms part of the vitamin B_{12} molecule. Symbol: Co. **cobalt-60 (radiocobalt)** a powerful emitter of gamma radiation, used in the radiation treatment of cancer (*see* radiotherapy, teletherapy).

cocaine (kŏ-kayn) *n.* an alkaloid, derived from the leaves of the coca plant (*Erythroxylon coca*) or prepared synthetically, formerly used as a local anaesthetic in ear, nose, and throat surgery. Since it may lead to psychological dependence, cocaine has been replaced by safer anaesthetics.

coccus (**kok**-ŭs) *n.* (*pl.* **cocci**) any spherical bacterium. *See* gonococcus, meningococcus, Micrococcus, pneumococcus, Staphylococcus, Streptococcus.

coccy- (coccyg-, coccygo-) *combining form denoting* the coccyx.

coccygodynia (coccydynia) (kok-si-goh-**din**-iă) *n.* pain in the coccyx and the neighbouring area, usually as a result of trauma.

coccyx (**kok**-siks) *n.* (*pl.* **coccyges** or **coccyxes**) the lowermost element of the backbone: the vestigial human tail. It consists of four rudimentary **coccygeal vertebrae** fused to form a triangular bone that articulates with the sacrum. *See also* vertebra. **—coccygeal** (kok-**sij**-iăl) *adj.*

cochlea (**kok**-liă) *n.* the spiral organ of the labyrinth of the ear, which is concerned with the reception and analysis of sound. **—cochlear** (**kok**-li-er) *adj.*

cochlear duct (scala media) *n. see* scala.

cochlear implant *n.* a device to improve the hearing of profoundly deaf people who derive no benefit from conventional hearing aids. It consists of an electrode that is permanently implanted into the inner ear (cochlea). An external battery-powered device with a microphone and an electronic processing unit passes information to the electrode using radio-frequency waves.

cochlear nerve (acoustic nerve, auditory nerve) *n.* the nerve connecting the cochlea to the brain and therefore responsible for transmitting the nerve impulses relating to hearing. It forms part of the vestibulocochlear nerve.

Cockayne's syndrome (kok-**aynz**) *n.* a hereditary disorder (inherited as an autosomal recessive condition) associated with trisomy of chromosome no. 20. Clinical features include epidermolysis bullosa, dwarfism, learning disability, and pigmentary degeneration of the retina. [E. A. Cockayne (1880–1956), British physician]

co-codamol (koh-**koh**-dă-mol) *n. see* codeine.

co-codaprin (koh-**koh**-dă-prin) *n. see* codeine.

codeine (**koh**-deen) *n.* an analgesic derived from morphine but less potent as a pain killer and sedative and less toxic. It is administered by mouth or intramuscular injection to relieve pain and by mouth to suppress dry coughs and treat diarrhoea. Codeine may also be administered orally in combination with paracetamol (as **co-codamol**) or aspirin (as **co-codaprin**) for pain relief.

cod liver oil (kod) *n.* a pale yellow oil, extracted from the livers of cod and related fish, that is rich in vitamins A and D and used in the treatment and prevention of deficiencies of these vitamins (e.g. rickets).

co-dydramol (koh-**dy**-dră-mol) *n. see* dihydrocodeine.

-coele *combining form denoting* **1.** a body cavity. **2.** *see* -cele.

coeli- (coelio-) *combining form denoting* the abdomen or belly.

coeliac (seel-i-ak) *adj.* of or relating to the abdominal region. **c. trunk** a branch of the abdominal aorta supplying the stomach, spleen, liver, and gall bladder.

coeliac disease *n.* a condition in which the small intestine fails to digest and absorb food. It is due to a permanent sensitivity of the intestinal lining to the protein gliadin, which is contained in gluten in the germ of wheat and rye and causes atrophy of the digestive and absorptive cells of the intestine. Symptoms, which include stunted growth, distended abdomen, and pale frothy foul-smelling stools, abate with a gluten-free diet. Medical name: **gluten-sensitive enteropathy**.

SEE WEB LINKS

- Website of Coeliac UK

coelioscopy (see-li-**os**-kŏpi) *n.* the technique of introducing an endoscope through an incision in the abdominal wall to examine the intestines and other organs within the abdominal cavity.

coenzyme (koh-**en**-zym) *n.* a non-protein organic compound that, in the presence of an enzyme, plays an essential role in the reaction that is catalysed by the enzyme.

coffee-ground vomit (**kof**-ee-grownd) *n.* vomit that has the appearance of ground coffee. It is composed of denatured oxidized blood and reflects bleeding in the upper gastrointestinal tract.

Coffin–Lowry syndrome (**kof**-in **low**-ri) *n.* an inherited disease, more severe in males, resulting in developmental delay and profound learning disability. It is characterized by distinctive facial anomalies, short stature, microcephaly, and kyphoscoliosis; some patients have episodes of collapse when startled or excited (**stimulus-induced drop episodes**; **SIDE**). [G. S. Coffin (1923–), US paediatrician; R. B. Lowry (1932–), British geneticist]

Cogan's syndrome (**koh**-gănz) *n.* a disorder in which keratitis and iridocyclitis (*see* uveitis) are associated with tinnitus, vertigo, and bilateral sensorineural deafness. [D. G. Cogan (1908–93), US ophthalmologist]

cognition (kog-**nish**-ŏn) *n.* a group of mental activities (including perception, recognition, and judgment) that leads to awareness of an object or situation. **—cognitive** (**kog**-ni-tiv) *adj.*

cognitive behavioural therapy (CBT) *n.* a cognitive therapy that is combined with behavioural elements (*see* behaviour therapy). The patient is encouraged to analyse his or her specific ways of thinking around a problem. The therapist then looks at the resulting behaviour and the consequences of that thinking and tries to encourage the patient to change his or her cognition in order to avoid adverse behaviour or its consequences.

cognitive psychology *n.* the school of psychology concerned with the ways in which knowledge is acquired, stored, correlated, and retrieved, by studying the mental processes underlying attention, concept formation, information processing, memory, and speech.

cognitive therapy *n.* a form of psychotherapy based on the belief that psychological problems are the products of faulty ways of thinking about the world. It may involve analysis and retraining of unhelpful behaviours (*see* cognitive behavioural therapy) or it may include an element of psychodynamic exploration of the problems (**cognitive analytical therapy**).

coitus (sexual intercourse, copulation) (koh-it-ŭs) *n.* sexual contact between a man and a woman during which the erect penis enters the vagina and is moved within it by pelvic thrusts until ejaculation occurs. **c. interruptus** an unreliable contraceptive method in which the penis is removed from the vagina before ejaculation of semen. *See also* orgasm. —**coital** *adj.*

col- (coli-, colo-) *combining form denoting* the colon.

colchicine (kol-chi-seen) *n.* a drug obtained from the meadow saffron (*Colchicum autumnale*), administered by mouth to relieve pain in attacks of gout and to prevent attacks of gout and hereditary polyserositis.

cold (common cold) (kohld) *n.* a widespread infectious virus disease causing inflammation of the mucous membranes of the nose, throat, and bronchial tubes. Symptoms include a sore throat, stuffy or runny nose, headache, cough, and general malaise.

cold sore *n. see* herpes (simplex).

colectomy (kŏ-lek-tŏmi) *n.* surgical removal of the colon (**total c.**) or a segment of the colon (**partial c.**). *See also* hemicolectomy, proctocolectomy.

colestipol (kŏ-les-ti-pol) *n.* a drug that binds bile acids (*see* bile-acid sequestrant). It is administered by mouth to lower cholesterol levels in the blood in patients with hyperlipidaemia and primary hypercholesterolaemia. Trade name: **Colestid**.

colestyramine (cholestyramine) (koli-sty-ră-meen) *n.* a drug that binds bile acids (*see* bile-acid sequestrant). It is administered by mouth to relieve conditions due to irritant effects of bile acids (such as the itching that occurs in obstructive jaundice), to treat diarrhoea, and to lower blood levels of cholesterol and other fats. Trade names: **Questran**, **Questran Light**.

colic (kol-ik) *n.* paroxysms of abdominal pain, usually of fluctuating severity. **infantile c.** colic that is common among babies, due to wind in the intestine associated with feeding difficulties. **intestinal c.** colic due to partial or complete obstruction of the intestine or to constipation. Medical name: **enteralgia**. **renal c.** excruciating pain caused by dilatation and spasm of the ureter when stones are present in the kidney, renal pelvis, or ureter. *See also* biliary (colic).

coliform bacteria (kol-i-form) *pl. n.* a group of Gram-negative rodlike bacteria that are normally found in the gastrointestinal tract and ferment the sugar lactose. It includes the genera *Enterobacter*, *Escherichia*, and *Klebsiella*.

colistimethate sodium (colistin) (kŏ-list-i-**mee**-thayt) *n.* an antibiotic administered by intravenous injection to treat resistant Gram-negative infections and by inhalation to treat infections associated with cystic fibrosis. Trade names: **Colobreathe**, **Colomycin**, **Promixin**.

colitis (kŏ-**ly**-tis) *n.* inflammation of the colon. **infectious c.** colitis due to viruses, bacteria, or protozoans (for example, **Entamoeba histolytica** causes amoebic colitis; *see* dysentery). **inflammatory c.** encompasses Crohn's disease, ulcerative colitis (which also involves the rectum; *see* proctitis), and microscopic colitis (which can only be seen under a microscope). Symptoms of inflammatory colitis may include diarrhoea, abdominal pain, and blood and mucus in the stools. **ischaemic c.** colitis caused by partial or temporary cessation of blood supply to the colon.

collagen (**kol**-ă-jin) *n.* a protein that is the principal constituent of white fibrous connective tissue (as occurs in tendons). Collagen is also found in skin, bone, cartilage, and ligaments.

collagen disease *n.* an obsolete term for connective-tissue disease.

collapsing pulse (kŏ-**laps**-ing) *n.* *see* Corrigan's pulse.

collar bone (**kol**-er) *n.* *see* clavicle.

collateral (kŏ-**lat**-er-ăl) **1.** *adj.* accessory or secondary. **2.** *n.* a branch (e.g. of a nerve fibre) that is at right angles to the main part.

collateral circulation *n.* **1.** an alternative route provided for the blood by secondary vessels when a primary vessel becomes blocked. **2.** the channels of communication between the blood vessels supplying the heart.

Colles' fracture (**kol**-iss) *n.* *see* fracture. [A. Colles (1773–1843), Irish surgeon]

collodion (kŏ-**loh**-diŏn) *n.* a syrupy solution of nitrocellulose in a mixture of alcohol and ether. When applied to minor wounds it evaporates to leave a thin clear transparent skin. Flexible collodion also contains camphor and castor oil, which allow the skin to stretch a little more.

colloid (**kol**-oid) *n.* a mixture in which particles of one component (diameter 10^{-6}–10^{-4} mm) are dispersed in a continuous phase of another component.—**colloidal** *adj.*

collyrium (ko-**leer**-iŭm) *n.* a medicated solution used to bathe the eyes.

coloboma (kolŏ-**boh**-mă) *n.* (*pl.* **colobomata**] a defect in the development of the eye causing abnormalities ranging in severity from a notch in the lower part of the iris, making the pupil pear-shaped, to defects in the retina, choroid, and optic nerve fundus.

colon (**koh**-lŏn) *n.* the main part of the large intestine, which consists of four sections – the **ascending**, **transverse**, **descending**, and **sigmoid colons** (see illustration). The colon absorbs large amounts of water and electrolytes from the undigested food passed on from the small intestine. At intervals strong peristaltic movements move the dehydrated contents (faeces)

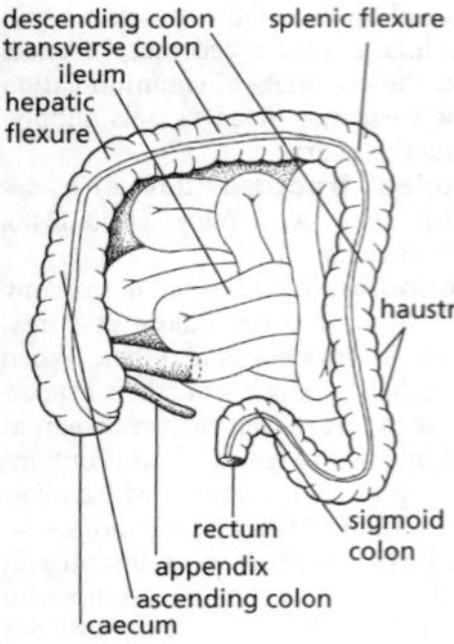

The colon

towards the rectum. **—colonic** (koh-**lon**-ik) *adj.*

colonic irrigation *n.* washing out the contents of the large bowel by means of copious enemas, using either water, with or without soap, or a liquid medication.

colonoscopy (koh-lŏn-**os**-kŏpi) *n.* an invasive endoscopic procedure for examining the interior of the colon and the terminal ileum. A **colonoscope** is a flexible steerable telescopic instrument that houses a high-definition digital video camera; it is introduced through the anus.

colony (**kol**-ŏni) *n.* a discrete population or mass of microorganisms, usually bacteria, all of which are considered to have developed from a single parent cell. *See also* culture.

colorectal cancer (ko-lĕ-**rek**-tăl) *n.* malignancy of the large intestine (colon, appendix, and rectum). Although it is the fourth most common cause of death from cancer, most cases should be preventable by screening and changes to lifestyle. Risk factors include older age, increased consumption of red meat, excessive alcohol intake, smoking, and sedentary life. Symptoms include change in bowel habit, rectal bleeding, loss of appetite and weight, anaemia, and gastrointestinal obstruction. Early localized disease is amenable to surgery, preoperative chemoradiation, and postoperative chemotherapy; advanced disease necessitates a palliative approach.

colorimeter (kul-ŏ-**rim**-it-er) *n.* an instrument for determining the concentration of a particular compound in a preparation by comparing the intensity of colour in it with that in a standard preparation of known concentration.

colostomy (kŏ-**lost**-ŏmi) *n.* a surgical operation in which a part of the colon is brought through the anterior abdominal wall and an artificial opening is created in order to drain or decompress the contents of the colon. The colostomy may be temporary, eventually being closed to restore intestinal continuity; or permanent, when the colon distal to the colostomy has been removed or is diseased.

SEE WEB LINKS

- Website of the British Colostomy Association

colostrum (kŏ-**los**-trŭm) *n.* the first secretion from the breast, occurring shortly after, or sometimes before, birth, prior to the secretion of true milk. It is a relatively clear fluid containing serum, white blood cells, and protective antibodies.

colour blindness (**kul**-er) *n.* any of various conditions in which certain colours are confused with one another. True lack of colour appreciation is extremely rare (*see* monochromat); the most common type of colour blindness is red-blindness (*see* Daltonism). *See also* deuteranopia, tritanopia.

colour flow ultrasound imaging *n. see* Doppler ultrasound.

colp- (colpo-) *combining form denoting* the vagina.

colpitis (kol-**py**-tis) *n.* inflammation of the vagina. *See* vaginitis.

colpohysterectomy (kol-poh-hiss-ter-**ek**-tŏmi) *n.* surgical removal of the uterus through the vagina. *See* hysterectomy.

colpoperineorrhaphy (kol-poh-pe-ri-ni-**o**-răfi) *n.* an operation to repair tears in the vagina and the muscles surrounding its opening.

colporrhaphy (perineal repair) (kol-**po**-răfi) *n.* an operation designed to remove lax and redundant vaginal tissue and so reduce the diameter of the vagina in cases of prolapse of the base of the bladder (**anterior c.**) or of the rectum (**posterior c.**).

colposcopy (kol-**pos**-kŏpi) *n.* examination of the cervix under low-power binocular magnification and an intense light source. Abnormalities are revealed as white areas after application of acetic acid and iodine to the cervix. —**colposcopic** (kol-pŏ-**skop**-ik) *adj.*

colposuspension (kol-poh-su-**spen**-shŏn) *n.* a surgical procedure for treating stress incontinence in women in which the upper part of the vaginal wall is fixed to the anterior abdominal wall by unabsorbable suture material. Performed through an abdominal incision (**Burch c.**) or using a laparoscope (**laparoscopic c.**), this operation has now been largely replaced by less invasive sling procedures.

column (**kol**-ŭm) *n.* (in anatomy) any pillar-shaped structure, especially any of the tracts of grey matter found in the spinal cord.

coma (**koh**-mă) *n.* a state of unrousable unconsciousness.

comatose (**koh**-mă-tohs) *adj.* in a state of coma; unconscious.

combined therapy (kŏm-**bynd**) *n.* therapy that combines several types of treatment in order to improve results. It is usually a combination of surgery with radiotherapy and/or chemotherapy for the treatment of malignant tumours (*see* adjuvant therapy). *See also* sandwich therapy.

comedo (**kom**-i-doh) *n.* (*pl.* **comedones**) *see* blackhead.

commando operation (kŏ-**mahn**-doh) *n.* a major operation performed to remove a malignant tumour from the head and neck. Extensive dissection, often involving the face, is followed by reconstruction to restore function and cosmetic acceptability.

commensal (kŏ-**men**-săl) *n.* an organism that lives in close association with another of a different species without either harming or benefiting it. *Compare* symbiosis. **—commensalism** *n.*

comminuted fracture (kom-i-new-tid) *n.* *see* fracture.

commissure (kom-iss-yoor) *n.* **1.** a bundle of nerve fibres that crosses the midline of the central nervous system, often connecting similar structures on each side. **2.** any other tissue connecting two similar structures.

commodification (kŏ-mod-ifi-**kay**-shŏn) *n.* the idea that objects or people that are not usually regarded as commodities can have an economic value. It suggests that the health care of a client is a product that can be bought or sold, and clients may be identified as healthcare consumers. However, there are practical and ethical issues in this approach, which suggest that health care should not be seen as a commodity.

common assessment framework (CAF) (kom-ŏn) *n.* a Department for Education initiative focused on assessing and meeting the needs of children and young people whose development is giving cause for concern. Children, their families, or professionals can initiate a four-step process that is voluntary and requires informed consent. It involves: (1) identifying the child's needs early; (2) assessing those needs; (3) delivering interventions to meet those needs via a multidisciplinary team of service practitioners whose work is coordinated by a lead professional; (4) reviewing progress. The CAF is a request for services, not a risk assessment tool.

commotio retinae (kŏ-**moh**-shi-oh **ret**-i-nee) *n.* swelling of the retina, usually resulting from blunt trauma to the eye.

communicable disease (contagious disease, infectious disease) (kŏ-**mew**-nik-ăbŭl) *n.* any disease that can be transmitted from one person to another. This may occur by direct physical contact, by common handling of a contaminated object (*see* fomes), through a disease carrier, or by spread of infected droplets exhaled into the air.

community-acquired pneumonia (CAP) *n.* *see* pneumonia.

community health (kŏ-**mew**-niti) *n.* preventive services, mainly outside the hospital, involving the surveillance of special groups of the population, such as preschool and school children, women, and the elderly, by means of routine clinical assessment and screening tests. *See also* child health clinic.

community hospital *n.* *see* hospital.

community interest group *n.* any of the groups that work with NHS foundation trusts to represent the views of patients and other interested parties. They are often formed around specific disease categories or patient groups (e.g. deaf patients, children in care).

community medicine *n.* *see* public health medicine.

community midwife (domiciliary midwife) *n.* (in Britain) a registered nurse with special training in midwifery (both hospital and domiciliary practice). The midwife must be registered with the Nursing and Midwifery Council in order to practise; this requires regular refresher courses to supplement the basic qualification of **registered midwife** (RM). Community midwives are attached to general practices or hospitals and their work includes home deliveries and antenatal and postnatal care in the community.

community nurses *pl. n.* (in Britain) a generic term for health visitors, community midwives, and district nurses. *See also* domiciliary services.

community paediatrician *n.* a consultant in paediatrics with special responsibility for the care of children outside the hospital. *See also* community health.

community services *pl. n. see* domiciliary services.

comparative study (kŏm-pa-ră-tiv) *n.* a study in which a participant is randomly assigned to one of two or more different treatment groups for purposes of comparing the effects of the treatments.

compartment (kŏm-part-mĕnt) *n.* any one of the spaces in a limb that are bounded by bone and thick sheets of fascia and contain the muscles and other tissues of the limb. **c. syndrome** swelling of the muscles in a compartment, which raises the pressure within so that the blood supply to the muscle is cut off, causing ischaemia and further swelling. It is caused by trauma, damage to blood vessels, reperfusion after ischaemia, or tight casts or bandages. *See also* Volkmann's contracture.

compassion *n.* the perception and, as far as is possible, understanding of another's suffering, important as a motivation in all caring professions. However, overwork may destroy fellow feeling (**compassion fatigue**): professionals should be aware of this possibility and make sure they are looking after themselves properly. Kindness and understanding are often undervalued as components of treatment by professionals but not by patients.

compatibility (kŏm-pati-**bil**-iti) *n.* the degree to which the body's defence systems will tolerate the presence of intruding foreign material, such as blood when transfused or a kidney when transplanted. *Compare* incompatibility. *See also* histocompatibility, immunity. **—compatible** *adj.*

compensation (kom-pen-say-shŏn) *n.* **1.** the act of making up for a functional or structural deficiency. For example, compensation for the loss of a diseased kidney is brought about by an increase in size of the remaining kidney, so restoring the urine-producing capacity. **2.** financial redress for injury or loss caused, for example, by negligence; the amount usually corresponds to the degree of harm suffered. **3.** (in psychoanalysis) the act of exaggerating an approved character trait to make up for a weakness in an opposite trait.

competence (**kom**-pĕt-ĕnss) *n. see* capacity.

complaints system (kŏm-**playnts**) *n.* a process that enables patients to voice concerns about the standard of care they receive In the UK, any complaints should be raised as soon as possible, in the first instance locally with the NHS provider involved. If a patient is not satisfied with the outcome the matter can be referred to the Health Service Ombudsman.

complement (**kom**-pli-mĕnt) *n.* a system of proteins that interact with one another to aid the body's defences when antibodies combine with antigens. *See also* immunity.

complementary medicine (kom-pli-**ment**-ări) *n.* various forms of therapy that are viewed as complementary to conventional medicine. Previously, complementary therapies were regarded as an alternative to conventional therapies, and the two types were considered to be mutually exclusive (hence the former names **alternative medicine** and **fringe medicine**). However, many practitioners now have dual training in conventional and complementary therapies. There is very limited provision for complementary medicine within the confines of the National Health Service. *See* acupuncture, aromatherapy, chiropractic, homeopathy, naturopathy, osteopathy, reflexology, reiki.

complement fixation *n.* the binding of complement to the complex that is formed when an antibody reacts with a specific antigen. Because complement is taken up from the serum only when such a reaction has occurred, testing for the presence of complement after mixing a suspension of a known organism with a patient's serum can give confirmation of infection with a suspected organism.

complex (**kom**-pleks) *n.* (in psychoanalysis) an emotionally charged and repressed group of ideas and beliefs that is capable of influencing an individual's behaviour.

complex partial seizure *n. see* epilepsy.

compliance (kŏm-**ply**-ĕnss) *n. see* adherence.

complication (kom-pli-**kay**-shŏn) *n.* a disease or condition arising during the course of or as a consequence of another disease.

compos mentis (**kom**-pŏs **men**-tis) *adj.* of sound mind; sane.

compress (**kom**-press) *n.* a pad of material soaked in hot or cold water and applied to an injured part of the body to relieve the pain of inflammation.

compressed air illness (caisson disease) (kŏm-**prest**) *n.* a syndrome occurring in people working under high pressure in diving bells or at great depths with breathing apparatus. On return to normal atmospheric pressure nitrogen dissolved in the bloodstream expands to form bubbles, causing pain (the **bends**) and blocking the circulation in small blood vessels in the brain and elsewhere (**decompression sickness**). Symptoms may be eliminated by returning the victim to a higher atmospheric pressure and reducing this gradually.

compression (kŏm-**presh**-ŏn) *n.* the state in which an organ, tissue, or part is subject to pressure. **cerebral c.** pressure on brain tissue from a cerebral tumour, intracranial haematoma, etc. **c. venography** *see* venography.

compulsion (kŏm-**pul**-shŏn) *n.* an obsession that takes the form of a motor act, such as repetitive washing based on a fear of contamination, as seen in obsessive–compulsive disorder.

compulsory admission (involuntary admission) (kŏm-**pul**-ser-i) *n.* (in Britain) the entry and detention of a person within an institution without his or her consent, either because of mental illness (*see* Mental Health Act) or severe social deprivation and self-neglect (*see* section 47 removal). *Compare* voluntary admission.

computer-assisted surgery (image-guided surgery, surgical navigation) *n.* a technique by which a virtual image of the patient is created from CT scans, MRI scans, X-rays, or ultrasound scans and loaded into a computer. Special instruments connected to the computer are then applied to certain reference points on the patient. The computer can thereafter produce a picture of the location of the instrument within the patient.

computerized tomography (CT) (kŏm-**pew**-tĕ-ryzd) *n.* a form of X-ray examination in which the X-ray source and detector (**CT scanner**) rotate around the object to be scanned and the information can be used to produce cross-sectional images by computer (a **CT scan**). A higher radiation dose is received by the patient than with some conventional X-ray techniques, but the diagnostic information obtained is far greater and should outweigh the risk. CT scanning can be used for all parts of the body.

conception (kŏn-**sep**-shŏn) *n.* **1.** (in gynaecology) the start of pregnancy, when a male germ cell (sperm) fertilizes a female germ cell (ovum) in the Fallopian tube. **2.** (in psychology) an idea or mental impression.

conceptus (kŏn-**sep**-tŭs) *n.* the products of conception: the developing fetus and its enclosing membrane at all stages in the uterus.

concha (**konk**-ă) *n.* (*pl.* **conchae**) (in anatomy) any part resembling a shell. **c. auriculae** a depression on the outer surface of the pinna (auricle), which leads to the external auditory meatus of the outer ear. *See also* nasal (concha).

concomitant (kŏn-**kom**-i-tănt) *adj.* at the same time: describing drugs that are administered together or symptoms that occur during the same period.

concordance (kŏn-**kor**-dănss) *n.* similarity of any physical characteristic that is found in both of a pair of twins.

concretion (kŏn-**kree**-shŏn) *n.* a stony mass formed within such an organ as the kidney, especially the coating of an internal organ or a foreign body with calcium salts. *See also* calculus.

concussion (kŏn-**kush**-ŏn) *n.* a condition caused by injury to the head, characterized by headache, confusion, and amnesia. These symptoms may be prolonged and constitute a **post-concussional syndrome**. *See also* (cerebral) contusion, punch-drunk syndrome.

condenser (kŏn-**den**-ser) *n.* (in microscopy) an arrangement of lenses beneath the stage of a microscope. It can be adjusted to provide correct focusing of light on the microscope slide.

conditioned reflex (kŏn-**dish**-ŏnd) *n.* a reflex in which the response occurs not to the sensory stimulus that normally causes it but to a separate stimulus, which has been learnt to be associated with it.

conditioning (kŏn-**dish**-ŏn-ing) *n.* the establishment of new behaviour by modifying the stimulus/response associations.

condom (**kon**-dŏm) *n.* a sheath made of latex rubber, plastic, or silk that is fitted over the penis during sexual intercourse. A condom is a reasonably reliable contraceptive; it also protects both partners against sexually transmitted diseases (including AIDS). **female c.** a similar device for women, designed to fit into the vagina.

conduct disorder (**kon**-dukt) *n.* a repetitive and persistent pattern of aggressive or otherwise antisocial behaviour. It is usually recognized in childhood or adolescence and can lead to antisocial personality disorder. Treatment is usually with behaviour therapy or family therapy.

conduction (kŏn-**duk**-shŏn) *n.* **1.** (in physics) the process in which heat is transferred through a substance from regions of higher to regions of lower temperature. **2.** (in physiology) the passage of a nerve impulse.

conductor (kŏn-**duk**-ter) *n.* **1.** (in physics) a substance capable of transmitting heat (e.g. copper, silver) or electricity. **2.** (in surgery) a grooved surgical director.

condyle (**kon**-dil) *n.* a rounded protuberance that occurs at the ends of some bones, e.g. the occipital bone, and forms an articulation with another bone.

condyloma (kon-di-**loh**-mă) *n.* (*pl.* **condylomata**) a raised wartlike growth. **c. acuminatum** (*pl.* **condylomata acuminata**) a wart, caused by human papillomavirus, found on the vulva, under the foreskin, or on the skin of the anal region. **c. latum** (*pl.* **condylomata lata**) a flat plaque occurring in the anogenital region in the secondary stage of syphilis.

cone (kohn) *n.* one of the two types of light-sensitive cells in the retina of the eye (*compare* rod). Cones are essential for acute vision and can also distinguish colours.

cone biopsy *n.* surgical removal, by knife or laser, of a cone-shaped segment of tissue from the cervix of the uterus. It may be performed if a cervical biopsy reveals evidence of carcinoma in situ (*see* CIN): the abnormal tissue is removed and examined microscopically for confirmation of the diagnosis.

confabulation (kŏn-fab-yoo-**lay**-shŏn) *n.* the invention of circumstantial but fictitious detail about events supposed to have occurred in the past. Usually this is to disguise a loss of memory; it typically occurs in Korsakoff's syndrome.

confection (kŏn-**fek**-shŏn) *n.* (in pharmacy) a sweet substance that is combined with a medicinal preparation to make it suitable for administration.

confidential enquiries (kon-fi-**den**-shăl) *pl. n.* special enquiries that seek to improve health and health care by collecting evidence on aspects of care, identifying any shortfalls in this, and disseminating recommendations based on these findings. They include **MBRRACE-UK** (Mothers and Babies: Reducing Risks through Audits and Confidential Enquires in the UK), which investigates maternal deaths, stillbirths, late fetal losses and terminations, and neonatal deaths; the **National Confidential Enquiry into Patient Outcome and Death**; and the **National Confidential Inquiry into Suicide and Homicide by People with Mental Illness**.

confidentiality (kon-fi-den-shi-**al**-iti) *n.* an ethical and legal obligation that requires health professionals to keep information about their patients private. Sometimes, however, it is permissible or even obligatory to breach a patient's confidence, e.g. for child protection or when a patient suffers from a notifiable disease. **—confidential** *adj.*

conflict (**kon**-flikt) *n.* (in psychology) the state produced when a stimulus produces two opposing reactions. Conflict has been used to explain the development of neurotic disorders, and the resolution of conflict remains an important part of psychoanalysis. *See also* conversion.

confounding (kŏn-**fown**-ding) *n.* the situation in which an apparent association between two variables is in fact explained by a third variable that correlates with both (a **confounding factor**). If confounding is not recognized, it can lead to the false assumption that two variables are directly related, known as a **spurious relationship**.

congenital (kŏn-**jen**-it'l) *adj.* describing a condition that is recognized at birth or that is believed to have been present since birth. Congenital malformations include all disorders present at birth whether they are inherited or caused by an environmental factor.

congenital adrenal hyperplasia (CAH) *n.* a family of autosomal recessive genetic disorders causing decreased activity of any of the enzymes involved in the synthesis of cortisol from cholesterol. Adrenal hyperplasia occurs due to excessive stimulation of the glands by ACTH (adrenocorticotrophic hormone) in response to the cortisol deficiency. The most serious consequence is adrenal crisis and/or severe salt wasting due to lack of cortisol and/or aldosterone. The condition is often easier to spot at birth in females, who may have indeterminate genitalia due to high levels of testosterone in utero.

congenital dislocation of the hip (CDH) *n.* an abnormality of the hip joint, present at birth, in which the head of the femur is displaced or easily displaceable from the acetabulum, which is poorly developed. It frequently affects both hip joints. *See also* Barlow's manoeuvre, Ortolani manoeuvre.

congenital heart disease *n.* a disorder of the heart, present at birth, that is due to malformation or dysfunction of the heart, its valves, or the great vessels.

congestion (kŏn-**jes**-chŏn) *n.* an accumulation of blood within an organ, which is the result of back pressure within its veins (for example congestion of the lungs and liver occurs in heart failure).

congestive cardiac failure (CCF, congestive heart failure) (kŏn-**jest**-iv) *n.* *see* heart failure.

Congo red (**kon**-goh) *n.* a dark-red or reddish-brown pigment that becomes blue in acidic conditions. It is used as a histological stain.

coning (**kohn**-ing) *n.* prolapse of the brainstem through the foramen magnum of the skull as a result of raised intracranial pressure: it is usually immediately fatal.

conization (ko-ny-**zay**-shŏn) *n.* surgical removal of a cone of tissue. The technique is commonly used in excising a portion of the cervix (neck) of the uterus (*see* cone biopsy) for the treatment of cervicitis or early cancer (carcinoma in situ).

conjoined twins (kŏn-**joind**) *pl. n.* identical twins that are physically joined together at birth. The condition ranges from twins joined only by the umbilical blood vessels to those in whom conjoined heads or trunk are inseparable.

conjugate (conjugate diameter, true conjugate) (**kon**-jŭg-it) *n.* the distance between the front and rear of the pelvis measured from the most prominent part of the sacrum to the back of the pubic symphysis. It is estimated by subtracting 1.3–1.9 cm from the distance between the lower edge of the symphysis and the sacrum (the **diagonal c.**). If the true conjugate is less than about 10.2 cm, delivery of an infant through the natural passages may be difficult or impossible.

conjunctiva (kon-junk-**ty**-vă) *n.* the delicate mucous membrane that covers the front of the eye and lines the inside of the eyelids. —**conjunctival** *adj.*

conjunctivitis (pink eye) (kŏn-junk-ti-**vy**-tis) *n.* inflammation of the conjunctiva, which becomes red and swollen and produces a watery or pus-containing discharge. Conjunctivitis is caused by infection by bacteria or viruses, allergy, or physical or chemical irritation. **allergic** (or **vernal**) **c.** conjunctivitis of allergic origin, often associated with hay fever or other forms of atopy. **inclusion c.** a sexually transmitted form of conjunctivitis caused by *Chlamydia trachomatis*. It can be acquired by newborn infants as they pass through an infected birth canal. *See also* ophthalmia (neonatorum), trachoma.

connective tissue (kŏ-**nek**-tiv) *n.* the tissue that supports, binds, or separates more specialized tissues and organs or functions as a packing tissue of the body. It consists of an amorphous matrix of mucopolysaccharides (**ground substance**) in which may be embedded white (collagenous), yellow (elastic), and reticular fibres, fat cells, fibroblasts, mast cells, and macrophages. Forms of connective tissue include bone, cartilage, tendons, ligaments, and adipose, areolar, and elastic tissues.

connective-tissue disease *n.* any one of a group of diseases that are characterized by inflammatory changes in connective tissue. They include dermatomyositis, systemic and discoid lupus erythematosus, morphoea, polyarteritis nodosa, and rheumatoid arthritis.

Conn's syndrome (konz) *n.* a condition resulting from overproduction of the hormone aldosterone due to disease of the adrenal cortex. *See* aldosteronism. [W. J. Conn (1907–94), US physician]

consanguinity (kon-sang-**win**-iti) *n.* relationship by blood; the sharing of a common ancestor within a few generations.

consensus management (kŏn-**sen**-sŭs) *n.* a style of management practised in the National Health Service, in which multidisciplinary management teams make decisions based on discussion and mutual agreement and commitment to the outcome.

consent (kŏn-**sent**) *n.* agreement to undergo medical treatment or to participate in medical research. Three criteria must be met for consent to be legally valid, namely that the patient must: (1) be given sufficient information about the treatment (*see* informed consent); (2) have capacity to make a choice; (3) be in a position to decide voluntarily, i.e. without external pressure or influence. In addition, the patient should be informed that they can change their mind about treatment at any time. The law requires consent to be evidenced in writing only in special cases, such as recruiting a subject to a clinical trial. Valid consent is not required in an emergency or when the patient lacks capacity.

consequentialism (kon-si-**kwen**-shăl-izm) *n.* an ethical approach arguing that the morality or otherwise of an action can be determined according to its outcome or consequences, rather than by its intrinsic nature. *Compare* deontology.

conservative treatment (kŏn-**ser**-vă-tiv) *n.* treatment aimed at preventing a condition from becoming worse, in the expectation that either natural healing will occur or progress of the disease will be so slow that no drastic treatment will be justified. *Compare* radical treatment.

consolidation (kŏn-soli-**day**-shŏn) *n.* **1.** the state of the lung in which the alveoli (air sacs) are filled with fluid produced by inflamed tissue, as in pneumonia. **2.** the stage of repair of a broken bone following callus formation, during which the callus is transformed by osteoblasts into mature bone.

constipation (kon-sti-**pay**-shŏn) *n.* a condition in which bowel evacuations occur infrequently, or in which the faeces are hard and small, or where passage of faeces causes difficulty or pain. Recurrent or long-standing constipation is treated by increasing dietary fibre (roughage), laxatives, or enemas.

constrictor (kŏn-**strik**-ter) *n.* any muscle that compresses an organ or causes a hollow organ or part to contract.

consultant (kŏn-**sul**-t'nt) *n.* a fully trained specialist in a branch of medicine who, in the United Kingdom, is responsible for the care of patients within a particular specialty.

consumption (kŏn-**sump**-shŏn) *n.* any disease causing wasting of tissues, especially (formerly) pulmonary tuberculosis. **—consumptive** *adj.*

contact (**kon**-takt) *n.* transmission of an infectious disease by touching or handling an infected person or animal (**direct c.**) or by inhaling airborne droplets, etc., containing the infective microorganism (**indirect c.**).

contact lenses *pl. n.* lenses worn directly against the eye, separated from it only by a film of tear fluid. They are made of a variety of materials; soft gas-permeable lenses have mostly replaced hard Perspex lenses. Contact lenses are used mainly in place of spectacles to correct errors of refraction, but soft lenses (**bandage lenses**) may be used for managing tiny perforations and other external eye disorders.

contagious disease (kŏn-**tay**-jŭs) *n.* originally, a disease transmitted only by direct physical contact: now usually taken to mean any communicable disease.

continent diversion (**kon**-ti-nĕnt dy-**ver**-shŏn) *n.* the diversion and collection of urine, usually after cystectomy, by constructing a reservoir or pouch from a section of small or large intestine or a combination of both. This can be emptied by catheterization via a small stoma; a urinary drainage bag is not required.

continuing professional development (CPD) (kŏn-**tin**-yoo-ing) *n.* the concept that learning continues throughout one's life, both through educational courses and work experience and practice. Individuals are encouraged to identify their personal learning needs and to assess their progress in dynamic ways.

continuity of care (kon-tin-**yoo**-iti) *n.* a continuous relationship between a patient and an identified health-care professional who is the sole source of care and information for the patient. However, as a patient's health-care needs over time can rarely be met by a single professional, multiprofessional pathways of continuity exist to achieve both quality of care and patient satisfaction.

continuous positive airways pressure (CPAP) (kŏn-tin-yoo-ŭs) *n.* an air pressure in the range 5–30 cm H_2O (1.2–7.5 mPa). It can be applied to the upper airways using a full face mask or a nasal mask only (nCPAP). It is used in high-dependency units to optimize oxygen delivery to patients who are being weaned from ventilators and on patients at home with obstructive sleep apnoea.

contra- *prefix denoting* against or opposite.

contraception (kon-tră-**sep**-shŏn) *n.* the prevention of unwanted pregnancy. *See* coitus (interruptus), condom, diaphragm, iucd, ius, oral contraceptive, postcoital (contraception), rhythm method, sterilization. —**contraceptive** *adj., n.*

contraction (kŏn-**trak**-shŏn) *n.* the shortening of a muscle in response to a motor nerve impulse. This generates tension in the muscle, usually causing movement.

contracture (kŏn-**trak**-cher) *n.* fibrosis of skeletal muscle or connective tissue producing shortening and resulting in deformity of a joint. *See also* Dupuytren's contracture, Volkmann's contracture.

contraindication (kon-tră-in-di-**kay**-shŏn) *n.* any factor in a patient's condition that makes it unwise to pursue a certain line of treatment.

contralateral (kon-tră-**lat**-er-ăl) *adj.* on or affecting the opposite side of the body.

contrast medium (contrast agent) (**kon**-trahst) *n.* a substance administered to enhance the visibility of structures (i.e. increase the contrast) during imaging. **positive c. m.** a contrast agent (e.g. barium sulphate) that increases the density of a structure in radiography. **negative c. m.** a contrast agent (e.g. gas) that decreases the density of a structure in radiography. **magnetic resonance c. m.** a contrast agent that contains either a positive contrast atom (usually gadolinium) to increase the signal or a negative contrast atom (such as iron) to decrease it. **ultrasound c. m.** a contrast medium consisting of tiny (1–10 μm diameter) bubbles of gas, which reflect back the sound waves strongly.

contrecoup (kon-trĕ-**koo**) *n.* injury of a part resulting from a blow on its opposite side. This may happen, for example, if a blow on the back of the head causes the front of the brain to be pushed against the inner surface of the skull.

controlled drug (CD) (kŏn-**trohld**) *n. see* Misuse of Drugs Act 1971.

controlled ovarian stimulation (COS) *n. see* superovulation.

controlled trial *n.* a study method in which one group of participants (the **experimental group**) is subjected to the experimental procedure and the other group (the **control group**) receives a standard or accepted treatment or procedure (or no active treatment). The participants should be randomly assigned to their groups (in a **randomized c. t.**).

control of substances hazardous to health (kŏn-**trohl**) *n. see* COSHH.

contusion (kŏn-**tew**-zhŏn) *n. see* bruise. **cerebral c.** bruising of the brain, resulting from head injury or surgery. Clinical signs range from concussion to coma, reflecting the severity of the trauma.

convection (kŏn-**vek**-shŏn) *n.* the transfer of heat through a liquid or gas by movement of the heated portions of the liquid or gas.

convergence (kŏn-**ver**-jĕns) *n.* inward turning of the eyes to achieve fusion of separate images during near vision.

conversion (kŏn-**ver**-shŏn) *n.* (in psychiatry) the expression of conflict as physical symptoms.

conversion disorder *n.* a psychological disorder, formerly known as **conversion hysteria**, in which a conflict or need manifests itself as an organic dysfunction or a physical symptom, such as blindness, deafness, loss of sensation, gait abnormalities, false memory, or paralysis of various parts of the body. None of these can be accounted for by organic disease.

convolution (kon-vŏ-**loo**-shŏn) *n.* a folding or twisting, such as one of the many that cause the fissures, sulci, and gyri of the surface of the cerebrum.

convulsion (kŏn-**vul**-shŏn) *n.* an involuntary contraction of the muscles producing contortion of the body and limbs. Rhythmic convulsions of the limbs are a feature of major epilepsy. **febrile c.** an epileptic-type seizure associated with a fever, which affects infants and young children and is usually caused by a viral infection.

Cooley's anaemia (**koo**-liz) *n. see* thalassaemia. [T. B. Cooley (1871–1945), US paediatrician]

Coombs' test (koomz) *n.* a means of detecting rhesus antibodies on the surface of red blood cells that precipitate proteins (globulins) in the blood serum. The test is used in the diagnosis of haemolytic anaemia. [R. R. A. Coombs (1921–2006), British immunologist]

COPD *n. see* chronic obstructive pulmonary disease.

co-phenotrope (koh-**fen**-ŏ-trohp) *n.* a drug administered by mouth in the treatment of diarrhoea. It consists of a mixture of diphenoxylate hydrochloride (an opioid that reduces peristalsis) and atropine (which relaxes the smooth muscle of the gut) in a ratio of 100 to 1. Trade name: **Lomotil**.

copper sulphate (**kop**-er) *n.* a salt of copper that, in solution, has been used as a fungicide and is a constituent of Fehling's and Benedict's solutions, used to test for the presence of glucose in the urine. Formula: $CuSO_4$.

copr- (copro-) *combining form denoting* faeces.

coprolalia (kop-rŏ-**lay**-liă) *n.* the repetitive speaking of obscene words. It can be involuntary, as part of Tourette's syndrome.

coprolith (kop-rŏ-lith) *n. see* faecalith.

coproporphyrin (kop-rŏ-**por**-fi-rin) *n.* a porphyrin compound that is formed during the synthesis of protoporphyrin IX. Coproporphyrin is excreted in the faeces in **hereditary coproporphyria**.

copulation (kop-yoo-**lay**-shŏn) *n. see* coitus.

cor (kor) *n.* the heart. **c. pulmonale** enlargement of the right ventricle of the heart resulting from disease of the lungs or pulmonary arteries.

coracoid process (**ko**-ră-koid) *n.* a beaklike process that curves upwards and forwards from the top of the scapula, over the shoulder joint.

cord (kord) *n.* any long flexible structure, which may be solid or tubular. Examples include the spermatic cord, spinal cord, umbilical cord, and vocal cord.

cordectomy (kor-**dek**-tŏmi) *n.* surgical removal of a vocal cord or, more usually, a piece of the vocal cord (**partial c.**).

cordocentesis (kor-doh-sen-**tee**-sis) *n.* the removal of a sample of fetal blood by inserting a fine hollow needle through the abdominal wall of a pregnant woman, under ultrasound guidance, into the umbilical vein. It is commonly performed for confirmation of fetal packed cell volume prior to intrauterine transfusion.

cordotomy (chordotomy) (kor-**dot**-ŏmi) *n.* a surgical procedure for the relief of severe and persistent pain in the pelvis or lower limbs, in which the tracts of the spinal cord transmitting the sensation of pain to consciousness are severed in the cervical (neck) region.

corium (**kor**-iŭm) *n. see* dermis.

corn (korn) *n.* an area of hard thickened skin on or between the toes or elsewhere on the foot: a type of callosity produced by ill-fitting shoes.

cornea (**korn**-iă) *n.* the transparent circular part of the front of the eyeball. It refracts the light entering the eye onto the lens, which then focuses it onto the retina. **—corneal** (**korn**-iăl) *adj.*

corneal arcus *n. see* arcus (senilis).

corneal graft *n. see* keratoplasty.

corneal topography *n. see* topography.

cornification (kor-ni-fi-**kay**-shŏn) *n. see* keratinization.

cornu (**kor**-new) *n.* (*pl.* **cornua**) (in anatomy) a horn-shaped structure. *See also* horn.

corona (kŏ-**roh**-nă) *n.* a crown or crownlike structure. **c. capitis** the crown of the head.

coronal (**ko**-rŏ-năl) *adj.* relating to the crown of the head or of a tooth. **c. plane** the plane that divides the body into dorsal and ventral parts. **c. suture** the immovable joint between the frontal and parietal bones (*see* skull).

coronary angiography (**ko**-rŏn-er-i) *n. see* angiography.

coronary arteries *pl. n.* the arteries supplying blood to the heart. They arise from the aorta, just above the aortic valve, and form branches that encircle the heart.

coronary artery bypass graft (CABG) *n.* an operation in which a segment of a coronary artery narrowed by atheroma is bypassed by an autologous section of healthy saphenous vein or internal mammary artery at thoracotomy. The improved blood flow resulting from one or more such grafts relieves angina pectoris and reduces the risk of myocardial infarction.

coronary care *n.* a type of intensive care developed in order to provide for the needs of critically ill and immediately postoperative patients with cardiac and coronary artery disease. **c. c. unit** (**CCU**) a designated ward in a hospital in which coronary care is given. *See* intensive care.

coronary heart disease (CHD) *n. see* ischaemic heart disease.

coronary thrombosis *n.* the formation of a blood clot (thrombus) in the coronary artery, which obstructs the flow of blood to the heart. *See* myocardial infarction.

coroner (ko-rŏn-er) *n.* the official who presides at an inquest, who must be either a medical practitioner or a lawyer of at least five years standing.

coronoid process (ko-rŏn-oid) *n.* **1.** a process on the upper end of the ulna. It forms part of the notch that articulates with the humerus. **2.** the process on the ramus of the mandible to which the temporalis muscle is attached.

corpus (kor-pŭs) *n.* (*pl.* **corpora**) any mass of tissue that can be distinguished from its surroundings. **c. callosum** the broad band of nervous tissue that connects the two cerebral hemispheres. **c. cavernosum** either of a pair of cylindrical blood sinuses that form the erectile tissue of the penis and clitoris. **c. luteum** the glandular tissue in the ovary that forms at the site of a ruptured Graafian follicle after ovulation. It secretes the hormone progesterone, which prepares the uterus for implantation. If implantation fails the corpus luteum degenerates. If an embryo becomes implanted the corpus luteum continues to secrete progesterone until the fourth month of pregnancy. **c. spongiosum** the blood sinus that surrounds the urethra of the male. Together with the corpora cavernosa, it forms the erectile tissue of the penis. **c. striatum** the part of the basal ganglia in the cerebral hemispheres of the brain consisting of the caudate nucleus and the lentiform nucleus.

corpuscle (kor-pŭs-ŭl) *n.* any small particle, cell, or mass of tissue.

corrective (kŏ-rek-tiv) *n.* any drug or agent that modifies the action of another substance.

Corrigan's pulse (collapsing pulse, water-hammer pulse) (ko-ri-gănz) *n.* a pulse characterized by an initial surge followed by a sudden collapse, usually due to aortic regurgitation. [Sir D. J. Corrigan (1802–80), Irish physician]

cortex (kor-teks) *n.* (*pl.* **cortices**) the outer part of an organ, situated immediately beneath its capsule or outer membrane. **—cortical** (kor-ti-kăl) *adj.*

cortical Lewy body disease *n.* *see* Lewy bodies.

corticosteroid (corticoid) (kor-ti-koh-**steer**-oid) *n.* any steroid hormone synthesized by the adrenal cortex. *See* glucocorticoid, mineralocorticoid.

corticotrophin (kor-ti-koh-**troh**-fin) *n.* *see* ACTH.

corticotrophin-releasing hormone (CRH) *n.* a peptide hypothalamic hormone stimulating the release of ACTH (adrenocorticotrophic hormone) from the anterior pituitary. **CRH test** a test in which CRH is administered intravenously to analyse the ACTH response, which is excessive in cases of primary adrenal failure and suppressed in cases of anterior hypopituitarism.

cortisol (**kor**-ti-sol) *n.* a steroid hormone: the major glucocorticoid synthesized and released by the human adrenal cortex. It is important for normal carbohydrate metabolism and for the normal response to any stress. *See also* hydrocortisone.

cortisone (**kor**-tiz-ohn) *n.* a naturally occurring corticosteroid that may be used to treat deficiency of corticosteroid hormones in Addison's disease and following surgical removal of the adrenal glands (hydrocortisone, to which it is converted in the body, is preferred). It is administered by mouth and may cause serious side-effects such as stomach ulcers, muscle and bone damage, and eye changes.

Corynebacterium (kŏ-ry-ni-bak-**teer**-iŭm) *n.* a genus of Gram-positive, mostly aerobic, nonmotile rodlike bacteria. **C. diphtheriae** (**Klebs-Loeffler bacillus**) the causative organism of diphtheria. It occurs in one of three forms: *gravis*, *intermedius*, and *mitis*.

coryza (cold in the head) (kŏ-**ry**-ză) *n.* a catarrhal inflammation of the mucous membrane in the nose caused by either a cold or hay fever. *See also* catarrh.

COS *see* controlled ovarian stimulation.

COSHH (control of substances hazardous to health) *n.* (in occupational health) legislation and resulting regulations concerning the duties and responsibilities of employers and employees to ensure that hazardous substances used in a workplace do not affect adversely the workforce or others. Employers must undertake risk assessment, training, and health surveillance.

cost- (costo-) *combining form denoting* the rib(s).

costal (**kos**-t'l) *adj.* of or relating to the ribs. **c. cartilage** a cartilage that connects a rib to the breastbone (sternum).

cot death (kot) *n. see* sudden infant death syndrome.

co-trimoxazole (koh-tri-**moks**-ă-zohl) *n.* an antibacterial drug consisting of sulfamethoxazole (a sulphonamide) and trimethoprim. Co-trimoxazole is taken by mouth or administered by intravenous infusion for treating *Pneumocystis* pneumonia, toxoplasmosis, and nocardiosis. Side-effects may be severe. Trade name: **Septrin**.

cotyledon (kot-i-lee-dŏn) *n.* any of the major convex subdivisions of the mature placenta. Each cotyledon contains a major branch of the umbilical blood vessels.

cotyloid cavity (kot-i-loid) *n.* *see* acetabulum.

coughing (kof-ing) *n.* a form of violent exhalation by which irritant particles in the airways can be expelled. Medical name: **tussis**.

cough suppressant (kof) *n.* *see* antitussive.

coulomb (koo-lom) *n.* the SI unit of electric charge, equal to the quantity of electricity transferred by 1 ampere in 1 second. Symbol: C.

counselling (kown-sĕl-ing) *n.* a method of approaching psychological difficulties in adjustment that aims to help the client work out his own problems.

counterextension (kownt-er-eks-ten-shŏn) *n.* traction on one part of a limb, while the remainder of the limb is held steady: used particularly in the treatment of a fractured femur.

counterirritant (kownt-er-i-ri-t'nt) *n.* an agent, such as methyl salicylate, that causes irritation when applied to the skin and is used in order to relieve more deep-seated pain or discomfort. —**counterirritation** *n.*

countertraction (kownt-er-trak-shŏn) *n.* the use of an opposing force to balance that being applied during traction, when a strong continuous pull is applied, for example, to a limb so that broken bones can be kept in alignment during healing.

covariate (covariable) (koh-vair-iăt) *n.* (in statistics) a continuous variable that is not part of the main experimental manipulation but has an effect on the dependent variable (*see* variable). The inclusion of covariates increases the power of the statistical test and removes the bias of confounding variables (*see* confounding factor).

Cowper's glands (bulbourethral glands) (kow-perz) *pl. n.* a pair of small glands that open into the urethra at the base of the penis. Their secretion contributes to the seminal fluid. [W. Cowper (1666–1709), English surgeon]

cowpox (kow-poks) *n.* a virus infection of cows' udders, transmitted to humans by direct contact, causing very mild symptoms similar to smallpox. An attack confers immunity to smallpox. Medical name: **vaccinia**.

cox- (coxo-) *combining form denoting* the hip.

coxa (koks-ă) *n.* (*pl.* **coxae**) **1.** the hip bone. **2.** the hip joint. **c. valga** a deformity of the hip joint in which the angle between the neck and shaft of the femur is abnormally increased. **c. vara** a deformity of the hip joint in which the angle between the neck and shaft of the femur is abnormally decreased.

coxalgia (koks-al-jiă) *n.* **1.** pain in the hip joint. **2.** disease of the hip joint.

COX-2 inhibitor *n.* an anti-inflammatory drug (*see* NSAID) that selectively blocks the action of the enzyme cyclo-oxygenase 2 (COX-2), which mediates the production of prostaglandin at sites of inflammation, especially in joints; such drugs are less likely than nonselective NSAIDs to cause gastrointestinal bleeding and ulceration. COX-2 inhibitors, including **etoricoxib** (Arcoxia), are used in the treatment of arthritis, ankylosing spondylitis, and acute gout. However, because their use is associated with an increased incidence of heart attack and stroke, they should only be taken by patients who are at high risk of peptic ulceration. *See also* celecoxib.

Coxsackie virus (kok-sak-i) *n.* one of a group of RNA-containing viruses that are able to multiply in the gastrointestinal tract (*see* enterovirus). Type A viruses generally cause less severe diseases, although some cause meningitis and severe throat infections. Type B viruses cause inflammation or degeneration of brain or heart tissue and they can also attack the muscles of the chest wall, the bronchi, pancreas, thyroid, and conjunctiva. *See also* Bornholm disease, hand, foot, and mouth disease.

CPAP *n.* *see* continuous positive airways pressure.

CPD *n.* *see* continuing professional development.

C-peptide *n.* a peptide (so-called because of its C shape) formed when insulin is produced from its precursor molecule, proinsulin. As it remains detectable in the plasma much longer than insulin, it can be more easily assayed as a marker of the degree of insulin secretion.

CPK *n.* creatine phosphokinase: *see* creatine (kinase).

CPN *n.* community psychiatric nurse. *See* community nurses.

CPR *n.* *see* cardiopulmonary resuscitation.

CQC *n.* *see* Care Quality Commission.

crab louse (krab) *n.* *see* Phthirus.

cradle (kray-d'l) *n.* a framework of metal strips or other material that forms a cage over an injured part of the body of a patient lying in bed, to protect it from the pressure of the bedclothes.

cradle cap *n.* a common condition in young babies in which crusty white or yellow scales form a 'cap' on the scalp. It is treated by applying oil or using a special shampoo and usually resolves in the first year of life, although it may represent the start of seborrhoeic eczema.

CRAFFT screening test (krarft) *n.* a screening tool for young people under the age of 21 to identify alcohol and drug use. The first part consists of three questions about drug or alcohol use over the past year. Participants giving positive answers to two or more questions proceed to the second part (from which the name derives), which contains six questions with the key words *c*ar, *r*elax, *a*lone, *f*amily/*f*riends, *f*orget, *t*rouble, used to assess the need for further input.

cramp (kramp) *n.* prolonged painful contraction of a muscle. It is sometimes caused by an imbalance of calcium and potassium in the body, but is more often a result of fatigue, imperfect posture, or stress. **occupational c.** spasm in the muscles making it impossible to perform a specific task but allowing the use of these muscles for any other movement. **writer's c.** *see* dystonia.

crani- (cranio-) *combining form denoting* the skull.

cranial nerves (kray-niăl) *pl. n.* the 12 pairs of nerves that arise directly from the brain and leave the skull through separate apertures. *Compare* spinal nerves.

craniometry (kray-ni-**om**-itri) *n.* the science or practice of measuring the differences in the size and shape of skulls.

craniopagus (dicephalus) (kray-ni-**op**-ăgŭs) *n.* conjoined twins united by their heads.

craniopharyngioma (kray-ni-oh-fă-rinj-i-**oh**-mă) *n.* a brain tumour derived from remnants of **Rathke's pouch**, the earliest detectable embryonic precursor of the pituitary gland.

craniostenosis (kray-ni-oh-sti-**noh**-sis) *n.* premature closing of the sutures and fontanelles between the cranial bones during development, resulting in the skull remaining abnormally small. *Compare* craniosynostosis.

craniosynostosis (kray-ni-oh-sin-os-**toh**-sis) *n.* premature fusion of some of the cranial sutures, usually before birth, so that the skull is unable to expand in certain directions to assume its normal shape under the influence of the growing brain. The skull may become elongated from front to back, broad and short, peaked (oxycephaly), or asymmetrical. *Compare* craniostenosis.

craniotabes (kray-ni-oh-**tay**-beez) *n.* abnormal thinness and brittleness of the bones of the vault of the skull, occurring in children with rickets.

craniotomy (kray-ni-**ot**-ŏmi) *n.* **1.** surgical removal of a portion of the cranium, performed to expose the brain and meninges for inspection or biopsy or to relieve excessive intracranial pressure (as in a subdural haematoma). **2.** surgical perforation of the skull of a dead fetus during difficult labour, so that delivery may continue.

cranium (**kray**-niŭm) *n.* the part of the skeleton that encloses the brain. It consists of eight bones connected together by immovable joints (*see* skull). **—cranial** *adj.*

C-reactive protein (CRP) *n.* a protein whose plasma concentrations are raised in infections and inflammatory states and in the presence of tissue damage or necrosis.

cream (kreem) *n.* a preparation for use on the skin consisting of an emulsion of oil in water, which may or may not contain medication. It rubs into the skin easily and contains preservatives, which may be allergenic. *Compare* ointment.

creatine (kree-ă-teen) *n.* a product of protein metabolism found in muscle. **c. kinase** (**CK**, **c. phosphokinase**, **CPK**) an enzyme involved in the breakdown of creatine to creatinine, isomers of which originate in the brain and thyroid, skeletal muscle, and heart. Damage to these tissues results in increased levels of the isomer in the serum. **c. phosphate** (**phosphocreatine**, **phosphagen**) the phosphate of creatine, which acts as a store of high-energy phosphate in muscle and serves to maintain adequate amounts of ATP.

creatinine (kree-**at**-i-neen) *n.* a substance derived from creatine and creatine phosphate in muscle. Creatinine is excreted in the urine.

creatinuria (kree-at-in-**yoor**-iă) *n.* an excess of the nitrogenous compound creatine in the urine.

credibility (kred-i-**bil**-iti) *n.* the extent to which a research study demonstrates effective analysis of a particular issue and hence its value to evidence-based practice. **—credible** (**kred**-ibŭl) *adj.*

Credit Accumulation Transfer Scheme (**kred**-it) *n. see* cats.

creeping eruption (larva migrans) (**kreep**-ing) *n.* a skin disease caused either by larvae of nematode worms (e.g. *Ancylostoma braziliense*) or by the maggots of certain flies. The larvae burrow within the skin tissues, their movements marked by long thin red lines that cause the patient intense irritation.

Creon (**kray**-on) *n. see* PERT.

crepitation (rale) (krep-i-**tay**-shŏn) *n.* a soft fine crackling sound heard in the lungs through the stethoscope. Crepitations are not normally heard in healthy lungs.

crepitus (**krep**-itŭs) *n.* **1.** a crackling sound or grating feeling produced by bone rubbing on bone or roughened cartilage, detected on movement of an arthritic joint. **2.** a similar sound heard with a stethoscope over an inflamed lung when the patient breathes in. **3.** a similar sound heard over an inflamed extensor tendon in the hand in scleroderma caused by thickening of the skin, or over a tendon injured by repetitive use in de Quervain's tendovaginitis.

cresol (**kree**-sol) *n.* a strong antiseptic effective against many microorganisms and used mostly in soap solutions as a general disinfectant. Cresol solutions irritate the skin and if taken by mouth are corrosive and cause pain, nausea, and vomiting.

crest (krest) *n.* a ridge or linear protuberance, particularly on a bone.

CREST syndrome (krest) *n.* a disease characterized by the association of *c*alcinosis, *R*aynaud's phenomenon, (o)*e*sophageal malfunction, *s*clerodactyly (tapering fingers), and *t*elangiectasia. It represents a variant of systemic sclerosis (**limited cutaneous systemic sclerosis**) and may be associated with severe pulmonary hypertension.

cretinism (**kret**-in-izm) *n.* a syndrome of dwarfism, learning disability, and coarseness of the skin and facial features due to congenital hypothyroidism.

Creutzfeldt-Jakob disease (CJD) (**kroits**-felt **yak**-ob) *n.* a disease in which rapid progressive degeneration of brain tissue results in dementia and eventually death. It is caused by an abnormal prion protein (*see* spongiform encephalopathy). Most cases occur sporadically but some forms of CJD are inherited and a few are acquired. **variant CJD** (**vCJD**) the human form of bovine spongiform encephalopathy (BSE): a form of CJD believed to be acquired by ingestion of infected beef products. [H. G. Creutzfeldt (1885–1964) and A. M. Jakob (1884–1931), German psychiatrists]

SEE WEB LINKS

- Website of the national CJD surveillance unit

CRF *n.* chronic renal failure.

CRH *n. see* corticotrophin-releasing hormone.

cribriform plate (**krib**-ri-form) *n. see* ethmoid bone.

cricoid cartilage (**kry**-koid) *n.* the cartilage, shaped like a signet ring, that forms part of the anterior and lateral walls and most of the posterior wall of the larynx.

cricoid pressure *n.* a technique in which a trained assistant presses downwards on the cricoid cartilage of a supine patient to aid endotracheal intubation.

cricothyroid membrane (kry-koh-**th'y**-roid) *n.* the fibrous tissue in the anterior aspect of the neck between the lower border of the thyroid cartilage (the 'Adam's apple') and the upper border of the cricoid cartilage, lying immediately below it. It is the site where certain emergency airway devices can be inserted.

cricothyroidotomy (kry-koh-th'y-roid-**ot**-ŏmi) *n.* a technique for obtaining an emergency airway through the cricothyroid membrane when standard airway techniques have failed. **needle c.** cricothyroidotomy in which a large-bore intravenous cannula is inserted directly through the membrane. **surgical c.** cricothyroidotomy in which a surgical hole is made in the membrane and a cuffed tube, similar to a short endotracheal tube is inserted directly.

cri-du-chat syndrome (kree-doo-**sha**) *n.* a congenital condition of severe learning disability associated with an abnormal facial appearance, spasticity, and a characteristic catlike cry in infancy. It results from an abnormality in chromosome no. 5.

Crigler-Najjar syndrome (**kry**-gler **nah**-jar) *n.* a genetic disease in which the liver enzyme glucuronyl transferase, responsible for dealing with bilirubin, is absent. Large amounts of bilirubin accumulate in the blood, and the child becomes progressively more jaundiced. The definitive treatment is a liver transplant; if left untreated, life expectancy is usually less than two years. [J. F. Crigler (1919–) and V. A. Najjar (1914–), US paediatricians]

crisis (**kry**-sis) *n.* (*pl.* **crises**) **1.** the turning point of a disease, after which the patient either improves or deteriorates. Since the advent of antibiotics, infections seldom reach the point of crisis. **2.** the occurrence of sudden severe pain in certain diseases. *See also* Dietl's crisis. **3.** a state of psychological or physiological disequilibrium in which normal coping strategies and mechanisms have been suspended. Intervention may be required.

crista (krist-ă) *n.* (*pl.* **cristae**) **1.** the sensory structure within the ampulla of a semicircular canal within the inner ear. **2.** one of the infoldings of the inner membrane of a mitochondrion. **3.** any anatomical structure resembling a crest.

critical incident (krit-i-kăl) *n.* an event or episode that deviates from the expected or desired course and could have potentially negative effects for patient care or safety. Such episodes may inform reflective practice and in the NHS should be reported.

critical realism *n.* a philosophical approach to science and the social sciences that explores the difference between physical reality and human perceptions and experiences. It has been increasingly influential since the 1970s.

Crohn's disease (krohnz) *n.* a condition in which segments of the gastrointestinal tract, commonly the small bowel and/or colon, become inflamed, thickened, ulcerated, and scarred. It usually affects the terminal ileum and may mimic acute appendicitis. Long-standing poorly controlled Crohn's disease may predispose to strictures, malabsorption, and internal obstruction. [B. B. Crohn (1884–1983), US physician]

cromoglicate (sodium cromoglicate, cromoglycate) (kroh-moh-gly-kayt) *n.* a drug used to prevent attacks of asthma and hay fever and to treat allergic conjunctivitis, food allergies, and other allergic conditions. It is administered as an aerosol inhalation, nasal spray, eye drops, or capsules. Trade names: **Catacrom**, **Intal**, **Nalcrom**, **Rynacrom**, **Vividrin**.

cross-dressing (kros-dres-ing) *n.* *see* transvestism.

cross-infection (kros-in-fek-shŏn) *n.* the transfer of infection from one patient to another in hospital.

cross-over trial (kros-oh-ver) *n.* a controlled trial in which the groups of participants exchange treatment after a prearranged period.

cross-sectional imaging (kros-sek-shŏn-ăl) *n.* any technique that produces an image in the form of a section through the body with the structures cut across. *See* computerized tomography, magnetic resonance imaging, positron emission tomography, SPECT scanning, ultrasonography.

crotamiton (kroh-tă-my-tŏn) *n.* a drug that is applied to the skin as a cream to relieve itching. Trade name: **Eurax**.

croup (kroop) *n.* acute inflammation and obstruction of the respiratory tract, involving the larynx and main air passages, in young children (usually aged between six months and three years). The usual cause is a virus infection but bacterial secondary infection can occur. The symptoms are those of laryngitis, accompanied by harsh difficult breathing (*see* stridor), a characteristic barking cough, a rising pulse rate, restlessness, and cyanosis.

crown (krown) *n.* **1.** the part of a tooth normally visible in the mouth and usually covered by enamel. **2.** a dental restoration that covers most or all of the natural crown. **3.** *see* corona.

crowning (**krown**-ing) *n.* the stage of labour when only the upper part of the infant's head is visible, encircled by, and just passing through, the vaginal opening.

CRP *n. see* C-reactive protein.

cruciate ligaments (krew-shi-ayt) *pl. n.* a pair (anterior and posterior) of ligaments inside each knee joint. Damage to the cruciate ligaments is a common sports injury, especially in football players.

crude rate (krood) *n.* the total number of events (e.g. cases of lung cancer) expressed as a rate per 1000 of the population.

crural (**kroor**-ăl) *adj.* **1.** relating to the thigh or leg. **2.** relating to the crura cerebri (*see* crus).

crus (kruus) *n.* (*pl.* **crura**) an elongated process or part of a structure. **c. cerebri** one of two symmetrical nerve tracts situated between the medulla oblongata and the cerebral hemispheres.

crush syndrome (krush) *n.* acute kidney injury caused by myoglobin that is released from damaged skeletal muscle. This is usually the result of trauma and was first recognized in victims trapped and crushed in the London Blitz. Medical name: **myoglobinuric acute renal failure**.

cry- (cryo-) *combining form denoting* cold.

cryaesthesia (kry-iss-**theez**-iă) *n.* **1.** exceptional sensitivity to low temperature. **2.** a sensation of coldness.

cryoprecipitate (kry-oh-pri-**sip**-i-tăt) *n.* a precipitate produced by freezing and thawing under controlled conditions, such as the residue obtained from fresh frozen blood plasma that has been thawed at 4°C. This residue is used in the control of bleeding in haemophilia.

cryopreservation (kry-oh-prez-er-**vay**-shŏn) *n.* preservation of tissues by freezing.

cryoprobe (**kry**-oh-prohb) *n.* an instrument used in cryosurgery, which has a fine tip cooled by allowing carbon dioxide or nitrous oxide gas to expand within it.

cryoretinopexy (kry-oh-**ret**-i-noh-peks-i) *n.* the use of extreme cold to freeze areas of weak or torn retina in order to cause scarring and seal breaks. It is used in cryosurgery for retinal detachment.

cryosurgery (kry-oh-**ser**-jer-i) *n.* the use of extreme cold in a localized part of the body to freeze and destroy unwanted tissues. Cryosurgery is commonly used for the treatment of retinal detachment, the destruction of certain bone tumours, and the obliteration of skin blemishes. *See* cryoprobe.

cryotherapy (kry-oh-**th'e**-ră-pi) *n.* treatment based on the use of extreme cold. *See* cryosurgery, hypothermia. *Compare* thermotherapy.

crypt (kript) *n.* a small sac, follicle, or cavity; for example, the crypts of Lieberkühn (*see* Lieberkühn's glands).

crypt- (crypto-) *combining form denoting* concealed.

cryptococcosis (torulosis) (krip-toh-kok-**oh**-sis) *n.* a disease caused by the fungus *Cryptococcus neoformans*, which attacks the lung, resulting in a solid tumour-like mass (**toruloma**). It may spread to the brain, leading to meningitis; this can occur as an opportunistic infection in those suffering from AIDS.

cryptogenic (krip-toh-**jen**-ik) *adj.* of obscure or unknown cause.

cryptomenorrhoea (krip-toh-men-ŏ-**ree**-ă) *n.* cyclical abdominal pain in association with amenorrhoea, usually about a year after the expected onset of menstruation and usually due to an imperforate hymen.

cryptorchidism (cryptorchism) (krip-**or**-kid-izm) *n.* the condition in which the testes fail to descend into the scrotum and are retained within the abdomen or inguinal canal. —**cryptorchid** *adj., n.*

cryptosporidiosis (krip-toh-sper-id-i-**oh**-sis) *n.* an intestinal infection of mammals and birds caused by parasitic protozoa of the genus *Cryptosporidium*, which is usually transmitted to humans via farm animals. Ingestion of water or milk contaminated with infective oocysts results in severe diarrhoea and abdominal cramps, caused by release of a toxin. Most patients recover in 7–14 days, but the disease can persist in the immunocompromised (including AIDS patients), the elderly, and young children.

CSF *n. see* cerebrospinal fluid.

CSI *n. see* Caregiver Strain Index.

CSOM *n.* chronic suppurative otitis media. *See* otitis (media).

CSSD *n.* Central Sterile Supplies Department (in a hospital).

CT scanner *n. see* computerized tomography.

cubital (kew-bit'l) *adj.* relating to the elbow or forearm. **c. fossa** the depression at the front of the elbow.

cuboid bone (**kew**-boid) *n.* the outer bone of the tarsus, which articulates with the fourth and fifth metatarsal bones in front and with the calcaneus (heel bone) behind.

cuirass ventilator (kwi-ras) *n. see* ventilator.

Cullen sign (**kul**-ĕn) *n.* a bluish bruiselike appearance around the umbilicus. Causes include a ruptured ectopic pregnancy and acute pancreatitis. [T. S. Cullen (1868–1953), US gynaecologist]

culture (**kul**-cher) **1.** *n.* a population of microorganisms, usually bacteria, grown in a solid or liquid laboratory medium (**c. medium**), which is usually agar, broth, or gelatin. **stock c.** a permanent bacterial culture, from which subcultures are made. *See also* tissue (culture). **2.** *vb.* to grow bacteria or other microorganisms in cultures.

cumulative action (kew-mew-lă-tiv) *n.* the toxic effects of a drug produced by repeated administration of small doses at intervals that are not long enough for it to be either broken down or excreted by the body.

cuneiform bones (kew-ni-form) *pl. n.* three bones in the tarsus that articulate with the first, second, and third metatarsal bones in front. All three bones articulate with the navicular bone behind.

cupola (kew-pŏ-lă) *n.* **1.** the small dome at the end of the cochlea. **2.** any of several dome-shaped anatomical structures.

curare (kew-rar-i) *n.* an extract from the bark of South American trees (*Strychnos* and *Chondodendron* species) that relaxes and paralyses voluntary muscle. Curare was formerly employed to control the muscle spasms of tetanus and as a muscle relaxant in surgical operations.

curettage (kewr-i-tij) *n.* the scraping of the skin or the internal surface of an organ or body cavity by means of a spoon-shaped instrument (**curette**). Curettage is usually performed to remove diseased tissue or to obtain a specimen for diagnostic purposes. *See also* dilatation and curettage.

curette (kewr-et) *n. see* curettage.

curie (kewr-ee) *n.* a former unit for expressing the activity of a radioactive substance. It has been replaced by the becquerel. Symbol: Ci.

Curling's ulcers (ker-lingz) *pl. n. see* stress (ulcers). [T. B. Curling (1811–88), British surgeon]

Cushing's syndrome (kuush-ingz) *n.* the condition resulting from excess amounts of corticosteroid hormones in the body. Symptoms include weight gain, reddening of the face and neck, excess growth of body and facial hair, raised blood pressure, loss of mineral from the bones (osteoporosis), raised blood glucose levels, and sometimes mental disturbances. The syndrome may be due to overstimulation of the adrenal glands by excessive amounts of the hormone ACTH, secreted either by a tumour of the pituitary gland (**Cushing's disease**) or by a malignant tumour in the lung or elsewhere. [H. W. Cushing (1869–1939), US surgeon]

cusp (kusp) *n.* **1.** any of the cone-shaped prominences on the teeth, especially the premolars and molars. **2.** a pocket or fold of the membrane lining the heart or of the layer of the wall of a vein, several of which form a valve. When the blood flows backwards the cusps fill up and become distended, so closing the valve.

cutaneous (kew-tay-niŭs) *adj.* relating to the skin.

cuticle (kew-ti-kŭl) *n.* **1.** the epidermis of the skin. **2.** a layer of solid or semisolid material that is secreted by and covers an epithelium. **3.** a layer of cells, such as the outer layer of cells in a hair.

cutis (kew-tis) *n. see* skin.

CVA *n. see* cerebrovascular accident.

CVAD *n. see* central venous access device.

CVP *n. see* central venous pressure.

CVS *n. see* chorionic villus sampling.

CXR *n.* chest X-ray.

cyan- (cyano-) *combining form denoting* blue.

cyanide (sy-ă-nyd) *n.* any of the notoriously poisonous salts of hydrocyanic acid. Cyanides combine with and render inactive the enzymes of the tissues responsible for cellular respiration, and therefore they kill extremely quickly.

cyanocobalamin (vitamin B_{12}) (sy-ă-noh-koh-**bal**-ă-min) *n. see* vitamin B.

cyanosis (sy-ă-**noh**-sis) *n.* a bluish discoloration of the skin and mucous membranes resulting from an inadequate amount of oxygen in arterial blood (**central c.**), due to reduced oxygenation of blood in the pulmonary circulation, or in venous blood (**peripheral c.**), due to excessive extraction of oxygen in the tissues. Cyanosis is associated with heart failure, lung diseases, the breathing of oxygen-deficient atmospheres, and asphyxia. Cyanosis is also seen in blue babies, because of congenital heart defects. **—cyanotic** *adj.*

cybernetics (sy-ber-**net**-iks) *n.* the science of communication processes and automatic control systems in both machines and living things: a study linking the working of the brain and nervous system with the functioning of computers and automated feedback devices. *See also* bionics.

cycl- (cyclo-) *combining form denoting* **1.** cycle or cyclic. **2.** the ciliary body.

cyclical vomiting (sy-klik-ăl) *n.* recurrent attacks of vomiting, often associated with acidosis, occurring in children but with no apparent cause.

cyclitis (sy-**kly**-tis) *n.* inflammation of the ciliary body of the eye (*see* uveitis).

cyclizine (sy-kliz-een) *n.* a drug with antihistamine properties, administered by mouth or injection to prevent and relieve nausea and vomiting in motion sickness, vertigo, disorders of the inner ear, and terminal illness. It is given by mouth or injection. Trade name: **Valoid**.

cycloablation (sy-kloh-ă-**blay**-shŏn) *n.* the destruction of part of the ciliary body of the eye to reduce the production of aqueous humour and hence reduce intraocular pressure. It is used in the treatment of advanced glaucoma resistant to other forms of treatment.

cyclocryotherapy (sy-kloh-kry-oh-**th'e**-ră-pi) *n.* the destruction of part of the ciliary body by freezing. It is used to reduce intraocular pressure in the control of glaucoma.

cyclodialysis (sy-kloh-dy-**al**-i-sis) *n.* separation of the ciliary body from its attachment to the sclera. This may result from trauma or it may be performed as part of an operation to treat glaucoma.

cyclopenthiazide (sy-kloh-pen-**th'y**-ă-zyd) *n.* a diuretic administered by mouth to treat oedema, high blood pressure, and heart failure. Trade name: **Navidrex**.

cyclopentolate (sy-kloh-**pen**-tŏ-layt) *n.* a drug, similar to atropine, that is used in eye drops to paralyse the ciliary muscles and dilate the pupil for treating uveitis. Trade names: **Minims Cyclopentolate Hydrochloride**, **Mydrilate**.

cyclophosphamide (sy-kloh-fos-fă-myd) *n.* an alkylating agent administered by mouth or injection to treat a variety of cancers, often in combination with other cytotoxic drugs. It also has immunosuppressant properties and is used in treating rheumatoid arthritis and other conditions requiring reduced immune response.

cyclophotoablation (sy-kloh-foh-toh-ă-**blay**-shŏn) *n.* the use of light or lasers to destroy the ciliary body of the eye in order to reduce production of aqueous humour and hence reduce intraocular pressure. It is used in the treatment of glaucoma.

cycloplegia (sy-kloh-**plee**-jiă) *n.* paralysis of the ciliary muscle of the eye (*see* ciliary body). This causes inability to alter the focus of the eye and is usually accompanied by paralysis of the muscles of the iris, resulting in fixed dilation of the pupil (mydriasis). It is induced by drugs to facilitate eye examination and to treat uveitis.

cycloserine (sy-kloh-**seer**-een) *n.* an antibiotic, active against a wide range of bacteria, that may be used as supporting treatment in tuberculosis resistant to first-line treatment. It is administered by mouth.

cyclosporin (sy-kloh-**spo**-rin) *n.* *see* ciclosporin.

cyclothymia (cyclothymic disorder) (sy-kloh-**th'y**-miă) *n.* the occurrence of mood swings from cheerfulness to misery. These fluctuations may represent a personality trait and are not as great as those of bipolar affective disorder.

cyclotomy (sy-**klot**-ŏmi) *n.* surgical incision of the ciliary body of the eye.

cyesis (sy-**ee**-sis) *n.* pregnancy. *See also* pseudocyesis.

cyproheptadine (sy-proh-**hep**-tă-deen) *n.* a potent antihistamine administered by mouth to treat allergies, such as hay fever and urticaria. Trade name: **Periactin**.

cyproterone (cyproterone acetate) (sy-**proh**-ter-ohn) *n.* a steroid drug that inhibits the effects of male sex hormones (*see* anti-androgen) and is used to treat hypersexuality disorders and advanced prostate cancer in men. A side-effect is liver damage. Combined with ethinylestradiol (as Dianette), it is used to treat severe acne and hirsutism in women. It is administered by mouth. Trade names: **Androcur**, **Cyprostat**.

cyst (sist) *n.* **1.** an abnormal sac or closed cavity lined with epithelium and filled with liquid or semisolid matter. There are many varieties of cysts occurring in different parts of the body. *See* dermoid cyst, fimbrial cyst, hydatid, ovarian cyst, retention cyst, sebaceous cyst. **2.** a dormant stage produced during the life cycle of certain protozoan parasites of the alimentary canal, including *Giardia* and *Entamoeba*. **3.** a structure formed by and surrounding the larvae of certain parasitic worms.

cyst- (cysto-) *combining form denoting* **1.** a bladder, especially the urinary bladder. **2.** a cyst.

cystadenoma (sis-tad-i-**noh**-mă) *n.* an adenoma showing a cystic structure.

cystalgia (sis-**tal**-jiă) *n.* pain in the urinary bladder. This is common in cystitis and when there are stones in the bladder and is occasionally present in bladder cancer.

cystectomy (sis-**tek**-tŏmi) *n.* surgical removal of the urinary bladder. Usually the ureters draining the urine from the kidneys are reimplanted into the ileum (*see* ileal conduit).

cysteine (**sis**-ti-een) *n.* a sulphur-containing amino acid that is an important constituent of many enzymes.

cystic (**sis**-tik) *adj.* **1.** of, relating to, or characterized by cysts. **2.** of or relating to the gall bladder or urinary bladder. **c. duct** *see* bile duct.

cysticercosis (sis-ti-ser-**koh**-sis) *n.* a disease caused by the presence of tapeworm larvae (*see* cysticercus) of the species *Taenia solium* in any of the body tissues. The presence of cysticerci in the muscles causes pain and weakness; in the brain the symptoms are more serious, including mental deterioration, paralysis, giddiness, epileptic attacks, and convulsions.

cysticercus (bladderworm) (sis-ti-**ser**-kŭs) *n.* a larval stage of some tapeworms in which the scolex and neck are invaginated into a large fluid-filled cyst. *See* cysticercosis.

cystic fibrosis (CF, fibrocystic disease of the pancreas, mucoviscidosis) *n.* a hereditary disease affecting cells of the exocrine glands; the faulty gene responsible for the most common form of CF has been identified as lying on chromosome no. 7 and is recessive, i.e. both parents of the patient can be carriers without being affected by the disease. The abnormality results in the production of thick mucus, which obstructs the intestinal glands (causing meconium ileus in newborn babies), pancreas (causing deficiency of pancreatic enzymes resulting in malabsorption and failure to thrive), and bronchi (causing bronchiectasis). Respiratory infections, which may be severe, are a common complication.

SEE WEB LINKS

• Website of the Cystic Fibrosis Trust

cystic hygroma *n. see* hygroma.

cystine (**sis**-teen) *n. see* amino acid.

cystinosis (sis-ti-**noh**-sis) *n.* an inborn defect in the metabolism of amino acids, leading to abnormal accumulation of the amino acid cystine in the blood, kidneys, and lymphatic system. *See also* Fanconi syndrome.

cystinuria (sis-tin-**yoor**-iă) *n.* an inborn error of metabolism resulting in excessive excretion of the amino acid cystine in the urine due to a defect of reabsorption by the kidney tubules. It may lead to the formation of cystine stones in the kidney.

cystitis (sis-**ty**-tis) *n.* inflammation of the urinary bladder, often caused by infection. It is usually accompanied by the desire to pass urine frequently, with a degree of burning.

cystitome (**sis**-ti-tohm) *n.* a fine curved needle with a hooked tip or a small knife with a tiny curved or hooked blade, used to create an opening in the lens capsule in some operations for cataract.

cystocele (sis-tŏ-seel) *n.* prolapse of the base of the bladder in women. It is usually due to weakness of the pelvic floor after childbirth and causes bulging of the anterior wall of the vagina on straining.

cystography (sis-**tog**-răfi) *n.* X-ray examination of the urinary bladder after filling it with a contrast medium. The X-ray photographs or films thus obtained are known as **cystograms**.

cystolithiasis (sis-toh-lith-**I**-ă-sis) *n.* the presence of stones (calculi) in the urinary bladder. The stones cause pain, the passage of bloody urine, and interruption of the urinary stream and should be removed surgically. *See* calculus.

cystometry (sis-**tom**-i-tri) *n.* measurement of the pressure within the bladder to assess filling and voiding phases of urination in a patient with incontinence. **—cystometer** *n.*

cystopexy (vesicofixation) (sis-toh-peksi) *n.* a surgical operation to fix the urinary bladder (or a portion of it) in a different position. It may be performed as part of the repair or correction of a prolapsed bladder.

cystoplasty (**sis**-toh-plasti) *n.* the operation to enlarge the capacity of and to decrease the pressure within the bladder by incorporating a segment of bowel. **clam c.** an operation in which the bladder is cut across longitudinally from one side of the neck to the other side through the dome (fundus) of the bladder and a length of ileum or colon is inserted as a patch. *See also* ileocaecocystoplasty, ileocystoplasty.

cystoscopy (sis-**tos**-kŏpi) *n.* examination of the bladder by means of an instrument (**cystoscope**) inserted via the urethra.

cystostomy (sis-**tost**-ŏmi) *n.* the operation of creating an artificial opening between the bladder and the anterior abdominal wall. This provides a temporary or permanent drainage route for urine.

cystotomy (sis-**tot**-ŏmi) *n.* surgical incision into the urinary bladder, usually by cutting through the abdominal wall above the pubic symphysis (**suprapubic c.**).

cyt- (cyto-) *combining form denoting* **1.** cell(s). **2.** cytoplasm.

cytarabine (sy-**ta**-ră-been) *n.* an antimetabolite that is used to suppress the symptoms of acute myeloblastic leukaemia and lymphomatous meningitis. It is administered by injection and can damage the normal bone marrow, leading to various blood cell disorders. Trade name: **DepoCyte**.

-cyte *combining form denoting* a cell.

cytochemistry (sy-toh-**kem**-istri) *n.* the study of chemical compounds and their activities in living cells.

cytogenetics (sy-toh-ji-**net**-iks) *n.* a science that links the study of inheritance (genetics) with that of cells (cytology); it is concerned mainly with the study of the chromosomes, especially their origin, structure, and functions.

cytokinesis (sy-toh-ki-**nee**-sis) *n.* *see* karyokinesis.

cytology (sy-**tol**-ŏji) *n.* the study of the structure and function of cells. **aspiration c.** the aspiration of specimens of cells from tumours or cysts through a hollow needle, using a syringe, and their subsequent examination under the microscope after suitable preparation (by staining, etc.). **cervical c.** the microscopic examination of cells obtained by scraping the cervix. *See* cervical (smear). **exfoliative c.** the microscopic examination of cells that have already been shed, used in the diagnosis of various diseases. *See also* liquid-based cytology. **—cytological** *adj.*

cytolysis (sy-**tol**-i-sis) *n.* the breakdown of cells, particularly by destruction of their outer membranes.

cytomegalovirus (CMV) (sy-toh-**meg**-ă-loh-vy-rŭs) *n.* a virus belonging to the herpesvirus group. It normally causes only mild symptoms, but in immunocompromised individuals its effects can be more severe; if contracted by a pregnant woman it may give rise to congenital handicap in her child.

cytometer (sy-**tom**-it-er) *n.* an instrument for determining the number of cells in a given quantity of fluid, such as blood, cerebrospinal fluid, or urine. *See* haemocytometer.

cytopenia (sy-toh-**pee**-niă) *n.* a deficiency of one or more of the various types of blood cells. *See* eosinopenia, erythropenia, lymphopenia, neutropenia, pancytopenia, thrombocytopenia.

cytoplasm (sy-toh-plazm) *n.* the jelly-like substance that surrounds the nucleus of a cell. *See also* protoplasm. **—cytoplasmic** *adj.*

cytosine (sy-toh-seen) *n.* one of the nitrogen-containing bases (*see* pyrimidine) that occurs in the nucleic acids DNA and RNA.

cytosome (sy-toh-sohm) *n.* the part of a cell that is outside the nucleus.

cytotoxic drug (sy-toh-**toks**-ik) *n.* a drug that damages or destroys cells and is used to treat various types of cancer. There are various classes of cytotoxic drugs, including alkylating agents, antimetabolites, anthracycline antibiotics, vinca alkaloids, platinum compounds (e.g. carboplatin), and taxanes. They destroy cancer cells by inhibiting cell division but also affect normal cells, causing side-effects, particularly in bone marrow (*see* myelosuppression), skin (causing hair loss), stomach lining (causing severe nausea and vomiting), and fetal tissue; dosage must therefore be carefully controlled.

cytotoxin (sy-toh-**toks**-in) *n.* any substance that has a toxic action on specific cells.

Dd

dacarbazine (da-**kah**-bă-zeen) *n.* a drug administered intravenously in the treatment of melanoma and (in combination with other cytotoxic drugs) of soft-tissue sarcomas and Hodgkin's disease.

dacry- (dacryo-) *combining form denoting* **1.** tears. **2.** the lacrimal apparatus.

dacryoadenitis (dak-ri-oh-ad-i-**ny**-tis) *n.* inflammation of the tear-producing gland. *See* lacrimal (apparatus).

dacryocystitis (dak-ri-oh-sis-**ty**-tis) *n.* inflammation of the lacrimal sac, usually occurring when the duct draining the tears into the nose is blocked. *See* lacrimal (apparatus).

dacryocystorhinostomy (DCR) (dak-ri-oh-sis-toh-ry-**nost**-ŏmi) *n.* an operation to relieve blockage of the nasolacrimal duct (which drains tears into the nose), in which a communication is made between the lacrimal sac and the nose by removing the intervening bone. *See* dacryocystitis, lacrimal (apparatus).

dacryolith (**dak**-ri-oh-lith) *n.* a stone in the lacrimal canaliculus or lacrimal sac. *See* lacrimal (apparatus).

dacryoma (dak-ri-**oh**-mă) *n.* a harmless tumour-like swelling obstructing any of the ducts associated with the lacrimal apparatus.

dactinomycin (actinomycin D) (dak-ti-noh-**my**-sin) *n.* a cytotoxic drug (an antibiotic) used mainly to treat cancers in children. It is administered intravenously.

dactyl- *combining form denoting* the digits (fingers or toes).

dactylion (dak-**til**-iŏn) *n. see* syndactyly.

dactylitis (dak-ti-**ly**-tis) *n.* inflammation of a finger or toe caused by bone infection (as in tuberculous osteomyelitis) or rheumatic disease or seen in infants with sickle-cell disease. The whole digit is swollen and may resemble a sausage (known as 'sausage digit').

dactylology (dak-ti-**lol**-ŏji) *n.* the representation of speech by finger movements: sign language.

DAFNE (dose adjustment for normal eating) (daf-ni) *n.* an education programme for patients with insulin-dependent diabetes. It teaches participants to adjust their insulin dosage according to their carbohydrate intake. Outcomes show improved glycaemic control and quality of life.

Daltonism (protanopia) (dawl-tŏn-izm) *n.* red-blindness: a defect in colour vision in which a person cannot distinguish between reds and greens. The term has been used to refer to colour blindness in general. [J. Dalton (1766–1844), British chemist]

danazol (**dan**-ă-zol) *n.* a synthetic progestogen that inhibits the secretion by the pituitary gland of gonadotrophins. Administered by mouth, it is used to treat endometriosis, severe pain associated with cystic tumours of the breast, and severe urticaria. Trade name: **Danol**.

D and C *n.* *see* dilatation and curettage.

dandruff (**dan**-druf) *n.* visible scaling from the surface of the scalp, associated with the presence of the yeast *Malassezia furfur*. It is the precursor of seborrhoeic eczema of the scalp, in which there is a degree of inflammation in addition to the greasy scaling. Dandruff can be controlled by shampoos containing tar, selenium sulphide, pyrithione zinc, or imidazole antifungals. Medical name: **pityriasis capitis**.

Dandy-Walker syndrome (**dan**-di **wawk**-er) *n.* a form of cerebral palsy in which the cerebellum is usually the part of the brain affected. It leads to unsteadiness of balance and an abnormal gait and may be associated with hydrocephalus. [W. E. Dandy (1886–1946) and A. E. Walker (1907–95), US surgeons]

dangerous drugs (**dayn**-jer-ŭs) *pl. n.* *see* Misuse of Drugs Act 1971.

dantrolene (**dan**-troh-leen) *n.* a muscle relaxant given by mouth to relieve spasticity in such conditions as cerebral palsy, multiple sclerosis, and spinal cord injury and intravenously to treat malignant hyperthermia, a serious complication of anaesthesia. Trade names: **Dantrium**, **Dantrium Intravenous**.

dapsone (**dap**-sohn) *n.* a drug (*see* sulphone) administered by mouth to treat leprosy and dermatitis herpetiformis and to prevent *Pneumocystis* pneumonia.

dark adaptation (dark) *n.* the changes that take place in the retina and pupil of the eye enabling vision in very dim light. *See* rod. *Compare* light adaptation.

daunorubicin (daw-noh-**roo**-bi-sin) *n.* an anthracycline antibiotic that interferes with DNA synthesis and is used in the treatment of acute leukaemias and AIDS-related Kaposi's sarcoma. It is administered by intravenous infusion. Trade name: **DaunoXome.**

dawn phenomenon (Somogyi effect) (dawn) *n.* the phenomenon of high fasting blood-sugar levels in the morning due to an unrecognized hypoglycaemic episode during the night in a person with diabetes. The episode has resulted in an outpouring of regulatory hormones (e.g. adrenaline, glucagon), which have increased the blood sugar to supernormal levels.

day blindness (hemeralopia) (day) *n.* comparatively good vision in poor light but poor vision in good illumination. The condition is usually congenital and associated with poor visual acuity and defective colour vision. *Compare* night blindness.

day-case surgery *n.* surgical procedures that can be performed in a single day, without the need to admit the patient for an overnight stay in hospital. Examples include removal of many breast lesions, dilatation and curettage, and operations for hernia and varicose veins. Special units are established in many hospitals.

day hospital *n.* *see* hospital.

DBS *n.* *see* deep brain stimulation.

D cells *pl. n.* the cells in the islets of Langerhans that produce somatostatin and pancreatic polypeptide. *Compare* alpha cells, beta cells.

DCIS *n.* *see* (ductal) carcinoma in situ.

DDT (chlorophenothane, dicophane) *n.* a powerful insecticide that was formerly widely used. The quantities now present in the environment – in the form of stores accumulated in animal tissues – have led to its use being restricted.

de- *prefix denoting* **1.** removal or loss. **2.** reversal.

dead space (ded) *n.* **1.** any part of the respiratory tract containing air that does not participate in the exchange of oxygen and carbon dioxide. **2.** a cavity that remains in an incompletely closed wound, in which blood may accumulate and delay healing.

deafness (**def**-nis) *n.* partial or total loss of hearing in one or both ears, now becoming more commonly called **hearing loss**. **conductive d.** deafness that is due to a defect in the conduction of sound from the external ear to the inner ear. This may be due to perforations of the eardrum, fluid or infection in the middle ear (*see* glue ear, otitis (media)), or disorders of the small bones in the middle ear (ossicles). **sensorineural d.** (**perceptive d.**) deafness that may be due to a lesion of the cochlea in the inner ear, the cochlear nerve, or the auditory centres in the brain. *See also* cochlear implant, hearing aid, hearing therapy, Rinne's test, Weber's test.

deamination (dee-ami-**nay**-shŏn) *n.* a process that occurs in the liver during the metabolism of amino acids. The amino group ($-NH_2$) is removed from an amino acid and converted to ammonia, which is ultimately converted to urea and excreted.

death (deth) *n.* absence of vital functions. **brain d.** permanent functional death of the centres in the brainstem that control breathing, heart rate, and other vital reflexes (including pupillary responses). Many decisions in medicine depend on death being clearly defined and objectively observed. Particular problems arise when a potential organ donor is being kept artificially alive. Legally, two independent medical opinions are required before brain death is agreed and organs can be removed.

death certificate *n.* a legal document, signed by a doctor, stating the immediate cause of a person's death followed by diseases underlying the condition.

debility (di-**bil**-iti) *n.* physical weakness; loss of strength and power.

debridement (di-**breed**-mĕnt) *n.* **1.** the process of cleaning an open wound by removal of foreign material and dead tissue, so that healing may occur without hindrance. **2.** (in dentistry) the cleaning of the root canal in root canal treatment.

dec- (deca-) *prefix denoting* ten.

decalcification (dee-kal-sifi-**kay**-shŏn) *n.* loss or removal of calcium salts from a bone or tooth.

decapitation (di-kapi-**tay**-shŏn) *n.* removal of the head, usually the head of a dead fetus to enable delivery to take place. This procedure is now very rare.

decapsulation (decortication) (dee-kaps-yoo-**lay**-shŏn) *n.* the surgical removal of a capsule from an organ; for example, the stripping of the membrane that envelops the kidney or of the inflammatory capsule that encloses a chronic abscess, as in the treatment of empyema.

decay (di-**kay**) *n.* (in bacteriology) the decomposition of organic matter due to microbial action.

deci- *prefix denoting* a tenth.

decidua (di-**sid**-yoo-ă) *n.* the modified mucous membrane that lines the wall of the uterus during pregnancy and is shed with the afterbirth at parturition (*see* endometrium). **d. basalis** the region of the decidua where the embryo is attached. **d. capsularis** the thin layer of the decidua that covers the embryo. **d. parietalis** the region of the decidua that is not in contact with the embryo. **—decidual** *adj.*

decompensation (dee-kom-pen-**say**-shŏn) *n.* inability of the heart to maintain an adequate circulation in the face of an increased workload or some structural defect.

decomposition (dee-kom-pŏ-**zish**-ŏn) *n.* the temperature-dependent gradual disintegration of dead organic matter, usually foodstuffs or tissues, by the chemical action of bacteria and/or fungi.

decompression (dee-kŏm-**presh**-ŏn) *n.* **1.** the reduction of pressure on an organ or part of the body by surgical intervention. Raised pressure in the fluid of the brain can be lowered by cutting into the dura mater; cardiac compression – the abnormal presence of blood or fluid round the heart – can be cured by cutting the pericardium. **2.** the gradual reduction of atmospheric pressure for deep-sea divers. *See* compressed air illness.

decompression sickness *n.* *see* compressed air illness.

decongestant (dee-kŏn-**jest**-ănt) *n.* an agent that reduces or relieves nasal congestion. Nasal decongestants are sympathomimetic or antimuscarinic drugs, which are applied locally in the form of nasal sprays or drops.

decongestive therapy (dee-kŏn-**jest**-iv) *n.* an approach that combines many of the different treatments (such as compression and physiotherapy) used to minimize the pain and swelling associated with lymphoedema following breast surgery and radiotherapy. There are two phases: reduction (which lasts up to twelve weeks) and maintenance (which continues for life).

decontamination (dee-kŏn-tam-i-**nay**-shŏn) *n.* the process of cleaning surgical instruments to remove adherent protein prior to sterilization in an autoclave.

decortication (dee-kor-ti-**kay**-shŏn) *n.* **1.** the removal of the outside layer (cortex) from an organ or structure, such as the kidney. **2.** an operation for removing the blood clot and scar tissue that forms after bleeding into the chest cavity. **3.** *see* decapsulation.

decubitus (di-**kew**-bit-ŭs) *n.* the recumbent position. **d. ulcer** *see* pressure sore.

decussation (dee-kus-**ay**-shŏn) *n.* a point at which two or more structures of the body cross to the opposite side. The term is used particularly for the point at which nerve fibres cross over in the central nervous system.

deep brain stimulation (DBS) *n.* a surgical treatment involving the implantation of a medical device that sends electrical impulses to specific parts of the brain. DBS can provide benefits for treatment-resistant movement disorders, such as Parkinson's disease and dystonia.

deep vein thrombosis (DVT) *n.* *see* phlebothrombosis.

defecation (def-i-**kay**-shŏn) *n.* the expulsion of faeces through the anus.

defence mechanism (di-**fenss**) *n.* the means whereby an undesirable impulse or emotion can be avoided or controlled. Defence mechanisms include repression, projection, reaction formation, sublimation, and splitting.

deferent (**def**-er-ĕnt) *adj.* **1.** carrying away from or down from. **2.** relating to the vas deferens.

defervescence (def-er-**ves**-ĕns) *n.* the disappearance of a fever, a process that may occur rapidly or take several days.

defibrillation (dee-fib-ri-**lay**-shŏn) *n.* administration of a controlled electric shock to restore normal heart rhythm in cases of cardiac arrest due to ventricular fibrillation. *See* defibrillator.

defibrillator (dee-**fib**-ri-lay-ter) *n.* the apparatus used for issuing a measured electrical current to a patient's heart in defibrillation. Defibrillators may be semi- or fully automated to recognize abnormal rhythms and to deliver the appropriate shock, fully operator-dependent, or implanted into the patient's body like a pacemaker.

defibrination (dee-fib-ri-**nay**-shŏn) *n.* the removal of fibrin, one of the plasma proteins that causes coagulation, from a sample of blood.

deficiency disease (di-**fish**-ĕn-si) *n.* any disease caused by the lack of an essential nutrient in the diet. Such nutrients include vitamins, minerals, essential amino acids, and essential fatty acids.

degeneration (di-jen-er-**ay**-shŏn) *n.* the deterioration and loss of specialized function of the cells of a tissue or organ. The changes may be caused by a defective blood supply or by disease. Degeneration may involve the deposition of calcium salts, of fat (*see* fatty degeneration), or of fibrous tissue in the affected organ or tissue. *See also* infiltration.

deglutition (dee-gloo-**tish**-ŏn) *n.* *see* swallowing.

dehiscence (di-**hiss**-ĕns) *n.* a splitting open, as of a surgical wound.

dehydration (dee-hy-**dray**-shŏn) *n.* loss or deficiency of water in body tissues. The condition may result from inadequate water intake and/or from excessive removal of water from the body; for example, by sweating, vomiting, or diarrhoea.

dehydroepiandrosterone (DHEA) (dee-hy-droh-epi-an-**dros**-ter-ohn) *n.* a weak androgen produced and secreted by the adrenal glands after adrenal maturation (*see* adrenarche). It is largely converted to dehydroepiandrosterone sulphate and androstenedione. All three of these molecules can cause a degree of mild androgenization but can also be converted in the circulation to the more potent androgens testosterone and dihydrotestosterone.

dehydrogenase (dee-hy-**droj**-ĕ-nayz) *n. see* oxidoreductase.

déjà vu (day-zha-**vew**) *n.* a vivid psychic experience in which immediately contemporary events seem to be a repetition of previous happenings. It is a symptom of some forms of epilepsy. *See also* jamais vu.

delayed suture (delayed primary closure) (di-**layd**) *n.* a technique used in the closure of contaminated wounds and wounds associated with tissue necrosis, such as those produced by missile injuries. The wound is partially closed after it has been cleaned sufficiently to allow adequate healing.

Delhi boil (**del**-i) *n. see* oriental sore.

deliberate self-harm (DSH) (di-**lib**-er-ăt) *n.* any attempt at self-injury or self-poisoning, without the intention to commit suicide, sometimes called **parasuicide**, which often occurs in the context of acute stress, personality disorder, depression, and alcoholism. *Compare* (attempted) suicide.

delirium (di-**li**-ri-ŭm) *n.* an acute disorder of the mental processes accompanying organic brain disease. It may be manifested by delusions, disorientation, hallucinations, or extreme excitement and occurs in metabolic disorders, intoxication, deficiency diseases, and infections. **d. tremens** an acute confusional state often seen as a withdrawal syndrome in chronic alcoholics and caused by sudden cessation of drinking alcohol. Features include anxiety, tremor, sweating, and vivid hallucinations.

delivery (di-**liv**-ĕri) *n. see* labour.

deltoid (**del**-toid) *n.* a thick triangular muscle that covers the shoulder joint. It is responsible for raising the arm from the side of the body. See illustration.

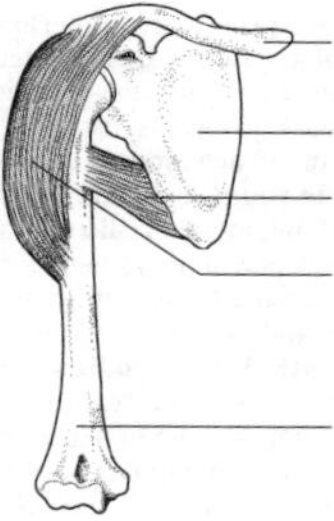

The deltoid muscle

delusion (di-**loo**-zhŏn) *n.* a belief that is held with unshakable conviction, cannot be altered by rational argument, and is outside the person's normal belief system. It may be a symptom of mania, schizophrenia, or an organic psychosis. *See also* paranoia.

delusion of reference *see* idea of reference.

Delusions Rating Scale (DRS) *n.* a tool to estimate the extent and effect of delusions in patients by means of a structured interview.

demarcation (dee-mar-**kay**-shŏn) *n.* the marking of a limit or boundary. **line of d.** a red or black line marking the boundary between necrotic and healthy tissue in gangrene.

demeclocycline (dee-mek-loh-**sy**-kleen) *n.* a tetracycline antibiotic that is administered by mouth to treat infections caused by *Chlamydia*, rickettsiae, and mycoplasmas.

dementia (di-**men**-shă) *n.* a chronic and progressive deterioration of behaviour and higher intellectual function due to organic brain disease, which is usually a condition of old age (**senile d.**) but can occur in youth or middle age. It is marked by memory disorders, changes in personality, deterioration in personal care, impaired reasoning ability, and disorientation. **d. with Lewy bodies** the third most common cause of dementia after Alzheimer's disease and vascular dementia resulting from a series of small strokes. *See* Lewy bodies. **vascular d.** any of various forms of dementia due to blockage of blood vessels, which interrupts blood supply to the brain. *See also* Alzheimer's disease, Pick's disease.

SEE WEB LINKS

- Information about dementia from the Alzheimer's Society

demi- *prefix denoting* half.

demography (di-**mog**-răfi) *n.* the study of the populations of the world, their racial make-up, movements, birth rates, death rates, and other factors affecting the quality of life within them.

demulcent (di-**mul**-sĕnt) *n.* a soothing agent that protects the mucous membranes and relieves irritation.

demyelination (dee-my-ĕ-li-**nay**-shŏn) *n.* damage to the myelin sheaths surrounding the nerve fibres in the central or peripheral nervous system. Demyelination may be a primary disorder, as in multiple sclerosis.

dendrite (**den**-dryt) *n.* one of the shorter branching processes of the cell body of a neuron, which makes contact with other neurons at synapses and carries nerve impulses from them into the cell body.

dendritic ulcer (den-**drit**-ik) *n.* a branching ulcer of the surface of the cornea caused by herpes simplex virus.

denervation (de-ner-**vay**-shŏn) *n.* interruption of the nerve supply to the muscles and skin. A denervated area of skin loses all forms of sensation and its subsequent ability to heal and renew its tissues may be impaired.

dengue (breakbone fever) (**deng**-i) *n.* a viral disease that occurs throughout the tropics and subtropics; it is transmitted to humans principally by the mosquito *Aëdes aegypti*. Symptoms include severe pains in the joints and muscles, headache, fever, and an irritating rash.

denial (di-**ny**-ăl) *n.* a psychological process in which an individual refuses to accept an aspect of reality despite robust evidence of this. It is seen particularly in dying patients who refuse to accept their impending death and in those who have problems with alcohol or drug dependency.

Denis Browne splint (**den**-iss brown) *n.* a splint used for the correction of club-foot in early infancy. [Sir Denis J. W. Browne (1892–1967), British orthopaedic surgeon]

denominator (di-**nom**-i-nay-ter) *n.* the part of the fetus that is used to describe positions for presentation. For vertex (back of the head) presentation, it is the occiput; for breech presentation, the sacrum; for face presentation, the mentum (chin).

dens (denz) *n.* a tooth or tooth-shaped structure.

dent- (denti-, dento-) *combining form denoting* the teeth.

dental care professional (**den**-t'l) *n.* any of several professionals supporting a dentist. A **dental hygienist** performs scaling and instruction in oral hygiene under the prescription of the dentist. A **dental nurse** helps the dentist at the chairside by preparing materials, passing instruments, and aspirating fluids from the patient's mouth. A **dental technician** constructs dentures, crowns, and orthodontic appliances in the laboratory for the dentist; a **clinical dental technician** provides dentures directly to patients. A **dental therapist** performs noncomplex treatment under the prescription of a dentist.

dental caries *n. see* caries.

dental nurse *n. see* dental care professional.

dentate (**den**-tayt) *adj.* **1.** having teeth. **2.** serrated; having toothlike projections.

dentifrice (**dent**-i-fris) *n.* a powder or paste for cleaning the teeth. Toothpastes contain a fine abrasive, flavouring materials, and (usually) fluoride. Some contain antimicrobials and whitening agents.

dentine (**den**-teen) *n.* a hard tissue that forms the bulk of a tooth. The dentine of the crown is covered by enamel and that of the root by cementum.

dentistry (**den**-tist-ri) *n.* the profession concerned with care and treatment of diseases of the teeth, gums, and jaws.

dentition (den-**tish**-ŏn) *n.* the number, type, and arrangement of the teeth as a whole in the mouth. **permanent d.** the 32 teeth usually present by the age of 21, made up of incisors, canines, premolars, and molars. **primary d.** the teeth of young children, which are progressively lost in preparation for the eruption of the permanent teeth. It consists of 20 teeth, made up of incisors, canines, and molars only. See illustration.

denture (den-cher) *n.* a removable plate or frame bearing one or more false teeth. **complete d.** a denture replacing all the teeth in one jaw. **partial d.** a denture replacing some teeth, designed to restore function to the remaining teeth.

deodorant (dee-**oh**-der-ănt) *n.* an agent that reduces or removes unpleasant body odours by destroying bacteria that live on the skin and break down sweat. Deodorant preparations often contain an antiseptic.

deontology (dee-on-**tol**-ŏji) *n.* an approach to ethics that is concerned with the question of what makes an action inherently right or wrong. This emphasis on rules and principles is at odds with the approach that judges actions by their outcomes (*see* consequentialism), and the tension between the two is central to many issues in medical ethics.

deoxycholic acid (dee-oks-i-**koh**-lik) *n. see* bile acids.

deoxycorticosterone (dee-oks-i-kor-ti-koh-**steer**-ohn) *n.* a hormone, synthesized and released by the adrenal cortex, that regulates salt and water balance. *See also* corticosteroid.

deoxyribonucleic acid (dee-oks-i-ry-boh-new-**klee**-ik) *n. see* DNA.

Department of Health (DH) (di-**part**-mĕnt) *n.* a department of central government that supports the Secretary of State for Health in meeting his or her obligations, which include the National Health Service and the promotion and protection of the health of the nation. Since April 2013, the Department of

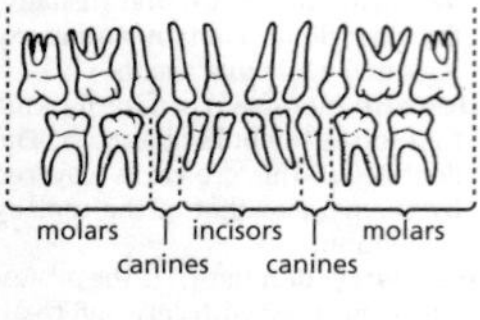

Primary dentition

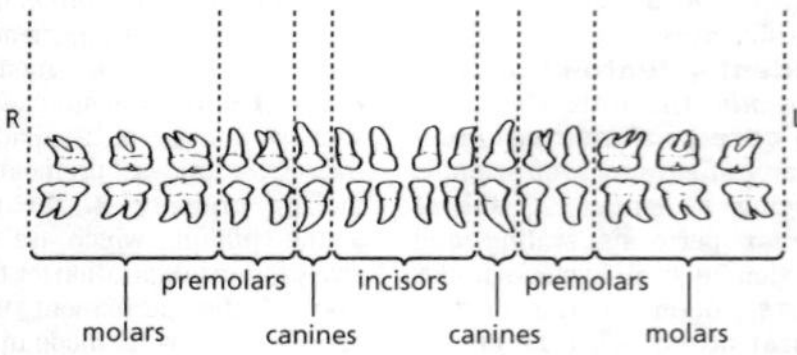

Permanent dentition

Health no longer has direct control of the NHS, which has passed to NHS England.

SEE WEB LINKS

- The Department of Health website

dependence (drug dependence) (di-**pen**-dăns) *n.* **1.** the physical and/or the psychological effects produced by the habitual taking of certain drugs, characterized by a compulsion to continue taking the drug. **physical d.** dependence in which withdrawal of the drug causes specific symptoms (**withdrawal symptoms**), such as sweating, vomiting, or tremors, that are reversed by further doses. It may be induced by alcohol, morphine, heroin, and cocaine. **psychological d.** dependence in which repeated use of a drug induces reliance on it for a state of wellbeing and contentment, but there are no physical withdrawal symptoms if use of the drug is stopped. It may be induced by nicotine in tobacco, cannabis, and such drugs as barbiturates and amphetamines. **2.** a state of reliance on others for aspects of self-care, sometimes used as a measure of nursing workload.

depersonalization (dee-per-sŏ-nă-ly-**zay**-shŏn) *n.* a state in which a person feels himself becoming unreal or strangely altered, or feels that his mind is becoming separated from his body. Severe feelings of depersonalization occur in conditions such as anxiety neurosis, schizophrenia, and epilepsy. *See also* derealization, out-of-body experience.

depilatory (di-**pil**-ă-ter-i) *n.* an agent applied to the skin to remove hair.

depolarization (dee-poh-lă-ry-**zay**-shŏn) *n.* the sudden surge of charged particles across the membrane of a nerve cell or of a muscle cell that accompanies a physicochemical change in the membrane and cancels out, or reverses, its resting potential to produce an action potential.

depot injection (**dep**-oh) *n.* the administration of a sustained-action drug formulation that allows slow release and gradual absorption, so that the active agent can act for much longer periods than is possible with standard injections. Depot injections are usually given deep into a muscle.

depressant (di-**pres**-ănt) *n.* an agent that reduces the normal activity of any body system or function. Drugs such as general anaesthetics, barbiturates, and opioids are depressants of the central nervous system and respiration.

depression (di-**presh**-ŏn) *n.* **1.** a mental state characterized by excessive sadness. **2.** a mental illness characterized by the pervasive and persistent presence of certain symptoms on most days for at least two weeks. These symptoms include low mood, loss or impairment of motivation, energy, interest, and enjoyment, impaired memory and concentration, loss of appetite and libido, insomnia, and early morning wakening. A single episode of these symptoms is known as a **major depressive episode**; more than one episode is called **major** (or **clinical**) **d.** Treatment for depression is usually with antidepressant drugs, cognitive behavioural therapy, and/or psychotherapy. *See also* postnatal (depression). **—depressive** *adj.*

SEE WEB LINKS

- Explanation of depression, including a short video, from the Royal College of Psychiatrists

depressor (di-pres-er) *n.* **1.** a muscle that causes lowering of part of the body. **2.** a nerve that lowers blood pressure.

Derbyshire neck (dar-bi-sher) *n.* endemic goitre that was once common in Derbyshire due to lack of iodine in the soil and water.

derealization (dee-riă-ly-zay-shŏn) *n.* a feeling of unreality in which the environment is experienced as unreal and strange. It occurs in association with depersonalization or with the conditions that cause depersonalization.

derm- (derma-, dermo-, dermat(o)-) *combining form denoting* the skin.

-derm *combining form denoting* **1.** the skin. **2.** a germ layer.

dermal (der-măl) *adj.* relating to or affecting the skin, especially the dermis.

dermatitis (der-mă-ty-tis) *n.* an inflammatory condition of the skin, especially one in which outside agents play a primary role (*compare* eczema). **allergic contact d.** dermatitis in which skin changes resembling those of eczema develop as a delayed reaction to contact with a particular allergen. Common examples include **nickel d.** from costume jewellery, clothing fasteners, etc., and fragrance allergy (from toiletries, deodorants, perfumes, etc.). **d. herpetiformis** an uncommon very itchy rash with symmetrical blistering, especially on the knees, elbows, buttocks, and shoulders. It is associated with gluten sensitivity. **primary irritant d.** a condition that may occur in anyone who has sufficient contact with such irritants as acids, alkalis, solvents, and (especially) detergents. It is the commonest cause of **occupational d.** in hairdressers, nurses, cooks, etc. *See also* napkin rash. **seborrhoeic d.** *see* (seborrhoeic) eczema.

dermatochalasis (der-mă-toh-kă-**lay**-sis) *n.* redundant eyelid skin, which may cause drooping of the upper lid. It usually occurs as a result of ageing. *Compare* blepharochalasis.

dermatoglyphics (der-mă-toh-**glif**-iks) *n.* **1.** the patterns of finger, palm, toe, and sole prints, which are unique to each individual. Abnormalities are found in those with chromosomal variants, e.g. Down's syndrome. **2.** the study of these patterns, which is of use in medicine, criminology, and anthropology.

dermatology (der-mă-**tol**-ŏji) *n.* the medical specialty concerned with the diagnosis and treatment of skin disorders. **—dermatological** *adj.* **—dermatologist** *n.*

SEE WEB LINKS

- Website of the British Association of Dermatologists

dermatology life quality index (DLQI) *n.* a validated questionnaire designed to assess the impact of skin diseases on psychological and social wellbeing. DLQI scores of more than 10 (indicating a severe impact on life) are required before biological treatments for psoriasis may be administered in the UK.

dermatome (**der**-mă-tohm) *n.* a surgical instrument used for cutting thin slices of skin in some skin grafting operations.

dermatomycosis (der-mă-toh-my-**koh**-sis) *n.* any infection of the skin caused by fungi.

dermatomyositis (der-mă-toh-my-oh-**sy**-tis) *n.* an inflammatory disorder of the skin and underlying tissues, including the muscles. A pink/purple skin eruption occurs on the face, scalp, neck, shoulders, and knuckles and is later accompanied by severe swelling. The condition is one of the connective-tissue diseases; it is often associated with internal cancer in adults, though not in children.

dermatophyte (**der**-mă-toh-fyt) *n.* any fungus belonging to the genera Microsporum, Epidermophyton, or Trichophyton, which cause ringworm (**dermatophytosis**). *See also* tinea.

dermatosis (der-mă-**toh**-sis) *n.* any disease of skin, particularly one without inflammation. **juvenile plantar d.** a condition in which the skin on the front of the sole becomes red, glazed, and symmetrically cracked. It affects children up to the age of 14 and is believed to be related to the wearing of trainers.

dermis (corium) (**der**-mis) *n.* the true skin: the thick layer of living tissue that lies beneath the epidermis. **—dermal** *adj.*

dermographism (der-moh-**graf**-izm) *n.* a common local reaction caused by pressure stroking the skin, which develops itchy weals. People with such highly sensitive skin can 'write' on it with a finger or blunt instrument, the pressure producing weals.

dermoid cyst (dermoid) (**der**-moid) *n.* a benign tumour (a type of teratoma) containing skin with hair follicles and sebaceous glands, and often sebum, blood, fat, bone, nails, teeth, and thyroid tissue, usually found at sites marking the fusion of developing sections of the body in the embryo. It is the most common benign ovarian tumour in girls.

Descemet's membrane (dess-ĕ-**mayz**) *n.* the membrane that forms the deepest layer of the stroma of the cornea of the eye. The endothelium lies between it and the aqueous humour. [J. Descemet (1732–1810), French anatomist]

descriptive statistics (dis-**kript**-iv) *n.* the use of statistics to organize and present data in a study in an informative way that describes the basic features of the data and enables analysis.

desensitization (dee-sen-si-ty-**zay**-shŏn) *n.* **1. (hyposensitization)** a method for reducing the effects of a known allergen by injecting, over a period, gradually increasing doses of the allergen, until resistance is built up. *See* allergy. **2.** a technique used in the behaviour therapy of phobic states. The thing that is feared is very gradually introduced to the patient, in conjunction with relaxation therapy, so that he or she is able to cope with progressively closer approximations to it.

desferrioxamine (dess-ferri-**oks**-ă-meen) *n.* a drug that combines with iron in body tissues and fluids and is administered by infusion to treat iron poisoning, iron overload, or diseases that involve iron storage in parts of the body (*see* haemochromatosis). Trade name: **Desferal**.

desmoid tumour (**dez**-moid) *n.* a dense connective-tissue tumour with a dangerous propensity for repeated local recurrence after treatment. Intra-abdominal desmoids have an association with familial adenomatous polyposis.

DESMOND (diabetes education and self-management for ongoing and newly diagnosed) (**dez**-mŏnd) *n.* a structured one-day education programme for patients with type 2 diabetes. Outcomes show an increase in participants' understanding of diabetes and risks factors associated with coronary heart disease.

desmopressin (dess-moh-**press**-in) *n.* a synthetic derivative of vasopressin that causes a decrease in urine output. It is taken orally, sublingually, intranasally, or by injection to treat diabetes insipidus, nocturnal enuresis, mild haemophilia, and von Willebrand's disease. Trade names: **DDAVP**, **DesmoMelt**, **Desmotabs**, **Desmospray**, **Octim**.

desogestrel (dess-oh-**jee**-strĕl) *n.* a progestogen used in various oral contraceptives, either alone (**Aizea**, etc.) or in combination with ethinylestradiol (**Gedarel**, **Marvelon**, **Mercilon**).

desquamation (dess-kwă-**may**-shŏn) *n.* the process in which the outer layer of the epidermis of the skin is removed by scaling.

detached retina (di-**tacht**) *n. see* retinal detachment.

detergent (di-**ter**-jĕnt) *n.* a synthetic cleansing agent that removes all impurities from a surface by reacting with grease and suspended particles, including bacteria and other microorganisms.

detoxification (detoxication) (dee-toksi-fi-**kay**-shŏn) *n.* **1.** the process by which toxic substances are removed or toxic effects neutralized. It is one of the functions of the liver. **2.** the period of withdrawal when a person stops long-term consumption of alcohol or some other drug.

detrition (di-**trish**-ŏn) *n.* the process of wearing away solid bodies (e.g. bones) by friction or use.

detritus (di-**try**-tŭs) *n.* particles of matter produced by disintegration, tissue death, etc.

detrusor muscle (di-**troo**-ser) *n.* the muscle of the urinary bladder wall. Its function is assessed by urodynamic investigation (*see* urodynamics).

detumescence (dee-tew-**mes**-ĕns) *n.* **1.** the reverse of erection, whereby the erect penis or clitoris becomes flaccid after orgasm. **2.** subsidence of a swelling.

deut- (deuto-, deuter(o)-) *combining form denoting* two, second, or secondary.

deuteranopia (dew-ter-ă-**noh**-piă) *n.* a defect in colour vision in which reds, yellows, and greens are confused. *Compare* tritanopia.

developmental delay (di-vel-ŏp-**men**-t'l) *n.* considerable delay in the physical or mental development of children when compared with their peers. There are many causes. **Global delay** describes the state of a child whose overall development is slow in all areas.

developmental disorder *n.* any one of a group of conditions that arise in infancy or childhood and are characterized by delays in biologically determined psychological functions, such as language. In **pervasive** conditions (e.g. autism) many types of development are involved; in **specific** disorders, (such as dyslexia) the handicap is an isolated problem.

developmental milestones *pl. n.* skills gained by a developing child, which should be achieved by a given age. Examples include smiling by six weeks and sitting unsupported by six months. Failure to achieve a particular milestone by a given age is indicative of developmental delay. See table.

deviation (dee-vi-**ay**-shŏn) *n.* **1.** (in ophthalmology) any abnormal position of one or both eyes. Deviations of both eyes may occur in brain disease. Deviations of one eye come into the category of squint (*see* strabismus). **dissociated vertical d.** an acquired condition, chiefly associated with infantile esotropia (convergent strabismus), in which one eye looks upwards when it is covered. **2.** *see* sexual deviation.

Devic's disease (**dev**-iks) *n. see* neuromyelitis optica. [E. Devic (1869–1930), French physician]

DEXA *n.* dual-energy X-ray absorptiometry: a method of measuring bone density based on the proportion of a beam of photons that passes through the bone. *See also* T score.

dexamethasone (deks-ă-**meth**-ă-zohn) *n.* a corticosteroid drug administered by mouth or injection or as eye drops principally to treat rheumatic and other inflammatory conditions and nausea and vomiting associated with cancer chemotherapy. Trade names: **Maxidex**, **Minims Dexamethasone**, **Ozurdex**.

dexamfetamine (dexamphetamine) (deks-am-**fet**-ămin) *n. see* amphetamines.

dextr- (dextro-) *combining form denoting* **1.** the right side. **2.** (in chemistry) dextrorotation.

dextran (**deks**-tran) *n.* a carbohydrate, consisting of branched chains of glucose units, that is a storage product of bacteria and yeasts. Preparations of dextran solution are used in transfusions, in order to increase the volume of plasma.

dextrin (**deks**-trin) *n.* a carbohydrate formed as an intermediate product in the digestion of starch by the enzyme amylase. Dextrin is

Developmental milestones

	6 weeks **Supine infant**	*6–9 months* **Sitting infant**	*1 year* **Standing/walking infant**	*18–24 months* **Mobile toddler**	*3–4 years* **Communicating child**
Gross motor	Symmetrical movements of all limbs When prone raises head	Supports head Sits unaided (6 m) Stands holding on (7 m) Pulls to standing (9m)	Walks holding onto furniture (9 m) Walks if led A few steps unsupported (12 m)	Walks with normal gait Climbs steps Kicks ball (20 m)	Hops on one foot
Fine motor/ vision	Fixes and follows gaze	Reaches for objects Palmar grasp Transfers objects hand to hand Bangs toys together	Pincer grip (10 m)	Scribbles (14 m) Builds tower of six blocks (24 m)	Copies circle (3 y) Copies square (4 y) Builds bridge or steps with blocks when shown

Language/ hearing	Normal cry Responds to sounds	Turns to a voice (7m) Nonspecific babble (10 m)	Understands simple commands: 'No' Says a few words appropriately: 'Mama' 'Dada' (13 m) Turns to own name	Combines two different words (20 m) Points to one named body part	Gives first and last name Recognizes colours (3 y) Speech fully comprehensible (4 y)
Social	Regards face Smiles responsively	Puts solid food in mouth (6 m) Waves goodbye (8 m)	Drinks from cup (12 m) Wary of strangers	Feeds self with spoon Removes clothing Asserts own wishes Symbolic play with miniature toys	Washes hands with help Eats with knife and fork Make-believe play Shows sympathy appropriately Likes hearing and telling stories

(Median ages of achievement of each skill in brackets)

used in the preparation of pharmaceutical products and surgical dressings.

dextrocardia (deks-troh-**kar**-diă) *n.* a congenital defect in which the position of the heart is a mirror image of its normal position, with the apex of the ventricles pointing to the right.

dextrose (**deks**-trohz) *n.* *see* glucose.

DH *n.* *see* Department of Health.

DHEA *n.* *see* dehydroepiandrosterone.

dhobie itch (**doh**-bi) *n.* an informal name for tinea cruris. *See* tinea.

DI *n.* donor insemination (*see* artificial insemination).

di- *prefix denoting* two or double.

dia- *prefix denoting* **1.** through. **2.** completely or throughout. **3.** apart.

diabetes (dy-ă-**bee**-teez) *n.* any disorder of metabolism causing excessive thirst and the production of large volumes of urine. **d. insipidus** a rare form of diabetes that is due to deficiency of the pituitary hormone vasopressin (antidiuretic hormone). **d. mellitus (DM)** a disorder of carbohydrate metabolism leading to an abnormally high blood sugar level (hyperglycaemia). As the blood sugar rises, the typical symptoms of urinary frequency and increased thirst emerge. Tiredness, blurring of vision, and weight loss are also common. The long-term complications of diabetes are damage to the eye, the kidney, and the nerve supply to the feet, as well as accelerated vascular disease leading to coronary heart disease or stroke. These can be delayed or avoided by control of blood glucose levels, combined with blood pressure control and a healthy lifestyle. **Type 1 d. Mellitus** is an autoimmune disease that typically starts in childhood or adolescence. Treatment with insulin injections needs to be started within a few weeks of the onset of symptoms and is almost invariably lifelong. **Type 2 d. Mellitus** is a genetically determined resistance to insulin action on target tissues and has become increasingly common in the developed world with the associated rise in obesity. People with type 2 diabetes outnumber those with type 1 diabetes by at least ten to one. The mainstay of treatment is a healthy diet, regular physical activity, and weight control in conjunction with oral hypoglycaemic drugs. Insulin treatment is often required after 5–10 years from diagnosis. The rarer forms of diabetes mellitus include **maturity-onset diabetes of the young (MODY)** and diabetes secondary to destruction of the pancreas (e.g. by pancreatitis). **gestational d.** diabetes mellitus or impaired glucose tolerance that is diagnosed during pregnancy. **pregestational d.** pre-existing diabetes mellitus in a woman who becomes pregnant. **—diabetic** (dy-ă-**bet**-ik) *adj., n.*

SEE WEB LINKS

- Website of Diabetes UK

diabetic amyotrophy *n.* *see* amyotrophy.

diabetic hand syndrome *n.* the combination of features, often found in the hands of long-standing diabetic subjects, consisting of Dupuytren's contractures, knuckle pads, carpal tunnel syndrome, cheiroarthropathy, and sclerosing tenosynovitis.

diabetic honeymoon period *n.* a well-recognized period just after the diagnosis of type 1 diabetes mellitus when only very low insulin doses are required to control the condition. It lasts for months to a few years.

diabetic ketoacidosis (DKA) *n.* *see* ketoacidosis.

diabetic nephropathy *n.* *see* nephropathy.

diabetic neuropathy *n.* *see* neuropathy.

diabetic retinopathy *n.* *see* retinopathy.

diabetologist (dy-ă-bĕ-**tol**-ŏ-jist) *n.* a doctor who specializes in the diagnosis and treatment of diabetes mellitus and the prevention of its long-term complications. In the UK most diabetologists are also endocrinologists.

diagnosis (dy-ăg-**noh**-sis) *n.* the process of determining the nature of a disorder by considering the patient's signs and symptoms, medical background, and – when necessary – results of laboratory tests and X-ray examinations. **differential d.** diagnosis of a condition whose signs and/or symptoms are shared by various other conditions. *See also* prenatal diagnosis. *Compare* prognosis. **—diagnostic** (dy-ăg-**noss**-tik) *adj.*

Diagnostic and Statistical Manual of Mental Disorders *n.* *see* DSM.

diagnostic peritoneal lavage *n.* the instillation of saline directly into the abdominal cavity and its subsequent aspiration a few minutes later. If the fluid is bloodstained on recovery an intra-abdominal haemorrhage is indicated. This is a useful diagnostic tool in trauma patients.

dialysate (dy-**al**-i-sayt) *n.* fluid used in dialysis. In haemodialysis the dialysate is purified tap water to which has been added a precise amount of electrolyte solution. In peritoneal dialysis the dialysate is a commercially produced fluid containing electrolytes with glucose, glucose polymers, or amino acids.

dialyser (**dy**-ă-ly-zer) *n.* a medical device designed to allow controllable transfer of solutes and water across a semipermeable membrane separating blood and dialysate solutions flowing counter-current to each other.

dialysis (dy-**al**-i-sis) *n.* a method of separating particles of different dimensions in a liquid mixture, using a thin semipermeable membrane (*see* dialyser). A solution of the mixture is separated from distilled water by the membrane; the solutes pass through the membrane into the water while the proteins, etc., are retained. The principle of dialysis is used in treating kidney failure (*see* haemodialysis). **peritoneal d.** the use of the peritoneum as a semipermeable membrane separating blood and dialysate by patients with kidney failure. It is either a temporary and emergency treatment, using a rigid cannula to deliver fluid into the peritoneal cavity, or a continuous treatment, in the form of chronic ambulatory peritoneal dialysis (*see* CAPD) or automated peritoneal dialysis (*see* APD).

diamorphine (dy-ă-**mor**-feen) *n.* a powerful opioid analgesic used for the relief of severe pain, especially in terminal illness, and pulmonary oedema.

diapedesis (dy-ă-pĕ-**dee**-sis) *n.* migration of cells through the walls of blood capillaries into the tissue spaces. Diapedesis is an important part of the reaction of tissues to injury (*see* inflammation).

diaphoresis (dy-ă-fer-**ee**-sis) *n.* the process of sweating, especially excessive sweating. *See* sweat.

diaphoretic (sudorific) (dy-ă-fer-**et**-ik) *n.* a drug that causes an increase in sweating. Antipyretic drugs have diaphoretic activity.

diaphragm (**dy**-ă-fram) *n.* **1.** (in anatomy) a thin musculomembranous dome-shaped muscle that separates the thoracic and abdominal cavities. It plays an important role in breathing. There are openings in the diaphragm through which the oesophagus, blood vessels, and nerves pass. **2.** a hemispherical rubber cap fitted inside the vagina over the neck (cervix) of the uterus as a contraceptive. When combined with the use of a chemical spermicide the diaphragm provides reasonably reliable contraception.

diaphysis (dy-**af**-i-sis) *n.* the body, or shaft, of a long bone, consisting of a thick cylinder of compact bone surrounding a large medullary cavity. *Compare* epiphysis. **—diaphyseal** (dy-ă-**fiz**-iăl) *adj.*

diarrhoea (dy-ă-**ree**-ă) *n.* frequent bowel evacuation or the passage of abnormally soft or liquid faeces. Its causes include intestinal infections, inflammation, anxiety, and irritable bowel syndrome. Severe or prolonged diarrhoea may lead to excessive loss of water, salts, and nutrients.

diarthrosis (synovial joint) (dy-arth-**roh**-sis) *n.* a freely movable joint. The ends of the adjoining bones are covered with a thin cartilaginous sheet, and the bones are linked by a ligament lined with synovial membrane, which secretes synovial fluid. See illustration.

diastase (**dy**-ă-stayz) *n.* an enzyme that hydrolyses starch in barley grain to produce maltose during

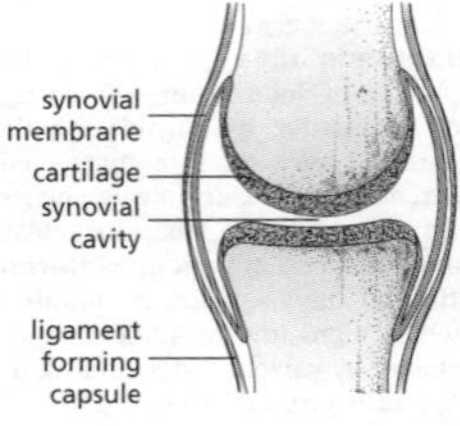

A diarthrosis

the malting process. It has been used to aid the digestion of starch in some digestive disorders.

diastasis (dy-**ast**-ă-sis) *n.* dislocation of bones at an immovable or slightly movable joint, as at the pubic symphysis.

diastema (dy-ă-**stee**-mă) *n.* a space between two teeth.

diastole (dy-**ast**-ŏ-li) *n.* the period between two contractions of the heart, when the muscle of the heart relaxes and allows the chambers to fill with blood. *See also* blood pressure, systole. —**diastolic** (dy-ă-**stol**-ik) *adj.*

diastolic pressure *n.* *see* blood pressure.

diathermy (**dy**-ă-therm-i) *n.* the production of heat in a part of the body by means of a high-frequency electric current passed between two electrodes. Diathermy is used to coagulate tissues and seal off blood vessels. Instruments used to deliver diathermy include various surgical instruments (e.g. **d. knives**, **forceps**, and **scissors**). A **d. snare** (or **needle**) is used to destroy unwanted tissue and to remove small superficial neoplasms. *See also* electrosurgery.

diathesis (dy-**ath**-i-sis) *n.* a higher than average tendency to acquire certain diseases, such as allergies, rheumatic diseases, or gout. Such diseases may run in families, but they are not inherited.

diazepam (dy-**az**-ĕ-pam) *n.* a long-acting benzodiazepine administered by mouth, injection, or rectally for the short-term relief of acute anxiety and insomnia and to treat delirium tremens, status epilepticus, and febrile convulsions. It is also used as a premedication.

diazoxide (dy-ă-**zok**-syd) *n.* a drug given by mouth to treat conditions in which the levels of blood sugar are chronically low. Trade name: **Eudemine**.

DIC *n.* *see* disseminated intravascular coagulation.

dicephalus (dy-**sef**-ă-lŭs) *n.* *see* craniopagus.

dichromatic (dy-kroh-**mat**-ik) *adj.* describing the state of colour vision of those who can appreciate only two of the three primary colours. *Compare* trichromatic.

diclofenac (dy-**kloh**-fen-ak) *n.* an anti-inflammatory drug (*see* NSAID) used to relieve joint pain in osteoarthritis, rheumatoid arthritis, acute gout, and actinic keratosis and also for postoperative pain relief. It is administered by mouth or injection or as suppositories, eye drops, or gel. Trade names: **Dyloject**, **Motifene**, **Solaraze**, **Voltarol**, etc.

dicophane (**dy**-koh-fayn) *n.* *see* DDT.

dicrotism (**dy**-krŏ-tizm) *n.* a condition in which the pulse is felt as a double beat for each contraction of the heart. It may be seen in typhoid fever. —**dicrotic** (dy-**krot**-ik) *adj.*

dicycloverine (dicyclomine) (dy-**sy**-klŏ-vĕ-reen) *n.* an antimuscarinic drug that reduces spasms of smooth muscle and is administered by mouth to relieve irritable bowel syndrome and related conditions.

didanosine (ddI) (dy-**dan**-ŏ-seen) *n.* an antiretroviral drug that is administered by mouth, in combination with other antiretroviral drugs, to treat AIDS and HIV infection. Possible side-effects include damage to nerves, severe pancreatitis, nausea, vomiting, and headache. Trade name: **Videx**.

didym- (didymo-) *combining form denoting* the testis.

diet (dy-ĕt) *n.* **1.** the mixture of foods that a person eats. **2.** a restrictive regime of food intake used by an individual to lose weight. **balanced d.** a diet that contains the correct proportions of all the nutrients.

dietary fibre (roughage) (dy-it-er-i) *n.* the part of food that cannot be digested and absorbed to produce energy. Foods with a high fibre content include wholemeal cereals and flour, root vegetables, nuts, and fruit. Dietary fibre is considered by some to be helpful in the prevention of such diseases as diverticulosis, constipation, appendicitis, obesity, and diabetes mellitus.

Dietary Reference Values (DRVs) *n.* a set of statistical terms used to describe nutritional requirements. **EAR** (estimated average requirement): the amount of a nutrient that will meet the needs of 50% of the population. **RDA** (recommended daily amount): the average amount that should be provided per head of a group of people if the needs of practically all members of the group are to be met. **LRNI** (lowest recommended nutrient intake): the amount of a nutrient that provides only 2.5% of the population with their requirements. **RNI** (reference nutrient intake): the amount that is sufficient for almost 97.5% of individuals in a population. It is the term generally used when expressing dietary requirements. **safe level**: used when there is insufficient data to determine the RNI, set as the average requirement plus 20%. **RI** (reference intake): a guide to how many calories and nutrients an average person can consume each day for a healthy balanced diet. This is used in labelling information for energy, protein, carbohydrate, sugars, fat, saturated fat, fibre, and salt.

dietetics (dy-i-**tet**-iks) *n.* the application of the principles of nutrition to the selection of food and the feeding of individuals and groups. *See also* dietitian.

SEE WEB LINKS

- Website of the British Dietetic Association

diethylcarbamazine (dy-eth-il-kar-**bam**-ă-zeen) *n.* an anthelmintic drug that is administered by mouth in the treatment of filariasis and loiasis.

diethylstilbestrol (dy-eth-il-stil-**bes**-trŏl) *n.* a synthetic female sex hormone (*see* oestrogen) that is licensed to treat breast cancer in postmenopausal women and prostate cancer but is now rarely used because of its toxicity. Prescribed in the 1950s to prevent miscarriage, it was subsequently found to increase the risk of cancers of the breast, genital tract, uterus, and ovary in daughters of patients who were treated with it.

dietitian (registered dietitian, RD) (dy-i-**tish**-ăn) *n.* (in the UK) a person with a degree in nutrition and dietetics, or a degree in nutrition and a postgraduate diploma in dietetics, who provides practical dietary advice, based on principles of food science and nutrition, for those on normal and therapeutic diets. A registered dietitian may also be involved in the diagnosis and dietary treatment of disease, working as a member of a multidisciplinary team in a hospital or the community.

Dietl's crisis (dee-t'lz) *n.* acute obstruction of a kidney causing severe pain in the loins. The obstruction usually occurs at the junction of the renal pelvis and the ureter, causing the kidney to become distended with accumulated urine (*see* hydronephrosis). [J. Dietl (1804–78), Polish physician]

differential diagnosis (dif-er-**en**-shăl) *n. see* diagnosis.

differential leucocyte count (differential blood count) *n.* a determination of the proportions of the different kinds of white cells (leucocytes) present in a sample of blood. The information often aids diagnosis of disease.

differentiation (dif-er-en-shi-**ay**-shŏn) *n.* **1.** (in embryology) the process in embryonic development during which unspecialized cells or tissues become specialized for particular functions. **2.** (in oncology) the degree of similarity of tumour cells to the structure of the organ from which the tumour arose. Tumours are classified as well, moderately, or poorly differentiated. *See also* grade.

diffusion (di-**few**-*zh*ŏn) *n.* the mixing of one liquid or gas with another by the random movement of their particles.

di George syndrome (dee-**jorj**) *n.* a hereditary condition resulting in an inability to fight infections (immunodeficiency) associated with absence of the parathyroid gland and thymus, abnormalities of the heart, and low levels of calcium. *See also* CATCH-22. [A. M. di George (1921–2009), US paediatrician]

digestion (dy-**jes**-chŏn) *n.* the process in which ingested food is broken down in the alimentary canal into a form that can be absorbed and assimilated by the tissues of the body.

digit (**dij**-it) *n.* a finger or toe.

digital (**dij**-it-ăl) *adj.* **1.** relating to a finger or toe. **2.** relating to or designating information that can be represented by a series of numbers. **d. hearing aid** *see* hearing aid. **d. image** an electronically produced image, such as an image produced by digital radiography, made up of pixels, each of which has numbers to represent its position and shade. *See* digitization. **d. radiography** *see* radiography. **d. subtraction** a radiological technique that enhances visualization of blood vessels. A digitized image is taken before the contrast medium is injected, and this is subtracted by computer from the images taken after contrast injection.

digitalis (dij-i-**tay**-lis) *n.* an extract from the dried leaves of foxgloves (*Digitalis* species), which contains various substances, including the glycoside digoxin, that stimulate heart muscle.

digitalization (dij-it-ă-ly-**zay**-shŏn) *n.* the administration of a derivative of digitalis to a patient with heart failure until the optimum level has been reached in the heart tissues.

digitization (dij-it-I-**zay**-shŏn) *n.* (in radiology) the representation of analogue images (i.e. images produced by X-ray machines, CT scanners, MRI scanners, or ultrasound probes) as a set of numerical values, which enables their electronic manipulation, storage, and transfer via computer links in the form of digital images.

dignity (**dig**-ni-ti) *n.* the feeling of patients that they are respected as individuals and not exposed unnecessarily to procedures they might find degrading. Its preservation is important whenever people are undressed or asked very personal questions, discussed in the third person, or involved in activities that are not essential (such as teaching). Clinical failures here may lead to lack of compliance with treatment or even complaint or depression. Dignity is vital in the care of any client group where help is needed with personal functions or when someone is dying. *See also* autonomy.

digoxin (di-**joks**-in) *n.* a drug derived from digitalis that increases the force of heart muscle contraction and decreases heart rate. It is administered by mouth or injection to control atrial fibrillation. Trade name: **Lanoxin**.

dihydrocodeine (dy-hy-drŏ-**koh**-deen) *n.* an opioid analgesic administered by mouth or injection to relieve moderate to severe pain. It is also administered orally in combination with paracetamol (as **co-dydramol**). Trade names: **DF118 Forte**, **DHC Continus**.

dihydrotestosterone (DHT) (dy-hy-droh-test-**ost**-er-ohn) *n.* a product formed from the action of the enzyme 5α-reductase on testosterone. DHT is an estimated 2.5 times more potent than testosterone but is present in much smaller amounts in the circulation.

dilatation (dy-lă-**tay**-shŏn) *n.* the enlargement or expansion of a hollow organ (such as a blood vessel) or cavity.

dilatation and curettage (D and C) *n.* an operation in which the cervix (neck) of the uterus is dilated, using a dilator, and the lining (endometrium) of the uterus is lightly scraped off with a manual curette (*see* curettage) or removed by suction using an aspirator. It is performed for a variety of reasons, including removal of any material remaining after miscarriage and obtaining an endometrial biopsy for histological examination.

dilator (dy-**lay**-ter) *n.* **1.** an instrument used to enlarge a body opening or cavity. **2.** a drug, applied either locally or systemically, that causes expansion of a structure. *See also* vasodilator. **3.** a muscle that, by its action, opens an aperture or orifice in the body.

dill water (dil) *n.* a preparation containing a volatile oil extracted from the dill plant (Anethum graveolens), used to treat flatulence in infants.

diltiazem (**dil**-ti-ă-zem) *n.* a calcium-channel blocker that is used in the prevention and treatment of angina and high blood pressure (hypertension). It acts as a vasodilator and is administered by mouth. Diltiazem may also be administered as a topical cream for chronic anal fissures. Trade names: **Adizem SR**, **Dilzem SR**, **Tildiem**, etc.

diluent (**dy**-loo-ĕnt) *n.* a substance, such as water, that is added to a solution or mixture to decrease its viscosity, enabling ease of administration, or to decrease its toxicity or potency.

dimeticone (dimethicone) (dy-**met**-i-kohn) *n.* a silicone preparation used as a lotion to treat head lice and also included as an ingredient in barrier creams to prevent undue drying of the skin and to protect it against irritating external agents. Trade name: **Hedrin**. *See also* simeticone.

dinoprostone (dy-noh-**prost**-ohn) *n.* a prostaglandin drug used mainly to induce labour. It is administered as pessaries or vaginal tablets or gel. Trade names: **Propess**, **Prostin E2**.

dioctyl sodium sulphosuccinate (dy-**ok**-tyl **soh**-di-ŭm sul-foh-**suk**-si-nayt) *n.* *see* docusate sodium.

diode laser (**dy**-ohd) *n.* *see* laser.

dioptre (dy-**op**-ter) *n.* the unit of measurement of the power of refraction of a lens. One dioptre is the power of a lens that brings parallel light rays to a focus at a point one metre from the lens, after passing through it.

diphtheria (dif-**theer**-iă) *n.* an acute highly contagious infection, caused by the bacterium *Corynebacterium diphtheriae*, that generally affects the throat but occasionally affects other mucous membranes and the skin. Early symptoms are a sore throat, weakness, and mild fever; later, a soft grey membrane forms across the throat, constricting the air passages and causing difficulty in breathing and swallowing. Bacteria multiply at the site of infection and release a toxin into the bloodstream, which damages heart and nerves. An effective immunization programme has now made diphtheria rare in most Western countries.

diphtheroid (**dif**-ther-oid) *adj.* resembling diphtheria (especially the membrane formed in diphtheria) or the bacteria that cause it.

diphyllobothriasis (dy-fil-oh-bo-**thry**-ă-sis) *n.* an infestation of the intestine with the broad tapeworm, *Diphyllobothrium latum*, which sometimes causes nausea, malnutrition, diarrhoea, and anaemia resulting from impaired absorption of vitamin B_{12} through the gut.

dipipanone (dy-**pip**-ă-nohn) *n.* a potent opioid analgesic administered by mouth in combination with cyclizine to relieve severe pain.

dipl- (diplo-) *combining form denoting* double.

diplacusis (dip-lă-**kew**-sis) *n.* perception of a single sound as double owing to a defect of the cochlea in the inner ear.

diplegia (dy-**plee**-jă) *n.* paralysis involving both sides of the body and affecting the legs more severely than the arms. **cerebral d.** a form of cerebral palsy in which there is widespread damage, in both cerebral hemispheres, of the brain cells that control the movements of the limbs. **—diplegic** *adj.*

diplococcus (dip-loh-**kok**-ŭs) *n.* any of a group of nonmotile parasitic spherical bacteria that occur in pairs. The group includes the pneumococcus.

diploë (**dip**-loh-ee) *n.* the lattice-like tissue that lies between the inner and outer layers of the skull.

diploid (**dip**-loid) *adj.* describing cells, nuclei, or organisms in which each chromosome except the Y sex chromosome is represented twice. *Compare* haploid. **—diploid** *n.*

diplopia (di-**ploh**-piă) *n.* double vision: the simultaneous awareness of two images of one object. It is usually due to limitation of movement of one eye, which may be caused by a defect of the nerves or muscles controlling eye movement or a mechanical restriction of eyeball movement in the orbit (**binocular d.**). Double vision that does not disappear on covering one eye (**monocular d.**) can be caused by early cataract (*see also* polyopia).

dipsomania (dip-sŏ-**may**-niă) *n.* morbid and insatiable craving for alcohol, occurring in paroxysms. A small proportion of alcoholics show this symptom.

dipyridamole (dy-py-**rid**-ă-mohl) *n.* a drug that dilates the blood vessels of the heart and reduces platelet aggregation. It is given by mouth to prevent thrombosis around prosthetic heart valves and recurrent stroke or transient ischaemic attacks. Trade names: **Persantin**, **Persantin Retard**.

directly observed therapy (DOT) (di-**rekt**-li) *n.* antituberculosis therapy in which a nurse practitioner watches the patient taking his or her drugs or administers the drugs.

director (di-**rek**-ter) *n.* an instrument used to guide the extent and direction of a surgical incision.

dis- *prefix denoting* separation.

disability (dis-ă-**bil**-iti) *n.* a loss or restriction of functional ability or activity as a result of impairment of the body or mind. *See also* handicap. **—disabled** (dis-**ay**-bŭld) *adj.*

disaccharide (dy-**sak**-ă-ryd) *n.* a carbohydrate consisting of two linked monosaccharide units. The most common disaccharides are maltose, lactose, and sucrose.

disarticulation (dis-ar-tik-yoo-**lay**-shŏn) *n.* separation of two bones at a joint. This may be the result of an injury or it may be done by the surgeon at operation in the course of amputation.

disc (disk) *n.* (in anatomy) a rounded flattened structure, such as an intervertebral disc or the optic disc.

discectomy (disk-**ek**-tŏmi) *n.* surgical removal of part (**partial d.**) or all (**total d.**) of a diseased or damaged intervertebral disc. *See also* microdiscectomy.

discoid lupus erythematosus (DLE) (dis-koid) *n.* *see* lupus (erythematosus).

discrete (dis-**kreet**) *adj.* composed of several parts: describing lesions that are separate and do not run into each other.

disease (di-**zeez**) *n.* a disorder with a specific cause and recognizable signs and symptoms; any bodily abnormality or failure to function properly, except that resulting directly from physical injury (the latter, however, may open the way for disease).

disease-modifying antirheumatic drug (DMARD) (anti-roo-**mat**-ik) *n.* a drug used in the treatment of rheumatic disease that affects the progression of the disease by suppressing the disease process. DMARDs include drugs affecting the immune response (immunomodulators), such as immunosuppressants (e.g. methotrexate) and infliximab; gold salts; penicillamine; sulfasalazine; and hydroxychloroquine.

disimpaction (dis-im-**pak**-shŏn) *n.* **1.** the process of separating the broken ends of a bone when they have been forcibly driven together during a fracture. **2.** (**faecal disimpaction**) *see* constipation.

disinfectant (dis-in-**fek**-tănt) *n.* an agent that destroys or removes bacteria and other microorganisms. In medicine disinfectants (e.g. cetrimide) are used to cleanse unbroken skin.

disinfection (dis-in-**fek**-shŏn) *n.* the process of eliminating infective microorganisms from contaminated instruments, skin, clothing, or surroundings by the use of physical means or chemicals (disinfectants).

disinfestation (dis-in-fes-**tay**-shŏn) *n.* the destruction of insect pests and other animal parasites. This generally involves the use of insecticides.

dislocation (luxation) (dis-lŏ-**kay**-shŏn) *n.* displacement from their normal position of bones meeting at a joint such that there is complete loss of contact of the joint surfaces. The bones are restored to their normal positions by manipulation under local or general anaesthesia (*see* reduction). *Compare* subluxation.

disopyramide (dy-soh-**py**-ră-myd) *n.* a drug administered by mouth, intravenous injection, or infusion to treat supraventricular and ventricular arrhythmias. Trade name: **Rythmodan**.

disorientation (dis-or-i-ĕn-**tay**-shŏn) *n.* the state produced by loss of awareness of space, time, or personality. It can occur as the result of drugs, mental illness, or organic disease.

dispensary (dis-**pen**-ser-i) *n.* a place where medicines are made up by a pharmacist according to the doctor's prescription and dispensed to patients.

dispensing practice (dis-**pen**-sing **prak**-tis) *n.* (in Britain) a general practice with a dispensary on site to issue prescribed medications to patients.

dissection (dis-**sek**-shŏn) *n.* the cutting apart and separation of the body tissues along the natural divisions of the organs and different tissues in the course of an operation. Dissection of corpses is carried out for the study of anatomy.

disseminated (dis-**sem**-in-ayt-id) *adj.* widely distributed in an organ (or organs) or in the whole body. The term may refer to disease organisms or to pathological changes.

disseminated intravascular coagulation (DIC) *n.* a condition resulting from overstimulation of the blood-clotting mechanisms in response to disease or injury, such as severe infection, malignancy, acute leukaemia, burns, severe trauma, or severe haemorrhage during childbirth. The overstimulation results in generalized blood coagulation and excessive consumption of coagulation factors. The resulting deficiency of these may lead to spontaneous bleeding.

disseminated sclerosis *n. see* multiple sclerosis.

dissociation (dis-soh-si-**ay**-shŏn) *n.* (in psychiatry) the process whereby thoughts and ideas can be split off from consciousness and may function independently, allowing conflicting opinions to be held at the same time about the same object. Dissociation may be the main factor in cases of dissociative fugue and multiple personalities (*see* dissociative disorder). **—dissociative** (dis-**soh**-shă-tiv) *adj.*

dissociative disorder *n.* any one of a group of mental disorders explained psychoanalytically as extreme defence mechanisms. Symptoms include amnesia, fugue, the assumption of a new identity, and trancelike states with severely reduced response to external stimuli. *See also* dissociation.

distal (**dis**-t'l) *adj.* (in anatomy) situated away from the origin or point of attachment or from the median line of the body. *Compare* proximal.

distichiasis (dis-ti-**ky**-ă-sis) *n.* a very rare condition in which there is an extra row of eyelashes behind the normal row. They may rub on the cornea.

distraction (dis-**trak**-shŏn) *n.* **1.** (in orthopaedics) increasing the distance between two joint surfaces or the two ends of a divided bone. **2.** (in therapy) a diversional therapy that can enable procedures to be carried out with the patient in a state of relaxation.

distraction test *n.* a hearing test used for screening infants between the ages of six and ten months. One examiner sits in front of the infant and gains its attention, while a second examiner, situated just behind the infant, makes a sound at the level of the infant's ear to one side or the other. If the infant can hear it turns in the direction of the sound.

district nurse (**dis**-trikt) *n.* (in Britain) a nurse with special training in domiciliary services. District nurses are usually employed by a primary care trust or health board but may also be allocated to a designated general practice (*see* attachment).

disulfiram (dy-**sul**-fi-ram) *n.* a drug administered by mouth in the treatment of chronic alcoholism. It acts as a deterrent by producing unpleasant effects, such as headache, nausea, and vomiting, when taken with alcohol. Trade name: **Antabuse**.

dithranol (**dith**-ră-nol) *n.* a drug applied to the skin as an ointment, paste, cream, or scalp gel to treat psoriasis. It may irritate the skin on application. Trade names: **Dithrocream**, **Micanol**, **Psorin**.

diuresis (dy-yoor-**ee**-sis) *n.* increased secretion of urine by the kidneys. This normally follows the drinking of more fluid than the body requires, but it can be stimulated by the administration of a diuretic.

diuretic (dy-yoor-**et**-ik) *n.* a drug that increases the volume of urine produced by promoting the excretion of salts and water from the kidney. Diuretics are used in the treatment of oedema and high blood pressure. **loop d.** a diuretic, such as furosemide, that acts by inhibiting reabsorption of sodium and potassium in Henle's loop. **potassium-sparing d.** a diuretic, such as amiloride, that prevents excessive loss of potassium at the distal convoluted tubules. **thiazide d.** a diuretic, such as bendroflumethiazide, that acts by preventing the reabsorption of sodium and potassium in the distal kidney tubules.

diurnal (dy-**ern**-ăl) *adj.* occurring during the day.

divarication (dy-va-ri-**kay**-shŏn) *n.* the separation or stretching of bodily structures. **rectus d.** stretching of the rectus abdominis muscle, a common condition associated with pregnancy or obesity.

divaricator (dy-va-ri-kay-ter) *n.* **1.** a scissor-like surgical instrument used to divide portions of tissue into two separate parts during an operation. **2.** a form of retractor used to open out the sides of an abdominal incision and facilitate access.

divergence (dy-ver-jĕns) *n.* (in ophthalmology) simultaneous movement of both the eyes away from the midline. **d. excess** a divergent squint in which the eyes are deviated outwards more when looking in the distance than for near objects. **d. insufficiency** a convergent squint in which the eyes are deviated slightly inwards only when looking in the distance.

diverticular disease (dy-ver-**tik**-yoo-ler) *n.* a condition in which there are diverticula (*see* diverticulum) in the colon associated with lower abdominal pain and altered stool frequency or consistency. The pain is often due to spasm of the muscle of the intestine (*compare* diverticulitis).

diverticulitis (dy-ver-tik-yoo-**ly**-tis) *n.* inflammation of a diverticulum, most commonly of one or more colonic diverticula. Symptoms include abdominal pain and fever with or without a change in bowel habit. A minority of patients may develop complications, including abscess formation, rectal bleeding, fistulae, strictures, and peritonitis. Surgery is often required in complicated diverticulitis. *Compare* diverticular disease.

diverticulosis (dy-ver-tik-yoo-**loh**-sis) *n.* the presence of non-inflamed diverticula (*compare* diverticulitis).

diverticulum (dy-ver-**tik**-yoo-lŭm) *n.* (*pl.* **diverticula**) a sac or pouch formed at weak points in the walls of the gastrointestinal tract. **colonic d.** a diverticulum that affects the colon. They are sometimes associated with abdominal pain or altered bowel habit (*see* diverticular disease, diverticulitis). **jejunal d.** a diverticulum that affects the small intestine. They are often multiple and may give rise to abdominal discomfort and malabsorption. **Meckel's d.** a diverticulum that occurs in the ileum as a congenital abnormality. It may become inflamed, mimicking appendicitis, or it may form a peptic ulcer, causing pain, bleeding, or perforation.

division (di-**vizh**-ŏn) *n.* the separation of an organ or tissue into parts by surgery.

dizygotic twins (dy-zy-**got**-ik) *pl. n. see* twins.

DKA *n. see* (diabetic) ketoacidosis.

DLE *n. see* (discoid) lupus erythematosus.

DLQI *n. see* dermatology life quality index.

DM *n. see* diabetes (mellitus).

DMARD *n. see* disease-modifying antirheumatic drug.

DMD *n.* Duchenne muscular dystrophy: *see* muscular dystrophy.

DMSA *n.* dimercaptosuccinic acid, which when labelled with technetium-99m is used as a tracer to obtain scintigrams of the kidney, by means of a gamma camera, particularly to show renal scarring resulting from infection and to assess the relative quantity of functioning tissue in each kidney.

DNA (deoxyribonucleic acid) *n.* the genetic material of nearly all living organisms, which controls heredity and is located in the cell nucleus (*see* chromosome, gene). DNA is a nucleic acid composed of two strands made up of units called nucleotides, wound around each other into a double helix. The DNA molecule can make exact copies of itself by the process of replication, thereby passing on the genetic information to the daughter cells when the cell divides.

DNAR order *n.* do not attempt resuscitation order: an instruction, usually made by a patient who has capacity and recorded in their notes, requesting that doctors desist from performing resuscitation in the event of physiological failure.

DNAse *n.* an enzyme that catalyses the cleavage of DNA. A genetically engineered form, recombinant human DNAse (**dornase alfa**), is administered by inhalation in the treatment of cystic fibrosis to reduce the viscosity of the sticky secretions in the lungs. Trade name: **Pulmozyme**.

dobutamine (doh-**bew**-tă-meen) *n.* an inotropic sympathomimetic drug used to increase the force of contraction of the ventricles and improve the heart output. It is administered by continuous intravenous drip.

docetaxel (dos-i-**taks**-ĕl) *n.* a cytotoxic anticancer drug (*see* taxane) administered by intravenous infusion for the treatment of breast cancer, non-small-cell lung cancer, prostate cancer, and (in combination with other drugs) for gastric adenocarcinoma and head and neck cancer. Trade name: **Taxotere**.

Doctor (**dok**-ter) *n.* **1.** the title given to a recipient of a higher university degree than a Master's degree, usually a Doctor of Philosophy (PhD or DPhil) degree. The degree Medicinae Doctor (MD) is awarded by some British universities as a research degree to those with a first degree in medicine. **2.** a courtesy title given to a qualified medical practitioner, i.e. one who has been registered by the General Medical Council.

docusate sodium (dioctyl sodium sulphosuccinate) (**dok**-yoo-sayt) *n.* a stimulant laxative and softening agent given by mouth or enema to relieve constipation or prepare the bowel for radiological examination and also included in ear drops to soften ear wax. Trade names: **Dioctyl**, **Docusol**, **Molcer**, **Norgalax Micro-enema**, **Waxsol**.

Döderlein's bacillus (**ded**-er-lynz) *n.* the bacterium *Lactobacillus acidophilus*, occurring normally in the vagina and its secretions. *See* lactobacillus. [A. S. G. Döderlein (1860–1941), German obstetrician and gynaecologist]

Doering rule (**der**-ing) *n.* identification of the first potential day of fertility during the menstrual cycle using body temperature measurement. This can be used as a means to prevent conception by avoiding intercourse on fertile days. It can also be used to facilitate conception by indicating the optimum time for intercourse to occur.

dolich- (dolicho-) *combining form denoting* long.

dolichocephaly (doli-koh-**sef**-ăli) *n.* the condition of having a relatively long narrow skull, with a cephalic index of 75 or less. —**dolichocephalic** *adj.*

dolor (**dol**-er) *n.* pain: one of the four classical signs of inflammation in a tissue. *See also* calor, rubor, tumor.

dolorimetry (dol-er-**im**-itri) *n.* the measurement of pain. *See* algesimeter.

domiciliary midwife (dom-i-**sil**-yeri) *n. see* community midwife.

domiciliary services *pl. n.* (in Britain) health and social services that are available in the home and are distinguished from hospital-based services.

dominant (**dom**-i-nănt) *adj.* (in genetics) describing a gene (or its corresponding characteristic) whose effect is shown in the individual whether its allele is the same or different. **autosomal d.** *see* autosomal (dominant). *Compare* recessive. —**dominant** *n.*

domperidone (dom-**pe**-ri-dohn) *n.* an antiemetic drug used to reduce the nausea and vomiting caused by other drugs (e.g. anticancer drugs) and to treat dyspepsia. It is administered by mouth or suppository. Trade name: **Motilium**.

donepezil (don-**ep**-i-zil) *n. see* acetylcholinesterase inhibitor.

donor (**doh**-ner) *n.* a person who makes his own tissues or organs available for use by someone else. For example, a donor may provide blood for transfusion or a kidney for transplantation. **d. insemination** *see* artificial insemination.

do not attempt resuscitation *see* DNAR order.

dopa (**doh**-pă) *n.* dihydroxyphenylalanine: a physiologically important compound that forms an intermediate stage in the synthesis of catecholamines from the essential amino acid tyrosine. The laevorotatory form, levodopa, is administered for the treatment of parkinsonism.

dopamine (**doh**-pă-meen) *n.* a catecholamine derived from dopa that functions as a neurotransmitter, acting on specific dopamine receptors and also on adrenergic receptors throughout the body; it also stimulates the release of noradrenaline from nerve endings. Dopamine is used to increase the strength of contraction of the heart in heart failure, shock, severe trauma, and septicaemia. It is administered by intravenous infusion in carefully controlled dosage.

Doppler ultrasound (**dop**-ler) *n.* a diagnostic technique utilizing the fact that the frequency of sound or light waves changes when they are reflected from a moving surface. It is used to study the flow in blood vessels (e.g. in deep vein thrombosis) and the movement of blood in the heart. The frequency detector may be part of the ultrasound imaging probe, which displays an image of the anatomy on a monitor. Simultaneously, the Doppler signal from a particular point on the image can be displayed superimposed on the anatomical position using a split screen (**duplex imaging**). Direction and velocity of blood flow can each be allocated different colours and displayed on a colour monitor over the anatomical image (**colour flow ultrasound imaging**). **MCA D.** Doppler measurement of the fetal middle cerebral artery, which can detect anaemia in cases of haemolytic disease of the newborn. [C. J. Doppler (1803–53), Austrian physicist]

dornase alfa (**dor**-nayz) *n. see* DNAse.

dors- (dorsi-, dorso-) *combining form denoting* **1.** the back. **2.** dorsal.

dorsal (**dor**-săl) *adj.* relating to or situated at or close to the back of the body or to the posterior part of an organ.

dorsiflexion (dor-si-**flek**-shŏn) *n.* backward flexion of the foot or hand or their digits; i.e. bending towards the upper surface.

dorsoventral (dor-soh-**ven**-trăl) *adj.* (in anatomy) extending from the back (dorsal) surface to the front (ventral) surface.

dorsum (**dor**-sŭm) *n.* **1.** the back. **2.** the upper or posterior surface of a part of the body.

dorzolamide (dor-**zol**-ă-myd) *n.* a carbonic anhydrase inhibitor used to reduce intraocular pressure in the treatment of glaucoma and ocular hypertension. It is administered as eye drops, sometimes in combination with timolol. Trade name: **Trusopt**.

dose (dohs) *n.* a carefully measured quantity of a drug that is prescribed by a doctor to be given to a patient at any one time.

dosimeter (doh-**sim**-it-er) *n.* **1.** a device to measure the intensity of a radiation source. **2.** a device to record the amount of radiation received by workers exposed to X-rays or other radiation.

dosimetry (doh-**sim**-itri) *n.* **1.** the calculation of appropriate radiation doses for treating given conditions, usually cancer in different parts of the body. **2.** the measurement of the dose received by a patient having a diagnostic technique involving ionizing radiation or by a radiation worker in his or her employment.

DOT *n. see* directly observed therapy.

double-blind trial (dub-ŭl-**blynd**) *n.* a controlled trial in which neither the participants nor the experimenter or observer are aware of which group each participant is assigned to.

double contrast *n.* a technique usually used in X-ray examinations of the bowel, to enhance the quality of the image. Barium sulphate contrast medium (first contrast) is used to coat the bowel wall; the bowel is then distended with gas (second contrast).

double vision *n. see* diplopia.

douche (doosh) *n.* a stream of water used for cleaning any part of the body, most commonly the vagina.

dowager's hump (**dow**-ă-jerz) *n.* curvature of the spine in the cervical (neck) and upper thoracic region caused by compression fractures from osteoporosis. *Compare* Buffalo hump.

Down's syndrome (downz) *n.* a condition resulting from a chromosomal abnormality, most commonly the presence of three no. 21 chromosomes (instead of the usual two), which is more likely to occur with advanced maternal age. Affected individuals share certain clinical features, including a characteristic flat facial appearance with slanting eyes (as in the Mongolian races, which gave the former name, **mongolism**, to the condition), broad hands with short fingers and a single crease across the palm, malformed ears, eyes with a speckled iris (**Brushfield spots**), and short stature. Many individuals also have a degree of learning disability, although the range of ability is wide. The incidence of congenital heart defects is 40–50%, and other structural malformations (e.g. duodenal atresia) and abnormalities (e.g. deafness, obesity, type 2 diabetes) may be present. Medical name: **trisomy 21**. [J. L. H. Down (1828–96), British physician]

SEE WEB LINKS

- Website of the Down's Syndrome Trust

doxapram (doks-ă-pram) *n.* a respiratory stimulant administered intravenously to raise the level of consciousness in patients recovering from surgery and to treat respiratory failure.

doxazosin (doks-az-oh-sin) *n.* an alpha-blocker drug used to treat high blood pressure and to relieve urinary retention due to an enlarged prostate gland. It is administered by mouth. Trade name: **Cardura**.

doxepin (doks-ĕ-pin) *n.* a drug administered by mouth to relieve depression, especially when associated with anxiety (*see* antidepressant), and applied topically as a cream to relieve itching associated with eczema. Trade names: **Sinepin**, **Xepin**.

doxorubicin (doks-oh-roo-bi-sin) *n.* an anthracycline antibiotic isolated from *Streptomyces peucetius caesius* and used mainly in the treatment of acute leukaemias, Hodgkin's disease, and non-Hodgkin's lymphoma. It is administered by injection or infusion and can be given as a lipid formulation to transport the drug to its target; side-effects are those of other cytotoxic drugs, and heart damage increases with cumulative dose of the drug. Trade names: **Caelyx**, **Myocet**.

doxycycline (doks-i-sy-kleen) *n.* a tetracycline antibiotic administered by mouth to treat infections caused by *Chlamydia*, rickettsiae, mycoplasmas, and *Brucella*, as well as Lyme disease. It is also used to treat periodontitis and aphthous ulcers and to prevent malaria. Trade names: **Efracea**, **Periostat**, **Vibramycin-D**.

DPT vaccine *n.* a combined vaccine against diphtheria, whooping cough (pertussis), and tetanus organisms, now replaced by the DTaP/IPV/Hib and DTaP/IPV vaccines.

DR *n. see* (digital) radiography.

dracontiasis (drak-on-ty-ă-sis) *n.* a tropical disease caused by the parasitic nematode *Dracunculus medinensis* (*see* guinea worm). The disease is transmitted to humans via contaminated drinking water. The worm migrates to the skin surface and eventually forms a large blister, usually on the legs or arms, which bursts and may ulcerate and become infected.

Dracunculus (dra-kunk-yoo-lŭs) *n. see* guinea worm.

dragee (dra-*zh*ay) *n.* a pill that has been coated with sugar.

drain (drayn) **1.** *n.* a device, usually a tube or wick, used to draw fluid from an internal body cavity to the surface. Suction can be applied through a tube drain to increase its effectiveness. **2.** *vb. see* drainage.

drainage (drayn-ij) *n.* the drawing off of fluid from a cavity in the body, usually fluid that has accumulated abnormally. *See also* drain.

drastic (dras-tik) *n.* any agent causing a major change in a body function.

draw-sheet (draw-sheet) *n.* a sheet placed beneath a patient in bed that may be pulled under the patient when one portion has been soiled or becomes uncomfortably wrinkled.

drepanocyte (sickle cell) (drep-ă-noh-syt) *n.* *see* sickle-cell disease.

drepanocytosis (drep-ă-noh-sy-toh-sis) *n.* *see* sickle-cell disease.

dressing (dres-ing) *n.* material applied to a wound or diseased part of the body, with or without medication, to give protection and assist healing.

drill (dril) *n.* (in dentistry) a rotary instrument used to remove tooth substance, particularly in the treatment of caries. It consists of a dental handpiece that takes variously shaped burs.

drip (intravenous drip) (drip) *n.* apparatus for the continuous infusion (transfusion) of blood, plasma, saline, glucose solution, or other fluid into a vein. The fluid flows under gravity from a suspended bottle through a cannula inserted into the patient's vein. Many infusions are now controlled by electronically regulated infusion pumps.

dropsy (drop-si) *n.* *see* oedema.

DRS *n.* *see* Delusions Rating Scale.

drug (drug) *n.* any substance that affects the structure or functioning of a living organism. Drugs are widely used for the prevention, diagnosis, and treatment of disease and for the relief of symptoms.

drug dependence *n.* *see* dependence.

drug intolerance *n.* a lowered threshold or heightened sensitivity to the normal pharmacological action and dosage of a drug. It is unpredictable but there is some evidence of familial history.

drusen (macular drusen) (droo-sĕn) *pl. n.* white or yellow deposits of hyalin in Bruch's membrane of the choroid. They are often associated with macular degeneration.

DRVs *n.* *see* Dietary Reference Values.

dry mouth (dry) *n.* a condition that occurs as a result of reduced salivary flow from a variety of causes, including therapeutic agents, Sjögren's syndrome, connective-tissue disease, diabetes, excision or absence of a major salivary gland, or radiotherapy to the head that destroys the salivary glands. Medical name: **xerostomia**.

DSH *n.* *see* deliberate self-harm.

DSM *n.* Diagnostic and Statistical Manual of Mental Disorders: an influential publication of the American Psychiatric Association in which psychiatric disorders are classified and defined. **DSM-5** is the current (2016) version.

DTaP/IPV (dTaP/IPV) *n.* a booster vaccine given to children between the ages of 3 years 4 months and 5 years. It tops up protection against diphtheria, tetanus, pertussis (whooping cough), and polio.

DTaP/IPV/Hib *n.* a primary immunization given to infants typically at 2, 3, and 4 months of age. It protects against diphtheria, tetanus, pertussis (whooping cough), polio (inactivated polio vaccine), and *Haemophilus influenzae* type b infection (*see* Hib vaccine).

DTPA *n.* diethylenetriaminepentaacetic acid, which when labelled with technetium-99m is used as a tracer to obtain scintigrams of the kidney over a period of time, by means of a gamma camera, to show function and reflux.

DU *n. see* duodenal ulcer.

Duchenne muscular dystrophy (DMD) (dew-**shen**) *n. see* muscular dystrophy. [G. B. A. Duchenne (1806–75), French neurologist]

Ducrey's bacillus (doo-**krayz**) *n.* the bacterium *Haemophilus ducreyi. See* Haemophilus. [A. Ducrey (1860–1940), Italian dermatologist]

duct (dukt) *n.* a tubelike structure or channel, especially one for carrying glandular secretions.

ductal carcinoma in situ (DCIS) (duk-t'l) *n. see* carcinoma in situ.

ductless gland (dukt-lis) *n. see* endocrine gland.

ductule (duk-tewl) *n.* a small duct or channel.

ductus arteriosus (duk-tŭs ar-teer-i-oh-sŭs) *n.* a blood vessel in the fetus connecting the pulmonary artery directly to the ascending aorta, so bypassing the pulmonary circulation. It normally closes after birth. **patent d. a. (PDA)** failure of the ductus to close, producing a

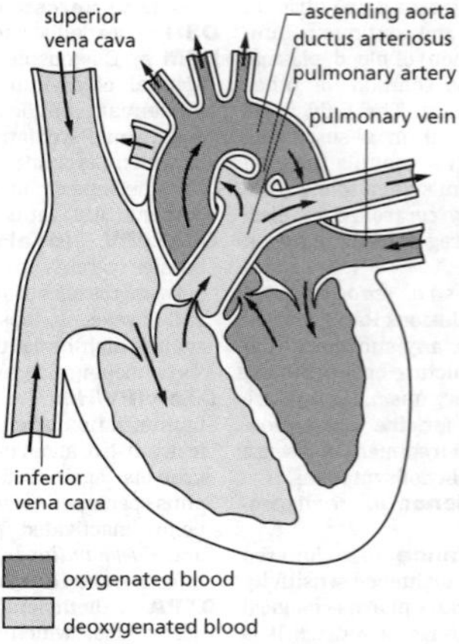

Patent ductus arteriosus

continuous murmur and consequences similar to those of a septal defect. See illustration.

duloxetine (dew-**loks**-ĕ-teen) *n. see* SNRI.

dumbness (**dum**-nis) *n. see* mutism.

Dumdum fever (**dum**-dum) *n. see* kala-azar.

dumping syndrome (**dump**-ing) *n.* a syndrome that may occur after stomach operations, particularly gastrectomy (**postgastrectomy syndrome**), owing to the precipitous transit of ingested food into the small intestine. In **early d. s.** abdominal cramps, flushing, sweating, and diarrhea start within 30 minutes of a meal. In **late d. s.** faintness, weakness, and nausea due to hyperglycaemia occur 1–2 hours after a meal. The patient has a rapid pulse and may sweat and become pale.

Duncan disease (**dun**-kăn) *n. see* X-linked lymphoproliferative syndrome. [Duncan family, in whom the disease was first studied]

duo- *combining form denoting* two.

duoden- (duodeno-) *combining form denoting* the duodenum.

duodenal ulcer (DU) (dew-ŏ-**deen**-ăl) *n.* an ulcer in the duodenum, caused by the action of acid and pepsin on the duodenal lining (mucosa) of a susceptible individual. Symptoms include chronic episodic pain in the upper abdomen; vomiting occurs infrequently. Complications include bleeding (*see* haematemesis), perforation, and obstruction due to scarring (*see* pyloric stenosis). *See also* Helicobacter.

duodenoscope (dew-ŏ-**deen**-ŏ-skohp) *n.* a fibreoptic or video instrument for examining the interior of the duodenum and for performing ERCP.

duodenostomy (dew-ŏ-di-**nost**-ŏmi) *n.* an operation in which the duodenum is brought through the abdominal wall and opened, usually in order to introduce food. *See also* gastroduodenostomy.

duodenum (dew-ŏ-**deen**-ŭm) *n.* the first of the three parts of the small intestine. It extends from the pylorus of the stomach to the jejunum. The duodenum receives bile from the gall bladder and pancreatic juice from the pancreas. **—duodenal** *adj.*

duplex imaging (**dew**-pleks) *n. see* Doppler ultrasound.

Dupuytren's contracture (dew-pwee-**trahnz**) *n.* a flexion deformity of the fingers (usually the ring and little fingers) caused by a nodular hypertrophy and contracture of the fascia in the palm and fingers. [Baron G. Dupuytren (1777–1835), French surgeon]

dura (dura mater, pachymeninx) (**dewr**-ă) *n.* the thickest and outermost of the three meninges surrounding the brain and spinal cord. **—dural** *adj.*

duty of care (**dew**-ti) *n.* the legal obligation of doctors and other health professionals to take reasonable care to avoid causing harm to their patients. If health-care support workers, registered nurses, or doctors fall short of their duty of care, they may be subject to a claim of negligence.

DVT *n.* deep vein thrombosis. *See* phlebothrombosis.

dwarfism (dworf-izm) *n.* abnormally short stature. The most common cause is achondroplasia (**achondroplastic d.**). Dwarfism may also be caused by a deficiency of growth hormone due to a defect in the pituitary gland (**pituitary d.**); a genetic defect in the response to growth hormone; thyroid deficiency (*see* cretinism); such chronic diseases as rickets; renal failure; and intestinal malabsorption.

dydrogesterone (dy-droh-**jest**-er-ohn) *n.* a synthetic female sex hormone (*see* progestogen) administered by mouth (in conjunction with estradiol) in hormone replacement therapy. Trade name: **Femoston**.

dying (dI-ing) *n.* the end stage of every person's life, lasting often for several days before death. Having a duty to save life, clinicians may fail to notice the moment when death becomes inevitable and they must provide the care appropriate for a dying patient. This point may be recognized by a change in demeanour, social involvement, and even vital signs. In the best care, treatments that may be burdensome are now stopped and symptom relief becomes the key factor. *See also* hospice, palliative.

dynamic splintage (dy-**nam**-ik **splint**-ij) *n.* a technique that retains the essentials of splinting but allows some controlled movement of the restrained body part.

dynamometer (dy-nă-**mom**-it-er) *n.* a device for recording the force of a muscular contraction. A small hand-held dynamometer may be used to record the strength of a patient's grip.

-dynia *combining form denoting* pain.

dys- *prefix denoting* difficult, abnormal, or impaired.

dysaesthesia (dis-iss-**theez**-i-ă) *n.* the abnormal and sometimes unpleasant sensation felt by a patient with partial damage to sensory nerve fibres when the skin is stimulated. *Compare* paraesthesia.

dysarthria (dis-**arth**-riă) *n.* a speech disorder in which the pronunciation is unclear although the language content and meaning are normal.

dysbarism (**dis**-bar-izm) *n.* any clinical syndrome due to a difference between the atmospheric pressure outside the body and the pressure of air or gas within a body cavity. *See* compressed air illness.

dyscalculia (dis-cal-**kyoo**-li-ă) *n.* a developmental disorder in which a child's ability to learn arithmetical facts and to process and manipulate numbers is significantly below normal for his or her age. Like dyslexia, with which it is associated, it is not caused by intellectual impairment.

dyschezia (dis-**kee**-ziă) *n.* a form of constipation resulting from a long period of voluntary suppression of the urge to defecate. The rectum becomes distended with faeces and bowel movements are difficult or painful.

dyschondroplasia (Ollier's disease) (dis-kon-droh-**play**-ziă) *n.* a condition due to faulty ossification of cartilage, resulting in development of many benign cartilaginous tumours (*see* chondroma). The bones involved may become stunted and deformed and there is a risk of developing malignant tumours (*see* chondrosarcoma).

dyschromatopsia (dis-kroh-mă-**top**-siă) *n.* any defect of colour vision.

dyscoria (dis-**kor**-iă) *n.* any abnormality in the shape of the pupil of the eye.

dyscrasia (dis-**kray**-ziă) *n.* an abnormal state of the body or part of the body, especially one due to abnormal development or metabolism.

dysdiadochokinesis (adiadochokinesis) (dis-dy-ad-ŏ-koh-ki-**nee**-sis) *n.* clumsiness in performing rapidly alternating movements. It indicates disease of the cerebellum or its intracerebral connections.

dysentery (**dis**-ĕn-tri) *n.* an infection of the intestinal tract causing severe diarrhoea with blood and mucus. **amoebic d. (amoebiasis)** dysentery caused by the protozoan *Entamoeba histolytica*. It is mainly confined to tropical and subtropical countries. **bacillary d.** dysentery caused by bacteria of the genus *Shigella*. Epidemics are common in overcrowded insanitary conditions. *Compare* cholera.

dysfunction (dis-**funk**-shŏn) *n.* impairment or abnormality in the functioning of an organ. **—dysfunctional** (dis-**funk**-shŏn-ăl) *adj.*

dysfunctional uterine bleeding *n.* excessively heavy, prolonged, or frequent uterine bleeding that is not due to pelvic or systemic disease.

dysgenesis (dis-**jen**-i-sis) *n.* faulty development.

dysgerminoma (germinoma, gonocytoma) (dis-jer-mi-**noh**-mă) *n.* a malignant tumour of the ovary, thought to arise from primitive germ cells; it is homologous to the seminoma of the testis. Treatment is by oophorectomy.

dysgraphia (dis-**graf**-iă) *n.* *see* agraphia.

dyshormonogenesis (dis-hor-moh-noh-**jen**-i-sis) *n.* a group of inherited disorders of thyroid hormone synthesis resulting in low levels of thyroxine and tri-iodothyronine and high levels of thyroid-stimulating hormone, with consequent goitre formation, resulting in cretinism or milder forms of hypothyroidism.

dyskaryosis (dis-ka-ri-**oh**-sis) *n.* the abnormal condition of a cell that has a nucleus showing the features characteristic of the earliest stage of malignancy. It may be seen, for example, in the squamous and columnar epithelial cells of a cervical smear.

dyskinesia (dis-ki-**nee**-ziă) *n.* a group of involuntary movements, including chorea, athetosis, and dystonia, that appear to be a fragmentation of the normal smoothly controlled limb and facial movements. **tardive d.** dyskinesia of the facial muscles, tongue, and limb muscles, associated with long-term medication with phenothiazines or certain other antipsychotic drugs.

dyslexia (dis-**leks**-ia) *n.* a developmental disorder selectively affecting a child's ability to learn to read and write. The condition can create serious educational problems. It is sometimes called **specific d.**, **developmental reading disorder**, or **developmental word blindness** to distinguish it from acquired difficulties with reading and writing. *Compare* alexia. **—dyslexic** *adj.*

dysmenorrhoea (dis-men-ŏ-**ree**-ă) *n.* menstruation associated with cramping low abdominal pain radiating into the lower back and thighs. **primary d.** dysmenorrhoea that begins with the onset of ovulatory cycles and is associated with increased production of prostaglandin $F_2\alpha$ by the endometrium. **secondary d.** dysmenorrhoea caused by organic pelvic disease, such as endometriosis or fibroids.

dysmetria (dis-**met**-riă) *n.* impaired coordination due to disorders of the cerebellum or its connections within the brainstem.

dysmorphic (dis-**mor**-fik) *adj.* describing a body characteristic that is abnormally formed. A dysmorphic feature can be a minor isolated feature, such as clinodactyly, or it may be found in association with other features in more serious syndromes, such as Down's syndrome.

dysostosis (dis-oss-**toh**-sis) *n.* the abnormal formation of bone or the formation of bone in abnormal places, such as a replacement of cartilage by bone.

dyspareunia (dis-pă-**roo**-niă) *n.* painful sexual intercourse experienced by a woman. It may be related to vaginismus or caused by underlying disease, such as endometriosis or pelvic inflammatory disease.

dyspepsia (indigestion) (dis-**pep**-siă) *n.* disordered digestion: usually applied to pain or discomfort in the lower chest or abdomen after eating and sometimes accompanied by nausea, vomiting, or a feeling of unease or fullness after eating. **—dyspeptic** *adj.*

dysphagia (dis-**fay**-jiă) *n.* difficulty in swallowing caused by either mechanical obstruction or neurological disease.

dysphasia (dis-**fay**-ziă) *n.* *see* aphasia.

dysphonia (dis-**foh**-niă) *n.* difficulty in voice production. This may be due to a disorder of the larynx, pharynx, tongue, or mouth, or it may be psychogenic. *Compare* aphasia, dysarthria.

dysplasia (alloplasia, heteroplasia) (dis-**play**-ziă) *n.* a premalignant condition characterized by abnormal development of epithelium, bone, or other tissues. **fibrous d.** dysplasia in which bony tissue is replaced by fibrous tissue, resulting in a tendency to pathological fracture. *See also* bronchopulmonary (dysplasia). **—dysplastic** (dis-**plas**-tik) *adj.*

dyspnoea (disp-**nee**-ă) *n.* laboured or difficult breathing. Dyspnoea can be due to obstruction to the flow of air into and out of the lungs (as in bronchitis and asthma), various diseases affecting the tissue of the lung, or heart disease.

dyspraxia (developmental coordination disorder) (dis-**praks**-iă) *n.* a lifelong developmental disorder affecting a patient's fine and/or gross motor coordination; it is often found in association with dyslexia and may significantly impair everyday skills in many aspects of life. *Compare* apraxia.

dysrhythmia (dis-**ri*th***-miă) *n.* abnormality in a rhythm, such as the rhythm of speech or of brain waves as recorded on an EEG.

dyssocial personality (dis-**soh**-shăl) *n.* *see* antisocial personality disorder.

dysthymia (dis-**th'**y-miă) *n.* a permanent state of mildly lowered mood. This never reaches the severity of clinical depression but it can impair the person's quality of life. **—dysthymic** *adj.*

dystocia (dis-**toh**-siă) *n.* difficult birth, caused by abnormalities in the fetus or the mother (*see* obstructed labour). **shoulder d.** an obstetric emergency in which the anterior fetal shoulder (most commonly) impacts on the maternal symphysis or sacral promontory.

dystonia (dis-**toh**-niă) *n.* muscle dysfunction characterized by spasms or abnormal muscle contraction. Forms of dystonia include torticollis, blepharospasm, and writer's cramp. Another form is a postural disorder often associated with disease of the basal ganglia in the brain. **—dystonic** *adj.*

dystrophia adiposogenitalis (dis-**troh**-fiă adi-poh-soh-jen-i-**tahl**-iss) *n.* *see* Fröhlich's syndrome.

dystrophia myotonica (myotonic dystrophy) (my-ŏ-**ton**-ikă) *n.* a type of muscular dystrophy in which the muscle weakness and wasting is accompanied by an unnatural prolongation of the muscular contraction after any voluntary effort (*see* myotonia). The disease can affect both sexes (as it is inherited as an autosomal dominant trait).

dystrophy (dystrophia) (dis-trŏ-fi) *n.* a disorder of an organ or tissue, usually muscle, due to impaired nourishment of the affected part. *See also* Becker muscular dystrophy, Fuchs' endothelial dystrophy, muscular dystrophy.

dysuria (dis-**yoor**-iă) *n.* difficult or painful urination. This is usually associated with urgency and frequency of urination if it is due to cystitis or urethritis.

Ee

Eagle-Barrett syndrome (ee-gĕl ba-rĕt) *n. see* prune belly syndrome.

ear (eer) *n.* the sense organ concerned with hearing and balance. Sound waves, transmitted from the outside into the external auditory meatus, cause the eardrum (tympanic membrane) to vibrate. The small bones (ossicles) of the middle ear – the malleus, incus, and stapes – transmit the sound vibrations to the fenestra ovalis, which leads to the inner ear (*see* labyrinth). Inside the cochlea the sound vibrations are converted into nerve impulses. Pressure within the ear is released through the Eustachian tube. The semicircular canals, saccule, and utricle – also in the inner ear – are all concerned with balance. See illustration.

earache (eer-ayk) *n. see* otitis, otalgia.

eardrum (eer-drum) *n. see* tympanic membrane.

early warning system (EWS) (er-li) *n.* a system to detect deteriorating patients on the ward. Certain physical parameters (e.g. blood pressure, respiratory and pulse rates, level of consciousness) are accorded

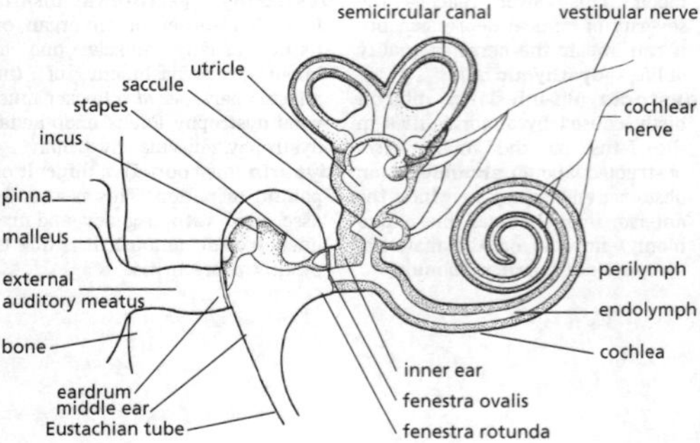

Structure of the ear

scores: the higher the scores for individual patients, the greater the deterioration in their condition.

earwax (eer-waks) *n.* *see* cerumen.

EB *n.* *see* epidermolysis bullosa.

EBM *n.* expressed breast milk.

Ebola virus (i-**boh**-lă) *n.* a virus responsible for an acute infection in humans with features similar to those of Marburg disease. Transmission is by contact with infected blood and other body fluids. The mortality rate is 53–88%, but intensive treatment (including rehydration) in the early stages of the disease can halt its rapid and usually irreversible progression to haemorrhaging of internal organs. A major epidemic of the disease started in West Africa at the end of 2013 and was not declared over until 2016. A vaccine is being developed.

EBP *n.* *see* evidence-based practice.

Ebstein's anomaly (**eb**-stynz) *n.* a form of congenital heart disease affecting the right side of the heart: the tricuspid valve is displaced towards the apex, resulting in impaired right ventricular function. It can cause breathlessness, failure to thrive, cyanosis, and abnormal heart rhythms. [W. Ebstein (1836–1912), German physician]

eburnation (ee-ber-**nay**-shŏn) *n.* the wearing down of the cartilage at the articulating surface of a bone, exposing the underlying bone and leading to bone sclerosis. This is an end result of osteoarthritis.

EBV (EB virus) *n.* *see* Epstein-Barr virus.

ec- *prefix denoting* out of or outside.

ecbolic (ek-**bol**-ik) *n.* an agent, such as oxytocin, that induces childbirth by stimulating contractions of the uterus.

ecchondroma (ek-kon-**droh**-mă) *n.* (*pl.* **ecchondromata**] a benign cartilaginous tumour (*see* chondroma) that protrudes beyond the margins of a bone. *Compare* enchondroma.

ecchymosis (eki-**moh**-sis) *n.* a bruise: an initially bluish-black mark on the skin, resulting from the release of blood into the tissues either through injury or through the spontaneous leaking of blood from the vessels.

eccrine (**ek**-ryn) *adj.* describing sweat glands that are distributed all over the body. They are densest on the soles of the feet and the palms of the hands. *Compare* apocrine.

ecdysis (ek-**dy**-sis) *n.* the act of shedding skin; desquamation.

ECF *n.* *see* extracellular (fluid).

ECG *n.* *see* electrocardiogram.

echinococciasis (echinococcosis) (i-ky-noh-kŏ-**ky**-ă-sis) *n.* *see* hydatid disease.

Echinococcus (i-ky-nŏ-**kok**-ŭs) *n.* a genus of small parasitic tapeworms. Adults are found in the intestines of dogs, wolves, or jackals. If the eggs are swallowed by humans, the resulting larvae may cause hydatid disease. Two species causing this condition are *E. granulosus* and *E. multilocularis.*

echocardiography (ek-oh-kar-di-**og**-răfi) *n.* the use of ultrasound waves to investigate and display the action of the heart as it beats. Used in the diagnosis and assessment of congenital and acquired heart diseases, it is safe, painless, and reliable. **2-D e.** a technique using a pulsed array of ultrasound beams to build up a moving image on a TV monitor of the chambers and valves of the heart. **Doppler e.** a technique for calculating blood flow and pressure within the heart and great vessels by observing the reflection of ultrasound from moving red blood cells. **M-mode e.** a technique using a single beam of ultrasound to produce a nonanatomical image that permits precise measurement of cardiac dimensions. **transoesophageal e.** echocardiography in which the ultrasound probe is mounted on an oesophageal endoscope, allowing the probe to be placed directly against the back of the heart and enabling improved visualization of posterior structures.

echolalia (ek-oh-**lay**-liă) *n.* pathological repetition of the words spoken by another person. It may be a symptom of language disorders, autism, catatonia, schizophrenia, dementia, or Tourette's syndrome.

echopraxia (echokinesis) (ek-oh-**praks**-iă) *n.* pathological imitation of the actions of another person. It may be a symptom of catatonia.

echovirus (**ek**-oh-vy-rŭs) *n.* one of a group of about 30 RNA-containing viruses originally isolated from the human intestinal tract. These viruses were termed *e*nteric *c*ytopathic *h*uman *o*rphan viruses and are the cause of some neurological disorders. *Compare* reovirus.

ECI *n. see* Experience of Caregiving Inventory.

eclabium (ek-**lay**-biŭm) *n.* the turning outward of a lip.

eclampsia (i-**klamp**-siă) *n.* the occurrence, in a woman with pre-eclampsia, of one or more convulsions not caused by other conditions, such as epilepsy or cerebral haemorrhage. The onset of convulsions may be preceded by a sudden rise in blood pressure and/or a sudden increase in oedema and development of oliguria. The convulsions are usually followed by coma. Eclampsia is a threat to the life of both mother and baby and must be treated immediately.

ecmnesia (ek-**nee**-ziă) *n.* loss of memory for recent events that does not extend to more remote ones: a common symptom of old age.

ECMO *n. see* extracorporeal (membrane oxygenation).

ECoG *n. see* electrocochleography.

ecology (bionomics) (ee-**kol**-ŏji) *n.* the study of the relationships between humans, plants and animals, and the environment. —**ecological** *adj.* —**ecologist** *n.*

econazole (ee-**kon**-ă-zohl) *n.* an antifungal drug used to treat ringworm and candidiasis. It is administered as a cream or vaginal pessary. Trade names: **Gyno-Pevaryl**, **Pevaryl**.

écraseur (ay-kra-**zer**) *n.* a surgical device, resembling a snare, that is used to sever the base of a tumour during its surgical removal.

ecstasy (**ek**-stă-si) *n.* a sense of extreme wellbeing and bliss. While not necessarily pathological, it can be caused by epilepsy (especially of the temporal lobe) or by schizophrenia or mania.

Ecstasy *n.* the street name for methylenedioxymethamphetamine (MDMA), a mildly hallucinogenic drug that generates feelings of euphoria in those who take it. Its most common side-effect is hyperthermia; drinking large quantities of water to combat the intense thirst produced by taking the drug may result in fatal damage to the body's fluid balance. Its manufacture, sale, use, and possession are illegal.

ECT *n. see* electroconvulsive therapy.

ect- (ecto-) *combining form denoting* outer or external.

ectasia (ectasis) (ek-tay-ziă) *n.* the dilatation of a tube, duct, or hollow organ.

ecthyma (ek-**th'y**-mă) *n.* an infection of the skin caused by *Streptococcus pyogenes*, *Staphylococcus aureus*, and other bacteria in which the full thickness of the epidermis is involved (*compare* impetigo). Ecthyma heals slowly and causes scarring.

ectoderm (**ek**-toh-derm) *n.* the outer of the three germ layers of the early embryo. It gives rise to the nervous system and sense organs, the teeth and lining of the mouth, and the epidermis and its associated structures (hair, nails, etc.). **—ectodermal** *adj.*

ectomorphic (ek-toh-**mor**-fik) *adj.* describing a body type that is relatively thin, with a large skin surface in comparison to weight. **—ectomorph** *n.* **—ectomorphy** *n.*

-ectomy *combining form denoting* surgical removal of a segment or all of an organ or part.

ectoparasite (ek-toh-**pa**-ră-syt) *n.* a parasite that lives on the outer surface of its host. *Compare* endoparasite.

ectopia (ek-**toh**-piă) *n.* **1.** the misplacement, due either to a congenital defect or injury, of a bodily part. **2.** the occurrence of something in an unnatural location (*see* ectopic beat, ectopic pregnancy). **—ectopic** (ek-**top**-ik) *adj.*

ectopic beat (extrasystole) *n.* a heartbeat due to an impulse generated somewhere in the heart outside the sinoatrial node. They may be produced by any heart disease, by nicotine from smoking, or by caffeine from excessive tea or coffee consumption; they are common in normal individuals. *See* arrhythmia.

ectopic pregnancy (extra-uterine pregnancy) *n.* the implantation of a fertilized egg cell at a site outside the uterus. The most common type of ectopic pregnancy occurs in Fallopian tubes that become blocked or inflamed (**tubal pregnancy**). The growth of the fetus may cause the tube to rupture and bleed. In such cases treatment is by laparoscopic surgery; otherwise medical treatment with methoxetrate, which preserves fertility, may be possible. Medical name: **eccyesis**.

ectro- *combining form denoting* congenital absence.

ectrodactyly (ek-troh-**dak**-ti-li) *n.* congenital absence of all or part of one or more fingers.

ectromelia (ek-troh-**mee**-liă) *n.* congenital absence or gross shortening (aplasia) of the long bones of one or more limbs. *See also* amelia, hemimelia, phocomelia.

ectropion (ek-**troh**-pi-ŏn) *n.* **1.** turning out of the eyelid, away from the eyeball. **2. (cervical ectopy)** the presence of columnar epithelium (which normally lines the endocervix) on the vaginal part of the cervix (ectocervix) as a result of exposure to higher levels of oestrogen (e.g. at puberty, in pregnancy, or with anovulation).

eczema (**eks**-imă) *n.* a common itchy skin disease characterized by reddening (erythema) and vesicle formation, which may lead to weeping and crusting. Outside agents do not play a primary role (*compare* dermatitis), but in some contexts the terms 'dermatitis' and 'eczema' are used interchangeably. **atopic e.** eczema that affects up to 20% of the population and is associated with asthma and hay fever. **discoid** (or **nummular**) **e.** a type of eczema that is characterized by coin-shaped lesions and occurs only in adults. **gravitational** (or **stasis**) **e.** eczema associated with poor venous circulation. **seborrhoeic e.** (**seborrhoeic dermatitis**) eczema that involves the scalp, eyelids, nose, and lips and is associated with the presence of *Malassezia* yeasts and may also be seen in HIV infection. *See also* pompholyx. **—eczematous** (eks-**em**-ă-tŭs) *adj.*

ED *n.* emergency department, also known as **A & E** (accident and emergency department): a hospital department that assesses and deals with the immediate problems of acutely ill and injured patients. *See also* A & E medicine.

EDD *n.* expected date of delivery.

edentulous (ee-**den**-choo-lŭs) *adj.* lacking teeth: usually applied to people who have lost some or all of their teeth.

edetate (ee-di-tayt) *n.* a salt of the compound **ethylenediaminetetraacetic acid** (EDTA), used as a chelating agent in the treatment of poisoning. **dicobalt e.** an antidote to cyanide, administered by intravenous injection as soon as possible after poisoning. **sodium calcium e.** a drug administered by intravenous infusion to treat poisoning by heavy metals, especially lead.

edrophonium (ed-roh-**foh**-niŭm) *n.* an anticholinesterase drug that is administered by intravenous injection after surgery to reverse the effects of some muscle relaxants and also used in a test for diagnosis of myasthenia gravis.

EDTA (ethylenediaminetetraacetic acid) *n. see* edetate.

EDV *n. see* end-diastolic volume.

Edwards' syndrome (**ed**-wădz) *n.* the condition of a baby born with multiple congenital abnormalities, including learning disability, due to trisomy of chromosome no. 18. [J. H. Edwards (1928–), British geneticist]

EEG (electroencephalogram) *n. see* electroencephalography.

effectiveness and efficiency (i-**fek**-tiv-něs i-**fi**-shěn-si) *pl. n.* measures that are used in health economics and ethics to assess treatments. A treatment that achieves its object is **effective**, but may do so at great cost. If it is also **efficient**, it achieves its aim at lower cost than other comparable treatments. Even effective and efficient treatments may work for patients only by depriving others of similar care, so a moral evaluation must take into account the overall aims and purposes of health care.

effector (i-**fek**-ter) *n.* any structure or agent that brings about activity in a muscle or gland. The term is also used for the muscle or gland itself.

efferent (**ef**-er-ěnt) *adj.* **1.** designating nerves or neurons that convey impulses from the brain or spinal cord to muscles, glands, and other effectors. **2.** designating vessels or ducts that drain fluid from an organ or part. *Compare* afferent.

efficacy (**ef**-i-kă-si) *n.* the ability to produce a beneficial or desired effect that may detect, relieve, or eliminate symptoms or a disease.

effleurage (ef-ler-**ahzh**) *n.* a form of massage in which the hands are passed continuously and rhythmically over a patient's skin in one direction only, with the aim of increasing blood flow in that direction and aiding the dispersal of any swelling due to oedema.

effusion (i-**few**-*zh*ŏn) *n.* **1.** the escape of pus, serum, blood, lymph, or other fluid into a body cavity. **2.** fluid that has escaped into a body cavity.

eformoterol (ef-or-**moh**-ter-ol) *n.* *see* formoterol.

egg cell (eg) *n.* *see* ovum.

ego (**eg**-oh) *n.* (in psychoanalysis) the part of the mind that develops from a person's experience of the outside world and is most in touch with external realities.

Ehlers-Danlos syndrome (**ay**-lerz **dan**-los) *n.* any one of a rare group of inherited (autosomal dominant or autosomal recessive) disorders of the connective tissue involving abnormal or deficient collagen. The skin is very elastic but also very fragile: it bruises easily and scars poorly, the scars often being paper-thin. The joints tend to be very mobile (double-jointed) and dislocate easily. In some types the uterus or bowel can rupture or the valves in the heart can be weaker than normal. [E. L. Ehlers (1863–1937), Danish dermatologist; H. A. Danlos (1844–1912), French dermatologist]

Ehrlich's theory (**air**-liks) *n.* an early theory of antibody production, postulating that receptor groups with side chains were carried on cells and combined with antigens. The receptors were then thrown off the cell and became antibodies in the circulation. [P. Ehrlich (1854–1915), German bacteriologist]

EIA *n.* exercise-induced asthma. *See* asthma.

eidetic (I-**det**-ik) *adj.* *see* imagery.

Eisenmenger reaction (Eisenmenger syndrome) (**I**-zěn-meng-er) *n.* a condition in which pulmonary hypertension is associated with a septal defect, so that blood flows from the right to the left side of the heart or from the pulmonary artery to the aorta. Oxygen-depleted blood enters the general circulation, which results in cyanosis and polycythaemia. [V. Eisenmenger (1864–1932), German physician]

ejaculation (i-jak-yoo-**lay**-shŏn) *n.* the discharge of semen from the erect penis at the moment of sexual climax (orgasm) in the male.

Ekbom's syndrome (**ek**-bomz) *n.* *see* restless legs syndrome. [K. A. Ekbom (1907–77), Swedish neurologist]

elastase (i-**la**-stayz) *n.* an enzyme that breaks down various proteins, including elastin. **Pancreatic elastase**, secreted by the pancreas, is not degraded in the small or large intestine: therefore, its concentration in the stools is the basis for the **faecal pancreatic elastase test**. In patients who have suspected pancreatic insufficiency, faecal pancreatic elastase is suppressed or absent.

elastic cartilage (i-**last**-ik) *n.* *see* cartilage.

elastic tissue *n.* strong extensible flexible connective tissue rich in yellow **elastic fibres**. Elastic tissue is found in the dermis of the skin, in arterial walls, and in the walls of the alveoli of the lungs.

elastin (i-**last**-in) *n.* protein forming the major constituent of elastic tissue fibres.

elastography (i-lasst-**og**-răfi) *n.* an ultrasonic imaging technique that displays the elasticity of soft tissues. It has been found useful in demonstrating abnormalities of muscle, liver, and breast tissue.

elation (i-**lay**-shŏn) *n.* a state of cheerful excitement and enthusiasm. Marked elation of mood is a characteristic of mania or hypomania.

elbow (**el**-boh) *n.* the joint in the arm formed between the ulna and part of the radius and the humerus.

Electra complex (i-**lek**-tră) *n.* (in Freudian psychoanalytic theory) the unconscious sexual feelings of a girl for her father, accompanied by aggressive feelings for her mother. *Compare* Oedipus complex.

electrocardiogram (ECG) (i-lek-troh-**kar**-di-oh-gram) *n.* a tracing of the electrical activity of the heart recorded by electrocardiography. It aids in the diagnosis of heart disease, which may produce characteristic changes in the ECG. See illustration.

electrocardiography (i-lek-troh-kar-di-**og**-răfi) *n.* a technique for recording the electrical activity of the heart. Electrodes connected to the recording apparatus (**electrocardiograph**) are placed on the skin of the four limbs and chest wall; the record itself is called an electrocardiogram (ECG). **intracardiac e.** the passage of a recording catheter into the heart for accurate mapping and analysis of arrhythmias.

electrocardiophonography (i-lek-troh-kar-di-oh-fŏ-**nog**-răfi) *n.* a technique for recording heart sounds and murmurs simultaneously

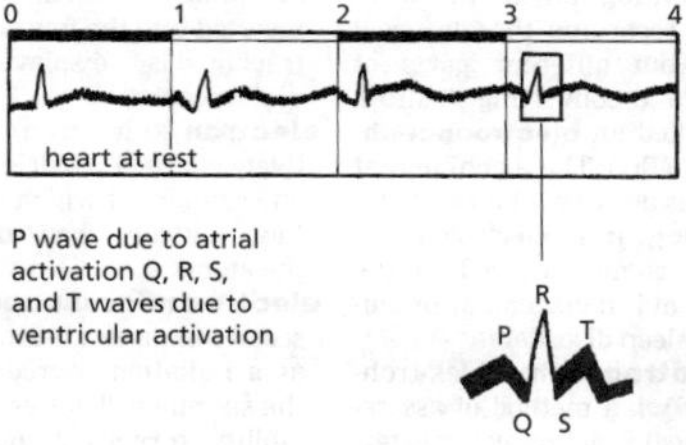

A typical electrocardiogram

with the ECG. The sound is picked up by a microphone placed over the heart. The tracing is a **phonocardiogram**.

electrocautery (i-lek-troh-kaw-ter-i) *n.* the destruction of diseased or unwanted tissue by means of a needle or snare that is electrically heated.

electrocoagulation (i-lek-troh-koh-ag-yoo-**lay**-shŏn) *n.* the coagulation of tissues by means of a high-frequency electric current concentrated at one point as it passes through them.

electrocochleography (ECoG) (i-lek-troh-kok-li-**og**-răfi) *n.* a test to measure electrical activity produced within the cochlea in response to a sound stimulus. It is used in the diagnosis of Ménière's disease and other forms of sensorineural deafness.

electroconvulsive therapy (ECT, electroplexy) (i-lek-troh-kŏn-**vul**-siv) *n.* a treatment for severe depression and occasionally for puerperal psychosis, catatonia, and mania. A convulsion is produced by passing an electric current through the brain; this is thought to induce stimulation, and is modified by giving a muscle relaxant drug and an anaesthetic. The treatment can cause short-term memory loss.

electrode (i-**lek**-trohd) *n.* any part of an electrical conductor or recording device that is used to apply electric current to a part of the body or collect electrical activity (e.g. from the heart or brain).

electrodesiccation (i-lek-troh-dess-i-**kay**-shŏn) *n.* *see* fulguration.

electroencephalogram (EEG) (i-lek-troh-en-**sef**-ă-lŏ-gram) *n.* *see* electroencephalography.

electroencephalography (i-lek-troh-en-sef-ă-**log**-răfi) *n.* the technique for recording the electrical activity from different parts of the brain and converting it into a tracing called an **electroencephalogram** (EEG). The machine that records this activity is known as an **encephalograph**. Electroencephalography is mostly used in the diagnosis and management of epilepsy and sleep disorders.

electroglottography (i-lek-troh-glot-**og**-răfi) *n.* a method of assessing laryngeal function using external recording electrodes.

electrolarynx (i-lek-troh-**la**-rinks) *n.* a battery-powered electrical vibrator that helps people to speak after laryngectomy.

electrolysis (i-lek-**trol**-i-sis) *n.* **1.** the chemical decomposition of a substance (*see* electrolyte) into positively and negatively charged ions (*see* anion, cation) when an electric current is passed through it. **2.** destruction of tissue, especially hair follicles (*see* epilation), by the passage of an electric current.

electrolyte (i-**lek**-trŏ-lyt) *n.* a solution that produces ions; for example, sodium chloride solution consists of free sodium and free chloride ions. In medical usage electrolyte usually means the ion itself; thus the **serum electrolyte level** is the concentration of separate ions (sodium, potassium, chloride, bicarbonate, etc.) in the circulating blood. *See also* anion, cation.

electromyography (EMG) (i-lek-troh-my-**og**-răfi) *n.* continuous recording of the electrical activity of a muscle by means of electrodes inserted into the muscle fibres. The tracing is displayed on an oscilloscope.

electron (i-**lek**-tron) *n.* a negatively charged particle in an atom, one or more of which orbit around the positively charged nucleus of the atom.

electron microscope *n.* a microscope that uses a beam of electrons as a radiation source for viewing the specimen. The resolving power (ability to register fine detail) is a thousand times greater than that of an ordinary light microscope.

electronvolt (i-**lek**-tron-vohlt) *n.* a unit of energy equal to the increase in the energy of an electron when it passes through a rise in potential of one volt. Symbol: eV.

electrooculography (i-lek-troh-ok-yoo-**log**-răfi) *n.* a method of recording eye movements and assessing the resting potential of the eye by means of tiny electrodes attached to the skin at the inner and outer corners of the eye. The recording is an **electrooculogram (EOG)**.

electroplexy (i-**lek**-troh-pleks-i) *n. see* electroconvulsive therapy.

electroretinography (i-lek-troh-ret-in-**og**-răfi) *n.* a method of recording changes in the electrical potential of the retina when it is stimulated by light; the recording is an **electroretinogram (ERG)**. One electrode is placed on the eye in a contact lens and the other is usually attached to the back of the head.

electrosurgery (i-lek-troh-**serj**-er-i) *n.* the use of a high-frequency electric current from a fine wire electrode (a diathermy knife) to cut tissue. The ground electrode is a large metal plate. When used correctly, little heat spreads to the surrounding tissues, in contrast to electrocautery.

electrotherapy (i-lek-troh-**th'e**-ră-pi) *n.* the passage of electric currents through the body's tissues to stimulate the functioning of nerves and the muscles that they supply. *See also* faradism, galvanism.

electuary (i-**lek**-tew-er-i) *n.* a pharmaceutical preparation in which the drug is made up into a paste with syrup or honey.

element (**el**-i-mĕnt) *n.* a substance, such as carbon, nitrogen, or oxygen, that cannot be decomposed into simpler substances. All the atoms of an element have the same number of protons. *See also* isotope, trace element.

elephantiasis (el-i-făn-**ty**-ă-sis) *n.* gross enlargement of the skin and underlying connective tissues caused by obstruction of the lymph vessels. Obstruction is commonly caused by the parasitic filarial worms *Wuchereria bancrofti* and *Brugia malayi*. The parts most commonly affected are the legs but the scrotum, breasts, and vulva may also be involved. *See also* filariasis.

elevator (**el**-i-vay-ter) *n.* **1.** an instrument that is used to raise a depressed broken bone. **periosteal e.** an instrument used in orthopaedics to strip the fibrous tissue (periosteum) covering bone. **2.** a lever-like instrument used to ease a tooth or root out of its socket during extraction.

elimination (i-lim-i-**nay**-shŏn) *n.* (in physiology) the process of excretion of metabolic waste products from the blood by the kidneys and urinary tract.

elimination diet (i-li-mi-**nay**-shŏn) *n.* a diet in which many foods suspected of not being tolerated are removed for a period of time and then reintroduced sequentially to identify any that then precipitate symptoms. An **exclusion diet** is a variant of this, in which a single food is excluded and symptoms monitored for any improvements.

ELISA *n. see* enzyme-linked immunosorbent assay.

elixir (i-**liks**-er) *n.* a preparation containing alcohol (ethanol) or glycerine, which is used as the vehicle for bitter or nauseous drugs.

elliptocytosis (i-lip-toh-sy-**toh**-sis) *n.* the presence of significant numbers of abnormal elliptical red cells (**elliptocytes**) in the blood.

em- *prefix. see* en-.

emaciation (i-may-si-**ay**-shŏn) *n.* wasting of the body, caused by such conditions as malnutrition or cancer.

emasculation (i-mas-kew-**lay**-shŏn) *n.* strictly, surgical removal of the penis. The term is often used to mean loss of male characteristics, as a result of castration or emotional stress.

embalming (im-**bahm**-ing) *n.* the preservation of a dead body by the introduction of chemical compounds that delay putrefaction.

embolectomy (em-bŏ-**lek**-tŏmi) *n.* surgical removal of an embolus in order to relieve arterial obstruction.

embolism (**em**-bŏl-izm) *n.* the condition in which an embolus becomes lodged in an artery and obstructs its blood flow. Treatment is by anticoagulant therapy; major embolism is treated by embolectomy or thrombolysis. **pulmonary e.** obstruction of the pulmonary artery by an embolus, usually a blood clot derived from phlebothrombosis of the leg veins. Large emboli result in acute heart failure. **systemic e.** embolism affecting any artery except the pulmonary artery. The embolus is often a blood clot formed in the heart in mitral valve disease or following myocardial infarction. *See also* air embolism.

embolization (therapeutic embolization) (em-bol-I-**zay**-shŏn) *n.* the introduction of any material in order to reduce or obstruct blood flow. Conditions such as varicocele, fibroids, hepatoma, congenital arteriovenous malformations, angiodysplasia, malignant tumours, or arterial rupture are commonly treated with embolization. **uterine artery e.** embolization of the uterine artery for the treatment of postpartum haemorrhage and fibroids and to terminate abdominal and cervical pregnancies.

embolus (**em**-bŏ-lŭs) *n.* (*pl.* **emboli**) material, such as a blood clot, fat, air, amniotic fluid, or a foreign body, that is carried by the blood from one point in the circulation to lodge at another point (*see* embolism).

embrocation (em-broh-**kay**-shŏn) *n.* a lotion that is rubbed onto the body for the treatment of sprains and strains.

embryo (**em**-bri-oh) *n.* an animal at an early stage of development, before birth (see illustration). In humans the term refers to the products of conception within the uterus up to the eighth week of development, during which time all the main organs are formed. *Compare* fetus. —**embryonic** (em-bri-**on**-ik) *adj.*

embryology (em-bri-**ol**-ŏji) *n.* the study of growth and development of the embryo and fetus from fertilization of the ovum until birth. —**embryological** *adj.*

emergency contraception (i-**mer**-jĕn-si) *n.* *see* postcoital contraception.

emesis (**em**-i-sis) *n.* *see* vomiting.

emetic (i-**met**-ik) *n.* an agent that causes vomiting, such as ipecacuanha or common salt.

EMG *n.* *see* electromyography.

emic (**em**-ik) *adj.* describing or based on the view of a culture from the perspective of members of that culture. Emic analysis is essential in qualitative research to ensure that culture-specific particularities are not suppressed. *Compare* etic.

eminence (**em**-in-ĕns) *n.* a projection, often rounded, on an organ or tissue, particularly on a bone.

emissary veins (**em**-iss-er-i) *pl. n.* a group of veins within the skull that drain blood from the venous

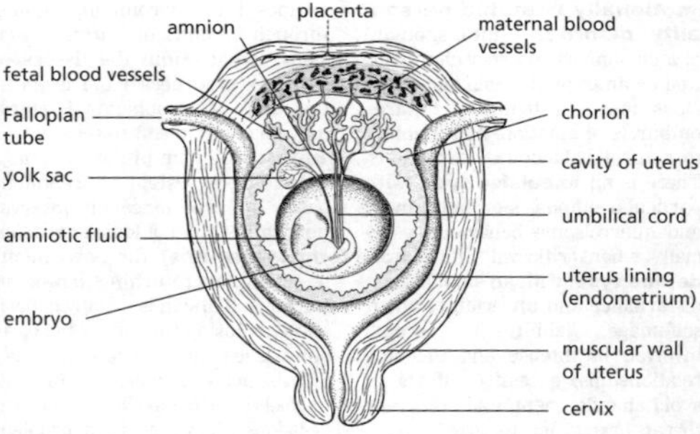

A developing embryo

sinuses of the dura mater to veins outside the skull.

emission (i-**mish**-ŏn) *n.* the flow of semen from the erect penis, usually occurring while the subject is asleep (**nocturnal e.**).

EMLA cream (em-lă) *n.* a cream containing a *e*utectic *m*ixture of *l*ocal *a*naesthetics (lidocaine and prilocaine). Applied to the skin as a thick coating and left for a maximum of 60 to 90 minutes, it gives a helpful degree of local anaesthesia, allowing blood samples to be taken and facilitating biopsy procedures in young children.

emmetropia (em-i-**troh**-piă) *n.* the state of refraction of the normal eye, in which parallel light rays are brought to a focus on the retina with the accommodation relaxed. *Compare* ametropia, hypermetropia, myopia.

emollient (i-**mol**-iĕnt) *n.* an agent that soothes and softens the skin, such as lanolin or liquid paraffin. Emollients are used alone as moisturizers to lessen the need for active drug therapy (such as corticosteroids for eczema) and in skin preparations as a base for more active drugs, such as antibiotics.

emotion (i-**moh**-shŏn) *n.* a state of arousal that can be experienced as pleasant or unpleasant. Emotions can have three components: for example, fear can involve an unpleasant subjective experience, an increase in physiological measures such as heart rate, and a tendency to flee from the situation provoking the fear.

emotionally unstable personality disorder (i-**moh**-shŏn-ăli) *n.* a personality disorder characterized by an unpredictable and capricious mood, a tendency towards outbursts of emotion, and inability to control behavioural explosions. There is an **impulsive type**, with particular emphasis on impulsivity and quarrelsome behaviour, especially when criticized; and a **borderline type**, with an emphasis on disturbance and uncertainty about self-image, liability to become involved in intense and unstable relationships, excessive efforts to avoid abandonment, and recurrent threats or acts of self-harm.

emotional touchpoints (i-**moh**-shŏn-ăl) *pl. n.* points at which a user has contact with or interacts with the service in order to share important emotional experiences and memories. Designating such points enables the delivery of compassionate, holistic, and insightful care, allowing staff to learn from users and to make changes to care delivery to improve their experience.

empathy (**em**-pă-thi) *n.* the ability to imagine and understand the thoughts, perspective, and emotions of another person.

emphysema (em-fi-**see**-mă) *n.* air in the tissues. **pulmonary e.** emphysema in which the alveoli of the lungs are enlarged and damaged, which reduces the surface area for the exchange of oxygen and carbon dioxide. Severe emphysema causes breathlessness, which is made worse by infections. **surgical e.** emphysema in which air escapes into surrounding tissues through wounds or surgical incisions, usually into the tissues of the chest and neck from leaks in the lungs or oesophagus. Bacteria may form gas in soft tissues.

empirical (im-**pi**-ri-kăl) *adj.* describing a system of treatment based on experience or observation, rather than of logic or reason.

empowerment (im-**powr**-mĕnt) *n.* giving or returning power to someone. Being ill is usually experienced as losing the ability to act as one wishes, and full recovery may only be achieved when the individual feels able to make his or her own decisions. This may be a problem where professionals insist on deciding for patients with certain conditions (e.g. mental illness) or offering explanations in a language or style that is not appropriate or easily understood. *See also* autonomy.

empyema (pyothorax) (em-py-**ee**-mă) *n.* pus in the pleural cavity, usually secondary to infection in the lung or in the space below the diaphragm.

emulsion (i-**mul**-shŏn) *n.* a preparation in which fine droplets of one liquid (such as oil) are dispersed in another liquid (such as water). In pharmacy medicines are prepared in the form of emulsions to disguise the taste of an oil, which is dispersed in a flavoured liquid.

EN *n. see* enrolled nurse.

en- (em-) *prefix denoting* in; inside.

enable (i-**nay**-bŭl) *vb.* to empower someone to undertake an action or to take responsibility for a situation. *See* empowerment.

enalapril (en-al-ă-pril) *n.* a drug administered by mouth for the treatment of high blood pressure (hypertension) and heart failure. It inhibits the action of angiotensin (*see* ACE inhibitor). Trade name: **Innovace**.

enamel (i-nam-ĕl) *n.* the extremely hard outer covering of the crown of a tooth, which consists of crystalline hydroxyapatite.

enarthrosis (en-arth-roh-sis) *n.* a ball-and-socket joint, e.g. the shoulder joint. Such a joint always involves a long bone, which is thus allowed to move in all planes.

encapsulated (in-kaps-yoo-layt-id) *adj.* (of an organ, tumour, bacterium, etc.) enclosed in a capsule.

encephal- (encephalo-) *combining form denoting* the brain.

encephalin (enkephalin) (en-sef-ă-lin) *n.* a peptide occurring naturally in the brain and having effects resembling those of morphine or other opiates. *See also* endorphin.

encephalitis (en-sef-ă-ly-tis) *n.* inflammation of the brain. It may be caused by a viral (e.g. herpes simplex) or bacterial infection, or it may be due to an abnormal autoimmune process, such as an allergic response to a systemic viral illness or vaccination (*see* encephalomyelitis), a remote response to malignancy, or a primary antibody-mediated autoimmune disorder. **e. lethargica** a form of viral encephalitis that is marked by headache and drowsiness, progressing to coma (hence its popular name – **sleepy sickness**). It can cause postencephalitic parkinsonism. *See also* Rasmussen's encephalitis.

encephalocele (en-sef-ă-loh-seel) *n.* protrusion of the brain through a defect in the bones of the skull. *See* neural tube defects.

encephalography (en-sef-ă-log-răfi) *n.* any of various techniques for recording the structure of the brain or the activity of the brain cells. *See* electroencephalography, pneumoencephalography.

encephaloma (en-sef-ă-loh-mă) *n.* a brain tumour.

encephalomalacia (en-sef-ă-loh-mă-lay-shiă) *n.* softening of the brain.

encephalomyelitis (en-sef-ă-loh-my-ĕ-ly-tis) *n.* an acute inflammatory disease affecting the brain and spinal cord. **acute disseminated e.** a form of delayed tissue hypersensitivity provoked by a mild infection or vaccination 7–10 days earlier.

encephalomyelopathy (en-sef-ă-loh-my-ĕ-lop-ă-thi) *n.* any condition in which there is widespread disease of the brain and spinal cord.

encephalon (en-sef-ă-lon) *n. see* brain.

encephalopathy (en-sef-ă-lop-ă-thi) *n.* any of various diseases that affect the functioning of the brain. *See* hepatic (encephalopathy), spongiform encephalopathy, Wernicke's encephalopathy.

enchondroma (en-kon-droh-mă) *n.* (*pl.* **enchondromata**] a benign cartilaginous tumour (*see* chondroma) occurring in the growing zone of a bone and not protruding beyond its margins. *Compare* ecchondroma.

encopresis (en-koh-**pree**-sis) *n.* incontinence of faeces. The term is used for faecal soiling in a child who has gained bowel control but passes formed stools in unacceptable places.

encysted (en-**sist**-id) *adj.* enclosed in a cyst.

end- (endo-) *combining form denoting* within or inner.

endarterectomy (end-ar-ter-**ek**-tŏmi) *n.* a surgical 're-bore' of an artery that has become obstructed by atheroma with or without a blood clot (thrombus); the former operation is known as **thromboendarterectomy**. The inner part of the wall is removed together with any clot that is present. **carotid e.** endarterectomy of one or more of the carotid arteries.

endarteritis (end-ar-ter-**I**-tis) *n.* chronic inflammation of the inner portion of the wall of an artery, which most often results from late syphilis. Thickening of the wall produces progressive arterial obstruction and symptoms from reduced blood supply to the affected part.

end artery (end) *n.* the terminal branch of an artery, which does not communicate with other branches.

endaural (end-**or**-ăl) *adj.* within the ear, especially relating to the external auditory meatus of the outer ear.

end-diastolic volume (EDV) (end-dy-ă-**stol**-ik) *n.* the volume of blood contained by the ventricles at the end of diastole when the chambers are full.

endemic (en-**dem**-ik) *adj.* occurring frequently in a particular region or population: applied to diseases that are generally or constantly found among people in a particular area. *Compare* epidemic, pandemic.

endemic syphilis *n. see* bejel.

endemiology (en-dee-mi-**ol**-ŏji) *n.* the study of endemic disease.

endocarditis (en-doh-kar-**dy**-tis) *n.* inflammation of the endocardium and heart valves. It is most often due to rheumatic fever or bacterial infection (**bacterial e.**). The main features are fever, changing heart murmurs, heart failure, and embolism. *See also* subacute bacterial endocarditis.

endocardium (en-doh-**kar**-diŭm) *n.* a delicate membrane that lines the heart and is continuous with the lining of arteries and veins. **—endocardial** *adj.*

endocervicitis (en-doh-ser-vi-**sy**-tis) *n.* inflammation of the mucous membrane lining the cervix (neck) of the uterus, usually caused by infection. The condition is accompanied by a thick mucoid discharge.

endocervix (en-doh-**ser**-viks) *n.* the mucous membrane lining the cervix of the uterus.

endochondral (en-doh-**kon**-drăl) *adj.* within the material of a cartilage.

endocrine gland (ductless gland) (**end**-oh-kryn) *n.* a gland that manufactures one or more hormones and secretes them directly into the bloodstream (and not through a duct to the exterior). Endocrine glands include the pituitary, thyroid, parathyroid, and adrenal glands, the ovary and testis, the placenta, and part of the pancreas.

endocrinology (en-doh-kri-**nol**-ŏji) *n.* the study of the endocrine glands and the hormones they secrete. —**endocrinologist** *n.*

endoderm (**end**-oh-derm) *n.* the inner of the three germ layers of the early embryo, which gives rise to the lining of most of the alimentary canal and its associated glands, the lining of the bronchi and alveoli of the lung, and most of the urinary tract. —**endodermal** (en-doh-**der**-măl) *adj.*

endodermal sinus tumour *n.* a rare tumour of fetal remnants of the ovaries or testes.

endogenous (en-**doj**-in-ŭs) *adj.* arising within or derived from the body. *Compare* exogenous.

endolymph (**end**-oh-limf) *n.* the fluid that fills the membranous labyrinth of the ear.

endolysin (en-**dol**-i-sin) *n.* a substance within a cell that has a specific destructive action against bacteria.

endometrial (en-doh-**mee**-tri-ăl) *adj.* relating to or affecting the lining of the uterus (endometrium). **e. ablation** an operation to remove the entire endometrium, usually to treat menorrhagia. It is performed under local anaesthetic by means of laser ablation, radiofrequency ablation (**NovaSure**), electrocoagulation, balloon thermal coagulation, or microwaves (**microwave e. a.**), which vaporize the endometrial tissue. **e. aspiration** the removal, by means of suction, of a sample of endometrial tissue for diagnostic purposes. **e. hyperplasia** an increase in the thickness of the cells of the endometrium, usually due to prolonged exposure to unopposed oestrogen (e.g. from HRT or an oestrogen-secreting tumour). Atypical cells may be present.

endometriosis (en-doh-mee-tri-**oh**-sis) *n.* the presence of endometrial tissue at sites in the pelvis outside the uterus or, rarely, throughout the body. Symptoms typically include pelvic pain, severe dysmenorrhoea, dyspareunia, and infertility.

endometritis (en-doh-mi-**try**-tis) *n.* inflammation of the endometrium due to acute or chronic infection. It may be caused by foreign bodies, bacteria, viruses, or parasites. Chronic endometritis may be responsible for the contraceptive action of IUCDs.

endometrium (en-doh-**mee**-tri-ŭm) *n.* the mucous membrane lining the uterus. It becomes thicker and more vascular during the latter part of the menstrual cycle and much of it breaks down and is lost in menstruation. If pregnancy becomes established the endometrium becomes the decidua.

endomorphic (en-doh-**mor**-fik) *adj.* describing a body type that is relatively fat, with highly developed viscera and weak muscular and skeletal development. —**endomorph** *n.* —**endomorphy** *n.*

endomyocarditis (en-doh-my-oh-kar-**dy**-tis) *n.* an acute or chronic inflammatory disorder of the muscle and lining membrane of the heart. The principal causes are rheumatic fever and virus infections. There is enlargement of the heart, murmurs, embolism, and frequently arrhythmias.

endomysium (en-doh-**miz**-iŭm) *n.* the fine connective tissue sheath that surrounds a single muscle fibre.

endoneurium (en-doh-**newr**-iŭm) *n.* the layer of fibrous tissue that separates individual fibres within a nerve.

endoparasite (en-doh-**pa**-ră-syt) *n.* a parasite that lives inside its host, for example in the liver, lungs, gut, or other tissues of the body. *Compare* ectoparasite.

endophthalmitis (end-off-thal-**my**-tis) *n.* inflammation, usually due to infection, within the eye.

endoplasmic reticulum (ER) (en-doh-**plaz**-mik) *n.* a system of membranes present in the cytoplasm of cells. It is the site of manufacture of proteins and lipids and is concerned with the transport of these products within the cell (*see also* Golgi apparatus).

end organ *n.* a specialized structure at the end of a peripheral nerve, such as the taste buds in the tongue, acting as a receptor for a particular sensation.

endorphin (en-**dor**-fin) *n.* one of a group of peptides that occur naturally in the brain and have pain-relieving properties similar to those of the opiates. *See also* encephalin.

endoscope (**end**-oh-skohp) *n.* any instrument, such as an auriscope or a gastroscope, used to obtain an interior view of a hollow organ or body cavity. Most endoscopes consist of a rigid or flexible tube, a light source, and an image-capturing system (either optical or digital) to deliver the images to the operator. *See also* fibrescope. **—endoscopic** (en-doh-**skop**-ik) *adj.* **—endoscopy** (en-**dos**-kŏ-pi) *n.*

endoscopic retrograde cholangiopancreatography *n. see* ERCP.

endoscopic sinus surgery (ESS) *n.* surgery of the paranasal sinuses using endoscopes. **functional e. s. s.** (**FESS**) surgery that clears inflamed tissue from routes of sinus drainage and aeration to allow the other sinuses to return to normal.

endospore (**end**-oh-spor) *n.* the resting stage of certain bacteria, particularly species of the genera *Bacillus* and *Clostridium*.

endostapler (**end**-oh-stay-pler) *n.* a stapling instrument (*see* staple) used endoscopically for purposes of fixing tissues or joining them together.

endosteum (en-**dos**-tiŭm) *n.* the membrane that lines the marrow cavity of a bone.

endothelioma (en-doh-th'ee-li-**oh**-mă) *n.* any tumour arising from or resembling endothelium.

endothelium (en-doh-**th'ee**-li-um) *n.* the single layer of cells that lines the heart, blood vessels, and lymphatic vessels. It is derived from embryonic mesoderm. *Compare* epithelium. **—endothelial** *adj.*

endotoxin (en-doh-**toks**-in) *n.* a poison generally harmful to all body tissues, contained within certain Gram-negative bacteria and released only when the bacterial cell is broken down or dies and disintegrates. *Compare* exotoxin.

endotracheal (ET) (en-doh-tray-ki-ăl) *adj.* within or through the trachea. **e. tube** a tube inserted into the trachea to maintain a patent airway. *See also* intubation.

endovascular (en-doh-vas-kew-ler) *adj.* describing procedures for imaging the circulation or for treating vascular disorders from within the circulation, including angioplasty, the placement of stents or coils in aneurysms, and embolization.

end-plate (end-playt) *n.* the area of muscle cell membrane immediately beneath the motor nerve ending at a neuromuscular junction.

end-stage renal failure (ESRF, CKD 5) (end-stayj) *n.* the most advanced stage of kidney failure, which is reached when the glomerular filtration rate (GFR) falls to 15 ml/min (normal GFR = 100 ml/min).

end-systolic volume (ESV) (end-sis-tol-ik) *n.* the volume of blood that remains in the ventricles after systole when the heart is fully contracted.

enema (en-im-ă) *n.* (*pl.* **enemata** or **enemas**] a quantity of fluid infused into the rectum through a tube passed into the anus. **barium e.** a radiological technique used to diagnose conditions of the large bowel using the combination of X-ray imaging and radiopaque contrast (barium sulphate). For double contrast, air is pumped through the tube to distend the large bowel before the radiographs are taken. **evacuant e.** an enema using soap or olive oil to remove faeces. **small-bowel e.** *see* small bowel. **therapeutic e.** an enema used to insert drugs into the rectum.

enervation (en-er-vay-shŏn) *n.* **1.** weakness; loss of strength. **2.** the surgical removal of a nerve.

engagement (in-gayj-mĕnt) *n.* (in obstetrics) the stage of pregnancy that occurs when the presenting part of the fetus has descended into the mother's pelvis. Engagement of the fetal head occurs when the widest part has passed through the pelvic inlet.

enhanced role (en-hahnst) *n.* (of the nurse) *see* extended role.

enkephalin (en-kef-ă-lin) *n.* *see* encephalin.

enophthalmos (en-off-thal-mŏs) *n.* a condition in which the eye is abnormally sunken into the socket.

enostosis (en-os-toh-sis) *n.* a benign growth within a bone.

enoximone (en-oks-i-mohn) *n.* an inotropic drug used in the treatment of heart failure to increase the force and output of the heart. It is administered by intravenous injection or infusion. Trade name: **Perfan**.

enrolled nurse (EN) (en-rohld) *n.* (in the UK) a nurse who completed a two-year programme of nursing education (*see* second-level nurse). Entry to the second-level part of the NMC register was in general, mental, or mental handicap nursing in England and Wales. In Scotland and Northern Ireland there was generic training for second-level qualification.

ensiform cartilage (en-si-form) *n. see* xiphoid process.

ENT *n.* ear, nose, and throat. *See* otorhinolaryngology.

Entamoeba (ent-ă-**mee**-bă) *n.* a genus of widely distributed amoebae. **E. coli** a harmless intestinal parasite. **E. gingivalis** a species found between the teeth; it is associated with periodontal disease and gingivitis. **E. histolytica** a species that invades the intestinal wall, causing amoebic dysentery and ulceration; infection of the liver with this species (amoebic hepatitis) is common in tropical countries.

enter- (entero-) *combining form denoting* the intestine.

enteral (**en**-ter-ăl) *adj.* of or relating to the intestinal tract. **e. feeding** *see* nutrition.

enteralgia (en-ter-**al**-jiă) *n. see* colic.

enterectomy (en-ter-**ek**-tŏmi) *n.* surgical removal of part of the intestine.

enteric (en-**te**-rik) *adj.* relating to or affecting the intestine. **e. fever** *see* paratyphoid fever, typhoid fever.

enteric-coated *adj.* describing tablets that are coated with a substance that enables them to pass through the stomach to the intestine unchanged.

enteritis (en-ter-**I**-tis) *n.* inflammation of the small intestine, usually causing diarrhoea. **infective e.** enteritis caused by infectious pathogens, such as viruses or bacteria. **radiation e.** a complication of radiation therapy for pelvic and abdominal malignancies. It can cause fistulae, strictures, and malabsorption. *See also* gastroenteritis.

enterobiasis (oxyuriasis) (en-ter-oh-**by**-ă-sis) *n.* a disease, common in children throughout the world, caused by the parasitic nematode *Enterobius vermicularis* (*see* threadworm) in the large intestine. The worms do not cause any serious lesions of the gut wall although, rarely, they may provoke appendicitis. Enterobiasis responds well to treatment with mebendazole.

Enterobius (Oxyuris) (en-ter-**oh**-biŭs) *n. see* threadworm.

enterocele (**en**-ter-oh-seel) *n.* a hernia of the pouch of Douglas (between the rectum and uterus) into the upper part of the posterior vaginal wall.

enteroclysis (en-ter-oh-**kly**-sis) *n.* small-bowel enema (*see* small bowel).

Enterococcus (en-ter-oh-**kok**-ŭs) *n.* a genus of bacteria that inhabit the human intestine. A few species (notably *E. faecalis* and *E. faecium*) are responsible for hospital-acquired infections that are difficult to treat, since the bacteria are able to survive under adverse conditions.

enterocolitis (en-ter-oh-kŏ-**ly**-tis) *n.* inflammation of the colon and small intestine. *See also* colitis, enteritis, necrotizing enterocolitis.

enterogenous (en-ter-**oj**-i-nŭs) *adj.* of intestinal origin.

enterokinase (en-ter-oh-**ky**-nayz) *n.* the former name for enteropeptidase.

enterolith (**en**-ter-oh-lith) *n.* a stone within the intestine. It usually builds up around a gallstone or a swallowed fruit stone.

enteron (**en**-ter-on) *n.* the intestinal tract.

enteropathy (en-ter-**op**-ă-thi) *n.* disease of the small intestine. *See also* coeliac disease (gluten-sensitive enteropathy).

enteropeptidase (en-ter-oh-**pep**-ti-dayz) *n.* an enzyme secreted by the glands of the small intestine that acts on trypsinogen to produce trypsin.

enterorrhaphy (en-ter-**o**-ră-fi) *n.* the surgical procedure of stitching an intestine that has either perforated or been divided during an operation.

enteroscope (**en**-ter-oh-skohp) *n.* an illuminated optical instrument used to inspect the interior of the small intestine. The image is transmitted through digital video technology. The double balloon **push-and-pull** type is introduced under direct vision and is the predominant type in current use. Inflation and deflation of the double balloon helps in progression of the enteroscope through the intestine. The enteroscope is useful in diagnosing the cause of obscure haemorrhage of the small intestine or of strictures. **—enteroscopy** (en-ter-**os**-kŏpi) *n.*

enterostomy (en-ter-**ost**-ŏmi) *n.* an operation in which the small intestine is brought through the abdominal wall and opened (*see* duodenostomy, jejunostomy, ileostomy) or is joined to the stomach (**gastroenterostomy**) or to another loop of small intestine (**enteroenterostomy**).

enterotomy (en-ter-**ot**-ŏmi) *n.* surgical incision into the intestine.

enterotoxin (en-ter-oh-**toks**-in) *n.* a poisonous substance that has a particularly marked effect upon the gastrointestinal tract, causing vomiting, diarrhoea, and abdominal pain.

enterovirus (en-ter-oh-**vy**-rŭs) *n.* any virus that enters the body through the gastrointestinal tract, multiplies there, and then (generally) invades the central nervous system. Enteroviruses include Coxsackie viruses and polioviruses.

enterozoon (en-ter-oh-**zoh**-on) *n.* any animal species inhabiting or infecting the gut of another. *See also* endoparasite.

enthesis (en-**th'ee**-sis) *n.* (*pl.* **entheses**) **1.** the site of insertion of tendons and ligaments into bones. **2.** insertion of synthetic inorganic material to replace lost tissue.

enthesopathy (en-theez-**op**-ă-thi) *n.* any rheumatic disease resulting in inflammation of entheses. Ankylosing spondylitis, psoriatic arthritis, and reactive arthritis are examples.

Entonox (**en**-tĕ-noks) *n. see* nitrous oxide.

entrapment neuropathy (en-**trap**-mĕnt) *n.* pain, muscle wasting, and paralysis resulting from pressure on a nerve in conditions in which it is subjected to compression by surrounding structures. *See* carpal tunnel syndrome.

entropion (en-**troh**-pi-on) *n.* inturning of the eyelid towards the eyeball. The lashes may rub against the eye and cause irritation (*see* trichiasis).

enucleation (i-new-kli-**ay**-shŏn) *n.* the complete removal of an organ, tumour, or cyst leaving surrounding structures intact. In ophthalmology it is an operation in which the eyeball is removed but the other structures in the socket are left in place when fitting an artificial eye.

enuresis (en-yoor-**ee**-sis) *n.* the involuntary passing of urine, especially bedwetting by children at night (**nocturnal e.**). *See also* incontinence. **—enuretic** (en-yoor-**et**-ik) *adj.*

environment (in-**vyr**-ŏn-mĕnt) *n.* any or all aspects of the surroundings of an organism, both internal and external, which influence its growth, development, and behaviour.

Environmental Health Officer (EHO) (in-vyr-ŏn-**men**-tăl) *n.* a person, employed by a local authority, who has special training in such aspects of environmental health as housing, pollution, and food safety (formerly known as a **Public Health Inspector**).

SEE WEB LINKS

- Website of the Chartered Institute for Environmental Health

environmental hearing aid *n. see* hearing aid.

enzyme (**en**-zym) *n.* a protein that, in small amounts, speeds up the rate of a biological reaction without itself being used up in the reaction (i.e. it acts as a catalyst). Enzymes are essential for the normal functioning and development of the body. Failure in the production or activity of a single enzyme may result in metabolic disorders; such disorders are often inherited and some have serious effects. **—enzymatic** *adj.*

enzyme-linked immunosorbent assay (ELISA) *n.* a sensitive technique for measuring the amount of a substance. An antibody that will bind to the substance is produced; the amount of an easily measured enzyme that then binds to the antibody complex enables accurate measurement.

EOG *n. see* electrooculography.

eosin (**ee**-oh-sin) *n.* a red acidic dye, produced by the reaction of bromine and fluorescein, used to stain biological specimens for microscopical examination.

eosinopenia (ee-oh-sin-oh-**pee**-niă) *n.* a decrease in the number of eosinophils in the blood.

eosinophil (ee-oh-**sin**-ŏ-fil) *n.* a variety of white blood cell (*see* polymorph) distinguished by the presence in its cytoplasm of coarse granules that stain orange-red with Romanowsky stains. Eosinophils are capable of ingesting foreign particles and are involved in allergic responses and host defence against parasites.

eosinophilia (ee-oh-sin-ŏ-**fil**-iă) *n.* an increase in the number of eosinophils in the blood. Eosinophilia occurs in response to certain drugs and in a variety of diseases, including allergies, parasitic infestations, and certain forms of leukaemia.

eparterial (ep-ar-**teer**-iăl) *adj.* situated on or above an artery.

ependyma (ep-**en**-dim-ă) *n.* the extremely thin membrane, composed of cells of the glia (**ependymal cells**), that lines the ventricles of the brain and the choroid plexuses. It is responsible for helping to form cerebrospinal fluid. **—ependymal** *adj.*

ependymoma (ep-en-di-**moh**-mă) *n.* a cerebral tumour derived from the glial ependymal cells. It may obstruct the flow of cerebrospinal fluid, causing a hydrocephalus.

ephebiatrics (hebiatrics) (i-fee-bi-**at**-riks) *n.* the branch of medicine concerned with the common disorders of adolescents. *Compare* paediatrics.

ephedrine (**ef**-i-drin) *n.* a drug that causes constriction of blood vessels and widening of the bronchial passages (*see* sympathomimetic). It is used mainly as a nasal decongestant, being administered as nose drops.

epi- *prefix denoting* above or upon.

epiblepharon (epi-**blef**-er-on) *n.* a fold of skin, present from birth, stretching across the eye just above the lashes of the upper eyelid or in front of them in the lower lid. It usually disappears within the first year of life.

epicanthus (epicanthic fold) (epi-**kanth**-ŭs) *n.* (*pl.* **epicanthi**) a vertical fold of skin from the upper eyelid that covers the inner corner of the eye. It occurs abnormally in certain congenital conditions, e.g. Down's syndrome. **—epicanthal, epicanthic** *adj.*

epicardium (epi-**kar**-diŭm) *n.* the outermost layer of the heart wall, enveloping the myocardium. It is a serous membrane that forms the inner layer of the serous pericardium. **—epicardial** *adj.*

epicondyle (epi-**kon**-dyl) *n.* the protuberance above a condyle at the end of an articulating bone.

epicranium (epi-**kray**-niŭm) *n.* the structures that cover the cranium, i.e. all layers of the scalp.

epicranius (epi-**kray**-ni-ŭs) *n.* the muscle of the scalp.

epicritic (epi-**krit**-ik) *adj.* describing or relating to sensory nerve fibres responsible for the fine degrees of sensation, as of temperature and touch. *Compare* protopathic.

epidemic (epi-**dem**-ik) *n.* a sudden outbreak of infectious disease that spreads rapidly through the population, affecting a large proportion of people. *Compare* endemic, pandemic. **—epidemic** *adj.*

epidemiology (epi-dee-mi-**ol**-ŏji) *n.* the study of the distribution of diseases and determinants of diseases in populations, including all forms of disease that relate to the environment and ways of life.

epidermis (epi-**der**-mis) *n.* the outer layer of the skin, which is divided into four layers (see illustration). The top three layers are continually renewed as cells from the continuously dividing Malpighian layer are gradually pushed outwards and become progressively impregnated with keratin (*see* keratinization). **—epidermal** *adj.*

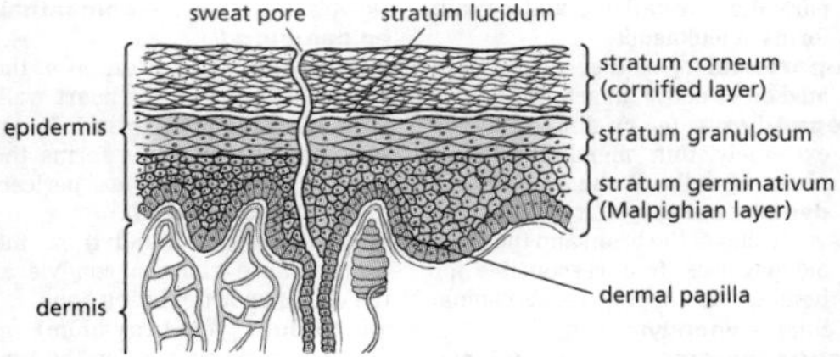

A section of epidermis

epidermoid cyst (epi-**der**-moid) *n. see* sebaceous cyst.

epidermolysis bullosa (EB) (epi-der-**mol**-i-sis buul-**oh**-să) *n.* any one of a group of genetically determined disorders characterized by blistering of skin and mucous membranes that occurs secondarily to minor mechanical trauma. The more serious (dystrophic) forms may be complicated by the development of skin squamous cell carcinomas; other serious types result in death in early childhood.

Epidermophyton (epi-der-**mof**-i-tŏn) *n.* a genus of fungi that grow on the skin, causing tinea (ringworm). *See also* dermatophyte.

epidiascope (epi-**dy**-ă-skohp) *n.* an apparatus for projecting a greatly magnified image of an object, such as a specimen on a microscope slide, on to a screen.

epididymectomy (epi-did-i-**mek**-tŏmi) *n.* the surgical removal or excision of the epididymis.

epididymis (epi-**did**-i-mis) *n.* (*pl.* **epididymides**] a highly convoluted tube, about seven metres long, that connects the testis to the vas deferens. The spermatozoa are moved along the tube and are stored in the lower part until ejaculation. **—epididymal** *adj.*

epididymitis (epi-did-i-**my**-tis) *n.* inflammation of the epididymis. The usual cause is infection spreading down the vas deferens from the bladder or urethra. The inflammation may spread to the testicle (**epididymo-orchitis**).

epididymovasostomy (epi-did-i-moh-vayz-**os**-tŏmi) *n.* the operation of connecting the vas deferens to the epididymis to bypass obstruction of the latter in an attempt to cure azoospermia caused by this blockage. It is also performed to reverse vasectomy as an alternative to vasovasostomy.

epidural (extradural) (epi-**dewr**-ăl) *adj.* on or over the dura mater. **e. anaesthesia** suppression of sensation in the lower part of the body by injecting a local anaesthetic into the epidural space, which anaesthetizes spinal nerve roots. It is used especially to provide pain relief during childbirth, to reduce the need for deep general anaesthesia, and for postoperative analgesia. **e. space** the space between the dura mater of the spinal cord and the vertebral canal.

epigastrium (epi-gas-tri-ŭm) *n.* the upper central region of the abdomen. **—epigastric** *adj.*

epigastrocele (epi-gas-troh-seel) *n.* a hernia through the upper central region of the abdominal wall.

epiglottis (epi-**glot**-iss) *n.* a thin leaf-shaped flap of cartilage, covered with mucous membrane, that is situated immediately behind the root of the tongue. It covers the entrance to the larynx during swallowing.

epiglottitis (epi-glot-**I**-tis) *n.* an infection of the epiglottis, which swells and causes obstruction of the upper airways. It usually occurs in children under seven years old, but is much less common since the Hib vaccine was introduced.

epikeratophakia (epi-ke-ră-toh-**fay**-kiă) *n.* eye surgery to correct errors of refraction in which the curvature of the cornea is altered using donor corneal tissue, which has been frozen and shaped using a lathe to produce a tissue lens that is then sutured onto the cornea.

epilation (epi-**lay**-shŏn) *n.* the removal of a hair by its roots. This can be done mechanically or by the use of topical creams, electrolysis, or lasers.

epilepsy (**ep**-i-lep-si) *n.* a disorder of brain function characterized by recurrent seizures that have a sudden onset and may be generalized or partial. **Generalized seizures**, which involve the entire brain, may take the form of tonic-clonic or absence seizures. In **tonic-clonic seizures** (formerly called **grand mal**) the patient falls to the ground unconscious with his muscles in a state of spasm (the tonic phase). This is replaced by the convulsive movements of the clonic phase, when the tongue may be bitten and urinary incontinence may occur. **Absence seizures** (formerly called **petit mal**) are brief spells of unconsciousness, lasting for a few seconds, during which posture and balance are maintained and the eyes stare blankly. They seldom appear before the age of three or after adolescence and often subside spontaneously in adult life, although they may be followed by the onset of tonic-clonic or partial seizures. **Partial** (or **focal**) **seizures** affect localized areas of the brain, causing motor, sensory, or autonomic effects. In a simple partial motor seizure convulsive movements may spread from the thumb to the hand, arm, and face (this spread of symptoms is called the **Jacksonian march**); there is no loss of awareness. The symptoms of **complex partial seizures** include hallucinations of smell, taste, sight, and hearing, paroxysmal disorders of memory, and automatism. Commonly caused by damage to the cortex of the temporal lobe or the adjacent parietal lobe of the brain, such seizures are often called **temporal lobe** (or **psychomotor**) **e.** —**epileptic** (epi-**lep**-tik) *adj., n.*

SEE WEB LINKS

- Website of Epilepsy Action

epileptiform (epi-**lep**-ti-form) *adj.* resembling an epileptic attack.

epileptogenic (epi-lep-toh-**jen**-ik) *adj.* having the capacity to provoke epileptic seizures.

epiloia (epi-**loi**-ă) *n. see* tuberous (sclerosis).

epinephrine (epi-**nef**-rin) *n. see* adrenaline.

epineurium (epi-**newr**-iŭm) *n.* the outer sheath of connective tissue that encloses the bundles (fascicles) of fibres that make up a nerve.

epiphenomenon (epi-fin-**om**-inŏn) *n.* an unusual symptom or event that may occur simultaneously with a disease but is not necessarily directly related to it. *Compare* complication.

epiphora (i-**pif**-er-ă) *n.* watering of the eye, in which tears flow onto the cheek. It is due to some abnormality of the tear drainage system: *see* lacrimal (apparatus).

epiphysis (i-**pif**-i-sis) *n.* (*pl.* **epiphyses**) **1.** the end of a long bone, which is initially separated by cartilage from the shaft (diaphysis) of the bone and develops separately. It eventually fuses with the diaphysis to form a complete bone. **2.** *see* pineal gland. —**epiphyseal** (epi-**fiz**-iăl) *adj.*

epiphysitis (ep-ifi-**sy**-tis) *n.* inflammation of the epiphysis of a long bone.

epiplo- *combining form denoting* the omentum.

epiplocele (i-**pip**-loh-seel) *n.* a hernia that contains omentum.

epiploon (i-**pip**-loh-on) *n. see* omentum.

episclera (epi-**skleer**-ă) *n.* the outermost covering of the sclera of the eye, which provides nutritional support to the sclera.

episcleritis (epi-skleer-**I**-tis) *n.* inflammation of the outermost layer of the sclera of the eyeball, resulting in a red painful eye that is sensitive to light.

episio- *combining form denoting* the vulva.

episiorrhaphy (ep-izi-**o**-răfi) *n.* stitching together the margins of a tear in the tissues around the vaginal opening.

episiotomy (ep-izi-**ot**-ŏmi) *n.* an incision into the perineum during a difficult birth. The aim is to make delivery easier and to avoid extensive tearing of adjacent tissues.

epispadias (epi-**spay**-di-ăs) *n.* a congenital abnormality in which the opening of the urethra is on the dorsal (upper) surface of the penis. Surgical correction is carried out in infancy.

epistaxis (epi-**staks**-iss) *n.* bleeding from the nose, which may be caused by low-grade bacterial infection of the front of the nose, hypertension, clotting disorders, or tumours of the nose or sinuses.

epithalaxia (epi-thal-aks-iă) *n.* loss of layers of epithelial cells from the lining of the intestine.

epithelialization (epi-th'ee-li-ă-ly-zay-shŏn) *n.* the growth of epithelium over the surface of a wound, which marks the final stage of healing.

epithelial pearls (epi-theel-i l) *n. see* Epstein's pearls.

epithelioma (epi-th'ee-li-**oh**-mă) *n.* a tumour of epithelium: a former name for carcinoma.

epithelium (epi-theel-iŭm) *n.* the tissue that covers the external surface of the body and lines hollow structures (except blood and lymphatic vessels). Epithelium may be either **simple**, consisting of a single layer of cells; **stratified**, consisting of several cell layers; or **pseudostratified**, in which the cells appear to be arranged in layers but in fact share a common basement membrane. See illustration. *See also* endothelium, mesothelium. **—epithelial** *adj.*

epoetin (recombinant human erythropoietin) (ep-oh-ee-tin) *n.* any of four forms of erythropoietin produced by genetic engineering – **e. alfa** (Binocrit, Eprex), **e. beta** (NeoRecormon), **e. theta** (Eporatio), or **e. zeta** (Retacrit) – administered by injection for treating anaemia associated with chronic renal failure or induced by chemotherapy.

eponym (ep-ŏ-nim) *n.* a disease, structure, or species named after a particular person, usually the person who first discovered or described it. **—eponymous** (i-pon-i-mŭs) *adj.*

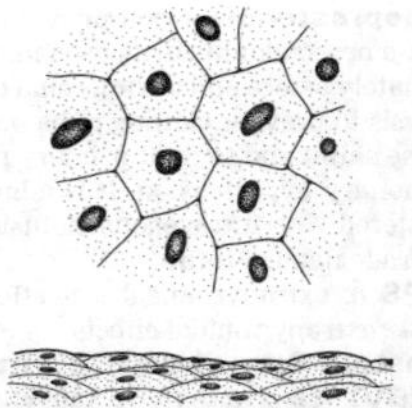
Stratified squamous epithelium, surface view above and sectional view below

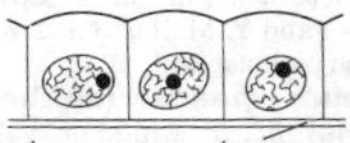

Simple cuboidal epithelium

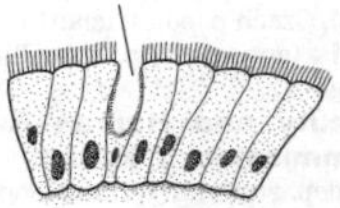

Ciliated columnar epithelium

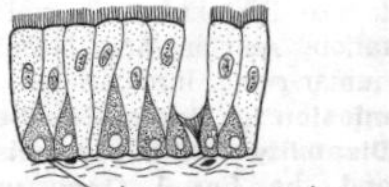

Pseudostratified ciliated epithelium

Types of epithelium

epoprostenol (ee-poh-**pros**-ti-nol) *n.* a prostaglandin drug used immediately before and during renal dialysis to prevent clotting of blood in the shunt and to treat primary pulmonary hypertension. It is administered by intravenous infusion. Trade name: **Flolan**.

EPS *n.* extrapyramidal side-effects (*see* extrapyramidal effects).

Epstein-Barr virus (EB virus, EBV) (**ep**-styn bar) *n.* the virus, belonging to the herpesvirus group, that is the causative agent of glandular fever. It is also implicated in Burkitt's lymphoma, Hodgkin's disease, and hepatitis. [Sir M. A. Epstein (1921–) and Y. M. Barr (1932–2016), British pathologists]

Epstein's pearls (epithelial pearls) *pl. n.* white or yellow cysts that are visible on the gums and hard palate of newborn babies. They spontaneously disappear at 1–2 weeks of age. [A. Epstein (1849–1918), Czech paediatrician]

epulis (ep-**yoo**-lis) *n.* a swelling on the gum.

Equality and Human Rights Commission (i-**kwol**-iti) *n.* a nondepartmental public body set up in 2007 to reduce discrimination and promote equality with regard to race, disability, sex, sexual orientation, religion and belief, and human rights. It replaced the **Commission for Racial Equality**, the **Disability Rights Commission**, and the **Equal Opportunities Commission**.

equi- *combining form denoting* equality.

equinia (i-**kwin**-iă) *n. see* glanders.

Erbitux (**er**-bi-tuks) *n. see* cetuximab.

Erb's palsy (erbz) *n.* weakness or paralysis of the shoulder and arm caused by injury to the upper roots of the brachial plexus during traumatic childbirth. The muscles of the shoulder and the flexors of the elbow are paralysed and the arm hangs at the side internally rotated at the shoulder. [W. H. Erb (1840–1921), German neurologist]

ERCP *n.* endoscopic retrograde cholangiopancreatography; a technique in which a catheter is passed through a duodenoscope into the ampulla of Vater of the common bile duct and injected with a radiopaque medium to outline the pancreatic duct and bile ducts radiologically. ERCP is used to confirm diagnosis of biliary and pancreatic disease and to facilitate various therapeutic interventions (e.g. removal of stones from the bile duct).

erectile (i-**rek**-tyl) *adj.* capable of causing erection or becoming erect. The penis is composed largely of erectile tissue.

erectile dysfunction *n.* inability in a male to obtain and/or maintain a penile erection sufficient to enable vaginal penetration for sexual intercourse. Often a combination of physical causes (e.g. peripheral vascular disease, diabetes mellitus, certain medications) and psychological factors is responsible for the condition. Treatments that work by increasing blood flow to the cavernous sinuses of the penis include oral sildenafil and injectable alprostadil. Penile prostheses are surgically inserted into the penis.

SEE WEB LINKS

- Factsheets about erectile dysfunction published by the Sexual Advice Association

erection (i-**rek**-shŏn) *n.* the sexually active state of the penis, which becomes enlarged and rigid (due to the erectile tissue being swollen with blood). The term is also applied to the clitoris.

erepsin (i-**rep**-sin) *n.* a mixture of protein-digesting enzymes (*see* peptidase) secreted by the intestinal glands. It is part of the succus entericus.

ERG *n. see* electroretinography.

erg- (ergo-) *combining form denoting* work or activity.

ergocalciferol (er-goh-kal-**sif**-er-ol) *n. see* vitamin D.

ergograph (er-gŏ-grahf) *n.* an apparatus for recording the work performed by the muscles of the body when undergoing activity.

ergometrine (er-goh-**met**-reen) *n.* a drug that stimulates contractions of the uterus. Combined with oxytocin (in **Syntometrine**), it is administered by intramuscular injection to assist the final stage of labour and to control bleeding following incomplete miscarriage.

ergonomics (er-gŏ-**nom**-iks) *n.* the study of humans in relation to their work and working surroundings.

ergosterol (er-**gos**-ter-ol) *n.* a plant sterol that, when irradiated with ultraviolet light, is converted to ergocalciferol (vitamin D_2). *See* vitamin D.

ergot (**er**-got) *n.* a fungus (Claviceps purpurea) that grows on rye. It produces several important alkaloids, including ergotamine and ergometrine. *See also* ergotism.

ergotamine (er-**got**-ă-meen) *n.* a drug that causes constriction of blood vessels and is used to relieve migraine. It is administered by mouth in combination with caffeine and cyclizine (in **Migril**).

ergotism (**er**-gŏ-tizm) *n.* poisoning caused by eating rye infected with the fungus ergot. The chief symptom is gangrene of the fingers and toes, with diarrhoea and vomiting, nausea, and headache.

erogenous (i-**roj**-in-ŭs) *adj.* describing certain parts of the body, the physical stimulation of which leads to sexual arousal.

erosion (i-**roh**-*zh*ŏn) *n.* an eating away of surface tissue by physical or chemical processes, including those associated with inflammation. **cervical e.** an abnormal area of epithelium that may develop at the cervix of the uterus. *See* ectropion. **dental e.** loss of surface tooth substance, usually caused by repeated application of acid. It may result from excessive intake of fruit juice, carbonated drinks, or acidic fruits or from regurgitation of acid from the stomach.

erot- (eroto-) *combining form denoting* sexual desire or love.

ERPC *pl. n.* evacuated retained products of conception.

error (**e**-rer) *n.* (in research) incorrectly rejecting a null hypothesis when it is true (**type I error**) or failing to reject a null hypothesis when it is false (**type II error**). *See* significance.

eructation (i-ruk-tay-shŏn) *n.* belching: the sudden raising of gas from the stomach.

eruption (i-rup-shŏn) *n.* **1.** the outbreak of a rash. **2.** (in dentistry) the emergence of a growing tooth from the gum into the mouth.

ERV *n. see* (expiratory) reserve volume.

erysipelas (e-ri-sip-ilăs) *n.* a streptococcal infection of the skin, especially the face, characterized by redness and swelling. The affected areas usually have sharply defined margins, which may differentiate erysipelas from the otherwise similar cellulitis.

erysipeloid (e-ri-sip-i-loid) *n.* an infection of the skin and underlying tissues with the bacterium *Erysipelothrix insidiosa*, developing usually in people handling fish, poultry, or meat. It is normally confined to a finger or hand, which becomes reddened; sometimes systemic illness develops.

erythema (e-ri-theem-ă) *n.* flushing of the skin due to dilatation of the blood capillaries in the dermis. **e. ab igne** a reticular pigmented rash on the lower legs or elsewhere caused by persistent exposure to radiant heat. **e. infectiosum** (**fifth disease**, **slapped cheek syndrome**) a common benign infectious viral disease of children, characterized by fever and a rash, first on the cheeks and later on the trunk and extremities, that disappears after several days. **e. multiforme** a condition characterized by so-called target lesions that may be recurrent and follow herpes simplex infection (especially in children) or medications (especially in adults). **e. nodosum** a condition characterized by tender bruiselike swellings on the shins. It is often associated with streptococcal infection. **e. toxicum neonatum** (**neonatal urticaria**) a self-limiting asymptomatic rash appearing in up to half of newborns, usually 2–5 days after birth.

erythr- (erythro-) *combining form denoting* **1.** redness. **2.** erythrocytes.

erythrasma (e-ri-thraz-mă) *n.* a chronic skin infection due to the bacterium *Corynebacterium minutissimum*, occurring in such areas as the armpits, where skin surfaces are in contact.

erythroblast (i-rith-roh-blast) *n.* any of a series of nucleated cells (*see* normoblast) that pass through a succession of stages of maturation to form red blood cells (erythrocytes). *See also* erythropoiesis.

erythroblastosis (i-rith-roh-blas-toh-sis) *n.* the presence in the blood of erythroblasts. **e. foetalis** a severe but rare haemolytic anaemia affecting newborn infants due to destruction of the infant's red blood cells by factors present in the mother's serum. It is usually caused by incompatibility of the rhesus blood groups between mother and infant (*see* rhesus factor).

erythrocyanosis (i-rith-roh-sy-ă-noh-sis) *n.* mottled purplish discoloration on the legs and thighs. The condition is worse in cold weather. Weight loss is the best treatment as it reduces the insulating effect of a thick layer of fat.

erythrocyte (red blood cell, RBC) (i-rith-roh-syt) *n.* a blood cell containing the pigment haemoglobin, the principal function of which is to transport oxygen. There are normally about 5×10^{12} erythrocytes per litre of blood.

erythrocyte sedimentation rate *n. see* ESR.

erythrocytosis (i-rith-roh-sy-**toh**-sis) *n.* an increase in the number of red blood cells (erythrocytes) in the blood. *See* polycythaemia.

erythroderma (exfoliative dermatitis) (i-rith-roh-**der**-mă) *n.* abnormal reddening, flaking, and thickening of the skin affecting a wide area of the body.

erythroedema (i-rith-ri-**dee**-mă) *n. see* pink disease.

erythromycin (i-rith-roh-**my**-sin) *n.* an antibiotic used to treat respiratory, skin, and other infections caused by a wide range of bacteria. It is administered by mouth or intravenous infusion or (for treating acne) topically. Trade names: **Erymax**, **Erythrocin**, **Erythroped**.

erythropenia (i-rith-roh-**pee**-niă) *n.* a reduction in the number of red blood cells (erythrocytes) in the blood.

erythroplasia (i-rith-roh-**play**-ziă) *n.* an abnormal red patch of skin that occurs particularly in the mouth or on the genitalia and is precancerous.

erythropoiesis (i-rith-roh-poi-**ee**-sis) *n.* the process of red blood cell (erythrocyte) production, which normally occurs in the blood-forming tissue of the bone marrow. *See also* haemopoiesis.

erythropoietin (EPO) (i-rith-roh-**poi**-ĕ-tin) *n.* a hormone secreted by certain cells in the kidney in response to a reduction in the amount of oxygen reaching the tissues. Erythropoietin increases and controls the rate of red cell production (erythropoiesis). *See also* epoetin.

erythropsia (e-ri-**throp**-siă) *n.* red vision: a symptom sometimes experienced after removal of a cataract and also in snow blindness.

Esbach's albuminometer (ess-bahks) *n.* a graduated glass tube used for measuring the amount of albumin in a specimen of urine. [G. H. Esbach (1843–90), French physician]

ESC *n. see* essential skills clusters.

eschar (**ess**-kar) *n.* a scab or slough, as produced by the action of heat or a corrosive substance on living tissue.

Escherichia (esh-er-**ik**-iă) *n.* a genus of Gram-negative, generally motile, rodlike bacteria that are found in the intestines of humans and many animals. **E. coli** a species that is usually not harmful but some strains of which cause gastrointestinal infections. **E. coli O157** a pathogenic serotype causing colitis, which may give rise to the complications of haemolytic uraemic syndrome or thrombocytopenic purpura.

Esmarch's bandage (ess-marks) *n.* a rubber or elastic bandage that is wound tightly around a limb in order to force blood out from an area in which an operation is to be performed in a blood-free field. [J. F. A. von Esmarch (1823–1908), German surgeon]

esotropia (ess-oh-**troh**-piă) *n.* convergent squint (*see* strabismus).

espundia (mucocutaneous leishmaniasis) (ess-**puun**-diă) *n.* a disease of the skin and mucous membranes caused by the parasitic protozoan *Leishmania braziliensis* (*see* leishmaniasis), occurring in South and Central America.

ESR (erythrocyte sedimentation rate) *n.* the rate at which red blood cells (erythrocytes) settle out of suspension in blood plasma, measured under standardized conditions. The ESR increases in rheumatic diseases, chronic infections, and malignant disease, and thus provides a valuable screening test for these conditions.

ESRF *n. see* end-stage renal failure.

essence (ess-ĕns) *n.* a solution consisting of an essential oil dissolved in alcohol.

essential (i-**sen**-shăl) *adj.* describing a disorder that is not apparently attributable to an outside cause.

essential amino acid *n.* an amino acid that is essential for normal growth and development but cannot be synthesized by the body and must therefore be obtained from protein in the diet. *See* amino acid.

essential fatty acids (omega fatty acids) *n.* two groups of polyunsaturated fatty acids that are essential for health but cannot be synthesized by the body. **Alpha-linolenic acid** (**ALA**) is the precursor for omega-3 (n-3) fatty acids. Good sources include walnuts, almonds, and pumpkin and flax seeds. **Linoleic acid** is the precursor for the omega-6 (n-6) fatty acids. Good sources include vegetable oils.

essential oil *n.* a volatile oil derived from an aromatic plant. Essential oils are used in various pharmaceutical preparations. *See also* aromatherapy.

essential skills clusters (**ESC**) *pl. n.* five groups of skills, knowledge, and professional behaviour that are identified as essential by the Nursing and Midwifery Council (NMC) for safe and effective nursing practice at the point of registration. See Appendix 9: Essential skills clusters.

ESV *n. see* end-systolic volume.

ESWL *n.* extracorporeal shockwave lithotripsy. *See* lithotripsy.

ET *adj. see* endotracheal.

etanercept (i-**tan**-er-sept) *n.* a disease-modifying antirheumatic drug that is administered by subcutaneous injection in the treatment of severe rheumatoid, juvenile, and psoriatic arthritis and severe psoriasis and ankylosing spondylitis that have not responded to other treatments. Trade name: **Enbrel**.

ethambutol (eth-**am**-bew-tol) *n.* a drug administered by mouth in the treatment of tuberculosis, in conjunction with other drugs.

ethanol (ethyl alcohol) (eth-ă-nol) *n. see* alcohol.

ether (ee-ther) *n.* a volatile liquid formerly used as an anaesthetic administered by inhalation.

ethics (eth-iks) *n.* the principles, values, virtues, or rules of conduct governing correct behaviour, which in the nursing profession includes behaviour towards patients and their families, visitors, and colleagues.

SEE WEB LINKS

- Website of the International Care Ethics Observatory

ethics committee *n.* a group including lay people, health-care practitioners, and other experts set up to review health care. **clinical e. c.** an ethics committee that deals with ethical issues in clinical practice other than those relating to research. **research e. c.** an ethics committee that reviews research involving the use of human subjects, including clinical trials of drugs.

ethinylestradiol (eth-i-nyl-ee-stră-**dy**-ol) *n.* a synthetic female sex hormone (*see* oestrogen) mainly used (in combination with a progestogen) in oral contraceptives.

ethmoid bone (eth-moid) *n.* a bone in the floor of the cranium that contributes to the nasal cavity and orbits. The part of the ethmoid forming the roof of the nasal cavity (the **cribriform plate**) is pierced with many small holes through which the olfactory nerves pass. *See also* nasal (concha), skull.

ethnology (eth-**nol**-ŏji) *n.* the comparative study of human racial, cultural, and religious groups, concerned mainly with differences between groups and how these are reflected in people's behaviour and attitudes.

ethosuximide (eth-oh-**suks**-i-myd) *n.* an anticonvulsant drug administered by mouth mainly to control absence seizures. Trade names: **Emeside**, **Zarontin**.

ethyl chloride (chloroethane) *n.* a volatile liquid used chiefly as a local anaesthetic applied topically to the skin before minor surgery. Formula: C_2H_5Cl.

etic (et-ik) *adj.* describing the view of a culture from the perspective of those outside it, based on cross-cultural generalizations. *Compare* emic.

etidronate (et-i-**droh**-nayt) *n. see* bisphosphonates.

etiology (ee-ti-**ol**-ŏji) *n. see* aetiology.

etoposide (e-**top**-oh-syd) *n.* a cytotoxic drug derived from an extract of the mandrake plant. It is administered intravenously or by mouth, primarily in the treatment of bronchial carcinoma, lymphomas, and testicular tumours. Trade names: **Etopophos**, **Vepesid**.

eu- *prefix denoting* **1.** good, well, or easy. **2.** normal.

EUA *n.* examination under anaesthetic.

eucalyptol (yoo-kă-**lip**-tol) *n.* a volatile oil that has a mild irritant effect on the mucous membranes of the mouth and digestive system. It is taken as pastilles or inhaled as vapour to relieve catarrh.

eugenics (yoo-**jen**-iks) *n.* the alleged science concerned with the improvement of the human race by means of the principles of genetics. —**eugenic** *adj.*

euglycaemia (yoo-gly-**see**-miă) *n.* *see* normoglycaemia.

eunuch (**yoo**-nŭk) *n.* a male who has undergone castration.

euphoria (yoo-**for**-iă) *n.* a state of cheerfulness and wellbeing. A morbid degree of euphoria is characteristic of mania and hypomania. *See also* ecstasy, elation.

euplastic (yoo-**plast**-ik) *adj.* describing a tissue that heals quickly after injury.

Eustachian tube (pharyngotympanic tube) (yoo-**stay**-shŏn) *n.* the tube that connects the middle ear to the pharynx. It allows the pressure on the inner side of the eardrum to remain equal to the external pressure. [B. Eustachio (1520–74), Italian anatomist]

euthanasia (yooth-ăn-**ay**-ziă) *n.* the act of deliberately taking life to relieve suffering. **involuntary (or compulsory) e.** termination of the life of a person (e.g. an infant) who cannot express his or her own wishes or has not given consent. **voluntary e.** euthanasia at the request of the patient, usually by the direct administration of drugs (as opposed to being provided with drugs in assisted suicide). Voluntary euthanasia is lawful in a number of European jurisdictions.

euthyroid (yoo-**th'y**-roid) *adj.* having a normally functioning thyroid gland. *Compare* hyperthyroidism, hypothyroidism. —**euthyroidism** *n.*

euthyroid sick syndrome (sick euthyroid syndrome) *n.* a syndrome in which the level of triiodothyronine is markedly reduced, thyroxine is slightly reduced, and thyroid-stimulating hormone is reduced or normal. It is commonly seen in nonthyroidal illness, due to altered metabolism and transport of the thyroid hormones.

evacuation (i-vak-yoo-**ay**-shŏn) *n.* removal of the contents of a cavity, especially the emptying of the bowels (defecation).

evacuator (i-**vak**-yoo-ay-ter) *n.* a device for sucking fluid out of a cavity. Evacuators may be used to empty the bladder of unwanted material during such operations as the removal of a calculus or transurethral prostatectomy.

evaluation (i-val-yoo-**ay**-shŏn) *n.* the final stage of the nursing process, in which the effects of nursing interventions are compared with the goals or objectives set in the care plan. *See* expected outcome.

eventration (ee-ven-**tray**-shŏn) *n.* **1.** protrusion of the intestines or omentum through the abdominal wall. **2.** abnormal elevation of part of the diaphragm due to congenital weakness.

eversion (i-**ver**-shŏn) *n.* a turning outward. **e. of the cervix** a condition in which the edges of the neck (cervix) of the uterus turn outward.

evidence-based practice (EBP) (ev-i-dĕns-bayst) *n.* the delivery of individualized health care on the basis of an awareness of the impact and strength of related evidence.

SEE WEB LINKS

- Website of the Centre for Evidence-Based Medicine, University of Oxford

evisceration (i-vis-er-ay-shŏn) *n.* **1.** (in surgery) the removal of the viscera. **2.** (in ophthalmology) an operation in which the contents of the eyeball are removed, the empty outer envelope (sclera) being left behind. *Compare* enucleation.

Ewing's tumour (Ewing's sarcoma) (yoo-ingz) *n.* a malignant bone tumour arising in the bone marrow. It usually affects the femur but is liable to spread to other bones and to the lung. It is most common in children and adolescents. [J. Ewing (1866–1943), US pathologist]

EWS *n. see* early warning system.

ex- (exo-) *prefix denoting* outside or outer.

exacerbation (eks-ass-er-**bay**-shŏn) *n.* an increase in the severity of a disorder, marked by an increase in the intensity of its symptoms and signs.

exanthem (exanthema) (eks-**anth**-ĕm) *n.* a rash or eruption, such as that occurring in measles. **e. subitum** *see* roseola (infantum). **—exanthematous** (eks-an-**th'em**-ătŭs) *adj.*

exchange transfusion (iks-**chaynj**) *n.* a technique for treating haemolytic disease in newborn infants. Blood is withdrawn from the baby (via the umbilical vein) and replaced by an equal amount of donor blood compatible with the mother's blood.

excimer laser (ek-sy-mer) *n. see* laser.

excise (ek-syz) *vb.* to cut out tissue, an organ, or a tumour from the body. **—excision** (ek-**si**-*zh*ŏn) *n.*

excitation (eks-i-**tay**-shŏn) *n.* (in neurophysiology) the triggering of a conducted impulse in the membrane of a muscle cell or nerve fibre.

exclusion diet (iks-**kloo**-*zh*ŏn) *n. see* elimination diet.

excoriation (iks-kor-i-**ay**-shŏn) *n.* the destruction and removal of the surface of the skin or the covering of an organ by scraping, the application of a chemical, or other means.

excrescence (iks-**kress**-ĕns) *n.* an abnormal outgrowth on the surface of the body, such as a wart.

excreta (iks-**kree**-tă) *n.* any waste material discharged from the body, especially faeces.

excretion (iks-**kree**-shŏn) *n.* the removal of the waste products of metabolism from the body, mainly through the action of the kidneys. Excretion also includes the loss of water, salts, etc. through the sweat glands, the loss of carbon dioxide and water vapour from the lungs, and the egestion of faeces.

executive dysfunction *n.* disruption of the cognitive processes that regulate, control, and manage other cognitive processes, leading to deficiencies in planning, abstract thinking, flexibility, and behavioural control. It can occur following stroke or brain injury, or in dementia.

exemestane (eks-i-**mess**-tayn) *n.* *see* aromatase inhibitor.

exenteration (eks-en-ter-**ay**-shŏn) *n.* (in ophthalmology) an operation in which all the contents of the eye socket (orbit) are removed, leaving only the bony walls intact.

exercise (**eks**-er-syz) *n.* any activity resulting in physical exertion that is intended to maintain physical fitness, to condition the body, or to correct a physical deformity. Exercises may be done actively by the person or passively by a therapist. **aerobic e.** an exercise intended to increase oxygen consumption (as in running) and to benefit the lungs and cardiovascular system. **isometric e.** an exercise in which the muscles contract but there is no movement; this is induced when a limb is made to push against something rigid and is designed to improve muscle tone. **isotonic e.** an exercise in which the muscles contract and there is movement, but the force remains the same; this improves joint mobility and muscle strength.

exfoliation (eks-foh-li-**ay**-shŏn) *n.* **1.** flaking off of the upper layers of the skin. **2.** separation of a surface epithelium from the underlying tissue. **3.** the natural shedding of primary teeth. **—exfoliative** *adj.*

exhalation (expiration) (eks-hă-**lay**-shŏn) *n.* the act of breathing air from the lungs out through the mouth and nose.

exhibitionism (eksi-**bish**-ŏn-izm) *n.* exposure of the genitals to another person, as a sexually deviant act. The word is often broadened to mean public flaunting of any quality of the individual.

exo- *prefix. see* ex-.

exocrine gland (**eks**-oh-kryn) *n.* a gland that discharges its secretion by means of a duct, which opens onto an epithelial surface. Examples of exocrine glands are the sebaceous and sweat glands. *See also* secretion.

exogenous (ek-**soj**-in-ŭs) *adj.* originating outside the body or part of the body: applied particularly to substances in the body that are derived from the diet rather than built up by the body's own processes of metabolism. *Compare* endogenous.

exomphalos (umbilical hernia) (ek-**som**-fă-lŭs) *n.* a congenital defect in which the abdominal wall fails to close during fetal development and peritoneum-covered bowel herniates through the umbilical cord.

exophthalmic goitre (Graves' disease) (eks-off-**thal**-mik) *n. see* thyrotoxicosis.

exophthalmos (eks-off-**thal**-mos) *n.* protrusion of the eyeballs in their sockets. This can result from injury or disease of the eyeball or socket but is most commonly associated with overactivity of the thyroid gland (*see* thyrotoxicosis). **—exophthalmic** *adj.*

exostosis (eks-os-**toh**-sis) *n.* a benign outgrowth of bone with a cap of cartilage, arising from the surface of a bone. It is a stalklike osteochondroma.

exotic (ig-**zot**-ik) *adj.* describing a disease occurring in a region of the world far from where it might be expected.

exotoxin (eks-oh-**toks**-in) *n.* a highly potent poison, often harmful to only a limited range of tissues, that is produced by a bacterial cell and secreted into its surrounding medium. Exotoxins are produced by the bacteria causing botulism, diphtheria, and tetanus. *Compare* endotoxin.

exotropia (eks-oh-**troh**-piă) *n.* divergent squint (*see* strabismus).

expected outcome (iks-**pekt**-id) *n.* a statement in the care plan of what the nursing intervention is intended to achieve, usually described in terms of the patient's expected behaviour. *See* behavioural objective.

expectorant (iks-**pek**-ter-ănt) *n.* a drug that enhances the expulsion of sputum from the air passages. *See* ipecacuanha, mucolytic.

expectoration (iks-pek-ter-**ay**-shŏn) *n.* the act of spitting out material brought into the mouth by coughing.

Experience of Caregiving Inventory (ECI) (iks-**peer**-i-ĕns) *n.* a tool used by mental health nurses and others to assess the burden of caring and the coping skills among members of a dependent's family.

experiential learning (iks-peer-i-**en**-shăl) *n.* learning by experiencing a situation or a simulated situation, as in role playing, and then reflecting on that experience.

experimental method (iks-pe-ri-**men**-t'l) *n.* a research method used to test a hypothesis by seeking to establish a causal relationship between dependent and independent variables (*see* variable). It involves manipulation of the independent variable, while trying to keep all other variables constant.

expiration (eks-per-**ay**-shŏn) *n.* **1.** the act of breathing out air from the lungs: exhalation. **2.** dying.

explant (**eks**-plahnt) **1.** *n.* live tissue transferred from the body (or any organism) to a suitable artificial medium for culture. **2.** *vb.* to transfer live tissue for culture outside the body. **—explantation** *n.*

exploration (eks-plŏ-**ray**-shŏn) *n.* (in surgery) an investigative operation on a wound, tissue, or cavity to determine the cause of symptoms. **—exploratory** (iks-**plo**-ră-ter-i) *adj.*

exposure (iks-**poh**-zher) *n.* (in behaviour therapy] a method of treating fears and phobias that involves confronting the individual with the feared object or situation, either gradually (*see* desensitization, graded self-exposure) or suddenly (*see* flooding).

expression (iks-**presh**-ŏn) *n.* **1.** the appearance of the face, reflecting the individual's physical or emotional state. **2.** expulsion by pressing or squeezing, as of milk from the breast after pregnancy or the fetus or placenta from the uterus at childbirth.

expressive aphasia (iks-**pres**-iv) *n. see* aphasia.

expulsive haemorrhage (eks-**pul**-siv) *n.* sudden bleeding from the choroid of the eye, usually during a surgical procedure or trauma. This may force the ocular tissue out of the wound and is potentially one of the most devastating intraoperative complications of ocular surgery.

exsanguination (iks-sang-win-**ay**-shŏn) *n.* **1.** depriving the body of blood; for example, as a result of an accident causing severe bleeding. **2.** a technique for providing a bloodless field to facilitate certain operative procedures. **3.** the removal of blood from a part (usually a limb) before stopping the inflow of blood (by tourniquet). **—exsanguinate** *vb.*

exsufflation (eks-suf-lay-shŏn) *n.* the forcible removal of secretions from the air passages by some form of suction apparatus.

extended role (enhanced role) (iks-ten-did) *n.* (of the nurse) activities concerned with patients, either in hospital or the community, that are appropriate for delegation by doctors to nurses. Agreement on the delegated responsibilities is reached locally by consultation between medical and nursing professions.

extension (iks-ten-shŏn) *n.* **1.** the act of extending or stretching, especially the muscular movement by which a limb is straightened. **2.** the application of traction to a fractured or dislocated limb in order to restore it to its normal position.

extensor (iks-ten-ser) *n.* any muscle that causes the straightening of a limb or other part.

exteriorization (iks-teer-i-er-I-zay-shŏn) *n.* a surgical procedure in which an organ is brought from its normal site to the surface of the body, as in colostomy.

external beam radiotherapy *n.* *see* teletherapy.

exteroceptor (eks-ter-oh-sep-ter) *n.* a sensory nerve, ending in the skin or a mucous membrane, that is responsive to stimuli from outside the body. *See also* chemoreceptor, receptor.

extinction (iks-tink-shŏn) *n.* (in psychology) the weakening of a conditioned reflex that takes place if it is not maintained by reinforcement.

extirpation (eks-ter-pay-shŏn) *n.* the complete surgical removal of tissue, an organ, or a growth.

extra- *prefix denoting* outside or beyond.

extracapsular (eks-tră-kaps-yoo-ler) *adj.* outside or not involving a capsule. **e. extraction** surgical removal of a cataract in which the capsule of the lens is left behind. **e. fracture** a fracture, especially of the hip, that does not involve the joint capsule.

extracellular (eks-tră-sel-yoo-ler) *adj.* situated or occurring outside cells. e. fluid (**ECF**) the fluid surrounding cells.

extracorporeal (eks-tră-kor-por-iăl) *adj.* situated or occurring outside the body. **e. circulation** the circulation of the blood outside the body, as through a heart-lung machine or haemodialysis. **e. membrane oxygenation (ECMO)** a rescue treatment for otherwise fatal respiratory failure in newborn babies or infants due to prematurity or overwhelming septicaemia. It involves prolonged cardiopulmonary bypass to support gas exchange.

extract (eks-trakt) *n.* a preparation containing the pharmacologically active principles of a drug, made by evaporating a solution of the drug in water, alcohol, or ether.

extraction (iks-**trak**-shŏn) *n.* **1.** the surgical removal of a part of the body. Extraction of teeth is usually achieved by applying elevators and extraction forceps to the crown or root of the tooth to dislocate it from its socket. **2.** the act of pulling out a baby from the body of its mother during childbirth.

extradural (eks-tră-**dewr**-ăl) *adj. see* epidural.

extraembryonic membranes (eks-tră-em-bree-**on**-ik) *pl. n.* the membranous structures that surround the embryo and contribute to the placenta and umbilical cord. They include the amnion, chorion, allantois, and yolk sac.

extrapleural (eks-tră-**ploor**-ăl) *adj.* relating to the tissues of the chest wall outside the parietal pleura.

extrapyramidal effects (extrapyramidal side-effects, EPS) (eks-tră-pi-**ram**-i-d'l) *pl. n.* symptoms caused by a reduction of dopamine activity in the extrapyramidal system due to the adverse effects of dopamine receptor antagonists, notably phenothiazine antipsychotic drugs. These effects include parkinsonism, akathisia, and dyskinesia.

extrapyramidal system *n.* the system of nerve tracts and pathways connecting the cerebral cortex, basal ganglia, thalamus, cerebellum, reticular formation, and spinal neurons in complex circuits not included in the pyramidal system. The extrapyramidal system is mainly concerned with the regulation of stereotyped reflex muscular movements.

extrasystole (eks-tră-**sis**-tŏ-li) *n. see* ectopic beat.

extrauterine (eks-tră-**yoo**-teryn) *adj.* outside the uterus.

extravasation (iks-trav-ă-**say**-shŏn) *n.* the leakage and spread of blood or fluid from vessels into the surrounding tissues, which follows injury, burns, inflammation, and allergy.

extraversion (eks-tră-**ver**-shŏn) *n. see* extroversion.

extrinsic factor (eks-**trin**-sik) *n.* an old name for vitamin B_{12}.

extrinsic muscle *n.* a muscle, such as any of those controlling movements of the eyeball, that has its origin some distance from the part it acts on.

extroversion (eks-trŏ-**ver**-shŏn) *n.* **1. (extraversion)** an enduring personality trait characterized by interest in the outside world rather than the self. People high in extroversion (**extroverts**) are gregarious and outgoing, prefer to change activities frequently, and are not susceptible to permanent conditioning. *Compare* introversion. **2.** a turning inside out of a hollow organ, such as the uterus (which sometimes occurs after childbirth).

extrovert (**eks**-trŏ-vert) *n. see* extroversion.

exudation (eks-yoo-**day**-shŏn) *n.* the slow escape of liquid (the **exudate**) that is rich in proteins and contains white cells through the walls of intact blood vessels, usually as a result of inflammation.

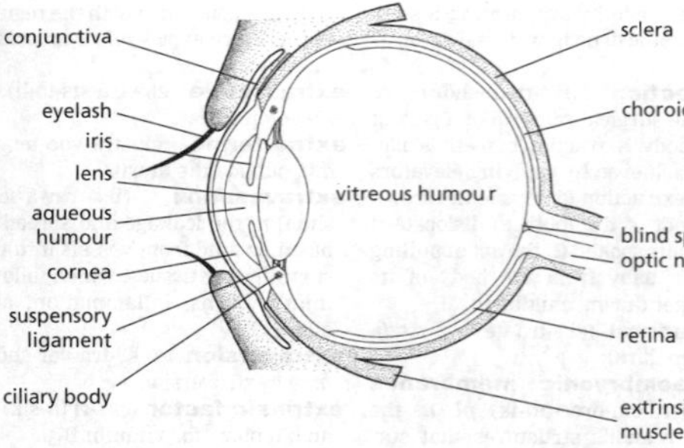

The eye (sagittal section)

Exudation is a normal part of the body's defence mechanisms.

eye (I) *n.* the organ of sight: a three-layered roughly spherical structure specialized for receiving and responding to light (see illustration). Light enters the eye through the cornea, which refracts it through the aqueous humour onto the lens. By accommodation light is focused through the vitreous humour onto the retina. Here light-sensitive cells (*see* cone, rod) send nerve impulses to the brain via the optic nerve.

eyeball (I-bawl) *n.* the body of the eye, which is roughly spherical, is bounded by the sclera, and lies in the orbit. Its movements are controlled by three pairs of extrinsic eye muscles.

eyelid (I-lid) *n.* the protective covering of the eye. Each eye has two eyelids consisting of skin, muscle, connective tissue (**tarsus**), and sebaceous glands (**meibomian** or **tarsal glands**). Each eyelid is lined with membrane (*see* conjunctiva) and fringed with eyelashes. Anatomical names: **blepharon**, **palpebra**.

eyestrain (I-strayn) *n.* a sense of fatigue brought on by use of the eyes for prolonged close work or in persons who have an uncorrected error of refraction. Symptoms are usually aching or burning of the eyes, accompanied by headache. Medical name: **asthenopia**.

eye tooth *n. see* canine.

Ff

F 1. *symbol for* Fahrenheit. **2.** *symbol for* farad.

face lift (fays-lift) *n.* plastic surgery designed to correct sagging facial tissues. Eyelid drooping can be corrected at the same procedure.

facet (fas-it) *n.* a small flat surface on a bone, especially a surface of articulation.

facet syndrome *n.* a syndrome caused by dislocation of the articulating surface of the vertebrae, resulting in pain and muscle spasm.

facial nerve (fay-shăl) *n.* the seventh cranial nerve (VII): a mixed sensory and motor nerve that supplies the muscles of facial expression, the taste buds of the front part of the tongue, the sublingual salivary glands, and the lacrimal glands.

-facient *suffix denoting* causing or making.

facies (fay-shi-eez) *n.* facial expression, often a guide to a patient's state of health as well as his emotions. **adenoid f.** a vacant look, with the mouth drooping open, seen in a patient with enlarged adenoids. **Hippocratic f.** the sallow face, sagging and with listless staring eyes, that indicates approaching death.

Factor IX (Christmas factor) *n.* a coagulation factor normally present in the blood. Deficiency of the factor results in haemophilia B.

Factor VIII (antihaemophilic factor, AHF) (fak-ter) *n.* a coagulation factor normally present in blood. Deficiency of the factor, which is inherited by males from their mothers, results in haemophilia A.

Factor V Leiden (ly-děn) *n.* an inherited mutation in the gene coding for coagulation Factor V, which results in an increased susceptibility to develop venous thrombosis.

Factor XI *n.* a coagulation factor normally present in blood. Deficiency of the factor is inherited, but rarely causes spontaneous bleeding. However, bleeding does occur after surgery or trauma to the blood vessels.

facultative (fak-ŭl-tă-tiv) *adj.* describing an organism, such as a parasite, that is not restricted to one way of life. *Compare* obligate.

faecalith (faecolith, coprolith) (fee-kă-lith) *n.* a hard mass of faeces in the colon, vermiform appendix, or rectum due to chronic constipation: a cause of inflammation.

faecal occult blood test (FOBT) *n.* a noninvasive test used to identify microscopic blood (*see* occult) in faeces. It is widely used as a screening test for colorectal cancer.

faeces (fee-seez) *n.* the waste material that is eliminated through the anus. It is formed in the colon and consists of a solid or semisolid mass of undigested food remains (chiefly cellulose) mixed with bile pigments (which are responsible for the colour), bacteria, various secretions (e.g. mucus), and some water. —**faecal** (fee-kăl) *adj.*

Fahrenheit temperature (fa-rĕn-hyt) *n.* temperature expressed on a scale in which the melting point of ice is assigned a temperature of 32° and the boiling point of water a temperature of 212°. The formula for converting from Fahrenheit (F) to Celsius (C) is: C = 5/9 (F − 32). *See also* Celsius temperature. [G. D. Fahrenheit (1686–1736), German physicist]

failure to thrive (FTT) (fayl-yer tŏ thryv) *n.* failure of an infant to grow satisfactorily compared with the average for that community. It is detected by regular measurements and plotting on centile charts. It can be the first indication of a serious underlying condition, such as kidney or heart disease or malabsorption, or it may result from problems at home, particularly nonaccidental injury.

fainting (faynt-ing) *n. see* syncope.

Fairbank's splint (fair-banks) *n.* a splint used for the correction of Erb's palsy in infants. It immobilizes the affected arm with the shoulder abducted and externally rotated, the elbow bent at 90°, and the forearm and wrist held in a supine position. [H. A. T. Fairbank (1876–1961), British orthopaedic surgeon]

falciform ligament (fal-si-form) *n.* a fold of peritoneum separating the right and left lobes of the liver and attaching it to the diaphragm and the anterior abdominal wall as far as the umbilicus.

Fallopian tube (oviduct, uterine tube) (fă-**loh**-piăn) *n.* either of a pair of tubes that conduct ova from the ovary to the uterus (*see* reproductive system). The ovarian end opens into the abdominal cavity via a funnel-shaped structure with fimbriae surrounding the opening. The ovum is fertilized near the ovarian end of the tube. [G. Fallopius (1523–63), Italian anatomist]

falloposcope (fă-**loh**-poh-skohp) *n.* a narrow flexible fibreoptic endoscope used to view the inner lining of the Fallopian tubes. —**falloposcopy** *n.*

Fallot's tetralogy (fal-**ohz**) *n. see* tetralogy of Fallot.

Falls Risk Assessment Tool (FRAT) (fawlz) *n.* a health-professional-directed or self-assessment tool that uses five key questions to identify the risk of falls: fall history, medication usage, balance, existence of Parkinson's disease or a previous cerebrovascular accident, and difficulty in rising from a chair. It enables assessment to be undertaken using a consistent approach and will act as a means of referral to appropriate specialist services.

false negative (fawls) *n.* a result of a diagnostic test or procedure that wrongly indicates the absence of a disease or other condition. *See* sensitivity.

false positive *n.* a result of a diagnostic test or procedure that wrongly indicates the presence of a disease or other condition. *See* sensitivity.

falx (falx cerebri) (falks) *n.* a sickle-shaped fold of the dura mater that dips inwards from the skull in the midline, between the cerebral hemispheres.

familial (fă-**mil**-iăl) *adj.* describing a condition or character that is found in some families but not in others. It is often inherited. **f. adenomatous polyposis** *see* polyposis.

family planning (fam-ili) *n.* **1.** the use of contraception to limit or space out the numbers of children born to a couple. **2.** provision of contraceptive methods within a community or nation.

SEE WEB LINKS

- Website of the Family Planning Association

family therapy *n.* a form of psychotherapy in which all family members are seen together in order to clarify and modify the ways they relate together.

famotidine (fam-**oh**-ti-deen) *n.* an H_2-receptor antagonist (*see* antihistamine) used for the treatment of gastric and duodenal ulcers and reflux oesophagitis. It is administered by mouth.

Fanconi's anaemia (fan-**koh**-niz) *n.* an autosomal recessive disorder characterized by severe aplastic anaemia and an increased predisposition to malignancy. It also causes learning disability, poor growth, skeletal abnormalities, and kidneys of an unusual shape or in an unusual position. [G. Fanconi (1892–1979), Swiss paediatrician]

Fanconi syndrome *n.* a disorder of the proximal kidney tubules, which may be inherited or acquired and is most common in children. It is characterized by the urinary excretion of large amounts of amino acids, glucose, and phosphates. Symptoms may include osteomalacia, rickets, muscle weakness, and cystinosis. [G. Fanconi]

fantasy (fan-tă-si) *n.* a complex sequence of imagination in which several imaginary elements are woven together into a story. An excessive preoccupation with one's fantasies may be symptomatic of a difficulty in coping with reality or part of a narcissistic personality disorder.

farad (fa-răd) *n.* the SI unit of capacitance, equal to the capacitance of a capacitor between the plates of which a potential difference of 1 volt appears when it is charged with 1 coulomb of electricity. Symbol: F.

faradism (fa-ră-dizm) *n.* the use of induced rapidly alternating electric currents to stimulate nerve and muscle activity. *See also* electrotherapy.

farcy (far-si) *n. see* glanders.

farinaceous (fa-ri-**nay**-shŭs) *adj.* starchy; describing foods rich in starch (e.g. flour, bread, cereals) or diets based on these foods.

farmer's lung (far-merz) *n.* an occupational lung disease caused by allergy to fungal spores that grow in inadequately dried stored hay, straw, or grain, which then becomes mouldy. An acute reversible form can develop a few hours after exposure; a chronic form, with the gradual development of irreversible breathlessness, occurs with or without preceding acute attacks.

FAS *n. see* fetal alcohol syndrome.

fascia (fash-iă) *n.* (*pl.* **fasciae**) connective tissue that envelops organs and tissues, forms sheaths for muscles, and is found immediately beneath the skin.

fasciculation (fă-sik-yoo-**lay**-shŏn) *n.* brief spontaneous contraction of a few muscle fibres, which is seen as a flicker of movement under the skin. It is most often associated with disease of the lower motor neurons (e.g. motor neuron disease).

fasciculus (fascicle) (fă-**sik**-yoo-lŭs) *n.* a bundle, e.g. of nerve or muscle fibres.

fasciitis (fash-i-**I**-tis) *n.* inflammation of fascia. It may result from bacterial infection or from a rheumatic disease, such as reactive arthritis or ankylosing spondylitis. *See* necrotizing fasciitis, plantar (fasciitis).

Fasciola (fas-i-**oh**-lă) *n.* a genus of flukes. **F. hepatica** the liver fluke, which normally lives as a parasite of sheep and other herbivorous animals but sometimes infects humans (*see* fascioliasis).

fascioliasis (fas-i-oh-**ly**-ă-sis) *n.* an infestation of the bile ducts and liver with the liver fluke, *Fasciola hepatica*. Symptoms include fever, dyspepsia, vomiting, loss of appetite, abdominal pain, and coughing; the liver may also be extensively damaged.

fastigium (fas-**tij**-iŭm) *n.* **1.** the period during which a fever or disease is fully developed. **2.** the highest point in the roof of the fourth ventricle of the brain.

fat (neutral fat) (fat) *n.* a substance that consists chiefly of triglycerides and is the principal form in which energy is stored by the body (*see* adipose tissue). It also serves as an insulating material beneath the skin and around certain organs. *See also* brown fat, fatty acid, lipid.

fatal familial insomnia (**fay**-t'l) *n.* an autosomal dominant disorder due to a mutation in the gene for the prion protein (PrP): it is an example of a spongiform encephalopathy. Patients present with intractable progressive insomnia, disturbances of the autonomic nervous system, and eventually dementia.

fatigue (fă-**teeg**) *n.* **1.** mental or physical tiredness, following prolonged or intense activity. Muscle fatigue may be due to the waste products of metabolism accumulating in the muscles faster than they can be removed by the venous blood. **2.** the inability of an organism, an organ, or a tissue to give a normal response to a stimulus until a certain recovery period has elapsed.

fatty acid (**fat**-i) *n.* an organic acid such as oleic acid or stearic acid. Fatty acids are the fundamental constituents of many important lipids, including triglycerides. Some fatty acids can be synthesized by the body; others (*see* essential fatty acid) must be obtained from the diet. **saturated f. a.** a fatty acid that cannot undergo reactions with other molecules, occurring mainly in animal and dairy products and associated with high serum cholesterol levels. **unsaturated f. a.** a fatty acid that can undergo reactions with other molecules, occurring in fish and plant-derived products and associated with low serum cholesterol levels. *See also* fat.

fatty degeneration *n.* deterioration in the health of a tissue due to the deposition of abnormally large amounts of fat in its cells. It may be caused by incorrect diet, excessive alcohol consumption, or a shortage of oxygen in the tissues.

fauces (faw-seez) *n.* the opening leading from the mouth into the pharynx. It is surrounded by the **glossopalatine arch** (which forms the anterior pillars of the fauces) and the **pharyngopalatine arch** (the posterior pillars).

favism (fay-vizm) *n.* an inherited defect in the enzyme glucose-6-phosphate dehydrogenase causing the red blood cells to become sensitive to a chemical in fava (broad) beans. Eating these beans results in destruction of red blood cells (haemolysis), which may lead to severe anaemia, requiring blood transfusion. Favism occurs most commonly in the Mediterranean and Middle East. *See also* glucose-6-phosphate dehydrogenase deficiency.

FBC *n.* *see* (full) blood count.

FBS *n.* *see* (fasting) blood sugar.

fear (feer) *n.* an emotional state evoked by threat of danger. It is usually characterized by unpleasant subjective experiences; physiological changes, such as increased heart rate and sweating; and behavioural changes, such as avoidance of fear-producing objects or situations. *See also* phobia.

Fear Questionnaire (FQ) *n.* a 16-item questionnaire used to assess anxiety utilizing a Likert scale. It can be self-administered.

febricula (fi-**brik**-yoo-lă) *n.* a fever of low intensity or short duration.

febrifuge (**feb**-ri-fewj) *n.* a treatment or drug that reduces or prevents fever. *See* antipyretic.

febrile (**fee**-bryl) *adj.* relating to or affected with fever.

feedback (**feed**-bak) *n.* the coupling of the output of a process to the input. Feedback mechanisms are important in regulating many physiological processes; for example, the output of hormones and neurotransmitters. **negative f.** a mechanism in which high levels of a substance (e.g. a circulating hormone) inhibit a further increase in its production (e.g. by reducing production of its releasing factors). **positive f.** a mechanism in which a rise in the output of a substance is associated with an increase in the output of another substance.

Fehling's test (fay-lingz) *n.* a test used for detecting the presence of sugar in urine; it has now been replaced by better and easier methods. [H. von Fehling (1812–85), German chemist]

Felty's syndrome (fel-tiz) *n.* enlargement of the spleen (*see* hypersplenism) associated with rheumatoid arthritis, characterized by a decrease in the numbers of white blood cells and frequent infections. [A. R. Felty (1895–1964), US physician]

female genital mutilation (female circumcision) *n.* removal of the clitoris, labia minora, and labia majora for cultural reasons. The anatomically least damaging form is **clitoridectomy** (removal of the clitoris); the most extensive, **infibulation**, also involves excision of the labia minora and labia majora. The vulval lips are sutured together, leaving a small passage for urine and menstrual fluid, meaning that episiotomy is usually required to allow delivery of a child. FGM removes most of the possibility of sexual pleasure for a woman, is unethical, and in children is a form of child abuse: it is prohibited under the Female Genital Mutilation Act 2003.

feminization (fem-i-ny-zay-shŏn) *n.* the development of female secondary sexual characteristics (enlargement of the breasts, loss of facial hair, and fat beneath the skin) in the male, either as a result of an endocrine disorder or of hormone therapy.

femoral (fem-er-ăl) *adj.* of or relating to the thigh or to the femur. **f. artery** an artery arising from the external iliac artery. It runs down the front medial aspect of the thigh, passing into the back of the thigh two-thirds of the way down. **f. epiphysis** the growth area of the upper end of the femur; partial dislocation leads to deformity of the head of the bone and premature degeneration of the hip joint. **f. neck** the narrowed end of the femur, which carries the head: the commonest site of fracture of the leg in elderly women. **f. nerve** the nerve that supplies the quadriceps muscle at the front of the thigh and receives sensation from the front and inner sides of the thigh. **f. triangle** (**Scarpa's triangle**) a triangular depression on the inner side of the thigh bounded by the sartorius and adductor longus muscles and the inguinal ligament. The pulse can be felt here as the femoral artery lies over the depression.

femur (thigh bone) (fee-mer) *n.* a long bone between the hip and the knee. The head of the femur articulates with the acetabulum of the hip bone; the lower end articulates with the tibia.

fenestra (fi-nes-tră) *n.* (in anatomy) an opening resembling a window. **f. ovalis** (**f. vestibuli**) the opening between the middle ear and the vestibule of the inner ear. **f. rotunda** (**f. cochleae**) the opening between the scala tympani of the cochlea and the middle ear.

fenestration (fen-i-stray-shŏn) *n.* a surgical operation in which a new opening is formed in the bony labyrinth of the inner ear as part of the treatment of deafness due to otosclerosis. It is now rarely performed, having been superseded by stapedectomy.

fenofibrate (fen-oh-**fy**-brayt) *n.* a drug used for treating hyperlipidaemia (*see* fibrate). It is administered by mouth. Trade names: **Lipantril**, **Supralip**.

fenoprofen (fen-oh-**proh**-fĕn) *n.* an analgesic drug that also reduces inflammation (*see* NSAID) and is administered by mouth to treat arthritic conditions and pain. Trade name: **Fenopron**.

fentanyl (**fen**-tă-nyl) *n.* a potent opioid analgesic (*see* opiate) used for the relief of severe pain and for pain relief during surgery. It is administered by mouth, nasal spray, in skin patches, or intravenously. Trade names: **Abstral**, **Actiq**, **Durogesic DTrans**, **Effentora**, **Instanyl**, **PecFent**, **Sublimaze**.

fermentation (fer-men-**tay**-shŏn) *n.* the biochemical process by which organic substances, particularly carbohydrates, are decomposed by the action of enzymes to provide chemical energy, as in the production of alcohol.

ferning (**fern**-ing) *n.* the appearance of a fernlike pattern in a dried specimen of cervical mucus, an indication of the presence of oestrogen, usually seen at the midpoint of the menstrual cycle. It can be helpful in the determination of ovulation. The same phenomenon occurs with premature rupture of the membranes.

ferri- (ferro-) *combining form denoting* iron.

ferrous sulphate (**fe**-rŭs) *n.* an iron salt administered by mouth to treat or prevent iron-deficiency anaemia. Similar preparations used to treat anaemia include **ferrous fumarate** and **ferrous gluconate**.

fertility rate (fer-**til**-iti) *n.* the number of live births occurring in a year per 1000 women of child bearing age (usually 15 to 44 years of age).

fertilization (fer-ti-ly-**zay**-shŏn) *n.* the fusion of a spermatozoon and an ovum to form a zygote.

FESS *n. see* functional endoscopic sinus surgery.

fester (**fes**-ter) *vb.* (of superficial wounds) to become inflamed, with the formation of pus.

festination (fes-ti-**nay**-shŏn) *n.* short tottering steps that become more rapid due to loss of postural reflexes and stooped posture: seen in patients with Parkinsonism.

fetal alcohol spectrum disorder (FASD, fetal alcohol syndrome, FAS) (**fee**-t'l) *n.* a condition of newborn babies caused by maternal over consumption of alcohol during pregnancy. Babies have a low birth weight and growth is retarded. They have a small head, facial abnormalities, and disturbances of behaviour and intellect.

fetal growth chart *n.* a graph, customized to a pregnant woman's height, weight, and other factors, that plots fundal height and estimated fetal weight on ultrasound against weeks of gestation. The graph, which shows centile lines (*see* centile chart), improves prediction of a baby who is small for gestational age.

fetal growth restriction *n. see* intrauterine (growth restriction).

fetal scalp electrode *n.* an electrical wire attached to the fetal scalp for direct measurement of fetal heart rate by electrical activity.

feticide (fee-ti-syd) *n.* the destruction of a fetus in the uterus by injection of potassium chloride into the fetal heart, usually to achieve a late-stage termination of pregnancy.

fetishism (fet-i-shizm) *n.* sexual attraction to an inappropriate object (known as a **fetish**). This may be a part of the body, clothing, or other objects (e.g. leather handbags or rubber sheets). Treatment can involve psychotherapy or behaviour therapy. *See also* sexual deviation.

feto- *combining form denoting* a fetus.

fetor (foetor) (fee-ter) *n.* an unpleasant smell. **f. oris** bad breath (*see* halitosis), which is most commonly caused by poor oral hygiene.

fetoscopy (fi-tos-kŏpi) *n.* direct visualization of a fetus by passing a special fibreoptic endoscope (a **fetoscope**) through the abdomen of a pregnant woman into the amniotic cavity. It is used to facilitate minimally invasive surgery on the fetus and placenta.

fetus (foetus) (fee-tŭs) *n.* a mammalian embryo during the later stages of development within the uterus; in humans it is an unborn child from its eighth week of development. **f. papyraceous** a twin fetus that has died in the uterus and become flattened and mummified. **—fetal** *adj.*

FEV *n.* *see* forced expiratory volume.

fever (pyrexia) (fee-ver) *n.* a rise in body temperature above the normal, i.e. above an oral temperature of 98.6° F (37° C) or a rectal temperature of 99° F (37.2° C), usually caused by bacterial or viral infection. Fever is generally accompanied by shivering, headache, nausea, constipation, or diarrhoea. **intermittent f.** a periodic rise and fall in body temperature, as in malaria. **remittent f.** a fever in which body temperature fluctuates but does not return to normal. *See also* relapsing fever.

FFP *n.* fresh frozen plasma.

fibr- (fibro-) *combining form denoting* fibres or fibrous tissue.

fibrate (fy-brayt) *n.* any of a class of drugs that reduce concentrations of triglycerides and possibly of low-density lipoproteins in the blood; they also tend to raise the levels of the beneficial high-density lipoproteins. Fibrates are used for treating hyperlipidaemia. *See* bezafibrate, ciprofibrate, fenofibrate, gemfibrozil.

fibre (fy-ber) *n.* **1.** (in anatomy) a threadlike structure, such as a muscle cell, a nerve fibre, or a collagen fibre. **2.** (in dietetics) *see* dietary fibre. **—fibrous** (fy-brŭs) *adj.*

fibre optics *n.* the use of fibres for the transmission of light images. Synthetic fibres with special optical properties can be used in instruments to relay pictures of the inside of the body for direct observation or photography. *See* fibrescope. **—fibreoptic** *adj.*

fibrescope (fy-ber-skohp) *n.* an endoscope that uses fibre optics for the transmission of images from the interior of the body. Being flexible, fibrescopes can be introduced into relatively inaccessible cavities of the body.

fibril (fy-bril) *n.* a very small fibre or a constituent thread of a fibre. —**fibrillar, fibrillary** *adj.*

fibrillation (fy-bril-ay-shŏn) *n.* chaotic electrical and mechanical activity of a heart chamber, which results in loss of synchronous contraction. The affected part of the heart then ceases to pump blood. **atrial f. (AF)** a common type of arrhythmia that results in a rapid and irregular pulse rate. The main causes are atherosclerosis, chronic rheumatic heart disease, and hypertensive heart disease. **ventricular f. (VF)** fibrillation that causes the ventricles to stop beating (*see* cardiac arrest). It is most commonly the result of myocardial infarction.

fibrin (fib-rin) *n.* the final product of the process of blood coagulation, produced by the action of the enzyme thrombin on a soluble precursor fibrinogen. Fibrin molecules link together to give a fibrous meshwork that forms the basis of a blood clot.

fibrinogen (fi-**brin**-ŏ-jĕn) *n.* a substance (*see* coagulation factors), present in blood plasma, that is acted upon by the enzyme thrombin to produce the insoluble protein fibrin in the final stage of blood coagulation.

fibrinolysin (fib-ri-**nol**-i-sin) *n. see* plasmin.

fibrinolysis (fib-ri-**nol**-i-sis) *n.* the process by which blood clots are removed from the circulation, involving digestion of the insoluble protein fibrin by the enzyme plasmin.

fibrinolytic (fib-rin-ŏ-**lit**-ik) *adj.* describing a group of drugs that are capable of breaking down the protein fibrin, which is the main constituent of blood clots, and are therefore used to disperse blood clots (thrombi) that have formed within the circulation. They include streptokinase, alteplase, **reteplase** (Rapilysin), **tenecteplase** (Metalyse), and **urokinase** (Syner-KINASE).

fibroadenoma (fy-broh-ad-in-**oh**-ma) *n. see* adenoma.

fibroblast (**fy**-broh-blast) *n.* a widely distributed cell in connective tissue that is responsible for the production of both the ground substance and the precursors of collagen, elastic fibres, and reticular fibres.

fibrocartilage (fy-broh-**kar**-ti-lij) *n.* a tough kind of cartilage in which there are dense bundles of fibres in the matrix.

fibrochondritis (fy-broh-kon-**dry**-tis) *n.* an inflammation of fibrocartilage.

fibrocyst (**fy**-broh-sist) *n.* a benign tumour of fibrous connective tissue containing cystic spaces. —**fibrocystic** (fy-broh-**sis**-tik) *adj.*

fibrocystic disease of the pancreas *n. see* cystic fibrosis.

fibrocyte (**fy**-broh-syt) *n.* an inactive cell present in fully differentiated connective tissue. It is derived from a fibroblast.

fibroelastosis (fy-broh-ee-las-**toh**-sis) *n.* overgrowth or disturbed growth of the yellow (elastic) fibres in connective tissue. **endocardial f.** overgrowth and thickening of the inner layer of the heart's left ventricle.

fibroid (fy-broid) **1. (leiomyoma, uterine fibroid)** *n.* a benign tumour of fibrous and muscular tissue, one or more of which may develop within or attached to the outside of the uterus. Large fibroids often cause pain and excessive menstrual bleeding and may cause problems with fertility and childbirth. Fibroids may be treated medically (e.g. with gonadorelin analogues or, more recently, ulipristal), by laser coagulation (**laparoscopic myolysis**) or uterine artery embolization, or surgically (by myomectomy or hysterectomy). **2.** *adj.* resembling or containing fibres.

fibroma (fy-**broh**-mă) *n.* (*pl.* **fibromas** or **fibromata**) a nonmalignant tumour of connective tissue.

fibromyalgia (fy-broh-my-**al**-jiă) *n.* a disorder characterized by pain in the fibrous tissue components of muscles without any inflammation (*compare* fibromyositis). Widespread aching and stiffness with specific tender points are accompanied by extreme fatigue and often associated with headache and various other symptoms. Fibromyalgia is frequently triggered by anxiety, stress, sleep deprivation, and straining or overuse of muscles; it appears to be closely related to CFS/ME/PVF.

fibromyoma (fy-broh-my-**oh**-mă) *n. see* fibroid.

fibromyositis (fy-broh-my-oh-**sy**-tis) *n.* general inflammation of fibromuscular tissue.

fibroplasia (fy-broh-**play**-ziă) *n.* the production of fibrous tissue, which is part of the normal healing process. *See also* retinopathy (of prematurity), retrolental fibroplasia.

fibrosarcoma (fy-broh-sar-**koh**-mă) *n.* a malignant tumour of connective tissue, derived from fibroblasts. Fibrosarcomas may arise in soft tissue or bone; they can affect any organ but are most common in the limbs, particularly the leg.

fibrosis (fy-**broh**-sis) *n.* thickening and scarring of connective tissue, most often a consequence of inflammation or injury. **pulmonary interstitial f.** thickening and stiffening of the lining of the alveoli causing progressive breathlessness. *See also* cystic fibrosis, retroperitoneal fibrosis. **—fibrotic** *adj.*

fibrositis (fy-brŏ-**sy**-tis) *n.* inflammation of fibrous connective tissue, especially an acute inflammation of back muscles and their sheaths, causing pain and stiffness.

fibula (**fib**-yoo-lă) *n.* the long thin outer bone of the lower leg. The head of the fibula articulates with the tibia just below the knee; the lower end projects laterally and articulates with one side of the talus.

field of vision (feeld) *n. see* visual field.

fifth disease (fifth) *n. see* erythema (infectiosum).

FIGO staging *n.* a classification drawn up by the International Federation of Gynaecology and Obstetrics to define the extent of spread of gynaecological cancers.

filament (fil-ă-mĕnt) *n.* a very fine threadlike structure, such as a chain of bacterial cells. **—filamentous** (fil-ă-ment-ŭs) *adj.*

filaria (fil-air-iă) *n.* (*pl.* **filariae**) any of the long threadlike nematode worms that, as adults, are parasites of the connective and lymphatic tissues of humans and capable of causing disease. They include the genera *Brugia*, *Loa*, *Onchocerca*, and *Wuchereria*. *See also* microfilaria. **—filarial** *adj.*

filariasis (fil-er-I-ă-sis) *n.* a disease, common in the tropics and subtropics, caused by the presence in the lymph vessels of the filariae *Wuchereria bancrofti* and *Brugia malayi*. The lymph vessels eventually become blocked, causing the surrounding tissues to swell (*see* elephantiasis).

filiform (fil-i-form) *adj.* shaped like a thread. **f. papillae** threadlike papillae on the tongue.

filipuncture (fil-i-punk-cher) *n.* the insertion of a fine wire thread into an aneurysm in order to cause clotting of the blood within it.

filling (fil-ing) *n.* (in dentistry) the operation of inserting a specially prepared substance into a cavity drilled in a tooth, often in the treatment of dental caries.

filtration (fil-tray-shŏn) *n.* the passage of a liquid through a porous filter in order to separate the solids or suspended particles within it.

filum (fy-lŭm) *n.* a threadlike structure. **f. terminale** the slender tapering terminal section of the spinal cord.

fimbria (fim-briă) *n.* (*pl.* **fimbriae**) a fringe or fringelike process, such as any of the finger-like projections that surround the opening of the ovarian end of the Fallopian tube. **—fimbrial** (fim-bri-ăl) *adj.*

fimbrial cyst *n.* a simple cyst of the fimbria of the Fallopian tube.

finasteride (fin-ass-tĕ-ryd) *n.* a drug that causes shrinkage of the prostate gland and is used both to relieve the symptoms of urinary retention caused by an enlarged gland obstructing the outflow of urine from the bladder and to reduce the risk of urinary retention. Administered by mouth, it is also used to treat baldness in men. Trade names: **Propecia**, **Proscar**.

fingerprint (fing-er-print) *n.* the distinctive pattern of minute ridges in the outer horny layer of the skin. Every individual has a unique pattern of loops, whorls, or arches. *See also* dermatoglyphics.

first aid (ferst) *n.* procedures used in an emergency to help a wounded or ill patient before the arrival of a doctor or admission to hospital.

SEE WEB LINKS

- St John's Ambulance website

first intention *n. see* intention.

first-level nurse *n.* a registered nurse who has completed a three-year programme of education leading to a nursing qualification and an academic qualification (a degree or diploma). *See also* nurse.

first-line treatment *n.* therapy that is the first choice for treating a particular condition; other (second-line) treatments are used only if first-line therapy has failed.

first-pass metabolism *n.* a process in which a drug administered by mouth is absorbed from the gastrointestinal tract and transported via the portal vein to the liver, where it is metabolized. As a result, in some cases only a small proportion of the active drug reaches the systemic circulation and its intended target tissue. First-pass metabolism can be bypassed by giving the drug via sublingual or buccal routes.

fission (fish-ŏn) *n.* a method of asexual reproduction in which the body of a protozoan or bacterium splits into two equal parts (**binary f.**), as in the amoebae, or more than two equal parts (**multiple f.**).

fissure (fish-er) *n.* **1.** (in anatomy) a groove or cleft. **2.** (in pathology) a cleftlike defect in the skin or mucous membranes. **anal f.** a break in the skin lining the anal canal, usually as a consequence of constipation, causing pain during bowel movements and sometimes bleeding. **3.** (in dentistry) a naturally occurring groove in the enamel on the surface of a tooth, especially a molar. It is a common site of dental caries. .

fistula (fiss-tew-lă) *n.* (*pl.* **fistulae**) an abnormal communication between two hollow organs connecting two mucosa-lined surfaces or between a hollow organ and the exterior. Many fistulae are caused by infection or injury, but there are a number of other causes. **anal f.** a break or rent of the mucosa of the anal canal, which commonly presents with anal pain during and immediately after defecation and the passage of bright red blood in the stools. *See also* ischiorectal abscess. **arteriovenous f.** a surgically created connection between an artery and a vein, usually in a limb, to create arterial and venous access for haemodialysis. **biliary f.** a fistula that may develop as a complication of gall bladder surgery. **gastrocolic f.** a fistula between the colon and the stomach that may result from malignant growth or ulceration. **rectovaginal f.** an opening between the rectum and vagina that occurs as a congenital abnormality. **urogenital f.** a fistula between the urinary and genital tracts, which may be congenital or acquired (e.g. as a result of complications of childbirth). **vesicovaginal f.** an opening between the bladder and the vagina causing urinary incontinence. It may result from damage during surgery, radiation damage following radiotherapy for pelvic malignancy, or prolonged obstructed labour.

fit (fit) *n.* a sudden attack. The term is commonly used specifically for the seizures of epilepsy but it is also used more generally, e.g. a fit of coughing.

fixation (fiks-ay-shŏn) *n.* **1.** (in psychoanalysis) a failure of psychological development, in which traumatic events prevent a child from progressing to the next developmental stage. *See also* psychosexual development. **2.** a procedure for the hardening and preservation of tissues or micro-organisms to be examined under a microscope.

fixator (fiks-ay-ter) *n.* an apparatus used to immobilize a fracture. **external f.** a rigid frame that connects pins passed through the skin into the bone above and below a fracture. It is used particularly to treat some open fractures and also for limb lengthening.

flaccid (flak-sid) *adj.* **1.** flabby and lacking in firmness. **2.** characterized by a decrease in or absence of muscle tone (e.g. **f. paralysis**). **—flaccidity** (flak-**sid**-iti) *n.*

flagellate (**flaj**-ĕl-ayt) *n.* a type of protozoan with one or more flagella projecting from its body surface, by means of which it is able to swim. Some flagellates are parasites of humans. *See* giardiasis, Leishmania, Trichomonas, trypanosomiasis.

flagellum (flă-**jel**-ŭm) *n.* (*pl.* **flagella**) a fine long whiplike thread attached to certain types of cell (e.g. spermatozoa and flagellates). Flagella are responsible for the movement of the organisms to which they are attached.

flail chest (flayl) *n.* instability of a segment of the ribcage due to fracture of two or more ribs in two or more places, resulting from trauma. It is often associated with underlying lung trauma or pneumothorax.

flap (flap) *n.* (in surgery) a strip of tissue dissected away from the underlying structures but left attached at one end so that it retains its blood and nerve supply in a pedicle. The flap is then used to repair a defect in another part of the body by suturing its free end into the area. When the flap has healed into its new site, the other end can be detached.

flare (flair) *n.* **1.** reddening of the skin that spreads outwards from a focus of infection or irritation in the skin. **2.** the red area surrounding an urticarial weal.

flashback (**flash**-bak) *n.* **1.** vivid involuntary reliving of the perceptual abnormalities experienced during a previous episode of drug intoxication (most commonly with LSD), including hallucinations and derealization. **2.** the reliving of a traumatic experience that occurs as a symptom of post-traumatic stress disorder.

flat-foot (**flat**-fuut) *n.* absence or collapse of the arch along the instep of the foot, so that the sole lies flat upon the ground. Common in children under 6 years, flat-foot that persists into adulthood may be due to an underlying bony disorder. Medical name: **pes planus**.

flatulence (**flat**-yoo-lĕns) *n.* **1.** the expulsion of intestinal gas by belching or by emission from the anus. **2.** a sensation of abdominal distension. **—flatulent** *adj.*

flatus (**flay**-tŭs) *n.* intestinal gas passed through the rectum, composed partly of swallowed air and partly of gas produced by bacterial fermentation of intestinal contents.

flatworm (platyhelminth) (**flat**-werm) *n.* any of the flat-bodied worms, including the flukes and tapeworms. Both these groups contain many parasites of medical importance.

flav- (flavo-) *combining form denoting* yellow.

flea (flee) *n.* a small wingless blood-sucking insect with a laterally compressed body and long legs adapted for jumping. Adult fleas are temporary parasites on birds and mammals and those species that attack humans (*Pulex*, *Xenopsylla*, and *Nosopsyllus*) may be important in the transmission of various diseases. Their bites may become a focus of infection.

flecainide (flek-ay-nyd) *n.* a drug used to control irregular heart rhythms. It is administered by mouth or intravenous injection. Trade name: **Tambocor**.

flexibilitas cerea (fleks-i-**bil**-i-tas seer-iă) *n.* a feature of catatonic patients in which the limbs may be moved passively by another person into positions that are then retained for hours on end. *See* catatonia.

flexion (**flek**-shŏn) *n.* the bending of a joint so that the bones forming it are brought towards each other. **plantar f.** the bending of the toes (or fingers) downwards, towards the sole (or palm). *See also* dorsiflexion.

Flexner's bacillus (**fleks**-nerz) *n.* the bacterium *Shigella flexneri*, which causes a form of bacillary dysentery. [S. Flexner (1863–1946), US pathologist]

flexor (**fleks**-er) *n.* any muscle that causes bending of a limb or other part.

flexure (**flek**-sher) *n.* a bend in an organ or part, such as the **hepatic** and **splenic flexures** of the colon. **—flexural** *adj.*

flight of ideas (flyt) *n.* accelerated thinking that occurs in psychosis, mania, hypomania, and attention-deficit/hyperactivity disorder. Speech is rapid, moving from one topic to another and reflecting casual associations between ideas.

floaters (**floh**-terz) *pl. n.* opacities in the vitreous humour of the eye, which cast a shadow on the retina and are therefore seen as shapes or spots (**muscae volitantes**) against a bright background in good illumination.

floccillation (carphology) (flok-si-**lay**-shŏn) *n.* plucking at the bedclothes by a delirious patient. This is often a sign of extreme exhaustion and may be the prelude to death.

flocculation (flok-yoo-**lay**-shŏn) *n.* a reaction in which normally invisible material leaves solution to form a coarse suspension or precipitate. *See also* agglutination.

flooding (**flud**-ing) *n.* **1.** excessive bleeding from the uterus, as in menorrhagia or miscarriage. **2.** (in psychology) a method of treating phobias in which the patient is exposed intensively and at length to the feared object, either in reality or fantasy.

floppy baby syndrome (**flop**-i) *n. see* amyotonia congenita.

flowmeter (**floh**-mee-ter) *n.* an instrument for measuring the flow of a liquid or gas. **laser Doppler f.** an instrument for measuring blood flow through tissue (e.g. skin) utilizing a laser beam.

flucloxacillin (floo-kloks-ă-sil-in) *n.* a semisynthetic penicillin administered by mouth, injection, or intravenous infusion to treat infections caused by penicillinase-producing staphylococci. Trade names: **Floxapen**, **Fluclomix**, **Ladropen**.

fluconazole (floo-kon-ă-zohl) *n.* an antifungal drug used to treat candidiasis and other fungal infections. It is administered by mouth or intravenous infusion. Trade name: **Diflucan**.

fluctuation (fluk-tew-ay-shŏn) *n.* the characteristic feeling of a wave motion produced in a fluid-filled part of the body by an examiner's fingers. If fluctuation is present when a swelling is examined, this is an indication that there is fluid within.

flucytosine (floo-sy-toh-seen) *n.* an antifungal drug that is effective against systemic infections, including cryptococcosis and candidiasis. It is administered by intravenous infusion. Trade name: **Ancotil**.

fludrocortisone (floo-droh-kor-tiz-ohn) *n.* a synthetic mineralocorticoid (*see* corticosteroid) administered by mouth to treat adrenal disorders caused by deficient production of aldosterone. Trade name: **Florinef**.

fluid balance (floo-id) *n.* the state in which the amount of fluid in the body is such as to enable normal physiological functioning. The volume of fluid taken in and excreted over 24 hours should be equal, so that the overall volume of body fluid remains constant. Accurate measurement of these volumes is an essential diagnostic tool and enables rapid intervention to correct any imbalance. **f. b. chart** a chart providing information on a patient's state of hydration, renal function, and cardiovascular function. **negative f. b.** the state in which the amount of fluid lost from the body is greater than that gained (e.g. because the patient is vomiting and/or has diarrhoea). **positive f. b.** the state in which the volume of fluid taken into the body is greater than that lost (e.g. because of a heart or kidney disorder).

fluke (flook) *n.* any of the parasitic flatworms that belong to the group Trematoda. Adult flukes are parasites of humans, occurring in the liver (*see* Fasciola), lungs (*see* paragonimiasis), gut (*see* heterophyiasis), and blood vessels (*see* Schistosoma) and often cause serious disease.

flumazenil (floo-maz-i-nil) *n.* a benzodiazepine antagonist drug, used to reverse the effects of benzodiazepines given during anaesthesia. It is administered by intravenous injection or infusion. Trade name: **Anexate**.

flunisolide (floo-nis-oh-lyd) *n.* an anti-inflammatory corticosteroid drug used in the prevention and treatment of hay fever. It is administered as a nasal spray. Trade name: **Syntaris**.

fluocinolone (floo-ŏ-sin-oh-lohn) *n.* a synthetic corticosteroid used topically to reduce inflammation in skin conditions, including eczema and psoriasis. It is applied as a cream, gel, or ointment. Administered as an implant into the vitreous humour, it is used to treat oedema associated with diabetic retinopathy. Trade names: **Iluvien**, **Synalar**.

fluorescein sodium (floo-er-ess-i-in) *n.* a water-soluble orange dye that glows with a brilliant green colour when blue light is shone on it. A dilute solution is used to detect defects in the surface of the cornea, since it stains areas where the epithelium is not intact. *See* angiography.

fluorescence (floo-er-ess-ĕns) *n.* the emission of light by a material as it absorbs radiation from outside. The radiation absorbed may be visible or invisible (e.g. ultraviolet rays or X-rays). *See* fluoroscope. **—fluorescent** *adj.*

fluoridation (floo-er-id-ay-shŏn) *n.* the addition of fluoride to drinking water in order to reduce dental caries. Drinking water with a fluoride ion content of one part per million is effective in reducing caries throughout life when given during the years of tooth development. *See also* fluorosis.

fluoride (floo-eryd) *n.* a compound of fluorine. The incorporation of fluoride ions in the enamel of teeth makes them more resistant to dental caries. Fluoride may be applied through fluoridation or topically in toothpaste or by a dentist.

fluoroscope (floo-er-ŏ-skohp) *n.* historically, an instrument by which X-rays were projected through a patient onto a fluorescent screen enabling the resultant image to be viewed directly by the radiologist. However, as this resulted in high radiation doses for the radiologist, for diagnostic purposes the screen has been replaced by an image intensifier and TV monitor. **—fluoroscopy** (floo-er-os-kŏ-pi) *n.*

fluorosis (floo-er-oh-sis) *n.* the effects of high fluoride intake. When the level of fluoride in the water supply is above 2 parts per million the enamel of teeth becomes mottled. At above 8 parts per million, calcification of ligaments may occur. *See also* fluoridation.

fluorouracil (floo-er-oh-yoor-ă-sil) *n.* a drug that prevents cell growth (*see* antimetabolite) and is used in the treatment of solid tumours, such as cancers of the digestive system and breast; it is usually administered by intravenous infusion or injection. Fluorouracil is also applied as a cream to treat certain skin conditions, including skin cancer.

fluoxetine (floo-oks-i-teen) *n.* an antidepressant drug (*see* SSRI) administered by mouth to treat depression, bulimia nervosa, and obsessive–compulsive disorder. Trade name: **Prozac**.

flupentixol (flupenthixol) (floo-pen-tiks-ol) *n.* an antipsychotic drug used to treat schizophrenia and other psychoses and depression. It is administered by mouth or depot injection. Trade names: **Depixol**, **Fluanxol**.

fluphenazine (floo-**fen**-ă-zeen) *n.* a phenothiazine antipsychotic drug used for the treatment of schizophrenia and other psychotic disorders. It is administered by depot injection. Trade name: **Modecate**.

flurazepam (floor-**az**-ĕ-pam) *n.* a benzodiazepine drug administered by mouth to treat insomnia and sleep disturbances (*see* hypnotic). Trade name: **Dalmane**.

flurbiprofen (fler-**bip**-roh-fen) *n.* an analgesic that relieves inflammation (*see* NSAID), given by mouth in the treatment of such conditions as rheumatoid arthritis, osteoarthritis, and dysmenorrhoea and as eye drops to prevent contraction of the pupil during eye surgery. Trade name: **Ocufen**.

flutamide (**floo**-tă-myd) *n.* a nonsteroidal anti-androgen commonly used in the treatment of advanced prostate cancer, either alone or in combination with gonadorelin analogues. It is taken by mouth.

flutter (**flut**-er) *n.* a disturbance of normal heart rhythm, less rapid and less chaotic than fibrillation.

fluvastatin (floo-**vas**-tă-tin) *n.* a drug used to reduce abnormally high levels of cholesterol and other lipids in the blood (*see* statin). It is taken by mouth. Trade name: **Lescol**.

fluvoxamine (floo-**voks**-ă-meen) *n.* an antidepressant drug (*see* SSRI) taken by mouth to treat depression and obsessive–compulsive disorder. Trade name: **Faverin**.

flux (fluks) *n.* an abnormally copious flow from an organ or cavity.

fly (fly) *n.* a two-winged insect belonging to the order Diptera. The mouthparts of flies are adapted for sucking and sometimes also for piercing and biting. Fly larvae (maggots) may infest human tissues and cause disease (*see* myiasis).

foam dressing (fohm) *n.* a dressing for exuding wounds that is absorbent and nonadherent and can take the shape of the wound cavity.

FOBT *n. see* faecal occult blood test.

focal distance (**foh**-kăl) *n.* (of the eye) the distance between the lens and the point behind the lens at which light from a distant object is focused.

focus (**foh**-kŭs) **1.** *n.* the point at which rays of light converge after passing through a lens. **2.** *n.* the principal site of an infection or other disease. **3.** *vb.* (in ophthalmology) to accommodate (*see* accommodation).

foetus (**fee**-tŭs) *n. see* fetus.

folate (**foh**-layt) *n.* a B vitamin that is important in the synthesis of nucleic acids. The metabolic role of folate is interdependent with that of vitamin B_{12} (both are required by rapidly dividing cells), and a deficiency of one may lead to deficiency of the other. A deficiency of folate results in megaloblastic anaemia. Good sources of folate include liver, green leafy vegetables, and brown rice; increased intake shortly before conception and during the first three months of pregnancy helps prevent spina bifida and other congenital malformations in the fetus.

folic acid (pteroylglutamic acid) (foh-lik) *n.* a synthetic form of folate, which can be added to foods or used as a supplement for treating folate-deficient states.

folie à deux (fol-i a der) *n.* a condition in which two people who are closely involved with each other share one or more delusions.

folinic acid (foh-lin-ik) *n.* a derivative of folic acid involved in purine synthesis. Administered by mouth or by injection or infusion (in the form of its calcium or disodium salts), it is used to reverse the biological effects of methotrexate, and so prevent excessive toxicity (**f. a. rescue**), and to potentiate the action of fluorouracil. Trade names: **Isovorin**, **Refolinon**, **Sodiofolin**.

follicle (fol-ikŭl) *n.* a small secretory cavity, sac, or gland. *See also* Graafian follicle, hair (follicle). **—follicular** (fŏ-lik-yoo-ler) *adj.*

follicle-stimulating hormone (FSH) *n.* a hormone (*see* gonadotrophin) synthesized and released by the anterior pituitary gland. FSH stimulates ripening of the follicles in the ovary and formation of sperm in the testes. Preparations of FSH (**follitropin alfa** and **beta**, Gonal-F, Puregon; and **urofollitropin**, Fostimon) are administered by injection to treat infertility caused by underactivity of the pituitary gland and to stimulate the ovaries in women undergoing fertility treatment.

folliculitis (fŏ-lik-yoo-ly-tis) *n.* inflammation of hair follicles in the skin, commonly caused by bacterial infection. *See also* sycosis.

fomentation (foh-men-tay-shŏn) *n. see* poultice.

fomes (foh-meez) *n.* (*pl.* **fomites**) any object that is used or handled by a person with a communicable disease and may therefore become contaminated with the infective organisms and transmit the disease to a subsequent user. Common fomites are towels, bed clothes, cups, and money.

fontanelle (fon-tă-nel) *n.* an opening in the skull of a fetus or young infant due to incomplete ossification of the cranial bones and the resulting incomplete closure of the sutures. **anterior f.** the opening at the junction of the coronal, frontal, and sagittal sutures. **posterior f.** the opening at the junction of the sagittal and lambdoidal sutures. See illustration.

food intolerance *n.* nonallergic food hypersensitivity: a non-life-threatening reaction (often delayed) to a food, drink, food additive, or compound that results in symptoms in the respiratory

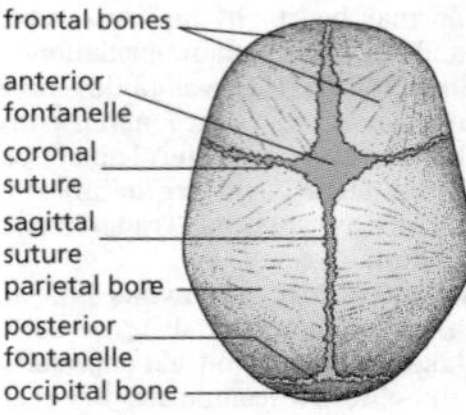

Fontanelles in the skull of a newborn infant (from above)

system, gut, or skin. It can result from metabolic reactions, pharmacological reactions, or malabsorption; treatment uses exclusion and elimination diets and the formation of tolerance over a period of time.

food poisoning (food) *n.* an illness affecting the digestive system that results from eating food contaminated by bacteria or bacterial toxins, viruses, or (less commonly) by poisonous chemicals such as lead or mercury. It can also be caused by eating poisonous fungi, berries, etc. Symptoms include nausea, vomiting, diarrhoea, and abdominal pain. Food-borne infections are caused by bacteria of the genus *Salmonella*, *Campylobacter*, and *Listeria* in foods of animal origin. Toxin-producing bacteria causing food poisoning include those of the genus *Staphylococcus*, which rapidly multiply in warm foods; pathogenic *Escherichia coli*; and the species *Clostridium perfringens*, which multiplies in reheated cooked meals. *See also* botulism, gastroenteritis.

foot (fuut) *n.* the terminal organ of the lower limb. It comprises the seven bones of the tarsus, the five metatarsal bones, and the phalangeal bones plus the surrounding tissues.

foot drop (fuut-drop) *n.* inability to keep the foot at right angles to the leg, caused by paralysis of the anterior leg muscles, pressure of bedclothes, or insufficient support for the sole of the foot when the leg is splinted.

footling (fuut-ling) *n.* a breech position in which the baby's feet are presented below its buttocks so that it will be delivered feet first.

foramen (fo-ray-men) *n.* (*pl.* **foramina**) an opening or hole, particularly in a bone. **apical f.** the small opening at the apex of a tooth. **f. magnum** a large hole in the occipital bone through which the spinal cord passes. **f. ovale** the opening between the two atria of the fetal heart, which allows blood to flow from the right to the left side of the heart by displacing a membranous valve.

forced expiratory volume (FEV) (forst iks-**pir**-ă-ter-i **vol**-yoom) *n.* the volume of air exhaled in a given period (usually limited to 1 second in tests of vital capacity). FEV is reduced in patients with obstructive airways disease and diminished lung volume.

forced vital capacity (FVC) *n. see* vital capacity.

forceps (**for**-seps) *n.* a pincer-like instrument designed to grasp an object so that it can be held firm or pulled. Specially designed forceps are used by surgeons and dentists in operations (see illustration).

forebrain (**for**-brayn) *n.* the furthest forward division of the brain, consisting of the diencephalon and the two cerebral hemispheres.

foregut (**for**-gut) *n.* the front part of the embryonic gut, which gives rise to the oesophagus, stomach, and part of the small intestine.

forensic medicine (fer-**en**-sik) *n.* the branch of medicine concerned with the scientific investigation of the causes of injury and death in unexplained circumstances,

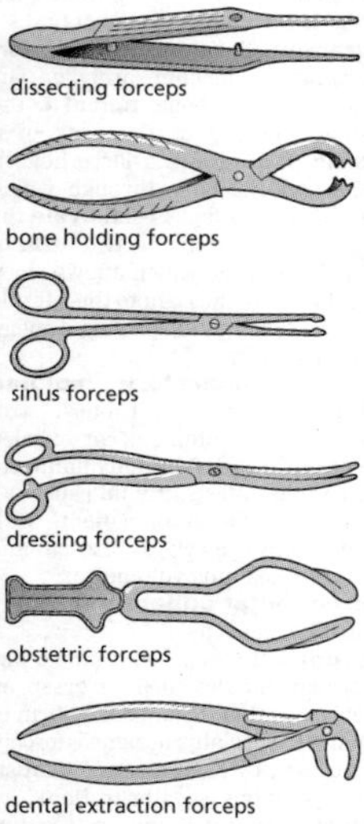

Types of forceps

particularly when criminal activity is suspected.

forequarter amputation (for-kwor-ter) *n.* an operation involving removal of an entire arm, including the scapula and clavicle. It is usually performed for soft tissue or bone sarcomas arising from the upper arm or shoulder. *Compare* hindquarter amputation.

foreskin (for-skin) *n. see* prepuce.

forewaters (for-waw-terz) *n.* the amniotic fluid that escapes from the uterus through the vagina when that part of the amnion lying in front of the presenting part of the fetus ruptures, either spontaneously or by amniotomy. Spontaneous rupture is usual in labour but rupture may occur before labour starts (premature rupture of membranes).

formaldehyde (for-**mal**-di-hyd) *n.* the aldehyde derivative of formic acid, formerly used as a vapour to sterilize and disinfect rooms and such items as mattresses and blankets. The toxic vapour is produced by boiling formalin in an open container or using it in a sealed autoclave.

formalin (**for**-mă-lin) *n.* a solution containing 40% formaldehyde in water, used as a sterilizing agent and, in pathology, as a fixative.

formication (for-mi-**kay**-shŏn) *n.* a prickling sensation said to resemble the feeling of ants crawling over the skin. It is sometimes a symptom of drug intoxication and can also be reported by patients with Parkinson's disease or multiple sclerosis.

formoterol (eformoterol) (for-**moh**-ter-ol) *n.* a sympathomimetic drug used as a long-acting bronchodilator to control chronic asthma and chronic obstructive pulmonary disease. Formoterol is formulated in powder or aerosol form for administration by inhaler. Trade names: **Atimos Modulite**, **Foradil**, **Oxis Turbohaler**.

formula (form-yoo-lă) *n.* **1.** a representation of the structure of a chemical compound using symbols and subscript numbers for the atoms it contains (e.g. H_2O for water; CO_2 for carbon dioxide). **2.** a prescription for a drug.

formulary (form-yoo-ler-i) *n.* a compendium of formulae used in the preparation of medicinal drugs.

fornix (for-niks) *n.* (*pl.* **fornices**) an arched or vaultlike structure. **f. cerebri** a triangular structure of white matter in the brain, situated between the hippocampus and hypothalamus. **f. of the conjunctiva** the upper or lower loose fold of conjunctiva between the posterior aspect of the eyelid and the eyeball. **f. of the vagina** any of three vaulted spaces at the top of the vagina, around the cervix of the uterus.

forward parachute reflex (for-wuud) *n.* a reflex action of the body that develops by five to six months and never disappears. If the body is held by the waist face down and lowered, the arms and legs extend automatically.

foscarnet (fos-kar-net) *n.* an antiviral drug used to treat herpes simplex that is resistant to aciclovir, and cytomegalovirus retinitis in patients with AIDS. It is administered by intravenous infusion.

fossa (fos-ă) *n.* (*pl.* **fossae**) a depression or hollow. **cubital f.** the triangular hollow at the front of the elbow joint. **iliac f.** the depression in the inner surface of the ilium. **pituitary f.** the hollow in the sphenoid bone in which the pituitary gland is situated. **tooth f.** a pit in the enamel on the surface of a tooth.

foundation trust (foundation hospital) (fownd-ay-shŏn) *n.* an NHS organization, established under the Health and Social Care Act 2003, that has greater freedom and more financial flexibility than NHS acute and mental health trusts; they are accountable to their local communities, commissioners, Parliament, and Monitor (an independent regulator). Foundation trusts are not under central government control but are subject to inspection by the Care Quality Commission. Under the Health and Social Care Act 2012 all NHS trusts were required to become foundation trusts (or part of a foundation trust) as soon as possible.

fourchette (foor-shet) *n.* a thin fold of skin at the back of the vulva.

four-layer system *n.* a continuous compression bandage consisting of four layers that are applied and left in situ for up to seven days to treat venous leg ulcers, increasing the chance of healing by up to 30%. Thorough assessment of the patient's status must be undertaken before the application.

fovea (foh-viă) *n.* (in anatomy) a small depression, especially the shallow pit in the retina at the back of the eye. It contains a large number of cones and is therefore the area of greatest acuity of vision. *See also* macula (lutea).

FQ *n. see* Fear Questionnaire.

fracture (frak-cher) *n.* breakage of a bone, either complete or incomplete. Treatment includes realignment of the bone ends and immobilization by external splints or internal fixation. **cervical f.** a fracture of a vertebra in the neck, with effects ranging from minor, requiring no treatment, to paralysis and instant death. **Colles' f.** a fracture of the distal (far) end of the radius, which is displaced backwards and upwards to produce a 'dinner fork' deformity. Avulsion of the ulnar styloid process usually takes place as well. **comminuted f.** a fracture in which the bone is broken into more than two pieces. **greenstick f.** an incomplete break in a bone occurring in children. **impacted f.** a fracture in which the bone ends are driven into each other. **march f.** a stress fracture in the distal section of the second or third metatarsal bone, associated with excessive walking. **open f.** a fracture in which the overlying skin is perforated and there is a wound extending to the fracture site. **pathological f.** fracture of a diseased or abnormal bone, usually resulting from a force insufficient to fracture a normal bone. **Pott's f.** a fracture of the lower end of the fibula accompanied by a fracture of the malleolus of the tibia. **simple f.** a clean break with little damage to surrounding tissues. **Smith's f.** a fracture just above the wrist, across the distal (far) end of the radius. The hand and wrist below the fracture are displaced forwards. **stress f.** a fracture occurring in a bone that has been subjected to excessive and repeated trauma resulting in cumulative microscopic fractures, as occurs in long-distance runners and others who undergo intensive training. See illustration.

fraenectomy (free-**nek**-tŏmi) *n.* *see* frenectomy.

fraenum (**free**-nŭm) *n.* *see* frenum.

fragile-X syndrome (fraj-yl-**eks**) *n.* a major genetic disorder caused by an abnormality in an X chromosome. The fragile-X syndrome is second only to Down's syndrome as a cause of learning disability. It predominantly affects males, but about one-third of the females with this mutation on one of their two X chromosomes also show developmental delay.

fragilitas (fră-**jil**-i-tas) *n.* abnormal brittleness or fragility. **f. crinium** brittleness of the hair. **f. ossium** brittleness of the bones (*see* osteogenesis (imperfecta)).

framboesia (fram-**bee**-ziă) *n.* *see* yaws.

Framingham risk score (**fram**-ing-hăm) *n.* an assessment tool that predicts a 10-year risk of developing cardiovascular disease based on gender, age, total and HDL cholesterol, blood pressure, and smoking, enabling preventative treatment. It does not incorporate the presence of diabetes or familial history of cardiovascular disease into the scoring.

Fraser guidelines (**fray**-zer) *pl. n.* *see* Gillick competence.

FRAT *n.* *see* Falls Risk Assessment Tool.

fraternal twins (fră-**ter**-năl) *pl. n.* *see* twins.

FRC *n.* *see* functional residual capacity.

freckle (**frek**-ĕl) *n.* a small harmless brown spot on the skin, commonly seen on exposed areas of fair-skinned people, due to excessive

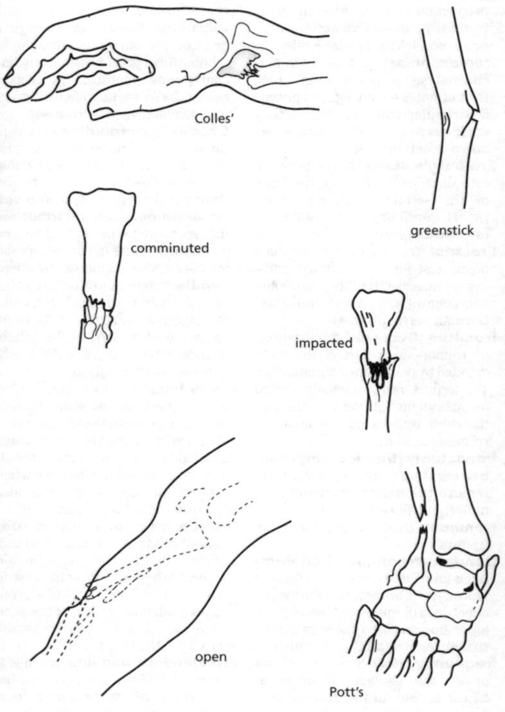

Types of fracture

production of melanin without an increase in melanocytes after exposure to sunlight. *Compare* lentigo.

free association (free) *n.* (in psychoanalysis) a technique in which the patient is encouraged to pursue a particular train of ideas as they enter his or her consciousness. *See also* association of ideas.

Freiburg's disease (**fry**-bergz) *n.* osteochondritis affecting the head of the second metatarsal bone. [A. H. Freiburg (1868–1940), US orthopaedic surgeon]

Frei test (fry) *n.* a rarely used diagnostic test for the sexually transmitted disease lymphogranuloma venereum. [W. S. Frei (1885–1943), German dermatologist]

fremitus (**frem**-i-tŭs) *n.* vibrations or tremors in a part of the body, detected by palpation or auscultation. The term is most commonly applied to vibrations perceived through the chest when a patient breathes, speaks (**vocal f.**), or coughs.

frenectomy (fraenectomy) (free-**nek**-tomi) *n.* an operation to remove the frenum, including the underlying fibrous tissue.

frenulum (**fren**-yoo-lŭm) *n. see* frenum.

frenum (fraenum, frenulum) (**free**-nŭm) *n.* **1.** any of the folds of mucous membrane under the tongue or between the gums and the upper or lower lips. **2.** any of several other structures of similar appearance.

frequency (**free**-kwĕn-si) *n.* (of urine) the passage of urine in excess of four to five times a day. *See* lower urinary tract symptoms.

frequency distribution *n.* (in statistics) presentation of the characteristics of a series of individuals (e.g. their heights, weights, or blood pressures; *see* variable) in tabular form or as a histogram (bar chart) so as to indicate the proportion of the series that have different measurements. A **normal** (or **Gaussian**) **distribution** is a continuous distribution that is symmetrical around the mean value and is defined by its mean and standard deviation; in a **skewed** (or **asymmetrical**) **distribution**, the measurements are clustered on one side of the mean and spread out over a wider range on the other.

Freudian (**froi**-di-ăn) *adj.* relating to or describing the work and ideas of Sigmund Freud (1856–1939): applied particularly to the school of psychiatry based on his teachings (*see* psychoanalysis).

friar's balsam (**fry**-erz) *n.* a tincture of benzoin, balsam of Tolu, storax, aloes, and various other plant extracts, the vapour of which is inhaled to relieve bronchitis. It provides a protective barrier when applied to the skin and also enhances adhesion of bandages.

friction murmur (friction rub) (**frik**-shŏn) *n.* a scratching sound, heard over the heart with the aid of the stethoscope, in patients who have pericarditis. It results from the two inflamed layers of the pericardium rubbing together during activity of the heart.

Friedländer's bacillus (**freed**-len-derz) *n.* a Gram-negative rodlike bacterium, *Klebsiella pneumoniae*, that causes a form of pneumonia. [K. Friedländer (1847–87), German pathologist]

Friedreich's ataxia (freed-ryks) *n. see* ataxia. [N. Friedreich (1825–82), German neurologist]

fringe medicine (frinj) *n. see* complementary medicine.

frog plaster (frog) *n.* a plaster of Paris splint used to maintain the legs in their correct position after a congenital dislocation of the hip has been corrected by manipulation.

Fröhlich's syndrome (frer-liks) *n.* a disorder of the hypothalamus affecting males: the boy is overweight with sexual development absent and disturbances of sleep and appetite. Medical name: **dystrophia adiposogenitalis**. [A. Fröhlich (1871–1953), Austrian neurologist]

Froin's syndrome (frwahnz) *n.* a condition in which the cerebrospinal fluid (CSF) displays a combination of yellow colour and high protein content. It is characteristic of a block to the spinal circulation of CSF often caused by a tumour. [G. Froin (1874–1932), French physician]

frontal (frun-t'l) *adj.* **1.** of or relating to the forehead. **f. bone** the bone forming the forehead and the upper parts of the orbits. **f. sinuses** *see* paranasal sinuses. **2.** denoting the anterior part of a body or organ. **f. lobe** the anterior part of each cerebral hemisphere, extending as far back as the deep central sulcus of its upper and outer surface.

frontotemporal dementia (FTD) (frun-toh-temp-er-ăl) *n.* a relatively rare neurodegenerative disease characterized by progressive loss of neurons in the frontal and/or temporal lobes. First described by A. Pick in 1892, it was originally called **Pick's disease**. Symptoms include lack of will and initiative and language deficits. It affects a younger population than Alzheimer's disease.

frostbite (frost-byt) *n.* damage to the tissues caused by freezing. The affected parts, usually the nose, fingers, or toes, become pale and numb. Ice crystals form in the tissues, causing destruction, and amputation may become necessary. Frostbitten skin is highly susceptible to bacterial infection.

frozen shoulder (adhesive capsulitis) (froh-zĕn) *n.* chronic painful stiffness of the shoulder joint, which has no clear single cause and usually resolves spontaneously over about 18 months. *See also* capsulitis.

frozen watchfulness *n.* the state of a child who is unresponsive to its surroundings but is clearly aware of them. Frozen watchfulness is usually a marker of child abuse.

fructose (fruk-tohz) *n.* a simple sugar found in honey and in such fruit as figs. Fructose is one of the two sugars in sucrose.

fructosuria (levulosuria) (fruk-tohz-yoor-iă) *n.* the presence of fructose (levulose) in the urine.

frusemide (frus-ĕ-myd) *n. see* furosemide.

FSH *n. see* follicle-stimulating hormone.

FTT *n. see* failure to thrive.

Fuchs' endothelial dystrophy (fooks) *n.* a hereditary condition in which the endothelium of the cornea fails to function with age; it may result in thickening and swelling of the cornea and thus affect vision. [E. Fuchs (1851–1913), German ophthalmologist]

fuchsin (magenta) (fook-sin) *n.* any one of a group of reddish to purplish dyes used in staining bacteria for microscopic observation and capable of killing various disease-causing microorganisms.

-fuge *combining form denoting* an agent that drives away, repels, or eliminates.

fugue (fewg) *n.* a period of memory loss during which the patient leaves his or her usual surroundings and wanders aimlessly or starts a new life elsewhere. It is often preceded by psychological conflict and associated with depression (*see* dissociative disorder), organic mental disease, or alcoholism.

fulguration (electrodesiccation) (ful-gewr-**ay**-shŏn) *n.* the destruction with a diathermy instrument of warts, growths, or unwanted areas of tissue, particularly inside the bladder.

fulminating (fulminant, fulgurant) (**ful**-min-ayt-ing) *adj.* describing a condition or symptom that is of very sudden onset, severe, and of short duration.

fumigation (few-mig-**ay**-shŏn) *n.* the use of gases or vapours, such as formaldehyde or chlorine, to bring about disinfestation of clothing, buildings, etc.

functional disorder (**funk**-shŏn-ăl) *n.* a condition in which a patient complains of symptoms for which no physical cause can be found. Such a condition is frequently an indication of a psychiatric disorder. *Compare* organic (disorder).

functional endoscopic sinus surgery (FESS) *n. see* endoscopic sinus surgery.

functional foods *n.* foods that contain a biologically active component that gives clinically proven health benefits in addition to the traditional nutrient value. For example, stanols and sterols added to margarine-type spreads lower cholesterol.

Functional Independence Measure (FIM) *n.* a table recommended by the WHO for assessing the degree of whole-person disability, being particularly useful for judging the extent of recovery from serious injury. It has five grades, ranging from 0 (fully independent) to 4 (completely dependent).

Functional Recovery Index *n.* an international index, published by the World Health Organization, that grades the degree of recovery after serious injury.

functional residual capacity (FRC) *n.* the volume of air that remains in the lungs after normal expiration.

fundal height (symphysis–fundal height) (**fun**-dăl) *n.* the distance, measured in centimetres, from the top of the symphysis pubis to the highest point in the midline at the top of the uterus (fundus). It is measured at each antenatal visit to assess fetal growth and development during pregnancy.

fundoplication (fun-doh-pli-**kay**-shŏn) *n.* a surgical operation for gastro-oesophageal reflux disease in which the upper part of the stomach is completely (**Nissen f.**) or partially (**toupe f.**) wrapped around the lower oesophagus.

fundoscopy (ophthalmoscopy) (fund-**os**-kŏpi) *n.* examination of the interior of the eye by means of an ophthalmoscope.

fundus (fun-dŭs) *n.* **1.** the base of a hollow organ: the part farthest from the opening. **2.** the interior concavity forming the back of the eyeball, opposite the pupil.

fungating wound (fun-gayt-ing) *n.* a mass of malignant tissue that has infiltrated the epithelium and broken through the skin surface. Often in the shape of a fungus, it may be infected, smell strongly, and cause pain. Such wounds are most likely to occur in the advanced stages of cancer, particularly of the breast, head, or neck.

fungicide (fun-ji-syd) *n.* an agent that kills fungi. *See also* antifungal.

fungoid (fung-oid) **1.** *adj.* resembling a fungus. **2.** *n.* a fungus-like growth.

fungus (fung-ŭs) *n.* (*pl.* **fungi**) a simple organism (formerly regarded as a plant) that lacks the green pigment chlorophyll. Fungi include the yeasts, rusts, moulds, and mushrooms. Some species infect and cause disease in humans. Some yeasts are a good source of vitamin B and many antibiotics are obtained from the moulds (*see* penicillin). *See also* yeast. —**fungal** *adj.*

funiculitis (few-nik-yoo-ly-tis) *n.* inflammation of the spermatic cord.

funiculus (few-nik-yoo-lŭs) *n.* **1.** any of the three main columns of white matter found in each lateral half of the spinal cord. **2.** a bundle of nerve fibres enclosed in a sheath. **3.** (formerly) the spermatic cord or umbilical cord.

funis (few-nis) *n.* (in anatomy) any cordlike structure, especially the umbilical cord.

funnel chest (fun-ĕl) *n.* a developmental abnormality in which the sternum is depressed and the ribs and costal cartilages curve inwards. Medical name: **pectus excavatum**.

funnelling (fun-ĕl-ing) *n.* a communication style that uses initial open questions and then concentrates on more focused questions with an increased amount of detail on specific points. It reflects the use of effective listening skills.

furosemide (frusemide) (fewr-os-ĕ-myd) *n.* a loop diuretic administered by mouth or injection to treat fluid retention (oedema) associated with heart failure or kidney disease and also high blood pressure. Trade name: **Lasix**.

furuncle (fewr-ung-kŭl) *n. see* boil.

furunculosis (fewr-unk-yoo-loh-sis) *n.* the occurrence of several boils (furuncles) at the same time, usually caused by *Staphylococcus aureus* infection.

fusidic acid (few-sid-ik) *n.* a steroid antibiotic used to treat staphylococcal skin and eye infections. It is administered topically. Trade name: **Fucidin**.

fusiform (few-zi-form) *adj.* spindle-shaped; tapering at both ends.

fusion (few-*zhŏn*) *n.* **1.** the joining together of two structures by surgery. For example, fusion of two or more vertebrae is performed to stabilize an unstable spine. **2.** the joining together of two structures by growth. Fusion of the epiphyses during development is the cause of arrested growth of stature.

FVC *n. see* (forced) vital capacity.

Gg

GABA *n.* *see* gamma-aminobutyric acid.

gabapentin (gab-ă-**pent**-in) *n.* an anticonvulsant drug administered by mouth to treat partial epilepsy and neuropathic pain, including peripheral neuropathy and post-herpetic neuralgia. **Pregabalin** (Lyrica) has similar uses and is also licensed to treat generalized anxiety disorder. Trade name: **Neurontin**.

GAD *n.* *see* glutamic acid decarboxylase.

GAD-7 (Generalized Anxiety Disorder Questionnaire) *n.* a self-administered screening tool to identify people who may suffer from anxiety disorders, consisting of seven questions based on DSM diagnostic criteria. Each item is scored from 0 (not at all) to 3 (nearly every day). Scores of 5, 10, and 15 are taken as the cut-off points for mild, moderate, and severe anxiety; a score of 10 indicates a reasonably high likelihood of generalized anxiety disorder.

gag (gag) *n.* (in medicine) an instrument that is placed between a patient's teeth to keep his mouth open.

gag reflex (pharyngeal reflex) *n.* a normal reflex action caused by contraction of pharynx muscles when the soft palate or posterior pharynx is touched. The reflex is used to test the integrity of the glossopharyngeal and vagus nerves.

gait (gayt) *n.* a manner of walking. **ataxic g.** an unsteady uncoordinated walk due to disease of the sensory nerves or cerebellum. *See* ataxia. **cerebellar g.** a staggering walk due to disease of the cerebellum. **spastic g.** a stiff shuffling walk in which the legs are held together.

galact- (galacto-) *combining form denoting* **1.** milk. **2.** galactose.

galactagogue (gă-**lak**-tă-gog) *n.* an agent that stimulates the secretion of milk or increases milk flow.

galactocele (gă-**lak**-toh-seel) *n.* **1.** a breast cyst containing milk, caused by closure of a milk duct. **2.** an accumulation of milky liquid in the sac surrounding the testis (*see* hydrocele).

galactorrhoea (gă-lak-tŏ-**ree**-ă) *n.* pathological secretion of breast milk by women or men, usually as a result of a benign pituitary tumour (prolactinoma).

galactosaemia (gă-lak-toh-**see**-miă) *n.* an inborn inability to utilize the sugar galactose, which in consequence accumulates in the blood. It is inherited as an autosomal recessive characteristic. Untreated, affected infants fail to thrive and show developmental delay, but if galactose is eliminated from the diet growth and development may be normal.

galactose (gă-**lak**-tohz) *n.* a simple sugar and a constituent of the milk sugar lactose. Galactose is converted to glucose in the liver.

galanin (gal-ă-nin) *n.* a peptide hormone having widespread effects on the central and peripheral nervous system and the gut. It is associated with the regulation of sleep, blood pressure, mood, and feeding, response to pain, physiological growth, and cognition.

galantamine (gă-lant-ă-meen) *n.* *see* acetylcholinesterase inhibitor.

galea (gay-liă) *n.* **1.** a helmet-shaped anatomical part. **2.** a type of head bandage.

galenical (gă-len-ikăl) *n.* a pharmaceutical preparation of a drug of animal or plant origin.

gall bladder (gawl) *n.* a pear-shaped sac (7–10 cm long), lying underneath the right lobe of the liver, in which bile is stored (see illustration). The gall bladder is a common site of stone formation (*see* gallstone).

Gallie's operation (gal-iz) *n.* an operation in which strips of fascia taken from the thigh are used as suturing material to repair a hernia. [W. E. Gallie (1882–1959), Canadian surgeon]

gallipot (gal-i-pot) *n.* a small pot for holding lotions or ointments.

gallium (gal-iŭm) *n.* a silvery metallic element. A radioisotope of gallium can be used for the detection of lymphomas and areas of infection (such as an abscess) following intravenous injection. Symbol: Ga.

gallstone (gawl-stohn) *n.* a hard mass composed of bile pigments, cholesterol, and calcium salts, in varying proportions, that can form in the gall bladder. They may cause severe pain (*see* biliary (colic)) or they may pass into the common

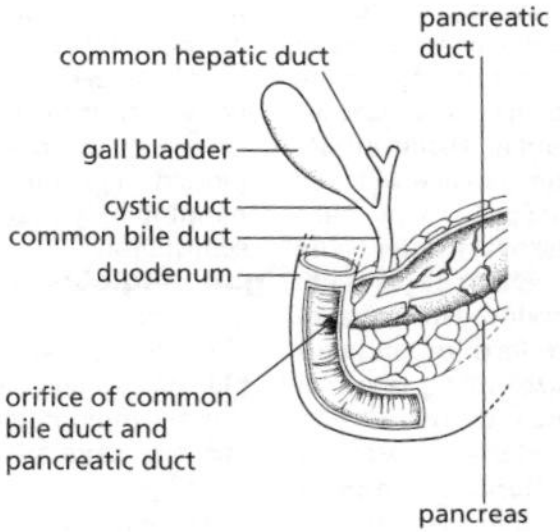

The gall bladder and pancreas and their associated ducts

bile duct and cause obstructive jaundice or cholangitis. Treatment of symptomatic gallstones is usually by surgical removal of the gall bladder (*see* cholecystectomy).

galvanism (gal-vă-nizm) *n.* (formerly) any form of medical treatment using electricity. **interrupted g.** a form of electrotherapy in which direct current is used to stimulate the activity of nerves or the muscles they supply. *See also* faradism.

galvanometer (gal-vă-**nom**-it-er) *n.* an instrument for measuring the strength of an electric current.

gamekeeper's thumb (gaym-keep-erz) *n.* *see* skier's thumb.

gamete (**gam**-eet) *n.* a mature sex cell: the ovum of the female or the spermatozoon of the male. Gametes are haploid, containing half the normal number of chromosomes.

gamete intrafallopian transfer (GIFT) (intră-fă-**loh**-piăn) *n.* a procedure for assisting conception, suitable for women whose Fallopian tubes are normal but in whom some other factor, such as endometriosis, prevents conception. Using needle aspiration, under laparoscopic or ultrasonic guidance, ova are removed from the ovary. After being mixed with the partner's spermatozoa, they are introduced into a Fallopian tube, where fertilization takes place. The fertilized ovum is subsequently implanted in the uterus. A similar procedure is used in **zygote intrafallopian transfer** (ZIFT), except that fertilization occurs in vitro and the zygote is introduced into a Fallopian tube.

gametocide (**gam**-i-toh-syd) *n.* a drug that kills gametocytes.

gametocyte (gă-**meet**-oh-syt) *n.* any of the cells that are in the process of developing into gametes by undergoing gametogenesis.

gametogenesis (gam-i-toh-**jen**-i-sis) *n.* the process by which spermatozoa and ova are formed. In both sexes the precursor cells undergo meiosis, which halves the number of chromosomes. *See* oogenesis, spermatogenesis.

gamgee tissue (**gam**-jee) *n.* a thick layer of absorbent cotton between two layers of gauze, used as a surgical dressing.

gamma-aminobutyric acid (GABA) (gam-ă-ă-meen-oh-bew-**ti**-rik) *n.* an amino acid found in the central nervous system, predominantly in the brain, where it acts as an inhibitory neurotransmitter.

gamma camera *n.* a piece of apparatus that detects radioactivity in the form of gamma rays emitted by radioactive isotopes that have been introduced into the body as tracers. The position of the source of the radioactivity can be plotted and displayed on a TV monitor or photographic film. *See* scintillator.

gammaglobulin (gam-ă-**glob**-yoo-lin) *n.* any of a class of proteins (*see* globulin) present in the blood plasma. Almost all gammaglobulins are immunoglobulins.

gamma rays *pl. n.* ionizing electromagnetic radiation of short wavelength, given off by certain radioactive substances, with equivalent properties to artificially produced X-rays. Gamma rays used in nuclear medicine have higher energy than diagnostic X-rays and greater penetration; higher energies are used in radiotherapy. Gamma rays are harmful to living tissues and can be used to sterilize certain materials and to kill bacteria as a means of food preservation.

gamo- *combining form denoting* marriage.

ganciclovir (gan-sy-kloh-veer) *n.* an antiviral drug used to treat severe cytomegalovirus infections in immunocompromised patients and also dendritic ulcers. It is administered by intravenous infusion or as an eye gel. Trade names: **Cymevene**, **Virgan**.

gangli- (ganglio-) *combining form denoting* a ganglion.

ganglion (gang-li-ŏn) *n.* (*pl.* **ganglia**) **1.** (in neurology) any structure containing a collection of nerve cell bodies and often also numbers of synapses. Ganglia are found in the sympathetic and parasympathetic nervous systems. Within the central nervous system certain well-defined masses of nerve cells are called ganglia (*see* basal ganglia). **2.** an abnormal but harmless swelling (cyst) that sometimes forms in tendon sheaths, especially at the wrist.

ganglionectomy (gang-li-ŏn-ek-tŏmi) *n.* surgical removal of a ganglion cyst.

gangrene (gang-reen) *n.* death and decay of part of the body due to deficiency or cessation of blood supply. The causes include disease, injury, or atheroma in major blood vessels, frostbite or severe burns, and diseases such as diabetes mellitus and Raynaud's disease. **dry g.** death and withering of tissues caused simply by a cessation of local blood circulation. **Fournier's g.** a rare but potentially life-threatening infection of the scrotum that can rapidly spread to involve the perineum, penis, and anterior abdominal wall. [J. A. Fournier (19th century), French venereologist]. **moist** (or **wet**) **g.** death and putrefactive decay of tissue caused by bacterial infection. *See also* gas gangrene.

Ganser syndrome (gan-ser) *n.* a syndrome characterized by approximate answers, i.e. the patient gives absurdly false replies to questions, but the reply shows that the question has been understood. The condition may be due to conversion disorder or to conscious malingering. [S. J. M. Ganser (1853–1931), German psychiatrist]

Gardnerella (gard-ner-el-ă) *n.* a genus of anaerobic bacteria. **G. vaginalis** a cause of bacterial vaginosis and, in pregnant women, of late miscarriage and premature labour.

Gardner's syndrome (gard-nerz) *n.* a variant form of familial adenomatous polyposis in which polyps in the colon are associated with fibromas, sebaceous cysts, and osteomas (benign tumours), especially of the skull and jaw. [E. J. Gardner (1909–89), US physician]

gargle (gar-gŭl) **1.** *n.* a medicated solution used for washing the mouth and throat. **2.** *vb.* to apply a gargle by holding it in the throat and exhaling through it.

gargoylism (gar-goil-izm) *n. see* Hunter's syndrome, Hurler's syndrome.

Garvin risk assessment scale (gar-vin) *n.* a pressure ulcer predictive risk assessment tool designed for use in the care of children. It uses four risk factors (mobility, sensory perception, nutrition, and moisture) to identify the potential for ulcer development.

gas (gas) *n.* a fluid whose physical state is such that the forces of attraction between its constituent atoms and molecules are very weak. It therefore has no definite shape or volume. **laughing g.** *see* nitrous oxide.

gas gangrene *n.* death and decay of wound tissue infected by the soil bacterium *Clostridium perfringens*. Toxins produced by the bacterium cause putrefactive decay of connective tissue with the generation of gas.

Gasserian ganglion (gas-eer-iăn) *n.* a ganglion on the sensory root of the trigeminal nerve, deep within the skull. [J. L. Gasser (1723–65), Austrian anatomist]

gastr- (gastro-) *combining form denoting* the stomach.

gastralgia (gas-tral-jiă) *n.* pain in the stomach.

gastrectomy (gas-trek-tŏmi) *n.* a surgical operation in which the whole or a part of the stomach is removed. **partial** (or **subtotal**) **g.** an operation in which the upper part of the stomach is joined to the duodenum or small intestine. *See also* Billroth's operation. **total g.** an operation usually performed for stomach cancer, in which the oesophagus is joined to the jejunum.

gastric (gas-trik) *adj.* relating to or affecting the stomach. **g. banding** bariatric surgery in which a band is placed around the stomach to reduce its size and therefore restrict the amount of food it can accommodate. **g. glands** tubular glands in the mucous membrane of the stomach wall that secrete gastric juice. **g. juice** the liquid secreted by the gastric glands, containing hydrochloric acid, mucin, rennin, and pepsinogen. The acid acts on pepsinogen to produce the digestive enzyme pepsin. The acidity of the stomach contents also kills unwanted bacteria and other organisms that have been ingested with the food. **g. ulcer** an ulcer in the stomach, caused by the action of gastric acid and pepsin on the stomach lining. Symptoms include vomiting and pain in the upper abdomen soon after eating, and such complications as bleeding (*see* haematemesis), perforation, and obstruction due to scarring may occur. *See also* Helicobacter.

gastrin (gas-trin) *n.* a hormone produced in the mucous membrane of the pyloric region of the stomach. Its secretion is stimulated by the presence of food. It is circulated in the blood to the rest of the stomach, where it stimulates the production of gastric juice.

gastrinoma (gas-tri-noh-mă) *n.* a rare tumour that secretes the hormone gastrin, which stimulates excessive gastric acid production.

Such tumours most frequently occur in the pancreas; about half of them are malignant. Patients present with intractable gastroduodenal ulceration, abdominal pain, and diarrhoea (the Zollinger–Ellison syndrome).

gastritis (gas-**try**-tis) *n.* inflammation of the lining (mucosa) of the stomach. **acute erosive (reactive) g.** gastritis in which vomiting occurs, caused by ingesting excess alcohol or other irritating or corrosive substances. **atrophic g.** gastritis in which the stomach lining is atrophied. **chronic g.** gastritis that is predominantly caused by the bacterium *Helicobacter pylori* but may be associated with smoking and chronic alcoholism or bile entering the stomach from the duodenum.

gastrocnemius (gas-trok-**nee**-miŭs) *n.* a muscle that forms the greater part of the calf of the leg. It flexes the knee and foot (so that the toes point downwards). See illustration.

gastrocolic reflex (gas-troh-**kol**-ik) *n.* a wave of peristalsis produced in the colon by introducing food into a fasting stomach.

gastroduodenoscopy (gas-troh-dew-ŏ-di-**nos**-kŏ-pi) *n. see* oesophagogastroduodenoscopy.

gastroduodenostomy (gas-troh-dew-ŏ-di-**nost**-ŏmi) *n.* a surgical operation in which the duodenum is joined to an opening made in the stomach in order to bypass an obstruction or to facilitate the exit of food from the stomach after vagotomy. *See also* duodenostomy.

gastroenteritis (gas-troh-enter-**I**-tis) *n.* inflammation of the stomach and intestine. It is usually due to acute viral or bacterial infection or to the ingestion of toxins in contaminated food. Symptoms are vomiting, diarrhoea, and fever. Fluid loss is sometimes severe, especially at the extremes of age, and intravenous fluid replacement may be necessary.

gastroenterology (gas-troh-enter-**ol**-ŏji) *n.* the study of gastrointestinal disease, which encompasses disease of any part of the digestive tract and also of the liver, biliary tract, and pancreas.

gastroenterostomy (gas-troh-enter-**ost**-ŏmi) *n.* a surgical operation in which the small intestine is joined to an opening made in the stomach. The usual technique is gastrojejunostomy.

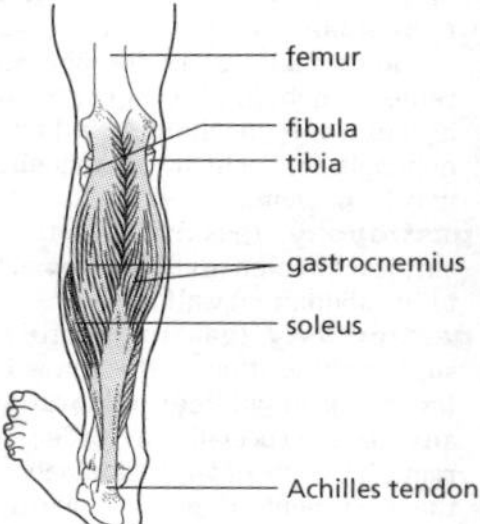

Gastrocnemius and soleus muscles

gastroileac reflex (gas-troh-**il**-i-ak) *n.* the relaxation of the ileocaecal valve caused by the presence of food in the stomach.

gastrointestinal (GI) (gas-troh-in-**test**-i-năl) *adj.* denoting, relating to, or affecting the stomach and intestines. **g. stromal tumour (GIST)** a tumour arising from the gastrointestinal tract that displays a wide range of malignancy.

gastrojejunostomy (gas-troh-ji-joo-**nost**-ŏmi) *n.* a surgical operation in which the jejunum is joined to an opening made in the stomach.

gastrolith (**gas**-trŏ-lith) *n.* a stone in the stomach, which usually builds up around a bezoar.

gastro-oesophageal reflux (GOR) (gas-troh-ee-sof-ă-**jee**-ăl) *n.* a condition in which the stomach contents reflux into the oesophagus because of impairment of the usual mechanisms preventing this. **g.-o. r. disease** the syndrome caused by abnormal gastro-oesophageal reflux, including symptoms of heartburn, regurgitation, and odynophagia, in which oesophagitis may be present.

gastropexy (**gas**-troh-peks-i) *n.* surgical attachment of the stomach to the abdominal wall.

gastroplasty (**gas**-troh-plasti) *n.* surgical alteration of the shape of the stomach without removal of any part, especially in order to reduce the size of the stomach in the treatment of morbid obesity. **vertical banded g.** *see* stomach stapling.

gastroschisis (gas-**tros**-ki-sis) *n.* a congenital defect in the abdominal wall, which during fetal development fails to close to the right of a normal umbilical cord. Bowel herniates through the defect and has no covering.

gastroscope (**gas**-trŏ-skohp) *n.* an illuminated optical endoscope used to inspect the interior of the oesophagus, stomach, and duodenum. Modern instruments house advanced digital systems to allow high-definition imaging of the stomach, oesophagus, and the first and second parts of the duodenum. Biopsies can be taken of visualized areas and therapeutic procedures may be performed. **—gastroscopy** (gas-**tros**-kŏ-pi) *n.*

gastrostomy (gas-**trost**-ŏmi) *n.* a procedure in which an opening is made through the anterior abdominal wall into the stomach to allow direct access for feeding or gastric decompression. It is performed when swallowing is considered unsafe or impossible due to a neurological condition or to obstruction by a tumour. **g. button** a device connecting the skin surface to the stomach to which feeding tubes are attached. Some buttons have a balloon inside the stomach to hold the device in place. (see illustration) **percutaneous endoscopic g. (PEG)** gastrostomy performed using an endoscope to guide insertion of the feeding tube.

gastrotomy (gas-**trot**-ŏmi) *n.* a procedure during abdominal

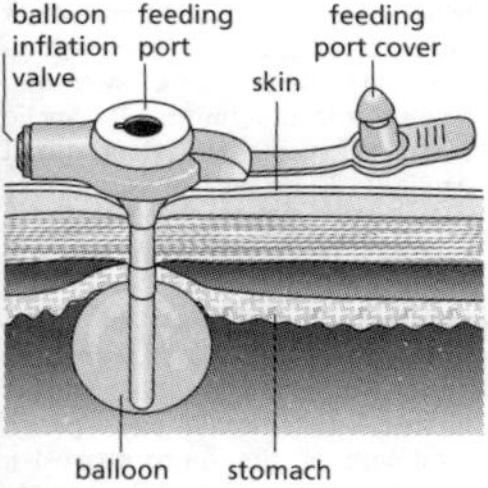

Gastrostomy button

surgery in which the stomach is opened, usually to allow inspection of the interior, to remove a foreign body, or to allow the oesophagus to be approached from below.

gastrula (gas-troo-lă) *n.* an early stage in the development of many animal embryos. The gastrula consists of a double-layered ball of cells formed by invagination and movement of cells in the preceding single-layered stage (blastula) in the process of **gastrulation**.

Gaucher's disease (goh-shayz) *n.* a genetically determined disease, inherited as a recessive condition, resulting from the deposition of fatty compounds in the brain and other tissues (especially bone). It results in learning disability, abnormal limb posture and spasticity, and difficulty with swallowing. [P. C. E. Gaucher (1854–1918), French physician]

gauze (gawz) *n.* thin open-woven material used in several layers for the preparation of dressings and swabs.

gavage (gav-ah*zh*) *n.* forced feeding: any means used to get an unwilling or incapacitated patient to take in food by mouth, especially via a stomach tube.

GCS *n. see* Glasgow Coma Scale.

GDS *n. see* Geriatric Depression Scale.

Geiger counter (gy-ger kownt-er) *n.* a device for detecting and measuring the level of radioactivity of a substance. [H. Geiger (1882–1945), German physicist]

gel (jel) *n.* a colloidal suspension that has set to form a jelly. Some insoluble drugs are administered in the form of gels.

gelatin (jel-ă-tin) *n.* a jelly-like substance formed when tendons, ligaments, etc. containing collagen are boiled in water. Gelatin has been used in medicine as a source of dietary protein, in pharmacy for the manufacture of capsules and suppositories, and in bacteriology for preparing culture media.

gemcitabine (jem-sit-ă-been) *n.* a cytotoxic drug that is administered intravenously in the treatment of advanced non-small-cell lung cancer and bladder, breast, and pancreatic cancers. Side-effects are less severe than those of other antimetabolites. Trade name: **Gemzar**.

gemeprost (jem-ĕ-prost) *n.* a prostaglandin drug, administered as a vaginal pessary to terminate pregnancy. It causes powerful contractions of the uterus at any stage of pregnancy.

gemfibrozil (jem-**fy**-broh-zil) *n.* a drug used to treat hyperlipidaemia that has not responded to diet, weight reduction, or exercise (*see* fibrate). It is administered by mouth. Trade name: **Lopid**.

gender identity disorder (GID)/gender dysphoria (**jen**-der) *n.* a condition in which an individual belongs to one gender on the basis of physical appearance and genetics but identifies psychologically with the other gender. *See also* transsexualism.

gene (jeen) *n.* the basic unit of genetic material, which is carried at a particular place on a chromosome. Originally it was regarded as the unit of inheritance and mutation but is now usually defined as a sequence of DNA or RNA that acts as the unit controlling the formation of a single polypeptide chain. In diploid organisms, including humans, genes occur as pairs of alleles (*see* dominant, recessive). *See also* (gene) clone, gene therapy.

General Health Questionnaire (GHQ) (**jen**-er-ăl) *n.* a reliable screening tool published in 1978 for identifying minor psychiatric disorders, still frequently used for research in the general population. The 28-question version (**GHQ28**) is most commonly used.

generalized anxiety disorder (**jen**-er-ă-lyzd) *n.* a state of anxiety, sometimes severe, without adequate cause, that lasts for at least six months. Symptoms affect all parts of the body: core symptoms are palpitations, sweating, tremor, and dry mouth. It can be diagnosed using the Generalized Anxiety Disorder questionnaire (*see* GAD-7). Treatment includes cognitive behavioural therapy and antidepressants.

general paralysis of the insane (GPI, general paresis) *n.* a stage of tertiary syphilis characterized by dementia and spastic weakness of the limbs (paresis). Deafness, epilepsy, and dysarthria may occur.

general practitioner (GP) (prak-**tish**-ŏn-er) *n.* a doctor who is the main agent of primary care, through whom patients make first contact with health services for a new episode of illness or fresh developments of chronic diseases. Advice and treatment are provided for those who do not require the expertise of a consultant or other specialist services of hospitals (*see* secondary care). *See also* group practice.

generic (jin-e-rik) **1.** *adj.* denoting a nonproprietary drug name, which is not protected by a trademark. **2.** *adj.* of or relating to a genus. **3.** *n.* a drug sold under its nonproprietary name.

-genesis *combining form denoting origin or development.*

gene therapy *n.* treatment directed to curing genetic disease by introducing normal genes into patients to overcome the effects of defective genes, using techniques of genetic engineering. At present, gene therapy is most feasible for treating disorders caused by a defect in a single recessive gene, such as adenosine deaminase (ADA) deficiency, severe combined immune deficiency, and cystic fibrosis. Gene therapy for certain types of cancer is also undergoing clinical trials.

genetic code (ji-**net**-ik) *n.* the code in which genetic information is carried by DNA and messenger RNA. This information determines the sequence of amino acids in every protein and thereby controls the nature of all proteins made by the cell.

genetic counselling *n.* the procedure by which patients and their families are given advice about the nature and consequences of inherited disorders, the possibility of becoming affected or having affected children, and the various options that are available to them for the prevention, diagnosis, and management of such conditions.

genetic engineering (recombinant DNA technology) *n.* the techniques involved in altering the characteristics of an organism by inserting genes from another organism into its DNA. This altered DNA is known as **recombinant DNA**. For example, the human genes for insulin, interferon, and growth hormone production have been incorporated into bacterial DNA to enable the commercial production of these substances.

genetics (ji-**net**-iks) *n.* the science of inheritance. It attempts to explain the differences and similarities between related organisms and the ways in which characters are passed from parents to their offspring. *See also* cytogenetics, Mendel's laws.

genetic screening *n.* screening tests to discover individuals whose genotypes are associated with specific diseases. Such individuals may later develop the disease itself or pass it on to their children (*see* carrier).

geni- (genio-) *combining form denoting* the chin.

-genic *combining form denoting* **1.** producing. **2.** produced by.

genicular (ji-**nik**-yoo-ler) *adj.* relating to the knee joint: applied to arteries that supply the knee.

genital (**jen**-i-t'l) *adj.* relating to the reproductive organs or to reproduction.

genitalia (jen-i-**tay**-liă) *pl. n.* the reproductive organs of either the male or the female, particularly the external parts of the reproductive system. *See also* vulva.

genito- *combining form denoting* the reproductive organs.

genitourinary (jen-i-toh-**yoor**-in-er-i) *adj.* of or relating to the organs of reproduction and excretion. g. medicine (GUM) the branch of medicine concerned with the study and treatment of sexually transmitted diseases.

genodermatosis (jen-oh-der-mă-**toh**-sis) *n.* any genetically determined skin disorder, such as ichthyosis, neurofibromatosis, or xeroderma pigmentosum.

genogram (**jen**-ŏ-gram) *n.* a diagram of a family tree that illustrates interpersonal (as well as familial) relationships. It can give a wealth of information about the traits, emotional relationships, health, and major life events of a patient and can be used as a therapeutic tool to analyse patterns that could have an impact on the patient.

genome (**jen**-ohm) *n.* the total genetic material of an organism, comprising the genes contained in its chromosomes; sometimes the term is used for the basic haploid set of chromosomes of an organism. The human genome comprises 23 pairs of chromosomes. *See also* Human Genome Project.

genotype (**jen**-oh-typ) *n.* **1.** the genetic constitution of an individual or group, as determined by the particular set of genes it possesses. **2.** the genetic information carried by a pair of alleles, which determines a particular characteristic. *Compare* phenotype.

gentamicin (jen-tă-**my**-sin) *n.* an aminoglycoside antibiotic used to treat serious infections caused by a wide range of bacteria. It can be administered by injection or infusion or as drops to the ears and eyes. Trade names: **Cidomycin**, **Genticin**.

gentian violet (**jen**-shăn **vy**-ŏ-lit) *n.* a dye used to stain tissues and microorganisms for microscopical study and also as a topically applied antiseptic.

genu (**jen**-yoo) *n.* **1.** the knee. **g. valgum** *see* knock-knee. **g. varum** *see* bow-legs. **2.** any bent anatomical structure resembling the knee. —**genual** *adj.*

genucubital position (knee-elbow position) (jen-yoo-**kew**-bit'l) *n.* the buttocks-up position assumed by patients undergoing anorectal examinations.

genupectoral position (knee-chest position) (jen-yoo-**pek**-ter-ăl) *n.* the position of a patient in which the weight of the body is supported on the knees and chest. *See* position.

genus (**jen**-ŭs) *n.* (*pl.* **genera**) a category used in the classification of animals and plants. A genus consists of several closely related and similar species; for example the genus *Canis* includes the dog, wolf, and jackal.

geographical tongue (jee-oh-**graf**-i-kăl) *n.* areas of erythema, reflecting benign loss of papillae, on the surface of the tongue that change from day to day.

ger- (gero-, geront(o)-) *combining form denoting* old age.

Geriatric Depression Scale (GDS) (je-ri-**at**-rik) *n.* a self-report tool to measure depression in adults aged 65 years or older. It consists of a 30-item questionnaire with yes–no answers; a score of 15 or above indicates the presence of depression but the test should be used in conjunction with other results from a comprehensive examination.

geriatrics (je-ri-**at**-riks) *n.* the branch of medicine concerned with the diagnosis and treatment of disorders that occur in old age and with the care of the aged. *See also* gerontology. **—geriatrician** (je-ri-ă-**trish**-ăn) *n.*

germ (jerm) *n.* any microorganism, especially one that causes disease. *See also* infection.

German measles (jer-măn) *n.* a mild highly contagious virus infection, mainly of childhood. Symptoms include headache, sore throat, and slight fever, followed by swelling and soreness of the neck and the eruption of a rash of minute pink spots, spreading from the face and neck to the rest of the body. German measles can cause fetal malformations during early pregnancy. Medical name: **rubella**. *Compare* scarlet fever.

germ cell (gonocyte) *n.* **1.** any of the embryonic cells that have the potential to develop into spermatozoa or ova. **g. c. tumour** a tumour arising in germ cells, most commonly in the testis and ovary. Examples are teratomas, seminomas, and dysgerminomas. They may be benign or malignant and typically occur in children and young adults. Tumour markers can be used to monitor disease. **2.** a gamete.

germicide (**jerm**-i-syd) *n.* an agent that destroys microorganisms, particularly those causing disease. *See* antibiotic, antifungal, antiseptic, disinfectant.

germinal (jer-min-ăl) *adj.* **1.** relating to the early developmental stages of an embryo or tissue. **2.** relating to a germ.

germ layer *n.* any of the three distinct types of tissue found in the very early stages of embryonic development (*see* ectoderm, endoderm, mesoderm).

gerontology (je-ron-**tol**-ŏji) *n.* the study of the changes in the mind and body that accompany ageing and the problems associated with them.

Gerstmann-Straussler-Scheinker syndrome (gerst-măn **strows**-ler **shyn**-ker) *n.* an autosomal dominant condition that is caused by a mutation in the prion protein gene and resembles Creutzfeldt-Jakob disease (CJD). Patients present with ataxia and dysarthria and later develop dementia. They continue to deteriorate over several years, in contrast with patients with CJD, who deteriorate rapidly over periods of less than 12 months. [J. G. Gerstmann (1887–1969), Austrian neurologist]

gestaltism (gestalt psychology) (gĕsh-**talt**-izm) *n.* a school of psychology that regards mental processes as wholes (**gestalt**) that cannot be broken down into constituent parts. From this was developed **gestalt therapy**, which aims at achieving a suitable gestalt within the patient that includes all facets of functioning.

gestation (jes-**tay**-shŏn) *n.* the period during which a fertilized egg cell develops into a baby that is ready to be delivered. *See also* pregnancy.

gestational diabetes (jes-tay-shŏn-ăl) *n. see* diabetes.

gestodene (jes-toh-deen) *n.* a progestogen used in oral contraceptives in combination with ethinylestradiol (an oestrogen). Trade names: **Femodene**, **Femodette**, **Katya 30/75**, **Millinette 20/75**, **Sunya 20/75**, **Triadene**.

GFR *n.* *see* glomerular filtration rate.

GH *n.* *see* growth hormone.

GHIH *n.* growth-hormone inhibiting hormone (*see* somatostatin).

Ghon's focus (gonz) *n.* the lesion produced in the lung of a previously uninfected person by tubercle bacilli. It is a small focus of granulomatous inflammation, which may become visible on a chest X-ray if it grows large enough or if it calcifies. [A. Ghon (1866–1936), Czech pathologist]

GHQ *n.* *see* General Health Questionnaire.

ghrelin (**grel**-in) *n.* a hormone produced by stomach cells that acts in the hypothalamus to increase appetite and stimulate secretion of growth hormone. Ghrelin levels are lower in obese individuals (suggesting that the hormone does not stimulate eating) and higher in patients with anorexia nervosa.

GI 1. *n.* *see* glycaemic index. **2.** *adj.* *see* gastrointestinal.

giant cell (**jy**-ănt) *n.* any large cell, such as a megakaryocyte. Giant cells may have one or many nuclei.

giant-cell arteritis *n.* *see* arteritis.

giardiasis (lambliasis) (jy-ar-**dy**-ă-sis) *n.* a disease caused by the parasitic protozoan *Giardia lamblia* in the small intestine. Symptoms include diarrhoea, nausea, bellyache, flatulence, and the passage of pale fatty stools (steatorrhoea). The disease is particularly common in children; it responds well to oral doses of metronidazole.

gibbus (gibbosity) (**gib**-ŭs) *n.* a sharply angled curvature of the backbone, resulting from collapse of a vertebra. Infection with tuberculosis was a common cause.

GIFT *n.* *see* gamete intrafallopian transfer.

gigantism (jy-**gan**-tizm) *n.* abnormal growth causing excessive height, most commonly due to oversecretion during childhood of growth hormone (somatotrophin) by the pituitary gland.

GIK regime *n.* *see* Alberti regime.

Gilbert's syndrome (***zh**eel*-bairz) *n.* familial unconjugated hyperbilirubinaemia: a condition caused by an inherited congenital deficiency of the enzyme UDP glucuronyl transferase in liver cells. Patients become mildly jaundiced, especially if they fast, overexert themselves, or have concomitant infection. [N. A. Gilbert (1858–1927), French physician]

Gilles de la Tourette syndrome (*zh*eel dĕ la toor-**et**) *n.* *see* Tourette's syndrome.

Gilliam's operation (**gil**-i-ămz) *n.* an operation to correct retroversion of the uterus in which the round ligaments are shortened. [D. T. Gilliam (1844–1923), US gynaecologist]

Gillick competence (**gil**-ik) *n.* the means by which to assess legal capacity in children under the age of 16 years, established in the case *Gillick v West Norfolk and Wisbech Area Health Authority* (1985) 2 A11 ER 402. Such children are deemed to be capable of giving valid consent to advice or treatment without parental knowledge or agreement provided they have sufficient understanding to fully appreciate the nature, purpose, and hazards of the proposed treatment. In the Gillick case the criteria for deciding competence, set out by Lord Fraser, related specifically to contraceptive treatment. In addition to the elements of Gillick competence, the **Fraser guidelines** specified that a health professional must be convinced that the child was likely to begin, or to continue having, sexual intercourse with or without contraceptive treatment, that his or her physical and/or mental health would probably suffer in the absence of treatment, and that it was in his or her best interests to provide treatment. The principle of Gillick competence applies to all treatment for those under the age of 16. **—Gillick-competent** *adj.*

SEE WEB LINKS

- Explanation of Gillick competence in the *British Medical Journal*

gingiv- (gingivo-) *combining form denoting* the gums.

gingiva (jin-jiv-ă) *n.* (*pl.* **gingivae**) the gum: the layer of dense connective tissue and overlying mucous membrane that covers the alveolar bone and necks of the teeth. **—gingival** *adj.*

gingivectomy (jin-ji-**vek**-tŏmi) *n.* the surgical removal of excess gum tissue. It is a specific procedure of periodontal surgery.

gingivitis (jin-ji-**vy**-tis) *n.* inflammation of the gums, which become swollen and bleed easily, caused by plaque at the necks of the teeth.

ginglymus (hinge joint) (**jing**-li-mŭs) *n.* a form of diarthrosis that allows angular movement in one plane only. Examples are the knee joint and the elbow joint.

girdle (**ger**-d'l) *n.* (in anatomy) an encircling or arching arrangement of bones. *See also* pelvic girdle, shoulder girdle.

Girdlestone's operation (**ger**-d'l-stohnz) *n.* an operation in which the head of the femur and part of the acetabulum are removed and a mass of muscle is sutured between the bone ends. It is performed for osteoarthritis. [G. R. Girdlestone (1881–1950), British surgeon]

GIST *n. see* gastrointestinal (stromal tumour).

glabella (glă-**bel**-ă) *n.* the smooth rounded surface of the frontal bone in the middle of the forehead, between the two eyebrows.

gladiolus (glad-i-**oh**-lŭs) *n.* the middle and largest segment of the sternum.

Glamorgan paediatric pressure ulcer scale (glă-**mor**-găn) *n.* a pressure ulcer predictive risk assessment tool developed specifically for the care of children (up to the age of 18). It uses a series of key areas to assess risk (including mobility, objects pressing against skin, anaemia or fever, and cold extremities), each area being accorded a score. The higher the score, the greater the risk. The tool incorporates preventive actions to diminish the potential for ulcer development.

gland (gland) *n.* an organ or group of cells that is specialized for synthesizing and secreting certain fluids, either for use in the body or for excretion. *See* endocrine gland, exocrine gland, secretion.

glanders (equinia) (**glan**-derz) *n.* an infectious disease of horses, donkeys, and mules that is caused by the bacterium *Pseudomonas mallei* and can be transmitted to humans. Symptoms include fever and inflammation of the lymph nodes (a form of the disease known as **farcy**), skin, and nasal mucous membranes. Administration of antibiotics is usually effective.

glandular fever (**glan**-dew-ler) *n.* an infectious disease, caused by the Epstein-Barr virus, that affects the lymph nodes in the neck, armpits, and groin. In the Western world, it mainly affects adolescents and young adults; in developing countries, young children are most affected. Symptoms include swelling and tenderness of the lymph nodes, fever, headache, a sore throat, lethargy, and loss of appetite. Glandular fever is diagnosed by the presence of large numbers of monocytes in the blood. Medical name: **infectious mononucleosis**.

glans (glans penis) (glanz) *n.* the acorn-shaped end part of the penis, formed by the expanded end of the corpus spongiosum. The term glans is also applied to the end of the clitoris.

glare (glair) *n.* the undesirable effects of scattered stray light on the retina, causing reduced contrast and visual performance as well as annoyance and discomfort.

Glasgow Coma Scale (GCS, Glasgow scoring system) (**glahz**-goh) *n.* a numerical system used to estimate a patient's level of consciousness after head injury. Each of the following are numerically graded: eye opening (1–4), motor response (1–6), and verbal response (1–5). The higher the score, the greater the level of consciousness: a score of 7 indicates a coma.

glatiramer (glă-**ti**-ră-mer) *n.* a drug that modifies the body's immune response and is used to treat multiple sclerosis and reduce the frequency of relapses in people with relapsing/remitting multiple sclerosis. It is administered by subcutaneous injection. Trade name: **Copaxone**.

glaucoma (glaw-**koh**-mă) *n.* a condition in which loss of retinal nerve fibres leads to loss of vision, the most significant risk factor being raised pressure in the eye. **angle-closure** (or **acute**) **g.** primary glaucoma in which there is a sudden rise in pressure due to blockage of the angle between the junction of the cornea and sclera and the margin of the iris, where aqueous humour usually drains from the eye. It is accompanied by sudden and severe pain and marked blurring of vision. **open-angle** (or **chronic simple**) **g.** a more common form of primary glaucoma in which the pressure increases gradually, usually without symptoms, and the visual loss is insidious. **primary g.** glaucoma that occurs without any other ocular disease. It is an important cause of blindness. **secondary g.** glaucoma that may occur when other ocular disease impairs the normal circulation of the aqueous humour and causes the intraocular pressure to rise.

Gleason grade (glee-sŏn) *n.* the grade (from one to five) given to an area of prostate cancer, reflecting the level of differentiation of the tumour. Higher grades indicate poorer differentiation. [D. F. Gleason (1920–2008), US pathologist]

Gleason score *n.* a numerical score from two to ten, which is the sum of the two Gleason grades given to the most common and second most common pattern of prostate cancer seen in the tumour. [D. F. Gleason]

gleet (gleet) *n.* a discharge of purulent mucus from the penis or vagina resulting from chronic gonorrhoea.

glenohumeral (glee-noh-**hew**-mer-ăl) *adj.* relating to the glenoid cavity and the humerus: the region of the shoulder joint.

glenoid cavity (glenoid fossa) (**glee**-noid) *n.* the socket of the shoulder joint: the pear-shaped cavity at the top of the scapula into which the head of the humerus fits.

gli- (glio-) *combining form denoting* **1.** glia. **2.** a glutinous substance.

glia (neuroglia) (glee-ă) *n.* the special connective tissue of the central nervous system. Glial cells outnumber the neurons by between five and ten to one, and make up some 40% of the total volume of the brain and spinal cord. **—glial** *adj.*

glibenclamide (gly-**ben**-klă-myd) *n.* a long-acting oral hypoglycaemic drug that reduces the level of sugar in the blood and is administered by mouth to treat type 2 diabetes (*see* sulphonylurea). It is not recommended for the elderly.

gliclazide (**gly**-klă-zyd) *n.* the most commonly prescribed sulphonylurea oral hypoglycaemic drug used in the treatment of type 2 diabetes. Trade name: **Diamicron**.

glioblastoma (glioblastoma multiforme) (gly-oh-blast-**oh**-mă) *n.* the most aggressive type of brain tumour derived from glial tissue. Its rapid enlargement destroys normal brain cells, with a progressive loss of function, and raises intracranial pressure, causing headache, vomiting, and drowsiness.

glioma (gly-**oh**-mă) *n.* any tumour of glial cells in the nervous system. The term is sometimes used for all tumours that arise in the central nervous system.

gliomyoma (gly-oh-my-**oh**-mă) *n.* a tumour composed of nervous and muscular tissue.

glipizide (**glip**-i-zyd) *n.* a short-acting drug used to control high blood-glucose levels (hyperglycaemia) in patients with type 2 diabetes after diet control has failed (*see* sulphonylurea). It is administered by mouth. Trade name: **Minodiab**.

Glivec (glee-vek) *n. see* imatinib.

globin (gloh-bin) *n.* a protein, found in the body, that can combine with iron-containing groups to form haemoglobin and myoglobin.

globulin (glob-yoo-lin) *n.* one of a group of simple proteins that are soluble in dilute salt solutions and can be coagulated by heat. **serum g.** any of the different globulins present in the blood, including gammaglobulins. Some have important functions as antibodies (*see* immunoglobulin). *See also* hormone-binding globulins.

globulinuria (glob-yoo-lin-yoor-iă) *n.* the presence in the urine of globulins.

globus (gloh-bŭs) *n.* a spherical or globe-shaped anatomical structure, such as the **g. pallidus** (*see* basal ganglia). **g. pharyngeus** (formerly **g. hystericus**) the sensation of having a lump in the throat, which is sometimes related to gastro-oesophageal reflux and tends to be worse during stress.

glomangioma (glomus tumour) (gloh-man-ji-oh-mă) *n. see* glomus.

glomerular filtration rate (GFR) (glom-e-roo-ler) *n.* the rate at which substances are filtered from the blood of the glomeruli into the Bowman's capsules of the nephrons. It is calculated by measuring the clearance of specific substances (e.g. creatinine) and is an index of renal function.

glomerulonephritis (glomerular nephritis, GN) (glom-e-roo-loh-ni-fry-tis) *n.* any of various conditions of the glomeruli (*see* glomerulus), not necessarily involving inflammation. It may be acute, with a nephritic or nephrotic syndrome; subacute, with rapidly declining renal function; or chronic.

glomerulus (glom-e-roo-lŭs) *n.* (*pl.* **glomeruli**) **1.** the network of blood capillaries contained within the cuplike end (Bowman's capsule) of a nephron. It is the site of primary filtration of waste products from the blood into the kidney tubule. **2.** any other small rounded mass. —**glomerular** *adj.*

glomus (gloh-mŭs) *n.* (*pl.* **glomera**) a small communication between a tiny artery and a vein that is well supplied with sensory receptors. For example, glomera in the skin of the limbs are concerned with temperature regulation. **g. jugulare** a collection of paraganglion cells in close relation to the internal jugular vein at its origin at the base of the skull.

glomus tumour *n.* **1.** a benign tumour arising from paraganglion cells associated with the vagus or glossopharyngeal nerves in the neck (*see* paraganglioma). In the middle ear they are called **glomus tympanicum tumours**; around the jugular vein they are called **glomus jugulare tumours**. **2. (glomangioma)** a harmless but often painful tumour produced by malformation and overgrowth of a glomus, usually in the skin at the ends of the fingers or toes.

gloss- (glosso-) *combining form denoting* the tongue.

glossa (glos-ă) *n. see* tongue.

glossectomy (glos-**ek**-tŏmi) *n.* surgical removal of the tongue, an operation usually carried out to remove a tumour.

glossitis (glos-**I**-tis) *n.* inflammation of the tongue.

glossodynia (glos-oh-**din**-iă) *n.* pain in the tongue.

glossopharyngeal nerve (glos-oh-fa-rin-**jee**-ăl) *n.* the ninth cranial nerve (IX), which supplies motor fibres to part of the pharynx and to the parotid salivary glands and sensory fibres to the posterior third of the tongue and the soft palate.

glossoplegia (glos-oh-**plee**-jiă) *n.* paralysis of the tongue.

glottis (**glot**-iss) *n.* the space between the two vocal folds. The term is often applied to the vocal folds themselves or to that part of the larynx associated with the production of sound.

gluc- (gluco-) *combining form denoting* glucose.

glucagon (**gloo**-kă-gon) *n.* a hormone, produced by the pancreas, that causes an increase in the blood sugar level. Glucagon is administered by injection to counteract diabetic hypoglycaemia. Trade name: **GlucaGen HypoKit**.

glucagonoma (gloo-kă-gŏn-**oh**-mă) *n.* a usually malignant pancreatic tumour that secretes glucagon and causes impaired glucose tolerance or diabetes, dermatitis, and weight loss.

glucagon stimulation test *n.* a test for phaeochromocytomas not displaying typically high levels of plasma catecholamines. An intravenous bolus of glucagon is administered and the test is positive when there is a threefold increase in plasma catecholamine levels with a consequent rise in blood pressure. The test is now rarely used.

glucocorticoid (gloo-koh-**kor**-ti-koid) *n.* any of a group of corticosteroids, including cortisone, that are essential for the utilization of carbohydrate, fat, and protein by the body. Naturally occurring and synthetic glucocorticoids have very powerful anti-inflammatory effects.

gluconeogenesis (gloo-koh-nee-oh-**jen**-i-sis) *n.* the biochemical process in which glucose is synthesized from non-carbohydrate sources, such as amino acids, when carbohydrate is not available in sufficient amounts in the diet.

glucose (dextrose) (**gloo**-kohz) *n.* a simple sugar containing six carbon atoms (a hexose). Glucose, an important source of energy, is one of the constituents of both sucrose and starch, both of which yield glucose after digestion. It is stored in the body in the form of glycogen. If the blood-glucose concentration falls below the normal level of around 5 mmol/l, neurological and other symptoms may result (*see* hypoglycaemia). If the blood-glucose level is raised to 10 mmol/l, the condition of hyperglycaemia develops. This is a symptom of diabetes mellitus. See illustration.

glucose-6-phosphate dehydrogenase deficiency *n.* a hereditary (X-linked) disorder in which absence of the enzyme

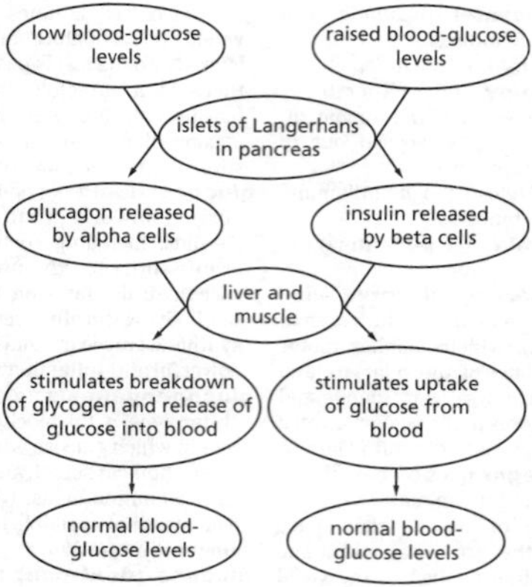

Regulation of blood-glucose levels

glucose-6-phosphate dehydrogenase (G6PD), which functions in carbohydrate metabolism, results in haemolysis, usually after exposure to oxidants (such as drugs) or infections. *See also* favism.

glucose tolerance test (oral glucose tolerance test, OGTT) *n.* the standard diagnostic test for diabetes mellitus and the related conditions, **impaired glucose tolerance (IGT)** and **impaired fasting glucose (IFG)** (known as **prediabetes** or **abnormal glucose regulation**). Blood-glucose level is measured after an overnight fast and again two hours after oral administration of 75 g glucose. Diabetes is diagnosed if the fasting level is above 7.0 mmol/l and/or the two-hour level is above 11.1 mmol/l. IGT is diagnosed when the fasting level is less than 7.0 nmol/1 and/or the two-hour level is 7.0–11.1 nmol/1, and IFG when the fasting level is 6.0–7.0 nmol/1 but the two-hour level is less than 7.8 nmol/1.

glucoside (gloo-koh-syd) *n.* *see* glycoside.

glucuronic acid (gloo-kewr-**on**-ik) *n.* a sugar acid derived from glucose. Glucuronic acid is an important constituent of chondroitin sulphate (found in cartilage) and hyaluronic acid (found in synovial fluid).

glue ear (gloo) *n.* a common condition in which viscous fluid accumulates in the middle ear, causing deafness. It is most frequently seen in children and is due to a malfunctioning of the Eustachian tube. Many cases resolve spontaneously; treatment, if required, consists of surgical incision of the eardrum (myringotomy), drainage of the fluid, and insertion of a grommet. Medical names: **otitis media with effusion**, **secretory otitis media**.

glutamic acid (glutamate) (gloo-**tam**-ik) *n. see* amino acid.

glutamic acid decarboxylase (GAD) *n.* a common enzyme that can provoke an autoimmune reaction against the beta cells of the pancreas progressing to type 1 diabetes mellitus.

glutamic oxaloacetic transaminase (GOT) *n. see* aspartate aminotransferase (AST).

glutamic pyruvic transaminase (GPT) *n. see* alanine aminotransferase (ALT).

glutaminase (gloo-**tam**-in-ayz) *n.* an enzyme, found in the kidney, that catalyses the breakdown of the amino acid glutamine to ammonia and glutamic acid: a stage in the production of urea.

glutamine (**gloo**-tă-meen) *n. see* amino acid.

gluten (**gloo**-tĕn) *n.* a mixture of the two proteins **gliadin** and **glutenin**. Gluten is present in wheat and rye and is important for its baking properties. Sensitivity to gluten leads to coeliac disease in children.

gluteus (gloo-**tee**-ŭs) *n.* one of three paired muscles of the buttocks (**g. maximus**, **g. medius**, and **g. minimus**). They are responsible for movements of the thigh. —**gluteal** *adj.*

glyc- (glyco-) *combining form denoting* sugar.

glycaemic index (GI) (glI-**see**-mik) *n.* a ranking system measuring the effect carbohydrate (CHO) ingestion has on blood glucose levels. Glucose is used as the reference value (50 g glucose has a GI of 100).

A portion of food containing 50 g CHO is ingested and the effect on blood glucose levels measured over a three-hour period and compared to the effect of 50 g of glucose. Foods with a low GI (<60) are slowly absorbed, causing a lower and more prolonged increase in blood glucose levels than foods with a high GI (<70). Low GI foods help with diabetes control and may be beneficial in the treatment of polycystic ovary syndrome.

glycated haemoglobin (glycosylated haemoglobin, HbA_{1c}) (gly-**kayt**-id) *n.* a derivative of haemoglobin in which a glucose molecule is attached to the haemoglobin molecule. Levels of HbA_{1c} are significantly increased in diabetes mellitus. The percentage of the haemoglobin molecules that become glycated is dependent on the general level of glucose in the plasma over the lifetime of the molecule (generally 3 months); HbA_{1c} values are therefore used as the standard measure of the degree of control of hyperglycaemia in a person with diabetes over this period.

glycerin (glycerol) (**glis**-er-in) *n.* a clear viscous liquid obtained by hydrolysis of fats and mixed oils and produced as a by-product in the manufacture of soap. It is used as an emollient in many skin preparations, as a laxative (particularly in the form of suppositories), and as a sweetening agent in the pharmaceutical industry.

glyceryl trinitrate (nitroglycerin) (**glis**-er-il try-**ny**-trayt) *n.* a drug that dilates blood vessels and is used mainly to prevent and treat angina (*see* vasodilator) but also to treat anal fissures. It is administered as sublingual tablets, a mouth spray, skin patches or ointment, a rectal ointment, or an intravenous infusion. Trade names: **Deponit**, **Glytrin Spray**, **Nitrolingual Pumpspray**, **Percutol**, **Rectogesic**, **Transiderm-Nitro**.

glycine (**gly**-seen) *n.* *see* amino acid.

glycocholic acid (gly-koh-**kol**-ik) *n.* *see* bile acids.

glycogen (**gly**-koh-jĕn) *n.* a carbohydrate consisting of branched chains of glucose units. Glycogen is the principal form in which carbohydrate is stored in the body (in liver and muscles); it may be readily broken down to glucose.

glycogenesis (gly-koh-**jen**-i-sis) *n.* the biochemical process, occurring chiefly in the liver and in muscle, by which glucose is converted into glycogen.

glycogenolysis (gly-koh-jĕ-**nol**-i-sis) *n.* a biochemical process, occurring chiefly in the liver and in muscle, by which glycogen is broken down into glucose.

glycolysis (gly-**kol**-i-sis) *n.* the conversion of glucose, by a series of ten enzyme-catalysed reactions, to lactic acid, with the production of energy in the form of ATP.

glycoprotein (gly-koh-**proh**-teen) *n.* one of a group of compounds consisting of a protein combined with a carbohydrate (such as galactose or mannose). Examples of glycoproteins are certain enzymes, hormones, and antigens.

glycoside (**gly**-koh-syd) *n.* a compound formed by replacing the hydroxyl group (–OH) of a sugar by another group. (If the sugar is glucose the compound is known as a **glucoside**.) Glycosides derived from plants include some pharmacologically important products. **cardiac g.** a drug, such as digoxin (derived from digitalis), that increases the force of heart muscle contraction.

glycosuria (gly-kohs-**yoor**-iă) *n.* the presence of glucose in the urine in abnormally large amounts. Glycosuria may be associated with diabetes mellitus, kidney disease, and some other conditions.

glycosylated haemoglobin (gly-**koh**-si-layt-id) *n.* *see* glycated haemoglobin.

GN *n. see* glomerulonephritis.

gnath- (gnatho-) *combining form denoting* the jaw.

gnathoplasty (nath-oh-plasti) *n.* plastic surgery of the jaw.

GnRH *n. see* gonadotrophin-releasing hormone.

GnRH analogue *n. see* gonadorelin analogue.

goal (gohl) *n.* a statement of what the nursing intervention is intended to achieve, usually expressed in terms of the patient's expected behaviour. *See* behavioural objective, expected outcome.

goblet cell (gob-lit) *n.* a column-shaped secretory cell found in the epithelium of the respiratory and intestinal tracts. Goblet cells secrete the principal constituents of mucus.

goitre (goi-ter) *n.* a swelling of the neck due to enlargement of the thyroid gland. This may be due to lack of dietary iodine, which is necessary for the production of thyroid hormone: the gland enlarges in an attempt to increase the output of hormone. Autoimmune thyroiditis can be associated with goitre (*see* Hashimoto's disease). **exophthalmic g.** (**Graves' disease**) *see* thyrotoxicosis. **sporadic g.** goitre due to simple overgrowth (hyperplasia) of the gland or to a tumour.

goitrogen (goi-troh-jen) *n.* any substance that causes goitre. **—goitrogenic** *adj.*

gold (gohld) *n.* (in pharmacology) a compound of the metal gold, used in the treatment of rheumatoid arthritis. **Sodium aurothiomalate** (Myocrisin) is administered by intramuscular injection.

GOLD (Global Initiative for Chronic Obstructive Lung Disease) *n.* a body that works with health-care professionals and public health officials around the world to raise awareness of chronic obstructive pulmonary disease (COPD) and to improve prevention and treatment of COPD.

Goldmann applanation tonometer (gohld-măn) *n. see* tonometer. [H. Goldmann (1899–1991), Swiss ophthalmologist]

golfer's elbow (golf-erz) *n.* inflammation of the origin of the common flexor tendon on the medial epicondyle of the humerus, caused by overuse of the forearm muscles. Treatment is by rest, a brace, anti-inflammatory medication, or steroid injection. *Compare* tennis elbow.

Golgi apparatus (gol-ji) *n.* a collection of vesicles and folded membranes in a cell. It stores and later transports the proteins manufactured in the endoplasmic reticulum. [C. Golgi (1844–1926), Italian histologist]

Golgi cells *pl. n.* types of neurons (nerve cells) within the central nervous system. **Golgi type I neurons** have very long axons that connect different parts of the system; **Golgi type II neurons** have only short axons or sometimes none.

gomphosis (gom-foh-sis) *n.* a form of synarthrosis (immovable joint) in which a conical process fits into a socket.

gonad (goh-nad) *n.* a male or female reproductive organ, which produces the gametes. *See* ovary, testis.

gonadarche (goh-năd-ar-ki) *n.* the period during which the gonads begin to secrete sex hormones, so triggering puberty. The timing for this event is controlled by the pituitary gland; gonadarche occurs usually between the ages of 10 and 11 in girls and 11 and 12 in boys.

gonadorelin analogue (GnRH analogue, LHRH analogue) (gon-ă-doh-rel-in) *n.* a synthetic analogue of gonadotrophin-releasing hormone, which stimulates the production of pituitary gonadotrophins (luteinizing hormone and follicle-stimulating hormone). Gonadorelin analogues include **goserelin** (Novgos, Zoladex), **leuprorelin** (Prostap), and **triptorelin** (Decapeptyl, Gonapeptyl Depot, Salvacyl). Administered by subcutaneous or intramuscular injection, nasal spray, or implant, they are used in the treatment of endometriosis, fibroids, some types of infertility, and advanced prostate cancer. *See also* buserelin.

gonadotrophin (gonadotrophic hormone) (gon-ă-doh-troh-fin) *n.* any of several hormones synthesized and released by the pituitary gland, such as follicle-stimulating hormone and luteinizing hormone, that act on the gonads to promote production of sex hormones and either sperm or ova. *See also* human chorionic gonadotrophin.

gonadotrophin-releasing hormone (GnRH, gonadorelin) *n.* a peptide hormone produced in the hypothalamus and transported via the bloodstream to the pituitary gland, where it controls the synthesis and release of other hormones, the pituitary gonadotrophins.

GnRH analogue *see* gonadorelin analogue.

gonagra (gon-ag-ră) *n.* gout in the knee.

goni- (gonio-) *combining form denoting* an anatomical angle or corner.

gonioscope (goh-ni-oh-skohp) *n.* a special lens used for viewing the structures around the edge of the anterior chamber of the eye (in front of the iris).

goniotomy (trabeculotomy) (goh-ni-**ot**-ŏmi) *n.* an operation for congenital glaucoma (*see* buphthalmos) in which a fine knife is used to make an incision into the blocked trabecular meshwork from within the eye.

gonococcus (gon-oh-**kok**-ŭs) *n.* (*pl.* **gonococci**) the causative agent of gonorrhoea: the bacterium *Neisseria gonorrhoeae*. **—gonococcal** *adj.*

gonocyte (gon-oh-syt) *n. see* germ cell.

gonorrhoea (gon-ŏ-ree-ă) *n.* a sexually transmitted disease, caused by the bacterium *Neisseria gonorrhoeae*, that affects the genital mucous membranes of either sex. Symptoms include pain on passing urine and discharge of gleet. In untreated cases, the infection may spread throughout the reproductive system, causing sterility; severe inflammation of the urethra in men can cause stricture. If a pregnant woman has gonorrhoea, her baby may contract ophthalmia neonatorum. Later complications can include arthritis, endocarditis, and infection of the eyes, causing conjunctivitis. Treatment with ciprofloxacin, ofloxacin, or cefotaxime is usually effective. —**gonorrhoeal** *adj.*

Goodpasture's syndrome (guud-pas-cherz) *n.* a haemorrhagic lung disorder, resulting in the coughing up of blood, associated with glomerulonephritis. [E. W. Goodpasture (1886–1960), US pathologist]

gooseflesh (goos-flesh) *n.* the reaction of the skin to cold or fear. The blood vessels contract and the small muscle attached to the base of each hair follicle also contracts, causing the hairs to stand up: this gives the skin an appearance of plucked goose skin.

GOR *n. see* gastro-oesophageal reflux.

Gordh needle (gord) *n.* an intravenous needle with an expanded base containing a rubber diaphragm, used to administer repeated injections. [T. Gordh, Swedish anaesthetist]

gorget (gor-jit) *n.* an instrument formerly used in the operation for removal of stones from the bladder. It is a director or guide with a wide groove.

goserelin (gos-ĕ-**rel**-in) *n. see* gonadorelin analogue.

gouge (gowj) *n.* a curved chisel used in orthopaedic operations to cut and remove bone.

gout (gowt) *n.* a disease in which a defect in purine metabolism causes an excess of uric acid and its salts (urates) to accumulate in the bloodstream and the joints respectively. It results in attacks of acute gouty arthritis and chronic destruction of the joints and deposits of urates (tophi) in the skin and cartilage, especially of the ears. Long-term treatment with uricosuric drugs or allopurinol can control the disease; acute attacks are treated with anti-inflammatory analgesics, colchicine, or corticosteroids. *See also* podagra.

GPI *n. see* general paralysis of the insane.

Graafian follicle (**grah**-fi-ăn) *n.* a mature follicle in the ovary prior to ovulation, containing a large fluid-filled cavity that distends the surface of the ovary. The oocyte develops inside the follicle, attached to one side. [R. de Graaf (1641–73), Dutch physician and anatomist]

grade (grayd) *n.* the severity of a malignant tumour according to its degree of differentiation. Low-grade tumours (grade 1) closely resemble normal tissues, are well differentiated, and have a good prognosis. High-grade tumours (grade 3) show a poor resemblance to normal tissues, are poorly differentiated, and have a poor prognosis.

graded self-exposure (gray-did self-iks-**poh**-*zh*er) *n.* a technique used in the behaviour therapy of phobias. A hierarchy of fears (increasingly fearful stimuli) is set up and the patients expose themselves to each level of the hierarchy in turn. Exposure continues until habituation occurs; the patient then proceeds to the next highest level of the hierarchy. The patient is ultimately able to cope with the feared object or situation.

Graefe's knife (gray-fiz) *n.* a knife with a narrow sharply pointed blade, used in operations for the removal of cataract. [A. von Graefe (1928–70), German ophthalmologist]

GRAF PIF (General Risk Assessment for Pediatric Inpatient Falls) *n.* a US predictive tool for assessing the risk of falls in hospitalized children. It assesses developmental, environmental, and situational risks to prevent falls and raise parental awareness of hazard.

graft (grahft) **1.** *n.* any organ, tissue, or object used for transplantation to replace a faulty part of the body. **bone g.** bone or a bonelike synthetic substance used to fill a defect in a bone or to augment bone formation. **corneal g.** *see* keratoplasty. *See also* coronary artery bypass graft, skin (graft), transplantation. **2.** *vb.* to transplant an organ or tissue.

graft-versus-host disease (GVHD) *n.* a condition that occurs following bone marrow transplantation and sometimes blood transfusion, in which lymphocytes from the graft attack specific tissues in the host. The skin, gut, and liver are the most severely affected. Drugs that suppress the immune reaction (such as steroids and ciclosporin) and antibodies directed against lymphocytes reduce the severity of the tissue damage.

grain (grayn) *n.* a unit of mass equal to 1/7000 of a pound (avoirdupois). 1 grain = 0.0648 gram.

gram (gram) *n.* a unit of mass equal to one thousandth of a kilogram. Symbol: g.

-gram *combining form denoting* a record; tracing.

Gram's stain (gramz) *n.* a method of staining bacterial cells, used as a primary means of identification. The bacterial cells are stained with a violet dye, treated with decolorizer (e.g. alcohol), and then counterstained with red dye. **Gram-negative** bacteria lose the initial stain but take up the counterstain, so that they appear red microscopically. **Gram-positive** bacteria retain the initial stain, appearing violet microscopically. [H. C. J. Gram (1853–1938), Danish physician]

grand mal (major epilepsy) (gron mal) *n. see* epilepsy.

grand multiparity (grand multi-pa-riti) *n.* the condition of a woman who has had five or more previous pregnancies. Such women are more prone to fetal malpresentations, postpartum haemorrhage, and rupture of the uterus.

granular cast (gran-yoo-ler) *n.* a cellular cast derived from a kidney tubule. Such casts are shed from the kidney in certain kidney diseases, notably acute glomerulonephritis. Their presence in the urine indicates continued activity of the disease.

granulation (gran-yoo-**lay**-shŏn) *n.* the formation of a multicellular mass of tissue (**g. tissue**) in response to an injury: this is an essential part of the healing process. The tissue contains many new blood vessels and many fibroblasts.

granulocyte (gran-yoo-loh-syt) *n.* any of a group of white blood cells that contain granules in their cytoplasm. They can be subclassified into neutrophils, eosinophils, and basophils.

granulocytopenia (gran-yoo-loh-sy-toh-**pee**-niă) *n.* a reduction in the number of granulocytes in the blood. *See* neutropenia.

granuloma (gran-yoo-**loh**-mă) *n.* (*pl.* **granulomata** or **granulomas**) a localized collection of cells, produced in response to chronic infection, inflammation, or a foreign body, that is characterized by the presence of epithelioid histiocytes. **g. annulare** a chronic skin condition, of unknown cause, in which there is a ring or rings of closely set papules, principally on the hands and arms. **g. inguinale** a sexually transmitted disease caused by the bacterium *Calymmatobacterium granulomatis*, marked by a pimply rash on and around the genital organs, which develops into a granulomatous ulcer. *See also* pyogenic (granuloma). **—granulomatous** *adj.*

granulomatosis (gran-yoo-loh-mă-**toh**-sis) *n.* any condition marked by multiple widespread granulomata. **g. with polyangiitis** (**GPA**) (po-li-an-gi-**I**-tis) an autoimmune disease, formerly known as **Wegener's granulomatosis**, affecting the sinuses, lungs, and kidneys and characterized by blood-vessel inflammation and the formation of necrotizing granulomas. Untreated, it is usually fatal but it can be controlled with corticosteroids, cyclophosphamide, or rituximab.

granulopoiesis (gran-yoo-loh-poi-**ee**-sis) *n.* the process of production of granulocytes, which normally occurs in the blood-forming tissue of the bone marrow. *See also* haemopoiesis.

graph- (grapho-) *combining form denoting* handwriting.

-graph *combining form denoting* an instrument that records.

grattage (grat-**ahzh**) *n.* the process of brushing or scraping the surface of a slowly healing ulcer or wound to remove granulation tissue, which may delay healing.

gravel (**grav**-ĕl) *n.* small stones formed in the urinary tract. The passage of gravel from the kidneys is usually associated with severe pain (ureteric colic) and may cause blood in the urine. *See also* calculus.

Graves' disease (exophthalmic goitre) (grayvz) *n. see* thyrotoxicosis. [R. J. Graves (1797–1853), Irish physician]

gravid (**grav**-id) *adj.* currently pregnant.

gravidity (gră-**vid**-iti) *n.* the status of a woman regarding the total number of pregnancies she has had (including the current one). *Compare* parity.

Grawitz tumour (**grah**-vits) *n. see* renal cell carcinoma. [P. A. Grawitz (1850–1932), German pathologist]

gray (gray) *n.* the SI unit of absorbed dose of ionizing radiation, being the absorbed dose when the energy per unit mass imparted to matter by ionizing radiation is 1 joule per kilogram. It has replaced the rad. Symbol: Gy.

green monkey disease *n. see* Marburg disease.

greenstick fracture (green-stik) *n. see* fracture.

grey matter (gray) *n.* the darker coloured tissues of the central nervous system, composed mainly of the cell bodies of neurons, branching dendrites, and glial cells. *Compare* white matter.

Grey Turner sign (gray ter-ner) *n.* a bluish bruiselike appearance around the flanks, which is seen in acute pancreatitis. [G. Grey Turner (1877–1951), British surgeon]

Griffith's types (grif-iths) *pl. n.* subdivisions of Lancefield group A streptococci (*see* Lancefield classification) on the basis of their agglutination reactions. [F. Griffith (1877–1941), British bacteriologist]

gripe (gryp) *n.* spasmodic abdominal pain or discomfort (*see* colic).

griseofulvin (griz-i-oh-**ful**-vin) *n.* an antifungal drug administered by mouth or topically to treat fungal infections of the hair, skin, and nails, such as ringworm. Trade names: **Fulsovin**, **Grisol AF**.

grocer's itch (groh-serz) *n.* dermatitis of the hands caused by frequent contact with flour and sugar.

groin (groin) *n.* the external depression on the front of the body that marks the junction of the abdomen with either of the thighs. *See also* inguinal.

grounded theory (grownd-id) *n.* a theory or hypothesis developed from data generated from interviews and observations of people in their own environment.

ground substance (grownd) *n. see* connective tissue.

group practice (groop) *n.* a partnership of two or more general practitioners who share such resources as premises and administrative and nursing staff. The premises from which they operate may be privately owned or a publicly owned health centre.

group therapy *n.* **1. (group psychotherapy)** psychotherapy involving at least two patients and a therapist. The patients are encouraged to understand and analyse their own and one another's problems. *See also* psychodrama. **2.** therapy in which people with the same problem, such as alcoholism or phobias, meet and discuss together their difficulties and possible ways of overcoming them.

growth factor (grohth) *n.* a polypeptide that is produced by cells and stimulates them to proliferate. Some are involved in the abnormal regulation of growth seen in cancer.

growth hormone (GH, somatotrophin) *n.* a hormone, synthesized and stored in the anterior pituitary gland, that promotes growth of the long bones in the limbs and increases protein synthesis (via somatomedin). Its release is controlled by the opposing actions of **growth-hormone releasing hormone** and somatostatin.

GTN *n. see* glyceryl trinitrate.

guanethidine (gwahn-**eth**-i-deen) *n.* a drug that is occasionally used (administered by intramuscular injection) to rapidly reduce very high blood pressure resistant to other treatments (*see* sympatholytic).

guanine (gwah-neen) *n.* one of the nitrogen-containing bases (*see* purine) that occurs in the nucleic acids DNA and RNA.

gubernaculum (gew-ber-**nak**-yoo-lŭm) *n.* (*pl.* **gubernacula**) either of a pair of fibrous strands of tissue that connect the gonads to the inguinal region in the fetus.

Guedel airway (gwed-ĕl) *n.* an oropharyngeal airway used in anaesthesia and resuscitation. [A. E. Guedel (20th century), US anaesthetist]

Guillain-Barré syndrome (post-infective polyneuropathy) (gee-**yan** ba-**ray**) *n.* a disease of the peripheral nerves in which there is numbness and weakness in the limbs. It usually develops 1–28 days after a respiratory or gastrointestinal infection: antibodies against the pathogen's cell surface antigens attack similar antigens on the myelin sheaths of the host's peripheral nerves. [G. Guillain (1876–1961) and A. Barré (1880–1967), French neurologists]

guillotine (gil-ŏ-teen) *n.* **1.** a surgical instrument used for removing the tonsils. **2.** an encircling suture to control the escape of fluid or blood from an orifice or to close a gap.

guinea worm (ginn-i) *n.* a parasitic nematode worm, *Dracunculus medinensis*. The adult female lives in the connective tissues beneath the skin and releases its larvae into a large blister on the legs or arms. *See also* dracontiasis.

Gulf War syndrome (gulf wor) *n.* a variety of symptoms, mainly neurological (including chronic fatigue, dizziness, amnesia, digestive upsets, and muscle wasting), that have been attributed to exposure of armed forces personnel to chemicals (e.g. insecticides) used during the Gulf War (1991) or possibly to the effects of vaccines and tablets given to protect personnel against the anticipated threat of chemical and biological warfare during the conflict.

gullet (**gul**-it) *n. see* oesophagus.

gum (gum) *n.* (in anatomy) *see* gingiva.

GUM *n. see* genitourinary (medicine).

gumboil (**gum**-boil) *n.* the opening on the surface of the gum of a sinus tract from a chronic abscess associated with the roots of a tooth. It may be accompanied by varying degrees of swelling, pain, and discharge.

gumma (**gum**-ă) *n.* a small soft tumour, characteristic of the tertiary stage of syphilis, that occurs in connective tissue, the liver, brain, testes, heart, or bone.

GUS *n.* genitourinary system. *See* genitourinary.

gustation (gus-**tay**-shŏn) *n.* the sense of taste or the act of tasting.

gustatory (**gus**-tă-ter-i) *adj.* relating to the sense of taste or to the organs of taste.

gut (gut) *n.* **1.** *see* intestine. **2.** *see* catgut.

Guthrie test (heel-prick blood test) (**guth**-ri) *n.* a blood test performed on all newborn babies at the end of the first week of life. It can detect several inborn errors of metabolism (including phenylketonuria), hypothyroidism, and cystic fibrosis (the last is not routinely offered). [R. Guthrie (1916–95), US paediatrician]

gutta (gut-ă) *n.* (*pl.* **guttae**) (in pharmacy) a drop. Drops are the form in which many medicines are applied to the eyes and ears.

gutta-percha (gut-ă-per-chă) *n.* the juice of an evergreen Malaysian tree, which is hard at room temperature but becomes soft and plastic when heated in hot water. On cooling gutta-percha will retain any shape imparted to it when hot; in dentistry it is used in root fillings.

gutter splint (gut-er) *n.* a splint formed from a casting material, moulded to conform to the shape of the limb but not encircling it, in which the limb rests as in a gutter.

GVHD *n.* *see* graft-versus-host disease.

gyn- (gyno-, gynaec(o)-) *combining form denoting* women or the female reproductive organs.

gynaecology (gy-ni-**kol**-ŏji) *n.* the study of diseases of women and girls, particularly those affecting the female reproductive system. *Compare* obstetrics. **—gynaecological** *adj.* **—gynaecologist** *n.*

SEE WEB LINKS
- Guidance from NICE focusing on gynaecological conditions
- Introduction to gynaecology from the GP Notebook website

gynaecomastia (gy-ni-koh-**mas**-tiă) *n.* enlargement of the breasts in the male, due either to hormone imbalance or to drug (e.g. hormone) therapy.

gypsum (jip-sŭm) *n.* *see* plaster of Paris.

gyr- (gyro-) *combining form denoting* **1.** a gyrus. **2.** a ring or circle.

gyrus (jy-rŭs) *n.* (*pl.* **gyri**) a raised convolution of the cerebral cortex, between two sulci (clefts).

Hh

H *symbol for* hydrogen.

habit (**hab**-it) *n.* a constant, almost automatic, practice acquired by frequent repetition. **h. training** teaching patients to learn or relearn habits of personal hygiene by repetition and encouragement.

habituation (hă-bit-yoo-**ay**-shŏn) *n.* **1.** (in psychology) a simple form of learning consisting of a gradual waning response by the subject to a continuous or repeated stimulus that is not associated with reinforcement. **2.** (in pharmacology) the condition of being psychologically dependent on a drug, following repeated consumption. It is marked by reduced sensitivity to its effects and a craving for the drug if it is withdrawn. *See also* dependence.

HADS *n. see* Hospital Anxiety and Depression Scale.

haem (heem) *n.* an iron-containing compound (a porphyrin) that combines with the protein globin to form haemoglobin.

haem- (haema-, haemo-, haemat(o)-) *combining form denoting* blood.

haemagglutination (heem-ă-gloo-tin-**ay**-shŏn) *n.* the clumping of red blood cells (*see* agglutination). It is caused by an antibody–antigen reaction of some viruses and other substances.

haemangioma (heem-an-ji-**oh**-mă) *n.* a benign tumour of blood vessels. It often appears on the skin as a type of birthmark (*see* naevus). *See also* angioma.

haemarthrosis (heem-arth-**roh**-sis) *n.* bleeding within a joint, which may follow injury or may occur spontaneously in bleeding disorders, such as haemophilia.

haematemesis (heem-ă-**tem**-i-sis) *n.* the act of vomiting fresh blood. The blood may have been swallowed but more often arises from bleeding in the oesophagus, stomach, or duodenum. Common causes are peptic ulcers and oesophageal varices (varicose veins).

haematin (**heem**-ă-tin) *n.* a chemical derivative of haemoglobin formed by removal of the protein part of the molecule and oxidation of the iron atom from the ferrous to the ferric form.

haematinic (heem-ă-**tin**-ik) *n.* a drug that increases the amount of haemoglobin in the blood, e.g. ferrous sulphate and other iron-containing compounds. Haematinics are administered to prevent and treat anaemia due to iron deficiency, particularly during pregnancy.

haematocele (**heem**-ă-toh-seel) *n.* a swelling caused by leakage of blood into a cavity, especially that of the membrane overlying the front and sides of the testis.

parametric (**pelvic**) **h.** a swelling near the uterus formed by the escape of blood, usually from a Fallopian tube in ectopic pregnancy.

haematocolpos (heem-ă-toh-**kol**-pos) *n.* distention of the vagina with blood due to an imperforate hymen. *See* cryptomenorrhoea.

haematocrit (heem-ă-toh-krit) *n. see* packed cell volume.

haematocyst (heem-ă-toh-sist) *n.* a cyst containing blood.

haematogenous (haematogenic) (heem-ă-**toj**-in-ŭs) *adj.* **1.** relating to the production of blood or its constituents. **2.** produced by, originating in, or carried by the blood.

haematology (heem-ă-**tol**-ŏji) *n.* the study of blood and blood-forming tissues and the disorders associated with them. **—haematological** (heem-ă-tŏ-**loj**-ik-ăl) *adj.* **—haematologist** *n.*

haematoma (heem-ă-**toh**-mă) *n.* an accumulation of blood within the tissues that clots to form a solid swelling. Injury, disease of the blood vessels, or a clotting disorder of the blood are the usual causative factors. **extradural h.** a haematoma caused by tearing of the middle meningeal artery, as a result of injury to the head. **intracerebral h.** a haematoma caused by bleeding into the brain resulting either from atherosclerosis of the cerebral arteries and high blood pressure or from severe head injury. subdural h. (SDH) a haematoma caused by tearing of the veins where they cross the space beneath the dura. *See also* perianal haematoma.

haematometra (heem-ă-toh-**mee**-tră) *n.* **1.** accumulation of menstrual blood in the uterus. **2.** abnormally copious bleeding in the uterus.

haematomyelia (heem-ă-toh-my-ee-liă) *n.* bleeding into the tissue of the spinal cord.

haematopoiesis (heem-ă-toh-poi-ee-sis) *n. see* haemopoiesis.

haematoporphyrin (heem-ă-toh-por-fi-rin) *n.* a type of porphyrin produced during the metabolism of haemoglobin.

haematosalpinx (haemosalpinx) (heem-ă-toh-**sal**-pinks) *n.* the accumulation of menstrual blood in the Fallopian tubes.

haematoxylin (heem-ă-**toks**-i-lin) *n.* a colourless crystalline compound extracted from logwood (*Haematoxylon campechianum*) and used in various histological stains.

haematozoon (heem-ă-toh-**zoh**-on) *n.* (*pl.* **haematozoa**) any animal parasite living in the blood.

haematuria (heem-a-**tewr**-ia) *n.* the passage of blood in the urine, which may be detected by the naked eye (**frank, macroscopic**, or **visible h.**), or urine microscopy or urine dipsticks (**microscopic** or **nonvisible h.**). Haematuria is associated with transitional cell carcinoma (the most common form of bladder cancer), kidney cancer, urinary-tract infections, stone disease, and some forms of glomerulonephritis.

haemin (heem-in) *n.* a chemical derivative of haemoglobin formed by removal of the protein part of the molecule, oxidation of the iron atom, and combination with an acid to form a salt. *Compare* haematin.

haemo- *combining form. see* haem-.

haemochromatosis (bronze diabetes, iron-storage disease) (heem-ŏ-kroh-mă-**toh**-sis) *n.* a hereditary (autosomal recessive) disorder in which there is excessive absorption and storage of iron. This leads to damage of many organs, including the liver, pancreas, and endocrine glands. The main features are a bronze colour of the skin, diabetes, and liver failure. *Compare* haemosiderosis.

haemoconcentration (hee-moh-kon-sĕn-**tray**-shŏn) *n.* an increase in the proportion of red blood cells relative to the plasma, brought about by a decrease in the volume of plasma or an increase in the concentration of circulating red blood cells (*see* polycythaemia). *Compare* haemodilution.

haemocytometer (hee-moh-sy-**tom**-it-er) *n.* a special glass chamber of known volume into which diluted blood is introduced. The numbers of the various blood cells present are then counted visually, through a microscope.

haemodialysis (hee-moh-dy-**al**-i-sis) *n.* a technique of removing waste materials or poisons from the blood using the principle of dialysis. Haemodialysis is performed on patients whose kidneys have ceased to function; the process takes place in a **dialyser**.

haemodilution (hee-moh-dy-**lew**-shŏn) *n.* a decrease in the proportion of red blood cells relative to the plasma, brought about by an increase in the total volume of plasma. *Compare* haemoconcentration.

haemoglobin (Hb) (hee-moh-**gloh**-bin) *n.* a substance contained within the red blood cells (erythrocytes) and responsible for their colour, composed of the pigment haem linked to the protein globin. Haemoglobin is the medium by which oxygen is transported within the body. Blood normally contains 115 to 180g/l of haemoglobin. *See also* myoglobin, oxyhaemoglobin.

haemoglobinaemia (heem-ŏ-gloh-bin-**ee**-miă) *n.* the presence of haemoglobin in the blood plasma.

haemoglobinometer (heem-ŏ-gloh-bin-**om**-it-er) *n.* an instrument for determining the concentration of haemoglobin in a sample of blood.

haemoglobinopathy (heem-ŏ-gloh-bin-**op**-ă-thi) *n.* any of a group of inherited diseases, including thalassaemia and sickle-cell disease, in which there is an abnormality in the production of haemoglobin.

haemoglobinuria (heem-ŏ-gloh-bin-**yoor**-iă) *n.* the presence in the urine of free haemoglobin. The condition sometimes follows strenuous exercise. It is also associated with certain infectious diseases, ingestion of certain chemicals, and injury.

haemogram (**hee**-moh-gram) *n.* the results of a routine blood test, including an estimate of the blood haemoglobin level, packed cell volume, and blood count.

haemolysin (hi-mol-i-sin) *n.* *see* lysin.

haemolysis (hi-mol-i-sis) *n.* the destruction of red blood cells (erythrocytes). Within the body, haemolysis may result from poisoning, infection, or the action of antibodies; it may occur in mismatched blood transfusions. It usually leads to anaemia. *See also* laking.

haemolytic (hee-moh-lit-ik) *adj.* causing, associated with, or resulting from destruction of red blood cells (erythrocytes). **h. anaemia** *see* anaemia.

haemolytic disease of the newborn *n.* the condition resulting from destruction (haemolysis) of the red blood cells of the fetus by antibodies in the mother's blood passing through the placenta. When an exchange occurs between fetal and maternal blood, the passage of red cells into the maternal circulation provokes an antibody response to the fetal red blood cell antigen in the mother. This most commonly happens when the red blood cells of the fetus are Rh positive (*see* rhesus factor) but the mother's red cells are Rh negative. If the mother is exposed in another pregnancy, maternal antibodies cross the placenta. This may result in very severe anaemia of the fetus or severe jaundice after birth. A blood test early in pregnancy enables the detection of antibodies in the mother's blood and the adoption of various precautions for the infant's safety. *See also* anti D.

haemolytic uraemic syndrome (HUS) *n.* a condition in which sudden rapid destruction of red blood cells (*see* haemolysis) causes acute renal failure due partly to obstruction of small arteries in the kidneys. The haemolysis also causes a reduction in the number of platelets, which can lead to severe haemorrhage. The syndrome may occur as a result of septicaemia following a respiratory or gastrointestinal infection (especially by pathogenic *Escherichia coli*), eclamptic fits in pregnancy (*see* eclampsia), or as a reaction to certain drugs.

haemopericardium (heem-ŏ-pe-ri-kar-diŭm) *n.* the presence of blood within the pericardium, which may result from injury, tumours, rupture of the heart, or a leaking aneurysm.

haemoperitoneum (heem-ŏ-pe-ri-tŏn-ee-ŭm) *n.* the presence of blood in the peritoneal cavity, between the lining of the abdomen or pelvis and the membrane covering the organs within.

haemophilia (hee-moh-fil-iă) *n.* a hereditary disorder in which the blood clots very slowly, due to a deficiency of either of two coagulation factors: Factor VIII (antihaemophilic factor), causing **haemophilia A**; or Factor IX (Christmas factor), causing **haemophilia B** (Christmas disease). Prolonged bleeding follows any injury or wound, and in severe cases there is spontaneous bleeding into muscles and joints. Bleeding in haemophilia may be treated by administration of recombinant-DNA-derived Factor VIII or concentrated freeze-dried Factor VIII or Factor IX. Haemophilia is controlled by a sex-linked gene and is almost exclusively restricted to males: women can carry the gene without being affected themselves. **—haemophiliac** *n.* **—haemophilic** *adj.*

Haemophilus (hi-**mof**-i-lŭs) *n.* a genus of Gram-negative aerobic nonmotile parasitic rodlike bacteria frequently found in the respiratory tract. Most species are pathogenic. **H. influenzae** a species associated with acute and chronic respiratory infections: a common secondary cause of influenza infections; type b is a primary cause of bacterial meningitis (*see* Hib vaccine).

haemophthalmia (heem-off-**thal**-miă) *n.* bleeding into the vitreous humour of the eye: vitreous haemorrhage.

haemopneumothorax (heem-ŏ-new-moh-**thor**-aks) *n.* the presence of blood and air in the pleural cavity, usually as a result of injury. *See also* haemothorax.

haemopoiesis (haematopoiesis) (hee-moh-poi-**ee**-sis) *n.* the process of production of blood cells and platelets which continues throughout life, replacing aged cells (which are removed from the circulation). In healthy adults, haemopoiesis is confined to the bone marrow. *See also* erythropoiesis, leucopoiesis, thrombopoiesis. **—haemopoietic** *adj.*

haemoptysis (hi-**mop**-ti-sis) *n.* the coughing up of blood.

haemorrhage (bleeding) (**hem**-er-ij) *n.* the escape of blood from a ruptured blood vessel, externally or internally. Arterial blood is bright red and emerges in spurts, venous blood is dark red and flows steadily, while damage to minor vessels may produce only an oozing. Rupture of a major blood vessel such as the femoral artery can lead to the loss of several litres of blood in a few minutes, resulting in shock, collapse, and death, if untreated. **primary h.** haemorrhage occurring immediately after injury or surgery. **secondary h.** haemorrhage occurring some time after injury, usually due to sepsis. *See also* haematemesis, haematuria, haemoptysis, splinter haemorrhage.

haemorrhagic (hem-er-**aj**-ik) *adj.* associated with or resulting from blood loss. *See* haemorrhage.

haemorrhagic disease of the newborn *n.* a transient disorder of newborn infants in which prolonged bleeding may result from the slightest injury. It is caused by deficiency of vitamin K and therefore of prothrombin, which is necessary for blood clotting.

haemorrhoidectomy (hem-er-oid-**ek**-tŏmi) *n.* the surgical operation for removing haemorrhoids, which are tied and then excised. The operation is usually performed only for second- or third-degree haemorrhoids.

haemorrhoids (piles) (hem-er-oidz) *pl. n.* enlargement of the normal spongy blood-filled cushions in the wall of the anus (**internal h.**), usually a consequence of prolonged constipation or, less often, diarrhoea. The main symptom is bleeding. **external h.** prolapsed internal haemorrhoids or perianal haematomas. **first-degree h.** haemorrhoids that never appear at the anus but cause bleeding at the end of defecation. **second-degree h.** haemorrhoids that protrude beyond the anus as an uncomfortable swelling but return spontaneously. **third-degree h.** haemorrhoids that remain outside the anus and need to be returned by manipulation. They often require surgery (*see* haemorrhoidectomy), especially if they become strangulated (producing severe pain and further enlargement).

haemosalpinx (hee-moh-sal-pinks) *n. see* haematosalpinx.

haemosiderosis (heem-ŏ-sid-er-**oh**-sis) *n.* the accumulation in various tissues of **haemosiderin**, an iron-storage compound normally found in the bone marrow, liver, and spleen.

haemostasis (hee-moh-stay-sis) *n.* the arrest of bleeding, involving the physiological processes of blood coagulation and the contraction of damaged blood vessels. The term is also applied to various surgical procedures used to stop bleeding.

haemostatic (styptic) (hee-moh-**stat**-ik) *n.* an agent that stops or prevents haemorrhage; for example, tranexamic acid or phytomenadione.

haemothorax (hee-moh-**thor**-aks) *n.* blood in the pleural cavity, usually due to injury.

HAI *n.* hospital-acquired infection (*see* nosocomial infection).

hair (hair) *n.* a threadlike keratinized outgrowth of the epidermis of the skin. The root of the hair, beneath the surface of the skin, is expanded at its base to form the bulb, which contains a matrix of dividing cells. As new cells are formed the older ones are pushed upwards and become keratinized to form the root and shaft. **h. follicle** a sheath of epidermal cells and connective tissue that surrounds the root of a hair. **h. papilla** a projection of the dermis that is surrounded by the base of the hair bulb. It contains the capillaries that supply blood to the growing hair.

hairball (**hair**-bawl) *n. see* trichobezoar.

hairy cell (**hair**-i) *n.* an abnormal white blood cell that has the appearance of an immature lymphocyte with fine hairlike cytoplasmic projections around the perimeter of the cell. It is found in a rare form of leukaemia (**h.-c. leukaemia**) most commonly occurring in young men.

half-life (**hahf**-lyf) *n.* **1.** the time taken for half the atoms of a radioactive isotope to decay: a measure of the radioactivity of the isotope. **2.** (in pharmacology) the time taken for the body to excrete half a given amount of a drug.

halibut liver oil (hal-i-bŭt) *n.* an oil extracted from the liver of halibut. It is rich in vitamins A and D.

halitosis (hal-i-**toh**-sis) *n.* bad breath. Causes of temporary halitosis include recently eaten strongly flavoured food; other causes include mouth breathing, periodontal disease, and infective conditions of the nose, throat, and lungs.

hallucination (hă-loo-sin-**ay**-shŏn) *n.* a false perception of something that is not really there. Hallucinations may be provoked by mental illness (such as schizophrenia or severe anxiety disorders) or physical disorders affecting the brain or they may be caused by drugs or sensory deprivation. *Compare* illusion.

Hallucinations Rating Scale (HRS) *n.* an 11-item scale to determine details of auditory hallucinations in patients.

hallucinogen (hă-**loo**-sin-ŏ-jen) *n.* a drug that produces hallucinations, e.g. cannabis and lysergic acid diethylamide. Hallucinogens were formerly used to treat certain types of mental illness. **—hallucinogenic** *adj.*

hallux (hal-ŭks) *n.* (*pl.* **halluces**) the big toe. **h. rigidus** painful stiffness and enlargement of the joint at the base of the big toe, resulting from osteoarthritis. **h. valgus** a deformity in which the big toe is displaced towards the other toes. It is associated with a bunion. **h. varus** displacement of the big toe away from the others.

halogen (hal-ŏ-jen) *n.* any one of the related elements fluorine, chlorine, bromine, or iodine.

haloperidol (hal-oh-**pe**-ri-dol) *n.* a butyrophenone antipsychotic drug that is administered by mouth or depot injection to relieve anxiety and tension in the treatment of schizophrenia and other psychiatric disorders and of tics. Trade names: **Haldol Decanoate**, **Serenace**.

hamate bone (unciform bone) (**ham**-ayt) *n.* a hook-shaped bone of the wrist (*see* carpus). It articulates with the capitate and triquetral bones at the sides, with the lunate bone behind, and with the fourth and fifth metacarpal bones in front.

hammer (**ham**-er) *n.* (in anatomy) *see* malleus.

hammer toe *n.* a deformity of a toe, most often the second, caused by fixed flexion of the proximal interphalangeal joint, which produces extension of the joints distal and proximal to it. A corn often forms over the deformity, which may be painful.

hamstring (**ham**-string) *n.* any of the tendons at the back of the knee. **h. muscles** the biceps femoris, semitendinosus, and semimembranosus, attached by the hamstrings to their insertions in the tibia and fibula.

hand (hand) *n.* the terminal organ of the upper limb. It comprises the eight bones of the carpus, the five metacarpal bones, and the phalangeal bones plus the surrounding tissues.

handedness (**han**-did-nis) *n.* the preferential use of one hand rather than the other in voluntary actions. Over 95% of right-handed people and 50–70% of left-handed people have left-hemisphere dominance for language.

hand, foot, and mouth disease *n.* a self-limiting disease, mainly affecting young children, caused by Coxsackie virus A16. A feeling of mild illness is accompanied by mouth ulcers and blisters on the hands and feet.

handicap (**han**-di-kap) *n.* partial or total inability to perform a social, occupational, or other activity that the affected person wants to do.

Hand-Schüller-Christian disease (hand **shew**-ler **kris**-chăn) *n. see* Langerhans cell histiocytosis. [A. Hand (1868–1949), US paediatrician; A. Schüller (1874–1958), Austrian neurologist; H. A. Christian (1876–1951), US physician]

Hansen's bacillus (**han**-sĕnz) *n. see* Mycobacterium. [A. G. H. Hansen (1841–1912), Norwegian bacteriologist]

Hansen's disease *n. see* leprosy.

hantavirus (**han**-tă-vy-rŭs) *n.* a virus that infects rats, mice, and voles and causes disease in humans when the secretions or excreta of these rodents are inhaled or ingested. The symptoms, which vary according to the strain of the infecting virus, range from those of a mild influenza-like illness to serious kidney or lung damage.

haploid (monoploid) (**hap**-loid) *adj.* describing cells, nuclei, or organisms with a single set of unpaired chromosomes. In humans the gametes are haploid following meiosis. *Compare* diploid, triploid. **—haploid** *n.*

happy puppet syndrome (**hap**-i **pup**-it) *n. see* Angelman syndrome.

hapt- (hapto-) *combining form denoting* touch.

hapten (**hap**-tĕn) *n.* a substance that becomes antigenic by combining with and modifying the body's own proteins.

harelip (**hair**-lip) *n. see* cleft lip.

harm (hahm) *n.* physical, mental, or moral damage. Although health service staff have a clear duty to benefit patients and avoid harming them (*see* nonmaleficence), in practice almost all medical actions run the risk of harm and in some no good effect can be achieved without a clearly harmful process (such as mastectomy for breast cancer). Therefore, all medical professionals should learn how to make a risk – benefit analysis at each point of care. The risk of harm should be explained to patients and agreed to at each appropriate point by them. Professional blame or litigation may result if this is not done and harm results.

Harrison's sulcus (**ha**-ri-sŏnz) *n.* a depression on both sides of the chest wall of a child between the pectoral muscles and the lower margin of the ribcage. It develops in conditions in which the airways are partially obstructed or when the lungs are abnormally congested due to some congenital abnormality of the heart. [E. Harrison (1789–1838), British physician]

Harris's operation (ha-ris-ĕz) *n.* an operation in which the prostate gland is removed through an incision above the pubic bone and through the bladder. *See* prostatectomy. [S. H. Harris (1880–1936), Australian surgeon]

Hartmann's pouch (hart-manz) *n.* a saclike dilatation of the gall-bladder wall near its outlet; it is a common site for finding gallstones. [R. Hartmann (1831–93), German anatomist]

Hartmann's solution *n.* a solution containing sodium, potassium, and calcium chlorides and sodium lactate, administered by infusion to treat dehydration. [A. Hartmann (1898–1964), US physician]

Hartnup disease (hart-nup) *n.* a rare hereditary defect in the absorption of the amino acid tryptophan, leading to learning disability, thickening and roughening of the skin on exposure to light, and lack of muscular coordination. The condition is similar to pellagra. Treatment with nicotinamide is usually effective. [Hartnup family, in whom it was first reported]

Hashimoto's disease (Hashimoto's thyroiditis) (hash-i-moh-tohz) *n.* chronic thyroiditis due to the formation of thyroid antibodies. Its features include a firm swelling of the thyroid and partial or total failure of secretion of thyroid hormones; often there are autoantibodies to other organs, such as the stomach. Women are more often affected than men and the condition often occurs in families. [H. Hashimoto (1881–1934), Japanese surgeon]

hashish (hash-eesh) *n. see* cannabis.

haustrum (how-strum) *n.* one of the pouches on the external surface of the colon.

HAV *n.* hepatitis A virus. *See* hepatitis.

Haversian canal (ha-ver-si-ăn) *n.* any one of the small canals that ramify throughout compact bone. *See also* bone. [C. Havers (1650–1702), English anatomist]

Haversian system *n. see* bone.

hay fever (hay) *n.* a form of allergy due to pollen, characterized by inflammation of the membrane lining the nose and sometimes of the conjunctiva (**vernal** or **allergic conjunctivitis**). The symptoms of sneezing, running or blocked nose, and watering eyes often respond to treatment with antihistamines. Medical name: **allergic rhinitis**.

Hb *n. see* haemoglobin.

HbA$_{1c}$ *n. see* glycated haemoglobin.

HC *n.* head circumference.

hCG *n. see* human chorionic gonadotrophin.

HCV *n.* hepatitis C virus. *See* hepatitis.

HD *n. see* Huntington's disease.

HDL *n. see* (high-density) lipoprotein.

HDU *n. see* high-dependency unit.

head (hed) *n.* **1.** the part of the body that contains the brain and the organs of sight, hearing, smell, and taste. **2.** the rounded portion of a bone, which fits into a groove of another to form a joint.

headache (hed-ayk) *n.* pain felt deep within the skull. Most headaches are caused by stress or fatigue but some are symptoms of serious intracranial disease. *See also* cluster headache, migraine.

head injury (in-jeri) *n.* an injury usually resulting from a blow to the head and often associated with traumatic brain injury. It may result in contusion or – if the blood vessels in the head are torn – a haematoma. The level of consciousness of a patient following a head injury can be monitored using the Glasgow Coma Scale.

head tilt/chin lift *n.* a manoeuvre for opening the airway of an unconscious patient. With the patient lying on his or her back, the neck is extended and the chin simultaneously pulled gently upwards to pull the tongue away from the back of the pharynx. *See also* jaw thrust.

Heaf test (heef) *n.* a skin test, no longer available, to determine whether or not an individual is immune to tuberculosis, carried out before vaccination. A spring-loaded gun mounted with very short needles produces a circle of six punctures in the forearm through which tuberculin is introduced. If the test is positive a reaction causes the skin to become red and raised, indicating that the individual is immune. [F. R. G. Heaf (1895–1973), British physician]

healing (heel-ing) *n.* making whole, both by restoring injured or diseased tissue and, more generally, by returning to full and independent function. The latter may take a lot longer than the former: this is one of the reasons for follow-up after a medical event and for convalescence and rehabilitation services.

health-adjusted life expectancy *n.* a measure developed by the World Health Organization to capture life expectancy in terms of both morbidity and mortality. The number of years lived with ill health, weighted according to severity, is subtracted from the overall life expectancy. Previously known as **disability-adjusted life expectancy**, it is sometimes referred to as **healthy life expectancy**.

Health and Safety Executive (HSE) (helth) *n.* (in Britain) a statutory body responsible for the health and safety of workers (including factory, office, and agricultural workers).

health authority *n. see* primary care trust, strategic health authority.

health care *n. see* primary care, secondary care, tertiary care.

health-care assistant *n.* a support worker in a clinical area who works under the supervision of a registered practitioner who is accountable for the support worker's standards and activities. A health-care assistant may be registered at level 1 or 2 of the National Council for Vocational Qualifications (NCVQ), having completed a recognized course. *See also* NCVQ, support worker.

health-care delivery *n.* the services provided by nurses and others in the health service.

health centre *n.* (in Britain) a building, usually owned or leased by a health authority, that houses personnel and/or services from one or more sections of the National Health Service. **GP-led h. c.** (**poly-clinic**) a health centre where a greater range of health and community services is available compared with a conventional GP practice.

health education *n.* methods used to inform people about health issues and to persuade and enable them to adopt lifestyles that the educators believe will improve health and to reject habits regarded as harmful to health.

Health Education England (HEE) *n.* a special health authority of the NHS responsible for leading education and training for the whole health-care and public health workforce. It was established following the Health and Social Care Act 2012.

SEE WEB LINKS

- HEE website

health impact assessment (HIA) *n.* a systematic process in which existing scientific literature and geographic and demographic knowledge are used to judge the potential impact of a project or policy on the health of a population.

Health Improvement Programme (HImP) *n.* a plan, developed by primary care trusts and acute trusts, patient groups, and the voluntary sector, to tackle inequalities in health care and its provision at a local level.

health needs assessment (HNA) *n.* a systematic assessment of the health needs of a given population, often with relation to a particular issue (e.g. alcohol consumption). It aims to lead to policy that allows heath resources to be used in the most efficient way.

Health of the Nation Outcome Scale (HoNOS) *n.* a 12-item scale, used in mental health care, that assesses risk behaviours, physical problems, deterioration or improvement in symptoms, and social functioning.

health promotion *n.* action to maintain the best possible health and quality of life of the members of the community and to encourage their involvement in their personal health. Programmes may include health education, immunization, screening tests, and environmental monitoring.

health service manager *n.* an administrator with special training and skills in management who is concerned with the planning and provision of health services and with managing performance. Doctors, nurses, and others may fill such posts, sometimes combining them with professional appointments.

health service planning *n.* balancing the health and health-care needs of a community, assessed by such indices as mortality, morbidity, and disability, with the resources available to meet these needs in terms of human resources (including ensuring the numbers in training grades meet future requirements) and technical resources, such as hospitals (capital planning), equipment, and medicines.

health visitor (specialist community public health nurse) *n.* a trained nurse with specialist qualifications in health promotion and public health. The health visitor works as a member of the primary health-care team, focusing on families with children under five years old, but the role can be extended to include other targeted groups (e.g. the elderly).

HealthWatch England *n.* the national consumer champion for health and social care, formed following the Health and Social Care Act 2012. In addition, there are 148 **local HealthWatch** groups, which have statutory representation on local health and wellbeing boards.

SEE WEB LINKS

- HealthWatch England website

hearing aid (heer-ing ayd) *n.* a device to improve hearing. **analogue h. a.** a battery-powered aid, consisting of a miniature microphone, an amplifier, and a tiny loudspeaker (or a vibrator in some cases of conductive deafness), that usually fits behind or within the ear. **bone-anchored h. a.** (BAHA) a hearing aid for those with certain forms of conductive deafness in which the vibrator is a small titanium screw fixed into the bone of the skull behind the external ear. **digital h. a.** a device similar to an analogue hearing aid but with the addition of a digital-to-analogue converter and a tiny computer, which improves sound quality. **environmental h. a.** a device for assisting those with hearing difficulties. *See* alerting device, assistive listening device. **implantable h. a.** a hearing aid in which a battery-powered device consisting of a microphone and electronic processing unit, fitted behind the ear, passes information to an electrical vibrator surgically attached to the ear ossicles.

hearing loss *n. see* deafness.

hearing therapy (th'e-ră-pi) *n.* the support and rehabilitation of people with hearing difficulties, tinnitus, or vertigo. It includes teaching lip-reading, advising on environmental hearing aids, and providing tinnitus retraining therapy.

heart (hart) *n.* a hollow muscular cone-shaped organ, lying between the lungs, with the apex directed downwards, forwards, and to the left. It is divided by a septum into separate right and left halves, each of which is divided into an upper atrium and a lower ventricle (see illustration). Deoxygenated blood is pumped to the lungs via the right atrium and ventricle; newly oxygenated blood is pumped out to the body via the left atrium and ventricle. The direction of blood flow within the heart is controlled by valves.

heart attack *n. see* myocardial infarction.

heart block *n.* a condition in which conduction of the electrical

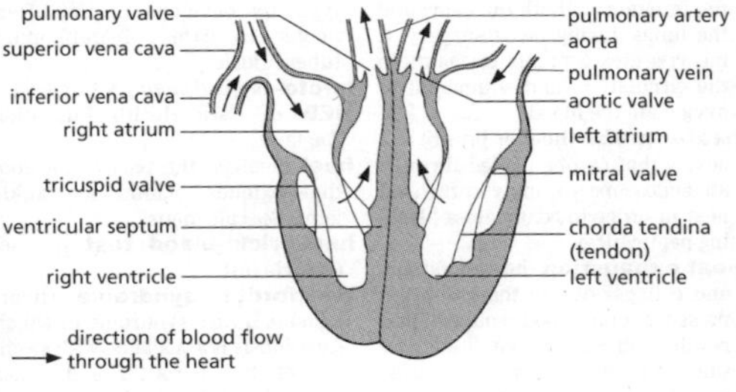

Vertical section through the heart

impulses generated by the sino-atrial node is impaired. Heart block may be congenital or it may be due to heart disease, myocarditis, cardiomyopathy, and disease of the valves. Symptoms may be abolished by the use of an artificial pacemaker. **first degree h. b.** heart block in which conduction between atria and ventricles is delayed. **second degree h. b.** heart block in which not all the impulses are conducted from the atria to the ventricles. **third degree h. b.** heart block in which no impulses are conducted and the ventricles beat at their own slow intrinsic rate (20–40 per minute).

heartburn (pyrosis) (hart-bern) *n.* discomfort or pain, usually burning in character, that is felt behind the breastbone. It may be accompanied by the regurgitation of saliva or gastric fluid in the mouth and is usually caused by reflux of stomach contents into the gullet.

heart failure *n.* a condition in which the pumping action of the heart is inadequate due to damaged heart valves, ventricular muscle, or both. This results in back pressure of blood, with congestion of organs. **congestive h. f.** (congestive cardiac failure, CCF) heart failure involving damage to both left and right ventricles. The patient suffers breathlessness (*see also* orthopnoea) and fluid accumulates in the lungs, legs, and/or abdominal cavity. There is reduced flow of arterial blood from the heart, which in extreme cases results in peripheral circulatory failure (*see* cardiogenic shock). Treatment includes diuretics, ACE inhibitors, and beta blockers.

heart-lung machine *n.* an apparatus for taking over temporarily the functions of both the heart and the lungs during heart surgery. It incorporates a pump, to maintain the circulation, and equipment to oxygenate the blood.

heater-probe (**heet**-er-prohb) *n.* a device that can be passed through an endoscope to apply controlled heat in order to coagulate a bleeding peptic ulcer.

heat exhaustion (heet) *n.* fatigue and collapse due to the low blood pressure and blood volume that result from loss of body fluids and salts after prolonged or unaccustomed exposure to heat.

heatstroke (sunstroke) (**heet**-strohk) *n.* raised body temperature (pyrexia), absence of sweating, and eventual loss of consciousness due to failure or exhaustion of the temperature-regulating mechanism of the body.

hebephrenia (hee-bi-**free**-niă) *n.* an obsolescent name for a chronic form of schizophrenia that typically starts in adolescence or young adulthood. The most prominent features are disordered thinking; inappropriate affect, thoughtless cheerfulness, apathy, or querulousness; and silly behaviour. **—hebephrenic** *adj.*

Heberden's node (**hee**-ber-děnz) *n.* a bony thickening arising at the terminal joint of a finger in osteoarthritis. It is often inherited, with women most commonly affected. [W. Heberden (1710–1801), British physician]

hebiatrics (hee-bi-**at**-riks) *n. see* ephebiatrics.

hectic (**hek**-tik) *adj.* occurring regularly. **h. fever** a fever that typically develops in the afternoons, in cases of pulmonary tuberculosis.

hecto- *prefix denoting* a hundred.

HEE *n. see* Health Education England.

heel (heel) *n.* the part of the foot that extends behind the ankle joint. *See* calcaneus.

heel-prick blood test *n. see* Guthrie test.

Heerfordt's syndrome (**heer**-forts) *n.* a rare syndrome in which sarcoidosis is associated with swelling of the parotitid and other salivary glands, uveitis, fever, and paralysis of the facial nerve. It can be treated with steroids but generally resolves spontaneously.

Hegar's sign (**hay**-garz) *n.* an indication of pregnancy detectable between the 6th and 12th weeks: used before modern urine tests for pregnancy were available. If the fingers of one hand are inserted into the vagina and those of the other are placed over the pelvic cavity, the lower part of the uterus feels very soft compared with the body of the uterus above and the cervix below. [A. Hegar (1830–1914), German gynaecologist]

Heimlich manoeuvre (**hym**-lik) *n. see* abdominal thrusts. [H. J. Heimlich (1920–2016), US physician]

helc- (helco-) *combining form denoting* an ulcer.

Helicobacter (hel-i-koh-**bak**-ter) *n.* a genus of spiral and flagellated Gram-negative bacteria. **H. pylori** (formerly *Campylobacter pylori*) a species that occurs in the stomach and may cause gastritis. It is nearly always present in duodenal ulceration and usually in gastric ulceration, and has been implicated in lymphomas of the stomach. It can be eradicated using various combinations of antibiotics and antisecretory drugs.

helicopter-based emergency medical services (hel-i-kopt-er-bayst i-**merj**-ĕn-si) *pl. n. see* HEMS.

helio- *combining form denoting* the sun.

heliotherapy (hee-li-oh-**th'e**-ră-pi) *n.* the use of sunlight to promote healing; sunbathing.

helium (**hee**-li-ŭm) *n.* a colourless inert gas that is used in combination with oxygen in respiratory tests and therapy and to prevent decompression sickness in deep-sea divers. Symbol: He.

helix (**hee**-liks) *n.* the outer curved fleshy ridge of the pinna of the outer ear.

Heller's operation (**hel**-erz) *n. see* cardiomyotomy. [E. Heller (1877–1964), German surgeon]

Heller's test *n.* a test for the presence of protein (albumin) in the urine. [J. F. Heller (1813–71), Austrian pathologist]

HELLP syndrome (help) *n.* a form of severe pre-eclampsia affecting many body systems and characterized by *h*aemolysis, *e*levated *l*iver enzymes, and a *l*ow *p*latelet count (hence the name). It constitutes an emergency requiring delivery as soon as the patient is stabilized.

helminth (**hel**-minth) *n.* any of the parasitic worms, including the flukes, tapeworms, and nematodes.

helminthiasis (hel-min-**th'y**-ă-sis) *n.* the diseased condition resulting from an infestation with parasitic worms (helminths).

helminthology (hel-min-**thol**-ŏji) *n.* the study of parasitic worms.

helper T cell (**help**-er) *n. see* T cell.

hemeralopia (hem-er-ă-**loh**-piă) *n. see* day blindness.

hemi- *prefix denoting* (in medicine) the right or left half of the body.

hemianopia (hemi-an-**oh**-piă) *n.* absence of half of the normal field of vision. **homonymous h.** hemianopia in which the same half of the visual field (right or left) is lost in both eyes.

hemiarthroplasty (hemi-**arth**-roh-plasti) *n.* replacement of the end of a bone on one side of a joint with a prosthesis (*see* arthroplasty). It is the treatment for some fractures of the hip and shoulder.

hemicolectomy (hemi-koh-**lek**-tŏmi) *n.* surgical removal of sections of the large bowel (colon), either the ascending colon (**right h.**) or the desending colon (**left h.**). An **extended h.** involves the additional excision of a section of the transverse colon. Such operations are performed in cases of inflammation (e.g. Crohn's disease) or cancer.

hemicrania (hemi-**kray**-niă) *n.* **1.** a headache affecting only one side of the head, usually migraine. **2.** absence of half of the skull in a developing fetus.

hemimelia (hemi-**mee**-liă) *n.* congenital absence or gross shortening (aplasia) of the distal portion of the arms or legs. *See also* ectromelia.

hemiparesis (hemi-pă-ree-sis) *n.* *see* hemiplegia.

hemiplegia (hemiparesis) (hemi-**plee**-jiă) *n.* paralysis of one side of the body. It is caused by disease of the opposite (contralateral) hemisphere of the brain.

hemisphere (**hem**-iss-feer) *n.* one of the two halves of the cerebrum, not in fact hemispherical but more nearly quarter-spherical.

hemlock (**hem**-lok) *n.* the plant *Conium maculatum,* found in Britain and central Europe. It is a source of the poisonous alkaloid coniine.

hemp (hemp) *n.* *see* cannabis.

HEMS *pl. n.* helicopter-based emergency medical services: a fast method for the provision of first aid and the rapid transport of the seriously injured (primary use) or the critically ill (secondary use) to a hospital.

Henderson's model (**hen**-der-sŏnz) *n.* a model for nursing that describes 14 components of basic nursing that define the unique function of the nurse, which is to act in the best interests of the patient when the patient lacks the ability to do so. *See also* nursing models. [V. Henderson (1897–1996), US nurse theorist]

Henle's loop (**hen**-liz) *n.* the part of a kidney tubule that forms a loop extending towards the centre of the kidney. It is surrounded by blood capillaries, which absorb water and selected soluble substances back into the bloodstream. [F. G. J. Henle (1809–85), German anatomist]

Henoch-Schönlein purpura (Schönlein-Henoch purpura, anaphylactoid purpura) (**hen**-ohk **shern**-lyn) *n.* a common and frequently recurrent form of purpura found especially (but not exclusively) in young children. It is characterized by red weals and a purple rash on the buttocks and lower legs due to bleeding into the skin from inflamed capillaries, together with arthritis, gastrointestinal symptoms, and (in some cases) nephritis. [E. H. Henoch (1820–1910), German paediatrician; J. L. Schönlein (1793–1864), German physician]

hepar (**hee**-par) *n.* the liver.

heparin (**hep**-er-in) *n.* an anticoagulant produced in liver cells, some white blood cells, and certain other sites, which acts by inhibiting the action of the enzyme thrombin in the final stage of blood coagulation. An extracted purified form of heparin is widely used for the treatment of deep vein thrombosis and the prevention of blood coagulation both in patients with deep vein thrombosis and similar conditions and in blood collected for examination. It is administered by intravenous or subcutaneous injection; the most important side-effect is bleeding. **low-molecular-weight h.** a type of heparin used to prevent and treat deep vein thrombosis following surgery or during kidney dialysis. It is more readily absorbed and requires less frequent administration than standard preparations.

hepat- (hepato-) *combining form denoting* the liver.

hepatalgia (hep-ă-tal-jiă) *n.* pain in or over the liver. It is caused by stretching of the outer covering (capsule) of the liver due to infection, an enlarging tumour, or swelling.

hepatectomy (hep-ă-tek-tŏmi) *n.* the operation of removing the liver. **partial h.** the removal of one or more lobes of the liver; it may be carried out after injury or to remove a localized tumour.

hepatic (hip-at-ik) *adj.* relating to the liver. **h. duct** *see* bile duct. **h. encephalopathy** (**portosystemic encephalopathy**) a condition in which brain function is impaired by the presence of toxic substances, absorbed from the colon, which are normally removed or detoxified by the liver. **h. flexure** the bend in the colon, just underneath the liver, where the ascending colon joins the transverse colon. **h. vein** one of several veins that drain blood from the liver directly into the inferior vena cava.

hepaticostomy (hip-at-i-kost-ŏmi) *n.* a surgical operation in which a temporary or permanent opening is made into the main duct carrying bile from the liver.

hepatitis (hep-ă-ty-tis) *n.* inflammation of the liver caused by viruses, toxic substances (including alcohol), autoimmune disease, metabolic disease, or excess deposition of fat. **chronic h.** hepatitis that continues for months or years, eventually leading to cirrhosis, caused by persistent infection with a hepatitis virus or by autoimmune disease. **h. A** infectious hepatitis transmitted by contaminated food or drink. After an incubation period of 15–40 days, the patient develops fatigue, anorexia, nausea, vomiting, joint pain, and fever. Yellow discoloration of the skin (*see* jaundice) appears about a week later and persists for up to three weeks. **h. B** (formerly **serum h.**) infectious hepatitis transmitted by infected blood or blood products, contaminated hypodermic needles, blood transfusions, etc., by unprotected sexual contact, or rarely by contact with other body fluids. Symptoms, which develop suddenly after an incubation period of 1–6 months, include headache, fever, chills, general weakness, and jaundice. **h. C** (formerly **non-A, non-B h.**) infectious hepatitis that has a mode of transmission similar to that of hepatitis B (predominantly intravenous drug abuse). **h. D** infectious hepatitis that can proliferate only when there is infection with hepatitis B; it is associated with severe chronic hepatitis. **h. E** hepatitis transmitted by infected food or drink. It can cause acute hepatitis. **infectious h.** hepatitis caused by viruses, several types of which have been isolated.

hepatization (hep-ă-ty-zay-shŏn) *n.* the conversion of lung tissue, which normally holds air, into a solid liver-like mass during the course of acute lobar pneumonia.

hepato- *combining form. see* hepat-.

hepatoblastoma (hep-ă-toh-blas-**toh**-mă) *n.* a malignant tumour of the liver occurring in children, made up of embryonic liver cells.

hepatocele (hip-at-oh-seel) *n.* a hernia of the liver.

hepatocellular (hep-ă-toh-**sel**-yoo-ler) *adj.* relating to or affecting the cells of the liver.

hepatocirrhosis (hep-ă-toh-si-**roh**-sis) *n.* cirrhosis of the liver. *See* cirrhosis.

hepatocyte (hip-**at**-oh-syt) *n.* the principal cell type in the liver: it has many functions, including protein synthesis and storage, carbohydrate and lipid metabolism detoxification, and bile production.

hepatoma (hepatocellular carcinoma) (hep-ă-**toh**-mă) *n.* the most common primary malignant tumour of the liver. In Western countries patients with chronic hepatitis B or C or cirrhosis are at the highest risk.

hepatomegaly (hep-ă-toh-**meg**-ă-li) *n.* enlargement of the liver. This may be due to inflammation, infiltration (e.g. by fat), congestion (due to congestive heart failure), or tumour.

hepatotoxic (hep-ă-toh-**toks**-ik) *adj.* damaging or destroying liver cells. Drugs such as paracetamol can be hepatotoxic at high doses or with prolonged use.

hepcidin (**hep**-si-din) *n.* a peptide hormone, secreted by the liver, that regulates the entry of iron into the circulation. It inhibits iron transfer through ferroportin channels (which transport iron from inside to outside the cells), enabling cellular iron storage.

hept- (hepta-) *prefix denoting* seven.

Herceptin (her-**sep**-tin) *n. see* trastuzumab.

herd immunity (herd) *n.* the immunity of a group, community, or population to an infectious disease as a result of mass vaccination. The higher the percentage of the population vaccinated, the greater will be the resistance to the spread of infection within the population.

hereditary (hi-**red**-it-er-i) *adj.* transmitted from parents to their offspring; inherited.

heredity (hi-**red**-iti) *n.* the process that causes the biological similarity between parents and their offspring. Genetics is the study of heredity.

heredo- *combining form denoting* heredity.

Hering-Breuer reflexes (h'e-ring **broi**-er) *pl. n.* the reflexes that maintain the normal rhythm of inflation and deflation of the lungs. [K. E. K. Hering (1834–1918), German physiologist; J. Breuer (1842–1925), German physician]

hermaphrodite (her-**maf**-rŏ-dyt) *n.* an individual in which both male and female sex organs are present or in which the sex organs contain both ovarian and testicular cells. **—hermaphroditism** *n.*

hermeneutics (her-mĕ-**newt**-iks) *n.* the practice of interpreting literary and historical texts in relation to one another and to their various contexts. By extension, interpreting an ill patient in terms of history taking, physical examination, diagnostic tests, and listening to the patient's account of their own experience.

hernia (her-niă) *n.* the protrusion of an organ or tissue out of the body cavity in which it normally lies. **diaphragmatic h.** the protrusion of an abdominal organ through the diaphragm into the chest cavity. **femoral h.** the protrusion of part of the bowel at the top of the thigh, through the point at which the femoral artery passes from the abdomen to the thigh. **hiatus h.** the most common type of diaphragmatic hernia, in which the stomach passes partly or completely into the chest cavity through the oesophageal opening. This hernia may be associated with gastro-oesophageal reflux, although most patients have no symptoms. **incarcerated h.** a hernia that is swollen and fixed within its sac. **incisional h.** a hernia that occurs through a defect at the site of a previous surgical incision. **inguinal h.** (or **rupture**) the protrusion of a sac of peritoneum, containing fat or part of the bowel, through the lower abdominal wall. **irreducible h.** a hernia that cannot be returned to its normal site. **strangulated h.** a hernia that is cut off from its blood supply, becoming painful and eventually gangrenous. **umbilical h.** *see* exomphalos.

hernio- *combining form denoting* a hernia.

hernioplasty (her-ni-oh-plasti) *n.* the surgical operation to repair a hernia, in which the sac is excised, the abnormal opening is sewn up, and the weakness strengthened, most commonly using a polypropylene mesh.

herniorrhaphy (her-ni-o-ră-fi) *n.* surgical repair of a hernia, which can be performed through a laparoscope. *See* hernioplasty.

herniotomy (her-ni-ot-ŏmi) *n.* an operation to repair a hernia that involves cutting the sac that contains it. *See* hernioplasty.

heroin (h'e-roh-in) *n.* a white crystalline powder derived from morphine that is a highly addictive drug of abuse.

herpangina (herp-an-jy-nă) *n.* an acute viral infection, predominantly affecting children, that causes fever of sudden onset associated with acute ulceration of the soft palate and tonsillar area. It usually lasts 2–5 days.

herpes (her-peez) *n.* inflammation of the skin or mucous membranes caused by herpesviruses and characterized by collections of small blisters. Treatment is with antiviral drugs (e.g. aciclovir). **genital h.** a sexually transmitted disease, usually caused by **herpes simplex virus** (**HSV**) type II, that is characterized by painful blisters in the genital region. It may be recurrent and is extremely contagious as the blisters burst to release viruses that infect the sexual partner. **h. simplex** (**cold sore**) herpes that affects the lips or surrounding area, caused by HSV type I. **h. zoster** (**shingles**) herpes caused by the varicella-zoster virus, which also causes chickenpox. Following an attack of chickenpox, the virus lies dormant in the spinal cord and later migrates down a sensory nerve to affect the skin in a band. One side of the face or an eye (**ophthalmic zoster**) may be involved. Shingles may be chronically painful, especially in the elderly.

herpesvirus (her-peez-**vy**-rŭs) *n.* one of a group of DNA-containing viruses causing latent infections in humans and animals. The herpesviruses are the causative agents of herpes and chickenpox. *See also* cytomegalovirus, Epstein-Barr virus.

Herxheimer reaction *n. see* Jarisch-Herxheimer reaction.

hesitation (hez-i-**tay**-shŏn) *n.* (in urology) a delay between being ready to pass urine and the actual flow of urine. *See* lower urinary tract symptoms.

heter- (hetero-) *combining form denoting* difference; dissimilarity.

heterochromia (het-er-oh-**kroh**-miă) *n.* colour difference in the iris of the eye, which is usually congenital but is occasionally secondary to inflammation of the iris. **—heterochromic** *adj.*

heterogeneous (het-er-oh-**jee**-niŭs) *adj.* having different properties or constituents. **—heterogeneity** (het-er-oh-jin-**ay**-iti) *n.*

heterogenous (het-er-**oj**-in-ŭs) *adj.* derived from a different source.

heterograft (**het**-er-oh-grahft) *n. see* xenograft.

heterologous (het-er-**ol**-ŏ-gŭs) *adj.* derived from a different species: describing tissue used for grafting, etc.

heterophoria (het-er-oh-**for**-iă) *n.* a tendency to squint. Normally both eyes work together, but if one eye is covered it will move out of alignment with the object the other eye is still viewing. When the cover is removed the eye immediately returns to its normal position. *See also* strabismus.

heterophyiasis (het-er-oh-fi-**I**-ă-sis) *n.* an infestation of the small intestine with the parasitic fluke *Heterophyes heterophyes*. Humans become infected on eating raw or salted fish that contains the larval stage of the fluke. Symptoms include abdominal pain and diarrhoea; if the eggs reach the brain, spinal cord, and heart they produce serious lesions.

heteropsia (het-er-**op**-siă) *n.* different vision in each eye.

heterosis (het-er-**oh**-sis) *n.* hybrid vigour: the increased sturdiness, resistance to disease, etc., of animals whose parents are genetically different.

heterotopia (heterotopy) (het-er-oh-**toh**-piă) *n.* the displacement of an organ or part of the body from its normal position.

heterotropia (het-er-oh-**troh**-piă) *n. see* strabismus.

heterozygous (het-er-oh-**zy**-gŭs) *adj.* describing an individual in whom the members of a pair of genes determining a particular characteristic are dissimilar. *See* allele. *Compare* homozygous. **—heterozygote** *n.*

hex- (hexa-) *prefix denoting* six.

hexamine (**heks**-ă-meen) *n. see* methenamine.

hexose (heks-ohz) *n.* a simple sugar with six carbon atoms. Hexose sugars are the sugars most frequently found in food. The most important hexose is glucose.

HFEA *n. see* Human Fertilization and Embryology Authority.

Hg *symbol for* mercury.

HGP *n. see* Human Genome Project.

HIA *n. see* health impact assessment.

5-HIAA *n. see* 5-hydroxyindoleacetic acid.

hiatus (hy-**ay**-tŭs) *n.* an opening or aperture. For example, the diaphragm contains hiatuses for the oesophagus and aorta. **h. hernia** *see* hernia.

Hib/MenC *n.* a combined vaccine that protects against *Haemophilus influenzae* type b infection (*see* Hib vaccine) and meningococcal disease (*see* meningitis C vaccine). *See also* immunization.

Hib vaccine (hib) *n.* a vaccine that gives protection against the bacterium *Haemophilus influenzae* type b, which is a common cause of meningitis in children under the age of two years. The vaccine is given with the primary vaccines at 2, 3, and 4 months of age and as a booster at 12 months. See Appendix 8: Immunization schedules.

hiccup (**hik**-up) *n.* abrupt involuntary lowering of the diaphragm and closure of the sound-producing folds at the upper end of the trachea, producing a characteristic sound as the breath is drawn in. Hiccups, which usually occur repeatedly, may be caused by indigestion or more serious disorders, such as alcoholism. Medical name: **singultus**.

Hickman catheter (**hik**-măn) *n.* a fine plastic cannula usually inserted into the subclavian vein in the neck to allow administration of drugs and repeated blood samples. The catheter is tunnelled for several centimetres beneath the skin to prevent infection entering the bloodstream. It is used most frequently in patients receiving long-term chemotherapy, particularly by infusion.

hidr- (hidro-) *combining form denoting* sweat.

hidradenitis suppurativa (hy-drad-ĕ-**ny**-tis sup-yoor-ă-**tee**-vă) *n.* a condition in which deep abscesses occur in the armpits, groin, and anogenital region. More common in women, it may be under androgen control.

hidrosis (hid-**roh**-sis) *n.* **1.** the excretion of sweat. **2.** excessive sweating.

hidrotic (hid-**rot**-ik) *n.* an agent that causes sweating. Parasympathomimetic drugs are hidrotics.

HIFU *n. see* (high-intensity focused) ultrasound.

Higginson's syringe (**hig**-in-sŏnz) *n.* a rubber syringe with a bulb in the centre that is compressed to force liquid in one direction to irrigate a body cavity. [A. Higginson (1808–84), British surgeon]

high-density lipoprotein (HDL) (hy-**den**-siti) *n. see* lipoprotein.

high-dependency unit (HDU) (hy-di-**pen**-dăn-si) *n.* a unit in a hospital that offers specialist nursing care and monitoring to seriously ill patients. It provides greater care than is available on general wards but less than is given to patients in intensive care.

hilar cell tumour (hy-ler) *n.* an androgen-producing tumour of the ovary found in older women and often resulting in virilization. Such tumours tend to occur around the area of the ovary where the blood vessels enter (the hilum).

hilum (hy-lŭm) *n.* (*pl.* **hila**) a hollow situated on the surface of an organ, at which structures such as blood vessels and nerve fibres enter or leave it. **—hilar** *adj.*

HImP *n. see* Health Improvement Programme.

hindbrain (rhombencephalon) (**hynd**-brayn) *n.* the part of the brain comprising the cerebellum, pons, and medulla oblongata.

hindgut (**hynd**-gut) *n.* the back part of the embryonic gut, which gives rise to part of the large intestine, the rectum, bladder, and urinary ducts. *See also* cloaca.

hindquarter amputation (**hynd**-kwort-er) *n.* an operation involving removal of an entire leg and part or all of the pelvis associated with it. It is usually performed for soft tissue or bone sarcomas arising from the upper thigh, hip, or buttock. *Compare* forequarter amputation.

hinge joint (hinj) *n. see* ginglymus.

hip (hip) *n.* the region of the body where the thigh bone (femur) articulates with the pelvis: the region on each side of the pelvis. **h. bone (innominate bone)** a bone formed by the fusion of the ilium, ischium, and pubis. It articulates with the femur at the hip joint. **h. girdle** *see* pelvic girdle. **h. joint** the ball-and-socket joint between the head of the femur and the acetabulum (socket) of the ilium. **h. replacement** a surgical procedure for replacing a diseased hip joint with a prosthesis. *See also* arthroplasty.

hippocampal formation (hip-oh-**kam**-păl) *n.* a curved band of cortex lying within each cerebral hemisphere. It forms a portion of the limbic system and is involved in the complex physical aspects of behaviour governed by emotion and instinct.

hippocampus (hip-oh-**kam**-pŭs) *n.* a swelling in the floor of the lateral ventricle of the brain. It contains complex foldings of cortical tissue and is involved in the workings of the limbic system. **—hippocampal** *adj.*

Hippocratic oath (hip-ŏ-**krat**-ik) *n.* an oath often assumed to be taken but actually rarely sworn by doctors to observe the code of behaviour and practice followed by the Greek physician Hippocrates (460–370 BC), called the 'Father of Medicine'.

Hirschsprung's disease (heersh-spruungz) *n.* a congenital condition in which the rectum and sometimes part of the lower colon have failed to develop a normal nerve network. The affected portion does not expand or conduct the contents of the bowel, which accumulate in and distend the colon. *See also* megacolon. [H. Hirschsprung (1830–1916), Danish physician]

hirsutism (herss-yoo-tizm) *n.* the presence of coarse pigmented hair on the face, chest, upper back, or abdomen in a female as a result of hyperandrogenism (excessive production of androgen). *See also* virilization.

hirudin (hi-**roo**-din) *n.* an anticoagulant, present in the salivary glands of leeches and in certain snake venoms, that prevents blood coagulation by inhibiting the action of the enzyme thrombin. **Bivalirudin** is a genetically engineered form of hirudin from the medicinal leech, used to treat myocardial infarction.

Hirudo (hi-**roo**-doh) *n.* a genus of leeches. *See* leech.

hist- (histio-, histo-) *combining form denoting* tissue.

histamine (**hist**-ă-meen) *n.* a compound derived from the amino acid histidine, found in nearly all tissues of the body. Histamine causes dilation of blood vessels and contraction of smooth muscle; it is an important mediator of inflammation and is released in large amounts after skin damage, producing flushing, a flare, and a weal. Histamine is also released in anaphylactic reactions. *See also* anaphylaxis, antihistamine.

histidine (**hist**-i-deen) *n.* an amino acid from which histamine is derived.

histiocyte (**hist**-i-ŏ-syt) *n.* a fixed macrophage, i.e. one that is stationary within connective tissue.

histiocytoma (hist-i-oh-sy-**toh**-mă) *n.* a tumour that contains macrophages or histiocytes.

histiocytosis (hist-i-oh-sy-**toh**-sis) *n.* any of a group of diseases in which there are abnormalities in histiocytes due to abnormal storage of fats, as in Gaucher's disease; inflammatory disorders, as in Langerhans cell histiocytosis; or malignant proliferation of histiocytes.

histocompatibility (hist-oh-kŏm-pat-i-**bil**-iti) *n.* the form of compatibility that depends upon tissue components, mainly specific glycoprotein antigens in cell membranes. A high degree of histocompatibility is necessary for a tissue graft or organ transplant to be successful. **—histocompatible** *adj.*

histogenesis (hist-oh-**jen**-i-sis) *n.* the formation of tissues.

histoid (**hist**-oid) *adj.* **1.** resembling normal tissue. **2.** composed of one type of tissue.

histology (hiss-**tol**-ŏji) *n.* the study of the structure of tissues by means of special staining techniques combined with light and electron microscopy. **—histological** *adj.*

histolysis (hiss-**tol**-i-sis) *n.* disintegration of tissue.

histone (**hist**-ohn) *n.* a simple protein that combines with a nucleic acid to form a nucleoprotein.

histoplasmin (hist-oh-**plaz**-min) *n.* a preparation of antigenic material from a culture of the fungus *Histoplasma capsulatum*, used to test for the presence of histoplasmosis by subcutaneous injection.

histoplasmosis (hist-oh-plaz-**moh**-sis) *n.* an infection caused by inhaling spores of the fungus *Histoplasma capsulatum*. The primary pulmonary form usually produces no symptoms or harmful effects. Occasionally, progressive histoplasmosis, which resembles tuberculosis, develops. The fungus may spread via the bloodstream to attack the liver, spleen, lymph nodes, or intestine. Symptomatic disease is treated with intravenous amphotericin.

histotoxic (hist-oh-**toks**-ik) *adj.* poisonous to tissues: applied to certain substances and conditions.

histrionic personality disorder (his-tree-**o**-nik) *n.* a type of personality disorder characterized by attention-seeking, self-dramatization, and an excessive need for approval. It affects more women than men. Classified as a specific personality disorder in DSM-IV-TR, in DSM-5 it is treated as a subtype of narcissistic personality disorder.

HIV (human immunodeficiency virus) *n.* a retrovirus responsible for AIDS. **HIV-1** the variety of HIV most common in Western countries. **HIV-2** the variety of HIV most common in Africa. *See also* HTLV.

SEE WEB LINKS

- Information about HIV from the National Aids Trust website

hives (hyvz) *n. see* urticaria.

HLA system *n.* human leucocyte antigen system: a series of four gene families (termed A, B, C, and D) that code for polymorphic proteins expressed on the surface of most nucleated cells. Individuals inherit from each parent one gene (or set of genes) for each subdivision of the HLA system. If two individuals have identical HLA types, they are said to be histocompatible. Successful tissue transplantation requires a minimum number of HLA differences between donor and recipient tissues.

HMG *n. see* human menopausal gonadotrophin.

H1N1 *n. see* influenza.

H5N1 *n.* a strain of influenza A virus that causes a virulent type of avian influenza (fowl plague). It is transmissible to humans by close contact with infected birds, causing a form of influenza with a high mortality rate; recent outbreaks occurred in Hong Kong (1997) and southeast Asia (starting in 2004).

HNA *n. see* health needs assessment.

hobnail liver (**hob**-nayl) *n.* the liver of a patient with cirrhosis, which has a knobbly appearance caused by regenerating nodules separated by bands of fibrous tissue.

Hodgkin's disease (Hodgkin's lymphoma) (**hoj**-kinz) *n.* a malignant disease of lymphatic tissues – a form of lymphoma – usually characterized by painless enlargement of one or more groups of lymph nodes in the neck, armpits, groin, chest, or abdomen; the spleen, liver, bone marrow, and bones may also be involved. Treatment may include surgery, radiotherapy, chemotherapy (using drugs such as procarbazine and prednisolone), or a combination of these. [T. Hodgkin (1798–1866), British physician]

hole in the heart (hohl) *n.* *see* septal defect.

holistic (hoh-**list**-ik) *adj.* describing an approach to patient care in which the physiological, psychological, and social factors of the patient's condition are taken into account, rather than just the diagnosed disease. The term is often used in relation to public health and is also applied to a range of orthodox and complementary methods of treatment. *See also* complementary medicine.

holo- *combining form denoting* complete or entire.

holocrine (**hol**-ŏ-kryn) *adj.* describing a gland or type of secretion in which the entire cell disintegrates when the product is released.

Homans' sign (**hoh**-mănz) *n.* pain felt in the calf when the foot is flexed backwards: a sign of phlebothrombosis. [J. Homans (1877–1954), US physician]

homeo- (homoeo-) *combining form denoting* similar; like.

homeopathic (homoeopathic) (hoh-mi-ŏ-**path**-ik) *adj.* **1.** of or relating to homeopathy. **2.** infinitesimally small, as applied to the dose of a drug.

homeopathy (homoeopathy) (hoh-mi-**op**-ă-thi) *n.* a complementary therapy based on the theory that 'like cures like'. It involves a belief that conditions may be treated with a tiny dose of a substance (so diluted as to be indistinguishable from pure water) that in larger doses would normally cause or aggravate that condition. A second principle is a process of dilution and shaking known as succussion. Homeopathy was developed in 1796 by a German doctor, Samuel Hahnemann (1755–1843). It was described as 'scientifically implausible' by the Chief Medical Officer in 2010 and is not recommended by NICE **—homeopathist** *n.*

SEE WEB LINKS

- Website of the Society of Homeopaths

homeostasis (hoh-mi-oh-**stay**-sis) *n.* the physiological process by which the internal systems of the body are maintained at equilibrium, despite variations in the external conditions. **—homeostatic** *adj.*

homo- *combining form denoting* the same or common.

homocysteine (hoh-moh-**sis**-ti-een) *n.* a sulphur-containing amino acid that is an intermediate in the synthesis of cysteine. Elevated levels of homocysteine in the blood are a risk factor for vascular disease independent of diabetes, hypertension, elevated levels of cholesterol in the blood, and smoking. *See also* homocystinuria.

homocystinuria (hoh-moh-sis-tin-**yoor**-iă) *n.* an inborn error of metabolism caused by an enzyme deficiency resulting in an excess of homocysteine in the blood and the presence of homocystine (an oxidized form of cysteine) in the urine. Clinically affected individuals have learning disability, are excessively tall with long fingers (due to overgrowth of bones), and have a tendency to form blood clots in the veins and arteries, leading to strokes.

homoeopathy (hoh-mi-**op**-ă-thi) *n. see* homeopathy.

homogenize (hŏ-**moj**-i-nyz) *vb.* to reduce material to a uniform consistency, e.g. by crushing and mixing. **—homogenization** *n.*

homogentisic acid (hoh-moh-jen-**tis**-ik) *n.* a product formed during the metabolism of the amino acids phenylalanine and tyrosine. In normal individuals homogentisic acid is oxidized by the enzyme **homogentisic acid oxidase**. In rare cases this enzyme is lacking and alcaptonuria results.

homograft (**hom**-ŏ-grahft) *n. see* allograft.

homoiothermic (hoh-moi-ŏ-**therm**-ik) *adj.* warm-blooded: able to maintain a constant body temperature independently of, and despite variations in, the temperature of the surroundings. *Compare* poikilothermic. **—homoiothermy** *n.*

homolateral (hoh-moh-**lat**-er-ăl) *adj. see* ipsilateral.

homologous (hoh-**mol**-ŏ-gŭs) *adj.* **1.** (in anatomy) describing organs or parts that have the same basic structure and evolutionary origin, but not necessarily the same function or superficial structure. *Compare* analogous. **2.** (in genetics) describing a pair of chromosomes of similar shape and size and having identical gene loci.

homonymous (hoh-**mon**-i-mŭs) *adj.* describing a visual defect in which the visual field to one side of the body is restricted in both eyes (*see* hemianopia).

homozygous (hoh-moh-**zy**-gŭs) *adj.* describing an individual in whom the members of a pair of genes determining a particular characteristic are identical. *See* allele. *Compare* heterozygous. **—homozygote** *n.*

honeycomb lung (**hun**-i-kohm) *n.* the honeycomb pattern seen on X-ray at the later stages of chronic lung conditions, in which the lungs become less elastic and more fibrotic and are likely to progress to respiratory failure.

HoNOS *n. see* Health of the Nation Outcome Scale.

hook (huuk) *n.* a surgical instrument with a bent or curved tip, used to hold, lift, or retract tissue at operation.

hookworm (**huuk**-werm) *n.* either of two nematode worms, *Necator americanus* or *Ancylostoma duodenale*, which live as parasites in the human intestine. **h. disease** a condition resulting from an infestation of the small intestine by hookworms. Heavy hookworm infections may cause considerable damage to the wall of the intestine, leading to severe anaemia. Mebendazole is used in treatment.

hordeolum (hor-**dee**-ŏ-lum) *n. see* stye.

horizontal transmission (ho-ri-**zon**-t'l) *n.* the spread of an infectious agent from one person or group to another, usually through contact with contaminated material, such as sputum or faeces. *Compare* vertical transmission.

hormone (hor-mohn) *n.* a substance that is produced by an endocrine gland in one part of the body, passes into the bloodstream, and is carried to other (distant) organs or tissues, where it acts to modify their structure or function. Examples of hormones are corticosteroids, adrenaline, growth hormone, androgens, oestrogens, thyroid hormone, and insulin.

hormone-binding globulins *pl. n.* a family of plasma proteins whose function is to bind free hormone molecules and thus reduce their function. Alterations in levels of the binding globulins, for example during pregnancy or ill health, can result in variations in assays of hormone levels in individuals.

hormone replacement therapy (HRT) *n.* the use of female hormones for the relief of symptoms resulting from cessation of ovarian function, either at the time of the natural menopause or following surgical removal of the ovaries. Oestrogenic hormones may be prescribed orally, by subcutaneous implant, or transdermally (as skin patches or gel); a combination of progestogen with oestrogen is preferred if the woman has retained her uterus.

horn (horn) *n.* (in anatomy) a process, outgrowth, or extension of an organ or other structure. It is often paired.

Horner's syndrome (hor-nerz) *n.* a syndrome consisting of a constricted pupil, ptosis, and an absence of sweating over the affected side of the face. The symptoms are due to a disorder of the sympathetic nerves in the brainstem or cervical (neck) region. [J. F. Horner (1831–86), Swiss ophthalmologist]

horseshoe kidney (hors-shoo) *n.* an anatomical variation in kidney development whereby the lower poles of both kidneys are joined together. This usually causes no trouble but it may be associated with impaired drainage of urine from the kidney by the ureters. The condition is associated with Turner's syndrome.

Horton's syndrome (hor-t'nz) *n.* a severe headache caused by the release of histamine. [B. T. Horton (20th century), US physician]

hospice (hos-pis) *n.* an institution that provides palliative or end-of-life care for people with terminal illnesses, specializing in symptom management and often also providing psychological and spiritual help.

hospital (hos-pi-t'l) *n.* an institution providing medical or psychiatric care and treatment of patients. **community h.** a small hospital, which may be staffed by general practitioners, providing care for patients for whom home care is not practicable. **day h.** a hospital at which patients are under clinical supervision during the day but do not stay overnight. **district general h.** a hospital that provides sufficient basic services for the population of a health district. *See also* trust.

hospital-acquired infection (HAI) *n.* *see* nosocomial infection.

Hospital Anxiety and Depression Scale (HADS) *n.* a screening and self-report device for measuring the severity of anxiety and depression separately. Consisting of a 14-item questionnaire, it can be used within hospital outpatient, primary-care, and community settings for all age groups from adolescence upwards.

host (hohst) *n.* an animal or plant in or upon which a parasite lives. **intermediate h.** a host in which the parasite passes its larval or asexual stages. **definitive h.** a host in which the parasite develops to its sexual stage.

hourglass contraction (ow-er-glahs) *n.* constriction of an organ at its centre as a result of abnormal muscular contraction. Hourglass contraction may be a complication of labour, tending to trap the placenta in the upper part of the constricted uterus and possibly leading to excessive blood loss after delivery.

hourglass stomach *n.* a deformity of the stomach in which the 'waist' is constricted by fibrosis caused by a chronic peptic ulcer, producing an upper and a lower cavity separated by a narrow channel.

housemaid's knee (prepatellar bursitis) (howss-maydz) *n.* inflammation and swelling of the bursa in front of the kneecap, usually due to repetitive friction and pressure over the kneecap, as from frequent kneeling. *See also* bursitis.

HPV *n. see* human papillomavirus.

HR *n.* heart rate.

H_2-receptor antagonist *n. see* antihistamine.

HRS *n. see* Hallucinations Rating Scale.

HRT *n. see* hormone replacement therapy.

HSDU *n.* Hospital Sterilization and Disinfection Unit.

HSE *n. see* Health and Safety Executive.

HSV *n.* herpes simplex virus: *see* herpes.

5HT *n.* 5-hydroxytryptamine: *see* serotonin.

$5HT_1$ agonist (triptan) *n.* a drug that stimulates serotonin receptors, causing constriction of cerebral blood vessels, and is used for the relief of migraine headaches. Such drugs include **sumatriptan** (Imigran), **almotriptan** (Almogran), **naratriptan** (Naramig), and **zolmitriptan** (Zomig).

HTLV (human T-cell lymphocytotrophic virus) *n.* a family of viruses. **HTLV-I** a cause of lymphoma. **HTLV-III** the former name for HIV (the AIDS virus).

Hughes syndrome (hewz) *n. see* antiphospholipid antibody syndrome. [G. Hughes (21st century), British physician]

human chorionic gonadotrophin (hCG) (hew-măn kor-i-on-ik) *n.* a hormone, similar to the pituitary gonadotrophins, that is produced by the placenta during pregnancy and maintains secretion of progesterone by the corpus luteum. Large amounts of hCG are excreted in the urine, and this is used as the basis for most pregnancy tests. Serum hCG monitoring is used for detecting ectopic pregnancies; the hormone is also a marker in prenatal screening tests (levels are high in Down's syndrome and hydatidiform mole) and for certain malignant tumours. A preparation of hCG is used to treat ovulation disorders and to induce superovulation for in vitro fertilization.

human chorionic somatomammotrophin (soh-mă-toh-mam-oh-**troh**-fin) *n.* *see* human placental lactogen.

Human Fertilization and Embryology Authority (HFEA) *n.* a body that controls, regulates, and reviews practice and research involving the use of embryos and issues licences for research and for treatment in assisted conception.

Human Genome Project (HGP) *n.* an international research project to isolate all the genes in human DNA and determine the sequence of genes on human chromosomes. The project began in 1988 and was completed in 2003. The human genome comprises some 3×10^9 nucleotide base pairs forming 22,000–25,000 genes. Knowledge of the human genome has already resulted in the identification of the genes associated with many hereditary disorders and revealed the existence of a genetic basis or component for many other diseases not previously known to have one.

human immunodeficiency virus *n.* *see* HIV.

humanism (hew-măn-izm) *n.* a way of thinking and living based on acceptance of the moral values of humanity. Humanists reject all religious and authoritarian beliefs, emphasizing rational and scientific inquiry, individual freedom and responsibility, and the need for tolerance and cooperation. —**humanist** *adj.*, *n.*

human leucocyte antigen system *n.* *see* HLA system.

human menopausal gonadotrophin (HMG, menotrophin) *n.* a gonadotrophin combining the actions of follicle-stimulating hormone and luteinizing hormone, which is extracted from the urine of postmenopausal women and administered by intramuscular or subcutaneous injection to treat infertility caused by underactivity of the pituitary gland and to stimulate the ovaries in women undergoing fertility treatment. Trade names: **Menopur**, **Merional**.

human papillomavirus (HPV) (pap-i-**loh**-mă-vy-rŭs) *n.* a virus – a member of the papovavirus group – that causes warts, including genital warts. Certain strains are considered to be causative factors in the development of anal and genital cancers, especially cervical cancer. HPV is one of the most common sexually transmitted infections. A vaccine that protects against strains of HPV associated with cervical cancer is now available.

human placental lactogen (human chorionic somatomammotrophin) (lak-tŏ-jĕn) *n.* a protein hormone produced by the placenta during most but not all pregnancies. Its exact function remains obscure, but it seems to contribute to the development of diabetes in some pregnancies.

human rights *pl. n.* a legal framework adopted by the United Nations after the Second World War that sought to define and promote fundamental entitlements, conditions, and freedoms to be afforded to all human beings. In the UK the Human Rights Act 1998 enacts the provisions of the 1950 European Convention on Human Rights, which set out, in 14 articles, an individual's rights, entitlements, and freedoms. See Appendix 11: The Human Rights Act.

SEE WEB LINKS

- Details of human rights from the United Nations website

humectant (hew-**mek**-tănt) **1.** *n.* a substance that is used for moistening. **2.** *adj.* causing moistening.

humerus (**hew**-mer-ŭs) *n.* the bone of the upper arm. The head of the humerus articulates with the scapula at the shoulder joint. At the lower end of the shaft the trochlea articulates with the ulna and part of the radius. See illustration.

humoral (**hew**-mer-ăl) *adj.* circulating in the bloodstream; humoral immunity requires circulating antibodies.

humour (**hew**-mer) *n.* a body fluid. *See* aqueous humour, vitreous humour.

hunger pain (**hung**-er) *n.* pain in the upper abdomen that is relieved by taking food. It is associated with a duodenal ulcer.

Hunner's ulcer (**hun**-erz) *n. see* interstitial cystitis. [G. L. Hunner (1868–1957), US urologist]

Hunter's syndrome (**hunt**-erz) *n.* a hereditary disorder caused by deficiency of an enzyme that results in the accumulation of protein–carbohydrate complexes and fats in the cells of the body. This leads to learning disability, enlargement of the liver and spleen, and prominent coarse facial features (**gargoylism**). Medical name: **mucopolysaccharidosis type II**. [C. H. Hunter (1872–1955), US physician]

Huntington's disease (HD, Huntington's chorea) (**hunt**-ing-tŏnz) *n.* a hereditary disease caused by a defect in a single gene that is inherited as an autosomal dominant characteristic, tending

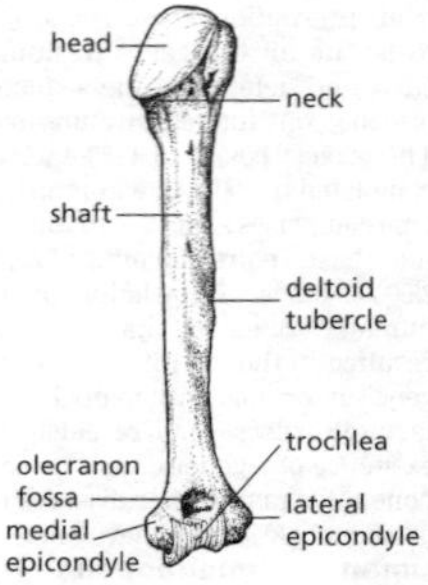

The humerus (posterior surface)

to appear in half of the children of the parents with this condition. Symptoms, which begin to appear in early middle age, include unsteady gait and jerky involuntary movements (*see* chorea), accompanied later by behavioural changes and progressive dementia. [G. Huntington (1850–1916), US physician]

Hurler's syndrome (hoor-lerz) *n.* a hereditary disorder caused by deficiency of an enzyme that results in the accumulation of protein–carbohydrate complexes and fats in the cells of the body. This leads to severe learning disability, enlargement of the liver and spleen, heart defects, deformities of the bones, and coarsening and thickening of the facial features (**gargoylism**). Medical name: **mucopolysaccharidosis type I**. [G. Hurler (1889–1965), Austrian paediatrician]

HUS *n. see* haemolytic uraemic syndrome.

Hutchinson's teeth (huch-in-sŏnz) *pl. n.* narrowed and notched permanent incisor teeth: a sign of congenital syphilis. [J. Hutchinson (1828–1913), British surgeon]

hyal- (hyalo-) *combining form denoting* **1.** glassy; transparent. **2.** hyalin. **3.** the vitreous humour of the eye.

hyalin (hy-ă-lin) *n.* a clear glassy material produced as the result of degeneration in certain tissues, particularly connective tissue and epithelial cells.

hyaline cartilage (hy-ă-lin) *n. see* cartilage.

hyaline membrane disease *n. see* respiratory distress syndrome.

hyalitis (hy-ă-ly-tis) *n.* inflammation of the vitreous humour of the eye. **asteroid h.** *see* asteroid hyalosis.

hyaloid membrane (hy-ă-loid) *n.* the transparent membrane that surrounds the vitreous humour of the eye, separating it from the retina.

hyaluronidase (hy-ăl-yoor-on-i-dayz) *n.* an enzyme that increases the permeability of connective tissue. Hyaluronidase is found in the testes, in semen, and in other tissues.

hybrid (hy-brid) *n.* the offspring of a cross between two genetically unlike individuals. A hybrid, whose parents are usually of different species or varieties, is often sterile.

HYCOSY (hysterosalpingo-contrast sonography) *n.* an out-patient technique that tests for blocked Fallopian tubes. Using transvaginal ultrasonography following the injection of an echo contrast medium through the cervix, flow along the tubes can be reliably visualized. *See also* Doppler ultrasound.

hydatid (hy-dă-tid) *n.* a bladder-like cyst formed in various human tissues following the growth of the larval stage of an *Echinococcus* tapeworm. **alveolar h.** an aggregate of small cysts, which enlarge by budding off external daughter cysts. **unilocular h.** a single large fluid-filled cyst, bound by a fibrous capsule, that gives rise internally to smaller daughter cysts. *See also* hydatid disease.

hydatid disease (hydatidosis, echinococciasis, echinococcosis) *n.* a condition resulting from the presence in the liver, lungs, or brain of hydatid cysts. Alveolar hydatids form malignant tumours; unilocular hydatids exert pressure as they grow and thereby damage surrounding tissues.

hydatidiform mole (hydatid mole, vesicular mole) (hy-dă-**tid**-i-form) *n.* a collection of fluid-filled sacs that develop when the chorion degenerates in early pregnancy. Complete moles show no evidence of fetal tissue; there is usually evidence of a fetus or fetal red blood cells with a partial mole.

hydatidosis (hy-dă-tid-**oh**-sis) *n.* *see* hydatid disease.

hydr- (hydro-) *combining form denoting* water or a watery fluid.

hydraemia (hy-**dree**-miă) *n.* the presence in the blood of more than the normal proportion of water.

hydralazine (hy-**dral**-ă-zeen) *n.* a vasodilator administered by mouth or intravenous injection or infusion, usually in conjunction with diuretics, in the treatment of hypertension. Trade name: **Apresoline**.

hydramnios (hy-**dram**-ni-ŏs) *n.* *see* polyhydramnios.

hydrargyria (hy-drar-**jy**-riă) *n.* *see* mercurialism.

hydrarthrosis (hy-drar-**throh**-sis) *n.* swelling at a joint caused by excessive synovial fluid. The condition usually involves the knees and may be recurrent.

hydrate (**hy**-drayt) **1.** *vb.* to undergo treatment or impregnation with water. **—hydration** *n.* **2.** *n.* a chemical compound in which one or more molecules of water are combined with a molecule of another substance.

hydrocalycosis (hy-droh-kal-i-**koh**-sis) *n.* *see* caliectasis.

hydrocele (**hy**-droh-seel) *n.* the accumulation of watery liquid in a sac, usually the sac surrounding the testes. This condition is characterized by painless enlargement of the scrotum.

hydrocephalus (hy-droh-**sef**-ă-lŭs) *n.* an abnormal increase in the amount of cerebrospinal fluid within the ventricles of the brain. In childhood, before the sutures of the skull have fused, hydrocephalus makes the head enlarge. In adults, hydrocephalus raises the intracranial pressure, with consequent drowsiness and vomiting. Spina bifida may be associated with hydrocephalus in childhood.

SEE WEB LINKS

- Website of Shine, the charity for people living with spina bifida and hydrocephalus

hydrochloric acid (hy-drŏ-**klor**-ik) *n.* a strong acid present, in a very dilute form, in gastric juice. The secretion of excess hydrochloric acid by the stomach results in the condition hyperchlorhydria.

hydrochlorothiazide (hy-drŏ-klor-oh-**th'y**-ă-zyd) *n.* a thiazide diuretic used in combination with other drugs (e.g. amiloride) to treat fluid retention (oedema) and high blood pressure.

hydrocolloid dressing (hy-droh-**kol**-oid) *n.* a dressing typically consisting of an absorbent layer of gel on a semipermeable film or foam that promotes rehydration and debridement of wounds, including infected wounds.

hydrocortisone (hy-droh-**kor**-tiz-ohn) *n.* a pharmaceutical preparation of the steroid hormone cortisol. Hydrocortisone is used to treat adrenal failure (Addison's disease), shock, and inflammatory, allergic, and rheumatic conditions (including rheumatoid arthritis, colitis, and eczema). It may be given by mouth, by intramuscular, intravenous, or intra-articular injection, or in the form of a cream, ointment, lotion, or eye or ear drops. Trade names: **Dioderm**, **Hydrocortistab**, **Locoid**, **Locoid Crelo**, **Mildison**, **Solu-Cortef**.

hydrocyanic acid (prussic acid) (hy-droh-sy-**an**-ik) *n.* an intensely poisonous volatile acid that can cause death within a minute if inhaled. It smells of bitter almonds. *See* cyanide.

hydroflumethiazide (hy-droh-floo-meth-**I**-ă-zyd) *n.* a diuretic administered by mouth to treat fluid retention (oedema) and high blood pressure.

hydrogel dressing (**hy**-droh-jel) *n.* a dressing consisting of a gel in the form of a sheet or an amorphous mass that can take the shape of the wound. Such dressings can be used for lightly exuding or granulating wounds but are not suitable for infected or heavily exuding wounds.

hydrogen (**hy**-drŏ-jĕn) *n.* a colourless gas that is combined with oxygen to form water (H_2O) and with various other molecules (chiefly carbon and oxygen) to form all organic compounds. Symbol: H. **h. ion concentration** *see* pH.

hydrogen peroxide (per-**ok**-syd) *n.* an oxidizing agent used (in the form of a solution or cream) as a skin disinfectant for cleansing wounds and treating superficial infections and as a deodorant mouthwash for treating oral infections. Trade names: **Crystacide**, **Peroxyl**.

hydrolysis (hy-**drol**-i-sis) *n.* any chemical reaction in which a compound and water react together to produce other compounds.

hydroma (hy-**droh**-mă) *n. see* hygroma.

hydrometer (hy-**drom**-it-er) *n.* an instrument for measuring the density or relative density of liquids. —**hydrometry** *n.*

hydrometra (hy-droh-**mee**-tră) *n.* an abnormal accumulation of watery fluid in the uterus.

hydronephrosis (hy-droh-ni-**froh**-sis) *n.* distension and dilatation of the pelvis of the kidney. This is due to an obstruction to the free flow of urine from the kidney. Surgical relief by pyeloplasty is advisable to avoid the back pressure atrophy of the kidney and the complications of infection and stone formation. —**hydronephrotic** *adj.*

hydropericarditis (hy-droh-pe-ri-kar-**dy**-tis) *n. see* hydropericardium.

hydropericardium (hy-droh-pe-ri-**kar**-di-ŭm) *n.* accumulation of a clear serous fluid within the membranous sac surrounding the heart. It occurs in many cases of pericarditis (**hydropericarditis**).

hydroperitoneum (hy-droh-pe-ri-tŏn-**ee**-ŭm) *n. see* ascites.

hydrophobia (hy-drŏ-**foh**-biă) *n. see* rabies.

hydrophthalmos (hy-drof-**thal**-mŏs) *n. see* buphthalmos.

hydropneumoperitoneum (hy-droh-new-moh-pe-ri-tŏn-**ee**-ŭm) *n.* the presence of fluid and gas in the peritoneal cavity.

hydropneumothorax (hy-droh-new-moh-**thor**-aks) *n.* air and fluid in the pleural cavity. An effusion of serous fluid commonly complicates a pneumothorax, and must be drained.

hydrops (**hy**-drops) *n.* an abnormal accumulation of fluid in body tissues or cavities. **corneal h.** the sudden painful accumulation of fluid in the cornea seen in keratoconus. It results in a sudden reduction of vision. *See also* hydrops fetalis, Ménière's disease (endolymphatic hydrops).

hydrops fetalis (fee-**tah**-lis) *n.* the accumulation of fluid in fetal tissues or body cavities. In its most severe form, excessive fluid collects in the peritoneal cavity (ascites), pleural and pericardial cavities, and soft tissues (oedema). The commonest cause is severe anaemia associated with haemolytic disease of the newborn; other causes include congenital heart defects and chromosomal abnormalities.

hydrorrhachis (hy-**dror**-ră-kis) *n.* an abnormal accumulation of watery fluid in the space surrounding the spinal cord.

hydrosalpinx (hy-droh-**sal**-pinks) *n.* the accumulation of fluid in one of the Fallopian tubes due to inflammation and subsequent obstruction.

hydrostatic accouchement (hy-droh-**stat**-ik) *n. see* accouchement.

hydrotherapy (hy-droh-**th'e**-ră-pi) *n.* the use of water in the treatment of disorders, such as exercising in remedial swimming pools as part of the rehabilitation of arthritic or partially paralysed patients.

hydrothorax (hy-droh-**thor**-aks) *n.* fluid in the pleural cavity. *See also* hydropneumothorax.

hydrotubation (hy-droh-tew-**bay**-shŏn) *n.* the introduction of a fluid (usually a dye) through the cervix (neck) of the uterus under pressure to allow visualization, by laparoscopy, of the passage of the dye through the Fallopian tubes. It is used to test whether or not the tubes are blocked in the investigation of infertility.

hydroureter (hy-droh-yoor-**ee**-ter) *n.* an accumulation of urine in one of the ureters, usually resulting from obstruction of the ureter by a stone or a pelvic mass.

hydroxocobalamin (hy-droks-oh-koh-**bal**-ă-min) *n.* a cobalt-containing drug administered by intramuscular injection to treat conditions involving vitamin B_{12} deficiency, such as pernicious anaemia. It is also given, by intravenous infusion, to treat cyanide poisoning. Trade names: **Cobalin-H**, **Cyanokit**, **Neo-Cytamen**.

hydroxyapatite (hy-droks-i-**ap**-ă-tyt) *n.* **1.** the crystalline component of bones and teeth, consisting of a complex form of calcium phosphate. Hydroxyapatite crystals may also occur in joints in association with arthritis. **2.** a biocompatible ceramic material that is a synthetic form of natural hydroxyapatite. It is used to coat some joint replacement prostheses, which encourages bone to grow onto the implant, and is also used in some forms of middle-ear surgery.

hydroxycarbamide (hydroxyurea) (hy-droks-i-**kar**-bă-myd) *n.* a drug that prevents cell growth and is administered by mouth to treat chronic myeloid leukaemia and to reduce the frequency of sickle-cell crises. Hydroxycarbamide may lower the white cell content of the blood due to its effects on the bone marrow. Trade names: **Hydrea**, **Siklos**.

hydroxychloroquine (hy-droks-i-**klor**-ŏ-kwin) *n.* a drug, similar to chloroquine, given by mouth mainly to treat lupus erythematosus and rheumatoid arthritis. Trade name: **Plaquenil**.

5-hydroxyindoleacetic acid (5-HIAA) (hy-droks-i-in-dohl-ă-**see**-tik) *n.* a metabolite of serotonin, the most common secretion product of carcinoid tumours. Measured over 24 hours in the urine, this is the most reliable screening test for such tumours.

hydroxyproline (hy-droks-i-**proh**-leen) *n.* a compound, similar in structure to the amino acids, found only in collagen.

5-hydroxytryptamine (hy-droks-i-**trip**-tă-meen) *n. see* serotonin.

hydroxyurea (hy-droks-i-yoor-**ee**-ă) *n. see* hydroxycarbamide.

hydroxyzine (hy-**droks**-i-zeen) *n.* an antihistamine drug with sedative properties, administered by mouth to treat pruritus. Trade names: **Atarax**, **Ucerax**.

hygiene (**hy**-jeen) *n.* the science of health and the study of ways of preserving it, particularly by promoting cleanliness.

hygr- (hygro-) *combining form denoting* moisture.

hygroma (hydroma) (hy-**groh**-mă) *n.* a type of cyst, which may develop from the liquified remains of a subdural haematoma (**subdural h.**). **cystic h.** a collection of fluid behind the neck of a fetus, which may be a diagnostic feature of a chromosomal abnormality. *See also* nuchal (translucency scanning).

hygrometer (hy-**grom**-i-ter) *n.* an instrument for measuring the relative humidity of the atmosphere, i.e. the ratio of the moisture in the air to the moisture it would contain if it were saturated at the same temperature and pressure.

hymen (**hy**-mĕn) *n.* the membrane that covers the opening of the vagina at birth but usually perforates spontaneously before puberty.

hymenectomy (hy-mĕn-**ek**-tŏmi) *n.* surgical removal of the hymen to enlarge the vaginal opening.

hymenotomy (hy-mĕn-**ot**-ŏmi) *n.* incision of the hymen. This operation may be performed in cases of imperforate hymen. It is also carried out to alleviate dyspareunia (painful intercourse).

hyo- *combining form denoting* the hyoid bone.

hyoid bone (**hy**-oid) *n.* a small isolated U-shaped bone in the neck, below and supporting the tongue. It is held in position by muscles and ligaments between it and the styloid process of the temporal bone.

hyoscine (scopolamine) (**hy**-ŏ-seen) *n.* an antimuscarinic drug that prevents smooth muscle spasm. **h. butylbromide** (**Buscopan**) a drug taken by mouth or injection for the treatment of bowel colic and irritable bowel syndrome or for painful menstruation. **h. hydrobromide (Joy Rides, Kwells, Scopoderm TTS)** a drug given by mouth, injection, or in skin patches for preoperative medication and motion sickness.

hyp- (hypo-) *prefix denoting* **1.** deficiency, lack, or small size. **2.** (in anatomy) below; beneath.

hypaemia (hy-**pee**-miă) *n.* a decrease in the blood supply to an organ or tissue. *Compare* hyperaemia.

hypalgesia (hy-pal-**jeez**-iă) *n.* an abnormally low sensitivity to pain.

hyper- *prefix denoting* **1.** excessive; abnormally increased. **2.** (in anatomy) above.

hyperacidity (hy-per-ă-**sid**-iti) *n.* an abnormally increased concentration of acid, especially in the stomach (*see* hyperchlorhydria).

hyperactivity (hy-per-ak-**tiv**-iti) *n.* *see* hyperkinesia.

hyperacusis (hy-per-ă-**kew**-sis) *n.* a form of reduced sound tolerance characterized by uncomfortable or even painful sensitivity to all sounds above a certain level.

hyperadrenalism (hy-per-ă-**dren**-ă-lizm) *n.* overactivity of the adrenal glands. *See* Cushing's syndrome.

hyperaemia (hy-per-**ee**-miă) *n.* the presence of excess blood in the vessels supplying a part of the body. **active h.** (**arterial h.**) hyperaemia that occurs when the arterioles are relaxed and there is an increased blood flow. **passive h.** hyperaemia that occurs when the blood flow from the affected part is obstructed.

hyperaesthesia (hy-per-ees-**theez**-iă) *n.* excessive sensibility, especially of the skin.

hyperaldosteronism (hy-per-al-**dos**-tĕ-rŏ-nizm) *n.* *see* aldosteronism.

hyperalgesia (hy-per-al-**jeez**-iă) *n.* an abnormal state of increased sensitivity to painful stimuli.

hyperandrogenism (hy-per-an-**droj**-in-izm) *n.* excessive secretion of androgen in women. It is associated with hirsutism, acne, sparse or infrequent menstruation (oligomenorrhoea), metrorrhagia, absent or infrequent ovulation, infertility, endometrial hyperplasia, hyperlipidaemia, hyperglycaemia, and hypertension. *See also* virilization.

hyperbaric (hy-per-**ba**-rik) *adj.* at a pressure greater than atmospheric pressure. **h. oxygenation** a technique for exposing a patient to oxygen at high pressure. It is used to treat compressed air illness, carbon monoxide poisoning, gas gangrene, and acute breathing difficulties.

hypercalcaemia (hy-per-kal-**see**-miă) *n.* the presence in the blood of an abnormally high concentration of calcium. The many causes include excessive ingestion of vitamin D, overactivity of the parathyroid glands, and malignant disease. It may also occur in association with other symptoms as a congenital condition. **malignant h.** hypercalcaemia resulting from the secretion by a tumour of substances that stimulate bone resorption or from bone metastases causing localized destruction and release of calcium into the bloodstream.

hypercalcinuria (hypercalcuria) (hy-per-kal-sin-**yoor**-iă) *n.* the presence in the urine of an abnormally high concentration of calcium.

hypercapnia (hypercarbia) (hy-per-**kap**-niă) *n.* the presence in the blood of an abnormally high concentration of carbon dioxide.

hypercatabolism (hy-per-kă-**tab**-ŏl-izm) *n.* an abnormally increased rate of metabolic breakdown of substances in the body. *See* catabolism. —**hypercatabolic** *adj.*

hyperchloraemia (hy-per-klor-**ee**-miă) *n.* the presence in the blood of an abnormally high concentration of chloride.

hyperchlorhydria (hy-per-klor-**hy**-driă) *n.* excess secretion of hydrochloric acid in the stomach, usually associated with a peptic ulcer.

hypercholesterolaemia (hy-per-kŏl-est-er-ol-**ee**-miă) *n.* *see* cholesterol.

hyperchromatism (hy-per-**kroh**-mă-tizm) *n.* the property of the nuclei of certain cells (for example, those of tumours) to stain more deeply than normal. —**hyperchromatic** *adj.*

hyperdactylism (polydactylism) (hy-per-**dak**-til-izm) *n.* the condition of having more than the normal number of fingers or toes.

hyperdynamia (hy-per-dy-**nay**-miă) *n.* excessive activity of muscles.

hyperemesis (hy-per-**em**-i-sis) *n.* severe vomiting. **h. gravidarum** persistent vomiting during pregnancy, which results in weight loss, greater than 5%, dehydration, ketosis, and electrolyte imbalances. In severe cases it may cause liver damage and Wernicke's encephalopathy, in which case it may be necessary to terminate the pregnancy.

hyperextension (hy-per-iks-**ten**-shŏn) *n.* extension of a joint or limb beyond its normal limit.

hyperflexion (hy-per-**flek**-shŏn) *n.* excessive and forceful flexion of a limb or other part.

hyperglycaemia (hy-per-gly-**see**-miă) *n.* an excess of glucose in the bloodstream. It may occur in a variety of diseases, most notably in diabetes mellitus.

hyperhidrosis (hyperidrosis) (hy-per-hy-**droh**-sis) *n.* excessive sweating, which may occur in certain diseases, such as fevers or thyrotoxicosis, or following the use of certain drugs, although more commonly there is no underlying cause.

hyperinsulinism (hy-per-**ins**-yoo-lin-izm) *n.* **1.** excessive secretion of the hormone insulin by the islet cells of the pancreas. **2.** metabolic disturbance due to administration of too much insulin.

hyperkalaemia (hy-per-kal-**ee**-miă) *n.* the presence in the blood of an abnormally high concentration of potassium, usually due to failure of the kidneys to excrete it. *See also* electrolyte.

hyperkeratosis (hy-per-ke-ră-**toh**-sis) *n.* thickening of the outer horny layer of the skin. It may occur as an inherited disorder, affecting the palms and soles. **hyperkeratotic** (hy-per-ke-ră-**to**-tik) *adj.*

hyperkinesia (hyperactivity) (hy-per-ki-**neez**-iă) *n.* a state of overactive restlessness in children. *See* attention-deficit/hyperactivity disorder. **—hyperkinetic** (hy-per-ki-**net**-ik) *adj.*

hyperlipidaemia (hyperlipaemia) (hy-per-lip-id-**ee**-miă) *n.* the presence in the blood of an abnormally high concentration of cholesterol and/or triglycerides in the form of lipoproteins, which is associated with an increased risk of atherosclerosis and coronary heart disease.

hypermetropia (long-sightedness) (hy-per-mi-**troh**-piă) *n.* the condition in which parallel light rays are brought to a focus behind the retina when the accommodation is relaxed. Normal vision can be restored by wearing spectacles with convex lenses (see illustration). *Compare* emmetropia, myopia.

hypermotility (hy-per-moh-**til**-iti) *n.* excessive movement or activity, especially of the stomach or intestine.

hypernatraemia (hy-per-nă-**tree**-miă) *n.* the presence in the blood of an abnormally high concentration of sodium. *See also* electrolyte.

hypernephroma (hy-per-ni-**froh**-mă) *n.* *see* renal cell carcinoma.

hyperopia (hy-per-**oh**-piă) *n.* the usual US term for hypermetropia.

hyperostosis (hy-per-os-**toh**-sis) *n.* excessive enlargement of the outer layer of a bone. It commonly affects the frontal bone of the skull

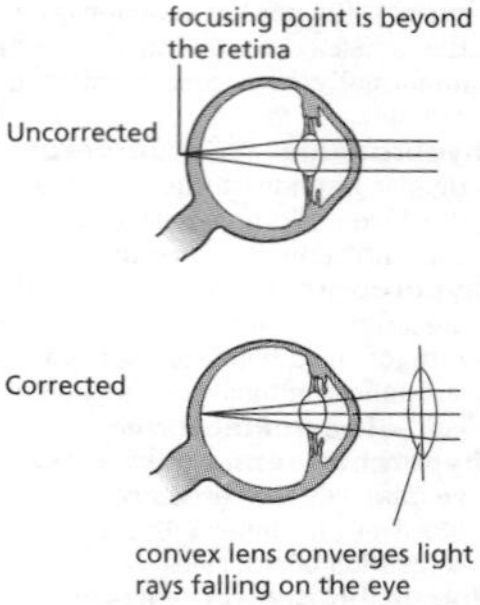

Hypermetropia (long-sightedness)

(**h. frontalis**). **infantile cortical h.** (**Caffey's disease**) periodic swelling of the long bones, jaw, and shoulder blade, associated with pain and fever, in infants under six months.

hyperparathyroidism (hy-per-pa-ră-**th'y**-roid-izm) *n.* excessive secretion of parathyroid hormone, usually due to a tumour in one of the parathyroid glands. *See* von Recklinghausen's disease.

hyperphagia (hy-per-**fay**-jiă) *n.* excessive overeating. *See* bulimia.

hyperpiesia (hy-per-py-**ee**-ziă) *n. see* hypertension.

hyperpituitarism (hy-per-pit-**yoo**-it-er-izm) *n.* overactivity of the pituitary gland, resulting in acromegaly or gigantism.

hyperplasia (hy-per-**play**-ziă) *n.* the increased production and growth of normal cells in a tissue or organ. **benign prostatic h.** *see* prostate gland. *See also* endometrial (hyperplasia). *Compare* hypertrophy, neoplasia.

hyperpnoea (hy-perp-**nee**-ă) *n.* an increase in the rate of breathing that is proportional to an increase in metabolism; for example, on exercise. *Compare* hyperventilation.

hyperprolactinaemia (hy-per-proh-lak-tin-**ee**-miă) *n.* raised serum levels of prolactin, usually due to the presence of a benign pituitary tumour (*see* prolactinoma); other causes include dopamine receptor antagonists (e.g. antipsychotic drugs) and chronic renal failure. Symptoms include loss of sexual drive, amenorrhoea or impotence, and secretion of breast milk in both women and men.

hyperpyrexia (hy-per-py-**reks**-iă) *n.* a rise in body temperature above 106° F (41.1° C). *See* fever.

hypersecretion (hy-per-si-**kree**-shŏn) *n.* excessive secretion, as of hydrochloric acid by the stomach (*see* hyperchlorhydria).

hypersensitive (hy-per-**sen**-si-tiv) *adj.* prone to respond abnormally to the presence of a particular antigen, which may cause a variety of tissue reactions ranging from serum sickness to an allergy (such as hay fever) or, at the severest, to anaphylactic shock (*see* anaphylaxis). *See also* allergy, immunity. **—hypersensitivity** *n.*

hypersplenism (hy-per-**splen**-izm) *n.* a decrease in the numbers of red cells, white cells, and platelets in the blood resulting from destruction or pooling of these cells by an enlarged spleen.

hypertension (hy-per-**ten**-shŏn) *n.* high blood pressure, i.e. elevation of the arterial blood pressure above the normal range expected in a particular age group. Hypertension may be of unknown cause (**essential h.** or **hyperpiesia**). It may also result from disease (**secondary** or **symptomatic h.**), as of the kidneys (**renovascular h.**), endocrine system, or arteries. Complications that may arise from hypertension include atherosclerosis, heart failure, cerebral haemorrhage, and kidney failure. Most cases of hypertension depend upon long-term drug therapy to lower the blood pressure and maintain it within the normal range. The drugs used include thiazide diuretics, ACE inhibitors, and calcium-channel blockers. *See also* portal hypertension, pulmonary (hypertension).

hyperthermia (hyperthermy) (hy-per-**therm**-iă) *n.* **1.** exceptionally high body temperature (about 41°C or above). *See* fever. **2.** treatment of disease by inducing fever. *Compare* hypothermia.

hyperthyroidism (hy-per-**th'y**-roid-izm) *n.* overactivity of the thyroid gland, either due to a tumour, overgrowth of the gland, or Graves' disease. **apathetic h.** a condition seen in patients with thyrotoxicosis, characterized by slow atrial fibrillation and depressive illness. *See* thyrotoxicosis.

hypertonia (hypertonicity) (hy-per-**toh**-niă) *n.* exceptionally high tension in muscles.

hypertonic (hy-per-**tonn**-ik) *adj.* **1.** describing a solution that has a greater osmotic pressure than another solution. *See* osmosis. **2.** describing muscles that demonstrate an abnormal increase in tonicity.

hypertrichosis (hy-per-trik-**oh**-sis) *n.* excessive growth of hair.

hypertrophic cardiomyopathy (hy-per-**trof**-ik) *n.* *see* cardiomyopathy.

hypertrophy (hypertrophia) (hy-**per**-trŏ-fi) *n.* increase in the size of a tissue or organ brought about by the enlargement of its cells rather than by cell multiplication. *See also* (hypertrophic) cardiomyopathy. *Compare* hyperplasia, neoplasia. **—hypertrophic** *adj.*

hypertropia (hy-per-**troh**-piă) *n.* strabismus in which one eye looks upwards.

hyperuricaemia (lithaemia) (hy-per-yoor-i-**see**-miă) *n.* the presence in the blood of an abnormally high concentration of uric acid. *See* gout.

hyperuricuria (lithuria) (hy-per-yoor-ik-**yoor**-iă) *n.* the presence in the urine of an abnormally high concentration of uric acid.

hyperventilation (hy-per-ven-ti-**lay**-shŏn) *n.* breathing at an abnormally rapid rate at rest. This causes a reduction of the carbon dioxide concentration of the arterial blood, leading to dizziness, tingling in the lips and limbs, tetanic cramps in the hands, and tightness across the chest. **h. syndrome** prolonged hyperventilation, often of psychogenic origin, which may lead to loss of consciousness.

hypervitaminosis (hy-per-vit-ă-min-**oh**-sis) *n.* the condition resulting from excessive consumption of vitamins. The fat-soluble vitamins A and D are toxic if taken in excessive amounts.

hypervolaemia (hy-per-vŏ-**lee**-miă) *n.* an increase in the volume of circulating blood.

hyphaema (hy-**fee**-mă) *n.* a collection of blood in the chamber of the eye that lies in front of the iris.

hypn- (hypno-) *combining form denoting* **1.** sleep. **2.** hypnosis.

hypnagogic (hip-nă-**goj**-ik) *adj.* relating to the period immediately before falling asleep. **h. imagery** the production of vivid mental images just before falling asleep.

h. hallucination a vivid and intense auditory or visual hallucination occurring at the beginning of sleep in 30–60% of patients with narcolepsy.

hypnosis (hip-**noh**-sis) *n.* a sleeplike state, artificially induced by a **hypnotist**, in which the mind is more than usually receptive to suggestion. Hypnotic suggestion may be used for a variety of therapeutic purposes.

hypnotherapy (hip-noh-**th'e**-ră-pi) *n.* any form of psychotherapy that utilizes hypnosis. **—hypnotherapist** *n.*

hypnotic (soporific) (hip-**not**-ik) *n.* a drug that produces sleep by depressing brain function and is used for the short-term treatment of insomnia. Hypnotics include benzodiazepines (e.g. nitrazepam, lorazepam) and drugs that act at benzodiazepine receptor sites, such as **zaleplon** (Sonata), **zolpidem** (Stilnoct), and **zopiclone** (Zimovane). Some hypnotics (e.g. nitrazepam, flurazepam) cause hangover effects in the morning.

hypnotism (**hip**-nŏ-tizm) *n.* the induction of hypnosis.

hypo- *prefix. see* hyp-.

hypoaesthesia (hy-poh-ees-**theez**-iă) *n.* a condition in which the sense of touch is diminished. This may rarely be extended to include other forms of sensation.

hypocalcaemia (hy-poh-kal-**see**-miă) *n.* the presence in the blood of an abnormally low concentration of calcium. *See* tetany. *Compare* hypercalcaemia.

hypocapnia (hy-poh-**kap**-niă) *n. see* acapnia.

hypochloraemia (hy-poh-klor-**ee**-miă) *n.* the presence in the blood of an abnormally low concentration of chloride.

hypochlorhydria (hy-poh-klor-**hy**-driă) *n.* reduced secretion of hydrochloric acid in the stomach. *See* achlorhydria.

hypochlorite (hy-poh-**klor**-ryt) *n.* any salt of hypochlorous acid (chloric(I) acid; HClO). Hypochlorites have antiseptic and disinfectant properties, e.g. Milton (sodium hypochlorite).

hypochondria (hy-poh-**kon**-driă) *n.* preoccupation with the physical functioning of the body and with imagined ill health. In the most severe form there are delusions of ill health, often associated with underlying illness, such as depression. **—hypochondriac** *n.* **—hypochondriacal** (hy-poh-kon-**dry**-ă-kăl) *adj.*

hypochondriacal disorder (hypochondriasis, illness anxiety disorder) (hy-poh-kon-**dry**-ă-sis) *n.* symptoms of hypochondria that have reached a level sufficient to be classified as a disorder.

hypochondrium (hy-poh-**kon**-dri-ŭm) *n.* the upper lateral portion of the abdomen, situated beneath the lower ribs. **—hypochondriac** *adj.*

hypochromic (hy-poh-**kroh**-mik) *adj.* **1.** deficient in pigmentation. **2.** (of red blood cells) deficient in haemoglobin.

hypocretin (hy-poh-**kree**-tin) *n.* a neuropeptide that originates in the hypothalamus. Low levels of hypocretin in the cerebrospinal fluid are found in most patients with narcolepsy and may also be found in patients who have suffered with stroke, brain tumours, head injuries, and infections of the nervous system.

hypodermic (hy-poh-**derm**-ik) *adj.* beneath the skin: usually applied to subcutaneous injections. The term is also applied to the syringe used for such injections.

hypofibrinogenaemia (fibrinogenopenia) (hy-poh-fi-brin-oh-jĕ-**nee**-miă) *n.* a deficiency of the clotting factor fibrinogen in the blood, which results in an increased tendency to bleed. It may occur as an inherited disorder or it may be acquired.

hypogammaglobulinaemia (hy-poh-gam-ă-glob-yoo-lin-**ee**-miă) *n.* a deficiency of the protein gammaglobulin in the blood, resulting in an increased susceptibility to infections. It may occur in a variety of inherited disorders or as an acquired defect.

hypogastrium (hy-poh-**gas**-triŭm) *n.* that part of the central abdomen situated below the region of the stomach. **—hypogastric** *adj.*

hypoglossal nerve (hy-poh-**glos**-ăl) *n.* the twelfth cranial nerve (XII), which supplies the muscles of the tongue and is therefore responsible for the movements of talking and swallowing.

hypoglycaemia (hy-poh-gly-**see**-miă) *n.* a deficiency of glucose in the bloodstream, causing muscular weakness and incoordination, mental confusion, and sweating. If severe it may lead to **hypoglycaemic coma**. Hypoglycaemia most commonly occurs in diabetes mellitus. It is treated by administration of glucose. **reactive h.** hypoglycaemia occurring after a meal, induced by excessive levels of insulin release from the pancreas. **—hypoglycaemic** (hy-poh-gly-**see**-mik) *adj.*

hypoglycaemic unawareness *n.* a serious condition in which a person with diabetes loses the earliest warning signs of an approaching hypoglycaemic episode and may thus suffer a severe attack, with confusion, seizures, or even coma and death. It is more common in long-standing diabetes and in those who experience frequent hypoglycaemic episodes.

hypohidrosis (hy-poh-hy-**droh**-sis) *n.* a reduction in sweating in the presence of an appropriate stimulus for sweating (such as heat). It may accompany disease or occur as a congenital defect.

hypoinsulinism (hy-poh-**ins**-yoo-lin-izm) *n.* a deficiency of insulin due either to inadequate secretion of the hormone by the pancreas or to inadequate treatment of diabetes mellitus.

hypokalaemia (hy-poh-kal-**ee**-miă) *n.* the presence of abnormally low levels of potassium in the blood: occurs in dehydration. *See* electrolyte.

hypomania (hy-poh-**may**-niă) *n.* a mild degree of mania. Elated mood leads to faulty judgment; behaviour lacks the usual social restraints and the sexual drive is increased;

there is a reduced need for sleep; speech is rapid and pressured; the individual is energetic but not persistent and tends to be irritable or possibly aggressive. **—hypomanic** (hy-poh-**man**-ik) *adj.*

hypomotility (hy-poh-moh-**til**-iti) *n.* decreased movement or activity, especially of the stomach or intestine.

hyponatraemia (hy-poh-nă-**tree**-miă) *n.* the presence in the blood of an abnormally low concentration of sodium: occurs in dehydration. *See* electrolyte.

hypoparathyroidism (hy-poh-pa-ră-**th'y**-roid-izm) *n.* subnormal activity of the parathyroid glands, causing a fall in the blood concentration of calcium and muscular spasms (*see* tetany).

hypopharynx (laryngopharynx) (hy-poh-**fa**-rinks) *n.* the part of the pharynx that lies below the level of the hyoid bone.

hypophysectomy (hy-pof-i-**sek**-tŏmi) *n.* the surgical removal or destruction (by radiotherapy) of the pituitary gland (hypophysis) in the brain.

hypophysis (hy-**pof**-i-sis) *n.* *see* pituitary gland.

hypopiesis (hy-poh-py-**ee**-sis) *n.* abnormally reduced blood pressure (*see* hypotension) in the absence of organic disease.

hypopituitarism (hy-poh-pit-**yoo**-it-er-izm) *n.* subnormal activity of the pituitary gland, causing dwarfism in childhood and a syndrome of impaired sexual function, pallor, and premature ageing in adult life (*see* Simmonds disease).

hypoplasia (hy-poh-**play**-ziă) *n.* underdevelopment of an organ or tissue. **—hypoplastic** (hy-poh-**plast**-ik) *adj.*

hypoplastic left heart *n.* a congenital heart disorder in which the left side of the heart, particularly the left ventricle, is underdeveloped. Affected babies usually develop severe heart failure within the first few days of life. Most babies die within the first few weeks, but milder cases may be amenable to surgery.

hypoplastic leukaemia *n.* a stage of leukaemia in which there is a decrease in the number of white cells, red cells, and platelets in the blood and reduced haemopoiesis in the bone marrow.

hypopnoea (hy-poh-**nee**-ă) *n.* an abnormal decrease in the rate and depth of breathing. **h. syndrome** a condition related to obstructive sleep apnoea, characterized by episodes of hypopnoea during sleep in which nasal airflow is between 30% and 50% of normal for more than 10 seconds.

hypoproteinaemia (hy-poh-proh-ti-**nee**-miă) *n.* a decrease in the quantity of protein in the blood, resulting in oedema and increased susceptibility to infections. It may result from malnutrition, impaired protein production, or increased loss of protein from the body. *See also* hypogammaglobulinaemia.

hypoprothrombinaemia (hy-poh-proh-throm-bin-**ee**-miă) *n.* a deficiency of the clotting factor prothrombin in the blood, which results in an increased tendency to bleed.

hypopyon (hy-**poh**-pi-ŏn) *n.* pus in the chamber of the eye that lies in front of the iris, seen in severe ocular infections.

hyposecretion (hy-poh-si-**kree**-shŏn) *n.* decreased secretion.

hyposensitive (hy-poh-**sen**-si-tiv) *adj.* less than normally responsive to the presence of antigenic material. *Compare* hypersensitive. **—hyposensitivity** *n.*

hyposensitization (hy-poh-sen-si-ty-**zay**-shŏn) *n. see* desensitization.

hypospadias (hy-poh-**spay**-di-ăs) *n.* a congenital abnormality in which the opening of the urethra is on the underside of the penis: either on the glans penis (**glandular h.**), at the junction of the glans with the shaft (**coronal h.**), on the shaft itself (**penile h.**), or in the perineum (**perineal h.**). *See* MAGPI operation.

hypostasis (hy-**pos**-tă-sis) *n.* accumulation of fluid or blood in a dependent part of the body in cases of poor circulation. **Hypostatic pneumonia** results from hypostatic congestion of the lung bases in debilitated patients who are confined to bed. **—hypostatic** (hy-poh-**stat**-ik) *adj.*

hyposthenia (hy-pos-**th'ee**-niă) *n.* a state of physical weakness or abnormally low muscular tension.

hypotension (hy-poh-**ten**-shŏn) *n.* a condition in which the arterial blood pressure is abnormally low, which is most commonly experienced when rising from a sitting or lying position (**postural** (or **orthostatic**) h.). Severe cases may manifest as shock.

hypothalamus (hy-poh-**thal**-ă-mŭs) *n.* the region of the forebrain in the floor of the third ventricle, linked with the thalamus above and the pituitary gland below. It contains several important centres controlling body temperature, thirst, hunger, and eating, water balance, and sexual function. It also functions as a centre for the integration of hormonal and autonomic nervous activity. **—hypothalamic** *adj.*

hypothenar (hy-**poth**-i-nar) *adj.* describing or relating to the fleshy prominent part of the palm of the hand below the little finger. *Compare* thenar.

hypothermia (hy-poh-**therm**-iă) *n.* **1.** accidental reduction of body temperature below the normal range. It is particularly liable to occur in babies and the elderly. **2.** deliberate lowering of body temperature for therapeutic purposes. This may be done during surgery, in order to reduce the patient's requirement for oxygen.

hypothyroidism (hy-poh-**th'y**-roid-izm) *n.* subnormal activity of the thyroid gland. If present at birth and untreated, it leads to cretinism. When acquired in later life, it causes mental and physical slowing and myxoedema. Treatment is through thyroid hormone replacement therapy.

hypotonia (hy-poh-**toh**-niă) *n.* a state of reduced tension in muscle.

hypotonic (hy-poh-**tonn**-ik) *adj.* **1.** describing a solution that has a lower osmotic pressure than another solution. *See* osmosis. **2.** describing muscles that demonstrate diminished tonicity.

hypotony (hy-poh-toh-ni) *n.* a very low intraocular pressure, usually as a result of trauma or surgery to the eye.

hypotrichosis (hy-poh-trik-**oh**-sis) *n.* a condition in which less hair develops than normal.

hypotropia (hy-poh-**troh**-piă) *n.* strabismus in which one eye looks downwards.

hypoventilation (hy-poh-ven-ti-**lay**-shŏn) *n.* breathing at an abnormally shallow and slow rate, which results in an increased concentration of carbon dioxide in the blood.

hypovitaminosis (hy-poh-vit-ă-min-**oh**-sis) *n.* a deficiency of a vitamin caused either through lack of the vitamin in the diet or from an inability to absorb or utilize it.

hypovolaemia (oligaemia) (hy-poh-vŏ-**lee**-miă) *n.* a decrease in the volume of circulating blood. *See* shock.

hypoxaemia (hy-poks-**ee**-miă) *n.* reduction of the oxygen concentration in the arterial blood, recognized clinically by the presence of central and peripheral cyanosis.

hypoxia (hy-**poks**-iă) *n.* a deficiency of oxygen in the tissues. *See also* anoxia, hypoxaemia. —**hypoxic** *adj.*

hypoxic-ischaemic encephalopathy *n.* *see* birth asphyxia.

hyster- (hystero-) *combining form denoting* **1.** the uterus. **2.** hysteria.

hysterectomy (hiss-ter-**ek**-tŏmi) *n.* the surgical removal of the uterus, either through an incision in the abdominal wall (**abdominal h.**) or through the vagina (**vaginal h.**). **subtotal h.** removal of the body of the uterus, leaving the neck (cervix) in place. **total h.** removal of the entire uterus. *See also* Wertheim's hysterectomy.

hysteria (hiss-**teer**-iă) *n.* **1.** formerly, a neurosis whose principal features consist of emotional instability, repression, dissociation, physical symptoms, and vulnerability to suggestion. **conversion h.** *see* conversion disorder. **dissociative h.** *see* dissociative disorder. **2.** a state of great emotional excitement.

hysterical (hiss-**te**-ri-kăl) *adj.* **1.** describing symptoms characteristic of conversion disorder. **2.** describing a kind of personality disorder characterized by instability and shallowness of feelings.

hysteroptosis (hiss-ter-op-**toh**-sis) *n.* prolapse of the uterus. *See* prolapse.

hysterosalpingography (hiss-ter-oh-sal-ping-**og**-răfi) *n.* X-ray imaging of the uterus and Fallopian tubes following the injection of water or a soluble contrast medium.

hysterosalpingosonography (hiss-ter-oh-sal-ping-oh-sonn-**og**-răfi) *n.* *see* hycosy.

hysteroscope (uteroscope) (**hiss**-ter-oh-skohp) *n.* a tubular instrument with a light source for observing the interior of the uterus. *See also* endoscope.

hysterotomy (hiss-ter-**ot**-ŏmi) *n.* an operation for removal of the fetus by incision of the uterus through the abdomen before the 24th week of gestation; after this time the operation is called Caesarean section. Hysterotomy is now rarely performed.

hysterotrachelorrhaphy (hiss-ter-oh-trak-el-o-răfi) *n.* the operation of stitching a tear in the cervix of the uterus.

Ii

-iasis *combining form denoting* a diseased condition.

iatro- *combining form denoting* **1.** medicine. **2.** doctors.

iatrogenic (I-at-roh-**jen**-ik) *adj.* describing a condition or disease that has resulted from treatment and/or the actions of health-care professionals, e.g. a side-effect, hospital-acquired infection, or post-operative complication.

IBD *n. see* inflammatory bowel disease.

IBS *n. see* irritable bowel syndrome.

ibuprofen (I-**bew**-proh-fen) *n.* an anti-inflammatory drug (*see* NSAID), administered by mouth or topically in the treatment of arthritic conditions, dysmenorrhoea, and migraine. Trade names: **Brufen**, **Fenbid**, **Nurofen**, etc.

IC *n. see* inspiratory capacity.

ICD *n. see* International Classification of Diseases. **ICD-10** the latest version, published in 1992.

ichor (**I**-kor) *n.* a watery material oozing from wounds or ulcers.

ichthammol (**ik**-tham-ol) *n.* a sulphur-containing drug with antibacterial properties, used in the form of an ointment or, combined with zinc paste, to impregnate bandages for treating eczema.

ichthyosis (ik-thi-**oh**-sis) *n.* any one of a group of genetically determined skin disorders in which there is abnormal scaling of the skin. Xeroderma is a very mild form of the disorder. **i. vulgaris** the most common form of the disease, which is inherited as an autosomal dominant condition.

ICP *n. see* intracranial (pressure).

ICSH (interstitial-cell-stimulating hormone) *n. see* luteinizing hormone.

ICSI (**ik**-si) *n.* intracytoplasmic sperm injection: a technique of assisted conception in some cases of male infertility in which a single spermatozoon is injected into the cytoplasm of an ovum in vitro. The fertilized ovum is then implanted into the uterus.

icterus (**ik**-ter-ŭs) *n. see* jaundice.

ictus (**ik**-tŭs) *n.* a stroke or any sudden attack. The term is often used for an epileptic seizure.

ICU *n. see* intensive care (unit).

id (id) *n.* (in psychoanalysis) a part of the unconscious mind governed by the instinctive forces of libido and the death instinct (governing aggression, etc.).

ID *adj. see* intradermal.

-id *suffix denoting* relationship or resemblance to.

IDDM *n.* insulin-dependent diabetes mellitus. *See* diabetes.

idea of reference (I-**dee**-ă) *n.* the sense that an everyday event experienced or object perceived by an individual has a special significance for him or her. For example, a person listening to the radio may believe that there is a special message in the broadcast directed specifically at him or her. Ideas of reference differ from **delusions of reference** in that insight is retained: the ideas are recognized by the individual as feelings that originate from within.

ideation (I-di-**ay**-shŏn) *n.* the process of thinking or of having imagery or ideas. **suicidal i.** thoughts or imagery of suicide.

identical twins (I-**den**-tik-ăl) *pl. n. see* twins.

ideo- *combining form denoting* **1.** the mind or mental activity. **2.** ideas.

idio- *combining form denoting* peculiarity to the individual.

idiopathic (idi-oh-**path**-ik) *adj.* denoting a disease or condition the cause of which is not known or that arises spontaneously. **i. thrombocytopenic purpura** *see* purpura. —**idiopathy** (idi-**op**-ă-thi) *n.*

idiosyncrasy (idi-oh-**sink**-răsi) *n.* an unusual and unexpected sensitivity exhibited by an individual to a particular drug or food. —**idiosyncratic** (idi-oh-sin-**krat**-ik) *adj.*

idioventricular (idi-oh-ven-**trik**-yoo-ler) *adj.* affecting or peculiar to the ventricles of the heart. **i. rhythm** the very slow beat of the ventricles under the influence of their own natural subsidiary pacemaker.

IDT *n. see* incident decision tree.

ifosfamide (I-**fos**-fă-myd) *n.* a cytotoxic drug used in the treatment of malignant disease, particularly sarcomas, testicular tumours, and lymphomas. It is administered intravenously by injection or infusion.

Ig *n. see* immunoglobulin.

IGT *n.* impaired glucose tolerance (*see* glucose tolerance test).

IHD *n. see* ischaemic heart disease.

IL-2 *n. see* interleukin.

ile- (ileo-) *combining form denoting* the ileum.

ileal conduit (**il**-i-ăl) *n.* a segment of small intestine (ileum) used to convey urine from the ureters to the exterior into an appliance (*see also* urinary diversion). The ureters are implanted into an isolated segment of bowel, one end of which is brought through the abdominal wall to the skin surface.

ileal pouch *n.* a reservoir made from loops of ileum to replace a surgically removed rectum, avoiding the need for a permanent ileostomy.

ileectomy (ili-**ek**-tŏmi) *n.* surgical removal of the ileum or part of the ileum.

ileitis (ili-**I**-tis) *n.* inflammation of the ileum. It may be caused by Crohn's disease, tuberculosis, the bacterium *Yersinia enterocolitica*, or typhoid or it may occur in association with ulcerative colitis.

ileocaecal (ili-oh-**see**-kăl) *adj.* relating to the ileum and caecum. **i. valve** a valve at the junction of the small and large intestines consisting of two membranous folds that close to prevent the backflow of food from the colon and caecum to the ileum.

ileocaecocystoplasty (ili-oh-see-koh-**sis**-toh-plasti) *n.* an operation in which the dome of the bladder is removed by cutting across the bladder transversely or sagittally above the openings of the ureters; the dome is replaced by an isolated segment of caecum and terminal ileum. *See* cystoplasty.

ileocolitis (ili-oh-kŏ-**ly**-tis) *n.* inflammation of the ileum and the colon. The most likely cause is Crohn's disease.

ileocolostomy (ili-oh-kŏ-**lost**-ŏmi) *n.* a surgical operation in which the ileum is joined to part of the colon.

ileocystoplasty (ili-oh-**sis**-toh-plasti) *n.* an operation in which the bladder is enlarged by an opened-out portion of small intestine. *See* cystoplasty.

ileoproctostomy (ili-oh-prok-**tost**-ŏmi) *n. see* ileorectal (anastomosis).

ileorectal (ili-oh-**rek**-t'l) *adj.* relating to the ileum and rectum. **i. anastomosis** (**ileoproctostomy**) a surgical operation in which the ileum is joined to the rectum, usually after surgical removal of the colon (*see* colectomy).

ileosigmoidostomy (ili-oh-sig-moid-**ost**-ŏmi) *n.* an operation in which an opening is created between the ileum and the sigmoid colon.

ileostomy (ili-**ost**-ŏmi) *n.* a surgical operation in which the ileum is brought through the abdominal wall to create an artificial opening (**stoma**) through which the intestinal contents can discharge, thus bypassing the colon. Various types of bag may be worn to collect the effluent.

SEE WEB LINKS

- Website of the Ileostomy Association

ileum (**il**-iŭm) *n.* the lowest of the three portions of the small intestine (*see* intestine). It runs from the jejunum to the ileocaecal valve. **—ileal, ileac** *adj.*

ileus (**il**-i-ŭs) *n.* intestinal obstruction, usually obstruction of the small intestine (ileum). **paralytic** or **adynamic i.** functional obstruction of the ileum due to loss of peristalsis, which may be caused by abdominal surgery, spinal injuries, electrolyte abnormalities, peritonitis, or ischaemia. Treatment consists of intravenous administration of fluid and nutrients and removal of excess stomach secretions by nasogastric tube until peristalsis returns.

ili- (ilio-) *combining form denoting* the ilium.

iliac (**il**-i-ak) *adj.* relating to the ilium. **i. arteries** the arteries that supply most of the blood to the lower limbs and pelvic region. **i. fossa** a concave depression on the inside of the pelvis. The right iliac fossa provides space for the vermiform appendix. **i. veins** the veins draining most of the blood from the lower limbs and pelvic region.

iliacus (i-**lee**-ă-kŭs) *n.* a flat triangular muscle situated in the area of the groin. This muscle acts in conjunction with the psoas muscle to flex the thigh.

iliococcygeal (ili-oh-kok-**sij**-iăl) *adj.* relating to the ilium and the coccyx.

iliopsoas (ili-oh-**soh**-ăs) *n.* a composite muscle made up of the iliacus and psoas muscles, which have a common tendon.

ilium (**il**-iŭm) *n.* the haunch bone: a wide bone forming the upper part of each side of the hip bone (*see also* pelvis). **—iliac** *adj.*

illness anxiety disorder *n. see* hypochondria.

illusion (i-**loo**-*zh*ŏn) *n.* a false perception due to misinterpretation of the stimuli arising from an object. Illusions can occur in normal people and may also occur in almost any psychiatric syndrome. *Compare* hallucination.

IM *adj. see* intramuscular.

image (**im**-ij) *n.* **1.** (in physiology) an optical reproduction of an object formed on the retina when light is refracted through the eye. **2.** (in radiology) a representation of the structure of an organ, tissue, etc., produced by radiography and used by physicians in diagnosis and in monitoring the effects of treatment. *See* imaging. **i. intensifier** an electronic device that provides a TV image from an X-ray source. It amplifies the signal from the original image, giving a brighter picture, so that the radiation dose can be reduced. **3.** (in psychology) a mental representation resulting from thought rather than from sensory perception. *See* body image, imagery.

image-guided surgery *see* computer-assisted surgery.

imagery (**im**-ij-er-i) *n.* the production of vivid mental representations by the normal processes of thought. **eidetic i.** the production of images of exceptional clarity, which may be recalled long after being first experienced.

imaging (**im**-ij-ing) *n.* the production of images of organs or tissues by a range of techniques. *See* computerized tomography, cross-sectional imaging, magnetic resonance imaging, real-time imaging, ultrasonography.

imago (i-**may**-goh) *n.* (in psychoanalysis) the internal unconscious representation of an important person in the individual's life, particularly a parent.

imatinib (i-**mat**-i-nib) *n.* a cytotoxic drug taken by mouth for the treatment of chronic myeloid leukaemia in which the Philadelphia chromosome is present, inoperable gastrointestinal stromal tumours, acute lymphoblastic leukaemia, and some myeloproliferative disorders. Trade name: **Glivec**.

imidazole (i-**mid**-ă-zohl) *n.* one of a group of chemically related antifungal drugs that are also effective against a wide range of bacteria; some (e.g. tiabendazole and mebendazole) are also used as anthelmintics. The group includes econazole, clotrimazole, ketoconazole, and miconazole.

imipramine (i-**mip**-ră-meen) *n.* a drug administered by mouth to treat depression (*see* antidepressant) and nocturnal enuresis.

immersion foot (i-mer-shŏn) *n.* *see* trench foot.

immiscible (i-**mis**-ibŭl) *adj.* incapable of being mixed to form a homogeneous substance. Oil and water are immiscible.

immobilization (i-moh-bi-ly-**zay**-shŏn) *n.* the procedure of making a normally movable part of the body, such as a joint, immovable. This helps infected, diseased, or injured tissue (bone, joint, or muscle) to heal.

immune (i-**mewn**) *adj.* protected against a particular infection by the presence of specific antibodies against the organisms concerned. **i. response** the reaction of the body to the presence of antigens (foreign tissues, bacteria, etc.), which are attacked and destroyed by antibodies. *See* antibody, antigen, immunity, lymphocyte. **i. system** the organs and tissues responsible for immunity, including the thymus, bone marrow, lymph nodes, spleen, and tonsils. *See also* lymphoid tissue.

immunity (i-**mewn**-iti) *n.* the body's ability to resist infection, afforded by the presence of circulating antibodies and white blood cells. **active i.** immunity that arises when the body's own cells produce, and remain able to produce, appropriate antibodies following an attack of a disease or deliberate stimulation (*see* immunization). **cell-mediated i.** immunity resulting from the action of T-lymphocytes. **humoral i.** immunity resulting from the action of circulating antibodies produced by B lymphocytes. **natural** (or **innate**) **i.** immunity resulting from the activity of phagocytic cells, natural killer cells, and other mechanisms present before exposure to infection. **passive i.** temporary immunity that may be provided by injecting ready-made antibodies in antiserum taken from another person or an animal already immune. Babies have passive immunity, conferred by antibodies from the maternal blood and colostrum, to common diseases for several weeks after birth. *See also* herd immunity.

immunization (im-yoo-ny-**zay**-shŏn) *n.* the production of immunity by artificial means. Passive immunity may be conferred by the injection of an antiserum, but the production of active immunity calls for the use of a vaccine (*see* vaccination). See Appendix 8: Immunization schedules.

SEE WEB LINKS

- Information on immunization from Public Health England

immuno- *combining form denoting* immunity or immunological response.

immunoassay (im-yoo-noh-**ass**-ay) *n.* any of various techniques for determining the levels of antigen and antibody in a tissue. *See* radioimmunoassay.

immunocompromised (im-yoo-noh-**kom**-prŏ-myzd) *adj.* describing patients in whom the immune response is reduced or defective due to immunosuppression. Such patients are vulnerable to opportunistic infections.

immunodeficiency (im-yoo-noh-di-**fish**-ĕn-si) *n.* deficiency in the immune response. This can be acquired, as in AIDS, but there are many varieties of primary immunodeficiency occurring as inherited disorders characterized by hypogammaglobulinaemia, defects in T-cell function, or both.

immunogenicity (im-yoo-noh-jĕn-**iss**-iti) *n.* the property that enables a substance to provoke an immune response, including foreignness (*see* antigen), size, route of entry into the body, dose, number and length of exposures to the antigen, and host genetic make-up.

immunoglobulin (Ig) (im-yoo-noh-**glob**-yoo-lin) *n.* one of a group of structurally related proteins (gammaglobulins) that act as antibodies.

immunological tolerance (im-yoo-nŏ-**loj**-ik-ăl) *n.* a failure of the body to distinguish between materials that are 'self', and therefore to be tolerated, and those that are 'not self', against which it mounts an immune response.

immunology (im-yoo-**nol**-ŏji) *n.* the study of immunity and all of the phenomena connected with the defence mechanisms of the body. **—immunological** *adj.*

immunosuppressant (im-yoo-noh-sŭ-**press**-ănt) *n.* a drug, such as azathioprine or ciclosporin, that reduces the body's resistance to infection and other foreign bodies by suppressing the immune system. Immunosuppressants are used to maintain the survival of organ and tissue transplants and to treat various autoimmune diseases (*see* disease-modifying antirheumatic drug). Side-effects include increased susceptibility to infection due to damage to the blood-forming cells of bone marrow.

immunosuppression (im-yoo-noh-sŭ-**presh**-ŏn) *n.* suppression of the immune response, usually by disease (e.g. AIDS) or by drugs (e.g. steroids, azathioprine, ciclosporin). **—immunosuppressed** *adj.*

immunotherapy (im-yoo-noh-**th'e**-ră-pi) *n.* the prevention or treatment of disease using agents that may modify the immune response. It is a largely experimental approach, studied most widely in the treatment of leukaemias, melanoma, and renal cell carcinoma.

immunotoxin (im-yoo-noh-**toks**-in) *n.* one of a class of compounds being studied for the treatment of certain cancers. Immunotoxins combine monoclonal antibodies, which specifically target cancerous cells, with a highly toxic compound (such as ricin) that inhibits protein synthesis.

immunotransfusion (im-yoo-noh-trans-**few**-*zhŏn*) *n.* the transfusion of an antiserum to treat or give temporary protection against a disease.

impacted (im-**pak**-tid) *adj.* firmly wedged. **i. faeces** faeces that are so hard and desiccated that they cannot pass spontaneously through the anus and require medical intervention. **i. fracture** *see* fracture. **i. tooth** a tooth, usually a wisdom tooth, that cannot erupt into a normal position because it is obstructed by other tissues. —**impaction** *n.*

impaired glucose tolerance (IGT) (im-**paird**) *n. see* glucose tolerance test.

impairment (im-**pair**-měnt) *n.* disruption of and reduction in the body's normal physiological or psychological functioning.

impalpable (im-**palp**-ăbŭl) *adj.* describing a structure within the body that cannot be detected by feeling with the hand.

imperforate (im-**per**-fer-it) *adj.* lacking an opening. **i. anus** (**proctatresia**) partial or complete obstruction of the anus: a congenital malformation in which the anal canal fails to develop correctly. Most mild cases of imperforate anus can be treated by a simple operation. **i. hymen** a condition in which the hymen completely closes the vagina and thus impedes the flow of menstrual blood.

impetigo (imp-i-**ty**-goh) *n.* a superficial bacterial infection of the skin, which usually responds to treatment with antibiotics. **bullous i.** impetigo caused by *Staphylococcus aureus*. It is characterized by blisters, is less contagious than the nonbullous form, and occurs at any age. **nonbullous i.** impetigo caused by *Staphylococcus aureus*, *Streptococcus* species, or both organisms; it mainly affects young children and is highly contagious, with yellowish-brown crusting.

implant (**im**-plahnt) *n.* a drug (such as a subcutaneous hormone implant), a prosthesis (such as an artificial hip), or a radioactive source (such as radium needles) that is put into the body. **breast i.** a prosthesis inserted subcutaneously to replace breast tissue that has been removed surgically during a simple mastectomy in the treatment of breast cancer or to augment existing breast tissue. The type of implant in current use is a silicone sac filled with silicone gel. **dental i.** a rigid structure that is embedded in the jawbone or under its periosteum to provide support for replacement teeth on a denture or a bridge. **heart i.** *see* artificial heart. **intraocular lens i.** a plastic lens placed inside the eye after cataract surgery. **osseointegrated i.** an implant that can be introduced into living bone without producing a foreign-body reaction (*see* osseointegration). *See also* cochlear implant.

implantation (im-plahn-**tay**-shŏn) *n.* **1.** (**nidation**) the attachment of the early embryo to the lining of the uterus, which occurs six to eight days after ovulation. **2.** the placing of a substance (e.g. a drug) or an object (e.g. an artificial pacemaker) within a tissue. **3.** the surgical replacement of damaged tissue with healthy tissue (*see* transplantation).

implementation (im-pli-men-**tay**-shŏn) *n.* the stage of the nursing process in which the patient's individual care plan is utilized and executed, in collaboration with other members of the health-care team.

impotence (**im**-pŏ-tĕns) *n.* inability of a man to have sexual intercourse. *See* erectile dysfunction.

impregnate (im-preg-nayt) *vb.* **1.** to make pregnant. **2.** to saturate with another substance. **—impregnation** *n.*

impression (im-presh-ŏn) *n.* (in dentistry) a mould made of the teeth and surrounding soft tissues or of a toothless jaw. An impression is used in the construction of orthodontic appliances, restorations, and dentures.

impulse (im-puls) *n.* (in neurology) *see* nerve impulse.

IMV *n. see* intermittent mandatory ventilation.

in- (im-) *prefix denoting* **1.** not. **2.** in; within; into.

inaccessible (in-ak-ses-ibŭl) *adj.* (in psychiatry) unresponsive to words and similar stimuli: describing the mental state of certain patients, e.g. schizophrenics. **—inaccessibility** *n.*

inanition (in-ă-nish-ŏn) *n.* a condition of exhaustion caused by lack of nutrients in the blood. This may arise through starvation, malnutrition, or intestinal disease.

in articulo mortis (in ar-tik-yoo-loh mor-tis) Latin: at the moment of death.

inborn error of metabolism (in-born e-rer) *n.* any one of a group of inherited conditions in which there is a disturbance in either the structure, synthesis, function, or transport of protein molecules. Examples are phenylketonuria, homocystinuria, and hypogammaglobulinaemia.

inbreeding (in-breed-ing) *n.* the production of offspring by parents who are closely related. *Compare* outbreeding.

incarcerated (in-kar-ser-ayt-id) *adj.* confined or constricted so as to be immovable: applied particularly to a type of hernia.

incest (in-sest) *n.* sexual intercourse between close relatives, e.g. brother and sister or father and daughter.

incidence rate (in-si-dĕns) *n.* a measure of morbidity based on the number of new episodes of illness arising in a population over a period of time. It can be expressed in terms of affected persons or episodes per 1000 individuals at risk. *Compare* prevalence.

incident decision tree (IDT) (in-si-dĕnt) *n.* a tool for managers to use when faced with a decision to suspend or exclude staff following a patient safety incident. It enables the identification of appropriate actions, the goal being to promote fairer and more consistent treatment of staff in these circumstances. It focuses on using a non-blame approach and can be used in conjunction with the RCA tool (*see* root cause analysis.) to ensure focus on the original situation.

incipient (in-sip-iĕnt) *adj.* coming into existence: describing a stage in a disease.

incision (in-si*zh*-ŏn) *n.* **1.** the surgical cutting of soft tissues, such as skin or muscle, with a knife or scalpel. **bladder neck i.** an incision through the bladder neck that is extended into the prostate to relieve lower urinary tract symptoms. **2.** the cut so made.

incisor (in-sy-zer) *n.* any of the four front teeth in each jaw, two on each side of the midline. *See also* dentition.

inclusion bodies (in-**kloo**-*zhŏn*) *pl. n.* particles occurring in the nucleus and cytoplasm of cells usually as a result of virus infection. Their presence can sometimes be used to diagnose such an infection.

inclusion conjunctivitis *n. see* conjunctivitis.

incompatibility (in-kŏm-pat-i-**bil**-iti) *n.* lack of compatibility. In cases of severe incompatibility, there are likely to be swift immune reactions to transplanted organs or tissues.

incompetence (in-**kom**-pi-tĕns) *n.* **1.** impaired function of the valves of the heart or veins, which allows backward leakage of blood. *See* aortic regurgitation, mitral regurgitation, varicose veins. **2.** (incapacity) impairment of mental functioning such that a person cannot understand, retain, or consider information so as to communicate a choice or preference. **3.** inability to fulfil the responsibilities and meet the standards of care expected of health-care professionals. *See also* capacity.

incontinence (in-**kon**-ti-nĕns) *n.* **1. (urinary incontinence)** the inappropriate involuntary passage of urine. **stress i.** the loss of urine on exertion (e.g. coughing or straining), which is common in women in whom the muscles of the pelvic floor are weakened after childbirth. **overflow i.** leakage from a full bladder, which occurs most commonly in elderly men with bladder outlet obstruction. **urge i.** leakage of urine that accompanies an intense desire to pass water with failure of restraint, frequently caused by instability of the detrusor muscle. *See also* enuresis. **2. (faecal (**or **anal) incontinence)** inability to control bowel movements, causing involuntary loss of faeces or flatus.

SEE WEB LINKS

- Website of the Continence Foundation

incoordination (in-koh-or-din-**ay**-shŏn) *n.* (in neurology) an impairment in the performance of precise movements. Incoordination may result from a disorder in any part of the nervous system. *See* apraxia, ataxia, dysmetria.

incretin (**in**-cree-tin) *n.* any one of a group of gastrointestinal hormones that cause a decrease in blood glucose levels by stimulating an enhanced release of insulin from the pancreatic beta cells after eating. Thus they help to regulate the rise in blood glucose levels after eating.

incubation (in-kew-**bay**-shŏn) *n.* **1.** the process of development of an egg or a culture of bacteria. **2.** the care of a premature baby in an incubator.

incubation period (latent period) *n.* the interval between exposure to an infection and the appearance of the first symptoms.

incubator (**ink**-yoo-bay-ter) *n.* a transparent container for keeping premature babies in controlled conditions and protecting them from infection. Other forms of incubator are used for cultivating bacteria and for hatching eggs.

incus (**ink**-ŭs) *n.* a small anvil-shaped bone in the middle ear that articulates with the malleus and the stapes. *See* ossicle.

Independent Mental Capacity Advocate (IMCA) (indi-**pend**-ĕnt) *n.* a person who must, by virtue of the Mental Capacity Act 2005, be contacted to represent the best interests of a patient who lacks capacity and has no family or friends, while acting as a proxy in medical decision-making. IMCAs are available via the local Independent Mental Capacity Advocacy Service.

independent nursing function *n.* any aspect of nursing practice for which the nurse alone is responsible, acting on his or her own initiative and without instructions from any other discipline.

Inderal-LA (**in**-der-al) *n.* *see* propranolol.

indican (**in**-di-kăn) *n.* a compound excreted in the urine as a detoxification product of indoxyl.

indicanuria (in-di-kăn-**yoor**-iă) *n.* the presence in the urine of an abnormally high concentration of indican. This may be a sign that the intestine is obstructed.

indication (indi-**kay**-shŏn) *n.* **1.** (in medicine) a strong reason for believing that a particular course of action is desirable. **2.** any of the conditions for which a particular drug treatment may be prescribed, as defined by its licence. *Compare* contraindication.

indigenous (in-**dij**-in-ŭs) *adj.* occurring naturally in a particular area, region, or country. Certain diseases are indigenous to particular regions.

indigestion (indi-**jes**-chŏn) *n.* *see* dyspepsia.

indigo carmine (in-dig-oh **kar**-myn) *n.* a blue dye that is administered by injection to test for kidney function.

indinavir (in-**din**-ă-veer) *n.* *see* protease inhibitor.

individualized nursing care (indi-**vid**-yoo-ă-lyzd) *n.* care that is planned to meet the particular needs of one patient, as opposed to a routine applied to all patients suffering from the same disease.

indole (**in**-dohl) *n.* a derivative of the amino acid tryptophan, excreted in the urine and faeces.

indolent (**in**-dŏl-ĕnt) *adj.* describing a disease process that is failing to heal or has persisted. The term is applied particularly to ulcers of skin or mucous membrane.

indometacin (indomethacin) (in-doh-**met**-ă-sin) *n.* an anti-inflammatory drug (*see* NSAID) administered by mouth or in suppositories mainly for the relief of pain and severe inflammation in the treatment of rheumatic disease and related disorders.

indoramin (in-**dor**-ă-min) *n.* an alpha blocker drug administered by mouth to treat high blood pressure and to relieve urinary retention in men with prostate enlargement. Trade name: **Doralese**.

indoxyl (in-**doks**-il) *n.* an alcohol derived from indole by bacterial action. It is excreted in the urine as indican.

induced abortion (in-**dewst**) *n.* *see* abortion.

induction (in-**duk**-shŏn) *n.* **1.** (in obstetrics) the artificial starting of childbirth, e.g. by injecting prostaglandins to prime the cervix and/or puncturing the amnion prior to using oxytocin to stimulate contractions. Labour is induced when pregnancy has continued considerably beyond the expected date of birth or if there is a risk to the health of mother or infant. **2.** (in anaesthetics) initiation of anaesthesia. General anaesthesia is usually induced by intravenous injection of short-acting anaesthetics (such as thiopental).

induration (in-dewr-**ay**-shŏn) *n.* abnormal hardening of a tissue or organ. *See also* sclerosis.

industrial disease (in-**dus**-tri-ăl) *n.* an occupational disease associated with a particular industry or group of industries.

inertia (in-**er**-shă) *n.* (in physiology) sluggishness or absence of activity in certain smooth muscles. **uterine i.** inertia of the muscular wall of the uterus during labour, making the process excessively long. It may be present from the start of labour or it may develop because of exhaustion following strong contractions.

in extremis (in iks-**tree**-mis) Latin: at the point of death.

infant (**in**-fănt) *n.* a child incapable of any form of independence from its mother: usually, a child under one year of age, especially a newborn child. **i. mortality rate** the number of deaths of children under one year of age per 1000 live births in a given year. Included are the **neonatal mortality rate** (calculated from deaths occurring in the first four weeks of life) and **postneonatal mortality rate** (from deaths in the remainder of the first year).

infanticide (in-**fant**-i-syd) *n.* (in Britain) under the terms of the Infanticide Act 1938, the killing of an infant by the natural mother within 12 months of birth. The crime is treated more leniently than murder because it is believed that the woman's balance of mind is disturbed due to childbirth and/or lactation.

infantile (**in**-făn-tyl) *adj.* **1.** denoting conditions occurring in adults that are recognizable in childhood, e.g. poliomyelitis (**i. paralysis**). **2.** of, relating to, or affecting infants. **i. spasms** (**salaam attacks**) a rare but serious form of epilepsy that usually begins between three and eight months of age. It is characterized by involuntary flexing movements of the arms, legs, neck, and trunk. It may be arrested by treatment with anti-epileptic drugs, corticosteroids, or ACTH.

infantilism (in-**fant**-il-izm) *n.* persistence of childlike physical or psychological characteristics into adult life.

infarct (in-**farkt**) *n.* a small localized area of dead tissue produced as a result of an inadequate blood supply.

infarction (in-**fark**-shŏn) *n.* the death of part or the whole of an organ that occurs when the artery carrying its blood supply is obstructed by a blood clot (thrombus) or an embolus. *See also* myocardial infarction.

infection (in-**fek**-shŏn) *n.* invasion of the body by harmful organisms (pathogens), such as bacteria, fungi, protozoa, rickettsiae, or viruses. The infective agent may be transmitted by a patient or carrier in airborne droplets or by direct contact; by animal or insect vectors; by ingestion of contaminated food or drink; or from an infected mother to the fetus. After an incubation period symptoms appear, usually consisting of either localized inflammation and pain or more remote effects. Treatment with drugs is usually effective against most infections, but there are few specific treatments for many common viral infections.

infectious disease (in-**fek**-shŭs) *n. see* communicable disease.

infectious mononucleosis *n. see* glandular fever.

inferential statistics (in-fer-**en**-shăl) *n.* the use of statistics to make inferences or predictions about a population based on the data collected from a small sample drawn from that population.

inferior (in-**feer**-i-er) *adj.* (in anatomy) lower in the body in relation to another structure or surface.

inferiority complex (in-feer-i-**o**-riti) *n.* **1.** an unconscious exaggeration of feelings of inferiority, which may be shown by compensatory behaviour, such as aggression. **2.** (in Freudian psychoanalysis) a complex said to result from the conflict between Oedipal wishes (*see* Oedipus complex) and the reality of the child's lack of power. This gives rise to repressed feelings of personal inferiority if not worked through.

infertility (in-fer-**til**-iti) *n.* inability of a woman to conceive or of a man to induce conception after regular unprotected sexual intercourse for two years. **primary i.** inability to conceive when there has been no previous conception or pregnancy. **secondary i.** failure to conceive after a previous conception or pregnancy. *See also* sterility.

infestation (in-fes-**tay**-shŏn) *n.* the presence of animal parasites either on the skin or inside the body.

infibulation (in-fib-yoo-**lay**-shŏn) *n.* excision of the clitoris, labia minora, and labia majora. *See* female genital mutilation.

infiltration (in-fil-**tray**-shŏn) *n.* **1.** the abnormal entry of a substance (**infiltrate**) into a cell, tissue, or organ. Examples of infiltrates are blood cells, cancer cells, fat, or starch. Infiltration can occur when a vein is damaged and the fluid being infused continues to leak out and accumulate in the surrounding tissue. **2.** the injection of a local anaesthetic solution into the tissues to cause local anaesthesia.

inflammation (in-flă-**may**-shŏn) *n.* the body's response to injury. **acute i.** the immediate defensive reaction of tissue to injury, which may be caused by infection, chemicals, or physical agents. It involves pain, heat, redness, swelling, and loss of function of the affected part. **chronic i.** the response that ensues when acute inflammation does not heal. **—inflammatory** (in-**flam**-ă-ter-i) *adj.*

inflammatory bowel disease (IBD) *n.* a group of inflammatory disorders of the gastrointestinal tract characterized by relapsing and remitting inflammation. The most common types are ulcerative colitis and Crohn's disease.

infliximab (in-**fliks**-i-mab) *n.* a monoclonal antibody that inhibits the activity of TNF-α (*see* tumour necrosis factor) and is used to treat severe Crohn's disease and ulcerative colitis and rheumatoid arthritis, ankylosing spondylitis, and psoriatic arthritis that have failed to respond to treatment with corticosteroids or immunosuppressants and antirheumatic drugs, respectively. It is administered by infusion. Trade name: **Remicade**.

influenza (in-floo-**en**-ză) *n.* a highly contagious virus infection that affects the respiratory system; types A and B are the forms that most commonly cause outbreaks in humans. Symptoms include headache, fever, loss of appetite, weakness, and general aches and pains. With bed rest and aspirin most patients recover, but a few go on to develop viral or bacterial pneumonia. **avian i.** a disease of poultry and other birds caused by influenza A viruses, some strains of which have been transmitted to humans to cause outbreaks of influenza with a high mortality rate. *See* H5N1. **swine i.** a very contagious disease of pigs caused by H1N1, a strain of influenza A virus, first seen in humans in 2009. It is not as virulent as avian influenza.

informed consent (in-**formd**) *n.* the principle that requires clinicians to provide sufficient information to patients or potential research participants in order to render their consent lawful. How much information is regarded as sufficient depends on the seriousness of what is proposed and on the understanding of those from whom consent is required. *See* consent.

infra- *prefix denoting* below.

infracolic omentectomy (in-fră-**col**-ik oh-men-**tek**-tŏ-mi) *n. see* omentectomy.

infrared radiation (in-fră-**red**) *n.* the band of electromagnetic radiation that is longer in wavelength than the red of the visible spectrum and is responsible for the transmission of radiant heat. It may be used in physiotherapy to warm tissues, reduce pain, and improve circulation.

infundibulum (in-fun-**dib**-yoo-lŭm) *n.* any funnel-shaped channel or passage, particularly the hollow conical stalk that extends downwards from the hypothalamus and is continuous with the posterior lobe of the pituitary gland.

infusion (in-**few**-*zhŏn*) *n.* **1.** the slow injection of a substance, usually into a vein (**intravenous i., IVI**). This is a common method for replacing water, electrolytes, and blood products and is also used for the continuous administration of drugs or nutrition. *See also* drip. **2.** the process whereby the active principles are extracted from plant material by steeping it in boiling water (as in the making of tea). **3.** the solution produced by this process.

ingesta (in-**jes**-tă) *pl. n.* food and drink that is taken into the alimentary canal through the mouth.

ingestion (in-**jes**-chŏn) *n.* the process by which food is taken into the alimentary canal. It involves chewing and swallowing.

ingrowing toenail (**in**-groh-ing) *n.* a toenail whose free margin grows or is pressed into the skin at the side of the nail, causing inflammation.

inguinal (**ing**-win-ăl) *adj.* relating to or affecting the region of the groin (inguen). **i. canal** either of a pair of openings that connect the abdominal cavity with the scrotum in the male fetus. **i. hernia** *see* hernia. **i. ligament** (**Poupart's ligament**) a ligament in the groin that extends from the anterior superior iliac spine to the pubic tubercle. It is part of the aponeurosis of the external oblique muscle of the abdomen.

INH *n. see* isoniazid.

inhalation (in-hă-**lay**-shŏn) *n.* **1. (inspiration)** the act of breathing air into the lungs through the mouth and nose. *See* breathing. **2.** a gas, vapour, or aerosol breathed in for the treatment of conditions of the respiratory tract.

inhaler (in-**hay**-ler) *n.* a device for the administration of inhalations. **metered-dose i.** an inhaler designed to deliver the correct dose of an inhalation to the appropriate section of the airway.

inherent (in-**heer**-ĕnt) *adj.* inborn; innate.

inhibin (in-**hi**-bin) *n. see* activin.

inhibition (in-hib-**ish**-ŏn) *n.* **1.** (in physiology) the prevention or reduction of the functioning of an organ, muscle, etc., by the action of certain nerve impulses. **2.** (in psychoanalysis) an inner command that prevents one from doing something forbidden.

inhibitor (in-**hib**-it-er) *n.* a substance that prevents the occurrence of a given process or reaction. *See also* MAO inhibitor.

injection (in-**jek**-shŏn) *n.* introduction into the body of drugs or other fluids by means of a syringe. Common routes for injection are into the skin (**intracutaneous** or **intradermal**); below the skin (**subcutaneous**); into a muscle (**intramuscular**), for drugs that are slowly absorbed; and into a vein (**intravenous**), for drugs to be rapidly absorbed. Enemas are also regarded as injections. See illustration.

injury scoring system (injury severity scale, ISS) (**in**-jer-i) *n.* a system used, particularly in triage, for grading the severity of an injury. *See also* abbreviated injury scale.

inlay (**in**-lay) *n.* a substance or piece of tissue inserted within a tissue, generally to replace a defect.

innate (in-**ayt**) *adj.* describing a condition or characteristic that is present in an individual at birth

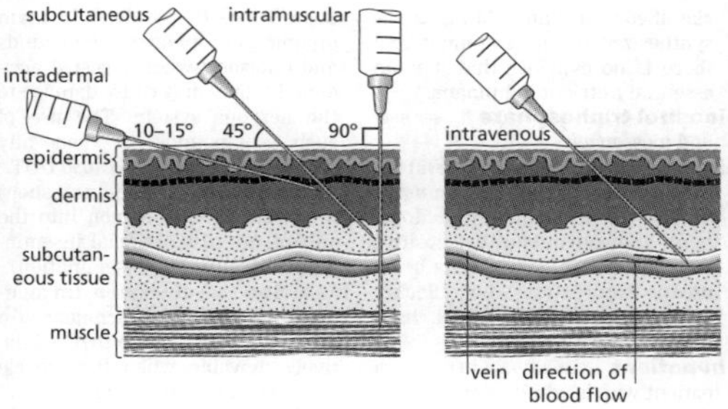

Common injection routes

and is inherited from his parents. *See also* congenital.

inner ear (in-er) *n. see* labyrinth.

innervation (in-er-vay-shŏn) *n.* the nerve supply to an area or organ of the body.

innominate artery (brachiocephalic artery) (in-**om**-in-it) *n.* a short artery originating as the first large branch of the aortic arch, which divides at the lower neck into the right common carotid and the right subclavian arteries.

innominate bone *n. see* hip (bone).

innominate vein (brachiocephalic vein) *n.* either of two veins, one on each side of the neck, formed by the junction of the external jugular and subclavian veins. The two veins join to form the superior vena cava.

INO *n. see* (internuclear) ophthalmoplegia.

ino- *combining form denoting* **1.** fibrous tissue. **2.** muscle.

inoculation (in-ok-yoo-**lay**-shŏn) *n.* the introduction of a small quantity of material, such as a vaccine, in the process of immunization: a more general name for vaccination.

inoculum (in-**ok**-yoo-lŭm) *n.* any material that is used for inoculation.

inorganic (in-or-**gan**-ik) *adj.* **1.** not of animal or vegetable origin. **2.** (in chemistry) describing or relating to compounds that do not contain carbon.

inositol (in-**oh**-sit-ol) *n.* a compound, similar to a hexose sugar, that is a constituent of some cell phospholipids; it is present in the bran of cereal grain. It is sometimes classified as a vitamin but it can be synthesized by most animals and there is no evidence that it is an essential nutrient in humans.

inositol triphosphate *n. see* second messenger.

inotropic (in-ŏ-**trop**-ik) *adj.* affecting the contraction of heart muscle. Such drugs as dobutamine, dopamine, and enoximone have positive inotropic action, stimulating heart muscle contractions. Beta-blocker drugs, such as propranolol, have negative inotropic action.

in-patient (**in**-pay-shĕnt) *n.* a patient who is admitted to a bed in a hospital ward and remains there for a period of time for treatment, examination, or observation. *Compare* out-patient.

inquest (**in**-kwest) *n.* an official judicial enquiry into the cause of a person's death: carried out when the death is sudden or takes place under suspicious circumstances. *See also* autopsy.

insanity (in-**san**-iti) *n.* a degree of mental illness such that the affected individual is not responsible for his actions. The term is a legal rather than a medical one.

insect (**in**-sekt) *n.* a member of a large group of mainly land-dwelling arthropods. Insects of medical importance include various blood-sucking insects transmitting tropical diseases; lice, whose bites can cause intense irritation and bacterial infection; and flies, which transmit organisms causing diarrhoea and dysentery to food. *See also* myiasis.

insecticide (in-**sekt**-i-syd) *n.* a preparation used to kill insects. Some insect powders contain organic phosphorus compounds and fluorides; when ingested accidentally they may cause damage to the nervous system. The use of such compounds is generally under strict control. *See also* DDT.

insemination (in-sem-i-**nay**-shŏn) *n.* introduction of semen into the vagina. *See also* artificial insemination, intrauterine (insemination).

insertion (in-**ser**-shŏn) *n.* (in anatomy) the point of attachment of a muscle (e.g. to a bone) that is relatively movable when the muscle contracts. *Compare* origin.

insidious (in-**sid**-iŭs) *adj.* describing a disease that develops gradually and imperceptibly.

insight (**in**-syt) *n.* **1.** (in medicine and psychiatry) a patient's awareness that he or she has an illness. Insight can be impaired by drug intoxication, physical or mental illness, brain damage, or dementia. **2.** (in psychology) a patient's accuracy of understanding the development of his or her personality and problems, which can be enhanced by psychotherapy.

in situ (in **sit**-yoo) *adj.* **1.** in the natural or original position. **2.** describing a cancer that has not undergone metastasis to invade surrounding tissue.

insolation (in-soh-**lay**-shŏn) *n.* exposure to the sun's rays. *See also* heatstroke.

insomnia (in-**som**-niă) *n.* inability to fall asleep or to remain asleep for an adequate length of time. Insomnia may be associated with physical disease or psychiatric illnesses, such as depression, anxiety, or mania. *See also* fatal familial insomnia.

inspiration (in-spi-ray-shŏn) *n. see* inhalation.

inspiratory capacity (IC) (in-spir-ă-teri) *n.* the maximum volume of air that can be inspired after normal expiration.

inspissated (in-spis-ayt-id) *adj.* thickened or hardened by absorption or evaporation. **i. sputum** a thick sputum produced in whooping cough, which is difficult to cough up.

instillation (in-stil-ay-shŏn) *n.* **1.** the application of liquid medication drop by drop, as into the eye. **2.** the medication applied in this way.

instinct (in-stinkt) *n.* **1.** a complex pattern of behaviour innately determined, which is characteristic of all individuals of the same species. **2.** an innate drive that urges the individual towards a particular goal.

institutionalization (in-sti-tyoo-shŏn-ăl-I-zay-shŏn) *n.* a condition produced by long-term residence in an unstimulating impersonal institution (such as some residential care homes). The individual adapts to the behaviour characteristic of the institution to such an extent that he or she is handicapped in other environments. The features often include apathy, dependence, social withdrawal or awkwardness, and a lack of personal responsibility.

insufficiency (in-sŭ-fish-ĕn-si) *n.* inability of an organ or part, such as the heart or kidney, to carry out its normal function.

insufflation (in-suf-lay-shŏn) *n.* the act of blowing gas or a powder, such as a medication, into a body cavity.

insulin (ins-yoo-lin) *n.* a protein hormone, produced in the pancreas by the beta cells of the islets of Langerhans, that is crucial in regulating the amount of sugar (glucose) in the blood. Lack of this hormone gives rise to diabetes mellitus, in which large amounts of sugar are present in the blood and urine. This condition may be treated successfully by subcutaneous injections or continuous subcutaneous infusion of insulin. **isophane i.** insulin combined with protamine, which reduces its rate of absorption from the injection site and hence prolongs its action in the bloodstream. **i. analogue** any of a group of insulin medications that are either rapidly absorbed from the subcutaneous injection site and have a short duration of action or are slowly absorbed at a constant rate. **i. pen** a user-friendly penlike device to inject a measured dose of insulin. For each injection a new disposable needle is applied. **i. shock** *see* shock. **i. stress test** a test of anterior pituitary gland function involving the induction of a hypoglycaemic episode with injected insulin and subsequent measurements of plasma cortisol and growth hormone.

insulinase (ins-yoo-lin-ayz) *n.* an enzyme, found in such tissues as the liver and kidney, that is responsible for the normal breakdown of insulin in the body.

insulinoma (ins-yoo-lin-**oh**-mă) *n.* an insulin-producing usually benign tumour of the beta cells in the islets of Langerhans of the pancreas. Symptoms include sweating, faintness, and other features of hypoglycaemia (*see* Whipple's triad).

insulin resistance *n.* diminution in the response of the body's tissues to insulin, so that higher concentrations of serum insulin are required to maintain normal circulating glucose levels. Eventually the islet cells can no longer produce adequate amounts of insulin for effective glucose lowering, resulting in hyperglycaemia. Insulin resistance is one of the risk factors for cardiovascular disease. *See also* metabolic syndrome.

insult (**in**-sult) *n.* an injury or physical trauma.

Intal (**in**-tal) *n. see* cromoglicate.

integrated care pathway (care pathway) (**in**-ti-gray-tid) *n.* a multidisciplinary plan for delivering health and social care to patients with a specific condition or set of symptoms. Such plans are often used for the management of common conditions and are intended to improve patient care by reducing unnecessary deviation from best practice.

integrity (in-**te**-gri-ti) *n.* moral honesty, consistency, and truthfulness. Integrity is particularly important in health care, where patients are vulnerable in all sorts of ways; it implies that someone can be trusted to behave well beyond their particular role.

integument (in-**teg**-yoo-měnt) *n.* **1.** the skin. **2.** a membrane or layer of tissue covering any organ of the body.

intelligence quotient (IQ) (in-**tel**-i-jěns **kwoh**-shěnt) *n.* an index of intellectual development. In childhood and adult life it represents intellectual ability relative to the rest of the population; in children it can also represent rate of development (mental age as a percentage of chronological age).

intelligence test *n.* a standardized assessment procedure for the determination of intellectual ability. The score produced is usually expressed as an intelligence quotient. Scores on intelligence tests are used for such purposes as the diagnosis of learning disability and the assessment of intellectual deterioration.

intensive care (intensive therapy) (in-**ten**-siv) *n.* specialized and monitored health care provided for critically ill and immediately postoperative patients by specialist multidisciplinary staff in a specially designed hospital unit (**i. c.** or **i. t. unit**, **ICU** or **ITU**). **neonatal i. c. unit** (**NICU**) a unit providing intensive care for preterm, very low-birth-weight, and seriously ill babies. **paediatric i. c. unit** (**PICU**) a unit providing intensive care for seriously ill children. *See also* coronary care.

intention (in-**ten**-shŏn) *n.* a process of healing. **first i.** healing in which the edges of a wound are brought together under aseptic conditions and granulation tissue forms. **second i.** healing in which the wound edges are separated and the cavity is filled with granulation tissue over which epithelial tissue grows from the wound edges. **third i.** healing in which the wound ulcerates, granulations are slow to form, and a scar forms at the wound site.

intention tremor *n. see* tremor.

inter- *prefix denoting* between.

intercalated (inter-kă-layt-id) *adj.* describing structures, tissues, etc., that are inserted or situated between other structures.

intercellular (inter-sel-yoo-ler) *adj.* situated or occurring between cells.

intercostal muscles (inter-kos-t'l) *pl. n.* muscles that occupy the spaces between the ribs and are responsible for controlling some of the movements of the ribs.

intercurrent (inter-ku-rĕnt) *adj.* going on at the same time: applied to an infection contracted by a patient who is already suffering from an infection or other disease.

interferon (inter-feer-on) *n.* a substance that is produced by cells infected with a virus and has the ability to inhibit viral growth. Particular interferons are effective only in the species that produces them. Preparations of human interferon produced by genetic engineering are used clinically in treating hepatitis B and certain leukaemias and lymphomas and other cancers (**i. alfa**), hepatitis C (i. alfa and **peginterferon alfa**), and multiple sclerosis (**i. beta**).

interkinesis (inter-ky-nee-sis) *n.* **1.** the resting stage between the two divisions of meiosis. **2.** *see* interphase.

interleukin (inter-lew-kin) *n.* any of a family of 12 proteins that control aspects of haemopoiesis and the immune response. **interleukin 2 (IL-2)** an interleukin that stimulates T lymphocytes to become natural killer cells. A recombinant form (**aldesleukin**, Proleukin), administered by subcutaneous injection, can be of benefit in the treatment of renal cell carcinoma.

intermediate care (inter-mee-di-ăt) *n.* health and social care, provided on a short-term basis, that aims to facilitate earlier discharge from hospital or prevent admission to hospital by providing support at a level between primary care and secondary care.

intermenstrual (inter-men-stroo-ăl) *adj.* between the menstrual periods.

intermittency (inter-mit-ĕn-si) *n.* a symptom in which the flow of urine is not continuous but stops and starts. *See* lower urinary tract symptoms.

intermittent claudication (inter-mit-ĕnt) *n. see* claudication.

intermittent fever *n.* a fever that rises, subsides, then returns again. *See* malaria.

intermittent mandatory ventilation (IMV) (man-dăt-eri) *n.* a form of assisted respiration in which the patient breathes at his or her normal rate but is assisted by a ventilator set to deliver a fixed volume of air at a specified rate.

IMV is often used to help patients to cease to rely on mechanical ventilation. **synchronized i. m. v.** (**SIMV**) intermittent mandatory ventilation synchronized with the patient's own efforts.

intermittent pneumatic compression (new-**mat**-ik) *n.* a technique to prevent thrombosis in bedridden patients. It uses an inflatable device that squeezes the calf when it inflates, preventing pools of blood forming behind the valves in the veins, thus mimicking the effects of walking.

intermittent self-catheterization (ISC, clean intermittent self-catheterization, CISC) *n.* a procedure in which the patient periodically passes a disposable catheter through the urethra into the bladder for the purpose of emptying it of urine. It is increasingly used in the management of patients of both sexes (including children) with chronic retention and large residual urine volumes, often due to neuropathic bladder. ISC may prevent back pressure and dilatation of the upper urinary tract with consequent infection and incontinence.

SEE WEB LINKS

- Introduction to ISC for people with continence problems

International Classification of Diseases (ICD) (inter-**nash**-ŏn-ăl) *n.* a list of all known diseases and syndromes published by the World Health Organization every ten years (approximately).

SEE WEB LINKS

- An outline of the ICD from the World Health Organization

interoceptor (inter-oh-**sep**-ter) *n.* any receptor organ composed of sensory nerve cells that respond to and monitor changes within the body, such as the stretching of muscles or the acidity of the blood.

interosseous (inter-**oss**-i-ŭs) *adj.* between two bones.

interparietal bone (inca bone, incarial bone) (inter-pă-**ry**-i-t'l) *n.* the bone lying between the parietal bones, at the back of the skull.

interphase (interkinesis) (**in**-ter-fayz) *n.* the period when a cell is not undergoing division (mitosis), during which activities such as DNA synthesis occur.

intersex (**in**-ter-seks) *n.* the condition of possessing the characteristics of both sexes, making it difficult to establish the sex of the individual at birth from the appearance of his or her genitals. **—intersexuality** *n.*

interstice (in-**ter**-stiss) *n.* a small space in a tissue or between parts of the body. **—interstitial** (inter-**stish**-ăl) *adj.*

interstitial cells *pl. n.* cells that form part of the connective tissue (**interstitium**) between other tissues, especially the cells interspersed between the seminiferous tubules of the testis (also called **Leydig cells**). They secrete androgens in response to stimulation by luteinizing hormone.

interstitial-cell-stimulating hormone *n. see* luteinizing hormone.

interstitial cystitis *n.* a chronic nonbacterial inflammation of the bladder accompanied by an urgent desire to pass urine frequently and bladder pain; it is usually associated with an ulcer in the bladder wall (**Hunner's ulcer**). The cause is unknown and contracture of the bladder eventually occurs.

intertrigo (inter-try-goh) *n.* superficial inflammation of two skin surfaces that are in contact. It is caused by friction and sweat.

interval data (in-ter-văl) *pl. n.* data on a scale of measurement (e.g. temperature on the Celsius scale) in which the intervals between points on the scale are equal but there is no absolute zero. Thus differences between data can be quantified but proportions cannot, since the scale reflects only relative positions in space, time, or magnitude.

interventional radiology (inter-ven-shŏn-al) *n. see* radiology.

intervention study (inter-ven-shŏn) *n.* a comparison of the outcome between two or more groups of patients that are deliberately subjected to different regimes to test a hypothesis, usually of treatment (in a **clinical trial**). *See* blind trial, controlled trial, cross-over trial, double-blind trial.

intervertebral disc (inter-ver-tib-răl) *n.* the flexible plate of fibrocartilage that connects any two adjacent vertebrae in the backbone. The intervertebral discs act as shock absorbers, protecting the brain and spinal cord from the impact produced by running and other movements. **i. d. tear** a tear in the fibrous outer portion of the disc, resulting in displacement of the inner gelatinous nucleus pulposus to varying degrees. *See also* prolapsed intervertebral disc.

intestinal flora (in-test-in-ăl) *pl. n.* bacteria normally present in the intestinal tract. Some are responsible for the synthesis of vitamin K.

intestinal glands *pl. n. see* Lieberkühn's glands.

intestinal juice *n. see* succus (entericus).

intestinal obstruction *n. see* obstruction.

intestine (bowel, gut) (in-test-in) *n.* the part of the alimentary canal that extends from the stomach to the anus. **large i.** the part that consists of the caecum, vermiform appendix, colon, and rectum. It is largely concerned with the absorption of water from the material passed from the small intestine. **small i.** the part of the intestine that consists of the duodenum, jejunum, and ileum. It is here that most of the processes of digestion and absorption of food take place. See illustration. **—intestinal** *adj.*

intima (tunica intima) (in-tim-ă) *n.* **1.** the inner layer of the wall of an artery or vein. It is composed of a lining of endothelial cells and an elastic membrane. **2.** the inner layer of various other organs or parts.

intolerance (in-tol-er-ăns) *n.* the inability of a patient to tolerate a particular drug, manifested by various adverse reactions.

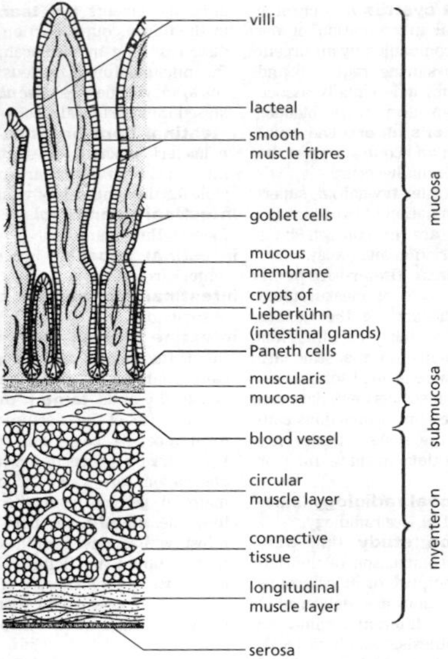

Intestine: A longitudinal section through the ileum

intoxication (in-toks-i-**kay**-shŏn) *n.* the symptoms of poisoning due to ingestion of any toxic material, including alcohol.

intra- *prefix denoting* inside; within.

intra-articular (intră-ar-**tik**-yoo-ler) *adj.* within or into a joint.

intracameral (intră-**kam**-ĕr-ăl) *adj.* within a chamber, such as the anterior or posterior chamber of the eye. **i. anaesthesia** injection of an anaesthetic agent into the anterior chamber of the eye, usually during surgery.

intracellular (intră-sel-yoo-ler) *adj.* situated or occurring inside a cell or cells. *Compare* extracellular.

intracorneal (intră-korn-iăl) *adj.* within the cornea.

intracranial (intră-kray-ni-ăl) *adj.* within the skull. **i. pressure (ICP)** the normal pressure within the skull. Causes of raised intracranial pressure include haemorrhage, oedema, haematoma, brain tumours, trauma, and disturbances to the flow of cerebrospinal fluid.

intracytoplasmic sperm injection (intr -sy-toh-plaz-mik) *n.* *see* ICSI.

intradermal (ID) (intră-derm-ăl) *adj.* within the skin. **i. injection** an injection that is made into the skin.

intradural (intră-dewr-ăl) *adj.* within or beneath the dura mater.

intramedullary (intră-mi-dul-er-i) *adj.* within the bone marrow.

intramuscular (IM) (intră-mus-kew-ler) *adj.* within a muscle. *See also* injection.

intraocular (intră-ok-yoo-ler) *adj.* of or relating to the area within the eyeball. **i. lens implant** *see* implant.

intraosseous (intră-oss-iŭs) *adj.* within a bone. **i. needle** a wide-bore needle for insertion directly into the bone marrow of (usually) the tibia in children, used only in emergencies to administer drugs and fluids to an unconscious patient when no other means of intravenous access can be gained. See illustration.

intrapartum (intră-par-tŭm) *adj.* occurring during labour or childbirth.

intrastromal (intra-stroh-măl) *adj.* within the stroma, especially of the cornea.

intrathecal (intră-th'ee-kăl) *adj.* **1.** within the meninges of spinal cord. **2.** within a sheath, e.g. a nerve sheath.

intrauterine (intră-yoo-teryn) *adj.* within the uterus. **i. contraceptive device** *see* IUCD. **i. growth restriction** (**IUGR**, fetal growth restriction) failure of a fetus to achieve its growth potential, resulting in the birth of a baby whose birth weight is abnormally low in relation to its gestational age (*see* small for gestational age). Causes include maternal disease (e.g. infection, malnutrition, high blood pressure, smoking, and alcoholism),

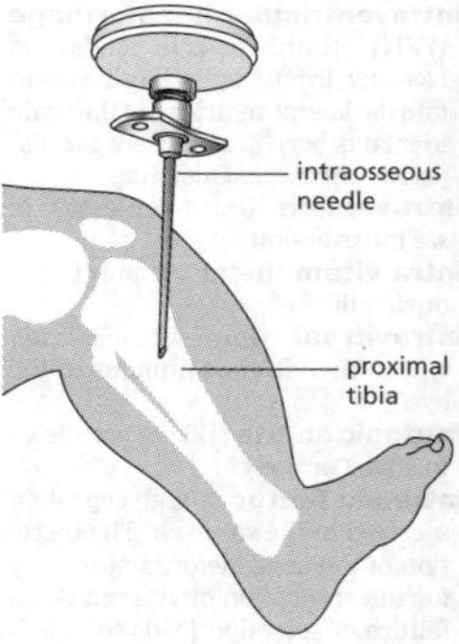

Intraosseous needle

poor socioeconomic conditions, multiple pregnancy, and fetal disease or chromosomal abnormalities. It may be associated with preterm birth. **i. insemination** a procedure for assisting conception in some cases of male infertility, and also used in donor insemination, in which spermatozoa are injected through the vagina into the uterus at the time of ovulation, under ultrasound monitoring and guidance. **i. system** *see* IUS.

intravascular (intră-vas-kew-ler) *adj.* within the blood vessels.

intravenous (IV) (intră-vee-nŭs) *adj.* into or within a vein. *See also* infusion, injection. **i. feeding** *see* nutrition. **i. pyelography** *see* pyelography. **i. urography (IVU)** *see* urography.

intraventricular haemorrhage (IVH) (intră-ven-**trik**-yoo-lă) *n.* bleeding from fragile blood vessels into the lateral ventricles of the brain in infants born prematurely. *See also* periventricular haemorrhage.

intraversion (intră-**ver**-shŏn) *n. see* introversion.

intra vitam (**in**-tră **vy**-tam) Latin: during life.

intravitreal (intră-**vit**-ri-ăl) *adj.* within the vitreous humour of the eye.

intrinsic (in-**trin**-sik) *adj.* exclusive to a part or body.

intrinsic factor *n.* a glycoprotein secreted in the stomach. The secretion of intrinsic factor is necessary for the absorption of vitamin B_{12}; a failure of secretion leads to a deficiency of the vitamin and the condition of pernicious anaemia.

intro- *prefix denoting* in; into.

introitus (in-**troh**-it-ŭs) *n.* (in anatomy) an entrance into a hollow organ or cavity.

introjection (intrŏ-**jek**-shŏn) *n.* (in psychoanalysis) the process of adopting, or of believing that one possesses, the qualities of another person. This can be a form of defence mechanism.

introspection (intrŏ-**spek**-shŏn) *n.* the study by an individual of his own mental processes, reactions, etc. —**introspective** *adj.*

introversion (intrŏ-**ver**-shŏn) *n.* **1. (intraversion)** an enduring personality trait characterized by interest in the self rather than the outside world. People high in introversion (**introverts**) tend to have a small circle of friends, like to persist in activities once they have started, and are highly susceptible to permanent conditioning. *Compare* extroversion. **2.** a turning inwards of a hollow organ (such as the uterus) on itself.

introvert (**in**-trŏ-vert) *n. see* introversion.

intubation (in-tew-**bay**-shŏn) *n.* the introduction of a tube into part of the body for the purpose of diagnosis or treatment. **endotracheal i.** introduction of an endotracheal tube to maintain an airway in an unconscious or anaesthetized patient. **gastric i.** intubation performed to keep the stomach empty during and after abdominal surgery or to provide feeding and drugs when the patient is unable to swallow.

intumescence (in-tew-**mes**-ĕns) *n.* a swelling or an increase in the volume of an organ.

intussusception (in-tŭs-sŭ-sep-shŏn) *n.* the telescoping (**invagination**) of one part of the bowel into another, resulting in intestinal obstruction. It is most common in young children under the age of four years. Symptoms include intermittent screaming and pallor, vomiting, and the passing of bloody mucus ('redcurrant jelly') with the stools; if the condition does not receive prompt surgical treatment, shock from gangrene of the bowel may result.

inulin (**in**-yoo-lin) *n.* a carbohydrate with a high molecular weight that is filtered from the bloodstream by the kidneys. **i. clearance** a test of kidney function in which inulin is injected into the blood. By measuring the amount that appears in the urine over a given period, it is possible to calculate how much filtrate the kidneys are producing.

inunction (in-**unk**-shŏn) *n.* the rubbing in with the fingers of an ointment or liniment.

invagination (in-vaj-i-**nay**-shŏn) *n.* **1.** the infolding of the wall of a solid structure to form a cavity. **2.** *see* intussusception.

invasion (in-vay-*zh*ŏn) *n.* **1.** the onset of a disease. **2.** the entry of bacteria into the body. **3.** the destruction of healthy tissue by a malignant tumour.

invasive (in-vay-ziv) *adj.* **1.** denoting tumours that spread into and destroy surrounding healthy tissue (*see* malignant). **2.** denoting a surgical or diagnostic procedure that involves penetration of the skin or underlying organs and tissues by needles or knives.

inversion (in-ver-shŏn) *n.* **1.** the turning inwards or inside-out of a part or organ: commonly applied to the state of the uterus after childbirth when its upper part is pulled through the cervical canal. **2.** a chromosome mutation in which a block of genes within a chromosome are in reverse order.

invertase (in-**ver**-tayz) *n.* an enzyme in intestinal juice that digest sugars.

in vitro (in **vee**-troh) Latin: describing biological phenomena that are made to occur outside the living body (traditionally in a test-tube).

in vitro fertilization (IVF) *n.* fertilization of an ovum outside the body, a technique used in women with infertility and also for purposes of surrogacy and egg donation. The woman is given hormone therapy causing a number of ova to mature at the same time (*see* superovulation). Several of them are then removed from the ovary through a laparoscope. The ova are mixed with spermatozoa and incubated in a culture medium until the blastocyst is formed. The blastocyst is then implanted in the mother's uterus and the pregnancy proceeds normally.

in vivo (in **vee**-voh) Latin: describing biological phenomena that occur within the bodies of living organisms.

involucrum (in-vŏ-**loo**-krŭm) *n.* a growth of new bone that sometimes surrounds a mass of infected and dead bone in osteomyelitis.

involuntary muscle (in-vol-ŭn-ter-i) *n.* muscle that is not under conscious control, such as the muscle of the gut, stomach, blood vessels, and heart. *See also* cardiac muscle, smooth muscle.

involution (in-vŏ-**loo**-shŏn) *n.* **1.** the shrinking of the uterus to its normal size after childbirth. **2.** degeneration of the corpus luteum, which occurs after pregnancy or if implantation of the embryo fails. **3.** atrophy of an organ in old age. **—involutional** (in-vŏ-**loo**-shŏn-ăl) *adj.*

iodine (I-ŏ-din) *n.* an element required in small amounts for healthy growth and development. The thyroid gland requires iodine to synthesize thyroid hormones; a deficiency of the element in adults leads to goitre and in a fetus leads to cretinism. **povidone-i**. (Betadine, Videne) an iodine-containing antiseptic and skin disinfectant, in the form of a powder spray, tincture, solution, or surgical scrub. **radioactive i.** the radioactive isotope iodine-131, which is administered as a drink to shrink the thyroid gland in the treatment of hyperthyroidism. Symbol: I. *See also* Lugol's solution.

iodism (I-ŏ-dizm) *n.* iodine poisoning. The main features are a characteristic staining of the mouth and odour on the breath. Emergency treatment includes administration of starch or flour in water and lavage with sodium thiosulphate solution.

ion (I-ŏn) *n.* an atom or group of atoms that has lost one or more electrons, making it electrically charged and therefore more chemically active. *See* anion, cation, electrolyte.

ionization (I-ŏ-ny-**zay**-shŏn) *n.* **1.** the dissociation of a substance into ions. Some molecules ionize in solution (*see* electrolyte). **2.** *see* iontophoresis.

iontophoresis (ionization) (I-on-toh-fer-**ee**-sis) *n.* the technique of introducing through the skin, by means of an electric current, charged particles of a drug, so that it reaches a deep site. *See also* cataphoresis.

IOUS *n.* *i*ntra*o*perative *u*ltra*s*ound examination. *See* ultrasonography.

IPD *n.* intermittent peritoneal dialysis. *See* (peritoneal) dialysis.

ipecacuanha (ipi-kak-yoo-**an**-ă) *n.* a plant extract used in small doses, usually in the form of tinctures and syrups, as an expectorant to relieve coughing and to induce vomiting.

IPPV *n.* intermittent positive-pressure ventilation. *See* positive-pressure ventilation.

ipratropium (ip-ră-**troh**-piŭm) *n.* an antimuscarinic drug used as a bronchodilator in the treatment of chronic reversible airways obstruction (*see* bronchospasm) and rhinorrhoea. It is administered by inhalation or nasal spray. Trade names: **Atrovent**, **Ipratropium Steri-Neb**, **Respontin**, **Rinatec**.

ipsilateral (ipselateral, homolateral) (ip-si-**lat**-er-ăl) *adj.* on or affecting the same side of the body. *Compare* contralateral.

IQ *n.* *see* intelligence quotient.

irbesartan (er-**bess**-ar-tan) *n. see* angiotensin II antagonist.

irid- (irido-) *combining form denoting* the iris.

iridectomy (i-ri-**dek**-tŏmi) *n.* an operation on the eye in which a part of the iris is removed.

iridocele (i-**rid**-oh-seel) *n.* the protrusion of part of the iris through a wound in the cornea.

iridocyclitis (i-ri-doh-sy-**kly**-tis) *n.* inflammation of the iris and ciliary body of the eye. *See* uveitis.

iridodialysis (i-ri-doh-dy-**al**-i-sis) *n.* a tear, caused by injury to the eye, in the attachment of the iris to the ciliary body.

iridoplegia (i-ri-doh-**plee**-jiă) *n.* paralysis of the iris, which is usually associated with cycloplegia and results from injury, inflammation, or the use of pupil-dilating eye drops.

iridoptosis (i-ri-**dop**-tŏ-sis) *n.* prolapse of the iris.

iridotomy (i-ri-**dot**-ŏmi) *n.* an operation on the eye in which an incision is made in the iris using a knife or a YAG laser.

irinotecan (i-rin-oh-**tee**-kăn) *n.* a cytotoxic drug administered by intravenous infusion for treating advanced colorectal cancer. Trade name: **Campto**.

iris (**I**-ris) *n.* the part of the eye that regulates the amount of light that enters. It forms a coloured muscular diaphragm across the front of the lens; light enters through a central opening (the pupil). Contraction of different sets of muscles of the iris causes the pupil to dilate in dim light and to contract in bright light. **i. bombé** an abnormal condition of the eye in which the iris bulges forward towards the cornea.

irisin (**I**-ris-in) *n.* a hormone that is released into the bloodstream from muscle during physical activity, which activates fat cells to increase energy turnover.

iritis (I-**ry**-tis) *n.* inflammation of the iris. *See* uveitis.

iron (**I**-ŏn) *n.* an element essential to life. The body of an adult contains on average 4 g of iron, over half of which is contained in haemoglobin in the red blood cells. Iron is an essential component in the transfer of oxygen in the body, as well as a component of enzymes involved in the immune function. A deficiency of iron may lead to anaemia. Many preparations of iron are used to treat iron-deficiency anaemia. Symbol: Fe.

iron dextran *n.* a drug containing iron (in the form of ferric hydroxide) and dextran, administered by intramuscular injection or intravenous infusion to treat iron-deficiency anaemia. Trade name: **CosmoFer**.

iron lung *n. see* ventilator.

iron-storage disease *n. see* haemochromatosis.

irradiation (i-ray-di-**ay**-shŏn) *n.* **1.** exposure of the body to ionizing radiation. The source may be background radiation, diagnostic X-rays, radiotherapy, or nuclear accidents. **2.** exposure of a substance or object to ionizing radiation. Irradiation of food with gamma rays to kill bacteria is a technique used in food preservation.

irreducible (i-ri-**dew**-sibŭl) *adj.* unable to be replaced in a normal position: applied particularly to a type of hernia.

irrigation (i-ri-**gay**-shŏn) *n.* the process of washing out a wound or hollow organ with a continuous flow of water or medicated solution. **whole-gut i.** washing out the entire intestinal tract as a prelude to surgery on the lower intestine.

irritability (i-ri-tă-**bil**-iti) *n.* (in physiology) the property of certain kinds of tissue that enables them to respond in a specific way to outside stimuli.

irritable bowel syndrome (IBS) (**i**-ri-tă-bŭl) *n.* a common disorder characterized by recurrent abdominal pain, altered stool consistency, and variable frequency of defecation.

irritable hip (transient synovitis of the hip) *n.* a self-limiting condition, affecting children between 3 and 10 years of age, due to inflammation of the synovial membrane of the hip joint. It is a common cause of sudden hip pain and limping in young children. Treatment is with NSAIDs and by limiting weight-bearing. It usually resolves in 7–10 days.

irritant (**i**-ri-tănt) *n.* any material that causes irritation of a tissue.

IRV *n. see* (inspiratory) reserve volume.

isch- (ischo-) *combining form denoting* suppression or deficiency.

ischaemia (isk-**ee**-miă) *n.* an inadequate flow of blood to a part of the body, caused by constriction or blockage of the blood vessels supplying it. **—ischaemic** (isk-**ee**-mik) *adj.*

ischaemic heart disease (IHD, coronary heart disease, CHD) *n.* a disease in which the supply of oxygen to the myocardium is inadequate, usually as a result of narrowing of the lumen of the coronary arteries by atheroma. The main symptom is chest pain of varying intensity. Untreated, it can lead to coronary thrombosis and myocardial infarction.

ischi- (ischio-) *combining form denoting* the ischium.

ischiorectal abscess (isk-i-oh-**rek**-t'l) *n.* an abscess in the space between the sheet of muscle that assists in control of the rectum and the pelvic bone. Symptoms are severe throbbing pain near the anus with swelling and fever; it may cause an anal fistula. Pus is drained from the abscess by surgical incision.

ischium (**isk**-iŭm) *n.* a bone forming the lower part of each side of the hip bone (*see also* pelvis). **—ischiac, ischial** *adj.*

islets of Langerhans (**I**-lits ŏv **lang**-er-hans) *pl. n.* small groups of endocrine cells, scattered through the material of the pancreas, that secrete insulin, glucagon, and other hormones. *See also* alpha cells, beta cells, D cells. [P. Langerhans (1847–88), German pathologist]

iso- *combining form denoting* equality, uniformity, or similarity.

isoantibody (alloantibody) (I-soh-**an**-ti-bodi) *n.* an antibody that occurs only in some individuals of a species against the components of foreign tissues from an individual of the same species.

isoantigen (alloantigen) (I-soh-**an**-ti-jĕn) *n.* an antigenic substance that occurs only in some individuals of a species.

isoimmunization (I-soh-im-yoo-ny-**zay**-shŏn) *n.* the development of antibodies (isoantibodies) within an individual against antigens from another individual of the same species.

isolation (I-sŏ-**lay**-shŏn) *n.* **1.** the separation of a person with an infectious disease from noninfected people. *See also* quarantine. **2.** (in surgery) the separation of a structure from surrounding structures by the use of instruments.

isolator (**I**-sŏ-lay-ter) *n.* a large transparent plastic bag in which a patient can be nursed or operated upon without the danger of contamination by infective agents.

isoleucine (I-soh-**loo**-seen) *n.* an essential amino acid. *See also* amino acid.

isometheptene (I-soh-meth-**ep**-teen) *n.* a sympathomimetic drug used in the treatment of migraine headaches, in combination with paracetamol (as **Midrid**). It is administered by mouth.

isometric (I-soh-**met**-rik) *adj.* of or denoting muscular contraction that does not cause muscle shortening. **i. exercise** *see* exercise.

isomorphism (I-soh-**mor**-fizm) *n.* the condition of two or more objects being alike in shape or structure. **—isomorphic, isomorphous** *adj.*

isoniazid (isonicotinic acid hydrazide, INH) [I-soh-**ny**-ă-zid] *n.* a drug used in the treatment of tuberculosis, usually taken by mouth. Because tuberculosis bacteria soon become resistant to isoniazid, it is given in conjunction with other antibiotics.

isophane insulin (I-soh-fayn) *n. see* insulin.

isosorbide dinitrate (I-soh-**sor**-byd dy-**ny**-trayt) *n.* a drug used for the prevention and treatment of angina (*see* vasodilator). It is administered orally (as a sublingual spray or tablets) or by intravenous infusion. Trade names: **Angitak**, **Isoket**, **Isoket Retard**.

isosorbide mononitrate (mon-oh-**ny**-trayt) *n.* an active form of isosorbide dinitrate, available as a preventative oral treatment for angina. Trade names: **Elantan LA**, **Imdur**, **Ismo**, **Isodur**, **Isotard**, **Monomax**, etc.

isosthenuria (I-sos-thĕn-**yoor**-iă) *n.* inability of the kidneys to produce either a concentrated or a dilute urine. This occurs in the final stages of renal failure.

isotonic (I-soh-**ton**-ik) *adj.* **1.** describing solutions that have the same osmotic pressure. *See* osmosis. **2.** describing muscles that have equal tonicity. **i. exercise** *see* exercise.

isotope (**I**-sŏ-tohp) *n.* any one of the different forms of an element, having the same atomic number but different atomic weights. Radioactive isotopes decay into other isotopes or elements, emitting alpha, beta, or gamma radiation.

Artificially produced radioactive isotopes are used extensively as tracers (*see also* gamma camera, scintigram) and in radiotherapy for the treatment of cancer.

isotretinoin (I-soh-tre-**tin**-oh-in) *n.* a drug related to vitamin A (*see* retinoid) administered by mouth or topically for the treatment of acne. Oral isotretinoin may cause fetal abnormalitites. Trade names: **Isotrex**, **Roaccutane**.

ispaghula husk (iss-pag-yoo-lă husk) *n.* a bulking agent (*see* laxative) used to treat constipation, diverticular disease, and irritable bowel syndrome. It is administered by mouth. Trade names: **Fybogel**, **Isogel**, **Ispagel Orange**, **Regulan**.

ISS *n. see* injury scoring system.

isthmus (iss-mŭs) *n.* a constricted or narrowed part of an organ or tissue.

itch (ich) *n.* discomfort or irritation of the skin, prompting the sufferer to scratch or rub the affected area. *See* pruritus.

-itis *combining form denoting* inflammation of an organ, tissue, etc.

itraconazole (I-tră-**kon**-ă-zohl) *n.* an antifungal drug that is administered by mouth or intravenous infusion to treat a wide variety of fungal infections, including candidiasis and ringworm. Trade name: **Sporanox**.

ITU *n.* intensive therapy unit. *See* intensive care.

IUCD (intrauterine contraceptive device) *n.* a plastic or metal coil, spiral, or other shape, about 25 mm long, that is inserted into the cavity of the uterus to prevent conception. Its exact mode of action is unknown but it is thought to interfere with implantation of the embryo. *See also* postcoital (contraception).

IUGR *n. see* intrauterine (growth restriction).

IUI *n. see* intrauterine (insemination).

IUS (intrauterine system) *n.* a removable hormonal contraceptive device that is inserted into the uterus. Consisting of a plastic T-shaped frame that carries a progestogen (levonorgestrel) in a sleeve around its stem, it provides a long-term method of contraception that is also reversible. Trade name: **Mirena**.

IV *adj. see* intravenous.

IVC *n. see* (inferior) vena cava.

ivermectin (I-ver-**mek**-tin) *n.* a drug administered by mouth in the treatment of onchocerciasis, creeping eruption, strongyloidiasis, and scabies.

IVF *n. see* in vitro fertilization.

IVI *n. see* (intravenous) infusion.

IVU *n. see* (intravenous) urography.

ixodiasis (iks-oh-**dy**-ă-sis) *n.* any disease caused by the presence of ticks.

Jj

Jacksonian march (jak-sohn-iăn) *n. see* epilepsy. [J. H. Jackson (1835–1911), British neurologist]

Jacquemier's sign (*zh*ak-mi-ayz) *n.* a bluish or purplish coloration of the vagina: a possible indication of pregnancy. [J. M. Jacquemier (1806–79), French obstetrician]

jactitation (jak-ti-tay-shŏn) *n.* restless tossing and turning of a person suffering from a severe disease, frequently one with a high fever.

Jaeger test types (yay-gĕr) *n.* a card with text printed in type of different sizes, used for testing acuity of near vision. [E. R. Jaeger von Jastthal (1818–84), Austrian ophthalmologist]

jamais vu (*zh*a-may-vew) *n.* one of the manifestations of temporal lobe epilepsy, in which there is a sudden feeling of unfamiliarity with everyday surroundings.

Jarisch-Herxheimer reaction (Herxheimer reaction) (yar-ish **herks**-hy-mer) *n.* exacerbation of the symptoms of syphilis that may occur on starting antibiotic therapy for the disease. The effect is transient and requires no treatment. [A. Jarisch (1850–1902), Austrian dermatologist; K. Herxheimer (1861–1944), German dermatologist]

jaundice (jawn-dis) *n.* a yellow discoloration of the skin or whites of the eyes, indicating excess bilirubin in the blood. **haemolytic j.** jaundice that occurs when there is excessive destruction of red cells in the blood (*see* haemolysis). **hepatocellular j.** jaundice due to disease of the liver cells, such as hepatitis. **obstructive j.** jaundice that occurs when bile made in the liver fails to reach the intestine due to obstruction of the bile ducts (e.g. by gallstones or a tumour) or to cholestasis. Medical name: **icterus**.

SEE WEB LINKS

- Details of the signs, symptoms, and differential diagnosis of jaundice

jaw (jaw) *n.* either the maxilla (upper jaw) or the mandible (lower jaw).

jaw thrust *n.* a manoeuvre for opening the airway of an unconscious patient. The flats of the hands are placed on the cheeks with the fingers hooked under the angles of the jaw so that the jaw can be pulled upwards to separate the tongue from the back of the pharynx. This method is particularly useful when spinal injury is suspected and movement of the neck is undesirable. *See also* head tilt/chin lift.

jejun- (jejuno-) *combining form denoting* the jejunum.

jejunal ulcer (ji-joo-năl) *n. see* peptic (ulcer), Zollinger-Ellison syndrome.

jejunectomy (ji-joo-**nek**-tŏmi) *n.* surgical removal of part or all of the jejunum.

jejunoileostomy (ji-joo-noh-ili-**ost**-ŏmi) *n.* an operation in which part of the jejunum is joined to the distal ileum (small intestine), following the removal or bypass of diseased segments of the small bowel.

jejunostomy (ji-joo-**nost**-ŏmi) *n.* a surgical operation in which the jejunum is brought through the abdominal wall as a stoma. It may enable the insertion of a catheter into the jejunum for short-term infusion of nutrients or other substances.

jejunotomy (ji-joo-**not**-ŏmi) *n.* surgical incision of the jejunum.

jejunum (ji-**joo**-nŭm) *n.* part of the small intestine. It comprises about two-fifths of the whole small intestine and connects the duodenum to the ileum. **—jejunal** *adj.*

jerk (jerk) *n.* the sudden contraction of a muscle in response to a nerve impulse. **ankle j.** reflex contraction of the calf muscles and plantar flexion of the ankle when the Achilles tendon is struck with a tendon hammer. The reflex may be increased or reduced if the spinal cord or first sacral spinal nerve, respectively, are compressed. **knee j.** *see* patellar reflex.

JIA *see* juvenile idiopathic arthritis.

joint (joint) *n.* the point at which two or more bones are connected. The opposing surfaces of bone are lined with cartilaginous, fibrous, or soft (synovial) tissue. *See also* amphiarthrosis, diarthrosis, synarthrosis.

joule (jool) *n.* the SI unit of work or energy, equal to the work done when the point of application of a force of 1 newton is displaced through a distance of 1 metre in the direction of the force. Symbol: J. *See also* calorie.

judgment (**juj**-mĕnt) *n.* the opinion of a clinician in the context of medical care. In spite of technical advances, few decisions in medicine are automatic. This is particularly true where there are critical differences of data interpretation or moral and procedural dilemmas.

jugular (**jug**-yoo-ler) *adj.* relating to or supplying the neck or throat. **j. vein** any one of several veins in the neck. j. venous pressure (JVP) the blood pressure in the internal jugular vein, which is an indirect measurement of pressure in the right atrium (central venous pressure). **internal j.** a very large paired vein running vertically down the side of the neck and draining blood from the brain, face, and neck into the subclavian vein.

jumper's knee (patellar tendinitis) (**jump**-erz) *n.* a form of tendinitis that occurs in athletes and dancers. Repeated sudden contracture of the quadriceps muscle at take-off causes inflammation of the attachment of the patellar tendon to the lower end of the patella.

junction (**junk**-shŏn) *n.* (in anatomy) the point at which two different tissues or structures are in contact. *See also* neuromuscular junction.

juvenile idiopathic arthritis (JIA, Still's disease) (joo-vě-nyl) *n.* any one of a group of conditions characterized by inflammation of the joints lasting longer than six weeks and occurring before the age of 16. JIA can affect either four or fewer joints (**pauciarticular JIA**) or more than four (**polyarticular JIA**).

juvenile polyp *n.* *see* polyp.

juxta- *combining form denoting* proximity to.

JVP *n.* *see* jugular (venous pressure).

Kk

K *symbol for* potassium.

Kahn reaction (kahn) *n.* a test for syphilis, in which antibodies specific to the disease are detected in a sample of the patient's blood by means of a precipitin reaction. This test is not as reliable as some. [R. L. Kahn (20th century), US bacteriologist]

kala-azar (visceral leishmaniasis, Dumdum fever) (kah-lă-ă-**zar**) *n.* a tropical disease caused by the parasitic protozoan *Leishmania donovani*, which is transmitted to humans by sandflies. Symptoms include enlargement and subsequent lesions of the liver and spleen; anaemia; a low leucocyte count; weight loss; and irregular fevers.

Kallmann's syndrome (**kal**-mănz) *n.* a familial condition that is the most common form of isolated gonadotrophin deficiency; it is combined with underdevelopment of the olfactory lobes, causing anosmia. [F. J. Kallmann (1897–1965), US geneticist]

kangaroo care (kan-gă-**roo**) *n.* an approach to neonatal care that encourages prolonged skin-to-skin contact between parents and their newborn baby to encourage the early development of attachment and bonding behaviours. The term refers to the way in which kangaroos carry their young. Kangaroo care can optimize breastfeeding and maintain physiological stability.

kaolin (**kay**-ŏ-lin) *n.* a white clay that contains aluminium and silicon and is purified and powdered for use as an adsorbent. An oral suspension of kaolin is available to treat chronic diarrhoea. Kaolin is also used in dusting powders and poultices.

Kaposi's sarcoma (**kap**-oh-siz) *n.* a malignant tumour arising from blood vessels in the skin and appearing as purple to dark brown plaques or nodules. It is common in Africa and in patients with HIV infection. The tumour evolves slowly; radiotherapy is the treatment of choice for localized lesions and chemotherapy may be of value in metastatic disease. First-line treatment for those with HIV infection is with highly active antiretroviral therapy (*see* antiretroviral). [M. Kaposi (1837–1902), Hungarian dermatologist]

Kardex (**kar**-deks) *n.* originally, the proprietary name for a filing system for nursing records and orders that was held centrally on the ward and contained all the nursing details and observations of patients that had been acquired during their stay in hospital. Although this system is no longer used for nursing records, since care plans are now held at the patient's bedside rather than centrally, the term 'kardex' continues to be used generically, for certain centrally held patient record systems.

Kartagener's syndrome (kar-tah-gay-nerz) *n.* a hereditary condition in which the heart and other internal organs lie on the opposite side of the body to the norm (i.e. the heart lies on the right; *see* dextrocardia); it is associated with chronic sinusitis and bronchiectasis. [M. Kartagener (1897–1975), German physician]

kary- (karyo-) *combining form denoting* a cell nucleus.

karyokinesis (ka-ri-oh-ky-**nee**-sis) *n.* division of the nucleus of a cell, which occurs during cell division before division of the cytoplasm (**cytokinesis**). *See* mitosis.

karyotype (ka-ri-ŏ-typ) **1.** *n.* the chromosome set of an individual or species described in terms of both the number and structure of the chromosomes. **2.** *n.* the representation of the chromosome set in a diagram. **3.** *vb.* to determine the karyotype of a cell, as by microscopic examination.

katathermometer (kat-ă-ther-**mom**-it-er) *n.* a thermometer used to measure the cooling power of the air surrounding it.

Kawasaki disease (Kawasaki syndrome, mucocutaneous lymph node syndrome) (kah-wă-**sah**-ki) *n.* a condition of unknown cause affecting young children, usually less than five years old, and characterized by fever, conjunctivitis, a sore throat, and a generalized rash and reddening of the palms and soles. This is followed by peeling of the fingers and toes. The fever usually persists for 1–2 weeks. Approximately one-fifth of children develop myocarditis and aneurysms of the coronary arteries. Treatment involves aspirin therapy, and gammaglobulin has recently been shown to reduce the risk of coronary artery disease. [T. Kawasaki (20th century), Japanese physician]

Kayser-Fleischer ring (ky-zer fly-sher) *n.* a brownish-yellow ring in the outer rim of the cornea of the eye. It is a deposit of copper granules and is diagnostic of Wilson's disease. [B. Kayser (1869–1954), German ophthalmologist; B. Fleischer (1848–1904), German physician]

Kegel exercises (pelvic-floor exercises, pelvic-floor muscle training) (keg-ĕl) *pl. n.* active rehabilitation of the pelvic-floor muscles by conscious contractions, which leads to a cure in 50–80% of patients with stress incontinence. [A. H. Kegel (20th century), US gynaecologist]

Kehr's sign (kairz) *n.* pain in the left shoulder caused by irritation of the undersurface of the diaphragm by blood leaking from a ruptured spleen. The pain impulses are referred along the phrenic nerve. [H. Kehr (1862–1913), German surgeon]

Kell antigens (kel) *pl. n.* a group of antigens that may or may not be present on the surface of red blood cells, forming the basis of a blood group. This group is important in blood transfusion reactions.

[Mrs Kell (20th century), patient in whom they were first demonstrated]

Keller's operation (kel-erz) *n.* a surgical operation to correct hallux valgus or hallux rigidus, in which the base of the first phalanx of the big toe is excised. [W. L. Keller (1874–1959), US surgeon]

keloid (kee-loid) *n.* an overgrowth of fibrous scar tissue following trauma to the skin. It does not resolve spontaneously but may be flattened by silicone gels, applied pressure, injections of potent corticosteroids, or excision. Keloid formation is particularly common at certain sites, such as the breastbone or ear lobe.

kerat- (kerato-) *combining form denoting* **1.** the cornea. **2.** horny tissue, especially of the skin.

keratectasia (ke-ră-tek-tay-ziă) *n.* bulging of the cornea at the site of scar tissue (which is thinner than normal corneal tissue).

keratectomy (ke-ră-tek-tŏmi) *n.* an operation in which a part of the cornea is removed, usually a superficial layer. This procedure is now frequently done by an excimer laser, to correct refractive errors (**photorefractive k.**) or remove diseased tissue (**phototherapeutic k.**), or by an automated keratome (**automated lamellar k.**).

keratin (ke-ră-tin) *n.* one of a family of proteins that are the major constituents of the nails, hair, and the outermost layers of the skin.

keratinization (cornification) (ke-ră-tin-I-zay-shŏn) *n.* the process by which cells become horny due to the deposition of keratin within them. It occurs in the epidermis of the skin and associated structures (hair, nails, etc.).

keratinocyte (ke-ra-tin-ō-syt) *n.* a type of cell that makes up 95% of the cells of the epidermis. Keratinocytes migrate from the deeper layers of the epidermis and are finally shed from the surface of the skin.

keratitis (ke-ră-ty-tis) *n.* inflammation of the cornea of the eye. The eye waters and is very painful and vision is blurred. It may be due to physical or chemical agents or result from infection. **disciform k.** inflammation within the cornea, usually as an immune response to viral infection, commonly herpes simplex virus.

keratoconjunctivitis (ke-ră-toh-kŏn-junk-ti-vy-tis) *n.* combined inflammation of the cornea and conjunctiva of the eye. **k. sicca** dryness of the cornea and conjunctiva due to deficient tear production, as occurs in Sjögren's syndrome, systemic lupus, systemic sclerosis, and sarcoidosis.

keratoconus (ke-ră-toh-koh-nŭs) *n.* conical cornea: a slowly progressive abnormality in the cornea, which changes from a gradual curve to a more conical shape causing distortion of vision.

keratocyte (ke-ra-to-sIt) *n.* *see* fibroblast.

keratoglobus (megalocornea) (ke-ră-toh-gloh-bŭs) *n.* a congenital disorder of the eye in which the whole cornea bulges forward in a regular curve. *Compare* keratoconus.

keratolytic (ke-ră-toh-**lit**-ik) *n.* an agent, such as salicylic acid, that breaks down the outer horny layer of epidermis and is used for treating warts.

keratomalacia (ke-ră-toh-mă-**lay**-shiă) *n.* a progressive nutritional disease of the eye due to vitamin A deficiency. The cornea softens and may even perforate. *See also* xerophthalmia.

keratome (**ke**-ră-tohm) *n.* any instrument designed for cutting the cornea.

keratometer (ophthalmometer) (ke-ră-**tom**-it-er) *n.* an instrument for measuring the radius of curvature of the cornea. It is used for assessing the degree of curvature of the cornea in different meridians. —**keratometry** *n.*

keratopathy (ke-ră-**top**-ă-thi) *n.* any disorder relating to the cornea.

keratoplasty (corneal graft) (**ke**-ră-toh-plasti) *n.* an eye operation in which any diseased part of the cornea is replaced by clear corneal tissue from a donor.

keratoprosthesis (ke-ră-toh-pros-**th'ee**-sis) *n.* an optically clear prosthesis that is implanted into the cornea to replace an area that has become opaque.

keratoscope (Placido's disc) (**ke**-ră-toh-skohp) *n.* an instrument for detecting abnormal curvature of the cornea. It consists of a black disc marked with concentric white rings. The examiner looks at the reflection of the rings in the patient's cornea; a cornea that is abnormally curved (for example in keratoconus) or scarred reflects distorted rings.

keratosis (ke-ră-**toh**-sis) *n.* a horny overgrowth of the skin. **actinic** (or **solar**) **k.** a red spot with a scaly surface, which may occasionally become a squamous cell carcinoma. These spots are found in older fair-skinned people who have been chronically overexposed to the sun. **seborrhoeic k.** (**seborrhoeic wart**) a superficial yellowish or brown spot, crusty or greasy looking, that never becomes malignant. Such spots occur especially on the trunk in middle age, slowly becoming warty over the years.

keratotomy (ke-ră-**tot**-ŏmi) *n.* an incision into the cornea. **arcuate k.** a curved incision in the periphery of the cornea to reduce astigmatism.

keratouveitis (ke-ră-toh-yoo-vi-**I**-tis) *n.* inflammation involving both the cornea (*see* keratitis) and the uvea (*see* uveitis).

kerion (**keer**-iŏn) *n.* an uncommon and severe form of tinea (ringworm) of the scalp consisting of a painful inflamed mass.

kernicterus (ker-**nik**-ter-ŭs) *n.* staining and subsequent damage of the brain by bile pigment (bilirubin), which may occur in severe cases of haemolytic disease of the newborn.

Kernig's sign (**ker**-nigz) *n.* a symptom of meningitis in which the patient is unable to extend his legs at the knee when the thighs are held at a right angle to the body. [V. Kernig (1840–1917), Russian physician]

ketoacidosis (kee-toh-asid-**oh**-sis) *n.* a potentially life-threatening condition in which acidosis is accompanied by ketosis, such as occurs in type 1 diabetes mellitus (**diabetic k.**, **DKA**). In DKA it results from dehydration and electrolyte inbalance due to potassium excretion via urine, usually as a result of infection or noncompliance with treatment and diet. Hyperglycaemia is present. Symptoms include nausea, vomiting, and extreme thirst.

ketoconazole (kee-toh-**kon**-ă-zohl) *n.* an antifungal drug (*see* imidazole) applied topically to treat fungal infections of the skin and anogenital region. Trade name: **Nizoral**.

ketogenesis (kee-toh-**jen**-i-sis) *n.* the production of ketone bodies. These are normal products of lipid metabolism and can be used to provide energy.

ketogenic diet (kee-toh-**jen**-ik) *n.* a diet that promotes the formation of ketone bodies in the tissues, in which the principal energy source is fat rather than carbohydrate. It can be used to control epileptic seizures and in the management of phenylketonuria (PKU).

ketonaemia (kee-toh-**nee**-miă) *n.* the presence in the blood of ketone bodies.

ketone (**kee**-tohn) *n.* any member of a group of organic compounds consisting of a carbonyl group (=CO) flanked by two alkyl groups. **k. bodies** (**acetone bodies**) the ketones acetoacetic acid, acetone, and β-hydroxybutyrate, produced during the metabolism of fats. *See also* ketosis.

ketonuria (**acetonuria**) (kee-tohn-**yoor**-iă) *n.* the presence in the urine of ketone bodies. This may occur in diabetes mellitus, starvation, or after persistent vomiting and results from the partial oxidation of fats.

ketoprofen (kee-toh-**proh**-fen) *n.* an anti-inflammatory drug (*see* NSAID) administered by mouth, rectal suppository, or topically to treat various arthritic and rheumatic diseases and to relieve pain. Trade names: **Orudis**, **Oruvail**, **Powergel**.

ketosis (kee-**toh**-sis) *n.* raised levels of ketone bodies in the body tissues, resulting from an imbalance in fat metabolism. Ketosis may result in severe acidosis. *See also* ketonuria.

ketosteroid (kee-toh-**steer**-oid) *n.* a steroid that contains one or more ketone groups (–C=O). 17-ketosteroids (having the oxygen at carbon 17) are normally excreted in the urine; excess 17-ketosteroids in the urine indicates overactivity of the adrenal glands and gonads.

keyhole surgery (**kee**-hohl) *n. see* minimally invasive surgery.

kidney (**kid**-ni) *n.* either of the pair of organs responsible for the excretion of nitrogenous wastes, principally urea, from the blood (see illustration). The active units of the kidney are the nephrons, which filter the blood under pressure and then reabsorb water and selected substances back into the blood. The urine thus formed is

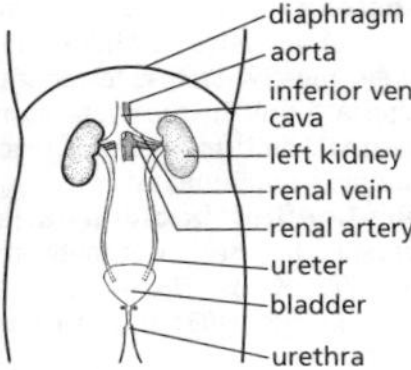

Position of the kidneys

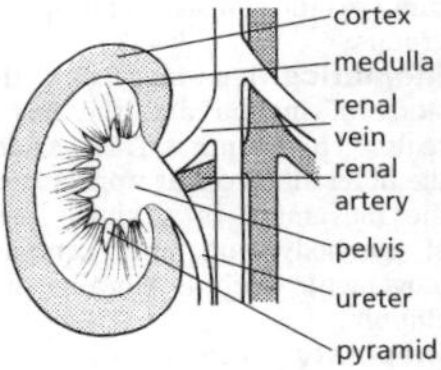

Section through a kidney

conducted via the renal tubules to the ureter, which leads to the bladder. *See also* haemodialysis, horseshoe kidney, renal (function tests).

Kienböck's disease (keen-berks) *n.* necrosis of the lunate bone of the wrist caused by interruption of its blood supply. It usually follows chronic stress or injury to the wrist. *See also* osteochondritis. [R. Kienböck (1871–1953), Austrian radiologist]

Kiesselbach's plexus (kees-ĕl-bahks) *n.* a collection of capillaries in the mucosa at the anterior part of the nasal septum. Nosebleeds frequently have their origin from this plexus. *See* epistaxis, Little's area. [W. Kiesselbach (1839–1902), German laryngologist]

killer cell (kil-er) *n. see* natural killer cell.

Killian's operation (kil-iănz) *n.* a surgical operation in which part of the frontal bone is removed to allow drainage of the frontal sinus (*see* paranasal sinuses), when this is filled with pus. [G. Killian (1860–1921), German otorhinolaryngologist]

kilo- *prefix denoting* a thousand.

kilogram (kil-ŏ-gram) *n.* the SI unit of mass equal to 1000 grams. Symbol: kg.

Kimmelstiel-Wilson disease (**kim**-ĕl-steel **wil**-sŏn) *n.* a disease in which diabetes mellitus is associated with the nephrotic syndrome, which results from breakdown of the glomeruli of the kidneys. [P. Kimmelstiel (1900–70), German-born pathologist; C. Wilson (1906–), British physician]

kin- (kine-) *combining form denoting* movement.

kinaesthesia (kin-iss-**theez**-iă) *n.* the sense that enables the brain to be constantly aware of the position and movement of muscles in different parts of the body.

kinanaesthesia (kin-anis-**theez**-iă) *n.* inability to sense the positions and movements of parts of the body, with consequent disordered physical activity.

kinase (ky-nayz) *n.* **1.** an agent that can convert the inactive form of an enzyme (*see* proenzyme) to the active form. **2.** an enzyme that catalyses the transfer of phosphate groups.

kinematics (kin-i-**mat**-iks) *n.* the study of motion and the forces required to produce it. This includes the different forces at work during the movement of a single part of the body, and more complex movements such as running and climbing.

kineplasty (**kin**-i-plasti) *n.* a method of amputation in which the muscles and tendons of the affected limb are arranged so that they can be integrated with a specially made artificial replacement.

-kinesis *combining form denoting* movement.

kinetochore (ky-**nee**-toh-kor) *n.* *see* centromere.

King's model (kingz) *n.* a model for nursing based on the view that individuals function in social systems through interpersonal relationships. Nursing is seen as a process of action, reaction, interaction, and transaction in order to set and achieve goals that meet the care needs of the patient. *See also* nursing models. [I. King (1923–2007), US nurse theorist]

kinin (**ky**-nin) *n.* one of a group of naturally occurring polypeptides that are powerful vasodilators, which lower blood pressure, and cause contraction of smooth muscle.

Kirschner's wire (**keersh**-nerz) *n.* a wire that can be inserted into a bone to exert skeletal traction or to fix fractures. [M. Kirschner (1879–1942), German surgeon]

kiss of life *n. see* mouth-to-mouth resuscitation.

Klebsiella (kleb-si-**el**-ă) *n.* a genus of Gram-negative rodlike nonmotile mostly lactose-fermenting bacteria found in the respiratory, intestinal, and urinogenital tracts of animals and humans.

Klebs-Loeffler bacillus (klebz-**lerf**-ler) *n. see* Corynebacterium. [T. Klebs (1834–1913) and F. A. J. Loeffler (1852–1915), German bacteriologists]

Kleine-Levin syndrome (klyn-**lev**-in) *n.* a rare episodic disorder characterized by periods (usually of a few days or weeks) in which sufferers eat enormously, sleep for most of the day and night, and may become more dependent or aggressive than normal. Between episodes they are usually quite unaffected. The disorder almost always resolves spontaneously. [W. Kleine (20th century), German neuropsychiatrist; M. Levin (20th century), US neurologist]

klepto- *combining form denoting* stealing.

kleptomania (kleptŏ-**may**-niă) *n.* a pathologically strong impulse to steal, often in the absence of any desire for the stolen object(s).

Klinefelter's syndrome (**klyn**-fel-terz) *n.* a genetic disorder in which there are three sex chromosomes, XXY, rather than the normal XX or XY. Affected individuals are apparently male, but have small testes, enlarged breasts, and absence of facial and body hair. [H. F. Klinefelter (1912–90), US physician]

Klumpke's paralysis (**kluump**-kĕz) *n.* a partial paralysis of the arm caused by injury to a baby's brachial plexus during birth. It results in weakness and wasting of the muscles of the hand. [A. Klumpke (1859–1927), French neurologist]

K-nail *n. see* Küntscher nail.

kneading (need-ing) *n. see* petrissage.

knee (nee) *n.* the hinge joint between the femur and the tibia. **k.-chest position** *see* genupectoral position. **k.-elbow position** *see* genucubital position. **k. jerk** *see* patellar reflex.

kneecap (nee-kap) *n. see* patella.

knock-knee (nok-nee) *n.* abnormal in-curving of the legs, resulting in a gap between the ankles when the knees are in contact. Medical name: **genu valgum**.

Kocher manoeuvre (kok-er) *n.* a method for reduction of an anteriorly dislocated shoulder by manipulation. [E. T. Kocher (1841–1917), Swiss surgeon]

Koch's bacillus (koks) *n. see* Mycobacterium. [R. Koch (1843–1910), German bacteriologist]

Köhler's disease (ker-lerz) *n.* osteonecrosis of the navicular bone of the foot (*see* osteochondritis). It occurs in children aged 3–7 years, causing pain and limping. [A. Köhler (1874–1947), German physician]

koilonychia (koi-loh-**nik**-iă) *n.* the development of brittle spoon-shaped nails, a common disorder that can occur with anaemia due to iron deficiency.

Koplik's spots (kop-liks) *pl. n.* small red spots with bluish-white centres that often appear on the mucous membranes of the mouth in measles. [H. Koplik (1858–1927), US paediatrician]

Korotkoff sounds (kor-ot-kof) *pl. n.* sounds heard (via a stethoscope) when the arterial pressure is occluded during manual blood pressure measurement. There are five phases to these sounds, which are used to determine systolic and diastolic blood pressure levels. [N. S. Korotkoff (1874–1920), Russian physician]

Korsakoff's syndrome (Korsakoff's psychosis) (kor-sak-offs) *n.* an organic disorder affecting the brain that results in impaired memory for recent events, disorientation in time and place, and confabulation. The commonest cause of the condition is untreated Wernicke's encephalopathy in the context of alcoholism. [S. S. Korsakoff (1854–1900), Russian neurologist]

kraurosis (kraw-**roh**-sis) *n.* shrinking of a body part, usually the vulva in elderly women (**k. vulvae**).

Krebs cycle (citric acid cycle) (krebz) *n.* a complex cycle of enzyme-catalysed reactions, occurring within the cells of all living animals, in which acetate is broken down to produce energy in the form of ATP and carbon dioxide. The cycle is the final step in the oxidation of carbohydrates, fats, and proteins. [Sir H. A. Krebs (1900–81), German-born biochemist]

Krukenberg tumour (kroo-kĕn-berg) *n.* a rapidly developing malignant growth in one or (more often) both ovaries. The tumour is secondary to a primary growth in the stomach or intestine. [F. E. Krukenberg (1871–1946), German pathologist]

krypton-81m (krip-ton) *n.* a radioactive gas that is the shortest-lived isotope in medical use (half-life 13 seconds). It can be used to investigate the ventilation of the lungs. *See also* rubidium-81.

KUB X-ray *n.* an abdominal plain X-ray film that is longer than normal to enable it to include the *k*idneys, *u*reters, and the entire *b*ladder.

Küntscher nail (K-nail) (koont-sher) *n.* a long steel nail that is inserted down the long axis of a long bone, into the marrow, in order to fix a fracture. See illustration. [G. Küntscher (1902–72), German orthopaedic surgeon]

Kupffer cells (kuup-fer) *pl. n.* phagocytic cells that line the sinusoids of the liver (*see* macrophage). They are particularly concerned with the formation of bile. [K. W. von Kupffer (1829–1902), German anatomist]

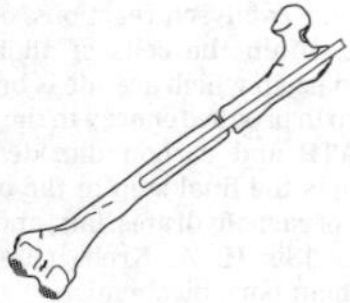

Küntscher nail

Kussmaul breathing (koos-mowl) *n.* the slow deep respiration associated with acidosis. [A. Kussmaul (1822–1902), German physician]

Kveim test (kvaym) *n.* a test used for the diagnosis of sarcoidosis. Tissue from a lymph node of a person suffering from the disease is injected intradermally; the development of a granuloma at the injection site indicates that the subject has sarcoidosis. [M. A. Kveim (20th century), Norwegian physician]

kwashiorkor (kwash-i-or-ker) *n.* a form of malnutrition due to a diet deficient in protein and energy-producing foods, common among young children in certain African tribes. The symptoms are oedema, loss of appetite, diarrhoea, general discomfort, and apathy; the child fails to thrive and there is usually associated gastrointestinal infection.

kymograph (ky-mŏ-grahf) *n.* an instrument for recording the flow and varying pressure of the blood within blood vessels. **—kymography** *n.*

kypho- *combining form denoting* a hump.

kyphos (ky-fos) *n.* a sharply localized posterior angulation of the spine, resulting in the appearance of a hump on the back (a hunchback deformity).

kyphoscoliosis (ky-foh-skoh-li-oh-sis) *n.* abnormal posterior and sideways curvature of the spine: kyphosis combined with scoliosis.

kyphosis (ky-foh-sis) *n.* outward curvature of the spine, which if pathological (excessive) causes hunching of the back. It may result from bad posture and be correctable by backward bending (**mobile k.**) or it may be congenital or result from such disorders as osteoporosis or ankylosing spondylitis (**fixed k.**). Treatment depends on the cause, and may include physiotherapy, bracing, and spinal osteotomy and fusion in severe cases. **adolescent k.** *see* Scheuermann's disease. *See also* kyphos, kyphoscoliosis.

L

labetalol (la-bee-tă-lol) *n.* a combined alpha- and beta-blocking drug, sometimes found to be more effective in the treatment of high blood pressure than beta blockers. It is administered by mouth or intravenously. Trade name: **Trandate**.

labia (lay-biă) *pl. n. see* labium.

labial (lay-bi-ăl) *adj.* **1.** relating to the lips or to a labium. **2.** designating the surface of a tooth adjacent to the lips.

labile (lay-byl) *adj.* unstable. The term is applied to drugs and other chemicals that readily undergo change in solution, when subjected to heat, etc., and also to emotions when there are rapid mood swings.

labio- *combining form denoting* the lip(s).

labioplasty (cheiloplasty) (lay-bi-oh-plasti) *n.* surgical repair of injury or deformity of the lips (cleft lip).

labium (lay-bi-ŭm) *n.* (*pl.* **labia**) a lip-shaped structure, especially either of the two pairs of skin folds that enclose the vulva. The larger outer pair are known as the **labia majora** and the smaller inner pair the **labia minora**.

labour (lay-ber) *n.* the sequence of actions by which a baby and the afterbirth (placenta) are expelled from the uterus at childbirth (see illustration). Labour usually starts spontaneously about 280 days after conception, but it may be started by artificial means (*see* induction). In the first stage the muscular wall of the uterus begins contracting while the cervix expands. The amnion ruptures releasing amniotic fluid to the exterior. In the second stage the baby passes through the vagina, assisted by contractions of the abdominal muscles and conscious pushing by the mother. When the whole infant has been eased clear of the vagina, the umbilical cord is cut. In the final stage the placenta and membranes are pushed out by the continuing contraction of the uterus. *See also* Caesarean section.

labrum (lay-brŭm) *n.* (*pl.* **labra**) a lip or liplike structure; occurring, for example, around the margins of the acetabulum.

labyrinth (inner ear) (lab-er-inth) *n.* a convoluted system of cavities and ducts comprising the organs of hearing and balance. **bony l.** the bony canals and chambers, embedded in the petrous part of the temporal bone, that surround the membranous labyrinth. **membranous l.** the membranous canals and chambers comprising the semicircular canals, utricle, saccule, and cochlea.

labyrinthectomy (lab-er-inth-**ek**-tŏmi) *n.* a surgical procedure to ablate (*see* ablation) the structures of the labyrinth, usually performed for cases of severe Ménière's disease.

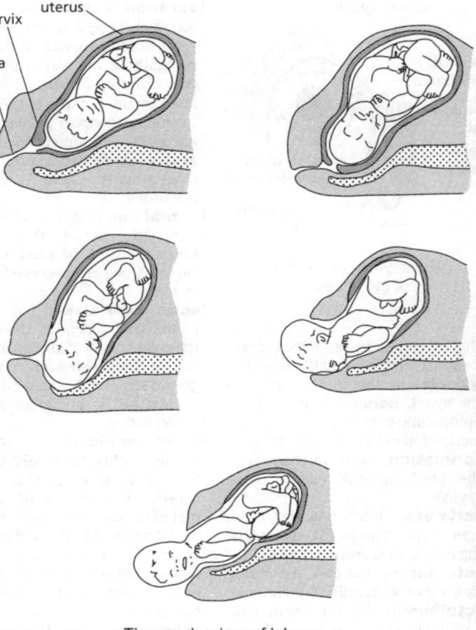

The mechanism of labour

labyrinthitis (lab-er-inth-I-tis) *n.* *see* otitis (interna).

laceration (las-er-ay-shŏn) *n.* a tear in the flesh caused by a blunt object producing a wound with irregular edges (such as a gunshot wound).

lacrimal (lak-rim-ăl) *adj.* relating to tears. **l. apparatus** the structures that produce and drain away fluid from the eye (see illustration). **l. bone** either of a pair of small rectangular bones that contribute to the orbits. **l. gland** the gland

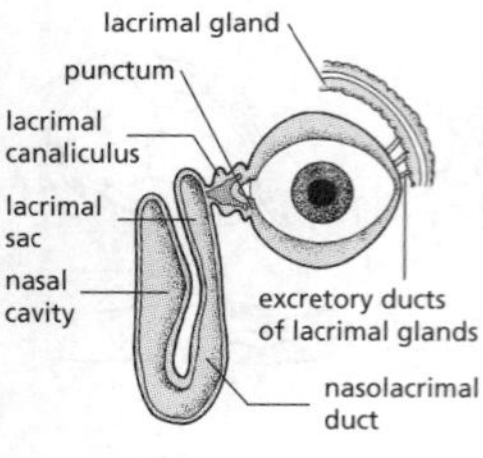

The lacrimal apparatus of the left eye

that secretes tears, which drain away through small openings (**puncta**) at the inner corner of the eye. **l. nerve** a branch of the ophthalmic nerve that supplies the lacrimal gland and conjunctiva.

lacrimation (lak-ri-**may**-shŏn) *n.* the production of excess tears; crying.

lacrimator (**lak**-rim-ay-ter) *n.* an agent that irritates the eyes, causing excessive secretion of tears.

lact- (lacti-, lacto-) *combining form denoting* **1.** milk. **2.** lactic acid.

lactalbumin (lak-**tal**-bew-min) *n.* a milk protein present in milk at a lower concentration than casein.

lactase (**lak**-tayz) *n.* an enzyme, secreted by the glands of the small intestine, that converts lactose (milk sugar) into glucose and galactose during digestion.

lactate (**lak**-tayt) **1.** *n.* any salt of lactic acid. **2.** *vb.* to secrete milk (*see* lactation).

lactation (lak-**tay**-shŏn) *n.* the secretion of milk by the mammary glands of the breasts, which begins normally at the end of pregnancy (*see also* colostrum) and is stimulated by the sucking of the baby at the nipple (*compare* galactorrhoea). Lactation is controlled by hormones (*see* oxytocin, prolactin); it stops when the baby is no longer breast-fed.

lacteal (**lak**-ti-ăl) *n.* a blind-ended lymphatic vessel that extends into a villus of the small intestine. Digested fats are absorbed into the lacteals.

lactic acid (**lak**-tik) *n.* a compound that forms in the cells as the end-product of glucose metabolism in the absence of oxygen (*see* glycolysis). Lactic acid (owing to its low pH) is an important food preservative.

lactic acidosis *n.* excessive plasma acidity due to an accumulation of lactic acid. This may be caused by a variety of illnesses, including heart failure or severe dehydration, or the accumulation of metformin used for treating type 2 diabetes mellitus, particularly when kidney failure is present.

lactiferous (lak-**tif**-er-ŭs) *adj.* transporting or secreting milk, as the ducts (**l. ducts**) of the breast.

lactifuge (**lak**-ti-fewj) *n.* a drug that reduces the secretion of milk. Some oestrogenic drugs have this effect.

Lactobacillus (lak-toh-bă-**sil**-ŭs) *n.* a genus of Gram-positive nonmotile rodlike bacteria that are capable of producing lactic acid from the fermentation of carbohydrates. They are found in fermenting animal and plant products, especially dairy products, and in the alimentary tract and vagina.

lactogenic hormone (lak-tŏ-**jen**-ik) *n. see* prolactin.

lactose (milk sugar) (**lak**-tohz) *n.* a sugar, consisting of one molecule of glucose and one of galactose, found only in milk. **l. intolerance** inability to absorb lactose, caused by absence or low activity of the enzyme lactase.

lactosuria (lak-tohs-**yoor**-iă) *n.* the presence of lactose in the urine. This often occurs during pregnancy and breast-feeding or if the milk flow is suppressed.

lactulose (**lak**-tew-lohz) *n.* a disaccharide sugar that acts as an osmotic laxative. Administered by mouth, it remains intact until it reaches the colon. There it is split by bacteria into simpler sugars that help to retain water, thereby softening the stools. Trade names: **Lactugal**, **Laevolac**.

lacuna (lă-**kew**-nă) *n.* (*pl.* **lacunae**) (in anatomy) a small cavity or depression.

Laënnec's cirrhosis (la-en-**neks**) *n.* alcoholic cirrhosis: the commonest type of cirrhosis. [R. T. H. Laënnec (1781–1826), French physician]

laevo- *combining form. see* levo-.

laevocardia (lee-voh-**kar**-di-ă) *n.* the normal position of the heart, in which its apex is directed towards the left. *Compare* dextrocardia.

laking (**layk**-ing) *n.* the physical or chemical treatment of blood to abolish the structure of the red cells and thus form a homogeneous solution. Laking is an important preliminary step in the analysis of haemoglobin or enzymes present in red cells.

-lalia *combining form denoting* a condition involving speech.

lallation (lalling) (la-**lay**-shŏn) *n.* an infantile form of speech characterized by the substitution of one consonant for another (e.g. 'l' for 'r').

lambda (**lam**-dă) *n.* the point on the skull at which the lambdoidal and sagittal sutures meet.

lambdoidal suture (**lam**-doi-d'l) *n.* the immovable joint between the parietal and occipital bones (*see* skull).

lambliasis (lam-**bly**-ă-sis) *n. see* giardiasis.

lamella (lă-**mel**-ă) *n.* (*pl.* **lamellae**) **1.** a thin membrane or layer of tissue. **2.** a thin gelatinous medicated disc used to apply drugs to the eye. The disc is placed on the eyeball; the gelatinous material dissolves and the drug is absorbed. **—lamellar** *adj.*

lamina (**lam**-in-ă) *n.* (*pl.* **laminae**) a thin membrane or layer of tissue, such as the bony plate forming part of a vertebral arch.

laminectomy (lam-in-**ek**-tŏmi) *n.* surgical cutting into the backbone to obtain access to the vertebral (spinal) canal. The operation is performed to remove tumours or prolapsed intervertebral discs or to relieve pressure on the spinal cord or roots.

lamivudine (lă-miv-yoo-deen) *n.* an antiviral drug administered by mouth for treating HIV infection and hepatitis B. Trade names: **Epivir**, **Zeffix**.

lamotrigine (lam-oh-try-geen) *n.* an antiepileptic drug used in the control of partial, tonic–clonic, and absence seizures, and for the prevention of depressive episodes in bipolar disorder. Lamotrigine is administered by mouth. Trade name: **Lamictal**.

Lancefield classification (lans-feeld) *n.* a classification of the *Streptococcus* bacteria based on the presence or absence of antigenic carbohydrate on the cell surface. Species are classified into the groups A–S. Most species causing disease in humans belong to groups A, B, and D. [R. C. Lancefield (1895–1981), US bacteriologist]

lancet (lahn-sit) *n.* a broad two-edged surgical knife with a sharp point.

lancinating (lahn-sin-ayt-ing) *adj.* describing a sharp stabbing or cutting pain.

Landau reflex (land-ow) *n.* a reflex seen in normal babies from three months until one year, when it disappears. If the baby is held horizontally, face down, it will straighten its legs and back and try to lift up its head. The presence of this reflex beyond one year may indicate a developmental disorder.

Langerhans cell histiocytosis (lang-er-hans) *n.* overgrowth of cells of the reticuloendothelial system. This includes disorders previously called **histiocytosis X**, including **eosinophilic granuloma**, **Hand-Schüller-Christian disease**, and **Letterer-Siwe disease**. [P. Langerhans (1847–88), German physician and anatomist]

Langer's lines (lahng-erz) *pl. n.* normal permanent skin creases. Incisions parallel to Langer's lines heal well and are less visible. [C. R. von E. Langer (1819–87), Austrian anatomist]

lanolin (lan-ŏ-lin) *n.* a fatty substance obtained from sheep's wool, used as an emollient and as a base for creams.

lanreotide (lan-ri-oh-tyd) *n.* an analogue of somatostatin that is administered by injection to treat acromegaly and hormone-secreting neuroendocrine tumours. Trade name: **Somatuline**.

lanugo (lă-new-goh) *n.* fine hair covering the body and limbs of the human fetus.

laparo- *combining form denoting* the loins or abdomen.

laparoscope (peritoneoscope) (lap-er-ŏ-skohp) *n.* *see* laparoscopy.

laparoscopy (abdominoscopy, peritoneoscopy) (lap-er-os-kŏpi) *n.* examination of the abdominal structures by means of a **laparoscope** (a type of endoscope). This is passed through a small incision in the wall of the abdomen after insufflation of carbon dioxide into the abdomen (creating a pneumoperitoneum). Laparoscopy enables visual assessment of abdominal organs, harvesting of biopsies, and cancer staging. Therapeutic uses include aspiration of cysts, division of adhesions, and surgery that would previously have required laparotomy. Examples include hysterectomy, cholecystectomy, prostatectomy, and the occlusion of Fallopian tubes for sterilization. *See also* minimally invasive surgery. **—laparoscopic** *adj.*

laparotomy (lap-er-**ot**-ŏmi) *n.* an incision to allow access to the abdominal cavity. All of the abdominal organs are examined to make a diagnosis and then proceed to treatment.

lardaceous (lar-**day**-shŭs) *adj.* resembling lard: often applied to tissue infiltrated with the starch-like substance amyloid (*see* amyloidosis).

Lariam (**la**-ri-am) *n. see* mefloquine.

larva (**lar**-vă) *n.* (*pl.* **larvae**) the preadult or immature stage hatching from the egg of some animal groups, e.g. insects and nematodes, which may be markedly different from the sexually mature adult. **l. migrans** *see* creeping eruption. **—larval** *adj.*

laryng- (laryngo-) *combining form denoting* the larynx.

laryngeal (la-rin-**jee**-ăl) *adj.* relating to the larynx. **l. mask** an airway tube for insertion into the mouth of a patient requiring artificial ventilation and designed to fit into the throat over the top of the laryngeal opening. **l. reflex** a cough produced by irritating the larynx. **l. stroboscopy** a method of studying the movements of the vocal folds of the larynx by using stroboscopic light (controlled intermittent flashes) to slow or freeze the movement.

laryngectomy (la-rin-**jek**-tŏmi) *n.* surgical removal of the whole or a part (**partial l.**) of the larynx in the treatment of laryngeal carcinoma. *See also* electrolarynx.

laryngismus (la-rin-**jiz**-mŭs) *n.* closure of the vocal folds by sudden contraction of the laryngeal muscles, followed by a noisy indrawing of breath. It occurs in young children when a foreign body has lodged in the larynx or in croup; in the past it was associated with low-calcium rickets.

laryngitis (la-rin-**jy**-tis) *n.* inflammation of the larynx and vocal folds, due to infection or irritation. The voice becomes husky or is lost completely; breathing is harsh and difficult (*see* stridor); and the cough is painful. Obstruction of the airways may occasionally be serious, especially in children (*see* croup).

laryngofissure (lă-ring-oh-**fish**-er) *n.* a surgical operation to open the larynx, enabling access for further procedures.

laryngology (la-ring-**ol**-ŏji) *n.* the study of diseases of the larynx and vocal folds. **—laryngologist** *n.*

laryngomalacia (lă-ring-oh-mă-**lay**-shiă) *n.* a condition characterized by paroxysmal attacks of breathing difficulty and stridor. It occurs in small children and is caused by flaccidity of the structure of the larynx. It usually resolves spontaneously by the age of two years.

laryngopharynx (lă-ring-oh-**fa**-rinks) *n. see* hypopharynx.

laryngoscope (lă-**ring**-ŏ-skohp) *n.* a device used to inspect the larynx for diagnostic purposes, to facilitate surgery on laryngeal structures, or to aid insertion of an endotracheal tube.

laryngoscopy (la-ring-**os**-kŏpi) *n.* examination of the larynx. This may be done indirectly using a small mirror or directly using a laryngoscope.

laryngospasm (lă-**ring**-oh-spazm) *n.* involuntary closure of the larynx, obstructing the flow of air to the lungs.

laryngostenosis (lă-ring-oh-sti-**noh**-sis) *n.* narrowing of the cavity of the larynx.

laryngotomy (la-ring-**ot**-ŏmi) *n.* surgical incision of the larynx. **inferior l.** surgical incision of the cricothyroid membrane beneath the larynx; a life-saving operation when there is obstruction to breathing at or above the larynx. *See* tracheostomy.

laryngotracheobronchitis (lă-ring-oh-trak-i-oh-brong-**ky**-tis) *n.* a severe and almost exclusively viral infection of the respiratory tract, especially of young children, in whom there may be a dangerous degree of obstruction either at the larynx (*see* croup) or bronchi.

larynx (**la**-rinks) *n.* the organ responsible for the production of vocal sounds, also serving as an air passage conveying air from the pharynx to the lungs. It is situated in the front of the neck, above the trachea. It is made up of a framework of nine cartilages, bound together by ligaments and muscles and lined with mucous membrane, and contains a pair of vocal folds. See illustration. **—laryngeal** *adj.*

LASEK (**lay**-sek) *n. la*ser in *s*itu *e*pithelial *k*eratomileusis: eye surgery used to correct both short sight and long sight. A flap of corneal epithelium is raised, the surface of the cornea is reshaped using an excimer laser, and the epithelium is then replaced.

laser (**lay**-zer) *n.* a device that produces a very thin beam of light in which high energies are concentrated. Lasers can be used to operate on small areas of abnormality without damaging delicate surrounding tissue. For example, they are used in eye surgery for operations on the lens (**femtosecond l.**), lens capsule (**YAG l.**), retina (**argon l.**, **diode l.**), and cornea (**excimer l.**). Lasers are also used to unblock coronary arteries

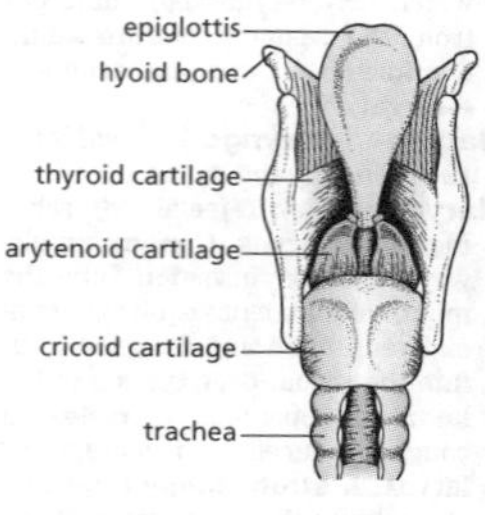

Cartilages of the larynx

narrowed by atheroma, to remove certain types of birthmark (*see* naevus), in the treatment of cervical intraepithelial neoplasia (*see* CIN) and varicose veins (**endovenous l. treatment**), and in endometrial ablation (**Nd:YAG l.**).

laser-assisted uvulopalatoplasty (LAUP) (yoov-yoo-loh-**pal**-ă-toh-plasti) *n.* laser surgery to the palate, used in the treatment of obstructive sleep apnoea.

LASIK (**lay**-sik) *n.* *la*ser in *si*tu *k*eratomileusis: eye surgery used to correct both short sight and long sight. A thin corneal flap (epithelium and stroma) is raised, the surface of the cornea reshaped using an excimer laser, and the flap then replaced.

Lasix (**las**-iks) *n.* *see* furosemide.

Lassa fever (**las**-ă) *n.* a serious virus disease confined to Central West Africa. Symptoms include headache, high fever, and severe muscular pains; difficulty in swallowing often arises. Death from kidney or heart failure occurs in over 50% of cases. Treatment with plasma from recovered patients is the best therapy.

Lassar's paste (**las**-arz) *n.* an ointment containing zinc oxide, starch, and salicylic acid in a soft paraffin base, used in the treatment of warts and calluses, scalp conditions, and other skin diseases. [G. Lassar (1849–1907), German dermatologist]

latent heat (**lay**-tĕnt) *n.* the quantity of heat absorbed or released when a substance changes state (e.g. from solid to liquid or from liquid to vapour) without any change in temperature.

late-onset schizophrenia (layt-**on**-set) *n.* a mental disorder, formerly called **paraphrenia**, characterized by systematic delusions and commonly auditory hallucinations, but without any other marked symptoms of mental illness. It is typically seen in the elderly and can also occur in people with severe hearing impediments.

lateral (**lat**-er-ăl) *adj.* **1.** situated at or relating to the side of an organ or organism. **2.** (in anatomy) relating to the region or parts of the body that are furthest from the median plane. **3.** (in radiology) in the sagittal plane.

lateroversion (lat-er-oh-**ver**-shŏn) *n.* a turning or displacement of an organ, for example the uterus (**uterine l.**), to one side.

laudanum (**lawd**-nŭm) *n.* a hydroalcoholic solution containing 1% morphine, prepared from macerated raw opium. It was formerly widely used as an opioid analgesic, taken by mouth.

laughing gas (**lahf**-ing) *n.* *see* nitrous oxide.

LAUP *n.* *see* laser-assisted uvulopalatoplasty.

Laurence-Moon-Biedl syndrome (**lo**-rĕns moon **bee**-d'l) *n.* an autosomal recessive condition characterized by obesity, short stature, learning disabilities, retinitis pigmentosa, impaired gonad development, and delayed puberty. [J. Z. Laurence (1830–74), British ophthalmologist; R. C. Moon (1844–1914), US ophthalmologist;

A. Biedl (1869–1933), Austrian physician]

lavage (lav-ah*zh*) *n.* washing out a body cavity, such as the colon or stomach, with water or a medicated solution. In cases of bowel obstruction the washing out can be done during the operation (**on-table l.**). *See also* bronchoalveolar lavage, diagnostic peritoneal lavage.

laxative (laks-ă-tiv) *n.* a drug used to treat constipation or to evacuate the bowel (e.g. before surgery). **bulk-forming l.** a laxative, such as methylcellulose, that encourages the passage of a softer or bulkier stool. **osmotic l.** a laxative, such as magnesium sulphate or lactulose, that acts by retaining water in the large bowel. **stimulant l.** (**cathartic**, **purgative**) a laxative, such as bisacodyl or senna, that stimulates or increases the frequency of bowel evacuation.

lazy eye (lay-zi) *n. see* amblyopia.

LBC *n. see* liquid-based cytology.

LDL *n.* low-density lipoprotein: *see* lipoprotein.

L-dopa *n. see* levodopa.

LE *n. see* lupus (erythematosus).

lead (led) *n.* a soft bluish-grey metallic element that forms several poisonous compounds. Acute lead poisoning causes abdominal pains, vomiting, diarrhoea, and sometimes encephalitis. In chronic poisoning a characteristic blue mark on the gums (**l. line**) is seen and the peripheral nerves are affected; there is also anaemia. Treatment is with edetate. The use of lead in paints is now strictly controlled. Symbol: Pb.

learning disability (learning difficulty) (lern-ing) *n.* delayed or incomplete intellectual development combined with social malfunction, such as educational or occupational failure or inability of individuals to look after themselves.

SEE WEB LINKS

- Website of the British Institute for Learning Disabilities

leather-bottle stomach (le*th*-er bot-t'l) *n. see* linitis plastica.

Leber's congenital amaurosis (lay-berz) *n.* a hereditary (autosomal recessive) condition causing severe visual loss in infants. [T. Leber (1840–1917), German ophthalmologist]

Leber's optic atrophy *n.* a rare hereditary disorder, usually affecting young males, that is characterized by rapid loss of central vision due to neuroretinal degeneration. [T. Leber]

lecithin (les-i-thin) *n.* one of a group of phospholipids that are important constituents of cell membranes and are involved in the metabolism of fat by the liver. An example is **phosphatidylcholine**. **l.-sphingomyelin ratio** (**LS ratio**) a measure of fetal lung maturity; an LS ratio below 2 indicates a higher risk of respiratory distress syndrome.

lecithinase (les-i-thin-ayz) *n.* an enzyme from the small intestine that breaks lecithin down into its constituents (i.e. glycerol, fatty acids, phosphoric acid, and choline).

leech (leech) *n.* a type of worm that possesses suckers at both ends of its body. Certain parasitic species suck blood from animals and humans, causing irritation and, occasionally, infection. Formerly widely used for bloodletting, the medicinal leech (*Hirudo medicinalis*) may now be used following microsurgery to restore patency to blocked or collapsed blood vessels. *See also* hirudin.

leflunomide (lĕ-**floo**-nŏ-myd) *n.* an immunosuppressant drug administered by mouth to treat rheumatoid and psoriatic arthritis that have not responded to methotrexate or other disease-modifying antirheumatic drugs. Trade name: **Arava**.

Legg-Calvé-Perthes disease (Perthes disease, pseudocoxalgia) (leg **kal**-vay **per**-tĕz) *n.* necrosis of the head of the femur due to interruption of its blood supply (*see* osteochondritis). It occurs most commonly in boys between the ages of 5 and 10, and causes aching and a limp. [A. T. Legg (1874–1939), US surgeon; J. Calvé (1875–1954), French orthopaedist; G. C. Perthes (1869–1927), German surgeon]

legionnaires' disease (lee-jŏn-**airz**) *n.* an infection of the lungs caused by the bacterium *Legionella pneumophila*. Symptoms include malaise and muscle pain, succeeded by a fever, dry cough, chest pain, and breathlessness. Erythromycin provides the most effective therapy.

legumin (lig-**yoo**-min) *n.* a protein (a globulin) obtained from the seeds of plants of the family Leguminosae, such as beans and peas.

Leininger's theory of transcultural nursing (lyn-in-gerz) *n. see* transcultural nursing.

leio- *combining form denoting* smoothness.

leiomyoma (ly-oh-my-**oh**-mă) *n.* a benign tumour of smooth muscle. Such tumours occur most commonly in the uterus (*see* fibroid) but can also arise in the digestive tract, walls of blood vessels, etc.

leiomyosarcoma (ly-oh-my-oh-sar-**koh**-mă) *n.* a malignant tumour of smooth muscle, most commonly found in the uterus, stomach, small bowel, and at the base of the bladder.

Leishman-Donovan body (**leesh**-măn **don**-ŏ-văn) *n. see* Leishmania. [Sir W. B. Leishman (1865–1926), British surgeon; C. Donovan (1863–1951), Irish physician]

Leishmania (leesh-**may**-niă) *n.* a genus of parasitic flagellate protozoans, several species of which cause disease in humans (*see* leishmaniasis). In humans, especially in kala-azar patients, the parasite is a small rounded structure called a **Leishman-Donovan body**, which is found within the cells of the lymphatic system, spleen, and bone marrow.

leishmaniasis (leesh-mă-**ny**-ă-sis) *n.* a disease, common in the tropics and subtropics, caused by parasitic protozoans of the genus *Leishmania*, which are transmitted by the bite of sandflies. **cutaneous l.** leishmaniasis that affects the tissues of the skin. *See* espundia, oriental sore. **visceral l.** leishmaniasis in which the cells of various internal organs are affected. *See* kala-azar.

lens (lenz) *n.* **1.** (in anatomy) the transparent crystalline structure situated behind the pupil of the eye. It helps to refract incoming light and focus it onto the retina. *See also* accommodation. **2.** (in optics) a piece of glass or other material shaped to refract rays of light in a particular direction. Lenses are worn to correct faulty eyesight. **l. implant** a plastic lens to replace a natural lens that has been removed because of cataract. *See also* bifocal lens, contact lenses, multifocal lens.

lenticular (len-**tik**-yoo-ler) *adj.* relating to or shaped like a lens.

lenticular nucleus (lentiform nucleus) *n. see* basal ganglia.

lentigo (len-**ty**-goh) *n.* (*pl.* **lentigines**) a flat dark brown spot found mainly in the elderly on skin exposed to light. **l. maligna** (**pre-invasive** or **in situ melanoma**) a form of lentigo that occurs on the cheeks of the elderly and has variable pigmentation.

leontiasis (lee-on-**ty**-ă-sis) *n.* a bilateral symmetrical hypertrophy of the bones of the face and cranium, said to resemble the appearance of a lion's head. It is a rare feature of untreated Paget's disease. Medical name: **leontiasis ossea**.

leproma (lep-**roh**-mă) *n.* a lump on the skin characteristic of leprosy.

leprosy (Hansen's disease) (**lep**-rŏ-si) *n.* a chronic disease, caused by the bacterium *Mycobacterium leprae*, that affects the skin, mucous membranes, and nerves. It is confined mainly to the tropics and is transmitted by direct contact. Symptoms mainly involve the skin and nerves. Leprosy should be treated with a combination of antibacterial drugs (including dapsone and rifampicin), to overcome the problem of resistance developing to a single drug, and reconstructive surgery can repair some of the damage caused by the disease. **indeterminate l.** a form of the disease in which the skin manifestations represent a combination of lepromatous and tuberculoid leprosy. **lepromatous** (or **multibacillary**) **l.** a contagious steadily progressive form of the disease characterized by the development of widely distributed lumps on the skin, thickening of the skin and nerves, and in serious cases by severe numbness of the skin, muscle weakness, and paralysis leading to disfigurement and deformity. Tuberculosis is a common complication. **paucibacillary l.** tuberculoid or indeterminate leprosy. **tuberculoid l.** a benign, often self-limiting, form of leprosy causing discoloration and disfiguration of patches of skin associated with localized numbness.

lept- (lepto-) *combining form denoting* **1.** slender; thin. **2.** small. **3.** mild; slight.

leptin (**lep**-tin) *n.* a protein, produced by adipose tissue (especially white fat), that has a role in regulating eating: an increase in adipose tissue results in higher concentrations of leptin and a reduction in appetite.

leptocyte (**lep**-toh-syt) *n.* a red blood cell (erythrocyte) that is wafer-thin and generally large in diameter, with the haemoglobin concentrated in a thin rim at the periphery. Leptocytes are seen in certain types of anaemia.

leptomeninges (lep-toh-min-**in**-jeez) *pl. n.* the inner two meninges: the arachnoid and pia mater.

leptomeningitis (lep-toh-men-in-**jy**-tis) *n.* inflammation of the leptomeninges. *See also* meningitis.

Leptospira (lep-toh-**spy**-ră) *n.* a genus of spirochaete bacteria, commonly bearing hooked ends. **L. icterohaemorrhagiae** a parasite that is the main causative agent of leptospirosis.

leptospirosis (Weil's disease) (lep-toh-spy-**roh**-sis) *n.* an infectious disease, caused by bacteria of the genus *Leptospira* (especially *L. icterohaemorrhagiae*), that is transmitted from rodents, dogs, and other mammals to humans. The disease begins with a high fever and headache and may affect the liver (causing jaundice) or kidneys (resulting in renal failure); in some cases meningitis may develop.

Leriche's syndrome (lĕ-**reesh**-ĕz) *n.* a condition in males characterized by absence of penile erection combined with absence of pulses in the femoral arteries and wasting of the buttock muscles. It is caused by occlusion of the abdominal aorta and iliac arteries. [R. Leriche (1879–1956), French surgeon]

Lesch-Nyhan disease (lesh-**ny**-hăn) *n.* a sex-linked hereditary disease caused by an enzyme deficiency resulting in overproduction of uric acid. Affected boys have learning disability, spasticity, and gouty arthritis. They also have a compulsion for self-mutilation. [M. Lesch (1939–) and W. L. Nyhan Jr. (1926–), US physicians]

lesion (**lee**-*zh*ŏn) *n.* a zone of tissue with impaired function as a result of damage by disease or wounding.

lethal gene (**lee**-thăl) *n.* a gene that, under certain conditions, causes the death of the individual carrying it. Lethal genes are usually recessive: an individual will die only if he or she receives the gene from both parents.

lethargy (**leth**-er-ji) *n.* mental and physical sluggishness: a degree of inactivity and unresponsiveness approaching or verging on the unconscious.

letrozole (**let**-rŏ-zohl) *n. see* aromatase inhibitor.

Letterer-Siwe disease (let-er-er **sy**-wĕ) *n. see* Langerhans cell histiocytosis. [E. Letterer (20th century) and S. A. Siwe (1897–1966), German physicians]

leuc- (leuco-, leuk-, leuko-) *combining form denoting* **1.** lack of colour; white. **2.** leucocytes.

leucine (**loo**-seen) *n.* an essential amino acid. *See also* amino acid.

leucocyte (white blood cell, WBC) (**loo**-kŏ-syt) *n.* any blood cell that contains a nucleus. In health there are three major subdivisions: granulocytes, lymphocytes, and monocytes, which are part of the immune system, being involved in protecting the body against foreign substances and in antibody production. In disease, a variety of other types may appear in the blood.

leucocytolysis (loo-koh-sy-**tol**-i-sis) *n.* destruction of white blood cells.

leucocytosis (loo-koh-sy-**toh**-sis) *n.* an increase in the number of leucocytes in the blood. *See* basophilia, eosinophilia, lymphocytosis, monocytosis.

leucocytospermia (loo-koh-sy-toh-**sperm**-iă) *n.* the presence of excess white blood cells (leucocytes) in the semen (more than 1 million/ml). It has an adverse effect on fertility.

leucoderma (loo-koh-**der**-mă) *n.* loss of pigment in areas of the skin, resulting in the appearance of white patches or bands.

leucolysin (loo-**kol**-i-sin) *n.* *see* lysin.

leucoma (loo-**koh**-mă) *n.* a white opacity in the cornea. Most leucomas result from scarring after corneal inflammation or ulceration.

leuconychia (loo-koh-**nik**-iă) *n.* white discoloration of the nails, which may be total or partial. There are many causes.

leucopenia (loo-koh-**pee**-niă) *n.* a reduction in the number of leucocytes in the blood. *See* eosinopenia, lymphopenia, neutropenia.

leucoplakia (loo-koh-**play**-kiă) *n.* *see* leukoplakia.

leucopoiesis (loo-koh-poi-**ee**-sis) *n.* the process of the production of leucocytes, which normally occurs in the blood-forming tissue of the bone marrow. *See also* granulopoiesis, haemopoiesis, lymphopoiesis, monoblast.

leucorrhoea (loo-kŏ-**ree**-ă) *n.* a whitish or yellowish discharge of mucus from the vaginal opening. An abnormally large discharge may indicate infection of the lower reproductive tract.

leucotomy (loo-**kot**-ŏmi) *n.* the surgical operation of interrupting the pathways of white nerve fibres within the brain: it involves stereotaxy to make selective lesions in small areas of the brain. The operation is very occasionally used for intractable pain, severe depression, obsessive–compulsive disorder, and chronic anxiety. **prefrontal l.** (**lobotomy**) the original form of the operation, which involved cutting through the nerve fibres connecting the frontal lobe with the thalamus and the association fibres of the frontal lobe; it has now been abandoned.

leukaemia (loo-**kee**-miă) *n.* any of a group of malignant diseases in which increased numbers of certain immature or abnormal leucocytes are produced. This leads to increased susceptibility to infection, anaemia, and bleeding. Other symptoms include enlargement of the spleen, liver, and lymph nodes. Leukaemias may be **acute** or **chronic** depending on the rate of progression of the disease. They are also classified according to the type of white cell that is proliferating abnormally, as in **lymphocytic l.** or **monocytic l.** (*see also* hairy cell, lymphoblast, myeloblast, myeloid (leukaemia)). Leukaemias are treated with cytotoxic drugs, monoclonal antibodies, or (occasionally) radiotherapy.

SEE WEB LINKS

- Website of Bloodwise (formerly Leukaemia and Lymphoma Research)

leukocidin (loo-koh-**sy**-din) *n.* a bacterial exotoxin that selectively destroys white blood cells (leucocytes).

leukoplakia (leucoplakia) (loo-koh-**play**-kiă) *n.* a thickened white patch on a mucous membrane, such as the mouth lining or vulva, that cannot be rubbed off. Occasionally leukoplakia can become malignant. **hairy l.** leukoplakia with a shaggy or hairy appearance, which is a marker of AIDS.

leukotriene receptor antagonist (loo-koh-**try**-een) *n.* one of a class of drugs that prevent the action of leukotrienes (chemicals involved in inflammatory reactions and the immune response) by blocking their receptors on cell membranes, such as those in the airways. These drugs are used in the treatment of asthma; they include **montelukast** (Singulair) and **zafirlukast** (Accolate), both of which are administered by mouth.

leuprorelin (loo-proh-**rel**-in) *n. see* gonadorelin analogue.

levator (li-**vay**-ter) *n.* **1.** a surgical instrument used for levering up displaced bone fragments in a depressed fracture of the skull. **2.** any muscle that lifts the structure into which it is inserted.

levo- (laevo-) *combining form denoting* **1.** the left side. **2.** (in chemistry) levorotation.

levobunolol (lee-voh-**boon**-ŏ-lol) *n.* a beta blocker used as eye drops in the treatment of open-angle glaucoma. Trade name: **Betagan**.

levodopa (L-dopa) (lee-voh-**doh**-pă) *n.* a naturally occurring amino acid (*see* dopa) used in the treatment of parkinsonism. It is administered by mouth in combination with benserazide in **co-beneldopa** (Madopar) or carbidopa in **co-careldopa** (Caramet CR, Duodopa, Sinemet), which prevent the breakdown of levodopa outside the brain, thus reducing its side-effects (e.g. nausea, vomiting, hypotension) and enabling lower doses to be given.

levodopa test *n.* a test of the ability of the pituitary to secrete growth hormone, in which levodopa is administered by mouth and plasma levels of growth hormone are subsequently measured (they should peak within the following hour).

levomepromazine (methotrimeprazine) (lee-voh-mĕ-**proh**-mă-zeen) *n.* a phenothiazine antipsychotic drug used in the treatment of schizophrenia and to relieve agitation, nausea and vomiting, and pain in terminally ill patients. It is administered by mouth or injection. Trade name: **Nozinan**.

levonorgestrel (lee-voh-nor-**jes**-trĕl) *n.* a synthetic female sex hormone – a progestogen – used mainly in oral contraceptives, either in combination with an oestrogen (e.g. **Logynon**, **Ovranette**) or as a progestogen-only preparation (**Norgeston**). It is also used in postcoital (emergency) contraception and in the IUS.

levothyroxine sodium (lee-voh-th'y-**roks**-een) *n.* a preparation of thyroxine administered orally for the treatment of hypothyroidism.

levulosuria (lev-yoo-lohs-**yoor**-iă) *n.* *see* fructosuria.

Lewy bodies (loo-i) *pl. n.* abnormal proteins found in the nerve cells of the cerebral cortex and basal ganglia in patients with **cortical Lewy body disease**, which is characterized by a combination of parkinsonism and dementia. [F. H. Lewy (1885–1950), German neurologist]

Leydig cells (ly-dig) *pl. n. see* interstitial cells. [F. von Leydig (1821–1908), German anatomist]

Leydig tumour *n.* a tumour of the interstitial (Leydig) cells of the testis. Such tumours often secrete testosterone, which in prepubertal boys causes virilization and precocious puberty.

LFTs *pl. n. see* liver function tests.

LGA *adj.* large for gestational age.

LH *n. see* luteinizing hormone.

Lhermitte's sign (lair-mits) *n.* a tingling shocklike sensation passing down the arms or trunk when the neck is flexed. It is a nonspecific indication of disease in the cervical (neck) region of the spinal cord. [J. Lhermitte (1877–1959), French neurologist]

LHRH analogue *n. see* gonadorelin analogue.

liaison psychiatry (lee-ay-zŏn) *n.* the speciality that provides an interface between medicine and psychiatry. Liaison teams, consisting of psychiatric nurses, psychiatrists, and sometimes psychologists or social workers, are usually located in general hospitals and see patients after deliberate self-harm and when a mental illness or delirium is suspected in order to diagnose and advise on treatment.

libido (lib-ee-doh) *n.* **1.** (in psychoanalytic theory) the life instinct or, more specifically, the sexual instinct. **2.** sexual desire.

Librium (**lib**-riŭm) *n. see* chlordiazepoxide.

lice (lys) *pl. n. see* louse, pediculosis.

licence (**ly**-sĕns) *n.* (in pharmaceutics) a document that allows a pharmaceutical company to market a particular drug. The company must apply for a licence to the regulatory body that issues them: in the UK this is the Medicines and Healthcare products Regulatory Agency. A drug is licensed only for defined uses (indications), which the health professional prescribing it should adhere to.

lichen (ly-kĕn) *n.* any of several types of skin disease. **l. planus** an extremely itchy skin disease of unknown cause. Shiny flat-topped mauve spots may occur anywhere but are characteristically found on the inside of the wrists. It may take the form of a white lacy pattern in the mouth, which usually produces no symptoms. **l. simplex chronicus** (**neurodermatitis**) thickened eczematous skin that develops at the site of constant rubbing, often at the nape of the neck (in women) or lower legs or scrotum (in men). **l. sclerosus** a chronic disease mainly affecting the anogenital area, especially the vulva in women and the foreskin in men, and characterized by sheets of ivory-white skin, which cause intense itching in women and loss of normal penile architecture in men.

lichenification (ly-ken-i-fi-**kay**-shŏn) *n.* thickening of the epidermis with exaggeration of the normal creases: a cardinal feature of chronic eczema. The cause is abnormal scratching or rubbing of the skin.

lichenoid (ly-kĕn-oid) *adj.* describing any skin disease that resembles lichen planus.

lidocaine (lignocaine) (ly-doh-kayn) *n.* a widely used local anaesthetic administered by injection or by direct application for minor surgery and dental procedures. For dental surgery it is normally used in combination with adrenaline. Lidocaine is also injected intravenously to treat conditions involving abnormal heart rhythm, particularly following myocardial infarction. Trade names: **Instillagel**, **Laryngojet**, **LMX 4**, **Minijet Lignocaine**, **Versatis**, **Xylocaine**.

lie (ly) *n.* the long axis of the fetus in relation to that of the mother. It may be longitudinal, transverse, or oblique.

Lieberkühn's glands (crypts of Lieberkühn, intestinal glands) (lee-ber-koonz) *pl. n.* simple tubular glands in the mucous membrane of the intestine. They are lined with columnar epithelium in which various types of secretory cells are found. [J. N. Lieberkühn (1711–56), German anatomist]

lien (ly-ĕn) *n. see* spleen.

lien- (lieno-) *combining form denoting* the spleen.

life expectancy *n.* the number of years after which half of the babies born today will have died, assuming mortality rates throughout their lifetime remain the same as they are today. It is the number of years that a person within a given population can expect, on average, to live.

ligament (lig-ă-mĕnt) *n.* **1.** a tough band of white fibrous connective tissue that links two bones together at a joint. Ligaments are inelastic but flexible; they strengthen the joint and limit its movements to certain directions. **2.** a sheet of peritoneum that supports or links together abdominal organs.

ligand (lig-ănd) *n.* a molecule that binds to another molecule, as in antigen–antibody and hormone–receptor bondings.

ligation (li-gay-shŏn) *n.* the application of a ligature.

ligature (lig-ă-cher) *n.* any material – for example, nylon, vicryl, or wire – that is tied firmly round a blood vessel or duct to prevent bleeding, the passage of materials, etc.

light adaptation (lyt) *n.* reflex changes in the eye to enable vision either in normal light after being in darkness or in very bright light after being in normal light. *See* iris. *Compare* dark adaptation.

lightening (ly-t'n-ing) *n.* the sensation experienced, usually after the 36th week of gestation, by many pregnant women, particularly those carrying their first child, as the presenting part of the fetus enters the pelvis. This reduces the pressure on the diaphragm and the woman notices that it is easier to breathe. *Compare* engagement.

lightning pains (lyt-ning) *pl. n.* severe stabbing pains in the legs experienced in tabes dorsalis.

light reflex *n. see* pupillary reflex.

lignocaine (lig-nŏ-kayn) *n. see* lidocaine.

likelihood ratio *n.* the degree to which a test result will change the odds that a patient has a disease. The likelihood ratio for a positive test expresses the degree to which the odds that a patient has a disease increase following a positive test. The likelihood ratio for a negative test expresses the degree to which the odds that a patient has a disease decrease following a negative test.

Likert scale (lik-ert) *n.* a tool used in questionnaires in which participants are asked to respond to statements on a scale ranging from "strongly agree" to "strongly disagree". [R. Likert (1903–81), US psychologist]

limbic system (lim-bik) *n.* a complex system of nerve pathways and networks in the brain that is involved in the expression of instinct and mood in activities of the endocrine and motor systems of the body. Among the brain regions involved are the amygdala, hippocampal formation, and hypothalamus.

limb lengthening (lim) *n.* an orthopaedic procedure for increasing the length of a limb (usually the leg). It involves division of the bone and the use of an external fixator to widen the gap between the divided ends. New bone is produced in the widening gap as the bone is stretched.

limbus (lim-bŭs) *n.* (in anatomy) an edge or border. **l. sclerae** the junction of the cornea and sclera of the eye.

limen (ly-men) *n.* (in anatomy) a border or boundary.

liminal (lim-in-ăl) *adj.* (in physiology) relating to the threshold of perception.

linac (ly-nak) *n. see* linear accelerator.

linctus (link-tŭs) *n.* a syrupy liquid medicine, particularly one used in the treatment of irritating coughs.

linea (lin-iă) *n.* (*pl.* **lineae**) (in anatomy) a line, narrow streak, or stripe. **l. alba** a tendinous line, extending from the xiphoid process to the pubic symphysis, where the flat abdominal muscles are attached. **l. nigra** a pigmented line, seen on the abdomen in pregnancy, extending from the umbilicus to the pubis.

linear accelerator (linac) (lin-ier) *n.* a machine that accelerates particles to produce high-energy radiation, used in the treatment (radiotherapy) of malignant disease.

linezolid (lini-**zoh**-lid) *n.* an antibiotic that is active against Gram-positive bacteria, including MRSA, and is used to treat pneumonia and soft-tissue infections caused by these organisms. It is administered by mouth or intravenous infusion. Trade name: **Zyvox**.

lingual (**ling**-wăl) *adj.* relating to, situated close to, or resembling the tongue (lingua).

lingula (**ling**-yoo-lă) *n.* a thin tongue-like projection of bone or other tissue.

liniment (**lin**-i-mĕnt) *n.* a medicinal preparation that is rubbed onto the skin or applied on a surgical dressing. Liniments often contain camphor and alcohol.

linitis plastica (leather-bottle stomach) (li-**ny**-tis **plas**-ti-kă) *n.* diffuse infiltration of the stomach submucosa with malignant tissue, producing rigidity, narrowing, and reduced capacity.

linoleic acid (lin-oh-**lee**-ik) *n. see* essential fatty acid.

linolenic acid (lin-oh-**len**-ik) *n. see* essential fatty acid.

lint (lint) *n.* a material used in surgical dressings, made of scraped linen or a cotton substitute. It is usually fluffy one side and smooth the other.

liothyronine (ly-oh-**th'y**-rŏ-neen) *n.* a preparation of the thyroid hormone triiodothyronine, administered by mouth or injection to treat conditions of thyroid deficiency.

lip- (lipo-) *combining form denoting* **1.** fat. **2.** lipid.

lipaemia (lip-**ee**-miă) *n.* the presence in the blood of an abnormally large amount of fat, such as cholesterol.

lipase (steapsin) (**lip**-ayz) *n.* an enzyme, produced by the pancreas and the glands of the small intestine, that breaks down fats into glycerol and fatty acids during digestion.

lipid (**lip**-id) *n.* one of a group of naturally occurring compounds that are soluble in solvents such as chloroform or alcohol, but insoluble in water. Lipids are important dietary constituents. The group includes fats, steroids, phospholipids, and glycolipids.

lipidosis (lipoidosis) (lip-i-**doh**-sis) *n.* (*pl.* **lipidoses**) any disorder of lipid metabolism within the cells of the body.

lipoatrophy (lip-oh-**at**-rŏ-fi) *n.* an immune reaction to insulin injections close to the site of injection, resulting in localized hollowing of the fat tissue. Formerly common with bovine insulin, it is now very rarely seen with human insulins and insulin analogues.

lipochondrodystrophy (lip-oh-kon-droh-**dis**-trŏ-fi) *n.* multiple congenital defects affecting lipid (fat) metabolism, cartilage and bone, skin, and the major internal organs, leading to learning disability, dwarfism, and deformities of the bones.

lipodystrophy (lip-oh-**dis**-trŏ-fi) *n.* any condition resulting in the loss and/or redistribution of fat tissue in part or all of the body. It may be congenital or acquired (e.g. as an adverse effect of antiretroviral drug therapy).

lipoedema (lip-i-**dee**-mă) *n.* a chronic progressive condition involving abnormal fat cell accumulation in the buttocks and lower limbs, which causes fluid retention, pain, reduced mobility, and psychological problems.

lipogenesis (lip-oh-**jen**-i-sis) *n.* the process by which glucose and other substances, derived from carbohydrate in the diet, are converted to fatty acids in the body.

lipohypertrophy (lip-oh-hy-**per**-trŏ-fi) *n.* a local build-up of fat tissue at the site of repeated insulin injections, which tends to alter the rate of absorption of further injections into the body. It is caused by the local action of the insulin, which promotes fat storage.

lipoid (**lip**-oid) *adj.* resembling a lipid.

lipoidosis (lip-oi-**doh**-sis) *n.* *see* lipidosis.

lipolysis (lip-**ol**-i-sis) *n.* the process by which lipids are broken down into their constituent fatty acids in the body by the enzyme lipase. —**lipolytic** *adj.*

lipoma (lip-**oh**-mă) *n.* (*pl.* **lipomas** or **lipomata**) a common benign tumour that is composed of well-differentiated fat cells.

lipomatosis (lip-oh-mă-**toh**-sis) *n.* **1.** the presence of an abnormally large amount of fat in the tissues. **2.** the presence of multiple lipomas.

lipoprotein (lip-oh-**proh**-teen) *n.* one of a group of compounds, found in blood plasma and lymph, each consisting of a protein (*see* apolipoprotein) combined with a lipid (cholesterol, a triglyceride, or a phospholipid). Lipoproteins are important for the transport of lipids in the blood and lymph. **high-density l.** (**HDL**) a type of lipoprotein that transports cholesterol from the tissues to the liver. **low-density l.** (**LDL**) a type of lipoprotein that is the main form in which cholesterol is transported in the bloodstream, from which it is taken into the cells by binding with LDL receptors. **very low-density l.** (**VLDL**) a type of lipoprotein that is the precursor of LDL.

liposarcoma (lip-oh-sar-**koh**-mă) *n.* a rare malignant tumour of fat cells. It is most commonly found in the thigh, usually in patients over the age of 30 years.

lipotropic (lip-oh-**trop**-ik) *adj.* describing a substance that promotes the transport of fatty acids from the liver to the tissues or accelerates the utilization of fat in the liver itself.

lipping (**lip**-ing) *n.* overgrowth of bone around a joint as seen on X-rays. This is a characteristic sign of degenerative joint disease, particularly osteoarthritis. *See also* osteophyte.

lipuria (adiposuria) (lip-**yoor**-iă) *n.* the presence of fat or oil droplets in the urine.

liquid-based cytology (LBC) (**lik**-wid) *n.* a technique used for analysing cervical smears taken for cervical screening. It yields specimens that are easier to screen and give more accurate results than those obtained by the traditional Pap test.

liquor (lik-er) *n.* **1.** (in pharmacy) any solution, usually an aqueous solution. **2.** the amniotic fluid surrounding a fetus.

Listeria (lis-teer-iă) *n.* a genus of Gram-positive aerobic motile rodlike bacteria that are parasites of warm-blooded animals. **L. monocytogenes** a species that, if transmitted to humans by eating infected animal products, may cause **listeriosis**, especially in the frail, ranging from influenza-like symptoms to meningoencephalitis. In pregnant women it may cause a miscarriage or damage the fetus.

lith- (litho-) *combining form denoting* a calculus (stone).

-lith *combining form denoting* a calculus (stone).

lithaemia (lith-ee-miă) *n. see* hyperuricaemia.

lithiasis (lith-I-ă-sis) *n.* formation of stones (*see* calculus) in an internal organ.

lithium (lith-iŭm) *n.* a drug given by mouth in the form of lithium carbonate or lithium citrate for the prevention and treatment of episodes of mania in patients with bipolar affective disorder and sometimes chronic or recurrent depression. Thyroid function can be impaired after many years of use and regular thyroid function tests are compulsory. Trade names: **Priadel**, etc.

litholapaxy (lithotripsy) (lith-ol-ă-paks-i) *n.* the operation of crushing a stone in the bladder, using an instrument called a **lithotrite**. The small fragments of stone can then be removed by irrigation and suction.

lithonephrotomy (lith-oh-ni-frot-ŏmi) *n.* surgical removal of a stone from the kidney. *See* nephrolithotomy, pyelolithotomy.

lithopaedion (lith-oh-pee-di-ŏn) *n.* a fetus that has died in the uterus or abdominal cavity and has become calcified.

lithotomy (lith-ot-ŏmi) *n.* the surgical removal of a stone (calculus) from the urinary tract. **l. position** an operating-table position that allows good access to the pelvis and perineum. The patient is placed supine so that the buttocks are at the edge of the table. The feet are placed in individual stirrups and the knees bent to allow the feet to be placed above or at the same level as the hips. *See* nephrolithotomy, pyelolithotomy, ureterolithotomy.

lithotripsy (lith-ŏ-trip-si) *n.* **1.** the process of breaking calculi (stones) into smaller fragments by means of shock waves. This will enable the stones to pass naturally. **extracorporeal shock-wave l.** (**ESWL**) a technique for destroying calculi in the upper urinary tract; it uses a specialized machine (a **lithotripter**) for generating and transmitting the shock waves and localizing the stones. **electrohydraulic l.** (**EHL**) a technique for destroying urinary calculi in which an electrically generated shock wave is transmitted to the stone by a contact probe delivered via a nephroscope or ureteroscope. **2.** *see* litholapaxy.

lithotripter (lith-oh-trip-ter) *n. see* lithotripsy.

lithotrite (lith-ŏ-tryt) *n. see* litholapaxy.

lithuresis (lith-yoor-ee-sis) *n.* the passage of small stones or gravel in the urine.

lithuria (lith-yoor-iă) *n. see* hyperuricuria.

litmus (lit-mŭs) *n.* a pigment used as an indicator of acids and alkalis. In the presence of acids it turns red; with alkalis it turns blue.

litre (lee-ter) *n.* a unit of volume equal to the volume occupied by 1 kilogram of pure water at 4°C and 760 mmHg pressure.

Little's area (li-t'lz) *n.* the anterior region of the nasal septum (*see* nose), which is richly supplied with capillaries (*see* Kiesselbach's plexus) and is a common site from which nosebleeds arise. [J. L. Little (1836–85), US surgeon]

Little's disease *n.* a form of cerebral palsy involving both sides of the body and affecting the legs more severely than the arms. [W. J. Little (1810–94), British surgeon]

Litzmann's obliquity (lits-manz) *n. see* asynclitism. [K. C. T. Litzmann (1815–90), German obstetrician]

livedo (liv-ee-doh) *n.* a discoloured area or spot on the skin, often caused by local congestion of the circulation.

liver (liv-er) *n.* the largest gland of the body, weighing 1200–1600 g. Situated in the top right portion of the abdominal cavity, the liver has a number of important functions. It synthesizes bile, which drains into the gall bladder before being released into the duodenum. The liver is an important site of metabolism of carbohydrates, proteins, and fats. It regulates the amount of blood sugar, removes excess amino acids, and stores and metabolizes fats. The liver also synthesizes fibrinogen, prothrombin, and heparin, and has an important role in the detoxification of poisonous substances. See illustration.

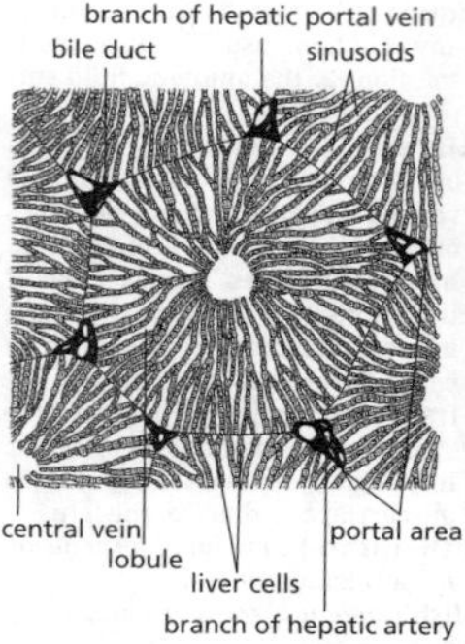

The microscopic structure of the liver

liver function tests (LFTs) *pl. n.* blood tests carried out to assess the functioning of the liver. These include tests for serum proteins, serum bilirubin, alanine aminotransferase, and alkaline phosphatase.

livid (liv-id) *adj.* denoting a bluish colour of the skin, such as that produced locally by a bruise or of the general complexion in cyanosis.

living will (liv-ing) *n. see* advance decision, directive, or statement.

SEE WEB LINKS

- Information about living wills from the NHS Choices website

LMP *n.* (date of) last menstrual period.

Loa (loh-ă) *n.* a genus of parasitic nematode worms (*see* filaria). **L. loa** the eye worm, which lives within the tissues beneath the skin and causes loiasis.

loading dose (lohd-ing) *n.* a high initial dose of a drug that is given to enable its therapeutic level in the bloodstream to be reached quickly. The loading dose is subsequently reduced to a lower **maintenance dose**.

lobe (lohb) *n.* a major division of an organ or part of an organ, especially one having a rounded form and often separated from other lobes by fissures or bands of connective tissue. **—lobar** *adj.*

lobectomy (loh-bek-tŏmi) *n.* the surgical removal of a lobe of an organ or gland, such as the lung, thyroid, or brain.

lobotomy (prefrontal leucotomy) (loh-bot-ŏmi) *n. see* leucotomy.

lobule (lob-yool) *n.* a subdivision of a part or organ, such as the liver or lung, that can be distinguished from the whole by boundaries, such as septa, that are visible with or without a microscope.

LOC *n.* level of consciousness.

localized (loh-kă-lyzd) *adj.* (of a lesion, eruption, etc.) restricted to a particular part of the body; not widespread.

lochia (lok-iă) *n.* the material eliminated from the uterus through the vagina after the completion of labour. The first discharge consists largely of blood (**l. rubra**). This is followed by a brownish mixture of blood and mucus (**l. serosa**), and finally a yellowish or whitish discharge containing microorganisms and cell fragments (**l. alba**). Each stage may last for several days. **—lochial** *adj.*

locked-in syndrome (lokt-in) *n.* a condition resulting from damage to the brainstem, in which the patient is conscious but unable to speak or to move any part of the body, except for blinking and upward eye movements. *Compare* vegetative state.

lockjaw (lok-jaw) *n. see* tetanus.

locomotor ataxia (loh-kŏ-moh-ter) *n. see* tabes dorsalis.

loculated (lok-yoo-layt-id) *adj.* divided into many cavities.

loculus (lok-yoo-lŭs) *n.* (in anatomy) a small space or cavity.

locum tenens (locum) (loh-kŭm teen-enz) *n.* a doctor who stands in temporarily for a colleague who is absent or ill.

locus (loh-kŭs) *n.* **1.** (in anatomy) a region or site. **2.** (in genetics) the region of a chromosome occupied by a particular gene.

lofepramine (loh-fep-ră-meen) *n.* a tricyclic antidepressant administered by mouth.

log- (logo-) *combining form denoting* words; speech.

LogMAR chart (**log**-mar) *n.* a chart for testing visual acuity in which the rows of letters vary in size in a logarithmic progression. This makes it more accurate than a Snellen chart and it is becoming increasingly used in testing vision. Most tests are done at a distance of 4 metres, allowing it to be used in smaller rooms.

logopaedics (log-ŏ-**pee**-diks) *n.* the scientific study of defects and disabilities of speech and of the methods used to treat them. *See also* speech and language therapy.

-logy (-ology) *combining form denoting* field of study.

loiasis (loh-**I**-ă-sis) *n.* a disease, occurring in West and Central Africa, caused by the eye worm *Loa loa*. The adult worms live and migrate within the skin tissues, causing inflammation and swellings, and often migrate across the eyeball just beneath the conjunctiva, producing irritation and congestion. Loiasis is treated with diethylcarbamazine.

loin (loin) *n.* the region of the back and side of the body between the lowest rib and the pelvis.

Lomotil (**lom**-ŏ-til) *n.* *see* co-phenotrope.

longitudinal study (long-i-**tew**-di-năl) *n.* a systematic study of a group of people over a period of time. *See also* prospective study, retrospective study.

long QT syndrome *n.* prolongation of the Q–T interval on the electrocardiogram. It indicates susceptibility to ventricular tachycardia, ventricular fibrillation, and sudden death. It may be familial or caused by certain drugs (e.g. sotalol, amiodarone, some antipsychotic drugs).

long-sightedness (long-**syt**-id-nis) *n.* *see* hypermetropia.

long-stretch bandage *n.* a bandage consisting of padding and/or crepe and material containing elastic fibres that can stretch to up 300% of their original length. It is used in the treatment of venous leg ulcers and may be applied dry or as a cohesive layer. The fibres provide constant pressure and should not be worn overnight or during extended periods of rest.

loop (loop) *n.* **1.** a bend in a tubular organ. **2.** one of the patterns of dermal ridges in fingerprints.

loperamide (loh-**per**-ă-myd) *n.* a drug used in the treatment of diarrhoea. It acts by reducing peristalsis of the digestive tract and is administered by mouth. Trade name: **Imodium**.

lopinavir (loh-**pin**-ă-veer) *n.* *see* protease inhibitor.

loprazolam (loh-**praz**-ŏ-lam) *n.* a short-acting benzodiazepine drug that is administered by mouth for the short-term treatment of insomnia. *See* hypnotic.

loratidine (lŏ-**rat**-i-deen) *n.* a non-sedating antihistamine administered by mouth to treat allergic conditions, such as hay fever and urticaria.

lorazepam (lor-**az**-ĕ-pam) *n.* a benzodiazepine administered by mouth or injection to relieve moderate or severe anxiety or insomnia, to treat status epilepticus, and for premedication. Trade name: **Ativan**.

lordosis (lor-**doh**-sis) *n.* forward curvature of the spine when viewed from the side. A certain degree of lordosis is normal in the lumbar and cervical regions of the spine. Exaggerated lordosis may occur through faulty posture or in disorders of vertebral development. *Compare* kyphosis.

losartan (**loh**-sar-tan) *n. see* angiotensin II antagonist.

loss (los) *n.* the state of not having some valued aspect of one's life, such as a relationship or a job, that one has previously enjoyed. The associated emotions may lead to symptoms that bring people to health care. Encouraging the patient to talk about the loss will require empathy, sensitivity, and judgment from the professional. *See also* bereavement.

lotion (**loh**-shŏn) *n.* a medicinal solution for external use. Lotions usually have a cooling, soothing, or antiseptic action.

Lou Gehrig's disease (loo ge-rigz) *n. see* (amyotrophic lateral) sclerosis. [Lou Gehrig (1903–41), US baseball player who suffered from it]

loupe (loop) *n.* **1.** a small magnifying hand lens used for examining the front part of the eye. **2.** (**loupes**) a binocular telescope system mounted on a spectacle frame or headband, used in microsurgery.

louse (lowss) *n.* (*pl.* **lice**) a small wingless bloodsucking insect that is an external parasite of humans and may transmit disease. Lice attach themselves to hair and clothing; they thrive in overcrowded and unhygienic conditions. *See also* pediculosis.

Løvset's manoeuvre (luv-setz) *n.* rotation of the trunk of the fetus during a breech birth to facilitate delivery of the arms and the shoulders. [J. Løvset (20th century), Norwegian obstetrician]

low-density lipoprotein (LDL) (loh-**den**-siti) *n. see* lipoprotein.

lower urinary tract symptoms (LUTS) (**loh**-er) *pl. n.* symptoms occuring during urine storage, voiding, or immediately after, including frequency, urgency, nocturia, incontinence, hesitation, intermittency, terminal dribble, dysuria, and postmicturition dribble. These symptoms may be due to benign prostatic hyperplasia (*see* prostate gland), detrusor overactivity, excessive drinking, diuresis due to poorly controlled diabetes, or a urethral stricture.

low-molecular-weight heparin (loh-mŏ-**lek**-yoo-ler-wayt) *n. see* heparin.

lozenge (**loz**-inj) *n.* a medicated tablet containing sugar.

LP *n. see* lumbar (puncture).

LRTI *n.* lower respiratory tract infection.

LSD *n. see* lysergic acid diethylamide.

lubb-dupp (lub-**dup**) *n.* a representation of the normal heart sounds as heard through the stethoscope. The first coincides with closure of the mitral and tricuspid valves; the second with closure of the aortic and pulmonary valves.

lucid interval (loo-sid in-ter-văl) *n.* temporary recovery of consciousness after a blow to the head, before relapse into coma. It is a sign of intracranial arterial bleeding.

Ludwig's angina (luud-vigz) *n.* severe inflammation caused by bacterial infection of the floor of the mouth, resulting in massive swelling of the neck. [W. F. von Ludwig (1790–1865), German surgeon]

lues (loo-eez) *n.* a serious infectious disease such as syphilis.

Lugol's solution (aqueous iodine solution) (loo-golz) *n.* an aqueous solution of iodine and potassium iodide used before thyroidectomy in the treatment of thyrotoxicosis. [J. G. A. Lugol (1786–1851), French physician]

lumbago (lum-bay-goh) *n.* pain in the lumbar region, of any cause or description. Severe lumbago, of sudden onset, can be due either to a slipped disc or to a strained muscle or ligament.

lumbar (lum-ber) *adj.* relating to the loin. **l. puncture** (**LP**) the insertion, under local anaesthetic, of a hollow needle into the subarachnoid space in the region of the lower back (usually between the third and fourth lumbar vertebrae). It may be performed to obtain and examine a sample of cerebrospinal fluid for diagnosis (e.g. of meningitis or multiple sclerosis) or to inject agents into the subarachnoid space. *See also* Queckenstedt test. **l. triangle** a weak area in the abdomen bounded by the iliac crest (below), the external oblique muscle (in front), and the erector spinae muscle (behind). **l. vertebrae** the five bones of the backbone that are situated between the thoracic vertebrae and the sacrum, in the lower part of the back. *See also* vertebra.

lumbo- *combining form denoting* the loin; lumbar region.

lumbosacral (lum-boh-say-krăl) *adj.* relating to the part of the spine composed of the lumbar vertebrae and the sacrum.

lumen (loo-min) *n.* **1.** the space within a tubular or saclike part. **2.** the SI unit of luminous flux. Symbol: lm.

luminescence (loo-min-ess-ĕns) *n.* the emission of light from a substance. Fluorescence is a type of luminescence after an object has been irradiated.

lumpectomy (lum-pek-tŏmi) *n.* an operation for breast cancer in which the tumour and surrounding breast tissue are removed: muscles, skin, and lymph nodes are left intact (*compare* mastectomy). The procedure, usually followed by radiation, is indicated for patients with a tumour less than 2 cm in diameter and who have no metastases to local lymph nodes or to distant organs.

lunate bone (loo-nayt) *n.* a bone of the wrist (*see* carpus). It articulates with the capitate and hamate bones in front, with the radius behind, and with the triquetral and scaphoid at the sides.

lung (lung) *n.* one of the pair of organs of respiration, situated in

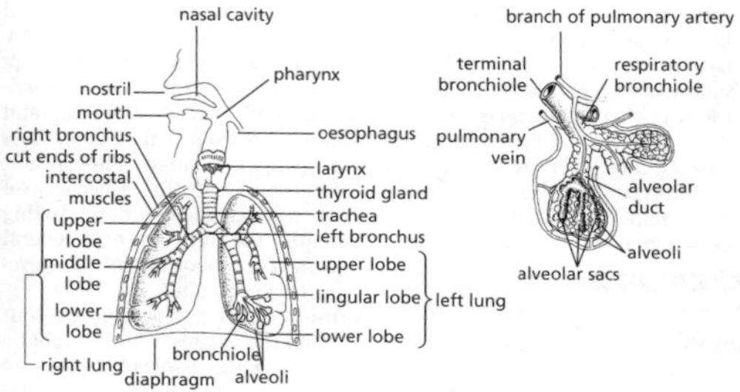

The lungs and main air passages with details of the alveoli

the chest cavity on either side of the heart. The lungs communicate with the atmosphere through the trachea, which opens into the pharynx. The trachea divides into two bronchi, which enter the lungs and branch into bronchioles. These divide further and terminate in minute air sacs (alveoli), the sites of gaseous exchange. (See illustrations.) Atmospheric oxygen is absorbed and carbon dioxide from the blood of the pulmonary capillaries is released into the lungs (*see* (pulmonary) circulation).

lung cancer *n.* cancer arising in the epithelium of the air passages (**bronchial cancer**) or lung. It is strongly associated with cigarette smoking and exposure to industrial air pollutants (including asbestos). Treatment includes surgical removal of the affected lobe or lung, radiotherapy, and chemotherapy. *See also* non-small-cell lung cancer, small-cell lung cancer.

lunula (**loon**-yoo-lă) *n.* the whitish crescent-shaped area at the base of a nail.

lupus (loo-pŭs) *n.* any of several chronic skin diseases. **l. erythematosus** (**LE**) an inflammatory autoimmune disease of connective tissue. In **systemic LE** (**SLE**) the skin and various internal organs are affected. Typically, there is a red rash on the nose and cheeks; arthritis; and progressive damage to the kidneys. Often the heart, lungs, and brain are also affected. In a milder form, known as **discoid LE** (**DLE**), only the skin is affected. LE is treated with corticosteroids or immunosuppressant drugs. **l. verrucosus** a rare tuberculous infection of the skin – commonly the arm or hand – typified by warty lesions. It occurs in those who have been reinfected with tuberculosis. **l. vulgaris** a tuberculous infection of the skin that often starts in childhood, with dark red patches on the nose or cheek. Unless treated with antituberculous drugs lupus vulgaris may spread, ulcerate, and cause extensive scarring.

SEE WEB LINKS

- Details of SLE from the Lupus Site

lutein (loo-ti-in) *n.* the yellow pigment of the corpus luteum.

luteinizing hormone (LH) (loo-ti-i-nyz-ing) *n.* a hormone (*see* gonadotrophin), synthesized and released by the anterior pituitary gland, that stimulates ovulation, corpus luteum formation, progesterone synthesis by the ovary, and androgen synthesis by the testes. Also called: **interstitial-cell-stimulating hormone (ICSH)**.

luteo- *combining form denoting* **1.** yellow. **2.** the corpus luteum.

luteotrophic hormone (luteotrophin) (loo-ti-oh-**trof**-ik) *n. see* prolactin.

LUTS *pl. n. see* lower urinary tract symptoms.

luxation (luks-ay-shŏn) *n.* **1.** *see* dislocation. **2.** extrusion of a tooth from its socket by trauma or pathology.

LVF *n.* left ventricular failure. *See* heart failure.

Lyme disease (lym) *n.* a disease caused by a spirochaete, *Borrelia burgdorferi*, and transmitted by certain ticks of the genus *Ixodes*. Following a 3–32-day incubation period, a slowly extending red rash develops in approximately 75% of cases; intermittent symptoms include fever, malaise, headache and neck stiffness, and muscle and joint pains. Later, 60% of patients suffer intermittent attacks of arthritis, especially of the knees, each attack lasting months and recurring over several years. Treatment is with doxycycline or a penicillin.

lymph (limf) *n.* the fluid present within the vessels of the lymphatic system, which is derived from the fluid that bathes the tissues. Lymph is similar in composition to plasma, but contains less protein and some cells, mainly lymphocytes. **l. node** one of a number of small swellings found at intervals along the lymphatic system. Groups of nodes occur in the groin and armpit, behind the ear, and in many other parts. They act as filters for the lymph and produce lymphocytes.

lymphaden- (lymphadeno-) *combining form denoting* lymph node(s).

lymphadenectomy (lim-fad-in-**ek**-tŏmi) *n.* surgical removal of lymph nodes.

lymphadenitis (lim-fad-in-**I**-tis) *n.* inflammation of lymph nodes, which become swollen, painful, and tender. The most commonly affected lymph nodes are those in the neck, in association with tonsillitis.

lymphadenopathy (lim-fad-in-**op**-ă-thi) *n.* enlargement of the lymph nodes. This is usually due to infection, when the nodes are painful and tender, but may alternatively be caused by malignancy (e.g. leukaemias, lymphomas), autoimmune disease (e.g. systemic lupus erythematosis), or adverse drug reactions.

lymphangi- (lymphangio-) *combining form denoting* a lymphatic vessel.

lymphangiectasis (lim-fan-ji-**ek**-tă-sis) *n.* dilatation of the lymphatic vessels, which is usually congenital. It may also be caused by obstruction of the lymphatic vessels (*see* lymphoedema).

lymphangiography (lymphography) (lim-fan-ji-**og**-răfi) *n.* X-ray examination of the lymphatic vessels and lymph nodes after a contrast medium has been injected into them (*see* angiography). Alternatively, the lymphatic system can be imaged using a gamma camera following the injection of a radioactive tracer.

lymphangioma (lim-fan-ji-**oh**-mă) *n.* a localized collection of distended lymphatic vessels, which may result in a large cyst in the neck or armpit.

lymphangioplasty (lim-fan-ji-oh-plasti) *n.* the surgical creation of artificial lymph channels when the lymphatic vessels are obstructed.

lymphangiosarcoma (lim-fan-ji-oh-sar-**koh**-mă) *n.* a rare malignant tumour of the lymphatic vessels. It is most commonly seen in the arms of women who have had a mastectomy for breast cancer and may be induced by radiation.

lymphangitis (lim-fan-**jy**-tis) *n.* inflammation of the lymphatic vessels, which can be seen most commonly as red streaks in the skin adjacent to a focus of streptococcal infection.

lymphatic (lim-**fat**-ik) **1.** *n.* a lymphatic vessel. *See* lymphatic system. **2.** *adj.* relating to or transporting lymph.

lymphatic system *n.* a network of vessels that conveys electrolytes, water, proteins, etc. – in the form of lymph – from the tissue fluids to the bloodstream. Lymph passes through fine capillaries into the lymphatic vessels, which have valves to prevent backflow of lymph. The lymphatics lead to two large channels – the **thoracic duct** and the **right lymphatic duct** – which return the lymph to the bloodstream via the innominate veins.

lympho- *combining form denoting* lymph or the lymphatic system.

lymphoblast (**lim**-foh-blast) *n.* an abnormal cell that is present in the blood and blood-forming organs in a type of leukaemia (**lymphoblastic leukaemia**). **—lymphoblastic** *adj.*

lymphocele (lymphocoele) (**lim**-foh-seel) *n.* a collection of lymph in the tissues, which follows injury to, or operations upon, lymph nodes or ducts.

lymphocyte (**lim**-foh-syt) *n.* a variety of white blood cell (leucocyte), present also in the lymph nodes, spleen, thymus gland, gut wall, and bone marrow. They are involved in immunity and can be subdivided into **B lymphocytes** (or **B cells**), which produce circulating antibodies, and **T lymphocytes**, which are primarily responsible for cell-mediated immunity (*see* T cell). **—lymphocytic** *adj.*

lymphocytopenia (lim-foh-sy-toh-**pee**-niă) *n. see* lymphopenia.

lymphocytosis (lim-foh-sy-**toh**-sis) *n.* an increase in the number of lymphocytes in the blood.

lymphoedema (lim-fee-**dee**-mă) *n.* an accumulation of lymph in the tissues, producing swelling; the legs are most often affected. It may be due to a congenital abnormality of the lymphatic vessels (as in Milroy's disease) or result from obstruction of the lymphatic vessels by a tumour, parasites, inflammation, or injury.

lymphogranuloma venereum (lim-foh-gran-yoo-**loo**-mă vi-**neer**-iŭm) *n.* a sexually transmitted disease that is caused by bacteria of the genus *Chlamydia* and is most common in tropical regions. An initial lesion on the genitals is followed by swelling and inflammation of the lymph nodes in the groin. Early treatment with sulphonamides or tetracyclines is usually effective.

lymphography (lim-**fog**-răfi) *n. see* lymphangiography.

lymphoid tissue (**lim**-foid) *n.* a tissue responsible for the production of lymphocytes and antibodies. It occurs in the form of the lymph nodes, tonsils, thymus, and spleen, and also as diffuse groups of cells. *See also* immune (system).

lymphokine (**lim**-foh-kyn) *n.* a substance produced by lymphocytes that has effects on other cells involved in the immune system. An example is interleukin 2 (IL-2).

lymphoma (lim-**foh**-mă) *n.* cancer of the lymph nodes, including Hodgkin's disease and other forms (**non-Hodgkin's l.**, **NHL**). Disease may be widespread, but in some cases is confined to a single area, which may be extranodal (such as the tonsil). Treatment is with such drugs as chlorambucil or with combinations of cyclophosphamide, vincristine, prednisolone, and rituximab. *See also* Burkitt's lymphoma.

lymphopenia (lymphocytopenia) (lim-foh-**pee**-niă) *n.* a decrease in the number of lymphocytes in the blood.

lymphopoiesis (lim-foh-poi-**ee**-sis) *n.* the process of the production of lymphocytes, which occurs in the bone marrow as well as in the lymph nodes, spleen, thymus gland, and gut wall.

lymphorrhagia (lim-fŏ-**ray**-jiă) *n.* the escape of the lymph from lymphatic vessels that have been injured.

lymphosarcoma (lim-foh-sar-**koh**-mă) *n.* a former name for non-Hodgkin's lymphoma.

lymphoscintigraphy (lim-foh-**sin**-tig-răfi) *n.* an imaging scan undertaken to identify the primary lymph nodes (or sentinel nodes), which receive lymph drainage from a tumour, and to differentiate these from disease-free nodes in order to plan treatment options, particularly for melanoma and breast cancer management.

lymphuria (limf-yoor-iă) *n.* the presence in the urine of lymph.

lyophilization (ly-ofi-ly-zay-shŏn) *n.* preservation of biological material (e.g. plasma, serum, skin) by rapid freezing followed by dehydration.

lys- (lysi-, lyso-) *combining form denoting* lysis; dissolution.

lysergic acid diethylamide (LSD) (ly-ser-jik ass-id dy-eth-il-ay-myd) *n.* an illegal hallucinogenic drug, formerly used to aid treatment of certain psychological disorders. Alterations in sight, hearing, and other senses occur, psychotic effects, depression, and confusion are common, and tolerance to the drug develops rapidly. Because of these toxic effects, LSD is no longer used clinically.

lysin (ly-sin) *n.* a specific complement-fixing antibody that is capable of bringing about the destruction (lysis) of whole cells. **Haemolysin** attacks red blood cells, **leucolysin** white cells, and a **bacteriolysin** bacterial cells.

lysine (ly-seen) *n.* an essential amino acid. *See also* amino acid.

lysis (ly-sis) *n.* **1.** the destruction of cells through damage or rupture of the plasma membrane, allowing escape of the cell contents. *See also* autolysis, lysozyme. **2.** gradual remission of the symptoms of a disease. **—lytic** *adj.*

-lysis *combining form denoting* lysis; dissolution.

lysosome (ly-sŏ-sohm) *n.* a particle in the cytoplasm of cells that contains enzymes responsible for breaking down substances in the cell. Lysosomes are especially abundant in liver and kidney cells.

lysozyme (ly-sŏ-zym) *n.* an enzyme found in tears and egg white. It catalyses the destruction of the cell walls of certain bacteria.

Mm

McArdle's disease (mă-ar-d'lz) *n.* an inborn error of metabolism in which a deficiency of the enzyme myophosphorylase prevents the breakdown of glycogen to lactate in exercising muscle. This results in fatigue, pain, and cramps in exercising muscles. [B. McArdle (20th century), British biochemist]

McBurney's point (măk-**ber**-niz) *n.* the point on the abdomen that overlies the anatomical position of the appendix and is the site of maximum tenderness in acute appendicitis. [C. McBurney (1845–1913), US surgeon]

maceration (mas-er-**ay**-shŏn) *n.* **1.** the softening of a solid by leaving it immersed in a liquid. **2.** (in obstetrics) the natural breakdown of a dead fetus within the uterus.

McGill Pain Questionnaire (MPQ) (mă-**gil**) *n.* an assessment tool that combines a list of questions about the nature and frequency of pain with a body-map diagram to pinpoint its location.

Mackenrodt's ligaments (mahk-ĕn-rohts) *pl. n. see* cardinal ligaments. [A. K. Mackenrodt (1859–1925), German gynaecologist]

macr- (macro-) *combining form denoting* large size.

macrocephaly (megalocephaly) (mak-roh-**sef**-ăli) *n.* abnormal largeness of the head. *Compare* microcephaly.

macrocheilia (mak-roh-**ky**-liă) *n.* hypertrophy of the lips: a congenital condition in which the lips are abnormally large. *Compare* microcheilia.

macrocyte (megalocyte) (**mak**-roh-syt) *n.* an abnormally large red blood cell (erythrocyte). *See also* macrocytosis. **—macrocytic** *adj.*

macrocytosis (mak-roh-sy-**toh**-sis) *n.* the presence of macrocytes in the blood. Macrocytosis is a feature of certain anaemias (known as **macrocytic anaemias**), including those due to deficiency of vitamin B_{12} or folate.

macrodactyly (mak-roh-**dak**-tili) *n.* abnormally large size of one or more of the fingers or toes.

macrogenitosoma (mak-roh-jen-it-oh-**soh**-mă) *n.* excessive bodily growth with marked enlargement of the genitalia.

macroglobulin (mak-roh-**glob**-yoo-lin) *n.* **1. (immunoglobulin M, IgM)** a protein of the globulin series that is present in the blood and functions as an antibody, forming an effective first-line defence against any bacteria that enter the bloodstream. *See also* immunoglobulin. **2.** an abnormal form of IgM produced by lymphoma cells or in other plasma-cell disorders.

macroglossia (mak-roh-**glos**-iă) *n.* an abnormally large tongue. It may be due to a congenital defect, to infiltration of the tongue with amyloid or a tumour, or to obstruction of the lymph vessels.

macrognathia (mak-roh-**nay**-thiă) *n.* a condition in which one or both jaws are unusually large.

macromelia (mak-roh-**mee**-liă) *n.* abnormally large size of the arms or legs. *Compare* micromelia.

macrophage (**mak**-roh-fayj) *n.* a large scavenger cell (*see* phagocyte) present in connective tissue and many major organs and tissues, including the bone marrow, spleen, lymph nodes, liver, and the central nervous system. *See also* histiocyte, reticuloendothelial system.

macropsia (mak-**rop**-siă) *n.* a condition in which objects appear larger than they really are. It is usually due to disease of the retina.

macroscopic (mak-roh-**skop**-ik) *adj.* visible to the naked eye. *Compare* microscopic.

macrosomia (mak-roh-**soh**-miă) *n.* abnormally large size. **fetal m.** large size in a baby associated with poorly controlled maternal diabetes; it is due to excessive production of fetal insulin (and thence to increased deposition of glycogen in the fetus) and maternal obesity.

macrotia (mak-**roh**-tiă) *n.* a congenital deformity of the external ear in which the pinna is larger than normal.

macula (**mak**-yoo-lă) *n.* (*pl.* **maculae**) a small anatomical area that is distinguishable from the surrounding tissue. **m. lutea** the yellow spot on the retina at the back of the eye, which surrounds the greatest concentration of cones (*see* fovea). **—macular** (**mak**-yoo-ler) *adj.*

macular degeneration *n.* a group of conditions affecting the macula lutea of the eye, resulting in a reduction or loss of central vision. **age-related m. d.** (**AMD**, **ARMD**) the most common cause of blindness in the elderly. **Atrophic** or **dry AMD** results from chronic choroidal ischaemia: small blood vessels of the choroid, which lies beneath the retina, become constricted, reducing the blood supply to the macula. This gives rise to degenerative changes in the retinal pigment epithelium (RPE; *see* retina). **Wet AMD** is associated with the growth of abnormal new blood vessels under the retina, derived from the choroid (*see* (choroidal) neovascularization). These can leak fluid and blood beneath the retina, which further reduces macular function.

SEE WEB LINKS

- Information about macular degeneration from the Royal National Institute of Blind People

macule (**mak**-yool) *n.* a flat circumscribed area of skin or an area of altered skin colour (e.g. a freckle). *Compare* papule. **—macular** *adj.*

maculopapular (mak-yoo-loh-**pap**-yoo-ler) *adj.* describing a rash that consists of both macules and papules.

maculopathy (mak-yool-**op**-ă-thi) *n.* any abnormality of the macula lutea of the eye. **bull's-eye m.** the appearance of the macula in some toxic conditions (e.g. chloroquine toxicity) and in some hereditary disorders of the macula.

Madopar (mad-ŏ-par) *n. see* levodopa.

Madura foot (mă-**dewr**-ă) *n.* an infection of the tissues and bones of the foot producing chronic inflammation (mycetoma), occurring in the tropics. Medical name: **maduromycosis**.

Madurella (mad-yoo-**rel**-ă) *n.* a genus of widely distributed fungi. The species *M. grisea* and *M. mycetomi* cause the tropical infection Madura foot.

maduromycosis (mă-dewr-oh-my-**koh**-sis) *n. see* Madura foot.

MAG3 *n. m*ercapto*a*cetyltri*g*lycine: a tracer used in nuclear medicine, during renography, when labelled with technetium-99m. It can be used to measure effective renal plasma flow and to give anatomical information. MAG3 is preferred to DTPA in patients with impaired renal function.

Magendie's foramen (ma-jen-deez) *n.* an opening in the roof of the fourth ventricle of the brain through which cerebrospinal fluid passes to the subarachnoid space. [F. Magendie (1783–1855), French physiologist]

magenta (mă-**jen**-tă) *n. see* fuchsin.

maggot (**mag**-ŏt) *n.* the wormlike larva of a fly, which occasionally infests human tissues (*see* myiasis).

Magill's forceps (mă-**gilz**) *n.* long angled forceps for use with a laryngoscope in removing foreign bodies from the mouth and throat of an unconscious patient. [Sir I. V. Magill (1888–1975), British anaesthetist]

magnesium (mag-**nee**-ziŭm) *n.* a metallic element essential to life. Magnesium is necessary for the proper functioning of muscle and nervous tissue. Symbol: Mg. **m. carbonate** a weak antacid used (often in combination with other compounds) to relieve indigestion. **m. hydroxide** a magnesium salt used as an osmotic laxative and also as an ingredient in antacid preparations. **m. sulphate** a magnesium salt used in the form of mixtures or powders for rapid evacuation of the bowel (*see* laxative). It is also administered intravenously to treat magnesium deficiency and serious arrhythmias and to prevent recurrent convulsions in eclampsia. **m. trisilicate** a compound of magnesium with antacid and absorbent properties, used in the treatment of indigestion.

magnetic resonance imaging (MRI) (mag-**net**-ik) *n.* a diagnostic imaging technique based on the emission of electromagnetic waves from the body when the patient is placed in a strong magnetic field and exposed to radiofrequency radiation (*see* nuclear magnetic resonance). Most images rely on the signal from hydrogen in water, which is particularly strong, although other elements can be used. A major advantage over computerized tomography is the lack of X-rays, which reduces exposure to ionizing radiation. **functional MRI (fMRI)** a type of MRI that measures the increased blood flow seen with neural activity in the brain or spinal cord.

MAGPI operation (**mag**-py) *n. m*eatal *a*dvancement and *g*lanulo*p*lasty operation: a simple surgical procedure that is designed to correct minor to moderate degrees of coronal or subcoronal hypospadias. This single-stage operation corrects any associated minor degrees of chordee and transfers the urethral opening to the glans, allowing normal urination.

MAI complex *n.* a group of bacteria comprising *Mycobacterium avium* and *M. intracellulare*, which are responsible for opportunistic infections of the lung that mimic tuberculosis but are resistant to many antituberculosis drugs. These bacteria are particularly liable to cause superimposed infection in AIDS patients. *See* Mycobacterium.

maintenance dose (**mayn**-tĕn-ans) *n. see* loading dose.

Makaton (**mak**-ă-ton) *n.* a language programme that uses sign language, speech, and graphical symbols to teach communication, language, and literacy skills to adults and children with communication and learning difficulties.

SEE WEB LINKS

- Website of the Makaton vocabulary development project

mal (mal) *n.* illness or disease.

mal- *combining form denoting* disease, disorder, or abnormality.

malabsorption (mal-ăb-**sorp**-shŏn) *n.* reduced or defective absorption of various nutrients in the small bowel. It commonly affects the absorption of fatty acids, fat-soluble vitamins, water-soluble vitamins, electrolytes, iron, and amino acids. Symptoms include weight loss, diarrhoea, failure to thrive, weakness and lethargy (due to anaemia), paraesthesia, swelling (oedema), and a propensity to bleeding. The commonest causes are coeliac disease, Crohn's disease, pancreatitis, cystic fibrosis, blind-loop syndrome, chronic infection, and previous surgery.

malacia (mă-**lay**-shiă) *n.* abnormal softening of a part, organ, or tissue, such as bone (*see* osteomalacia).

-malacia *combining form denoting* abnormal softening of a tissue.

maladie de Roger (Roger's disease) (ma-la-**di** dĕ ro-*zh***ay**) *n.* a form of congenital heart disease in which there is a small ventricular septal defect that produces a loud heart murmur. [H. L. Roger (1809–91), French physician]

malaise (mal-**ayz**) *n.* a general feeling of being unwell. The feeling may be accompanied by identifiable physical discomfort and may indicate the presence of disease.

malar bone (**may**-ler) *n. see* zygomatic bone.

malaria (ague, marsh fever, periodic fever, paludism) (mă-**lair**-iă) *n.* an infectious disease due to the presence of parasitic protozoa of the genus *Plasmodium* within the red blood cells. The disease is transmitted by the

Anopheles mosquito and is confined mainly to tropical and subtropical areas. After an incubation period varying from 12 days to 10 months parasites invade, multiply within, and eventually destroy the red blood cells, releasing new parasites. This causes a short bout of shivering, fever, and sweating, and the loss of healthy red cells results in anaemia. When the next batch of parasites is released symptoms reappear. The interval between fever attacks varies in different types of malaria. Preventive and curative treatment relies on such drugs as chloroquine and proguanil. **benign m.** malaria caused by *P. vivax*, *P. malariae*, or *P. ovale*, with intervals of 2–3 days between fever attacks. **falciparum** (or **malignant**) **m.** the most severe form of malaria, in which the interval between fever attacks varies from a few hours to 2 days.

Malassezia (Pityrosporum) *n.* a genus of yeasts producing superficial infections of the skin. **M. furfur** the cause of pityriasis versicolor.

malathion (mal-ă-th'y-on) *n.* an organophosphorous insecticide used to treat head and pubic lice and scabies. It is applied externally in the form of a liquid. Trade name: **Derbac-M.**

malformation (mal-for-may-shŏn) *n.* any variation from the normal physical structure, due either to congenital or developmental defects or to disease or injury.

malignant (mă-lig-nănt) *adj.* **1.** describing a tumour that invades and destroys the tissue in which it originates and has the potential to spread to other sites in the body. *See* cancer, metastasis. **2.** describing any disorder that becomes life threatening if untreated. *Compare* benign.

malignant melanoma *n. see* melanoma.

malignant pustule *n. see* anthrax.

malingering (mă-ling-er-ing) *n.* pretending to be ill, usually in order to avoid work or to gain attention. It may be a sign of mental disorder (*see* Munchausen's syndrome).

malleolus (mă-lee-ŏ-lŭs) *n.* either of the two protuberances on each side of the ankle: at the lower end of the fibula (**lateral m.**) and at the lower end of the tibia (**medial m.**).

mallet finger (mal-it fing-er) *n.* a condition in which a finger (usually the index finger) is bent downwards at the tip, due to avulsion of the long extensor tendon from the bone.

malleus (mal-iŭs) *n.* a hammer-shaped bone in the middle ear that articulates with the incus and is attached to the eardrum. *See* ossicle.

Mallory bodies (mal-eri) *pl. n.* large irregular masses abnormally located in the hepatocytes of the liver. They are found in patients with alcoholic hepatitis, alcoholic cirrhosis, Wilson's disease, primary biliary cirrhosis, clinical obesity, and hepatocellular carcinoma. [F. B. Mallory (1862–1941), US pathologist]

Mallory-Weiss syndrome (mal-eri-**vys**) *n.* trauma of the mucosal lining at the junction of the oesophagus (gullet) and stomach following protracted vomiting and retching. It is associated with haematemesis and (rarely) perforation of the oesophagus. [G. K. Mallory (1900–86), US pathologist; S. Weiss (1899–1942), US physician]

malnutrition (mal-new-**trish**-ŏn) *n.* a condition in which there is an imbalance between the nutrients the body receives and what is required to maintain health. This can result from eating too little (**undernutrition**) but may also be due to dietary excess (**overnutrition**).

malnutrition universal screening tool *n. see* MUST.

malocclusion (mal-ŏ-**kloo**-zhŏn) *n.* a condition in which there is an abnormal arrangement of the teeth or discrepancy in the relationship of the jaws.

Malpighian body (mal-**pig**-iăn) *n.* the part of a nephron comprising the blood capillaries of the glomerulus and its surrounding Bowman's capsule. [M. Malpighi (1628–94), Italian anatomist]

Malpighian layer *n.* the stratum germinativum: one of the layers of the epidermis.

malposition (mal-pŏ-**zish**-ŏn) *n.* (in obstetrics) an abnormal position of the fetal head when this is the presenting part in labour (e.g. the occipitoposterior position), such that the diameter of the skull in relation to the pelvic opening is greater than normal. This is likely to result in a prolonged and complicated labour.

malpractice (mal-**prak**-tis) *n.* professional misconduct: treatment falling short of the standards of skill and care that can reasonably be expected from a qualified medical practitioner.

malpresentation (mal-prez-ĕn-**tay**-shŏn) *n.* the condition in which the presenting part of the fetus (*see* presentation) is other than the crown of the head (e.g. the brow, face, shoulder, or buttocks).

malt (mawlt) *n.* a mixture of carbohydrates, predominantly maltose, produced by the breakdown of starch contained in barley or wheat grains. Malt is used for brewing and distilling; it has been used as a source of nutrients in wasting diseases.

Malta fever (**mawl**-tă) *n. see* brucellosis.

maltase (**mawl**-tayz) *n.* an enzyme, present in saliva and pancreatic juice, that converts maltose into glucose during digestion.

maltose (**mawl**-tohz) *n.* a sugar consisting of two molecules of glucose. Maltose is formed from the digestion of starch and glycogen.

malt-worker's lung *n.* a form of extrinsic allergic alveolitis seen in people who work with barley.

malunion (mal-**yoon**-yŏn) *n.* union of the fragments of a fracture in an unsatisfactory position. Osteotomy may be needed to correct it.

mamilla (mă-**mil**-ă) *n. see* nipple.

mamma (mam-ă) *n.* *see* breast.

mammary gland (mam-er-i) *n.* the milk-producing gland of female mammals. *See* breast.

mammography (mam-og-răfi) *n.* the study of the breast by imaging techniques, most commonly by X-ray examination: used particularly to enable the early diagnosis of breast cancer.

SEE WEB LINKS

- Explanation of the procedure in the diagnosis of breast cancer

mammoplasty (mam-ŏ-plasti) *n.* plastic surgery of the breasts, in order to alter their shape or increase or decrease their size.

mammothermography (mam-oh-ther-mog-răfi) *n.* the technique of examining the breasts for the presence of abnormalities by thermography.

mandible (man-dib-ŭl) *n.* the lower jawbone. It consists of a horseshoe-shaped body, the upper surface of which bears the lower teeth, and two vertical parts (rami). *See also* temporomandibular joint. **—mandibular** (man-dib-yoo-ler) *adj.*

mandibular advancement splint (MAS) *n.* an orthodontic device used to advance the mandible to improve the airway in the pharynx during sleep in the treatment of obstructive sleep apnoea.

manganese (mang-ă-neez) *n.* a greyish metallic element, the oxide of which, when inhaled by miners in underventilated mines, causes brain damage. It is a trace element. Symbol: Mn.

mania (may-niă) *n.* a state of mind characterized by excessive cheerfulness and increased activity. The mood is euphoric and can change rapidly to irritability. Thought and speech are pressured and rapid to the point of incoherence and the connections between ideas may be impossible to follow. Treatment is usually with medication such as lithium, benzodiazepines, or antipsychotics. *See also* bipolar affective disorder. **—manic** (man-ik) *adj.*

-mania *combining form denoting* obsession, compulsion, or exaggerated feeling for.

manic depression *n.* a former (but still quite commonly used) term for bipolar affective disorder.

manipulation (mă-nip-yoo-lay-shŏn) *n.* the use of the hands to produce a desired movement or therapeutic effect in part of the body.

mannitol (man-i-tol) *n.* a diuretic administered by intravenous infusion mainly to reduce intracranial pressure in brain injuries, and in the emergency treatment of glaucoma. Mannitol powder is inhaled to treat cystic fibrosis. Trade name: **Bronchitol**.

mannosidosis (man-oh-si-doh-sis) *n.* a progressive autosomal recessive disorder causing deficiency of the enzyme mannosidase, which results in errors of carbohydrate metabolism and lysosomal function, leading to a spectrum of learning difficulties and muscle weakness.

Mann–Whitney U test (man-wit-ni) *n.* *see* parametric test.

manometer (mă-**nom**-it-er) *n.* a device for measuring pressure in a liquid or gas. *See also* sphygmomanometer.

manometry (mă-**nom**-itri) *n.* measurement of pressures within organs of the body. The technique is used to record changes within fluid-filled chambers (e.g. cerebral ventricles) or to indicate muscular activity in motile tubes, such as the oesophagus, rectum, or bile duct.

mantle (**man**-t'l) *adj.* (in radiotherapy) *see* treatment field.

Mantoux test (man-**too**) *n.* a test for immunity to tuberculosis. Tuberculin is injected beneath the skin and a patch of inflammation appearing in the next 48–72 hours indicates that a degree of immunity is present. [C. Mantoux (1877–1947), French physician]

manual lymphatic drainage (**man**-yoo-al) *n.* a series of therapeutic movements, using massage, developed to enhance lymph drainage, alleviate swelling, and improve wound healing.

manubrium (mă-**new**-bri-ŭm) *n.* (*pl.* **manubria**) **1.** the upper section of the breastbone (*see* sternum). It articulates with the clavicles and the first costal cartilage. **2.** the handle-like part of the malleus, attached to the eardrum. —**manubrial** *adj.*

manuka honey (mă-**noo**-kă) *n.* a honey, produced in Australia and New Zealand, from nectar of the manuka (or tea) tree, that is reported to have antibacterial and antioxidant properties and is used to promote wound healing. The thickness of the honey acts as a moist protective barrier.

MAO *n. see* monoamine oxidase.

MAO inhibitor (MAOI) *n.* a drug that prevents the activity of the enzyme monoamine oxidase (MAO). The use of irreversible MAOA inhibitors, such as phenelzine (Nardil), as antidepressants is now restricted because their side-effects include interactions with other drugs and foods containing tyramine (e.g. cheese) to produce a sudden and dangerous increase in blood pressure. *See also* moclobemide, selegiline.

MAP *n. see* mean arterial pressure.

maple syrup urine disease (aminoacidopathy) (may-pŭl **si**-rŭp) *n.* an inborn defect of amino acid metabolism causing an excess of valine, leucine, isoleucine, and alloisoleucine in the urine, which has an odour like maple syrup. Treatment is dietary; if untreated, the condition leads to learning disability and death in infancy.

marasmus (mă-**raz**-mŭs) *n.* mixed deficiency of both protein and calories, resulting in severe wasting in infants. Body weight is below 60% of that expected for age; the infant looks 'old', has thin sparse hair, is pallid and apathetic, lacks skin fat, and has subnormal temperature. The condition may be due to malabsorption, wrong feeding, metabolic disorders, repeated vomiting, diarrhoea, or disease.

marble-bone disease (**mar**-bŭl bohn) *n. see* osteopetrosis.

Marburg disease (green monkey disease) (**mar**-berg) *n.* a virus disease of vervet (green) monkeys transmitted to humans by contact with blood or tissues from an infected animal. Symptoms include fever, malaise, severe headache, vomiting, diarrhoea, and bleeding from mucous membranes. Treatment with antiserum and measures to reduce the bleeding are sometimes effective.

Marcus Gunn jaw-winking syndrome (mar-kŭs gun) *n.* a congenital condition characterized by drooping (ptosis) of one eyelid. On opening or moving the mouth, the droopy lid elevates momentarily, resembling a wink. [R. Marcus Gunn (1850–1909), British ophthalmologist]

Marfan's syndrome (mar-fahnz) *n.* an inherited disorder of connective tissue characterized by excessive height, abnormally long and slender fingers and toes (**arachnodactyly**), heart defects, and partial dislocation of the lenses of the eyes. [B. J. A. Marfan (1858–1942), French physician]

marijuana (ma-ri-**hwah**-nă) *n. see* cannabis.

Marion's disease (**ma**-ri-ŏnz) *n.* obstruction of the outlet of the bladder caused by enlargement of the muscle cells in the neck of the bladder. [J. B. C. G. Marion (1869–1960), French surgeon]

Marjolin's ulcer (mar-*zh*oh-lanz) *n.* a carcinoma that develops at the edge of a chronic ulcer of the skin, usually a venous ulcer in the ankle region. [J. N. Marjolin (1780–1850), French surgeon]

marrow (**ma**-roh) *n. see* bone marrow.

marsupialization (mar-soo-piăl-I-zay-shŏn) *n.* an operative technique for curing a cyst. The cyst is opened, its contents removed, and the edges then stitched to the skin incision. This technique is commonly used for the treatment of vulval abscesses.

MAS *n. see* mandibular advancement splint.

masculinization (mas-kew-lin-I-zay-shŏn) *n.* development of excess body and facial hair, deepening of the voice, and increase in muscle bulk in a female due to a hormone disorder or to hormone therapy. *See also* virilism, virilization.

Maslow's hierarchy of human needs (**maz**-lohz) *n.* a listing of human needs in order of priority, from basic physiological needs (e.g. eating and drinking) to self-actualization. It is held that the individual does not consider meeting each level of need until the previous level has been at least partly satisfied. *See* self-actualization. [A. H. Maslow (1908–70), US psychologist]

massage (**mas**-ahz*h*) *n.* manipulation of the soft tissues of the body with the hands. Massage is used to improve circulation, prevent adhesions in tissues after injury, and reduce muscular spasm. *See also* effleurage, petrissage, tapotement.

masseter (ma-**see**-ter) *n.* a thick muscle in the cheek extending from the zygomatic arch to the outer corner of the mandible. It is important for mastication and acts by closing the jaws.

mast- (masto-) *combining form denoting* the breast.

mastalgia (mas-**tal**-jiă) *n.* pain in the breast.

mastatrophy (mastatrophia) (mas-**tat**-rŏfi) *n.* atrophy of the breasts.

mast cell (mahst) *n.* a large cell in connective tissue. Mast cells contain heparin, histamine, and serotonin, which are released during inflammation and allergic responses.

mastectomy (mas-**tek**-tŏmi) *n.* surgical removal of a breast. **radical m.** surgical removal of the breast with the skin and all the lymphatic tissue of the armpit. In modern surgical practice the underlying pectoral muscles are usually preserved. It is performed when breast cancer has spread to involve the lymph nodes. **simple m.** surgical removal of the breast retaining the skin and, if possible, the nipple. It is performed for extensive but not necessarily invasive tumours. *See also* lumpectomy.

mastication (mas-ti-**kay**-shŏn) *n.* the process of chewing food.

mastitis (mas-**ty**-tis) *n.* inflammation of the breast, usually caused by bacterial infection via damaged nipples. **cystic m.** chronic mastitis in which the breast feels lumpy due to the presence of cysts. **puerperal m.** acute mastitis that develops during the period of breastfeeding.

mastoid (**mas**-toid) *adj.* relating to the mastoid process. **m. antrum** an air-filled channel connecting the mastoid process to the cavity of the middle ear. **m. cells** air spaces in the mastoid process. **m. process** a nipple-shaped process on the temporal bone that extends downward and forward behind the ear canal.

mastoidectomy (mas-toi-**dek**-tŏmi) *n.* an operation to remove some or all of the mastoid cells when they have become infected (*see* mastoiditis) or invaded by cholesteatoma.

mastoiditis (mas-toi-**dy**-tis) *n.* inflammation of the mastoid process and antrum, usually caused by bacterial infection that spreads from the middle ear. *See* otitis (media).

masturbation (mas-ter-**bay**-shŏn) *n.* physical self-stimulation of the genitalia in order to produce sexual pleasure, often resulting in orgasm.

materia medica (mă-**teer**-iă **med**-ik-ă) *n.* the study of drugs used in medicine and dentistry, including pharmacognosy, pharmacy, pharmacology, and therapeutics.

maternal deprivation (mă-**ter**-năl) *n.* the condition said to result if infants are deprived of the opportunity to form a close relationship with a single parental figure, who may or may not be the child's natural parent. It is characterized by distress and depression, leading to an inability to form lasting relationships.

maternal mortality rate *n.* the number of deaths due to complications of pregnancy, childbirth, and the puerperium per 100,000 live births.

matrix (**may**-triks) *n.* the substance of a tissue or organ in which more specialized structures are embedded.

mattress suture (mat-ris) *n.* a suture in which a loop is made on each side of the incision, which may be parallel with the incision (**horizontal m. s.**) or at right angles to it (**vertical m. s.**).

maturation (mat-yoor-ay-shŏn) *n.* the process of attaining full development.

maturity-onset diabetes of the young (MODY) (mă-tyoor-iti-on-set) *n. see* diabetes.

maxilla (maks-il-ă) *n.* (*pl.* **maxillae**) **1.** (loosely) the upper jaw. **2.** either of the pair of bones contributing to the upper jaw, the orbits, the nasal cavity, and the roof of the mouth (*see* palate). **—maxillary** (maks-il-er-i) *adj.*

maxillary sinus (maxillary antrum) *n. see* paranasal sinuses.

maxillofacial (maks-il-oh-fay-shăl) *adj.* describing or relating to the region of the face, jaws, and related structures.

maximum breathing capacity (MBC) (maks-i-mŭm) *n.* the volume of gas exchanged per minute when breathing at maximum rate and depth.

MBC *n. see* maximum breathing capacity.

MBRRACE-UK *n. see* confidential enquiries.

MCI *n. see* mild cognitive impairment.

MCS *n. see* minimally conscious state.

MCU *n. see* micturating cystourethrogram.

MDT *n. see* multidisciplinary team.

ME *n.* myalgic encephalomyelitis. *See* CFS/ME/PVF.

mean (arithmetic mean) (meen) *n.* the average of a group of observations calculated by adding their values and dividing by the number in the group. *See also* median, mode.

mean arterial pressure (MAP) *n.* a reflection of the average blood pressure of a patient during a single cardiac cycle. It is regulated by systemic vascular resistance and cardiac output and can be calculated using a range of different formulae. An average MAP is between 70 and 110 mmHg but a value of 60 mmHg is considered necessary to maintain essential organ perfusion.

measles (mee-zŭlz) *n.* a highly infectious virus disease that mainly affects children. Early symptoms are those of a cold accompanied by a high fever, and Koplik's spots may appear on the inside of the cheeks. On the third to fifth day a blotchy slightly elevated pink rash develops; it lasts 3–5 days. The patient is infectious throughout this period. In most cases the symptoms soon subside but patients are susceptible to pneumonia and middle ear infections. Medical names: **rubeola**, **morbilli**.

SEE WEB LINKS

- More information about measles from the NHS Choices website

meat- (meato-) *combining form denoting* a meatus.

meatus (mee-ay-tŭs) *n.* (in anatomy) a passage or opening. **external auditory m.** the auditory canal: the passage leading from the pinna of the outer ear to the eardrum. **nasal m.** one of three groovelike parts of the nasal cavity beneath each of the nasal conchae. **urethral m.** the external opening of the urethra.

mebendazole (mi-**ben**-dă-zohl) *n.* an anthelmintic drug used to get rid of roundworms, hookworms, threadworms, and whipworms. Trade name: **Vermox**. *See also* imidazole.

mechanism of labour (**mek**-ă-nizm) *n.* the sum of the forces that act to expel a fetus from the uterus together with those that resist its expulsion and affect its position during birth. *See* labour.

mechanotherapy (mek-ă-noh-**th'e**-ră-pi) *n.* the use of mechanical equipment during physiotherapy to produce regularly repeated movements in part of the body.

Meckel's diverticulum (**mek**-ĕlz) *n. see* diverticulum. [J. F. Meckel (1781–1833), German anatomist]

meconism (**mek**-oh-nizm) *n.* poisoning from the effects of eating or smoking opium or the products derived from it, especially morphine.

meconium (mi-**koh**-niŭm) *n.* the first stools of a newborn baby, which are sticky and dark green and composed of cellular debris, mucus, and bile pigments. **m. aspiration** a condition in which a baby inhales meconium into the lungs during delivery, which can cause plugs in the airway; the baby may become hypoxic. **m. ileus** obstruction of the ileum caused by thickened meconium in babies with cystic fibrosis.

media (tunica media) (**meed**-iă) *n.* **1.** the middle layer of the wall of a vein or artery. **2.** the middle layer of various other organs or parts.

medial (**mee**-di-ăl) *adj.* **1.** relating to or denoting parts of the body that are closest to the median plane of the body. **2.** relating to or situated in the central region of an organ, tissue, or the body.

median (**mee**-di-ăn) **1.** *adj.* (in anatomy) situated in or denoting the plane that divides the body into right and left halves. **2.** *n.* (in statistics) the middle observation of a series arranged in ascending order. *See also* mean.

mediastinitis (mee-di-asti-**ny**-tis) *n.* inflammation of the mediastinum, usually complicating a rupture of the oesophagus (gullet).

mediastinoscopy (mee-di-asti-**nos**-kŏpi) *n.* examination of the mediastinum, usually by means of an endoscope inserted through a small incision in the neck region. It can be used to assess the spread of intrathoracic tumours and for lymph node biopsy.

mediastinum (mee-di-ă-**sty**-nŭm) *n.* the space in the thorax between the two pleural sacs. The mediastinum contains the heart, aorta, trachea, oesophagus, and thymus gland.

medical (**med**-ik-ăl) *adj.* **1.** of or relating to the science or practice of medicine. **2.** of or relating to conditions that require the attention of a physician rather than a surgeon.

medical assistant *n.* a health service worker who is not a registered medical practitioner (often in the armed forces) working in association with a doctor to undertake minor treatments and preliminary assessments.

medical certificate *n.* a certificate stating a doctor's diagnosis of a patient's medical condition, disability, or fitness to work.

medical emergency team (MET) *n.* a team, usually consisting of a group of physicians, anaesthetists, and senior nurses, that can be summoned urgently to attend to patients with deteriorating medical conditions. The aim is to prevent further deterioration and to decide if enhanced levels of care are appropriate (e.g. on the high-dependency or intensive care units). The team will also assume the role of the cardiac-arrest team.

medical jurisprudence *n.* the study or practice of the legal aspects of medicine. *See* forensic medicine.

medicated (**med**-i-kayt-id) *adj.* containing or impregnated with a medicinal drug: applied to dressings, lotions, soaps, sweets, etc.

medication (med-i-**kay**-shŏn) *n.* **1.** a substance administered by mouth, applied to the body, or introduced into the body for the purpose of treatment. *See also* premedication. **2.** treatment of a patient using drugs.

medicine (**med**-sin) *n.* **1.** the science or practice of the diagnosis, treatment, and prevention of disease. **2.** the science or practice of nonsurgical methods of treating disease. **3.** any drug or preparation used for the treatment or prevention of disease, particularly a preparation that is taken by mouth.

Medicines and Healthcare products Regulatory Agency (MHRA) *n.* a UK government agency that regulates the use of medicinal drugs and medical devices. The agency regulates and issues licences for the clinical trial, manufacture, and marketing of new products. It also applies the regulations governing the collection, storage, and use of human blood and blood products.

SEE WEB LINKS

• The MHRA website

medicochirurgical (med-i-koh-ky-**rer**-jik-ăl) *adj.* of or describing matters that are related to both medicine and surgery.

medicolegal (med-i-koh-**lee**-găl) *adj.* relating to the legal aspects of the practice of medicine.

Mediterranean fever (med-it-er-ay-ni-ăn) *n.* **1.** *see* brucellosis. **2.** *see* polyserositis.

medium (**meed**-iŭm) *n.* **1.** any substance, usually a broth, agar, or gelatin, used for the culture of microorganisms or tissue cells. **2.** *see* contrast medium.

medroxyprogesterone (med-roks-i-proh-**jes**-ter-ohn) *n.* a synthetic female sex hormone (*see* progestogen) administered by mouth to treat menstrual disorders (including endometriosis) and certain cancers (especially breast and endometrial cancer) and in hormone replacement therapy (in **Indivina**). It is also given by depot injection as a long-term contraceptive. Trade names: **Climanor**, **Depo-Provera**, **Provera**, **Sayana Press**.

medulla (mi-**dul**-ă) *n.* **1.** the inner region of any organ or tissue, particularly the inner part of the kidney, adrenal glands, or lymph nodes. **m. oblongata** (**myelencephalon**) the extension within the skull of the upper end of the spinal cord, containing centres responsible for the regulation of the heart and blood vessels, respiration, salivation, and swallowing. **2.** the myelin layer of certain nerve fibres. **—medullary** *adj.*

medullated nerve fibre (myelinated nerve fibre) (**med**-ŭl-ayt-id) *n. see* myelin.

medulloblastoma (mi-dul-oh-blas-**toh**-mă) *n.* a malignant brain tumour that occurs during childhood and develops in the cerebellum. Symptoms include headaches, dizziness, and unsteadiness; the flow of cerebrospinal fluid may become obstructed, causing hydrocephalus. Treatment involves surgery followed by radiotherapy.

mefenamic acid (me-fen-**am**-ik) *n.* an anti-inflammatory drug (*see* NSAID) administered by mouth to treat rheumatic conditions and relieve pain. Trade name: **Ponstan**.

mefloquine (**mef**-loh-kween) *n.* a drug used mainly for the prevention of malaria that is resistant to chloroquine. It is administered by mouth but should not be taken during pregnancy, by psychiatric patients, or with beta blockers. Trade name: **Lariam**.

mega- *combining form denoting* **1.** large size or abnormal enlargement or distension. **2.** a million.

megacolon (meg-ă-**koh**-lŏn) *n.* pathological dilatation of the colon. It is caused by chronic obstruction of the colon (e.g. due to Hirschsprung's disease) or long-standing constipation.

megakaryocyte (meg-ă-**ka**-ri-oh-syt) *n.* a cell in the bone marrow that produces platelets. *See also* thrombopoiesis.

megal- (megalo-) *combining form denoting* abnormal enlargement.

megaloblast (**meg**-ă-loh-blast) *n.* an abnormal form of erythroblast. Megaloblasts are unusually large and their nuclei fail to mature in the normal way; they are seen in the bone marrow in certain anaemias (**megaloblastic anaemias**) due to deficiency of vitamin B_{12} or folate. **—megaloblastic** *adj.*

megalocephaly (meg-ă-loh-**sef**-ăli) *n.* **1.** *see* macrocephaly. **2.** overgrowth and distortion of the skull bones (*see* leontiasis).

megalocyte (**meg**-ă-loh-syt) *n. see* macrocyte.

megalomania (meg-ă-loh-**may**-niă) *n.* an obsolete word for delusions of grandeur. It may be a feature of a schizophrenic or manic illness.

-megaly *combining form denoting* abnormal enlargement.

megaureter (meg-ă-yoor-**ee**-ter) *n.* gross dilatation of the ureter. This occurs above the site of a long-standing obstruction in the ureter, which blocks the free flow of urine from the kidney.

megestrol (mi-**jes**-trohl) *n.* a synthetic female sex hormone (*see* progestogen) that is taken by mouth mainly in the treatment of metastatic endometrial cancer. Trade name: **Megace**.

megophthalmia (meg-off-**thal**-miă) *n.* an abnormally large eyeball.

meibomian cyst (my-**boh**-mi-ăn) *n. see* chalazion. [H. Meibom (1638–1700), German anatomist]

meibomian glands (tarsal glands) *pl. n.* small sebaceous glands that lie under the conjunctiva of the eyelids.

meibomianitis (my-boh-mi-ăn-**I**-tis) *n.* inflammation of the meibomian glands of the eyelids.

Meigs' syndrome (mIgz) *n.* the rare combination of a benign ovarian fibroma with ascites and a right-sided pleural effusion. [J. V. Meigs (1892–1963), US gynaecologist]

meiosis (reduction division) (my-**oh**-sis) *n.* a type of cell division that produces four daughter cells, each having half the number of chromosomes of the original cell. It occurs before the formation of sperm and ova and the normal (diploid) number of chromosomes is restored after fertilization. *Compare* mitosis. **—meiotic** (my-**ot**-ik) *adj.*

Meissner's plexus (submucous plexus) (**my**-snerz) *n.* a fine network of parasympathetic nerve fibres in the wall of the alimentary canal, supplying the muscles and mucous membrane. [G. Meissner (1829–1905), German physiologist]

melaena (mi-**lee**-nă) *n.* black tarry faeces discoloured by the presence of digested blood. Melaena usually reflects significant bleeding in the upper gastrointestinal tract but may be due to disease in the small bowel or proximal large bowel (such as carcinoma or angiodysplasia). It may be associated with vomiting blood (*see* haematemesis) or coffee-ground vomit. *See also* haemorrhagic disease of the newborn.

melan- (melano-) *combining form denoting* **1.** black coloration. **2.** melanin.

melancholia (mel-ăn-**koh**-liă) *n.* an obsolete name for depression not triggered by any stressor.

melanin (**mel**-ăn-in) *n.* a dark-brown to black pigment occurring in the hair, the skin, and in the iris and choroid layer of the eyes.

melanism (melanosis) (**mel**-ăn-izm) *n.* an unusually pronounced darkening of body tissues caused by excessive production of the pigment melanin. Melanism may affect the skin after sunburn, during pregnancy, or in Addison's disease.

melanocyte (**mel**-ă-noh-syt) *n.* a cell within the epidermis of skin that produces melanin.

melanocyte-stimulating hormone (MSH) *n.* a hormone synthesized and released by the pituitary gland. In humans it stimulates production and dispersal of melanin in the melanocytes. **α-MSH** a hormone released by the hypothalamus that suppresses appetite, regulates energy balance, stimulates sexual activity, and helps regulate heart rate and blood pressure.

melanoma (malignant melanoma) (mel-ă-**noh**-mă) *n.* a highly malignant tumour of melanocytes. Such tumours usually occur in the skin (pale skin, genetic predisposition, and repeated episodes of sunburn are the most important factors) and may arise from a pre-existing mole or apparently normal skin. They are usually dark but may be free of the pigment (**amelanotic m.**). Superficial melanomas can often be successfully treated by surgical excision.

melanophore (**mel**-ă-noh-for) *n.* a cell that contains melanin.

melanoplakia (mel-ă-noh-**play**-kiă) *n.* pigmented areas of melanin in the mucous membrane lining the inside of the cheeks.

melanosis (mel-ă-**noh**-sis) *n.* **1.** *see* melanism. **2.** a disorder in the body's production of the pigment melanin. **3.** cachexia associated with the spread of the skin cancer melanoma. **—melanotic** *adj.*

melanuria (mel-ăn-**yoor**-iă) *n.* the presence of dark pigment in the urine. This may occur in some cases of melanoma; it may alternatively be caused by metabolic disease, such as porphyria.

melasma (mi-**laz**-mă) *n. see* chloasma.

melatonin (mel-ă-**toh**-nin) *n.* a hormone produced by the pineal gland in darkness but not in bright light. Melatonin is a derivative of serotonin, with which it works to regulate the sleep cycle.

melioidosis (mee-li-oi-**doh**-sis) *n.* a disease of wild rodents caused by the bacterium *Pseudomonas pseudomallei*. It can be transmitted to humans, causing pneumonia, multiple abscesses, and septicaemia.

melphalan (**mel**-fă-lan) *n.* an alkylating agent administered by mouth or intravenous injection or infusion to treat various types of cancer, particularly myeloma. Trade name: **Alkeran**.

membrane (**mem**-brayn) *n.* **1.** a thin layer of tissue surrounding an organ or tissue, lining a cavity, or separating adjacent structures or cavities. *See also* basement membrane, mucous membrane, serous membrane. **2.** the lipoprotein envelope surrounding a cell (**cell m.**). **—membranous** (**mem**-brăn-ŭs) *adj.*

membranous labyrinth *n. see* labyrinth.

men- (meno-) *combining form denoting* menstruation.

menarche (men-**ar**-ki) *n.* the start of the menstrual periods and other physical and mental changes associated with puberty. The menarche occurs when the reproductive organs become functionally active and may take place at any time between 10 and 19 years of age. *Compare* gonadarche.

Mendel's laws (**men**-d'lz) *pl. n.* rules of inheritance based on the breeding experiments of Gregor Mendel, which showed that the inheritance of characteristics is controlled by particles now known as genes. In modern terms they are as follows. (1) Each somatic cell of an individual carries two factors (genes) for every characteristic and each gamete carries only one.

(2) Each pair of factors segregates independently of all other pairs at meiosis, so that the gametes show all possible combinations of factors. *See also* dominant, recessive. [G. J. Mendel (1822–84), Austrian monk]

Mendelson's syndrome (men-d'l-sŏnz) *n.* inhalation of regurgitated stomach contents by an anaesthetized patient, which may result in death from anoxia or cause extensive lung damage or pulmonary oedema with severe bronchospasm. It may be prevented by giving gastric-acid inhibitors (e.g. cimetidine, ranitidine) or sodium citrate before inducing anaesthesia. [C. L. Mendelson (1913–2002), US obstetrician]

Ménétrier's disease (may-nay-tri-ayz) *n.* a rare disorder caused by hypertrophy of the mucous membrane lining the stomach. It may lead to anaemia, protein loss, and peripheral oedema. [P. Ménétrier (1859–1935), French physician]

menidrosis (menhidrosis) (men-id-**roh**-sis) *n.* the production of sweat, sometimes containing blood, instead of the normal menstrual flow.

Ménière's disease (mayn-**yairz**) *n.* a disease of the inner ear characterized by episodes of deafness, buzzing in the ears (tinnitus), and vertigo. Symptoms last for several hours and between attacks the affected ear may return to normal. It is thought to be caused by the build-up of fluid in the inner ear and is treated by drugs or surgery. Medical name: **endolymphatic hydrops**. [P. Ménière (1799–1862), French physician]

mening- (meningo-) *combining form denoting* the meninges.

meninges (min-**in**-jeez) *pl. n.* (*sing.* **meninx**) the three connective tissue membranes that line the skull and vertebral canal and enclose the brain and spinal cord: the dura mater, arachnoid mater, and pia mater. **—meningeal** *adj.*

meningioma (min-in-ji-**oh**-mă) *n.* a benign tumour arising from the meninges. It is usually slow-growing and produces symptoms by pressure on the underlying nervous tissue. Treatment of the majority of cases is by surgical removal if the tumour is accessible.

meningism (**men**-in-jizm) *n.* stiffness of the neck that is found in meningitis.

meningitis (men-in-**jy**-tis) *n.* an inflammation of the meninges due to viral, bacterial, or fungal infection. Meningitis causes an intense headache, fever, loss of appetite, intolerance to light (photophobia) and sound (phonophobia), rigidity of muscles, especially those in the neck (*see also* Kernig's sign), and in severe cases convulsions, vomiting, and delirium leading to death. Bacterial meningitis is treated with antibiotics administered as soon as possible after diagnosis. **meningococcal m.** a serious form of bacterial meningitis, caused by the meningococcus (most importantly, strains B and C), that can lead to widespread infection and meningococcal septicaemia. **pneumococcal m.** a form of bacterial meningitis caused by the pneumococcus. *See also* Hib vaccine, meningitis C vaccine, pneumococcal vaccine.

SEE WEB LINKS

- Website of the Meningitis Research Foundation

meningitis C vaccine (MenC) *n.* a vaccine that provides protection against the C strain of the bacterium *Neisseria meningitidis* (the meningococcus), which accounts for approximately 50% of all cases of meningococcal meningitis and tends to occur in clusters. The vaccine is given to all babies with their primary immunizations at 3 and 4 months of age and as a booster at 12 months (see Appendix 8: Immunization schedules). It can also be given as a single vaccine and is currently offered to everyone under the age of 24.

meningocele (min-**ing**-oh-seel) *n.* protrusion of the meninges through a gap in the spine. *See* neural tube defects.

meningococcus (min-ing-oh-**kok**-ŭs) *n.* (*pl.* **meningococci**) the bacterium *Neisseria meningitidis*, which can cause a serious form of septicaemia and is a common cause of meningitis. **—meningococcal** *adj.*

meningoencephalitis (min-ing-oh-en-sef-ă-**ly**-tis) *n.* inflammation of the brain and the meninges caused by bacterial, viral, fungal, or amoebic infection.

meningoencephalocele (min-ing-oh-en-**sef**-ă-loh-seel) *n.* protrusion of the meninges and brain through a defect in the skull. *See* neural tube defects.

meningomyelocele (myelocele, myelomeningocele) (min-ing-oh-**my**-ĕ-loh-seel) *n.* protrusion of the meninges, spinal cord, and nerve roots through a gap in the spine, accompanied by paralysis of the legs and urinary incontinence. *See* neural tube defects.

meningovascular (min-ing-oh-**vas**-kew-ler) *adj.* relating to or affecting the meninges and the blood vessels that penetrate them to supply the underlying neural tissues.

meniscectomy (men-i-**sek**-tŏmi) *n.* surgical removal of a cartilage (meniscus) in the knee. This is carried out when the meniscus has been torn or is diseased and is causing pain, swelling, locking, or other symptoms. The operation is routinely performed through an arthroscope.

meniscus (min-**isk**-ŭs) *n.* (in anatomy) a crescent-shaped structure, such as the fibrocartilaginous disc that divides the cavity of a synovial joint.

Menkes kinky-hair disease (**men**-kis) *n.* a genetic disorder characterized by severe learning disability, seizures, poor vision, colourless fragile hair, and chubby red cheeks. Affected infants usually die before the age of three. [J. H. Menkes (1928–), US neurologist]

menopause (climacteric) (**men**-ŏ-pawz) *n.* the time in a woman's life when ovulation and menstruation cease and the woman is no longer able to bear children. The menopause can occur at any age between the middle thirties and the middle fifties, but occurs most commonly between 45 and 55; it can only be established in retrospect after 12 consecutive months of amenorrhoea. It is associated with a change in the balance of sex hormones in the body, which sometimes leads to hot flushes and other vasomotor symptoms, palpitations, and emotional disturbances. **—menopausal** *adj.*

menorrhagia (men-ŏ-**ray**-jiă) *n.* abnormally heavy bleeding at menstruation. Menorrhagia may be associated with pelvic inflammatory disease, tumours (especially fibroids) in the pelvic cavity, endometriosis, or the presence of an IUCD. *See also* dysfunctional uterine bleeding.

MENS *pl. n.* multiple endocrine neoplasia syndromes, which involve tumour formation or hyperplasia in various combinations of endocrine glands. Type 1 (**Wermer's syndrome**) involves the parathyroid, pituitary, and pancreas, whereas type 2A (**Sipple's syndrome**) involves the thyroid medullary cells, the adrenal medulla (phaeochromocytoma), and the parathyroids. Type 2B is similar to 2A, but patients tend to resemble people with Marfan's syndrome and have multiple neuromas on their mucous membranes.

menses (**men**-seez) *n.* **1.** the blood and other materials discharged from the uterus at menstruation. **2.** *see* menstruation.

menstrual cycle (**men**-stroo-ăl) *n.* the periodic sequence of events in sexually mature nonpregnant women by which an egg cell (ovum) is released from a follicle in the ovary at four-weekly intervals until the menopause (see

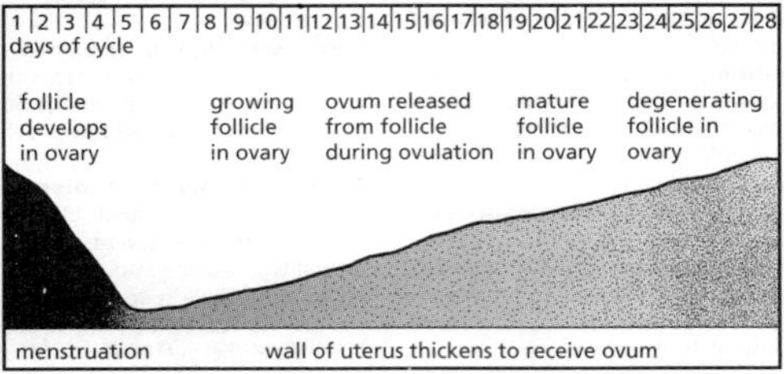

The menstrual cycle

illustration). The secretion of progesterone in the ruptured follicle causes the lining of the uterus (endometrium) to become thicker and richly supplied with blood in preparation for pregnancy. If the ovum is not fertilized the endometrium is shed at menstruation.

menstruation (menses) (men-stroo-**ay**-shŏn) *n.* the discharge of blood and fragments of endometrium from the vagina at intervals of about four weeks in women of childbearing age (*see* menarche, menopause). The normal duration of discharge varies from three to seven days. **anovular m.** discharge that takes place without previous release of an egg cell from the ovary. **vicarious m.** bleeding from a mucous membrane other than the endometrium when normal menstruation is due. *See also* amenorrhoea, dysmenorrhoea, menorrhagia, oligomenorrhoea.

mental[1] (**men**-t'l) *adj.* relating to or affecting the mind.

mental[2] *adj.* relating to the chin.

mental age *n.* a measure of the intellectual level at which an individual functions; for example, someone described as having a mental age of 6 years would be functioning at the level of an average 6-year-old child. *See also* intelligence quotient, intelligence test.

Mental Capacity Act 2005 *n.* legislation for England and Wales, which came into force in October 2007, to govern the treatment of people who lack capacity to make decisions. It gives legal force to the importance of autonomy in health care and to advance directives, decisions, or statements. It also provides statutory legislation for medical and social decision-makers to act in the patient's best interests should he or she lose capacity (*see* Independent Mental Capacity Advocate). It allows proportionate force to implement decisions made in a patient's best interests. For Scotland the current legislation is the Adults with Incapacity (Scotland) Act 2000.

mental handicap *n.* a former name for learning disability.

Mental Health Act *n.* (in England and Wales) legislation that governs the treatment of people with a mental disorder, which is defined as covering mental illness, personality disorder, and learning disability. For England and Wales the Mental Health Act 1983 has been amended by the Mental Health Act 2007. The legislation provides for the voluntary and compulsory admission of patients with a diagnosis or symptoms of a mental disorder; the purposes of the latter are both to provide treatment for patients who have lost insight into their condition and to manage the risks that such patients pose to themselves or to others. For Scotland the current legislation is the Mental Health (Care and Treatment) (Scotland) Act 2003. **MHA Commission** a body that was responsible for reviewing psychiatric care, now subsumed under the Care Quality Commission.

SEE WEB LINKS

- A summary of the Mental Health Act 1983 from the National Archives

Mental Health Review Tribunal (MHRT) *n.* a tribunal, now operating under the Mental Health Act 2007, to which applications may be made for the discharge from hospital of a person compulsorily detained there under provisions of the Act (*see* compulsory admission).

mental illness *n.* a disorder of one or more of the functions of the mind, which causes suffering to the patient or others. Mental illnesses are broadly categorized as psychoses, in which the capacity for appreciating reality is lost, or neuroses, in which it is preserved.

mental impairment *n.* (mostly in legal usage) the condition of significant or severe impairment of intellectual and social functioning.

mental retardation *n.* a former name for learning disability.

menthol (**men**-thol) *n.* a compound extracted from peppermint oil, used in inhalants to relieve cold symptoms, in ointments and liniments, and to relieve itching. Formula: $C_{10}H_{20}O$.

mento- *combining form denoting* the chin.

mentor (**men**-tor) *n.* a person with the experience and knowledge to fulfil the role of a trusted friend and adviser. The mentor guides, counsels, and supports a student or junior in a clinical or educational area. This role can be formal or informal. **sign-off m.** a mentor who supports students on a range of nursing programmes in their final placement before registration, enabling them to achieve the skills, behaviour, and knowledge to become effective practitioners. This role requires training and experience to make a judgment that students are fit to practise and to enter the register. Midwifery students are supported by sign-off mentors on a continuous basis, throughout their programme.

mentum (**men**-tŭm) *n.* the chin.

mepacrine (**mep**-ă-kreen) *n.* a drug administered by mouth to treat giardiasis.

meralgia paraesthetica (mi-**ral**-jiă pa-ris-**thet**-ik-ă) *n.* painful tingling and numbness felt over the lateral surface of the thigh when the lateral cutaneous nerve is trapped as it passes through the muscular tissues of the groin.

mercaptopurine (mer-kap-tŏ-**pewr**-een) *n.* a drug that prevents the growth of cancer cells and is administered by mouth, chiefly in the treatment of acute leukaemias and chronic myeloid leukaemia but also in severe Crohn's disease (*see* antimetabolite). Trade names: **Puri-Nethol**, **Xaluprine**.

mercurialism (hydrargyria) (mer-**kewr**-iă-lizm) *n.* mercury poisoning. Acute poisoning causes vomiting, diarrhoea, and kidney damage. Treatment is with dimercaprol. Chronic poisoning causes mouth ulceration, loose teeth, and intestinal and renal disturbances. Treatment is removing the patient from further exposure.

mercury (**mer**-kewr-i) *n.* a silvery metallic element that is liquid at room temperature. Its toxicity has caused a decline in the use of its compounds in medicine. The main use of mercury today is as a component of amalgam fillings in dentistry. Symbol: Hg. *See also* mercurialism, pink disease.

mes- (meso-) *combining form denoting* middle or medial.

mesaortitis (mes-ay-or-**ty**-tis) *n.* inflammation of the middle layer (media) of the wall of the aorta, generally the result of late syphilis.

mesarteritis (mes-ar-ter-**I**-tis) *n.* inflammation of the middle layer (media) of an artery, which is often combined with inflammation in all layers of the artery wall.

mescaline (**mesk**-ă-leen) *n.* an alkaloid present in the dried tops of the cactus *Lophophora williamsii* that produces inebriation and hallucinations when ingested.

mesencephalon (mes-en-**sef**-ă-lon) *n. see* midbrain.

mesentery (**mes**-ĕn-ter-i) *n.* a double layer of peritoneum attaching the stomach, small intestine, pancreas, spleen, and other abdominal organs to the posterior wall of the abdomen. **—mesenteric** (mes-ĕn-**te**-rik) *adj.*

mesial (**mee**-zi-ăl) *adj.* **1.** medial. **2.** relating to or situated in the median line or plane. **3.** designating the surface of a tooth towards the midline of the jaw.

mesmerism (**mez**-mer-izm) *n.* hypnosis based on the ideas of Franz Mesmer, sometimes employing magnets and a variety of other equipment. [F. A. Mesmer (1734–1815), Austrian physician]

mesna (**mez**-nă) *n.* a drug administered by mouth or intravenous injection to prevent the toxic effect of alkylating agents, particularly ifosfamide and cyclophosphamide, on the bladder. It binds with the toxic metabolite acrolein in the urine.

mesoappendix (mes-oh-ă-**pen**-diks) *n.* the mesentery of the appendix.

mesocolon (mes-oh-**koh**-lon) *n.* the fold of peritoneum by which the colon is fixed to the posterior abdominal wall.

mesoderm (**mes**-oh-derm) *n.* the middle germ layer of the early embryo. It gives rise to cartilage, muscle, bone, blood, kidneys, gonads and their ducts, and connective tissue. **—mesodermal** *adj.*

mesometrium (mes-oh-**mee**-tri-ŭm) *n.* the broad ligament of the uterus: a sheet of connective tissue that carries blood vessels to the uterus and attaches it to the abdominal wall.

mesomorphic (mes-oh-**mor**-fik) *adj.* describing a body type characterized by a well developed skeletal and muscular structure and a sturdy upright posture. **—mesomorph** *n.* **—mesomorphy** *n.*

mesonephros (Wolffian body) (mes-oh-**nef**-ross) *n.* kidney tissue that is functional only in the embryo. Its duct – the **Wolffian** (or **mesonephric**) **duct** – persists in males as the epididymis and vas deferens. **—mesonephric** *adj.*

mesosalpinx (mes-oh-**sal**-pinks) *n.* a fold of peritoneum that surrounds the Fallopian tubes. It is the upper part of the broad ligament that surrounds the uterus.

mesotendon (mes-oh-**ten**-dŏn) *n.* the delicate connective tissue membrane that surrounds a tendon.

mesothelioma (mes-oh-th'ee-li-**oh**-mă) *n.* a tumour of the pleura, peritoneum, or pericardium. The occurrence of pleural mesothelioma is often due to exposure to asbestos dust (*see* asbestosis).

mesothelium (mes-oh-**th'ee**-liŭm) *n.* the single layer of cells that lines serous membranes. It is derived from embryonic mesoderm. *Compare* epithelium.

mesovarium (mes-oh-**vair**-iŭm) *n.* the mesentery of the ovaries.

messenger RNA (**mes**-in-jer) *n.* a type of RNA that carries the information of the genetic code of the DNA from the cell nucleus to the ribosomes, where the code is translated into protein. *See* transcription, translation.

mestranol (**mes**-tră-nol) *n.* a synthetic female sex hormone (*see* oestrogen) used, in combination with norethisterone (a progestogen), as an oral contraceptive. Trade name: **Norinyl-1**.

MET *n.* *see* medical emergency team.

met- (meta-) *prefix denoting* **1.** distal to; beyond; behind. **2.** change; transformation.

meta-analysis (met-ă-ă-**nal**-i-sis) *n.* a statistical technique for combining and analysing the results of a number of different studies on the same topic to enable identification of trends and patterns and more accurate estimation of significant effects.

metabolic syndrome (insulin resistance syndrome, syndrome X) (met-ă-**bol**-ik) *n.* a very common condition in which impaired glucose tolerance, impaired fasting glucose, or type 2 diabetes is combined with central obesity (increased fat within the abdomen), raised blood pressure (hypertension), and hyperlipidaemia. It is associated with a risk of premature vascular disease (heart attack and stroke). The principal underlying cause is insulin resistance, which is genetically determined.

metabolism (mi-**tab**-ŏl-izm) *n.* **1.** the sum of all the chemical and physical changes that take place within the body and enable its continued growth and functioning. Metabolism involves the breakdown of complex organic constituents of the body (*see* catabolism) and the building up of complex substances from simple ones (*see* anabolism). *See also* basal metabolism. **2.** the sum of the biochemical changes undergone by a particular constituent of the body. **—metabolic** *adj.*

metabolite (mi-**tab**-ŏ-lyt) *n.* a substance that takes part in the process of metabolism.

metacarpal (met-ă-**kar**-păl) **1.** *adj.* relating to the metacarpus. **2.** *n.* any of the bones forming the metacarpus.

metacarpophalangeal (met-ă-kar-poh-fal-ăn-**jee**-ăl) *adj.* relating to the metacarpal bones and the phalanges, especially to the joints between these bones.

metacarpus (met-ă-**kar**-pŭs) *n.* the five bones of the hand that connect the carpus (wrist) to the phalanges (digits).

metamorphopsia (met-ă-mor-**fop**-siă) *n.* a condition in which objects appear distorted. It is usually due to a disorder of the retina affecting the macula.

metamorphosis (met-ă-**mor**-fŏ-sis) *n.* a structural change, especially the change from one developmental stage to another that occurs in certain animals (e.g. in amphibians from larval to adult form).

metaphase (**met**-ă-fayz) *n.* the second stage of mitosis and of each division of meiosis, in which the spindle forms and the chromosomes line up at the centre of the spindle, with their centromeres attached to the spindle fibres.

metaphysis (mi-**taf**-i-sis) *n.* the growing portion of a long bone that lies between the epiphyses and the diaphysis.

metaplasia (met-ă-**play**-ziă) *n.* an abnormal change in the nature of a tissue, usually in response to an environmental factor. **myeloid m.** the development of bone marrow elements in organs such as the spleen and liver. This may occur after bone marrow failure. **—metaplastic** *adj.*

metaraminol (met-ă-**ram**-i-nol) *n.* a sympathomimetic drug that stimulates alpha receptors and is used as a vasoconstrictor to treat acute hypotension. It is administered by intravenous injection or infusion.

metastasis (mi-**tas**-tă-sis) *n.* (*pl.* **metastases**) the spread of disease, especially of a malignant tumour, from its site of origin. This occurs by three main routes: (1) through the bloodstream; (2) through the lymphatic system; (3) across body cavities. **—metastatic** (met-ă-**stat**-ik) *adj.*

metastasize (mi-**tas**-tă-syz) *vb.* (of a malignant tumour) to spread by metastasis.

metatarsal (met-ă-**tar**-săl) **1.** *adj.* relating to the metatarsus. **2.** *n.* any of the bones forming the metatarsus.

metatarsalgia (met-ă-tar-**sal**-jiă) *n.* aching pain in the metatarsal bones of the foot. Repeated injury, arthritis (particularly rheumatoid), and deformities of the foot are common causes, and corrective footwear and insoles may be prescribed.

metatarsus (met-ă-**tar**-sŭs) *n.* the five bones of the foot that connect the tarsus (ankle) to the phalanges (toes).

meteorism (**meet**-i-er-izm) *n.* *see* tympanites.

-meter *combining form denoting* an instrument for measuring.

metformin (met-**for**-min) *n.* a biguanide drug that is used to treat type 2 diabetes. Trade names: **Bolamyn SR**, **Glucinet SR**, **Glucophage**, **Metabet SR**. *See also* oral hypoglycaemic drug.

methadone (**meth**-ă-dohn) *n.* a potent opioid (*see* opiate) administered by mouth or injection to relieve severe pain and as a linctus to suppress coughs. It can also be substituted for heroin to prevent withdrawal symptoms in people with heroin dependence. Trade names: **Methadose**, **Physeptone**, **Synastone**.

methaemalbumin (met-heem-**al**-bew-min) *n.* a chemical complex of the pigment portion of haemoglobin (haem) with the plasma protein albumin. It is formed in the blood in conditions (e.g. blackwater fever) in which red blood cells are destroyed and free haemoglobin is released into the plasma.

methaemoglobin (met-hee-mŏ-**gloh**-bin) *n.* a substance formed when the iron atoms of haemoglobin have been oxidized from the ferrous to the ferric form (*compare* oxyhaemoglobin). Methaemoglobin cannot bind molecular oxygen and therefore cannot transport oxygen round the body.

methaemoglobinaemia (met-hee-mŏ-gloh-bin-**ee**-miă) *n.* the presence of methaemoglobin in the blood, which may result from ingestion of oxidizing drugs. Symptoms are fatigue, headache, dizziness and cyanosis.

methanol (**meth**-ă-nol) *n. see* methyl alcohol.

methenamine (hexamine) (meth-**en**-ă-meen) *n.* a drug taken by mouth to prevent and treat chronic or recurrent infections of the lower urinary tract. Trade name: **Hiprex**.

methicillin (meth-i-**sil**-in) *n. see* meticillin.

methionine (meth-**I**-ŏ-neen) *n.* a sulphur-containing essential amino acid. *See also* amino acid.

methotrexate (meth-oh-**treks**-ayt) *n.* a drug that interferes with cell growth and is administered by mouth, injection, or infusion to treat many types of cancer, including leukaemia in children and various solid tumours (*see* antimetabolite). It also affects the immune response and may be used in the treatment of rheumatoid arthritis, severe Crohn's disease, and severe psoriasis. Trade names: **Ebetrex**, **Metoject**.

methotrimeprazine (meth-oh-try-**mep**-ră-zeen) *n. see* levomepromazine.

methyl alcohol (methanol) (**mee**-thyl) *n.* wood alcohol: an alcohol that is oxidized in the body much more slowly than ethyl alcohol and forms poisonous products. As little as 10 ml of pure methyl alcohol can produce permanent blindness, and 100 ml is likely to be fatal. *See also* methylated spirits.

methylated spirits (**meth**-il-ayt-id) *n.* a mixture consisting mainly of ethyl alcohol with methyl alcohol and petroleum hydrocarbons. It is used as a solvent, cleaning fluid, and fuel.

methylcellulose (mee-thyl-**sel**-yoo-lohz) *n.* a compound that absorbs water and is administered by mouth as a bulk laxative to treat constipation, to control diarrhoea, and in patients with a colostomy. Trade name: **Celevac**.

methyldopa (mee-thyl-**doh**-pa) *n.* a drug that is administered by mouth to treat hypertension. Trade name: **Aldomet**.

methylphenidate (mee-thyl-fen-id-ayt) *n.* a drug that stimulates the central nervous system. It is administered by mouth to treat attention-deficit/hyperactivity disorder in children. Trade names: **Concerta XL**, **Equasym XL**, **Medikinet XL**, **Ritalin**.

methylprednisolone (mee-thyl-pred-**nis**-ŏ-lohn) *n.* a glucocorticoid that is used in the treatment of inflammatory conditions and allergic states. It is administered by mouth, by intravenous injection or infusion, or by intramuscular injection. Trade names: **Depo-Medrone**, **Medrone**, **Solu-Medrone**.

methyl salicylate *n.* oil of wintergreen: a liquid with counterirritant and analgesic properties, included in preparations applied to the skin to relieve pain in lumbago, sciatica, and rheumatic conditions.

methysergide (meth-i-**ser**-jyd) *n.* a drug administered by mouth to prevent severe migraine attacks and cluster headaches and to control diarrhoea associated with carcinoid syndrome. It is administered under supervision in hospital because it carries a risk of dangerous fibrotic reactions. Trade name: **Deseril**.

meticillin (methicillin) (met-i-**sil**-in) *n.* a semisynthetic penicillin formerly used to treat infections caused by staphylococci that destroy natural penicillin but now replaced by newer antibiotics. It is still used to test the drug sensitivity of staphylococci. **m.-resistant Staphylococcus aureus** *see* MRSA.

metoclopramide (met-oh-**kloh**-pră-myd) *n.* a drug that antagonizes the actions of dopamine. It is administered by mouth or injection to treat nausea and vomiting, including that associated with migraine. Trade name: **Maxolon**.

metolazone (met-**oh**-lă-zohn) *n.* a diuretic administered by mouth to treat fluid retention (oedema) and high blood pressure.

metoprolol (met-oh-**proh**-lol) *n.* a drug that controls the activity of the heart (*see* beta blocker) and is administered by mouth or intravenous injection to treat high blood pressure, angina, and arrhythmias. Trade names: **Betaloc**, **Lopresor**.

metr- (metro-) *combining form denoting* the uterus.

metralgia (mi-**tral**-jiă) *n.* pain in the uterus.

metre (**mee**-ter) *n.* the SI unit of length that is equal to 39.37 inches. Symbol: m.

metritis (mi-**try**-tis) *n.* inflammation of the uterus. *See also* endometritis, myometritis.

metronidazole (met-roh-**ny**-dă-zohl) *n.* a drug administered by mouth, infusion, topically, or in suppositories to treat infections of the urinary, genital, and digestive systems (such as *Helicobacter pylori* infection, trichomoniasis, amoebic dystentery, giardiasis), acute ulcerative gingivitis, fungating wounds, and rosacea. Trade names: **Acea**, **Anabact**, **Flagyl**,

Metrogel, **Metrolyl**, **Metrosa**, **Rosiced**, **Rozex**, **Zyomet**.

-metry *combining form denoting* measuring or measurement.

metyrapone (mi-**ty**-ră-pohn) *n.* a drug that interferes with the production of the hormones cortisol and aldosterone and is used in the diagnosis and treatment of Cushing's syndrome. It is administered by mouth. Trade name: **Metopirone**.

MEWS *n.* modified early warning score (*see* national early warning score).

MHRA *n. see* Medicines and Healthcare products Regulatory Agency.

MI *n. see* myocardial infarction.

mianserin (mi-**an**-ser-in) *n.* a drug, related to the tricyclic antidepressants, administered by mouth to relieve moderate or severe depression and anxiety.

Michel's clips (mee-**shelz**) *pl. n.* small metal clips used for suturing surgical wounds. [G. Michel (1875–1937), French surgeon]

miconazole (mi-**kon**-ă-zohl) *n.* a drug used to treat fungal infections, such as ringworm of the scalp, body, and feet, and oral and vaginal candidiasis. It is administered by mouth, intravaginally, or topically. Trade names: **Daktarin**, **Gyno-Daktarin**, **Loramyc**.

micr- (micro-) *combining form denoting* **1.** small size. **2.** one millionth part.

microaneurysm (my-kroh-**an**-yoor-izm) *n.* a minute localized swelling of a capillary wall, which is found in the retina of patients with diabetic retinopathy.

microangiopathy (my-kroh-an-ji-**op**-ă-thi) *n.* damage to the walls of the smallest blood vessels. It may result from a variety of diseases, including diabetes mellitus, connective-tissue diseases, infections, and cancer.

microbe (**my**-krohb) *n. see* microorganism.

microbiology (my-kroh-by-**ol**-ŏji) *n.* the science of microorganisms. Microbiology in relation to medicine is concerned mainly with the isolation and identification of the microorganisms that cause disease. **—microbiological** *adj.* **—microbiologist** *n.*

microcephaly (my-kroh-**sef**-ăli) *n.* abnormal smallness of the head: a congenital condition in which the brain is not fully developed. *Compare* macrocephaly.

microcheilia (my-kroh-**ky**-liă) *n.* abnormally small size of the lips. *Compare* macrocheilia.

Micrococcus (my-kroh-**kok**-ŭs) *n.* a genus of spherical Gram-positive bacteria occurring in colonies. They are saprophytes or parasites. **M. tetragenus** a species that can cause arthritis, endocarditis, meningitis, or abscesses in tissues.

microcyte (**my**-kroh-syt) *n.* an abnormally small red blood cell (erythrocyte). *See also* microcytosis. **—microcytic** *adj.*

microcytosis (my-kroh-sy-**toh**-sis) *n.* the presence of microcytes in the blood. Microcytosis is a feature of certain anaemias (**microcytic anaemias**), including those due to iron deficiency.

microdactyly (my-kroh-**dak**-tili) *n.* abnormal smallness or shortness of the fingers.

microdiscectomy (my-kroh-disk-**ek**-tŏmi) *n.* surgical removal of all or part of a prolapsed intervertebral disc using an operating microscope. It is a form of minimally invasive surgery.

microdissection (my-kroh-dis-**sek**-shŏn) *n.* the process of dissecting minute structures under the microscope. Using this technique it is possible to dissect the nuclei of cells and even to separate individual chromosomes. *See also* microsurgery.

microdochectomy (my-kroh-dok-**ek**-tŏmi) *n.* excision of a single mammary duct that is causing nipple discharge. The duct is sent for histology to determine the presence of a papilloma or carcinoma.

microdontia (my-kroh-**don**-tiă) *n.* a condition in which the teeth are unusually small.

microfilaria (my-kroh-fil-**air**-iă) *n.* (*pl.* **microfilariae**) the slender motile embryo of certain nematodes (*see* filaria). Microfilariae are commonly found in the circulating blood or lymph of patients suffering an infection with any of the filarial worms.

microglossia (my-kroh-**glos**-iă) *n.* abnormally small size of the tongue.

micrognathia (my-kroh-**nay**-thiă) *n.* a condition in which one or both jaws are unusually small.

microgram (**my**-kroh-gram) *n.* one millionth of a gram. Symbol: μg.

micrograph (photomicrograph) (**my**-kroh-graf) *n.* a photograph of an object viewed through a microscope. **electron m.** a micrograph that is photographed through an electron microscope. **light m.** a micrograph that is photographed through a light microscope.

micromanipulation (my-kroh-mă-nip-yoo-**lay**-shŏn) *n.* the manipulation of extremely small structures under the microscope, as in microdissection or microsurgery.

micromelia (my-kroh-**mee**-liă) *n.* abnormally small size of the arms or legs. *Compare* macromelia.

micrometastasis (my-kroh-mi-**tas**-tă-sis) *n.* (*pl.* **micrometastases**) a secondary tumour that is undetectable by clinical examination or diagnostic tests but is visible under the microscope.

micrometer (my-**krom**-it-er) *n.* an instrument for making extremely fine measurements of thickness or length.

micrometre (**my**-kroh-mee-ter) *n.* one millionth of a metre (10^{-6} m). Symbol: μm.

microorganism (microbe) (my-kroh-**or**-găn-izm) *n.* any organism too small to be visible to the naked eye. Microorganisms include bacteria, some fungi, mycoplasmas, protozoa, rickettsiae, and viruses.

microphthalmos (my-krof-**thal**-mos) *n.* a congenitally small eye, usually associated with a small eye socket.

micropsia (my-**krop**-siă) *n.* a condition in which objects appear smaller than they really are. It is usually due to disease of the retina.

microscope (**my**-krŏ-skohp) *n.* an instrument for producing a greatly magnified image of an object, which may be so small as to be invisible to the naked eye. *See also* electron microscope, operating microscope. **—microscopical** *adj.* **—microscopy** (my-**kros**-kŏ-pi) *n.*

microscopic (my-krŏ-**skop**-ik) *adj.* **1.** too small to be seen clearly without the use of a microscope. **2.** of, relating to, or using a microscope.

Microsporum (my-kroh-**spor**-ŭm) *n.* a genus of fungi causing tinea (ringworm). *See also* dermatophyte.

microsurgery (my-kroh-**ser**-jer-i) *n.* the branch of surgery in which extremely intricate operations are performed through highly refined operating microscopes using miniaturized precision instruments. The technique enables surgery of previously inaccessible parts of the eye, inner ear, spinal cord, and brain.

microtia (my-**kroh**-tiă) *n.* a congenital deformity of the external ear in which the pinna is small or absent. The ear canal may also be absent, giving a conductive deafness.

microtome (**my**-krŏ-tohm) *n.* an instrument for cutting extremely thin slices of material that can be examined under a microscope.

microvascular (my-kroh-**vas**-kew-ler) *adj.* involving small vessels. The term is often applied to techniques of microsurgery for reuniting small blood vessels (the same techniques are applied frequently to nerve suture).

microwave therapy (**my**-kroh-wayv) *n.* a form of diathermy using electromagnetic waves of extremely short wavelength.

micturating cystourethrogram (MCU) (**mik**-tewr-ayt-ing sist-oh-yoor-**ee**-throh-gram) *n.* an X-ray recording of the bladder and urethra taken during the voiding of water-soluble contrast material that has been previously inserted into the bladder. It demonstrates disorders of micturition.

micturition (mik-tewr-**ish**-ŏn) *n.* *see* urination.

midazolam (mid-**az**-oh-lam) *n.* a benzodiazepine drug used as a sedative before and after surgery and to induce general anaesthesia. It is administered by injection or buccal application. Trade names: **Buccolam**, **Hypnovel**.

midbrain (mesencephalon) (**mid**-brayn) *n.* the small portion of the brainstem, excluding the pons and the medulla, that joins the hindbrain to the forebrain.

middle ear (tympanic cavity) (**mi**-d'l) *n.* the air-filled part of the ear that transmits vibrations from the eardrum to the inner ear via three small bones (*see* ossicle). It is connected to the pharynx by the Eustachian tube.

midgut (**mid**-gut) *n.* the middle portion of the embryonic gut, which gives rise to most of the small intestine and part of the large intestine.

midstream specimen of urine (MSU) (**mid**-streem) *n.* a specimen of urine that is subjected to examination for the presence of microorganisms. In order to obtain a specimen that is free of contamination, the periurethral area is cleansed and the patient is requested to discard the initial flow of urine before collecting the specimen in a sterile container.

midwife (**mid**-wyf) *n.* (in Britain) a health-care professional who, having undertaken a three-year period of study, is qualified to provide advice, care, and support for women and their families during the antenatal, intranatal, and postnatal periods. Midwives work in a variety of care settings. *See also* community midwife. **—midwifery** (mid-**wif**-ri) *n.*

mifepristone (mi-**fep**-ris-tohn) *n.* a drug used to produce a medical abortion; it acts by blocking the action of progesterone, which is essential for maintaining pregnancy. It is taken by mouth, followed after 36–48 hours by gemeprost intravaginally. Trade name: **Mifegyne**.

migraine (**mee**-grayn) *n.* a neurovascular disorder in a genetically predisposed individual in which an instability in the brainstem is triggered by a variety of stimuli (e.g. foods, light, stress). This results in a recurrent throbbing headache that characteristically affects one side of the head. The headache is often accompanied by prostration, nausea and vomiting, and photophobia. The patient sometimes has forewarning of an attack (*see* aura). **—migrainous** *adj.*

Mikulicz's disease (**mik**-oo-lich-iz) *n.* swelling of the lacrimal and salivary glands as a result of infiltration with lymphoid tissue. [J. von Mikulicz Radecki (1850–1905), Polish surgeon]

Milan criteria (mi-**lan**) *pl. n.* criteria used to select patients with cirrhosis and hepatoma for liver transplantation. Transplantation can be considered if patients have a single tumour under 5 cm in size or no more than three tumours that are less than 3 cm in size and show no evidence of extrahepatic symptoms and no vascular invasion.

mild cognitive impairment (MCI) *n.* cognitive impairment beyond that expected for age that does not interfere with normal daily function. When memory loss is the predominant symptom, it is termed **amnestic MCI** and is frequently seen as an early stage of Alzheimer's disease.

miliaria rubra (mili-**air**-iă **roo**-bră) *n. see* prickly heat.

miliary (**mil**-yer-i) *adj.* describing or characterized by very small nodules or lesions, resembling millet seed. **m. tuberculosis** *see* tuberculosis.

milium (**mil**-iŭm) *n.* (*pl.* **milia**) a white nodule in the skin, particularly on the face. Up to 2 mm in diameter, milia are tiny keratin cysts occurring just beneath the epidermis. Milia are commonly seen in newborn babies around the nose; they may disappear without active treatment.

milk (milk) *n.* the liquid food secreted by female mammals from the mammary gland. Milk is a complete food in that it has most of the nutrients necessary for life: protein, carbohydrate, fat, minerals, and vitamins. Cows' milk is comparatively deficient in vitamins C and D. Human milk contains more sugar (lactose) and less protein than cows' milk.

milk rash *n.* a spotty red facial rash that is common during the first few months of life; it disappears without treatment.

milk sugar *n.* *see* lactose.

milk teeth *pl. n.* the primary teeth of children. *See* dentition.

Miller-Abbott tube (**mil**-er **ab**-ŏt) *n.* a double-channel rubber tube used to relieve obstruction of the small intestine. One channel terminates in a balloon that is inflated when the tube reaches the duodenum; the other is used for suction of the obstructing material. [T. G. Miller (1886–1981) and W. O. Abbott (1902–43), US physicians]

milli- *prefix denoting* one thousandth part.

milliampere (milliamp) (mili-**am**-pair) *n.* one thousandth of an ampere (10^{-3} A). Symbol: mA.

milligram (**mil**-i-gram) *n.* one thousandth of a gram. Symbol: mg.

millilitre (**mil**-i-lee-ter) *n.* one thousandth of a litre. Symbol: ml.

millimetre (**mil**-i-mee-ter) *n.* one thousandth of a metre (10^{-3} m). Symbol: mm.

millimole (**mil**-i-mohl) *n.* one thousandth of a mole (*see* mole[1]). The concentration of a solution is expressed in millimoles per litre. Symbol: mmol.

Milroy's disease (**mil**-roiz) *n.* congenital lymphoedema of the legs. *See* lymphoedema. [W. F. Milroy (1855–1942), US physician]

Milton (**mil**-tŏn) *n. Trademark.* a solution of sodium hypochlorite, used especially for sterilizing babies' feeding bottles.

mineralocorticoid (min-er-ăl-oh-**kor**-ti-koid) *n.* any of a group of corticosteroids, such as aldosterone, that are necessary for the regulation of salt and water balance.

miner's elbow (**my**-nerz) *n.* inflammation of the bursa over the elbow, caused by pressure on the olecranon process.

minim (**min**-im) *n.* a unit of volume used in pharmacy, equivalent to one sixtieth part of a fluid drachm.

minimally conscious state (MCS) *n.* a disorder of consciousness distinct from persistent vegetative state (PVS) and locked-in syndrome (*see* vegetative state). Patients with MCS have partial preservation of conscious awareness although the level of awareness frequently fluctuates over time.

minimally invasive surgery (minimal-access surgery) (**min**-i-măli) *n.* surgical intervention involving the least possible physical trauma to the patient, particularly surgery performed using an operating laparoscope or other endoscope (*see* laparoscopy) passed through tiny incisions; it is known popularly as **keyhole surgery**. Several types of abdominal surgery, including gall bladder removal (*see* cholecystectomy), are now commonly performed in this way.

SEE WEB LINKS

- Explanation of minimally invasive surgery from the Patient.co website

Mini-Mental State Examination (MMSE) *n.* a 30-point questionnaire used to screen for cognitive impairment in the diagnosis of dementia. It is also used to estimate the severity of any impairment and to document response to treatment. It tests functions including arithmetic, memory, and orientation.

Mini Nutritional Assessment (MNA) *n.* a validated nutritional screening tool that enables the identification of malnourishment or the risk of malnourishment in elderly patients. It can be used in a variety of settings and reviews appetite, weight loss, mobility, neuropsychological problems, and body mass index, allocating a score to indicate potential risk status.

minitracheostomy (min-i-tray-ki-**ost**-ŏmi) *n.* temporary tracheostomy using a needle or fine-bore tube inserted through the skin.

minocycline (min-oh-**sy**-kleen) *n.* a tetracycline antibiotic active against a wide range of bacteria, including *Chlamydia*, meningococcus, rickettsiae, and mycoplasmas. It is administered by mouth. Trade names: **Acnamino MR**, **Minocin MR**, **Sebomin MR**.

minoxidil (min-**oks**-i-dil) *n.* a peripheral vasodilator used in the treatment of high blood pressure (hypertension) when other drugs are not effective; it is administered by mouth in conjunction with a diuretic and a beta blocker. It is also applied to the scalp, in the form of a solution, to restore hair growth. Trade names: **Loniten**, **Regaine**.

mio- *combining form denoting* **1.** reduction or diminution. **2.** rudimentary.

miosis (myosis) (my-**oh**-sis) *n.* constriction of the pupil. This occurs in bright light (normally) and in Horner's syndrome, but persistent miosis is most commonly caused by certain types of eye drops used to treat glaucoma. *See also* miotic. *Compare* mydriasis.

miotic (myotic) (my-**ot**-ik) *n.* **1.** a drug, such as pilocarpine, that causes the pupil of the eye to contract by constricting the ciliary muscle. **2.** *adj.* showing miosis.

miscarriage (mis-**ka**-rij) *n.* spontaneous loss of pregnancy before 24 weeks, formerly known as **spontaneous abortion**. **complete m.** miscarriage in which the cervix has closed and ultrasound scanning shows an empty uterus. **incomplete m.** miscarriage in which some fetal tissue remains in the uterus and the cervix is open. **inevitable m.** vaginal bleeding associated with crampy pelvic pain and a closed cervix, which precedes expulsion of the fetus from the uterus. **late m.** miscarriage occurring after 20–24 weeks. **recurrent m.** the loss of three or more pregnancies consecutively. **silent** (or **missed**) **m.** failure of a nonviable fetus to be expelled from the uterus.

miso- *combining form denoting* hatred.

misophonia (mis-oh-**foh**-niă) *n.* dislike of or aversion to particular sounds, irrespective of the level of that sound. *See* hyperacusis, phonophobia.

misoprostol (mis-**op**-rŏ-stol) *n.* a prostaglandin drug administered by mouth for the prevention and treatment of peptic ulcer, especially when caused by nonsteroidal anti-inflammatory drugs (*see* NSAID). Trade name: **Cytotec**.

Misuse of Drugs Act 1971 *n.* (in the UK) an Act of Parliament that, together with the Misuse of Drugs Regulations 2001, restricts the prescription, dispensing, sale, and possession of dangerous drugs. These **controlled drugs** include the natural opiates and their synthetic substitutes, cocaine, and LSD (class A drugs), amphetamines, barbiturates, and cannabis (class B drugs), and most benzodiazepines (class C drugs).

mite (myt) *n.* a free-living or parasitic arthropod belonging to a group (Acarina) that also includes the ticks. Medically important mites include the many species causing dermatitis. **house-dust m.** a mite of the genus *Dermatophagoides*, the waste products of which produce an allergic response in susceptible people that is an important trigger for some forms of rhinitis and asthma.

mitochondrion (my-toh-**kon**-dri-ŏn) *n.* (*pl.* **mitochondria**) a structure, occurring in varying numbers in the cytoplasm of every cell, that is the site of the cell's energy production. Mitochondria contain ATP and the enzymes involved in the cell's metabolic activities, and also their own DNA; mitochondrial genes are inherited through the female line. **—mitochondrial** *adj.*

mitomycin (my-toh-**my**-sin) *n.* an anthracycline antibiotic that inhibits the growth of cancer cells. It causes severe marrow suppression but is of use in the treatment of stomach, breast, and bladder cancers. It is administered by intravenous injection or by bladder instillation. Trade name: **Mitomycin C Kyowa**.

mitosis (my-**toh**-sis) *n.* a type of cell division in which a single cell produces two genetically identical daughter cells. It is the way in which new body cells are produced for both growth and repair. *Compare* meiosis. **—mitotic** (my-**tot**-ik) *adj.*

mitoxantrone (mi-**toks**-an-trohn) *n.* an anthracycline antibiotic given by intravenous infusion in the treatment of certain cancers, including metastatic breast cancer, leukaemia, and non-Hodgkin's lymphoma. Trade name: **Onkotrone**.

mitral regurgitation (mitral incompetence) (**my**-trăl) *n.* failure of the mitral valve to close, allowing a reflux of blood from the left ventricle of the heart to the left atrium. Its manifestations include breathlessness, atrial fibrillation, embolism, enlargement of the left ventricle, and a systolic murmur.

mitral stenosis *n.* narrowing of the opening of the mitral valve: a result of chronic scarring that follows rheumatic fever. Mild cases need no treatment, but severe cases are treated by reopening the stenosis or by inserting an artificial valve (**mitral prosthesis**).

mitral valve (bicuspid valve) *n.* a valve in the heart consisting of two cusps attached to the walls at the opening between the left atrium and left ventricle. It allows blood to pass from the atrium to the ventricle, but prevents any backward flow.

mittelschmerz (**mit**-ĕl-shmairts) *n.* pain in the lower abdomen experienced about midway between successive menstrual periods, i.e. at ovulation.

ml *symbol for* millilitre.

MLD *n.* minimal lethal dose: the smallest quantity of a toxic compound that is recorded as having caused death.

MMR vaccine *n.* a combined vaccine against measles, mumps, and German measles (rubella). It is currently recommended that this vaccine is given to all children at 13 months of age, with a subsequent booster dose. See Appendix 8: Immunization schedules.

MMSE *n. see* Mini-Mental State Examination.

MNA *n. see* Mini Nutritional Assessment.

MND *n. see* motor neuron disease.

Mobitz type I and type II (**moh**-bitz) *pl. n.* types of abnormality on an electrocardiogram (ECG) tracing that indicate forms of heart block. [W. Mobitz (20th century), German cardiologist]

moclobemide (mok-**loh**-bi-myd) *n.* an antidepressant drug that reversibly inhibits the enzyme monoamine oxidase A. It is less likely to cause the adverse effects associated with irreversible MAO inhibitors. Trade name: **Manerix**.

modality (moh-**dal**-iti) *n.* **1.** a form of sensation, such as smell, hearing, tasting, or detecting temperature. **2.** one form of therapy as opposed to another, such as the modality of physiotherapy contrasted with that of radiotherapy.

mode (mohd) *n.* (in statistics) the observation (or group of observations when these occur as a continuous quantitative variable) that occurs most often in a series of observations. *Compare* mean.

Modecate (**mod**-i-kayt) *n. see* fluphenazine.

modelling (**mod**-ĕl-ing) *n.* **1.** a technique used in behaviour modification, whereby an individual learns a behaviour by observing someone else doing it. **2.** An element of normal social learning and development whereby children learn through emulating other people's behaviour.

modified early warning score (MEWS) (**mod**-i-fId) *see* national early warning score.

modiolus (moh-**dy**-oh-lŭs) *n.* the conical central pillar of the cochlea in the inner ear.

MODS *n. see* multiple organ dysfunction syndrome.

MODY *n. see* maturity-onset diabetes of the young.

MOF *n. see* multi-organ failure.

Mogadon (mog-ă-don) *n. see* nitrazepam.

molar (**moh**-ler) *n.* the fourth or fifth tooth (in the primary dentition) or the sixth, seventh, or eighth tooth (in the permanent dentition) from the midline on each side of each jaw. *See also* dentition.

molarity (mol-a-ri-ti) *n.* the strength of a solution, expressed as the weight of dissolved substance in grams per litre divided by its molecular weight, i.e. the number of moles per litre.

mole[1] (mohl) *n.* the SI unit of amount of substance. One mole of a compound has a mass equal to its molecular weight expressed in grams. Symbol: mol.

mole[2] *n.* a nonmalignant collection of pigmented cells in the skin. Moles vary widely in appearance, being flat or raised, smooth or hairy. Changes in the shape, colour, etc., of moles in adult life may be an early sign of malignant melanoma. Medical name: **pigmented naevus**.

molecular biology (mŏ-**lek**-yoo-ler) *n.* the study of the molecules that are associated with living organisms, especially proteins and nucleic acids.

molecule (**mol**-i-kewl) *n.* a particle consisting of two or more atoms held together by chemical bonds. It is the smallest unit of an element or compound capable of existing independently. **—molecular** *adj.*

molluscum contagiosum (mol-**usk**-ŭm kon-ta-**joh**-sŭm) *n.* a common disease of the skin, mainly affecting children. Characterized by papules less than 5 mm in diameter, each with a central depression, the disease is caused by a poxvirus and is spread by direct contact. Untreated, the papules generally disappear in 6–9 months. Widespread disease in adults may be a sign of HIV infection.

mon- (mono-) *combining form denoting* one, single, or alone.

Mongolian blue spots (mong-**oh**-liăn) *pl. n.* blue-black pigmented areas seen at the base of the back and on the buttocks of babies. They are more common in dark-skinned babies and usually fade during the first year of life.

Monilia (moh-**nil**-iă) *n.* the former name of the genus of yeasts now known as *Candida*.

moniliasis (mon-i-**ly**-ă-sis) *n.* an obsolete name for candidiasis.

Monitor (**mon**-i-ter) *n. see* quality assurance (tool).

monitoring (**mon**-i-ter-ing) *n.* the periodic observation of a patient's condition, which may be by visual, manual, or electronic means.

monoamine oxidase (MAO) (mon-oh-**ay**-meen) *n.* either of two enzymes, MAO A and MAO B, that catalyse the oxidation of a large variety of monoamines, including noradrenaline and serotonin (MAO A) and dopamine (MAO B). Monoamine oxidase is found in most tissues, particularly the gastrointestinal and nervous systems. *See also* MAO inhibitor.

monoblast (**mon**-oh-blast) *n.* the earliest identifiable cell that gives rise to a monocyte. It is normally found in the blood-forming tissue of the bone marrow but may appear in the blood in certain diseases, most notably in **acute monoblastic leukaemia**.

monochromat (mon-oh-**kroh**-mat) *n.* a person who is completely colour-blind. The condition is probably inherited.

monochromatic (mon-oh-krŏ-**mat**-ik) *adj.* denoting radiation, especially light, of the same frequency or wavelength.

monoclonal antibody (mon-oh-**kloh**-năl) *n.* an antibody produced artificially from a cell clone and therefore consisting of a single type of immunoglobulin. Monoclonal antibodies are used in research, are valuable diagnostic tools, and have been developed as pharmaceutical agents for treating a variety of conditions, including some cancers.

monocular (mon-**ok**-yoo-ler) *adj.* relating to or used by one eye only. *Compare* binocular.

monocyte (**mon**-oh-syt) *n.* a variety of white blood cell with a kidney-shaped nucleus. Its function is the ingestion of foreign particles, such as bacteria and tissue debris. **—monocytic** *adj.*

monocytosis (mon-oh-sy-**toh**-sis) *n.* an increase in the number of monocytes in the blood. Monocytosis occurs in a variety of diseases, including monocytic leukaemias.

monodactylism (mon-oh-**dak**-til-izm) *n.* the congenital absence of all but one digit on each hand and foot.

monomania (mon-oh-**may**-niă) *n.* the state in which a particular delusion or set of delusions is present in an otherwise normally functioning person. *See also* paranoia.

mononeuritis (mon-oh-newr-**I**-tis) *n.* disease affecting a single peripheral nerve. *See* (peripheral) neuropathy.

mononuclear (mon-oh-**new**-kli-er) *adj.* (of a cell) having one nucleus.

mononucleosis (mon-oh-new-kli-**oh**-sis) *n.* the condition in which the blood contains an abnormally high number of mononuclear leucocytes (monocytes and lymphocytes). *See* glandular fever (infectious mononucleosis).

monoplegia (mon-oh-**plee**-jiă) *n.* paralysis of one limb. **—monoplegic** *adj.*

monoploid (**mon**-ŏ-ploid) *adj. see* haploid.

monorchism (**mon**-or-kizm) *n.* the absence of one testis. This is usually due to failure of one testicle to descend into the scrotum before birth.

monosaccharide (mon-oh-**sak**-ă-ryd) *n.* a simple sugar having the general formula $(CH_2O)_n$. The most abundant monosaccharide is glucose.

monosomy (**mon**-ŏ-soh-mi) *n.* a condition in which there is one chromosome missing from the normal (diploid) set. *Compare* trisomy. **—monosomic** *adj.*

monozygotic twins (mon-oh-zy-**got**-ik) *pl. n. see* twins.

mons (monz) *n.* (in anatomy) a rounded eminence. **m. pubis** the mound of fatty tissue lying over the pubic symphysis.

montelukast (mon-ti-**loo**-kăst) *n.* *see* leukotriene receptor antagonist.

Montgomery's glands (mŏnt-**gom**-er-iz) *pl. n.* sebaceous glands on the areola surrounding the nipple of a woman's breast. They enlarge during pregnancy and their secretions lubricate and protect the breast during breast feeding. [W. F. Montgomery (1797–1859), Irish obstetrician]

mood disorder (mood) *n.* *see* affective disorder.

mood stabilizer (**stay**-bi-lyz-er) *n.* a drug used in the treatment of bipolar affective disorder to reduce the severity of manic and depressive episodes. Mood stabilizers include lithium and antiepileptics.

Mooren's ulcer (**moor**-ĕnz) *n.* a rare chronic progressive ulceration of the cornea, occurring in the elderly. It is typically very painful and difficult to control. [A. Mooren (1829–99), German ophthalmologist]

morbid (**mor**-bid) *adj.* diseased or abnormal; pathological.

morbidity (mor-**bid**-iti) *n.* the state of being ill or having a disease.

morbilli (mor-**bil**-I) *n.* *see* measles.

morbilliform (mor-**bil**-i-form) *adj.* describing a skin rash resembling that of measles. A morbilliform rash is usually caused by viral infection, medications, or both.

morbus (**mor**-bŭs) *n.* disease. The term is usually used as part of the medical name of a specific disease.

moribund (**mo**-ri-bund) *adj.* dying.

morning sickness (**mor**-ning) *n.* nausea and vomiting during early pregnancy. *Compare* hyperemesis (gravidarum).

Moro reflex (startle reflex) (**moh**-roh) *n.* the normal reaction of a newborn baby to a sudden loud noise. The infant flings its arms and legs wide and appears to stiffen; the limbs are then drawn back into flexion. [E. Moro (1874–1951), German paediatrician]

morphine (**mor**-feen) *n.* a potent analgesic (*see* opiate) administered by mouth, injection, or in suppositories to relieve severe and persistent pain, particularly in terminally ill patients; it also induces feelings of euphoria. Trade names: **Morphgesic SR**, **Oramorph**, **Sevredol**, **Zomorph**, etc.

morpho- *combining form denoting* form or structure.

morphoea (mor-**fee**-ă) *n.* a localized form of scleroderma characterized by firm ivory-coloured waxy plaques in the skin without any internal sclerosis.

morphogenesis (mor-foh-**jen**-i-sis) *n.* the development of form and structure of the body and its parts.

morphology (mor-**fol**-ŏji) *n.* the study of differences in form between species.

-morphous *combining form denoting* form or structure (of a specified kind).

Morquio-Brailsford disease (mor-**kee**-oh **braylz**-ferd) *n.* a defect of mucopolysaccharide metabolism that causes dwarfism with a kyphosis, knock-knee, and an angulated sternum. Intelligence is normal. [L. Morquio (1867–1935), Uruguayan physician; J. F. Brailsford (20th century), British radiologist]

Morse fall scale (morss) *n.* a systematic tool that can be used to assess a patient's risk of falling. It reviews six areas, each accorded a score, including history of recent falls, mental status, and the use of aids to assist mobility. The higher the score, the greater the risk of falling.

mortality rate (mor-**tal**-iti) *n.* the incidence of death in the population in a given period. **annual m. r.** the number of registered deaths in a year, multiplied by 1000 and divided by the population at the middle of the year. *See also* infant (mortality rate), maternal mortality rate.

mortification (mor-ti-fi-**kay**-shŏn) *n. see* necrosis.

morula (**mo**-roo-lă) *n.* an early stage of embryonic development formed by cleavage of the fertilized ovum. It consists of a solid ball of cells and is an intermediate stage between the zygote and blastocyst.

mosaicism (mŏ-**zay**-i-sizm) *n.* a condition in which the cells of an individual do not all contain identical chromosomes; there may be two or more genetically different populations of cells. **—mosaic** *adj.*

mosquito (mos-**kee**-toh) *n.* a small winged bloodsucking insect belonging to a large group – the Diptera. Female mosquitoes transmit the parasites responsible for several major infectious diseases, such as malaria. The mosquito-borne zika virus has recently been shown to cause microcephaly. The mosquito-borne zika virus has recently been shown to cause microcephaly. *See* Aëdes, Anopheles.

motile (**moh**-tyl) *adj.* being able to move spontaneously, without external aid: usually applied to a microorganism or a cell.

motilin (**moh**-til-in) *n.* a polypeptide hormone, secreted in the small intestine, that controls smooth muscle contractions in the stomach and small intestine, increasing gut motility and promoting the production of pepsin.

motions (**moh**-shŏnz) *pl. n.* the products of bowel evacuation.

motion sickness (travel sickness) (**moh**-shŏn) *n.* nausea, vomiting, and headache caused by motion during travel by sea, road, or air. The symptoms are due to overstimulation of the balance organs in the inner ear. Sedative antihistamine drugs are used for prevention and treatment.

motor cortex (**moh**-ter) *n.* the region of the cerebral cortex that is responsible for initiating nerve impulses that bring about voluntary activity in the muscles of the body.

motor nerve *n. see* nerve.

motor neuron (motor neurone) *n.* one of the units (neurons) that goes to make up the nerve pathway between the brain and an effector organ, such as a skeletal muscle. **lower m. n.** a motor neuron that has a cell body in the spinal cord or brainstem and an axon that extends outwards to reach an effector. **upper m. n.** a motor neuron that has a cell body in the brain and an axon that extends into the spinal cord, where it ends in synapses.

motor neuron disease (motor neurone disease, MND) *n.* a progressive degenerative disease of the motor system occurring in middle age and causing muscle weakness and wasting. It primarily affects the cells of the anterior horn of the spinal cord, the motor nuclei in the brainstem, and the corticospinal fibres. Some forms of the disease are familial (inherited).

mould (mohld) *n.* any multicellular filamentous fungus that commonly forms a rough furry coating on decaying matter.

moulding (mohld-ing) *n.* the changing of the shape of an infant's head during labour, due to movement of the bones of the skull, brought about by the pressures to which it is subjected when passing through the birth canal.

mountain sickness (mownt-in) *n. see* altitude sickness.

mouth-to-mouth resuscitation (mowth) *n.* emergency artificial respiration, performed mouth-to-mouth, by blowing air into the victim's lungs to inflate them, while the nostrils are pinched shut, and then allowing exhalation to occur automatically. It is commonly known as the **kiss of life**.

mouthwash (mowth-wosh) *n.* an aqueous solution used for rinsing of the mouth and teeth. **m. test** a test for detecting carriers of single-gene defects (e.g. cystic fibrosis) in which cells from the buccal cavity are obtained from a saline mouthwash and their DNA is isolated and genetically analysed.

MPQ *n. see* McGill Pain Questionnaire.

MR *n.* magnetic resonance: relating to magnetic resonance imaging, as in **MR scan**.

MRI *n. see* magnetic resonance imaging.

MRSA *n.* meticillin- or multiple-resistant *Staphylococcus aureus*: an increasingly common dangerous bacterium that is resistant to many antibiotics and is responsible for many infections in already ill people in hospitals. **community-associated MRSA (CA-MRSA)** infections, especially skin infections, caused by MRSA outside the hospital environment.

SEE WEB LINKS

- Overview of MRSA from the NHS Choices website

MS *n. see* multiple sclerosis.

MSA *n. see* multiple system atrophy.

MSH *n. see* melanocyte-stimulating hormone.

MSP *n. see* Munchausen's syndrome (by proxy).

MSU *n. see* midstream specimen of urine.

mucilage (mew-si-lij) *n.* (in pharmacy) a thick aqueous solution of a gum used as a lubricant in skin preparations, for the production of pills, and for the suspension of insoluble substances.

mucin (mew-sin) *n.* the principal constituent of mucus. Mucin is a glycoprotein.

muco- *combining form denoting* **1.** mucus. **2.** mucous membrane.

mucociliary transport (mew-koh-**sil**-i-er-i) *n.* the process by which cilia move a thin film of mucus from the upper and lower respiratory tracts towards the digestive tract. Particles of dust and microorganisms are trapped on the mucus and thereby removed from the respiratory tract.

mucocoele (**mew**-koh-seel) *n.* a space or organ distended with mucus. It may occur in the gall bladder when the exit duct becomes obstructed.

mucocutaneous (mew-koh-kew-**tay**-niŭs) *adj.* relating to or affecting mucous membrane and skin.

mucoid (**mew**-koid) *adj.* resembling mucus.

mucolytic (mew-koh-**lit**-ik) *n.* an agent, such as dornase alfa (*see* DNAse), that breaks down mucus in sputum, making it easier to cough up. Mucolytics are used to treat chest conditions involving excessive or thickened mucus secretions.

mucopolysaccharide (mew-koh-poli-**sak**-er-yd) *n.* one of a group of complex carbohydrates functioning mainly as structural components in connective tissue.

mucopolysaccharidosis (mew-koh-poli-sak-er-I-**doh**-sis) *n.* any one of a group of rare inborn errors of metabolism in which the storage of complex carbohydrates is disordered. *See* Hunter's syndrome, Hurler's syndrome.

mucoprotein (mew-koh-**proh**-teen) *n.* one of a group of proteins found in the globulin fraction of blood plasma. Mucoproteins are globulins combined with a carbohydrate group (an amino sugar).

mucopurulent (mew-koh-**pewr**-oo-lĕnt) *adj.* containing mucus and pus. *See* mucopus.

mucopus (**mew**-koh-pus) *n.* a mixture of mucus and pus.

mucosa (mew-**koh**-să) *n. see* mucous membrane. **—mucosal** *adj.*

mucous membrane (mucosa) (**mew**-kŭs) *n.* the moist membrane lining many tubular structures and cavities, including the nasal sinuses, respiratory tract, gastrointestinal tract, biliary, and pancreatic systems. The surface layer of the membrane contains glands that secrete mucus.

mucoviscidosis (mew-koh-vis-i-**doh**-sis) *n. see* cystic fibrosis.

mucus (**mew**-kŭs) *n.* a viscous fluid secreted by mucous membranes. Mucus acts as a protective barrier over the surfaces of the membranes, as a lubricant, and as a carrier of enzymes. **—mucous** *adj.*

MUGA scan (multiple-gated acquisition scan) (**mug**-ă) *n.* a technique used in nuclear medicine for studying left ventricular function and wall motion of the heart by injecting the patient's red cells with radioactive technetium-99m to form an image of the blood pool within the heart at specific points in the cardiac cycle, using an ECG, gamma camera, and computer.

Müllerian duct (paramesonephric duct) (mew-**leer**-iăn) *n.* either of a pair of ducts in the embryo that in females develop into the Fallopian tubes, uterus, and part of the vagina. [J. P. Müller (1801–58), German physiologist]

multi- *prefix denoting* many; several.

multidisciplinary team (MDT) (multi-dis-i-**plin**-ări) *n.* a group of health-care professionals with different areas of expertise who unite to plan and carry out treatment of complex medical conditions. *See also* integrated care pathway.

multifactorial (multi-fak-**tor**-iăl) *adj.* describing a condition, such as spina bifida, that is believed to have resulted from the interaction of genetic factors, usually polygenes, with an environmental factor or factors.

multifocal lens (multi-**foh**-kăl) *n.* a lens containing more than one segment made to different prescriptions for visual correction. *See also* bifocal lens.

multigravida (multi-**grav**-id-ă) *n.* a woman who has been pregnant at least twice.

multi-organ failure (multiple-organ failure, **MOF**) (multi-**or**-găn) *n.* the terminal stage of serious illness.

multipara (mul-**tip**-er-ă) *n.* a woman who has given birth to a live child after each of at least two pregnancies. *See also* grand multiparity.

multiple myeloma (**mul**-ti-pŭl) *n. see* myeloma.

multiple organ dysfunction syndrome (MODS) *n.* a common cause of death following severe injury, overwhelming infection, or immune deficiency states.

multiple personality disorder *n.* a controversial psychiatric disorder (the vast majority of psychiatrists deny its existence) in which the affected person is alleged to have two or more distinct, and often contrasting, personalities. As each personality assumes dominance, it determines attitudes and behaviour and usually appears to be unaware of the other personality (or personalities).

multiple sclerosis (MS, disseminated sclerosis) *n.* a chronic disease of the nervous system affecting young and middle-aged adults. The myelin sheaths surrounding nerves in the brain and spinal cord are damaged, which affects the function of the nerves involved. The course of the illness is usually characterized by recurrent relapses followed by remissions but a proportion of patients run a chronic progressive course. Symptoms include ataxia, abnormal eye movements (e.g. nystagmus), dysarthria, spastic weakness, and retrobulbar neuritis.

SEE WEB LINKS

- Website of the Multiple Sclerosis Society

multiple system atrophy (MSA) *n.* a condition that results from degeneration of cells in the basal ganglia (resulting in parkinsonism), the cerebellum (resulting in ataxia), the pyramidal system, and the autonomic nervous system.

multisystem (multi-**sis**-tĕm) *adj.* describing a disease that affects many systems of the body.

mummification (mum-i-fi-**kay**-shŏn) *n.* the conversion of dead tissue into a hard shrunken mass, chiefly by dehydration.

mumps (mumps) *n.* a common virus infection mainly affecting children. Symptoms appear 2–3 weeks after exposure: fever, headache, and vomiting may precede a typical swelling of the parotid salivary glands. The infection may spread to other salivary glands and to the pancreas, brain, and testicles (*see* orchitis). *See also* MMR vaccine. Medical name: **infectious parotitis**.

Munchausen's syndrome (**muunch**-how-zĕnz) *n.* a very rare mental disorder in which the patient persistently feigns symptoms in order to obtain invasive hospital treatment, especially surgery. **M. s. by proxy (MSP)** a condition in which the patient (usually a mother) presents false health information about her child or inflicts harm on the child in order to attract medical attention. [Baron von Munchausen, a fictional character who told exaggerated stories]

murmur (**mer**-mer) *n.* a noise, heard with the aid of a stethoscope, that is generated by turbulent blood flow within the heart or blood vessels produced by damaged valves, septal defects, narrowed arteries, or arteriovenous communications. **continuous m.** murmur heard throughout systole and diastole. **diastolic m.** murmur heard during diastole. **innocent m.** heart murmur heard in normal individuals. **systolic m.** murmur heard during systole.

Murphy's sign (**mer**-fiz) *n.* an indication of an inflamed gall bladder: continuous pressure over the gall bladder while the patient is taking a deep breath will cause pain at the peak of inhalation. [J. B. Murphy (1857–1916), US surgeon]

muscae volitantes (**mus**-kee vol-i-**tan**-teez) *pl. n. see* floaters.

muscarine (**musk**-er-in) *n.* a highly poisonous alkaloid occurring in certain mushrooms, such as fly agaric (*Amanita muscaria*).

muscle (**mus**-ŭl) *n.* a tissue whose cells have the ability to contract, producing movement or force. The major functions of muscles are to produce movements of the body and of structures within it and to alter pressures or tensions of internal organs. There are three types of muscle (*see* cardiac muscle, smooth muscle, striated muscle). See illustration. **—muscular** (**mus**-kew-ler) *adj.*

muscle relaxant *n.* an agent that reduces tension in voluntary muscles. Drugs such as baclofen and diazepam are used to relieve skeletal muscular spasms. Other drugs, e.g. atracurium besilate and suxamethonium, are used to relax voluntary muscles during the administration of anaesthetics in surgical operations.

muscular dystrophy *n.* a group of muscle diseases, marked by weakness and wasting of selected muscles, in which there is a recognizable pattern of inheritance. The affected muscle fibres degenerate and are replaced by fatty tissue. The most common form is **Duchenne muscular dystrophy**, which is nearly always restricted

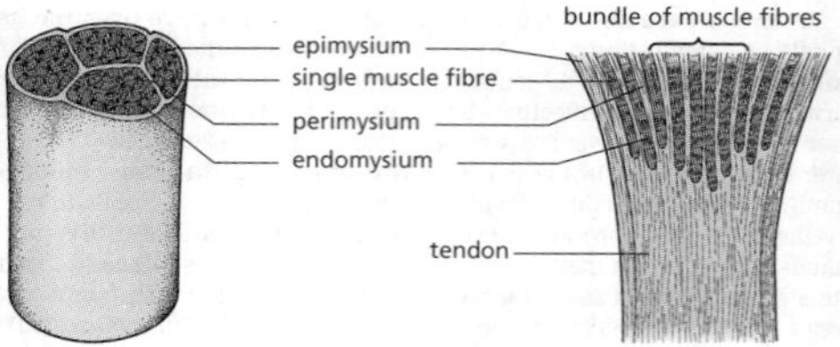

A voluntary muscle in transverse section (left) and in longitudinal section at its junction with a tendon (right)

to boys and usually begins before the age of four. The child has a waddling gait and lordosis of the lumbar spine. The calf muscles – and later the shoulders and upper limbs – often become firm and bulky. *See also* Becker muscular dystrophy, dystrophia myotonica (myotonic dystrophy).

muscularis (mus-kew-**lar**-is) *n.* a muscular layer of the wall of a hollow organ (such as the stomach) or a tubular structure (such as the ureter or intestine).

musculo- *combining form denoting* muscle.

musculocutaneous nerve (mus-kew-loh-kew-**tay**-niŭs) *n.* a nerve of the brachial plexus that supplies some muscles of the arm and the skin of the lateral part of the forearm.

musculoskeletal (mus-kew-loh-**skel**-i-t'l) *adj.* relating to both the muscles and the bones.

mushroom (**mush**-room) *n.* the spore-producing body of various fungi. Great care must be taken in identifying edible mushrooms, as many species are poisonous, including *Amanita phalloides* (death cap) and *A. muscaria* (fly agaric).

MUST (malnutrition universal screening tool) *n.* a screening tool that can be applied to the care of adult patients to identify the potential risks of under- or over-nutrition through the use of a check list. It promotes multidisciplinary working and reflects key initiatives in UK practice. Its use is recommended by NICE (2006).

mutant (mew-tănt) *adj.* affected by or showing the effects of a mutation. **—mutant** *n.*

mutation (mew-**tay**-shŏn) *n.* a change in the amount or structure of the genetic material (DNA) of a cell, or the change this causes in a characteristic of the individual. A mutation affecting developing sex cells can be inherited. Mutations may occur spontaneously or be caused by external agents (e.g. radiation or certain viruses).

mutism (mewt-izm) *n.* inability or refusal to speak. Innate speechlessness most commonly occurs in those who have been totally deaf since birth (**deaf m.**). Mutism may also result from brain damage (*see* aphasia) or be caused by depression, anxiety, psychosis, or psychological trauma, in which case the patient may speak only in particular situations or to particular people (**selective m.**). **—mute** *adj., n.*

my- (myo-) *combining form denoting* muscle.

myalgia (my-al-jiă) *n.* pain in the muscles. **—myalgic** (my-al-jik) *adj.*

myalgic encephalomyelitis (myalgic encephalopathy, **ME**) *n.* *see* CFS/ME/PVF.

myasthenia (my-ăs-th'ee-niă) *n.* weakness of the muscles. **m. gravis** a chronic disease marked by abnormal fatigability and weakness of selected muscles, initially those around the eyes, mouth, and throat, resulting in drooping of the upper eyelid (ptosis), double vision, dysarthria, and dysphagia. It is an autoimmune disease in which the ability of the neurotransmitter acetylcholine to induce muscular contraction is impaired. Treatment with anticholinesterase drugs and surgical removal of the thymus in patients under the age of 45 lessen the severity of the symptoms. Steroid therapy, intravenous immunoglobulins, or plasma exchange may be used to treat the more severely affected patients.

myc- (myco-, mycet(o)-) *combining form denoting* a fungus.

mycelium (my-see-liŭm) *n.* (*pl.* **mycelia**) the tangled mass of fine branching threads that make up the feeding and growing part of a fungus.

mycetoma (my-si-toh-mă) *n.* a chronic inflammation of tissues caused by a fungus. *See* Madura foot.

Mycobacterium (my-koh-bak-teer-iŭm) *n.* a genus of rodlike aerobic Gram-positive bacteria. Several species are responsible for opportunistic infections of the lung (*see* MAI complex). **M. leprae** (**Hansen's bacillus**) the species that causes leprosy. **M. tuberculosis** (**Koch's bacillus**) the species that causes tuberculosis.

mycology (my-kol-ŏji) *n.* the science of fungi. *See also* microbiology. **—mycologist** *n.*

mycoplasma (my-koh-plaz-mă) *n.* one of a group of minute non-motile bacteria that lack a rigid cell wall and hence display a variety of forms. The species *Mycoplasma pneumoniae* causes atypical pneumonia.

mycosis (my-koh-sis) *n.* any disease caused by a fungus, including actinomycosis, aspergillosis, cryptococcosis, rhinosporidiosis, ringworm, and sporotrichosis.

mycosis fungoides (fung-oid-eez) *n.* the most common form of cutaneous T-cell lymphoma, with patches, plaques, and later nodules on the skin. It progresses very slowly and can be treated with topical corticosteroids, phototherapy, radiotherapy, or other agents.

Mycota (my-**koh**-ta) *n. see* undecenoates.

mydriasis (mid-ry-ă-sis) *n.* widening of the pupil, which occurs normally in dim light. The commonest cause of prolonged mydriasis is drug therapy (*see* mydriatic) or injury to the eye. *See also* cycloplegia. *Compare* miosis.

mydriatic (mid-ri-**at**-ik) *n.* a drug, such as atropine or phenylephrine, that causes the pupil of the eye to dilate and is used to aid examination of the eye and to treat some eye inflammations.

myectomy (my-**ek**-tŏmi) *n.* a surgical operation to remove part of a muscle.

myel- (myelo-) *combining form denoting* **1.** the spinal cord. **2.** bone marrow. **3.** myelin.

myelencephalon (my-ĕl-en-**sef**-ă-lon) *n. see* medulla (oblongata).

myelin (**my**-ĕ-lin) *n.* a complex material formed of protein and phospholipid that is laid down as a sheath surrounding and insulating the axons of certain neurons, known as **myelinated** (or **medullated**) **nerve fibres**.

myelination (my-ĕ-lin-**ay**-shŏn) *n.* the process in which myelin is laid down as an insulating layer around the axons of certain nerves.

myelitis (my-ĕ-**ly**-tis) *n.* **1.** an inflammatory disease of the spinal cord. The most usual kind (**transverse m.**) most often occurs during the development of multiple sclerosis. The inflammation spreads across the tissue of the spinal cord, resulting in paralysis of the legs and lower trunk. **2.** inflammation of the bone marrow. *See* osteomyelitis.

myeloblast (**my**-ĕ-loh-blast) *n.* the earliest identifiable cell that gives rise to a granulocyte. It is normally found in the blood-forming tissue of the bone marrow, but may appear in the blood in a variety of diseases, most notably in **acute myeloblastic leukaemia**. *See also* granulopoiesis. **—myeloblastic** *adj.*

myelocele (**my**-ĕ-loh-seel) *n. see* meningomyelocele.

myelocyte (**my**-ĕ-loh-syt) *n.* an immature form of granulocyte. It is normally found in the blood-forming tissue of the bone marrow, but may appear in the blood in a variety of diseases, including infections, infiltrations of the bone marrow, and certain leukaemias. *See also* granulopoiesis.

myelofibrosis (my-ĕ-loh-fy-**broh**-sis) *n.* a chronic but progressive disease characterized by fibrosis of the bone marrow, which leads to anaemia; enlargement of the spleen; and the presence of myeloid tissue in abnormal sites, such as the spleen and liver. Its cause is unknown.

myelography (my-ĕ-**log**-răfi) *n.* a specialized method of X-ray examination to demonstrate the spinal canal that involves injection of a radiopaque contrast medium into the subarachnoid space by lumbar puncture. The X-rays obtained are called **myelograms**.

myeloid (**my**-ĕ-loid) *adj.* **1.** like, derived from, or relating to bone marrow. **m. leukaemia** a variety of leukaemia in which the type of blood cell that proliferates abnormally originates in the blood-forming tissue of the bone marrow. *See also* Philadelphia chromosome. **m. tissue** a tissue in the bone marrow in which the various classes of blood cells are produced. *See also* haemopoiesis. **2.** resembling a myelocyte. **3.** relating to the spinal cord.

myeloma (multiple myeloma, myelomatosis) (my-ĕ-**loh**-mă) *n.* a malignant disease of the bone marrow, characterized by two or more of the following: (1) the presence of an excess of abnormal malignant plasma cells in the bone marrow; (2) lytic deposits in the bones, giving the appearance of holes on X-ray; (3) the presence in the serum of an abnormal gammaglobulin, usually IgG. The patient may complain of tiredness due to anaemia and of bone pain and may develop pathological fractures. Treatment is usually with drugs, such as steroids, melphalan, cyclophosphamide, or thalidomide, withlocal radiotherapy to particular areas of pain. *See also* plasmacytoma.

myelomalacia (my-ĕ-loh-mă-**lay**-shiă) *n.* softening of the tissues of the spinal cord, most often caused by an impaired blood supply.

myelomatosis (my-ĕ-loh-mă-**toh**-sis) *n. see* myeloma.

myelomeningocele (my-ĕ-loh-min-**ing**-oh-seel) *n. see* meningomyelocele.

myelosuppression (my-ĕ-loh-sŭ-**presh**-ŏn) *n.* a reduction in blood-cell production by the bone marrow. It commonly occurs after chemotherapy and may result in anaemia, infection, and abnormal bleeding (*see* neutropenia, thrombocytopenia). **—myelosuppressive** *adj.*

myenteron (my-**en**-ter-on) *n.* the muscular layer of the intestine, consisting of a layer of circular muscle inside a layer of longitudinal muscle. These muscles are used in peristalsis. **—myenteric** (my-en-**te**-rik) *adj.*

myiasis (**my**-ă-sis) *n.* an infestation of a living organ or tissue by maggots. Treatment of external myiases involves the destruction and removal of maggots followed by the application of antibiotics to wounds and lesions.

myo- *combining form. see* my-.

myoblast (**my**-oh-blast) *n.* a cell that develops into a muscle fibre. **—myoblastic** *adj.*

myocardial infarction (MI) (my-oh-**kar**-di-ăl) *n.* death of a segment of heart muscle, which follows interruption of its blood supply (*see* coronary thrombosis). The patient typically experiences a 'heart attack': sudden severe chest pain, which may spread to the arms and throat. The main danger is that of ventricular fibrillation, which accounts for most of the fatalities. Other complications include heart failure, rupture of the heart, phlebothrombosis, pulmonary embolism, pericarditis, shock, mitral regurgitation, and perforation of the septum between the ventricles.

SEE WEB LINKS

- Guide to MI from the British Heart Foundation

myocarditis (my-oh-kar-**dy**-tis) *n.* acute or chronic inflammation of the heart muscle. It may be seen alone or as part of endomyocarditis.

myocardium (my-oh-**kar**-diŭm) *n.* the middle of the three layers forming the wall of the heart (*see also* endocardium, epicardium). It is composed of cardiac muscle and forms the greater part of the heart wall. **—myocardial** *adj.*

myocele (**my**-oh-seel) *n.* protrusion of a muscle through a rupture in its sheath.

myoclonus (my-oh-**kloh**-nŭs) *n.* a sudden spasm of the muscles. Myoclonus is a major feature of some progressive neurological illnesses with extensive degeneration of brain cells. **nocturnal m.** spasm of the muscles on falling asleep, which occurs in normal individuals. **—myoclonic** (my-oh-**klon**-ik) *adj.*

myocyte (**my**-oh-syt) *n.* a muscle cell.

myofibrosis (my-oh-fy-**broh**-sis) *n.* the replacement of muscle tissue by fibrous tissue, with consequent loss of muscle function.

myogenic (my-oh-**jen**-ik) *adj.* originating in muscle: applied to the inherent rhythmicity of contraction of some muscles (e.g. cardiac muscle), which does not depend on neural influences.

myoglobin (myohaemoglobin) (my-oh-**gloh**-bin) *n.* an iron-containing protein, resembling haemoglobin, found in muscle cells. Like haemoglobin it contains a haem group, which binds reversibly with oxygen, and so acts as an oxygen reservoir within the muscle fibres.

myoglobinuria (myohaemoglobinuria) (my-oh-gloh-bin-**yoor**-iă) *n.* the presence in the urine of the pigment myoglobin.

myogram (**my**-ŏ-gram) *n.* a recording of the activity of a muscle. *See* electromyography.

myograph (**my**-ŏ-graf) *n.* an instrument for recording the activity of muscular tissues. *See* electromyography.

myohaemoglobin (my-oh-hee-moh-**gloh**-bin) *n. see* myoglobin.

myohaemoglobinuria (my-oh-hee-moh-gloh-bin-**yoor**-iă) *n. see* myoglobinuria.

myokymia (my-oh-**ky**-miă) *n.* prominent quivering of a few muscle fibres. It is usually a benign condition. *See also* fasciculation.

myology (my-**ol**-ŏji) *n.* the study of the structure, function, and diseases of the muscles.

myolysis (my-**ol**-i-sis) *n. see* fibroid.

myoma (my-**oh**-mă) *n.* a benign tumour of muscle. It may originate in smooth muscle (*see* leiomyoma) or in striated muscle.

myomectomy (my-oh-**mek**-tŏmi) *n.* surgical removal of one or more fibroids from the uterus.

myometritis (my-oh-mi-**try**-tis) *n.* inflammation of the myometrium.

myometrium (my-oh-**mee**-tri-ŭm) *n.* the muscular tissue of the uterus, which surrounds the endometrium. It is composed of smooth muscle that undergoes small regular spontaneous contractions.

myoneural junction (my-oh-**newr**-ăl) *n.* *see* neuromuscular junction.

myopathy (my-**op**-ă-thi) *n.* any disease of the muscles. The myopathies are usually subdivided into those that are inherited (*see* muscular dystrophy) and those that are acquired. All are typified by weakness and wasting of the muscles, which may be associated with pain and tenderness.

myopia (short-sightedness) (my-**oh**-piă) *n.* the condition in which parallel light rays are brought to a focus in front of the retina. The condition is corrected by wearing spectacles with concave lenses or contact lenses, and can also be treated surgically. *Compare* emmetropia, hypermetropia. See illustration. **—myopic** (my-**op**-ik) *adj.*

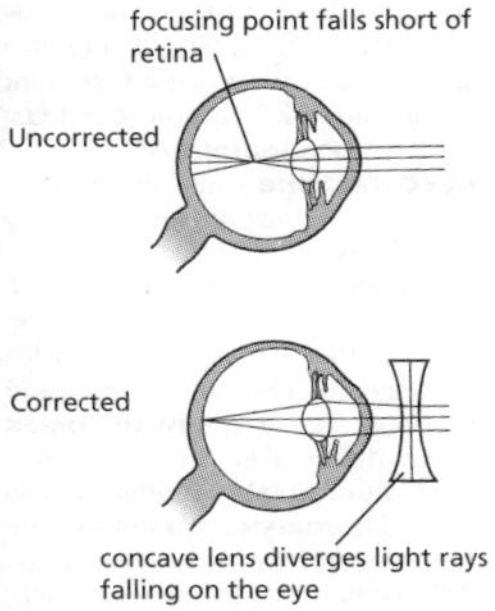

Myopia (short-sightedness)

myoplasm (**my**-oh-plazm) *n.* *see* sarcoplasm.

myoplasty (**my**-oh-plasti) *n.* the plastic surgery of muscle, in which part of a muscle is used to repair tissue defects or deformities in the vicinity of the muscle.

myosarcoma (my-oh-sar-**koh**-mă) *n.* a malignant tumour of muscle. *See also* leiomyosarcoma, rhabdomyosarcoma.

myosin (**my**-oh-sin) *n.* the most abundant protein in muscle fibrils, having the important properties of elasticity and contractility. *See* striated muscle.

myosis (my-**oh**-sis) *n.* *see* miosis.

myositis (my-oh-**sy**-tis) *n.* any of a group of muscle diseases in which inflammation and degenerative changes occur. Polymyositis is the most commonly occurring example. **m. ossificans** the formation of bone within a muscle, which most commonly occurs after dislocations or severe muscle bruising, especially around the elbow, shoulder, hip, or knee.

myotactic (my-oh-**tak**-tik) *adj.* relating to the sense of touch in muscles. **m. reflex** *see* stretch reflex.

myotic (my-**ot**-ik) *n.* *see* miotic.

myotomy (my-**ot**-ŏmi) *n.* the dissection or surgical division of a muscle. *See also* cardiomyotomy.

myotonia (my-oh-**toh**-niă) *n.* a disorder of the muscle fibres that results in abnormally prolonged contractions. It is a feature of a hereditary condition starting in infancy or early childhood (**m. congenita**) and of a form of muscular dystrophy (dystrophia myotonica).

myotonic (my-oh-**ton**-ik) *adj.* **1.** relating to muscle tone. **2.** relating to myotonia.

myotonus (my-oh-**toh**-nŭs) *n.* **1.** a tonic muscular spasm. **2.** muscle tone.

myringa (mi-**ring**-ă) *n.* the eardrum (*see* tympanic membrane).

myringitis (mi-rin-**jy**-tis) *n.* inflammation of the eardrum, often due to a viral infection.

myringoplasty (tympanoplasty) (mi-**ring**-oh-plasti) *n.* surgical repair of a perforated eardrum by grafting.

myringotome (mi-**ring**-oh-tohm) *n.* a surgical knife used to pierce the eardrum in myringotomy.

myringotomy (mi-ring-**ot**-ŏmi) *n.* incision of the eardrum to create an artificial opening, either to allow infected fluid to drain from the middle ear in acute otitis media or to remove fluid in glue ear and permit the insertion of a grommet.

myx- (myxo-) *combining form denoting* mucus.

myxoedema (miks-i-**dee**-mă) *n.* **1.** a dry firm waxy swelling of the skin and subcutaneous tissues found in patients with underactive thyroid glands (*see* hypothyroidism). **2.** the clinical syndrome due to hypothyroidism in adult life, including coarsening of the skin, intolerance to cold, weight gain, and mental dullness. **m. coma** a life-threatening condition due to severe hypothyroidism, often precipitated by an acute event, such as surgery, prolonged exposure to cold, infection, trauma, or sedative drugs. **—myxoedematous** *adj.*

myxofibroma (miks-oh-fy-**broh**-mă) *n.* a benign tumour of fibrous tissue that contains myxomatous elements or has undergone mucoid degeneration.

myxoid cyst (**miks**-oid) *n.* a small and often painful cyst containing a thick sticky fluid that develops over the end joint of a finger or toe. It may be in communication with the underlying joint.

myxoma (miks-**oh**-mă) *n.* a benign gelatinous tumour of connective tissue. **atrial m.** a tumour of the heart, usually of the left side, arising from the septum dividing the two upper chambers. Symptoms may include fever, lassitude, joint pains, and sudden loss of consciousness. **—myxomatous** *adj.*

myxosarcoma (miks-oh-sar-**koh**-mă) *n.* a sarcoma containing mucoid material.

myxovirus (**miks**-oh-vy-rŭs) *n.* one of a group of RNA-containing viruses that are associated with various diseases in animals and humans. The **orthomyxoviruses** cause diseases of the respiratory tract, most notably influenza. The related **paramyxoviruses** include the respiratory syncytial virus (RSV) and the agents causing measles, mumps, and parainfluenza.

Nn

N *symbol for* nitrogen or newton.

Na *symbol for* sodium.

nabilone (nab-i-lohn) *n.* a drug related to cannabis, administered by mouth to control severe nausea and vomiting caused by anticancer drugs.

nabothian follicle (nabothian cyst, nabothian gland) (nă-boh-thi-ăn) *n.* one of a number of retention cysts on the cervix of the uterus. The sacs, which contain mucus, form when the ducts of the glands in the cervix are blocked by a new growth of epithelium over an area damaged because of infection. [M. Naboth (1675–1721), German anatomist]

NAD *n.* nicotinamide adenine dinucleotide: a coenzyme that acts as a hydrogen acceptor in oxidation-reduction reactions, particularly in the electron transport chain in cellular respiration. NAD and the closely related coenzyme **NADP** (nicotinamide adenine dinucleotide phosphate) are derived from nicotinic acid; they are reduced to **NADH** and **NADPH**, respectively.

nadolol (nad-ŏ-lol) *n.* a beta blocker administered by mouth mainly for the treatment of angina pectoris and arrhythmias and to prevent migraine headaches. Trade name: **Corgard**.

Naegele rule (nay-gi-li) *n.* a method used to calculate the estimated date of delivery: nine months and seven days are added to the date of the start of the last menstrual period. A correction is required if the woman does not have 28-day menstrual cycles. [F. K. Naegele (1777–1851), German obstetrician]

Naegele's obliquity *n. see* asynclitism.

naevus (nee-vŭs) *n.* (*pl.* **naevi**) a birthmark: a clearly defined malformation of the skin, present at birth. **capillary n. (port-wine stain)** a permanent purplish discoloration, composed of small blood vessels, that may occur anywhere but usually appears on the upper half of the body. Laser treatment can reduce the discoloration. Occasionally it may be associated with a malformation of blood vessels over the brain, for example in the Sturge-Weber syndrome. **spider n.** a collection of distended blood capillaries radiating out from a central point: a sign of liver cirrhosis, hepatitis, or thyrotoxicosis and also a feature of normal pregnancy. **strawberry n. (strawberry mark)** a raised red lump, composed of small blood vessels, usually appearing on the face and growing rapidly in the first month of life. It slowly resolves and spontaneously disappears between the ages of 5 and 10. *See also* mole[2].

Naga sore (nah-gă) *n. see* tropical ulcer.

NAI *n.* *see* nonaccidental injury.

nail (nayl) *n.* a horny structure, composed of keratin, formed from the epidermis on the dorsal surface of each finger and toe. Growth of the nail occurs at the end of the nail root, behind the exposed nail, by division of the germinative layer of the underlying epidermis. Anatomical name: **unguis**.

nalidixic acid (nal-i-**diks**-ik) *n.* a quinolone antibiotic active against various bacteria and administered by mouth to treat infections of the urinary tract.

naloxone (nal-**oks**-ohn) *n.* a drug that is a specific antidote to morphine and other opioids. Administered by injection or intravenous infusion, it is used in the emergency treatment of opioid overdosage and to reverse the respiratory depression induced by opioid analgesics during surgery. As it is short-acting, repeated doses may be necessary. Trade names: **Minijet Naloxone**, **Prenoxad**.

naltrexone (nal-**treks**-ohn) *n.* an opioid antagonist drug used to prevent relapse in formerly opioid- and alcohol-dependent patients. It is administered by mouth. Trade names: **Adepend**, **Nalorex**, **Opizone**.

named nurse (naymd) *n.* a nurse designated as being responsible for a patient's nursing care during a hospital stay and who is identified by name as such to the patient. The concept of the named nurse stresses the importance of continuity of care. *See also* primary nursing.

nandrolone (**nan**-droh-lohn) *n.* a synthetic male sex hormone with anabolic effects. It is administered by deep intramuscular injection in the treatment of aplastic anaemia. Trade name: **Deca-Durabolin**.

nano- *prefix denoting* **1.** extremely small size. **2.** one thousand-millionth part (10^{-9}).

nanometre (**nan**-oh-mee-ter) *n.* one thousand-millionth of a metre (10^{-9}m). One nanometre is equal to 10 angstrom. Symbol: nm.

nanophthalmos (nan-off-**thal**-mŏs) *n.* a congenitally small eye in which all the structures are proportionally reduced.

nape (nayp) *n.* *see* nucha.

napkin rash (nappy rash) (**nap**-kin) *n.* a red skin rash within the napkin area, usually caused by chemical irritation (ammoniacal dermatitis) or fungal infection with *Candida*. Ammoniacal dermatitis is caused by skin contact with wet soiled nappies; treatment involves exposure to air, application of barrier creams, and frequent nappy changes. Candidal nappy rash is treated with antifungal creams. Other causes of napkin rash include eczema and psoriasis.

naproxen (nă-**proks**-ĕn) *n.* an analgesic drug that also reduces inflammation and fever (*see* NSAID). It is administered by mouth to treat rheumatoid arthritis, gout, and dysmenorrhoea. It may be used in combination with misoprostol (as **Napratec**) to prevent gastrointestinal bleeding. Trade name: **Naprosyn**.

naratriptan (na-ră-**trip**-tan) *n. see* 5HT$_1$ agonist.

narcissism (**nar**-sis-izm) *n.* an excessive involvement with oneself and one's self-importance, often to cover insecurity. In Freudian terms it is a state in which the ego has taken itself as a love object. An extreme degree of narcissism may become a personality disorder. —**narcissistic** *adj.*

narco- *combining form denoting* narcosis; stupor.

narcoanalysis (nar-koh-ă-**nal**-i-sis) *n.* a type of psychotherapy during which the patient is in a relaxed or sleeplike state induced by drugs.

narcolepsy (**nar**-kŏ-lep-si) *n.* a brain disorder involving poor control of sleep–wake cycles; the patient experiences overwhelming urges to sleep that have an impact on daily activities. Patients can fall asleep during any habitual activity, such as eating or typing, for a few seconds or longer. Although they can be woken with ease and may feel refreshed, their memory of the period is impaired. Cataplexy, sleep paralysis, and hallucinations are associated but less common. —**narcoleptic** *adj., n.*

narcosis (nar-**koh**-sis) *n.* a state of diminished consciousness or complete unconsciousness caused by the use of narcotic (i.e. opioid) drugs. The body's normal reactions to stimuli are diminished and the body may become sedated or completely anaesthetized.

narcotic (nar-**kot**-ik) *n.* a drug that relieves pain and also induces stupor and insensibility. Now largely obsolete in medical contexts, the term was used particularly for morphine and other derivatives of opium (*see* opiate) but also referred to other drugs that depress brain function (e.g. general anaesthetics and hypnotics).

nares (**nair**-eez) *pl. n.* (*sing.* **naris**) openings of the nose. **external** (or **anterior**) **n.** the nostrils, which lead from the nasal cavity to the outside. **internal** (or **posterior**) **n.** (**choanae**) the openings leading from the nasal cavity into the pharynx.

nasal (**nay**-zăl) *adj.* relating to the nose. **n. bone** either of a pair of narrow oblong bones that together form the bridge and root of the nose. **n. cavity** the space inside the nose that lies between the floor of the cranium and the roof of the mouth. **n. concha** (**turbinate bone**) any of three thin scroll-like bones that form the sides of the nasal cavity.

naso- *combining form denoting* the nose.

nasogastric (NG) (nay-zoh-**gas**-trik) *adj.* relating to the nose and stomach. **n. tube** a tube inserted into the stomach through the nose (*see* intubation).

nasolacrimal (nay-zoh-**lak**-ri-măl) *adj.* relating to the nose and the lacrimal (tear-producing) apparatus. **n. duct** the duct that drains the tears away from the lacrimal apparatus into the inferior meatus of the nose.

nasopharyngeal airway (nay-zoh-fă-**rin**-ji-ăl) *n.* a curved tube to be slotted down one nostril of an unconscious patient, to sit behind the tongue, to create a patent airway. *See also* oropharyngeal airway.

nasopharynx (postnasal space, rhinopharynx) (nay-zoh-fa-rinks) *n.* the part of the pharynx that lies above the level of the junction of the hard and soft palates. It connects the nasal cavity to the oropharynx. **—nasopharyngeal** *adj.*

nates (nay-teez) *pl. n.* the buttocks. **—natal** (nay-t'l) *adj.*

National Council for Vocational Qualifications (nash-ŏn-ăl) *n.* *see* NCVQ.

national early warning score (NEWS) *n.* a national system for detecting deteriorating patients on the ward. Six physiological parameters – systolic blood pressure, respiratory and pulse rates, temperature, oxygen saturation, and level of consciousness – are accorded scores that are aggregated: the higher the aggregated scores of individual patients, the greater the deterioration in their condition. NEWS is designed to replace the various systems currently used in different hospitals (e.g. the **modified early warning score**, or **MEWS**) and thus standardize the assessment of acutely ill patients.

National Health Service (NHS) *n.* (in the UK) a comprehensive service offering therapeutic and preventive medical and surgical care, including the prescription and dispensing of medicines, spectacles, and medical and dental appliances. Exchequer funds pay for the services of doctors, nurses, and other professionals, as well as residential costs in NHS hospitals, and meet a substantial part of the cost of the medicines and appliances.

National Institute for Health and Care Excellence *see* NICE.

national service frameworks (NSFs) *pl. n.* national standards of care published for a variety of conditions and patient groups, which are designed to improve and reduce variations in quality of care by defining long-term strategies for delivery of the standards and by setting specific goals.

SEE WEB LINKS

- Details of NSFs for specific conditions from the National Archives

natriuretic (nay-tri-yoor-**et**-ik) *n.* an agent that promotes the excretion of sodium salts in the urine. Most diuretics are natriuretics.

natriuretic peptide *n.* any of several peptides that stimulate diuresis and vasodilatation. They act on the kidney tubules to promote excretion of sodium (natriuresis) and water. **atrial n. p.** (**ANP**) a peptide produced in the atria of the heart in response to a rise in atrial pressure. **brain n. p.** (**BNP**) a peptide produced in the brain and the ventricles of the heart, mainly in response to stretching of the ventricular muscle (as occurs in congestive heart failure). *See* BNP (test).

natural childbirth (nach-ĕr-ăl) *n.* labour and delivery that relies largely on the efforts of the mother alone, with the minimum of medical intervention.

natural killer cell *n.* a type of lymphocyte that can kill virus-infected cells and cancerous cells and mediates rejection of bone-marrow grafts. These cells are a part of natural immunity.

naturopathy (nay-cher-**op**-ă-thi) *n.* a system of medicine that relies upon the use of only 'natural' substances for the treatment of disease, rather than drugs.

nausea (**naw**-ziă) *n.* the feeling that one is about to vomit, as experienced in seasickness. Actual vomiting often occurs subsequently.

navel (**nay**-vĕl) *n. see* umbilicus.

navicular bone (nă-**vik**-yoo-ler) *n.* a boat-shaped bone of the ankle (*see* tarsus) that articulates with the three cuneiform bones in front and with the talus behind.

NBM *n.* nothing (or nil) by mouth.

NCVQ *n.* (in the UK) National Council for Vocational Qualifications: a body set up by the government to achieve a coherent national framework for vocational qualifications in England, Wales, and Northern Ireland. Five levels of National Vocational Qualification (NVQ) are currently accredited by the council.

NDU *n.* (in the UK) Nursing Development Unit: a centre for creative nursing managed directly by nurses, who are responsible for controlling the budget and appointing staff. The unit can be based in hospital or the community in either the public or the private sector. NDUs are committed to practising research-based patient-centred care.

nearthrosis (nee-arth-**roh**-sis) *n. see* pseudarthrosis.

nebula (**neb**-yoo-lă) *n.* a faint opacity of the cornea that remains after an ulcer has healed.

nebulizer (**neb**-yoo-ly-zer) *n.* an instrument used for applying a liquid in the form of a fine spray.

NEC *n. see* necrotizing enterocolitis.

Necator (ni-**kay**-ter) *n.* a genus of parasitic nematodes that live in the small intestine (*see* hookworm). **N. americanus** the species that infests humans.

necessity (nĕ-**ses**-iti) *n.* the ethical and legal doctrine that provides justification for doing something that might otherwise be seen as blameworthy, when the consequences of not doing so would be worse. For example, doctors have no right to touch a patient without consent, yet might be considered lacking in duty of care if they did not restrain patients who were about to kill themselves.

neck (nek) *n.* **1.** a narrowed region of the body connecting the head to the trunk. It contains the cervical vertebrae. **2.** any other constricted region of an organ or part, such as the narrow section of the femur between the head and shaft. *See* cervix.

necro- *combining form denoting* death or dissolution.

necrobiosis (nek-roh-by-**oh**-sis) *n.* a gradual process by which cells lose their function and die.

necrology (nek-**rol**-ŏji) *n.* the study of the phenomena of death, involving determination of the moment of death and the different changes that occur in the tissues of the body after death.

necropsy (**nek**-rop-si) *n.* *see* autopsy.

necrosis (mortification) (nek-**roh**-sis) *n.* the death of some or all of the cells in an organ or tissue, caused by disease, physical or chemical injury, or interference with the blood supply (*see* gangrene). **—necrotic** *adj.*

necrospermia (nek-roh-**sper**-miă) *n.* the presence of either dead or motionless spermatozoa in the semen. *See* infertility.

necrotizing enterocolitis (NEC) (**nek**-rŏ-tyz-ing) *n.* a serious disease affecting the bowel during the first three weeks of life; it is much more common in preterm formula milk-fed babies. The abdomen distends and blood and mucus appear in the stools; the bowel may perforate.

necrotizing fasciitis *n.* a life-threatening bacterial infection of the layer of fascia beneath the skin, usually by *Streptococcus*. Tissue necrosis and toxin production can result in shock and multi-organ failure. It is often associated with vascular disease, especially in diabetics, and the elderly and those who have recently undergone surgery are also vulnerable to the infection, which requires prompt treatment with intravenous antibiotics and excision of the involved tissue.

nedocromil (ned-oh-**kroh**-mil) *n.* a drug used to prevent asthma attacks and treat allergic conjunctivitis. It is administered by metered-dose aerosol inhaler or as eye drops. Trade names: **Rapitil**, **Tilade**.

needle (**nee**-d'l) *n.* a slender sharp-pointed instrument. Most needles used for stitching tissue during surgery have the suture material fused onto them. Hollow needles are used to inject substances into the body, to obtain specimens of tissue (*see* puncture), or to withdraw fluid from a cavity. **intraosseous n.** *see* intraosseous. *See also* stop needle.

needle-stick injury *n.* a common accidental injury to the fingers and hands of nurses and doctors by contaminated injection needles. It can result in transmitted infections (e.g. hepatitis, HIV, AIDS).

needling (**need**-ling) *n.* the use of a sharp needle to make a hole in the capsule surrounding the lens of the eye. This technique has now largely been replaced by use of the YAG laser.

needs deprivation *n.* an unhealthy state said to exist if an individual is unable to meet basic human needs.

negative feedback (**neg**-ă-tiv) *n.* *see* feedback.

negative symptom *n.* (in psychiatry) a symptom of schizophrenia characterized by a deficiency in or absence of some aspect of functioning, such as social withdrawal, loss of initiative, or blunted affect. *Compare* positive symptom.

negativism (**neg**-ă-tiv-izm) *n.* uncooperative or obstructive behaviour. **active n.** negativism in which the individual does the opposite of what is asked for. This is usually associated with other features of catatonia. **passive n.** negativism in which the person fails to cooperate, occurring in schizophrenia and depression.

negligence (neg-li-jĕns) *n.* failure by a health-care professional to exercise a reasonable standard of care, as defined in the UK by the Bolam and Bolitho tests. In order to establish negligence a claimant must show that the professional had a duty of care, that he or she breached this duty by falling below the expected standard of care, and that foreseeable harm was caused as a result of the professional's conduct.

Neisseria (ny-**seer**-iă) *n.* a genus of spherical Gram-negative aerobic nonmotile bacteria characteristically grouped in pairs. **N. gonorrhoeae** (the **gonococcus**) the species that causes gonorrhoea, found within pus cells of urethral and vaginal discharge. **N. meningitidis** (the **meningococcus**) the species that causes meningococcal meningitis. Meningococci are found within pus cells of infected cerebrospinal fluid and blood or in the nasal passages of carriers.

nematode (roundworm) (**nem**-ă-tohd) *n.* any one of a large group of worms having an unsegmented cylindrical body, tapering at both ends. Some nematodes, including hookworms, filariae, pinworms, and guinea worms, are parasites of humans.

neo- *combining form denoting* new or newly formed.

neoadjuvant chemotherapy (nee-oh-**aj**-oo-vănt) *n.* chemotherapy given before (usually) surgical treatment of a primary tumour with the aim of improving the results of surgery or radiotherapy and preventing the development of metastases. *Compare* adjuvant therapy.

neocerebellum (nee-oh-se-ri-**bel**-ŭm) *n.* the middle lobe of the cerebellum, excluding the pyramid and uvula.

neologism (ni-**ol**-ŏ-jizm) *n.* (in psychiatry) the invention of words that do not exist in one's language. It may be a symptom of a psychotic illness, such as schizophrenia.

neomycin (nee-oh-**my**-sin) *n.* an aminoglycoside antibiotic used to treat infections caused by a wide range of bacteria, mainly those affecting the skin, ears, and eyes. It is usually applied in creams, ointments, or drops (with steroids for ear infections), but can be given by mouth to sterilize the bowel before surgery.

neonatal early warning score *n.* an assessment tool for newborn babies, consisting of a chart in which a combination of vital signs, neurological involvement, observation of blue skin and lips, and level of behavioural response indicates the appropriate level of concern. It is colour-coordinated from red to green to enable standardized escalation of concerns about the sick baby.

neonatal intensive care unit (NICU) (nee-oh-**nay**-t'l) *n.* *see* intensive care.

neonatal mortality rate *n.* *see* infant (mortality rate).

neonatal screening *n.* screening tests carried out on newborn babies to detect diseases that appear in the neonatal period, such as phenylketonuria (*see* Guthrie test). Early detection enables treatment to be instigated before irreversible damage occurs to the baby.

neonatal urticaria (er-ti-**kair**-iă) *n.* *see* erythema (toxicum neonatorum).

neonate (**nee**-oh-nayt) *n.* an infant at any time during the first 28 days of life. The word is particularly applied to infants just born or in the first week of life. —**neonatal** *adj.*

neoplasia (nee-oh-**play**-ziă) *n.* abnormal growth of cells that is purposeless, independent of the body's growth-regulating mechanisms, and continues after the initiating stimulus has been removed. *See* CIN, MENS, prostatic intraepithelial neoplasia. *Compare* hyperplasia, hypertrophy. —**neoplastic** (nee-oh-**plast**-ik) *adj.*

neoplasm (**nee**-oh-plazm) *n.* any new and abnormal growth: a benign or malignant tumour. —**neoplastic** *adj.*

neosphincter (**nee**-oh-sfink-ter) *n.* a substituted muscle or an implant for an absent or ineffective sphincter (*see* artificial sphincter).

neostigmine (nee-oh-**stig**-meen) *n.* an anticholinesterase drug used mainly to treat myasthenia gravis and to reverse the action of some muscle-relaxant drugs used during surgery. It is administered by mouth or injection.

neovascularization (nee-oh-vas-kew-ler-I-**zay**-shŏn) *n.* the abnormal formation of new and fragile blood vessels, usually in response to ischaemia. **choroidal n.** the formation of abnormal vessels, derived from the choroid, in the space between the retinal pigment epithelium (*see* retina) and the choroid. This occurs, for example, in macular degeneration.

nephr- (nephro-) *combining form denoting* the kidney(s).

nephralgia (ni-**fral**-jiă) *n.* pain in the kidney, which is felt in the loin and can be caused by a variety of kidney complaints.

nephrectomy (ni-**frek**-tŏmi) *n.* surgical removal of a kidney. **radical n.** removal of the entire organ together with its surrounding fat and the adjacent adrenal gland, performed for cancer of the kidney.

nephritis (Bright's disease) (ni-**fry**-tis) *n.* inflammation of the kidney. Nephritis is a nonspecific term used to describe a condition resulting from a variety of causes. *See* glomerulonephritis.

nephroblastoma (Wilms' tumour) (nef-roh-blas-**toh**-mă) *n.* a malignant tumour arising from the embryonic kidney and found in young children (usually between the ages of three and eight). In some cases it is associated with a chromosome abnormality, when aniridia and other abnormal features are present. Treatment is by nephrectomy followed by chemotherapy and sometimes radiotherapy.

nephrocalcinosis (nef-roh-kal-sin-**oh**-sis) *n.* the presence of calcium deposits in the kidneys. This can be caused by excess calcium in the blood, due to overactivity of the parathyroid glands, or it may result from an underlying abnormality of the kidney.

nephrocapsulectomy (nef-roh-kaps-yoo-**lek**-tŏmi) *n.* surgical removal of the fibrous capsule around a kidney.

nephrolithiasis (nef-roh-lith-**I**-ă-sis) *n.* the presence of stones in the kidney (*see* calculus). Such stones can cause pain and blood in the urine, but they may produce no symptoms.

nephrolithotomy (nef-roh-lith-**ot**-ŏmi) *n.* the surgical removal of a stone from the kidney by an incision into the kidney substance. **percutaneous n.** nephrolithotomy that is performed via a nephroscope passed into the kidney through a tract from the skin surface.

nephrology (ni-**frol**-ŏji) *n.* the branch of medicine concerned with the study, investigation, and management of diseases of the kidney. *See also* urology. **—nephrologist** *n.*

nephroma (ni-**froh**-mă) *n.* a tumour of the kidney.

nephron (**nef**-ron) *n.* the active unit of excretion in the kidney (see illustration). Blood is filtered through the glomerulus into the Bowman's capsule so that water, nitrogenous waste, and many other substances pass into the renal tubule. Here most of the substances are reabsorbed back into the blood, the remaining fluid (urine) passing into the collecting duct, which drains into the ureter.

nephropathy (ni-**frop**-ă-thi) *n.* disease of the kidney. **diabetic n.** progressive damage to the kidneys seen in some people with long-standing diabetes mellitus.

nephropexy (**nef**-roh-peks-i) *n.* an operation to fix a mobile kidney.

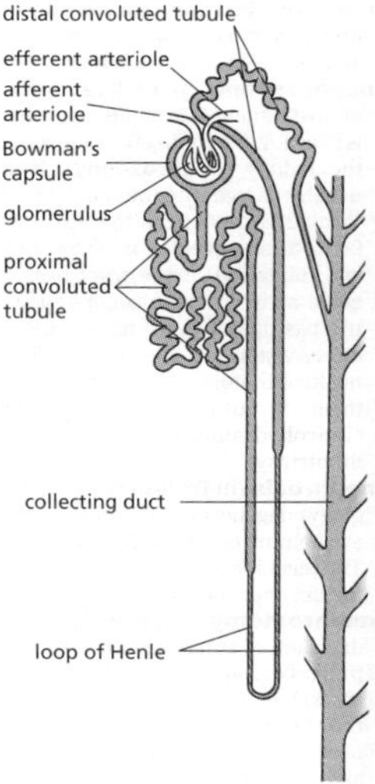

A single nephron

The kidney is fixed to the twelfth rib and adjacent posterior abdominal wall. It is now usually performed laparoscopically.

nephroptosis (nef-rop-**toh**-sis) *n.* abnormal descent of a kidney into the pelvis on standing. If this is accompanied by pain and obstruction to free drainage of urine by the kidney, nephropexy may be advised.

nephrosclerosis (nef-roh-skleer-**oh**-sis) *n.* hardening of the arteries and arterioles of the kidneys.

nephroscope (**nef**-roh-skohp) *n.* an instrument (*see* endoscope) that is used for examining the interior of the kidney (**nephroscopy**). It is usually passed into the renal pelvis through a track from the skin surface after needle nephrostomy and dilatation of the tract over a guide wire. The nephroscope allows the passage of instruments under direct vision to remove calculi (*see* nephrolithotomy) or disintegrate them by ultrasound probes or electrohydraulic shock waves (*see* lithotripsy).

nephrosis (ni-**froh**-sis) *n.* (in pathology) degenerative changes in the epithelium of the kidney tubules. The term is sometimes used loosely for the nephrotic syndrome.

nephrostomy (ni-**frost**-ŏmi) *n.* drainage of urine from the kidney by a tube (catheter) passing through the kidney into the renal pelvis via the skin surface. This is commonly used as a temporary procedure to alleviate renal obstruction.

nephrotic syndrome (ni-**frot**-ik) *n.* a condition characterized by heavy loss of protein in the urine (>3.5 g/day), reduced levels of albumin in the blood (usually <25 g/l), and peripheral oedema. It can be caused by a variety of disorders; the most common cause in adults is diabetic nephropathy.

nephrotomy (ni-**frot**-ŏmi) *n.* surgical incision into the substance of the kidney. This is usually undertaken to remove a kidney stone (*see* nephrolithotomy).

nephrotoxic (nef-roh-**toks**-ik) *adj.* liable to cause damage to the kidneys. Nephrotoxic drugs include aminoglycoside antibiotics, sulphonamides, and gold compounds. **—nephrotoxicity** *n.*

nephroureterectomy (ureteronephrectomy) (nef-roh-yoor-i-ter-**ek**-tŏmi) *n.* surgical removal of a kidney together with its ureter. This operation is performed for cancer of the kidney pelvis or ureter.

nerve (nerv) *n.* a bundle of nerve fibres enclosed in a connective tissue sheath (see illustration). **motor n.** a nerve that transmits impulses from the brain or spinal cord to the muscles and glands. **sensory n.** a nerve that transmits impulses inwards from the sense organs to the brain and spinal cord.

nerve block *n.* a method of producing anaesthesia in part of the body by blocking the passage of pain impulses in the sensory nerves supplying it. A local anaesthetic, such as lidocaine, is injected into the tissues in the region to be anaesthetized. *See also* ring block.

nerve cell *n.* *see* neuron.

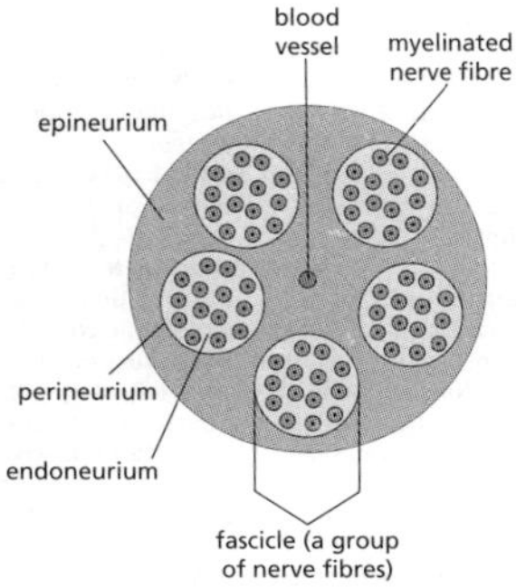

Transverse section through a peripheral nerve with five fascicles

nerve conduction study *n.* a test done to assess the peripheral nervous system. It involves activating the nerves with electrical pulses and measuring the responses obtained.

nerve ending *n.* the final part (terminal) of one of the branches of a nerve fibre, where a neuron makes contact either with another neuron or with a muscle or gland cell.

nerve entrapment syndrome (in-**trap**-mĕnt) *n.* any syndrome resulting from pressure on a nerve from surrounding structures. Examples include the carpal tunnel syndrome and meralgia paraesthetica.

nerve fibre *n.* the long fine process that extends from the cell body of a neuron and carries nerve impulses. Bundles of nerve fibres running together form a nerve.

nerve gas *n.* any gas that disrupts the normal functioning of nerves and thus of the muscles they supply.

nerve impulse *n.* the electrical activity in the membrane of a neuron that is the means by which information is transmitted within the nervous system along the axons of the neurons.

nerve regeneration *n.* the growth of new nerve tissue, which occurs at a very slow rate (1–2 mm per day) after a nerve has been severed and is often partially or totally incomplete. *See also* axonotmesis, neurotmesis.

nervous breakdown (**ner**-vŭs **brayk**-down) *n.* a lay term applied to a range of emotional crises varying from a brief attack of 'hysterical' behaviour to a major mental illness. The term is also sometimes used as a euphemism for a frank psychiatric illness, such as schizophrenia.

nervous system *n.* the vast network of cells specialized to carry information (in the form of nerve impulses) to and from all parts of the body in order to bring about bodily activity. *See* autonomic nervous system, central nervous system, peripheral nervous system.

Nesbit's operation (**nez**-bits) *n.* an operation originally devised to surgically straighten a congenitally curved penis but now more frequently employed to correct the penile curvature caused by Peyronie's disease. [R. M. Nesbit (20th century), US surgeon]

nesidioblastosis (nes-idi-oh-blas-**toh**-sis) *n.* a rare condition of childhood in which abnormal cells in the pancreas secrete a selection of hormones (including insulin) in an uncontrolled manner. This causes a variety of problems, including recurrent hypoglycaemia.

nettle rash (**ne**-t'l) *n. see* urticaria.

Neuman's model (**new**-mănz) *n.* a systems model for nursing that can be interpreted to include various social and physiological systems. The goal of nursing is seen as maintaining equilibrium within these systems, which should lead to the 'whole' person being restored to health. *See also* nursing models. [B. Neuman (1924–), US nurse theorist]

neur- (neuro-) *combining form denoting* nerves or the nervous system.

neural (**newr**-ăl) *adj.* relating to a nerve or nerves. **n. arch** *see* vertebra.

neuralgia (newr-**al**-jă) *n.* a severe burning or stabbing pain often following the course of a nerve. **post-herpetic n.** intense debilitating pain felt at the site of a previous attack of shingles. **trigeminal n.** (**tic douloureux**) neuralgia in which brief paroxysms of searing pain are felt in the distribution of one or more branches of the trigeminal nerve in the face.

neural tube *n.* a hollow tube of tissue in the embryo from which the brain and spinal cord develop. It is formed when two edges of a groove in a plate of primitive neural tissue (**neural plate**) come together and fuse.

neural tube defects *pl. n.* a group of congenital abnormalities involving defects in the spine or skull caused by failure of the neural tube to form normally. They include spina bifida, in which the bony arches of the spine fail to close, and more severe defects of bone fusion involving herniation of neural tissue and consequent mental and physical disorders, such as meningocele, meningomyelocele, and meningoencephalocele.

neurapraxia (newr-ă-**praks**-iă) *n.* temporary loss of nerve function resulting in tingling, numbness, and weakness. It is usually caused by compression of the nerve.

neurasthenia (newr-ăs-**th'ee**-niă) *n.* a set of psychological and physical symptoms, including fatigue, irritability, headache, and dizziness. It can be caused by organic damage, such as a head injury, or it can be due to anxiety. —**neurasthenic** *adj., n.*

neurectasis (newr-**ek**-tă-sis) *n.* the surgical procedure for stretching a peripheral nerve.

neurectomy (newr-**ek**-tŏmi) *n.* the surgical removal of the whole or part of a nerve.

neurilemma (neurolemma) (newr-i-**lem**-ă) *n.* the sheath of the axon of a nerve fibre. The neurilemma of a medullated fibre contains myelin. —**neurilemmal** *adj.*

neurilemmoma (neurinoma) (newr-i-lem-**oh**-mă) *n.* a benign slow-growing tumour that arises from the neurilemma of a nerve fibre.

neurinoma (newr-i-**noh**-mă) *n. see* neurilemmoma.

neuritis (newr-**I**-tis) *n.* a disease of the peripheral nerves showing the pathological changes of inflammation. The term is also used in a less precise sense as an alternative to neuropathy. *See also* retrobulbar neuritis.

neuroanatomy (newr-oh-ă-**nat**-ŏmi) *n.* the study of the structure of the nervous system.

neuroblast (**newr**-oh-blast) *n.* any of the nerve cells of the embryo that give rise to neurons.

neuroblastoma (newr-oh-blas-**toh**-mă) *n.* a malignant tumour, usually of childhood, composed of embryonic nerve cells. It may originate in any part of the sympathetic nervous system, most commonly in the medulla of the adrenal gland.

neurocranium (newr-oh-**kray**-niŭm) *n.* the part of the skull that encloses the brain.

neurodermatitis (newr-oh-der-mă-**ty**-tis) *n. see* lichen (simplex chronicus).

neuroendocrine system (newr-oh-**end**-ŏ-kryn) *n.* the system of dual control of certain activities of the body by means of both nerves and circulating hormones. It can give rise to **neuroendocrine tumours**, which secrete active hormones. *See* neurohormone, neurosecretion.

neuroepithelioma (newr-oh-epi-th'ee-li-**oh**-mă) *n.* a malignant tumour of the retina of the eye. It is a form of glioma and may spread into the brain if not treated early.

neuroepithelium (newr-oh-epi-**th'ee**-liŭm) *n.* a type of epithelium associated with organs of special sense. It contains sensory nerve endings and is found in the retina, the membranous labyrinth, and the taste buds. —**neuroepithelial** *adj.*

neurofibroma (newr-oh-fy-**broh**-mă) *n.* a benign tumour growing from the fibrous coverings of a peripheral nerve. *See also* schwannoma.

neurofibromatosis (newr-oh-fy-broh-mă-**toh**-sis) *n.* an autosomal dominant condition characterized by multiple benign tumours growing from peripheral nerves. **n. type I** (**von Recklinghausen's**

disease) a form of neurofibromatosis in which numerous neurofibromas can be felt beneath the skin along the course of the nerve; they may become large, causing disfigurement, and are commonly associated with café au lait spots. **n. type II** a form of neurofibromatosis characterized by vestibular schwannomas (acoustic neuromas) arising on both vestibular nerves (causing hearing loss) and meningiomas.

neurogenesis (newr-oh-**jen**-i-sis) *n.* the growth and development of nerve cells.

neurogenic (newr-oh-**jen**-ik) *adj.* **1.** caused by disease or dysfunction of the nervous system. **2.** arising in nervous tissue. **3.** caused by nerve stimulation.

neuroglia (newr-**og**-liă) *n. see* glia.

neurohormone (newr-oh-**hor**-mohn) *n.* a hormone, such as vasopressin or noradrenaline, that is produced within specialized nerve cells and is secreted from the nerve endings into the circulation.

neurohypophysis (newr-oh-hy-**pof**-i-sis) *n. see* pituitary gland.

neurolemma (newr-oh-**lem**-ă) *n. see* neurilemma.

neuroleptic (newr-oh-**lep**-tik) *n.* any drug that induces an altered state of consciousness, such as an antipsychotic drug.

neurology (newr-**ol**-ŏji) *n.* the study of the structure, functioning, and diseases of the nervous system (including the brain, spinal cord, peripheral nerves, and muscles). **—neurological** *adj.* **—neurologist** *n.*

neuroma (newr-**oh**-mă) *n.* any tumour derived from cells of the nervous system, now usually categorized more specifically (e.g. neurofibroma, neurilemmoma). **acoustic n.** *see* (vestibular) schwannoma.

neuromuscular junction (myoneural junction) (newr-oh-**mus**-kew-ler) *n.* the meeting point of a motor nerve fibre and the muscle fibre that it supplies. It consists of a minute gap across which a neurotransmitter must diffuse from the nerve to trigger contraction of the muscle.

neuromyelitis optica (Devic's disease) (newr-oh-my-ĕ-**ly**-tis **op**-tik-ă) *n.* a condition that resembles multiple sclerosis. Typically there is a transverse myelitis, producing paralysis and numbness of the limbs and trunk below the inflamed spinal cord, and retrobulbar (optic) neuritis affecting both optic nerves.

neuron (neurone, nerve cell) (**newr**-on) *n.* one of the basic functional units of the nervous system: a cell specialized to transmit electrical nerve impulses and so carry information from one part of the body to another (see illustration). Impulses enter the neuron through branches of the dendrites and are carried away from the cell body through the axon (nerve fibre). They are transmitted to adjacent neurons or to effector organs through minute gaps (*see* neuromuscular junction, synapse). *See also* motor neuron.

neuropathic arthritis *n. see* Charcot's joint.

neuropathic bladder *n.* a malfunctioning bladder due to partial

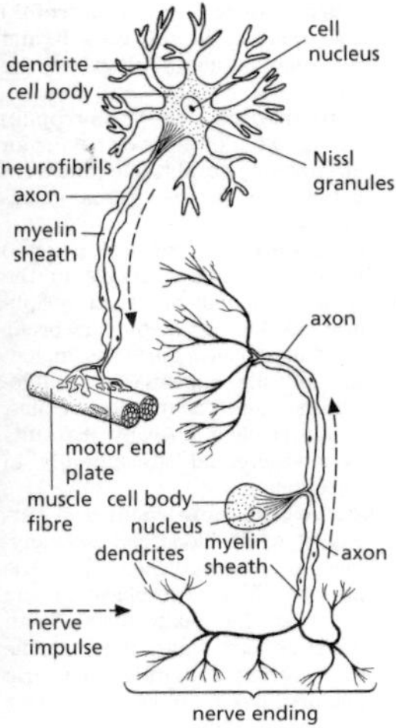

Types of neuron: motor (left) and sensory (right)

or complete interruption of its nerve supply. Causes include injury to the spinal cord, spina bifida, multiple sclerosis, and diabetic neuropathy.

neuropathy (newr-**op**-ă-thi) *n.* disease of one or more of the peripheral nerves, usually causing weakness and numbness. **diabetic n.** neuropathy seen in some people with long-standing diabetes, most commonly affecting the legs. **peripheral n.** (**polyneuritis**, **polyneuropathy**) neuropathy affecting sensory and/or motor nerves and tending to start in the fingers and toes and progress proximally. Causes include diabetes, alcohol, certain drugs, infections (e.g. HIV), and Charcot-Marie-Tooth disease. **—neuropathic** (newr-oh-**path**-ik) *adj.*

neurophysiology (newr-oh-fiz-i-**ol**-ŏji) *n.* the study of the complex chemical and physical changes that are associated with the activity of the nervous system.

neuroplasty (**newr**-oh-plasti) *n.* reconstructive surgery for damaged or severed peripheral nerves.

neuropsychiatry (newr-oh-si-**ky**-ă-tri) *n.* the branch of medicine concerned with the psychiatric effects of disorders of neurological function or structure. It investigates the relationship between demonstrable brain changes and the resulting effects on the mind.

neurorrhaphy (newr-**o**-răfi) *n.* the operation of suturing a cut nerve.

neurosecretion (newr-oh-si-**kree**-shŏn) *n.* any substance produced within, and secreted by, a nerve cell. Important examples are the hormone-releasing factors produced by the cells of the hypothalamus.

neurosis (newr-**oh**-sis) *n.* (*pl.* **neuroses**) any long-term mental or behavioural disorder in which contact with reality is retained and the condition is recognized by the sufferer as abnormal. A neurosis essentially features anxiety or behaviour that, according to Freudian theory, is exaggeratedly designed to avoid anxiety. Such defence mechanisms against anxiety take various forms and may appear as phobias, obsessions, compulsions, or sexual dysfunctions. Behaviour therapy and antidepressants (SSRIs) are effective in many cases. In accordance with the DSM-IV classification, the disorders formerly included under the neuroses have been renamed **anxiety disorders**. *See also* anxiety, conversion disorder, dissociative disorder, obsession. **—neurotic** *adj.*

neurosurgery (newr-oh-**ser**-jer-i) *n.* the surgical or operative treatment of diseases of the brain and spinal cord.

neurosyphilis (newr-oh-**sif**-i-lis) *n.* syphilis affecting the nervous system.

neurotmesis (newr-ot-**mee**-sis) *n.* an injury in which a nerve is severed. Nerve regeneration is slow.

neurotomy (newr-**ot**-ŏmi) *n.* the surgical procedure of severing a nerve.

neurotoxic (newr-oh-**toks**-ik) *adj.* poisonous or harmful to nerve cells and dental pulp cells. **—neurotoxicity** *n.*

neurotransmitter (newr-oh-tranz-**mit**-er) *n.* a chemical substance, such as acetylcholine, noradrenaline, dopamine, or serotonin, that is released from nerve endings to transmit impulses across synapses to other nerves and across the minute gaps between the nerves and the muscles or glands that they supply.

neurotrophic (newr-oh-**trof**-ik) *adj.* relating to the growth and nutrition of neural tissue in the body.

neurotropic (newr-oh-**trop**-ik) *adj.* growing towards or having an affinity for neural tissue. The term may be applied to viruses, chemicals, or toxins.

neutropenia (new-troh-**pee**-niă) *n.* an abnormal decrease in the number of neutrophils in peripheral blood. Neutropenia may occur in a wide variety of diseases, including aplastic anaemias, agranulocytosis, and acute leukaemias, and after chemotherapy. It results in an increased susceptibility to infections.

neutrophil (**new**-trŏ-fil) *n.* a variety of white blood cell (*see* polymorph) distinguished by the presence in its cytoplasm of fine granules that stain purple with Romanowsky stains. It is capable of ingesting and killing bacteria and provides an important defence against infection.

NEWS *n. see* national early warning score

newton (**new**-t'n) *n.* the SI unit of force, equal to the force required to impart to 1 kilogram an acceleration of 1 metre per second per second. Symbol: N.

nexus (**neks**-ŭs) *n.* (in anatomy) a connection or link.

NG *adj. see* nasogastric.

NGU *n. see* (nongonococcal) urethritis.

NHL *n. see* (non-Hodgkin's) lymphoma.

NHS *n. see* National Health Service.

NHS 111 *n.* a nonemergency telephone helpline number operating in England. The service is available 24 hours a day to give health-care advice to patients with urgent but not life-threatening problems, or to direct them to the most appropriate local service. It is staffed by trained call handlers, supported by nurses and paramedics. NHS 111 replaced the **NHS Direct** phone service.

NHS Direct *n. see* NHS 111.

NHS England *n.* a nondepartmental public body that oversees the day-to-day operation of the NHS in England. It is also responsible for commissioning GP services and some specialized health-care services. In addition to a central team, there are four **NHS England Regional Teams** and twenty-five **NHS England Area Teams**. NHS England was previously known as the **NHS Commissioning Board** and the **NHS Commissioning Board Authority**.

SEE WEB LINKS

- NHS England website

NHS walk-in centre *n.* a medical centre offering free and fast access to health-care advice and treatment. Centres provide advice and treatment for minor injuries and illnesses and guidance on how to use NHS services.

niacin (ny-ă-sin) *n. see* nicotinic acid.

nicardipine (ni-kar-di-peen) *n.* a calcium-channel blocker used to prevent angina and treat hypertension. It is administered by mouth. Trade name: **Cardene**.

NICE *n.* **(National Institute for Health and Care Excellence)** a nondepartmental public body that provides national guidance and advice to improve health and social care. NICE was originally set up in 1999 as the **National Institute for Clinical Excellence**, a special health authority, to reduce variation in the availability and quality of NHS treatments and care. In 2005 it began developing public health guidance and in 2013 took on responsibility for developing guidance and quality standards in social care.

SEE WEB LINKS

- Details of recommendations and guidance from the NICE website

niclosamide (ni-**kloh**-să-myd) *n.* an anthelmintic drug used to remove tapeworms. It is administered by mouth and is relatively free of side-effects.

nicorandil (nik-or-**and**-il) *n. see* potassium-channel activator.

nicotinamide (nik-ŏ-**tin**-ă-myd) *n.* a B vitamin: the amide of nicotinic acid.

nicotine (**nik**-ŏ-teen) *n.* a poisonous alkaloid derived from tobacco, responsible for the dependence of regular smokers on cigarettes. In small doses nicotine has a stimulating effect on the autonomic nervous system. Large doses cause paralysis of the autonomic ganglia.

nicotinic acid (niacin) (nik-ŏ-**tin**-ik) *n.* a B vitamin. Nicotinic acid is required in the diet but can also be synthesized from the essential amino acid tryptophan.

A deficiency of the vitamin leads to pellagra. Good sources of nicotinic acid are meat, yeast extracts, and pulses.

nictitation (nik-ti-tay-shŏn) *n.* exaggerated and frequent blinking or winking of the eyes.

NICU *n.* neonatal intensive care unit: *see* intensive care.

nidation (ny-**day**-shŏn) *n.* *see* implantation.

nidus (**ny**-dŭs) *n.* a place in which bacteria have settled and multiplied because of particularly suitable conditions: a focus of infection.

Niemann-Pick disease (nee-man pik) *n.* a rare inherited disease of phospholipid metabolism in which sphingomyelin and lecithin accumulate in the bone marrow, spleen, and lymph nodes. It is characterized by enlargement of the liver and the spleen and by physical and learning disability. [A. Niemann (1880–1921), German paediatrician; F. Pick (1868–1935), German physician]

nifedipine (ny-**fed**-i-peen) *n.* a calcium-channel blocker used to prevent angina and treat hypertension and Raynaud's phenomenon. It is administered by mouth. Trade names: **Adalat**, **Adipine MR** and **XL**, **Coracten SR** and **XL**, **Fortipine LA 40**, **Nifedipress**, **Tensipine MR**, **Valni XL.**

night blindness (nyctalopia) (nyt) *n.* the inability to see in dim light or at night. It is due to a disorder of the rods in the retina and can result from dietary deficiency of vitamin A. This deficiency may progress to include xerophthalmia and keratomalacia. Night blindness may be caused by other retinal diseases, e.g. retinitis pigmentosa. *Compare* day blindness.

Nightingale ward (**nyt**-in-gayl) *n.* a large open-plan ward that provides dormitory-style accommodation for hospital in-patients. This now outdated design offers patients little personal privacy or peace, and the closure of Nightingale wards for elderly patients was mandated by the National Service Framework for Older People in 2001.

night sweat *n.* copious sweating during sleep. Night sweats may be an early indication of tuberculosis, AIDS, or other disease.

night terror *n.* the condition in which a young child, soon after falling asleep, starts screaming and appears terrified. The attack ceases when the child wakes up fully and is never remembered.

nihilistic (ny-i-**lis**-tik) *adj.* (in psychiatry) describing or relating to the state of patients who believe that they and things about them do not exist.

nipple (mamilla, papilla) (**nip**-ŭl) *n.* the protuberance at the centre of the breast. In females the milk ducts open at the nipple.

NIPPV *n.* noninvasive intermittent positive-pressure ventilation (*see* noninvasive ventilation).

Nippy (**nip**-i) *n.* trade name for a brand of noninvasive positive-pressure ventilator that delivers air through a close-fitting nasal mask (*see* noninvasive ventilation).

Nissl granules (**nis**-ŭl) *pl. n.* collections of dark-staining material, containing RNA, seen in the cell bodies of neurons on microscopic examination. [F. Nissl (1860–1919), German neuropathologist]

nit (nit) *n.* the egg of a louse. The eggs of head lice are firmly cemented to the hair; those of body lice are fixed to the clothing.

nitrates (**ny**-trayts) *pl. n.* a class of drugs used as coronary vasodilators for the treatment and prevention of angina attacks. They include glyceryl trinitrate, isosorbide dinitrate, and isosorbide mononitrate.

nitrazepam (ny-**traz**-ĕ-pam) *n.* a benzodiazepine drug administered by mouth to treat short-term insomnia (*see* hypnotic). Morning drowsiness, lightheadedness, and confusion may occur. Trade name: **Mogadon**.

nitric acid (**ny**-trik) *n.* a strong corrosive mineral acid, the concentrated form of which is capable of producing severe burns of the skin. Swallowing the acid leads to intense burning pain and ulceration of the mouth and throat. Treatment is by immediate administration of alkaline solutions. Formula: HNO_3.

nitric oxide *n.* an important gaseous mediator that is involved in the manifestations of sepsis and septic shock. Formula: NO.

nitrofurantoin (ny-troh-fewr-**ant**-oh-in) *n.* a drug administered by mouth to treat bacterial infections of the urinary system. Trade name: **Macrobid**.

nitrogen (**ny**-trŏ-jĕn) *n.* a gaseous element and a major constituent of air (79%). Nitrogen is an essential constituent of proteins and nucleic acids and is obtained by humans in the form of protein-containing foods. Nitrogenous waste is excreted as urea. Liquid nitrogen is used to freeze some specimens before pathological examination. Symbol: N.

nitrogen balance *n.* the relationship between the nitrogen taken into the body and that excreted, denoting the balance between the manufacture and breakdown of the body mass. A negative nitrogen balance, when excretion exceeds intake, is usual after injury or operations as the energy requirements of the body are met disproportionately from endogenous sources.

nitroglycerin (ny-troh-**glis**-er-in) *n. see* glyceryl trinitrate.

nitroprusside (sodium nitroprusside) (ny-troh-**prus**-syd) *n.* a cyanide-containing drug used in the emergency treatment of high blood pressure. Given by controlled infusion into a vein, its effects and level in the blood must be closely monitored.

nitrous oxide (**ny**-trŭs) *n.* a colourless gas used as an anaesthetic with good analgesic properties, administered by inhalation during surgery in combination with oxygen and other agents for the maintenance of anaesthesia. A mixture of nitrous oxide and oxygen (**Entonox**, **Equanox**) is used for pain relief, particularly in childbirth. Because it tends to excite the patient when used alone, nitrous oxide was formerly known popularly as **laughing gas**. Formula: N_2O.

NIV *n. see* noninvasive ventilation.

nizatidine (ny-**zat**-i-deen) *n.* an H_2-receptor antagonist (*see* antihistamine) used to treat gastric and duodenal ulcers and prevent their recurrence and to treat gastro-oesophageal reflux disease. It is administered by mouth.

nm *symbol for* nanometre.

NMC *n. see* Nursing and Midwifery Council.

NMR *n. see* nuclear magnetic resonance.

Nocardia (noh-**kar**-diă) *n.* a genus of rodlike or filamentous Gram-positive nonmotile bacteria found in the soil. **N. asteroides** the species that causes nocardiosis. **N. madurae** the species associated with the disease Madura foot.

nocardiosis (noh-kar-di-**oh**-sis) *n.* a disease caused by bacteria of the genus *Nocardia*, primarily affecting the lungs, skin, and brain, resulting in the formation of abscesses.

noci- *combining form denoting* pain or injury.

nociceptive (noh-si-**sep**-tiv) *adj.* describing nerve fibres, endings, or pathways that are concerned with the condition of pain.

nociceptor (noh-si-**sep**-ter) *n.* a receptor that responds to the stimuli responsible for the sensation of pain. Nociceptors may be interoceptors, responding to such stimuli as inflammation, or exteroceptors, sensitive to heat, etc.

noct- (nocti-) *combining form denoting* night.

nocturia (nokt-**yoor**-iă) *n.* the passage of urine at night. Nocturia usually occurs in elderly people, since the normal rhythm of making less urine at night is lost with age.

nocturnal enuresis (nok-**ter**-năl) *n. see* enuresis.

node (nohd) *n.* a small swelling or knot of tissue. *See* atrioventricular node, lymph (node), sinoatrial node. **n. of Ranvier** one of the gaps that occur at regular intervals in the myelin sheath of medullated nerve fibres, between adjacent Schwann cells. [L. A. Ranvier (1835–1922), French pathologist]

nodule (**nod**-yool) *n.* a small swelling or aggregation of cells.

noma (**noh**-mă) *n.* a gangrenous infection of the mouth that spreads to involve the face. It is a severe form of ulcerative gingivitis that is usually found in debilitated or undernourished individuals.

nominal data (**nom**-i-năl) *pl. n.* data assigned to different categories that are in no particular order.

nonaccidental injury (NAI) (non-aks-i-**den**-t'l) *n.* injury inflicted on babies and young children; the perpetrator is usually an adult – often a parent or step-parent. Known colloquially as the **battered baby** (or **battered child**) **syndrome**, it is most commonly seen in babies aged six months or less. It usually takes the form of bruising, particularly on the face; bite marks; burns or scalds, particularly cigarette burns; and bone injuries, especially spiral fractures of the long bones in the limbs and skull fractures. Internal injuries may be fatal. Careful examination often reveals several injuries of different ages, indicating long-term abuse. NAI usually has serious consequences for the child, including failure to thrive and behavioural problems.

nonadherence (non-ăd-**heer**-ĕnss) *n.* not following medical advice. **intentional n.** nonadherence that involves the patient making a decision not to follow medical advice. **unintentional n.** nonadherence in which the patient forgets or misunderstands the advice.

non compos mentis (non **kom**-pŏs **men**-tis) *adj.* Latin: mentally incapable of managing one's own affairs.

nondeclarative memory (non-di-**kla**-ră-tiv **mem**-ĕ-ri) *n.* a collection of intuitive or implicit memories that enable a person to demonstrate a skill for which they have no previous recollection. It cannot be accessed consciously.

noninvasive (non-in-**vay**-siv) *adj.* **1.** denoting techniques of investigation or treatment that do not involve penetration of the skin by needles or knives. **2.** denoting tumours that do not spread into surrounding tissues (*see* benign).

noninvasive ventilation (NIV) mechanical assistance with breathing that does not require the insertion of an endotracheal tube (*see* intubation). In **noninvasive intermittent positive-pressure ventilation (NIPPV)** air is blown into the lungs through a close-fitting mask: designs range from helmet-like devices to nasal cushions and full-face or nasal masks (*see also* BiPAP, continuous positive airways pressure, Nippy). **Negative-pressure ventilation** involves the use of devices that draw air into and out of the lungs noninvasively by applying negative pressure in a cyclical way (*see* ventilator).

nonmaleficence (non-mal-**ef**-i-sĕns) *n.* (in ethics) the duty to avoid causing harm to patients.

nonparametric test (non-pa-ră-**met**-rik) *n.* *see* parametric test.

non-small-cell lung cancer (NSCLC) *n.* any type of lung cancer other than small-cell lung cancer. Such cancers include adenocarcinoma of the lung, large-cell carcinomas, and squamous-cell carcinoma of the lung.

nonsteroidal anti-inflammatory drug (non-steer-**oi**-d'l) *n.* *see* NSAID.

Noonan syndrome (**noo**-năn) *n.* an autosomal dominant condition that is associated with a wide range of health problems and other physical features, the most common being cardiovascular defects, restricted growth, abnormalities of the bones of the chest, and a characteristic facial appearance. It is sometimes associated with mild learning disabilities. [J. Noonan (1921–), US paediatrician]

noradrenaline (norepinephrine) (nor-ă-**dren**-ă-lin) *n.* a hormone, closely related to adrenaline, secreted by the medulla of the adrenal gland and also released as a neurotransmitter by sympathetic nerve endings. Among its many actions are constriction of small blood vessels leading to an increase in blood pressure, increase in the rate and depth of breathing, and relaxation of the smooth muscle in intestinal walls.

norepinephrine (nor-epi-**nef**-rin) *n. see* noradrenaline.

norethisterone (nor-eth-**ist**-er-ohn) *n.* a synthetic female sex hormone (*see* progestogen) administered by mouth to treat menstrual disorders, including endometriosis. Its main use, however, is in contraceptives, either alone (oral or injectable) or in combination with an oestrogen (oral); it is also used in hormone replacement therapy. Trade names: **Micronor**, **Noriday**, **Noristerat**, **Primolut N**, **Utovlan**.

norfloxacin (nor-**floks**-ă-sin) *n.* a quinolone antibiotic given by mouth for treating urinary-tract infections.

normal distribution (**nor**-măl) *n. see* frequency distribution.

normalization (nor-mă-ly-**zay**-shŏn) *n.* (in psychiatry) the process of making the living conditions of people with learning disabilities as similar as possible to those of people who are not handicapped. This includes moves to living outside institutions and encouragement to cope with work, pay, social life, sexuality, and civil rights.

normo- *combining form denoting* normality.

normoblast (**nor**-moh-blast) *n.* a nucleated cell that forms part of the series giving rise to the red blood cells and is normally found in the blood-forming tissue of the bone marrow. *See also* erythroblast, erythropoiesis.

normocyte (**nor**-moh-syt) *n.* a red blood cell of normal size. **—normocytic** *adj.*

normoglycaemia (euglycaemia) (nor-moh-gly-**see**-miă) *n.* the state of having normal blood glucose levels, which – depending on when food was last eaten – are generally between 4 and 7 mmol/l.

normotension (nor-moh-**ten**-shŏn) *n.* the state in which the arterial blood pressure is within the normal range. *Compare* hypertension, hypotension. **—normotensive** *adj.*

norovirus (Norwalk virus) (**no**-roh-vy-rŭs) *n.* an RNA virus that causes acute gastroenteritis in humans. The faecal–oral route is the typical mode of transmission and symptoms appear after an incubation period of between 24 and 48 hours. Noroviruses are highly contagious and are implicated in over 50% of all gastroenteritis outbreaks.

Norton scale (**nor**-tŏn) *n.* a predictive tool developed in the UK in 1962 to identify patients at risk of developing pressure ulcers through the assessment of five key risk factors – physical condition, mental condition, activity level, mobility, and continence – each of which is accorded a score from 1 (very bad) to 4 (good): the lower the total score, the greater the risk. A review of the tool added nutritional status as a potential risk factor. [D. Norton (1922–2007), British nurse]

nortriptyline (nor-**trip**-ti-leen) *n.* a tricyclic antidepressant drug that is administered by mouth to relieve depression and also to treat pain resulting from nerve damage. Trade name: **Allegron**.

nose (nohz) *n.* the organ of olfaction, which also acts as an air passage that warms, moistens, and filters the air on its way to the lungs. It consists of a triangular cartilaginous projection in the front of the face that contains the nostrils (*see* nares). It leads to the nasal cavity, which is lined with mucous membrane containing olfactory cells.

nosebleed (**nohz**-bleed) *n.* *see* epistaxis.

noso- *combining form denoting* disease.

nosocomial infection (hospital-acquired infection, HAI) (nos-oh-**koh**-mi-ăl) *n.* an infection that originates in a hospital, such as one developing in a hospitalized patient or a member of the hospital staff or acquired in hospital and developing after discharge. Such infections include fungal and bacterial infections and are aggravated by factors favouring the spread of organisms (cross-contamination) or by the reduced resistance of individual patients.

nosology (nos-**ol**-ŏji) *n.* the naming and classification of diseases.

nostrils (**nos**-trilz) *pl. n.* *see* nares.

notch (noch) *n.* (in anatomy) an indentation, especially one in a bone.

notifiable disease (noh-ti-**fy**-ăbŭl) *n.* a disease that must be reported to a proper officer of the local authority so that prompt control and preventive action may be undertaken if necessary. The 'proper officer' duty is often delegated by local authorities to a consultant in communicable disease control within Public Health England. In Great Britain notifiable diseases include anthrax, diphtheria, food poisoning, malaria, measles, rabies, tetanus, tuberculosis, and whooping cough.

NPF *n.* *see* nurse prescribers' formulary.

NSAID (nonsteroidal anti-inflammatory drug) *n.* any one of a large group of drugs used for pain relief, particularly in rheumatic disease associated with inflammation. NSAIDs act by inhibiting the enzymes controlling the formation of prostaglandins, which are important mediators of inflammation. They include aspirin, ibuprofen, ketoprofen, and naproxen. Adverse effects include gastric bleeding and ulceration. *See also* COX-2 inhibitor.

NSFs *pl. n.* *see* national service frameworks.

NSU *n.* *see* (nonspecific) urethritis.

nucha (**new**-kă) *n.* the nape of the neck.

nuchal (**new**-kăl) *adj.* relating to the nape of the neck. **n. fold** the fold of skin at the back of the neck of the fetus. **n. translucency scanning** a screening test performed during pregnancy at 11 weeks of gestation that measures the thickness of the translucent area overlying the neck region of the spine of the fetus, as observed on ultrasound scanning. Increased thickness is associated with an increased risk of chromosomal abnormalities and structural (e.g. heart) defects. *See also* ultrasound marker.

nucle- (nucleo-) *combining form denoting* a cell nucleus.

nuclear magnetic resonance (NMR) (new-kli-er) *n.* the absorption and emission of high-frequency radio waves by the nuclei of certain elements when placed in a strong magnetic field. The strongest signal is obtained from hydrogen atoms, which are abundant in the water and organic molecules in the body. NMR has important applications in noninvasive diagnostic techniques. *See* magnetic resonance imaging.

nuclear medicine *n.* the use of radionuclides (especially technetium-99m) as tracers to study the structure and function of organs of the body, often using a gamma camera. *See also* cardiology.

nuclease (new-kli-ayz) *n.* an enzyme that catalyses the breakdown of nucleic acids by cleaving the bonds between adjacent nucleotides.

nucleic acid (new-klee-ik) *n.* either of two organic acids, DNA or RNA, present in the nucleus and in some cases the cytoplasm of all living cells.

nucleolus (new-kli-oh-lŭs) *n.* (*pl.* **nucleoli**) a dense spherical structure within the cell nucleus that disappears during cell division. The nucleolus contains RNA for the synthesis of ribosomes.

nucleoprotein (new-kli-oh-proh-teen) *n.* a compound that occurs in cells and consists of nucleic acid and protein tightly bound together.

nucleoside (new-kli-ŏ-syd) *n.* a compound that consists of a nitrogen-containing base (a purine or pyrimidine) linked to a sugar. *See also* nucleotide.

nucleotide (new-kli-ŏ-tyd) *n.* a compound that consists of a nitrogen-containing base (a purine or pyrimidine) linked to a sugar and a phosphate group. Nucleic acids are long chains of linked nucleotides.

nucleus (new-kli-ŭs) *n.* (*pl.* **nuclei**) **1.** the part of a cell that contains the genetic material, DNA. The nucleus also contains RNA, most of which is located in the nucleolus. **2.** an anatomically and functionally distinct mass of nerve cells within the brain or spinal cord. **3.** the central part of the lens of the eye, which is harder than the outer cortex.

nucleus pulposus (pul-poh-sŭs) *n.* the central part of an intervertebral disc, which consists of a soft pulpy material.

null hypothesis (nul hy-poth-i-sis) *n.* *see* significance.

nullipara (nul-ip-er-ă) *n.* a woman who has never given birth.

nurse (ners) *n.* a person who has completed a programme of basic nursing education and is qualified and authorized in his or her country to practise nursing. In Britain, student nurses gain a diploma or degree in nursing and must undertake a specified period of training in a hospital approved by the Nursing and Midwifery Council to qualify as a **registered n.** (adult health, child health, mental health, or learning disabilities). *See* district nurse, health visitor, midwife, nurse practitioner, occupational health nurse, practice nurse, school nurse.

nurse-led clinic *n.* a clinic in which a nurse organizes his or her own patient workload and makes decisions about the organization of the care of a group of patients. This can include assessment, monitoring, and medicines prescription and reflects the ability to undertake advanced high-level practice care.

nurse practitioner *n.* a nurse specialist with advanced skills in physical diagnosis, psychosocial assessment, and management of patients' needs in primary care. A key member of the health-care team, a nurse practitioner can be based in a group practice or a health centre. Patients may present to the nurse or be referred to her for direct consultation about health problems. The nurse practitioner has the authority to prescribe drugs and other treatments within agreed policies.

nurse prescribers' formulary (NPF) *n.* a formulary from which nurses who have completed an appropriate course are required to prescribe. It covers a limited range of drugs that relate to an individual specialist practice area.

Nursing and Midwifery Council (NMC) (ners-ing) *n.* a statutory body that regulates the nursing and midwifery professions in the public interest.

SEE WEB LINKS

- The NMC website

nursing audit *n.* the process of collecting information from nursing reports and other documented evidence about patient care and assessing the quality of care by the use of quality assurance programmes. *See* performance indicators, quality assurance.

nursing home *n.* a residential facility that provides nursing supervision and limited medical care to individuals who do not require hospitalization.

nursing intervention *n.* an act to implement the nursing care plan as part of the nursing process. *See* planning.

nursing models *pl. n.* abstract frameworks, linking facts and phenomena, that assist nurses to plan nursing care, investigate problems related to clinical practice, and study the outcomes of nursing actions and interventions. Most of the nursing models in current usage are of North American origin but some have gained acceptance in the UK and are used in conjunction with the nursing process. *See* Casey's model, Henderson's model, King's model, Neuman's model, Orem's model, Peplau's model, Roper, Logan, and Tierney model, Roy's model.

nursing process *n.* an individualized problem-solving approach to the nursing care of patients. It involves four stages: assessment (of the patient's problems), planning (how to resolve them), implementation (of the plans), and evaluation (of their success).

nursing standard *n.* a measure or measures by which nursing care can be judged or compared; the measures used are agreed upon by common consent. Standards for an agreed level of care for a particular purpose should be derived and set in a democratic way, with the participation of all those involved. *See also* quality circle.

nutation (new-**tay**-shŏn) *n.* the act of nodding the head.

nutrient (**new**-tri-ĕnt) *n.* a substance that must be consumed in order to provide the essential components needed for growth and the maintenance of life. Nutrients include carbohydrates, proteins, fats, vitamins, and certain minerals, including the trace elements.

nutrition (new-**trish**-ŏn) *n.* **1.** the study of food in relation to the physiological processes that depend on its absorption by the body. The science of nutrition includes the study of diets and deficiency diseases. **2.** the intake of nutrients and their subsequent absorption and assimilation by the tissues. Patients who cannot be fed in a normal way can be given either nutrients by tubes into the gastrointestinal tract (**enteral n.** or **feeding**) or a nutrient solution that does not require digesting by infusion into a vein (**parenteral n.** or **feeding**). total parenteral n. (TPN) the delivery of all the essential nutrients to a patient directly into the bloodstream via a catheter in a vein. This may be via a vein in the upper arm for short-term use or into the subclavian vein in the neck for longer than two weeks. TPN has a risk of complications and should only be used when the gastrointestinal tract is not functioning.

SEE WEB LINKS

- Independent evidence-based advice on healthy eating from the British Nutrition Foundation

nyct- (nycto-) *combining form denoting* night or darkness.

nyctalopia (nik-tă-**loh**-piă) *n. see* night blindness.

nyctohemeral (nik-toh-**hem**-er-ăl) *adj.* denoting a cyclical event occurring both in the day and the night.

nympho- *combining form denoting* **1.** the labia minora. **2.** female sexuality.

nystagmus (nis-**tag**-mŭs) *n.* rapid involuntary movements of the eyes that may be from side to side, up and down, rotatory, or a combination of these. Nystagmus may be congenital and associated with poor sight; it also occurs in disorders of the part of the brain responsible for eye movements and in disorders of the organ of balance in the ear.

nystatin (**nis**-tă-tin) *n.* an antifungal drug used especially to treat infections caused by *Candida*. It is formulated, often in combination with other drugs, as a cream for skin infections and as a suspension for oral infections. Trade names: **Nystan**, **Nystaform**.

Oo

O *symbol for* oxygen.

OAE *pl. n. see* otoacoustic emissions.

oat-cell carcinoma (oht-sel) *n. see* small-cell lung cancer.

obesity (oh-**beess**-iti) *n.* the condition in which excess fat has accumulated in the body, in both the subcutaneous and visceral tissues. Clinical obesity is defined as a body mass index of 30 or over. *See also* leptin. **—obese** *adj.*

objective (ŏb-**jek**-tiv) **1.** *n.*(in microscopy) the lens or system of lenses in a light microscope that is nearest to the object under examination and furthest from the eyepiece. **2.** *n. see* behavioural objective. **3.** *adj.* existing independently of a patient's perception: applied particularly to the signs of a disease.

objective structured clinical examination (OSCE) *n.* a type of examination used increasingly in the health sciences (medicine, dentistry, nursing, physiotherapy, pharmacy) to assess clinical skills in examination, communication, medical procedures, and interpretation of results. The examination usually takes the form of a circuit of stations, with interactive and noninteractive tasks, around which each candidate moves after a specified time (5–10 minutes) at each station. Each station has a different examiner and the stations are standardized with specific marking criteria, thus enabling fairer comparison with peers.

obligate (**ob**-lig-ayt) *adj.* describing an organism that is restricted to one particular way of life. *Compare* facultative.

obscure auditory dysfunction (ŏb-**skyoor**) *n.* hearing difficulty, especially in noisy environments, in an individual with a normal audiogram; a form of auditory processing disorder. Treatment includes hearing therapy.

observations (ob-ser-**vay**-shŏns) *pl. n.* (in nursing) the frequent and systematic collection of data relevant to a patient's condition. As well as monitoring the patient's vital signs (pulse, blood pressure, respiratory rate, temperature, etc.), observations may include careful attention to (and noting of) the patient's interactions, verbal and nonverbal behaviour, and reactions to the physical surroundings. The data are analysed to determine the level of care the patient requires and must be clearly documented to prevent ambiguous interpretation.

obsession (ŏb-**sesh**-ŏn) *n.* a recurrent thought, feeling, or impulse that is unpleasant and provokes anxiety but cannot be eliminated. Although an obsession dominates the person, he or she realizes its senselessness and struggles to resist it, which causes anxiety. Obsessions are a feature of **obsessive–compulsive disorder** (**OCD**) and sometimes of depression and of organic states, such as encephalitis. *See also* compulsion, neurosis. **—obsessional** *adj.*

obsessive–compulsive disorder (OCD) (ŏb-ses-iv kŏm-**pul**-siv) *n.* a mental illness prevalent in about 1% of the adult population but more common in children. The affected person has obsessions or compulsions he or she recognizes as senseless; resisting the obsession causes anxiety, which is relieved by giving in to the compulsion. The obsession may be a fear or an impulse (e.g. to wash the hands repetitively). In severe cases obsessions and rituals can take over many hours of a person's life each day. The condition can be treated with behaviour therapy and antidepressant medication, particularly clomipramine and SSRIs.

obstetrics (ŏb-**stet**-riks) *n.* the branch of medical science concerned with the care of women during pregnancy, childbirth, and the period of about six weeks following the birth. *Compare* gynaecology. **—obstetric** *adj.* **—obstetrician** (ob-stit-**rish**-ăn) *n.*

obstructed labour *n.* failure of the presenting part to descend during delivery in spite of uterine contractions. Obstruction is usually due to (1) an abnormality in the woman's pelvis; (2) an abnormality in her baby; or (3) an abnormality in the relationship between them, either an abnormal lie (e.g. transverse) or malpresentation, or the state in which the diameter of the fetal head is greater than the pelvic outlet.

obstruction (ŏb-**struk**-shŏn) *n.* the condition of being blocked, which may affect any tubular organ or structure. **intestinal o.** blockage of the bowel, producing symptoms of vomiting, distension, and abdominal pain due to failure to pass intestinal contents. Acute obstruction may be caused by incarcerated hernias, adhesions, or malignancy; chronic obstruction may be due to tumours, strictures, anatomical abnormality, or neurological disease. **—obstructive** (ŏb-**struk**-tiv) *adj.*

obstructive sleep apnoea *n. see* sleep apnoea.

obturation (ob-tewr-**ay**-shŏn) *n.* obstruction of a bodily passage, usually by impaction of a foreign body, viscid secretions, or hardened faeces.

obturator (**ob**-tewr-ay-ter) *n.* **1.** a wire or rod within a cannula or hollow needle for piercing tissues or fitting aspirating needles. **2.** a removable form of denture that both closes a defect in the palate and also restores the dentition. **3.** (**o. muscle**) either of two muscles that cover the outer surface of the anterior wall of the pelvis and are responsible for lateral rotation of the thigh and movements of the hip. **o. foramen** a large opening in the hip bone, below and slightly in front of the acetabulum. *See also* pelvis.

obtusion (ŏb-tew-zhŏn) *n.* the weakening or blunting of normal sensations. This may be associated with disease.

occipital bone (ok-**sip**-i-t'l) *n.* a saucer-shaped bone of the skull that forms the back and part of the base of the cranium. At the base of the occipital are two condyles that articulate with the first (atlas) vertebra of the backbone. Between the condyles is the foramen magnum.

occipitoanterior (ok-sip-i-toh-an-**teer**-i-er) *adj.* describing the most favourable position of a baby at the time of delivery, in which the back of the head is towards the front of the mother's pelvis.

occipitoposterior (ok-sip-i-toh-pos-**teer**-i-er) *adj.* describing a malposition of a baby at the time of delivery in which the back of the head is towards the posterior aspect of the mother's pelvis. *See* malposition.

occipitotransverse (ok-sip-i-toh-**tranz**-vers) *adj.* describing a malposition of a baby at the time of delivery in which the back of the head is towards the lateral aspect of the mother's pelvis. *See* malposition.

occiput (**oks**-ip-ut) *n.* the back of the head. **—occipital** *adj.*

occlusion (ŏ-**kloo**-zhŏn) *n.* **1.** the closing or obstruction of a hollow organ or part. **2.** (in dentistry) the relation of the upper and lower teeth when they are in contact. *See also* malocclusion.

occult (ŏ-**kult**) *adj.* not apparent to the naked eye; not easily detected. **o. blood** blood present in such small quantities that it can only be detected microscopically or by chemical testing. *See* faecal occult blood test.

occupational disease (ok-yoo-**pay**-shŏn-ăl) *n.* any disease to which workers in certain occupations are particularly prone. Examples include the various forms of pneumoconiosis, cataracts in glassblowers, decompression sickness in divers, and infectious diseases contracted from animals by farm workers, such as woolsorter's disease (*see* anthrax). *See also* industrial disease, prescribed disease.

occupational health nurse *n.* (in the UK) a nurse who has undergone a specialized course of study (full or part time) in the health care of people at work. An occupational health nurse is responsible for promoting a high degree of physical and mental health in industrial and commercial settings and in the NHS.

occupational therapy *n.* the treatment of physical and psychiatric conditions through specific activities in order to help people reach their maximum level of function and independence in all aspects of daily life.

OCD *n. see* obsessive–compulsive disorder.

oct- (octa-, octi-, octo-) *combining form denoting* eight.

octreotide (**ok**-tri-oh-tyd) *n.* an analogue of somatostatin that is administered by injection to treat acromegaly and hormone-secreting neuroendocrine tumours. Trade name: **Sandostatin**.

ocular (**ok**-yoo-ler) *adj.* of or concerned with the eye or vision. **o. hypertension (OHT)** a constantly raised intraocular pressure (greater than 21mmHg by Goldmann applanation tonometry) registered on two or more occasions in one or both eyes with the absence of evidence of optic nerve damage or visual field defect. Intraocular pressure increases slowly with age and OHT can increase the risk of developing glaucoma. It is treated with eye drops and surgery if indicated. **o. pemphigoid** *see* pemphigoid.

oculo- *combining form denoting* the eye(s).

oculogyric (ok-yoo-loh-**jy**-rik) *adj.* causing or concerned with movements of the eye. **o. crisis** a spasmodic deviation of the eyes upwards when the head is tilted backwards, which occurs in patients with postencephalitic parkinsonism or who are taking phenothiazines.

oculomotor (ok-yoo-loh-**moh**-ter) *adj.* concerned with eye movements. **o. nerve** the third cranial nerve (III), which supplies muscles in and around the eye, including those responsible for altering the size of the pupil and those that turn the eyeball in different directions.

oculonasal (ok-yoo-loh-**nay**-zăl) *adj.* concerned with the eye and nose.

oculoplastics (ok-yoo-loh-**plast**-iks) *n.* a surgical specialty concerned with reconstructive and cosmetic surgery around the eye (including the orbit, eyelids, lacrimal apparatus, and other accessory structures).

oculoplethysmography (ok-yoo-loh-pleth-iz-**mog**-răfi) *n.* measurement of the pressure inside the eyeball. A rising or above-normal pressure is an important indication of the presence of glaucoma.

o.d. (omni die) Latin: daily, used as a direction in prescriptions.

odont- (odonto-) *combining form denoting* a tooth.

odontalgia (od-on-**tal**-jiă) *n.* toothache.

odontoid process (od-**ont**-oid) *n.* a toothlike process from the upper surface of the axis vertebra.

odontology (od-on-**tol**-ŏji) *n.* the study of the teeth.

odontome (od-**ont**-ohm) *n.* an abnormal mass of calcified dental tissue, usually representing a developmental abnormality.

-odynia *combining form denoting* pain in (a specified part).

odynophagia (od-i-noh-**fay**-jiă) *n.* painful swallowing. This may be due to severe inflammation of the gullet (*see* oesophagitis), or to infection, as by cytomegalovirus, candidiasis, or herpes simplex virus.

oedema (ee-**dee**-mă) *n.* excessive accumulation of fluid in the body tissues: historically known as **dropsy**. The resultant swelling may be local, as with an injury or inflammation, or more general. In generalized oedema there may be collections of fluid within the chest cavity, abdomen (*see* ascites), or within the air spaces of the lung (**pulmonary o.**). It may result from heart or kidney failure, cirrhosis of the liver, acute nephritis, the nephrotic syndrome, starvation, allergy, or certain drugs. Diuretics are administered to get rid of the excess fluid. **angio-o.** *see* urticaria. **subcutaneous o.** oedema that commonly occurs in the legs and ankles; the swelling subsides with rest and elevation of the legs. **—oedematous** *adj.*

Oedipus complex (ee-dip-ŭs) *n.* in Freudian theory, repressed sexual feelings of a child for its opposite-sexed parent, combined with rivalry towards the same-sexed parent: said to be a normal stage of development. Arrest of development at the Oedipal stage is said to be responsible for sexual deviations and other neurotic behaviour.

oesophag- (oesophago-) *combining form denoting* the oesophagus.

oesophageal ulcer (ee-sof-ă-**jee**-ăl) *n.* a peptic ulcer in the oesophagus, associated with reflux oesophagitis.

oesophageal varices *pl. n.* dilated veins in the lower oesophagus due to portal hypertension. Varices have a high risk of bleeding, resulting in life-threatening haematemesis. Bleeding may be arrested by band ligation, an endoscopic technique in which rubber bands are applied; if this fails, it may be necessary to insert a Sengstaken tube.

oesophagectomy (ee-sof-ă-**jek**-tŏmi) *n.* surgical removal of part or the whole of the oesophagus.

oesophagitis (ee-sof-ă-**jy**-tis) *n.* inflammation of the oesophagus. **corrosive o.** oesophagitis caused by the ingestion of caustic acid or alkali. **infective o.** oesophagitis caused by infection with *Candida* or, more rarely, by viruses. It is common in AIDS patients. **reflux o.** the commonest form of oesophagitis, caused by frequent regurgitation of acid and peptic juices from the stomach. It may be associated with a hiatus hernia. The main symptoms are heartburn, acid regurgitation, odynophagia, and sometimes difficulty in swallowing; complications include bleeding, narrowing (stricture) of the oesophageal canal, and Barrett's oesophagus.

oesophagocele (ee-**sof**-ă-goh-seel) *n.* protrusion of the lining (mucosa) of the oesophagus through a tear or weakness in its muscular wall.

oesophagogastroduodenoscopy (OGD) (ee-sof-ă-goh-gas-troh-dew-ŏ-di-**nos**-kŏpi) *n.* endoscopic examination of the upper gastrointestinal tract using a fibreoptic or video instrument. *See also* gastroscope.

SEE WEB LINKS

- Information about this procedure from BUPA

oesophagoscope (ee-**sof**-ă-goh-skohp) *n.* an illuminated optical instrument that is used to inspect the interior of the oesophagus, dilate strictures, obtain material for biopsy, or remove a foreign body. **—oesophagoscopy** (ee-sof-ă-**gos**-kŏ-pi) *n.*

oesophagostomy (ee-sof-ă-gost-ŏmi) *n.* a surgical operation in which the oesophagus is opened onto the neck. It is usually performed after operations on the throat as a temporary measure to allow feeding.

oesophagotomy (ee-sof-ă-**got**-ŏmi) *n.* surgical opening of the oesophagus in order to inspect its interior or to remove or insert something.

oesophagus (ee-**sof**-ă-gŭs) *n.* the gullet: a muscular tube, about 23 cm long, that extends from the pharynx to the stomach. It is lined with mucous membrane, whose secretions lubricate food as it passes from the mouth to the stomach. —**oesophageal** *adj.*

oestradiol (ees-tră-**dy**-ol) *n.* the major female sex hormone produced by the ovary. *See* oestrogen.

oestriol (**ees**-tri-ol) *n.* one of the female sex hormones produced by the ovary. *See* oestrogen.

oestrogen (**ees**-trŏ-jĕn) *n.* one of a group of steroid hormones (including oestriol, oestrone, and oestradiol) that control female sexual development. Oestrogens are synthesized mainly by the ovary; small amounts are also produced by the adrenal cortex, testes, and placenta. Naturally occurring and synthetic oestrogens are administered by mouth or injection to treat amenorrhoea, menopausal symptoms (*see* hormone replacement therapy), and androgen-dependent cancers. Synthetic oestrogens are a major constituent of oral contraceptives. —**oestrogenic** *adj.*

oestrone (**ees**-trohn) *n.* one of the female sex hormones produced by the ovary. *See* oestrogen.

ofloxacin (oh-**floks**-ă-sin) *n.* a quinolone antibiotic used to treat infections of the genitourinary and respiratory tracts, skin, and eye. It is administered by mouth, intravenous infusion, or as eye drops. Trade names: **Exocin**, **Tarivid**.

OGD *n.* *see* oesophagogastroduodenoscopy.

Ogilvie's syndrome (**oh**-gil-viz) *n.* *see* pseudo-obstruction.

ohm (ohm) *n.* the SI unit of electrical resistance, equal to the resistance between two points on a conductor when a constant potential difference of 1 volt applied between these points produces a current of 1 ampere. Symbol: Ω.

OHT *see* ocular hypertension.

-oid *suffix denoting* like; resembling.

ointment (**oint**-mĕnt) *n.* a greasy preparation, which may or may not contain a medication, applied to the skin or mucous membranes.

olanzapine (oh-**lanz**-ă-peen) *n.* *see* antipsychotic.

olecranon process (oh-**lek**-ră-non) *n.* the large process of the ulna that projects behind the elbow joint.

oleic acid (oh-**lee**-ik) *n.* *see* fatty acid.

oleo- *combining form denoting* oil.

oleum (**oh**-li-ŭm) *n.* (in pharmacy) an oil.

olfaction (ol-**fak**-shŏn) *n.* **1.** the sense of smell. **2.** the process of smelling. Sensory cells in the mucous membrane that lines the nasal cavity are stimulated by the presence of chemical particles dissolved in the mucus. **—olfactory** (ol-**fak**-ter-i) *adj.*

olfactory nerve *n.* the first cranial nerve (I): the special sensory nerve of smell. Fibres of the nerve run upwards from smell receptors in the nasal mucosa and join to form the olfactory tract to the brain.

olig- (oligo-) *combining form denoting* **1.** few. **2.** a deficiency.

oligaemia (ol-ig-**ee**-miă) *n. see* hypovolaemia.

oligodactylism (ol-i-goh-**dak**-til-izm) *n.* the congenital absence of some of the fingers and toes.

oligodipsia (ol-i-goh-**dip**-siă) *n.* a condition in which thirst is diminished or absent.

oligohydramnios (ol-i-goh-hy-**dram**-ni-os) *n.* a decrease in the amount of amniotic fluid surrounding the fetus, which may occur in the second and third trimesters and is usually associated with restricted fetal growth.

oligomenorrhoea (ol-i-goh-men-ŏ-**ree**-ă) *n.* menstruation at intervals of between 35 days and 6 months.

oligospermia (ol-i-goh-**sper**-miă) *n.* a reduced number of spermatozoa in the semen (*see* seminal analysis). In oligospermia there are less than 20 million spermatozoa per ml with poor motility and often including many bizarre and immature forms. It is a cause of male infertility.

oliguria (ol-ig-**yoor**-iă) *n.* the production of an abnormally small volume of urine. This may be a result of copious sweating, kidney disease, oedema, loss of blood, diarrhoea, or poisoning.

olive (**ol**-iv) *n.* a smooth oval swelling in the upper part of the medulla oblongata on each side. It contains a mass of nerve cells, mainly grey matter (**olivary nucleus**). **—olivary** *adj.*

Ollier's disease (ol-i-ayz) *n. see* dyschondroplasia.
[L. L. X. E. Ollier (1830–1900), French surgeon]

-ology *combining form. see* -logy.

olsalazine (ol-**sal**-ă-zeen) *n.* a salicylate preparation used to treat mild ulcerative colitis. It is administered by mouth. Trade name: **Dipentum**.

o.m. (omni mane) Latin: in the morning, used as a direction in prescriptions.

om- (omo-) *combining form denoting* the shoulder.

-oma *combining form denoting* a tumour.

omalizumab (oh-**mal**-i-zoo-mab) *n.* a monoclonal antibody administered by subcutaneous injection for the prevention of severe allergic asthma that has not responded to standard therapy and is also a highly effective treatment for chronic urticaria. Trade name: **Xolair**.

omentectomy (oh-men-**tek**-tŏmi) *n.* the surgical removal of all or part of the omentum. **infracolic o.** excision of the lower section of the greater omentum as part of the management of ovarian or bowel cancer.

omentum (epiploon) (oh-**men**-tŭm) *n.* a double layer of peritoneum attached to the stomach and linking it with other abdominal organs. **greater o.** a highly folded portion of the omentum that covers the intestines in an apron-like fashion. It acts as a heat insulator and prevents friction between abdominal organs. **lesser o.** a portion of the omentum that links the stomach with the liver. **—omental** *adj*.

omeprazole (oh-**mep**-ră-zohl) *n.* a drug used to treat gastric and duodenal ulcers, gastro-oesophageal reflux disease, and the Zollinger-Ellison syndrome (*see* proton-pump inhibitor). Administered by mouth or intravenously, it is long-acting and need only be taken once a day. Trade name: **Losec**.

omphal- (omphalo-) *combining form denoting* the navel or umbilical cord.

omphalitis (om-fă-**ly**-tis) *n.* inflammation of the navel, especially in newborn infants.

omphalocele (**om**-fă-loh-seel) *n.* an umbilical hernia.

omphalus (**om**-fă-lŭs) *n.* *see* umbilicus.

o.n. (omni nocte) Latin: at night, used as a direction in prescriptions.

Onchocerca (onk-oh-**ser**-kă) *n.* a genus of parasitic worms (*see* filaria) occurring in central Africa and central America. **O. volvulus** the cause of onchocerciasis.

onchocerciasis (onk-oh-ser-**ky**-ă-sis) *n.* a tropical disease of the skin and underlying connective tissue caused by the parasitic worm *Onchocerca volvulus*. Fibrous nodular tumours grow around the adult worms in the skin; the migration of the larvae into the eye can cause total or partial blindness (**river blindness**). Ivermectin is used in treatment.

onco- *combining form denoting* **1.** a tumour. **2.** volume.

oncogene (**onk**-oh-jeen) *n.* a gene in viruses and mammalian cells that can cause cancer; it results from the mutation of a normal gene (a proto-oncogene) and is capable of both initiation and continuation of malignant transformation of normal cells. Oncogenes probably produce peptides (growth factors) regulating cell division that, under certain conditions, become uncontrolled and may transform a normal cell to a malignant state.

oncogenesis (onk-oh-**jen**-i-sis) *n.* the development of a new abnormal growth (a benign or malignant tumour).

oncogenic (onk-oh-**jen**-ik) *adj.* describing a substance, organism, or environment that is known to be a causal factor in the production of a tumour. Some viruses are oncogenic. *See also* carcinogen.

oncology (onk-**ol**-ŏji) *n.* the study and practice of treating tumours. It is often subdivided into medical, surgical, clinical, and radiation oncology. **—oncologist** *n.*

oncolysis (onk-**ol**-i-sis) *n.* the destruction of tumours and tumour cells. This may occur spontaneously or, more usually, in response to treatment with drugs or radiotherapy.

oncometer (onk-**om**-it-er) *n.* *see* plethysmography.

oncotic (onk-ot-ik) *adj.* **1.** characterized by a tumour or swelling. **2.** relating to an increase in volume or pressure.

ondansetron (on-**dan**-si-tron) *n.* a drug administered by mouth, injection, or infusion, or as rectal suppositories to control severe nausea and vomiting, especially when this is caused by chemotherapy and radiotherapy. Trade name: **Zofran**.

ontogeny (on-**toj**-ĕ-ni) *n.* the history of the development of an individual from the fertilized egg to maturity.

onych- (onycho-) *combining form denoting* the nail(s).

onychogryphosis (on-i-koh-grif-**oh**-sis) *n.* gross thickening and hardening of a nail, which becomes elongated and deformed.

onycholysis (on-i-**kol**-i-sis) *n.* separation or loosening of part or all of a nail from its bed. The condition may be due to psoriasis, fungal infections of the skin or nail bed, trauma, or drugs.

onychomycosis (on-i-koh-my-**koh**-sis) *n.* fungal infection of the nails caused by dermatophytes or *Candida*. The nails become discoloured, opaque, and thickened. *See also* tinea.

O'nyong nyong fever (joint-breaker fever) (oh-**n'yong**-n'yong) *n.* an African disease caused by an arbovirus and transmitted by mosquitoes of the genus *Anopheles*. Symptoms include rigor, severe headache, an irritating rash, fever, and pains in the joints.

oo- *combining form denoting* an egg; ovum.

oocyte (**oh**-ŏ-syt) *n.* a cell in the ovary that undergoes meiosis to form an ovum. *See* oogenesis.

oocyte donation *n.* the transfer of oocytes from one woman to another. It allows the recipient, who is unable to ovulate, to achieve a normal pregnancy.

oogenesis (oh-ŏ-**jen**-i-sis) *n.* the process by which mature ova are produced in the ovary (see illustration). Primordial germ cells multiply to form oogonia, which start their first meiotic division to become oocytes in the fetus and complete it at ovulation. Fertilization stimulates the completion of the second meiotic division, which produces a mature ovum.

oogonium (oh-ŏ-**goh**-niŭm) *n.* (*pl.* **oogonia**) a cell produced at an

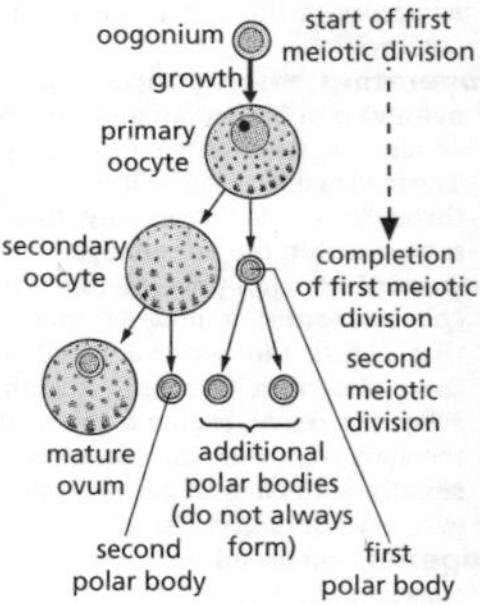

Oogenesis

early stage in the formation of an ovum. *See* oogenesis.

oophor- (oophoro-) *combining form denoting* the ovary.

oophorectomy (ovariectomy) (oh-ŏ-fŏ-**rek**-tŏmi) *n.* surgical removal of an ovary.

oophoritis (ovaritis) (oh-ŏ-fŏ-**ry**-tis) *n.* inflammation of an ovary, either on the surface or within the organ. Oophoritis may be associated with infection of the Fallopian tubes (*see* salpingitis) or the lower part of the abdominal cavity.

oophoropexy (oh-**off**-ŏ-roh-peks-i) *n.* the stitching of a displaced ovary to the wall of the pelvic cavity.

oophorosalpingectomy (oh-off-ŏ-roh-sal-pin-**jek**-tŏmi) *n.* surgical removal of an ovary and its associated Fallopian tube.

opacity (ŏ-**pas**-iti) *n.* **1.** lack of transparency. **2.** an opaque area, as occurs in the lens of the eye in cataract.

operating microscope (**op**-er-ayt-ing) *n.* a binocular microscope commonly used in microsurgery. The field of operation is illuminated through the objective lens by a light source within the microscope.

operculum (oh-**per**-kew-lŭm) *n.* (*pl.* **opercula**) a plug of mucus that blocks the cervical canal of the uterus in a pregnant woman. When the cervix begins to dilate at the start of labour, the operculum, slightly stained with blood, comes away as a discharge ('show').

operon (**op**-er-on) *n.* a group of closely linked genes that regulate the production of enzymes in bacteria.

ophthalm- (ophthalmo-) *combining form denoting* the eye or eyeball. Examples: **ophthalmectomy** (surgical removal of); **ophthalmorrhexis** (rupture of).

ophthalmia (off-**thal**-miă) *n.* inflammation of the eye, particularly the conjunctiva (*see* conjunctivitis). **o. neonatorum** conjunctivitis occurring in newborn infants, who contract the disease as they pass through an infected birth canal. The two most common infections are gonorrhoea and *Chlamydia*. Unless both mother and baby are treated (with antibiotics), the infection may cause lasting damage to the eye. **sympathetic o.** a granulomatous uveitis affecting all parts of the uveal tract of both eyes that may develop after perforating trauma or (more rarely) intraocular surgery.

ophthalmic (off-**thal**-mik) *adj.* concerned with the eye.

ophthalmitis (off-thal-**my**-tis) *n.* inflammation of the eye. *See* conjunctivitis, uveitis.

ophthalmologist (off-thal-**mol**-ŏ-jist) *n.* a doctor who specializes in the diagnosis and treatment of eye diseases.

ophthalmology (off-thal-**mol**-ŏji) *n.* the branch of medicine that is devoted to the study and treatment of eye diseases. **—ophthalmological** *adj.*

ophthalmometer (off-thal-**mom**-it-er) *n. see* keratometer.

ophthalmoplegia (off-thal-moh-**plee**-jiă) *n.* paralysis of the muscles of the eye. It may accompany exophthalmos due to thyrotoxicosis. **external o.** ophthalmoplegia affecting the muscles that move the eye. **internal o.** ophthalmoplegia affecting the iris and ciliary muscle. **internuclear o.** ophthalmoplegia due to a lesion in the brainstem, seen in patients with multiple sclerosis or stroke.

ophthalmoscope (off-**thal**-mŏ-skohp) *n.* an instrument for examining the interior of the eye. **—ophthalmoscopy** (off-thal-**mos**-kŏ-pi) *n.*

ophthalmotonometer *n. see* tonometer.

-opia *combining form denoting* a defect of the eye or of vision.

opiate (**oh**-piăt) *n.* one of a group of drugs derived from opium. Synthetic drugs with similar effects are called **opioids**, a term often used to include both the natural and synthetic drugs. This group includes morphine, codeine, diamorphine (heroin), methadone, and buprenorphine. They depress the central nervous system and are used to relieve moderate to severe pain and suppress coughing. Side-effects include drowsiness, nausea and vomiting, constipation, and depression of breathing; prolonged use can lead to tolerance and dependence.

opioid (**oh**-pi-oyd) *n. see* opiate.

opisth- (opistho-) *combining form denoting* **1.** dorsal; posterior. **2.** backwards.

opisthorchiasis (op-iss-thor-**ky**-ă-sis) *n.* a condition caused by the presence of the parasitic fluke *Opisthorchis* in the bile ducts. Heavy infections can damage the tissues of the bile duct and liver and may progress to cirrhosis. The disease is treated with praziquantel.

Opisthorchis (op-iss-**thor**-kis) *n.* a genus of parasitic flukes occurring in E Europe, India, Japan, and SE Asia. The adult flukes, which live in the bile ducts, can cause opisthorchiasis.

opisthotonos (op-iss-**thot**-oh-nŏs) *n.* the position of the body in which the head, neck, and spine are arched backwards. It is assumed involuntarily by patients with tetanus and strychnine poisoning.

opium (**oh**-piŭm) *n.* an extract from the poppy *Papaver somniferum*, which contains a number of alkaloids, principally morphine (which accounts for its analgesic, euphoric, and addictive effects). *See also* opiate.

opponens (oh-**poh**-nenz) *n.* one of a group of muscles in the hand that bring the digits opposite to other digits. **o. pollicis** the principal muscle causing opposition of the thumb.

opportunistic (op-er-tew-**nis**-tik) *adj.* denoting a disease that occurs when the patient's immune system is impaired by, for example, an infection, another disease, or drugs. The infecting organism rarely causes the disease in healthy persons. Opportunistic infections, such as *Pneumocystis* pneumonia and those caused by *Mycobacterium* (*see* MAI complex), are common in patients with AIDS.

-opsia *combining form denoting* a condition of vision.

opsoclonus (op-soh-**kloh**-nŭs) *n.* a series of erratic eye movements resembling a large-amplitude nystagmus, which is seen in people with disease of the cerebellum or other parts of the brain.

opsonin (op-sŏn-in) *n.* a serum complement component that attaches itself to invading bacteria and apparently makes them more susceptible to phagocytosis.

opt- (opto-) *combining form denoting* vision or the eye.

optic (op-tik) *adj.* concerned with the eye or vision. **o. atrophy** degeneration of the optic nerve. **o. chiasm** (**o. commissure**) the X-shaped structure formed by the two optic nerves as nerve fibres from the nasal side of the retina of each eye cross over to join fibres from the lateral side of the retina of the opposite eye (see illustration). **o. disc** (**o. papilla**) the start of the optic nerve, where nerve fibres from the rods and cones leave the eyeball. *See* blind spot. **o. nerve** the second cranial nerve (II), which is responsible for vision. It passes into the skull behind the eyeball to reach the optic chiasm, after which the visual pathway continues to the occipital lobe. **o. neuritis** *see* retrobulbar neuritis.

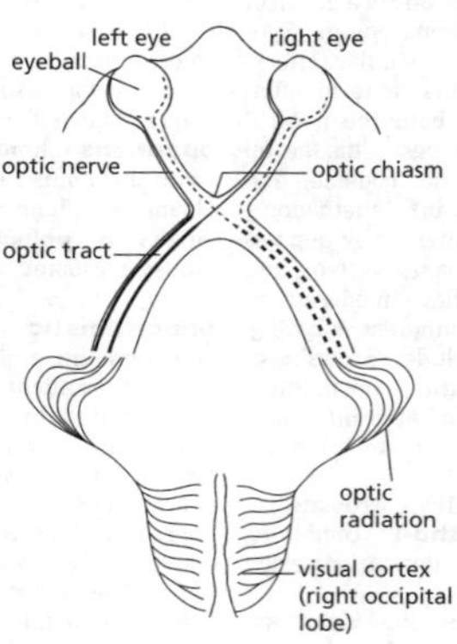

The visual (or optic) pathway

optician (op-**tish**-ăn) *n.* a person who either makes and fits glasses (**dispensing o.**) or who can both test people for glasses and dispense glasses (**ophthalmic o.** or **optometrist**).

opticokinetic (op-tik-oh-ky-**net**-ik) *adj.* relating to the movements of the eye.

optometer (refractometer) (op-**tom**-it-er) *n.* an instrument for measuring the refraction of the eye.

optometrist (op-**tom**-i-trist) *n. see* optician.

optometry (op-**tom**-itri) *n.* the practice of testing the visual acuity of eyes and prescribing lenses to correct defects of vision.

oral (**or**-ăl) *adj.* **1.** relating to the mouth. **2.** taken by mouth: applied to medicines, etc.

oral contraceptive *n.* the Pill: a tablet, containing one or more synthetic female sex hormones, taken by women to prevent conception. Most oral contraceptives are combined pills, consisting of an oestrogen, which blocks the normal process of ovulation, and a progestogen, which acts on the pituitary gland to block the normal control of the menstrual cycle.

oral hypoglycaemic drug (oral antihypoglycaemic drug) (hy-poh-gly-**see**-mik) *n.* one of the group of drugs that reduce the level of glucose in the blood and are taken by mouth for the treatment of type 2 (noninsulin-dependent) diabetes mellitus. They include the sulphonylurea drugs, metformin (a biguanide), alpha-glucosidase inhibitors, meglitinides, thiazolidinediones, DPP-IV inhibitors, and SGLT-2 inhibitors.

oral rehydration therapy (ORT) (ree-hy-**dray**-shŏn) *n.* the administration of an isotonic solution of various sodium salts, potassium chloride, glucose, and water to treat acute diarrhoea, particularly in children. In developing countries it is the mainstay of treatment for cholera. Preparations in clinical use include **Dioralyte** and **Electrolade**.

orbicularis (or-bik-yoo-**lar**-iss) *n.* either of two circular muscles of the face. **o. oculi** the muscle around each orbit that is responsible for closing the eye. **o. oris** the muscle around the mouth that closes and compresses the lips.

orbit (**or**-bit) *n.* the cavity in the skull that contains the eye. It is formed from parts of the frontal, sphenoid, zygomatic, lacrimal, ethmoid, palatine, and maxillary bones. **—orbital** *adj.*

orbitotomy (or-bit-**ot**-ŏmi) *n.* surgical removal of part of the orbital bones to gain access to the orbital space.

orchi- (orchido-, orchio-) *combining form denoting* the testis or testicle.

orchidalgia (or-kid-**al**-jiă) *n.* pain in the testicle, often due to a varicocele, orchitis, or torsion of the testis.

orchidectomy (or-kid-**ek**-tŏmi) *n.* surgical removal of a testis. A **radical orchidectomy** is performed for malignant tumours within the testis (usually germ-cell tumours such as seminoma and teratoma).

orchidometer (or-kid-**om**-it-er) *n.* a calliper device for measuring the size of the testicles. **Prader o.** a collection of testicle-shaped beads of different sizes, each of known volume, for direct comparison to and sizing of the testicles, enabling the precise charting of testicular growth.

orchidopexy (or-kid-oh-peks-i) *n.* the operation of mobilizing an undescended testis in the groin and fixing it in the scrotum.

orchidotomy (or-kid-**ot**-ŏmi) *n.* an incision into the testis, usually done to obtain biopsy material for histological examination.

orchis (**or**-kis) *n.* the testis or testicle.

orchitis (or-**ky**-tis) *n.* inflammation of the testis. This causes pain, redness, and swelling of the scrotum, and may be associated with inflammation of the epididymis (**epididymo-orchitis**). The condition is usually caused by infection spreading down the vas deferens but can develop in mumps (**mumps o.**).

ordinal data (or-di-năl) *pl. n.* data measured on a scale in which the scale points reflect order of magnitude and differences between data cannot be quantified.

Orem's model (or-ĕmz) *n.* a model for nursing based on the self-care deficit theory of nursing, in which patients are seen as able, when they are well, to initiate and perform activities on their own behalf, in order to maintain life, health, and wellbeing. Infants, children, the elderly, the disabled, and the ill may require assistance or complete care with these activities. *See also* nursing models. [D. Orem (1914–2007), US nurse theorist]

orf (orf) *n.* an infectious disease of sheep and goats caused by a parapoxvirus. Those bottle-feeding infected lambs may develop a painful nodule on the fingers or hands; it resolves spontaneously.

organ (**or**-găn) *n.* a part of the body, composed of more than one tissue, that forms a structural unit responsible for a particular function (or functions). **o. of Corti** (**spiral o.**) the sense organ of the cochlea, which converts sound signals into nerve impulses that are transmitted to the brain via the cochlear nerve. [A. Corti (1822–88), Italian anatomist]

organelle (or-gă-**nel**) *n.* a structure within a cell that is specialized for a particular function.

organic (or-**gan**-ik) *adj.* **1.** relating to any or all of the organs of the body. **o. disorder** a disorder associated with changes in the structure of an organ or tissue. *Compare* functional disorder. **2.** describing chemical compounds containing carbon, found in all living systems.

organism (**or**-găn-izm) *n.* any living thing, which may consist of a single cell (*see* microorganism) or a group of differentiated but interdependent cells.

organo- *combining form denoting* organ or organic.

orgasm (**or**-gazm) *n.* the climax of sexual excitement.

oriental sore (Baghdad boil, Delhi boil, Aleppo boil)

(or-i-**en**-t'l) *n.* a skin disease, occurring in tropical and subtropical Africa and Asia, caused by the parasitic protozoan *Leishmania tropica*. The disease takes the form of a slow-healing open sore or ulcer, which sometimes becomes secondarily infected with bacteria.

orientation (or-i-en-**tay**-shŏn) *n.* (in psychology) awareness of oneself in time, space, and place. Orientation may be disturbed in such conditions as organic brain disease, toxic drug states, mental illness, and concussion. *See also* reality orientation.

orifice (**o**-ri-fis) *n.* an opening in an anatomical part. *See* ostium.

origin (**o**-ri-jin) *n.* (in anatomy) **1.** the point of attachment of a muscle that remains relatively fixed during contraction of the muscle. *Compare* insertion. **2.** the point at which a nerve or blood vessel branches from a main nerve or blood vessel.

orlistat (**or**-lis-tat) *n.* a drug that reduces the absorption of fat in the stomach and small intestine by inhibiting the action of pancreatic lipases. It is administered by mouth to treat clinical obesity, in conjunction with dietary control; side-effects include the production of copious oily stools and flatulence. Trade names: **Alli**, **Xenical**.

ornithine (**or**-ni-theen) *n.* an amino acid produced in the liver as a by-product during the conversion of ammonia to urea.

ornithosis (or-ni-**thoh**-sis) *n. see* psittacosis.

oro- *combining form denoting* the mouth.

oropharyngeal airway (o-roh-fă-**rin**-ji-ăl) *n.* a curved tube designed to be placed in the mouth of an unconscious patient, behind the tongue, to create a patent airway. *See also* nasopharyngeal airway.

oropharynx (o-roh-**fa**-rinks) *n.* the part of the pharynx that lies between the level of the junction of the hard and soft palates above and the hyoid bone below. It contains the tonsils. **—oropharyngeal** *adj.*

orphenadrine (or-**fen**-ă-dreen) *n.* an antimuscarinic drug that relieves spasm in muscle, administered by mouth to treat drug-induced parkinsonism. Trade names: **Biorphen**, **Disipal**.

ORT *n. see* oral rehydration therapy.

ortho- *combining form denoting* **1.** straight. **2.** normal.

orthodontics (orthŏ-**don**-tiks) *n.* the branch of dentistry concerned with the growth and development of the face and jaws and the treatment of irregularities of the teeth by means of various **orthodontic appliances**. **—orthodontic** *adj.*

orthokeratology (orthŏ-ke-ră-**tol**-ŏji) *n.* the use of contact lenses designed to reshape the cornea in the treatment of refractive errors, such as myopia (short sight).

orthopaedics (orthŏ-**pee**-diks) *n.* the science or practice of correcting deformities caused by disease of or damage to the bones and joints of the skeleton. **—orthopaedic** *adj.*

orthopnoea (or-thop-**nee**-ă) *n.* breathlessness that prevents the patient from lying down, so that he or she has to sleep propped up in bed or sitting in a chair. **—orthopnoeic** *adj*.

orthoptics (or-**thop**-tiks) *n*. the practice of using nonsurgical methods, particularly eye exercises, to treat abnormalities of vision and of coordination of eye movements (most commonly strabismus and amblyopia). **—orthoptic** *adj*. **—orthoptist** *n*.

orthoptoscope (or-**thop**-toh-skohp) *n*. *see* amblyoscope.

orthosis (or-**thoh**-sis) *n*. (*pl*. **orthoses**) a surgical appliance that exerts external forces on part of the body to support joints or correct deformity. **—orthotic** *adj*.

orthostatic (orthŏ-**stat**-ik) *adj*. relating to the upright position of the body: used when describing this posture or a condition caused by it.

orthotics (or-**thot**-iks) *n*. the science and practice of fitting orthoses to improve the mechanical functioning of a limb, part of a limb, or the trunk.

Ortolani manoeuvre (or-toh-**lah**-ni mà-**noo**-ver) *n*. a test for congenital dislocation of the hip in which, with the baby lying supine and the pelvis steadied with one hand, the examiner attempts to relocate a dislocated hip by gently abducting the hip while simultaneously pushing upwards on the greater trochanter. If the hip is dislocated, it will relocate with a detectable and sometimes audible clunk. [M. Ortolani (20th century), Italian orthopaedic surgeon]

os[1] (oss) *n*. (*pl*. **ossa**) a bone.

os[2] *n*. (*pl*. **ora**) the mouth or a mouthlike part.

OSA (OSAS) *n*. *see* (obstructive) sleep apnoea (syndrome).

osche- (oscheo-) *combining form denoting* the scrotum.

oscillation (oss-i-**lay**-shŏn) *n*. a regular side-to-side movement; vibration.

oscilloscope (oss-**il**-ŏ-skohp) *n*. a cathode-ray tube designed to display electronically a wave form corresponding to the electrical data fed into it. Oscilloscopes are used to provide a continuous record of many different measurements, such as the activity of the heart and brain. *See* electrocardiography, electroencephalography.

osculum (**osk**-yoo-lŭm) *n*. (in anatomy) a small aperture.

oseltamivir (oss-el-**tam**-i-veer) *n*. an antiviral drug that is administered orally for the prevention and treatment of influenza A and B. To be effective, the drug must be taken within 48 hours of exposure to influenza (for prophylaxis) or onset of symptoms (for treatment). Trade name: **Tamiflu**.

Osgood-Schlatter disease (Schlatter's disease) (oz-guud **shlat**-er) *n*. inflammation and swelling of the tibial tuberosity (*see* tibia), to which the tendon of the quadriceps muscle is attached just below the kneecap (*see* apophysitis). It occurs in adolescence as a result of excessive physical activity causing excessive pull of the tendon. [R. B. Osgood (1873–1956), US orthopaedist; C. Schlatter (1864–1934), Swiss surgeon]

Osiander's sign (oss-i-**an**-derz) *n*. an early indication of pregnancy (at eight weeks) in which pulsation can be felt through the lateral vaginal fornix. [J. F. Osiander (1787–1855), German obstetrician]

-osis *suffix denoting* **1.** a diseased condition. **2.** any condition. **3.** an increase or excess.

Osler's nodes (ohss-lerz) *pl. n.* small tender swellings in or beneath the skin at the ends of the fingers and toes, seen in subacute bacterial endocarditis. [Sir W. Osler (1849–1919), Canadian physician]

osm- (osmo-) *combining form denoting* **1.** smell or odour. **2.** osmosis or osmotic pressure.

osmolality (oz-moh-**lal**-iti) *n.* the osmotic pressure of a substance expressed in terms of osmoles of substance per kg of water. *Compare* osmolarity.

osmolarity (oz-moh-**la**-riti) *n.* the osmotic pressure of a substance expressed in terms of osmoles of substance per kg of solution.

osmole (**oz**-mohl) *n.* a unit of osmotic pressure equal to the molecular weight of a solute in grams divided by the number of ions or other particles into which it dissociates in solution.

osmoreceptor (oz-moh-ri-**sep**-ter) *n.* a group of cells in the hypothalamus that monitor blood concentration.

osmosis (oz-**moh**-sis) *n.* the passage of a solvent from a less concentrated to a more concentrated solution through a semipermeable membrane. In living organisms, the process of osmosis plays an important role in controlling the distribution of water. —**osmotic** (oz-**mot**-ik) *adj.*

osmotic pressure *n.* the pressure by which water is drawn into a solution through a semipermeable membrane; the more concentrated the solution, the greater its osmotic pressure.

osseointegration (oss-i-oh-in-ti-**gray**-shŏn) *n.* the process by which certain materials, such as titanium, may be introduced into living bone without producing a foreign-body reaction. This allows a very tight and strong joint between the two structures. Osseointegration is used, for example, to fix some dental implants and bone-anchored hearing aids.

osseous (**oss**-iŭs) *adj.* bony: applied to the bony parts of the inner ear.

ossicle (**oss**-i-kŭl) *n.* a small bone. **auditory o.** any of the three small bones (the incus, malleus, and stapes) in the middle ear.

ossification (osteogenesis) (oss-i-fi-**kay**-shŏn) *n.* the formation of bone, which takes place in three stages by the action of osteoblasts. A meshwork of collagen fibres is deposited in connective tissue, followed by the production of a cementing polysaccharide. Finally the cement is impregnated with minute crystals of calcium salts. The osteoblasts become enclosed within the matrix as osteocytes.

ost- (oste-, osteo-) *combining form denoting* bone.

ostectomy (oss-**tek**-tŏmi) *n.* the surgical removal of a bone or a piece of bone. *See also* osteotomy.

osteitis (osti-**I**-tis) *n.* inflammation of bone, due to infection, damage, or metabolic disorder. **o. deformans**

see Paget's disease. **o. fibrosa cystica** the characteristic cystic changes that occur in bones during long-standing hyperparathyroidism.

osteo- *combining form. see* ost-.

osteoarthritis (osteoarthrosis) (osti-oh-arth-**ry**-tis) *n.* a degenerative disease of joints resulting in loss of the articular cartilage, remodelling of adjacent bone, and inflammation. The joints become painful and stiff, with restricted movement. The condition may be primary or may result from abnormal load to the joint or damage to the cartilage from inflammation or trauma. Treatment consists of analgesics, reducing the load to the joint (by weight loss or use of a walking stick), or surgery (osteotomy, arthrodesis, or arthroplasty).

SEE WEB LINKS

- Information on osteoarthritis from Arthritis Care

osteoarthropathy (osti-oh-arth-**rop**-ă-thi) *n.* any disease of the bone and cartilage adjoining a joint.

osteoarthrosis (osti-oh-arth-**roh**-sis) *n. see* osteoarthritis.

osteoarthrotomy (osti-oh-arth-**rot**-ŏmi) *n.* surgical excision of the bone adjoining a joint.

osteoblast (oss-ti-oh-blast) *n.* a cell, originating in the mesoderm of the embryo, that is responsible for the formation of bone. *See also* ossification.

osteochondritis (osti-oh-kon-**dry**-tis) *n.* any one of a group of conditions affecting areas of growth at the epiphyses and apophyses of bones before skeletal maturity, usually during early adolescence. It is characterized as crushing (*see* Kienböck's disease, Köhler's disease, Legg-Calvé-Perthes disease), pulling (*see* Osgood-Schlatter disease, Sever's disease), or splitting (e.g. osteochondritis dissecans). **o. dissecans** the development of a small area of avascular bone on the surface of a joint, most commonly the knee, with resulting pain, swelling, and limitation of movement. The area and its overlying cartilage can become loose and may detach.

osteochondroma (osti-oh-kon-**droh**-mă) *n.* (*pl.* **osteochondromata**) a bony protuberance covered with a cap of cartilage arising from the end of a bone, most commonly around the knee or shoulder. It may be stalklike (an exostosis) or flattened.

osteochondrosis (osti-oh-kon-**droh**-sis) *n. see* osteochondritis.

osteoclasia (osteoclasis) (osti-oh-**klay**-ziă) *n.* **1.** (osteoclasty) the deliberate breaking of a malformed or malunited bone, carried out by a surgeon to correct deformity. **2.** *see* osteolysis.

osteoclasis (osti-**ok**-lă-sis) *n.* **1.** remodelling of bone by osteoclasts, during growth or the healing of a fracture. **2.** *see* osteoclasia.

osteoclast (oss-ti-oh-klast) *n.* **1.** a large multinucleate cell that resorbs calcified bone. **2.** a device for fracturing bone for therapeutic purposes.

osteoclastoma (osti-oh-klas-**toh**-mă) *n.* a rare tumour of bone, caused by proliferation of osteoclast cells.

osteocyte (oss-ti-oh-syt) *n.* a bone cell. *See also* ossification.

osteodystrophy (osti-oh-**dis**-trŏ-fi) *n.* any generalized bone disease resulting from a metabolic disorder.

osteogenesis (osti-oh-**jen**-i-sis) *n. see* ossification. **o. imperfecta** (**fragilitas ossium**) a congenital disorder of connective tissue formation, of varying degrees of severity, in which the bones are unusually brittle and fragile; the teeth and soft tissues are also affected.

osteogenic (osti-oh-**jen**-ik) *adj.* originating in or composed of bone tissue. **o. sarcoma** *see* osteosarcoma.

osteology (osti-**ol**-ŏji) *n.* the study of the structure and function of bones and related structures.

osteolysis (osteoclasia) (osti-**ol**-i-sis) *n.* dissolution of bone through disease, commonly by infection or loss of the blood supply (ischaemia) to the bone. **—osteolytic** *adj.*

osteoma (osti-**oh**-mă) *n.* a benign bone tumour. **compact o.** (**ivory exostosis**) a relatively uncommon slow-growing tumour occurring usually in the skull and facial bones. **osteoid o.** a small relatively common tumour, most commonly occurring in the shaft of the femur or tibia, that causes nocturnal pain.

osteomalacia (osti-oh-mă-**lay**-shiă) *n.* softening of the bones due to inadequate mineralization: the adult counterpart of rickets. Causes include insufficient calcium absorption from the intestine due to dietary deficiency or vitamin D deficiency; common symptoms are bone pain, backache, and muscle weakness. The usual treatment is large doses of vitamin D.

osteomyelitis (osti-oh-my-ĕ-**ly**-tis) *n.* inflammation of bone due to infection. It can cause fracture and deformity of the bone. **acute o.** osteomyelitis occurring when bacteria enter the bone via the bloodstream; it is more common in children. There is severe pain and redness over the involved bone, accompanied by general illness and high fever. **chronic o.** osteomyelitis that may develop from partially treated acute osteomyelitis or after open fractures or surgery during which the bone is contaminated.

osteopathy (osti-**op**-ă-thi) *n.* a system of diagnosis and treatment based on the theory that many diseases are associated with disorders of the musculoskeletal system. Diagnosis and treatment of these disorders involves palpation, manipulation, and massage. Osteopathy provides relief for many disorders of bones and joints. **—osteopath** (**ost**-i-ŏ-path) *n.* **—osteopathic** (osti-ŏ-**path**-ik) *adj.*

osteopetrosis (Albers-Schönberg disease, marble-bone disease) (osti-oh-pi-**troh**-sis) *n.* a congenital abnormality in which bones become abnormally dense and brittle and tend to fracture. *See also* osteosclerosis.

osteophyte (oss-ti-ŏ-fyt) *n.* a projection of bone, usually shaped like a rose thorn, that occurs at sites of cartilage degeneration or destruction near joints and intervertebral discs.

osteoplasty (oss-ti-ŏ-plasti) *n.* plastic surgery of bones.

osteoporosis (osti-oh-por-**oh**-sis) *n.* a bone disease characterized by a decrease in bone mineral density and bone mass, resulting in bones that are liable to fracture. Infection, injury, and synovitis can cause localized osteoporosis. Generalized osteoporosis is common in older people, and in women it often follows the menopause. Increased calcium and vitamin D intake and exercise are preventative, and drugs (e.g. bisphosphonates, parathyroid hormone, and denosumab) can reduce the risk of fracture. **—osteoporotic** *adj.*

osteosarcoma (osteogenic sarcoma) (osti-oh-sar-**koh**-mă) *n.* a highly malignant tumour arising from within a bone. In children the usual site for the tumour is the leg, particularly the femur. Secondary growths (metastases) are common, most frequently in the lungs (though other sites, such as the liver, may also be involved). Treatment of disease localized to the primary site is now usually by limb-sparing surgery after neoadjuvant chemotherapy, with replacement of the diseased bone by a metal prosthesis.

osteosclerosis (osti-oh-skleer-**oh**-sis) *n.* an abnormal increase in the density of bone, as a result of poor blood supply, chronic infection, or tumour. *See also* osteopetrosis.

osteotome (oss-ti-ŏ-tohm) *n.* a surgical chisel designed to cut bone. See illustration.

osteotomy (osti-**ot**-ŏmi) *n.* a surgical operation to cut a bone into two parts, followed by realignment of the ends to allow healing. The operation may be performed to reduce pain and disability in an arthritic joint.

ostium (oss-tiŭm) *n.* (*pl.* **ostia**) (in anatomy) an opening. **o. abdominale** the opening of the Fallopian tube into the abdominal cavity.

-ostomy *combining form. see* -stomy.

ot- (oto-) *combining form denoting* the ear.

otalgia (oh-**tal**-jiă) *n.* pain in the ear.

OTC drug *n. see* over-the-counter drug.

otic (**oh**-tik) *adj.* relating to the ear.

otitis (oh-**ty**-tis) *n.* inflammation of the ear. **o. externa** inflammation of the canal between the eardrum and the external opening of the ear. **o. interna (labyrinthitis)** inflammation of the inner ear resulting in dizziness, vertigo, and hearing loss. **o. media** acute or chronic inflammation of the middle ear. Acute inflammation, usually due to bacterial or viral infection, causes pain and a high fever; treatment is usually with antibiotics. Chronic inflammation is associated with perforations of the eardrum; treatment involves surgical repair. **secretory o. media** *see* glue ear.

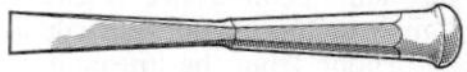

An osteotome

otoacoustic emissions (OAE) (oh-toh-ă-**koo**-stik) *pl. n.* tiny sounds that emerge from the inner ear either spontaneously or shortly after the ear is exposed to an external sound. An objective screening test for newborn children detects otoacoustic emissions in response to a small sound.

otoconium (oh-toh-**koh**-niŭm) *n. see* otolith.

otolaryngology (oh-toh-la-ring-**ol**-ŏji) *n.* the study of diseases of the ears and larynx. **—otolaryngologist** *n.*

otolith (otoconium) (**oh**-toh-lith) *n.* one of the small particles of calcium carbonate associated with a macula in the saccule or utricle of the inner ear.

otology (oh-**tol**-ŏji) *n.* the study of diseases of the ear. **—otologist** *n.*

-otomy *combining form. see* -tomy.

otomycosis (oh-toh-my-**koh**-sis) *n.* a fungus infection of the ear, causing irritation and inflammation of the canal between the eardrum and the external opening of the ear.

otoplasty (pinnaplasty) (**oh**-toh-plasti) *n.* surgical repair or reconstruction of the ears after injury or in the correction of a congenital defect (such as bat ears).

otorhinolaryngology (oh-toh-ry-noh-la-ring-**ol**-ŏji) *n.* the study of ear, nose, and throat diseases (i.e. ENT disorders). **—otorhinolaryngologist** *n.*

otorrhagia (oh-toh-**ray**-jiă) *n.* bleeding from the ear.

otorrhoea (oh-toh-**ree**-ă) *n.* any discharge from the ear, commonly a purulent discharge in chronic middle ear infection (otitis media).

otosclerosis (otospongiosis) (oh-toh-skleer-**oh**-sis) *n.* a disorder causing conductive deafness in adult life. An overgrowth of the bone of the inner ear leads to the stapes becoming fixed to the fenestra ovalis, so that sounds cannot be conducted to the inner ear.

otoscope (**oh**-toh-skohp) *n. see* auriscope.

otospongiosis (oh-toh-spunji-**oh**-sis) *n. see* otosclerosis.

ototoxic (oh-toh-**toks**-ik) *adj.* having a toxic effect on the organs of balance or hearing in the inner ear or on the vestibulocochlear nerve. Ototoxic drugs may be used in the treatment of Ménière's disease.

outbreeding (**owt**-breed-ing) *n.* the production of offspring by parents who are not closely related. *Compare* inbreeding.

outer ear (**owt**-er) *n.* the pinna and the external auditory meatus of the ear.

out-of-body experience *n.* a form of derealization in which there is a sensation of leaving one's body, sometimes accompanied by visions of travel. It typically occurs after anaesthesia or severe illness and is often attributed to anoxia of the brain.

out-patient (**owt**-pay-shĕnt) *n.* a patient who receives treatment at a hospital but is not admitted to a bed in a hospital ward. Large hospitals have clinics at which out-patients can be given specialist treatment. *Compare* in-patient.

oval window (**oh**-văl) *n. see* fenestra (ovalis).

ovari- (ovario-) *combining form denoting* the ovary.

ovarian cancer (oh-**vair**-iăn) *n.* a malignant tumour of the ovary, usually a carcinoma. The incidence of the disease reaches a peak in postmenopausal women; treatment involves surgery and most cases also require combined chemotherapy and/or radiotherapy.

ovarian cyst *n.* a benign tumour of the ovary, of which there are many varieties. Although most ovarian cysts are not malignant, they may reach a very large size and rotate on their stalks, thus cutting off their blood supply and causing severe abdominal pain and vomiting; in such cases the cysts require urgent surgical removal.

ovarian hyperstimulation syndrome *n.* a potentially life-threatening condition classically associated with ovarian stimulation using gonadotrophins in assisted conception procedures (*see* superovulation). It is characterized by gross enlargement of the ovaries resulting in pain, bloating, nausea, vomiting, haemoconcentration, and ascites.

ovariectomy (oh-vair-i-**ek**-tŏmi) *n. see* oophorectomy.

ovariotomy (oh-vair-i-**ot**-ŏmi) *n.* literally, incision of an ovary. However, the term commonly refers to surgical removal of an ovary (oophorectomy).

ovaritis (oh-vă-**ry**-tis) *n. see* oophoritis.

ovary (**oh**-ver-i) *n.* the main female reproductive organ, which contains follicles that produce ova and steroid hormones in a regular cycle (*see* menstrual cycle). There are two ovaries, situated in the lower abdomen, one on each side of the uterus (*see* reproductive system). **—ovarian** *adj.*

overcompensation (oh-ver-kom-pen-**say**-shŏn) *n.* (in psychology) the situation in which a person tries to overcome a disability by making greater efforts than are required.

overt (**oh**-vert) *adj.* plainly to be seen or detected: applied to diseases with observable signs and symptoms.

over-the-counter drug (OTC drug) (oh-ver-*thĕ*-**kownt**-er) *n.* a drug that may be purchased directly from a pharmacist without a doctor's prescription. Current government policy is to extend the range of OTC drugs: a number have already been derestricted (e.g. ibuprofen, ranitidine) and this trend is expected to increase.

ovi- (ovo-) *combining form denoting* an egg; ovum.

oviduct (**oh**-vi-dukt) *n. see* Fallopian tube.

ovulation (ov-yoo-**lay**-shŏn) *n.* the process by which an ovum is released from a mature Graafian follicle. The fluid-filled follicle distends the surface of the ovary until a thin spot breaks down and the ovum floats out and starts to travel down the Fallopian tube to the uterus.

ovulation induction *n.* a procedure to enhance ovarian follicle stimulation resulting in multiple egg production within a menstrual cycle. Drugs used include clomifene tablets or injections of gonadotrophins containing follicle-stimulating hormone. These drugs also affect the timing of egg release to enhance the likelihood of successful pregnancy. *See also* superovulation.

ovum (egg cell) (oh-vŭm) *n.* (*pl.* **ova**) the mature female sex cell (*see* gamete). See illustration.

oxalate (oks-ă-layt) *n.* a salt of oxalic acid. **balanced o.** a mixture of ammonium and potassium oxalates (an anticoagulant) in which blood specimens are stored before laboratory examination.

oxalic acid (oks-al-ik) *n.* an extremely poisonous acid found in many plants, including sorrel and the leaves of rhubarb, and in some bleaching powders. When swallowed it produces burning sensations in the mouth and throat, vomiting of blood, breathing difficulties, and circulatory collapse. Treatment is with calcium lactate or other calcium salts, lime water, or milk. Formula: $C_2H_2O_4$.

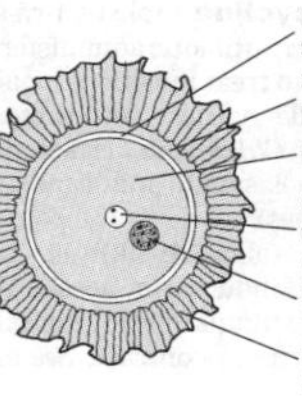

A mature ovum (magnification about × 600)

oxaliplatin (oks-al-i-**plat**-in) *n.* a third-generation analogue of cisplatin that is administered by intravenous infusion in the treatment of advanced colorectal cancer. It has less toxic side-effects than cisplatin.

oxaluria (oks-ăl-**yoor**-iă) *n.* the presence in the urine of oxalic acid or oxalates, especially calcium oxalate.

oxazepam (oks-**az**-ĕ-pam) *n.* a benzodiazepine drug administered by mouth for the short-term relief of severe anxiety and tension.

oxidant (**oks**-i-dănt) *n.* (in biological systems) a molecule that serves as an electron acceptor. In human disease oxidants are derived from normal intracellular processes and released by inflammatory cells. They are counteracted by antioxidants, such as beta-carotene.

oxidase (**oks**-i-dayz) *n. see* oxidoreductase.

oxidation (oks-i-**day**-shŏn) *n.* a reaction in which an atom or molecule loses electrons. Many biological oxidations are effected by the removal of hydrogen atoms, which combine with an **oxidizing agent**. For example, glucose is oxidized during cellular respiration: $C_6H_{12}O_6 + 6O_2 \rightarrow 6CO_2 + 6H_2O$.

oxidoreductase (oks-i-doh-ri-**duk**-tayz) *n.* one of a group of enzymes that catalyse oxidation-reduction reactions. This class includes the enzymes formerly known either as **dehydrogenases** or as **oxidases**.

oximeter (oks-**im**-it-er) *n.* an instrument for measuring the proportion of oxyhaemoglobin in the blood. *See* pulse oximetry.

oxprenolol (oks-**pren**-ŏ-lol) *n.* a drug that controls the activity of the heart (*see* beta blocker), administered by mouth mainly to treat angina, high blood pressure, abnormal heart rhythm, and anxiety. Trade name: **Slow-Trasicor**.

oxybutynin (oksi-**bew**-tin-in) *n.* an antimuscarinic drug administered orally or in skin patches to reduce frequency and urgency of passing urine associated with instability of the detrusor muscle of the bladder wall. Trade names: **Cystrin**, **Ditropan**, **Kentera**, **Lyrinel XL**.

oxycephaly (turricephaly) (oksi-**sef**-ăli) *n.* a deformity of the bones of the skull giving the head a pointed appearance. *See also* craniosynostosis. **—oxycephalic** (oksi-si-**fal**-ik) *adj.*

oxycodone (oks-i-**koh**-dohn) *n.* an opioid analgesic (*see* opiate) used to treat moderate or severe pain, primarily in terminally ill patients. It is administered orally, intravenously, or subcutaneously. Trade names: **Dolocodon PR**, **Longtec**, **OxyContin**, **OxyNorm**.

oxygen (**oks**-i-jĕn) *n.* an odourless colourless gas that makes up one-fifth of the atmosphere. Oxygen is essential to most forms of life; in humans, it is absorbed into the blood from air breathed into the lungs. Oxygen is administered therapeutically in various conditions in which the tissues are unable to obtain an adequate supply through the lungs. Symbol: O. **o. deficit** a physiological condition that exists in cells during periods of temporary oxygen shortage. **o. tent** *see* tent.

oxygenation (oksi-ji-**nay**-shŏn) *n.* the process of becoming saturated with oxygen, such as occurs in the lungs during inhalation of air.

oxygenator (**oks**-i-ji-nay-ter) *n.* a machine that oxygenates blood outside the body. *See also* heart-lung machine.

oxyhaemoglobin (oksi-hee-moh-**gloh**-bin) *n.* the bright-red substance formed when the pigment haemoglobin in red blood cells combines reversibly with oxygen. Oxyhaemoglobin is the form in which oxygen is transported from the lungs to the tissues. *Compare* methaemoglobin.

oxyntic cells (oks-**in**-tik) *pl. n. see* parietal cells.

oxytetracycline (oksi-tet-ră-**sy**-kleen) *n.* an antibiotic administered by mouth to treat infections caused by a wide variety of bacteria (including *Chlamydia*, rickettsiae, and mycoplasmas) and acne (*see* tetracyclines).

oxytocic (oksi-**toh**-sik) *n.* any agent that induces or accelerates labour by stimulating the muscles of the uterus to contract. *See also* oxytocin.

oxytocin (oksi-**toh**-sin) *n.* a hormone, released by the pituitary gland, that causes contraction of the uterus during labour and stimulates milk flow from the breasts by causing contraction of muscle fibres in the milk ducts. Intravenous infusions or injections of oxytocin (Syntocinon) are used to induce labour and to control or prevent postpartum haemorrhage. *See also* ergometrine.

oxyuriasis (oksi-yoor-I-ă-sis) *n.* *see* enterobiasis.

Oxyuris (oksi-yoor-iss) *n.* *see* threadworm.

ozaena (oh-zee-nă) *n.* a disorder of the nose in which the mucous membranes inside the nose become atrophied, with the production of an offensive discharge and crusts.

ozone (**oh**-zohn) *n.* a poisonous gas containing three oxygen atoms per molecule. Ozone is a very powerful oxidizing agent. Ozone in the troposphere (the atmospheric layer closest to the earth's surface), as found in photochemical smog, can cause health problems. At very high altitudes (the **ozone layer**) it is responsible for absorbing a large proportion of the sun's ultraviolet radiation.

Pp

P *symbol for* **1.** phosphorus. **2.** (in statistics) probability (*see* significance).

Pacchionian body (pak-i-**oh**-ni-ăn) *n. see* arachnoid. [A. Pacchioni (1665–1726), Italian anatomist]

pacemaker (payss-mayk-er) *n.* **1.** a device used to produce and maintain a normal heart rate in patients who have a slow heart rate. It consists of a battery that stimulates the heart through one or more insulated electrode wires (leads) attached to the surface of the ventricle (**epicardial p.**) or lying in contact with the lining of the heart (**endocardial p.**). **demand p.** a pacemaker that stimulates the heart when it senses a fall in the heart rate. A pacemaker may be temporary, with an external battery, or it may be permanent, when the whole apparatus is surgically implanted under the skin. **2.** the part of the heart that regulates the rate at which it beats: the sinoatrial node.

pachy- *combining form denoting* **1.** thickening of a part or parts. **2.** the dura mater.

pachydactyly (pak-i-**dak**-tili) *n.* abnormal enlargement of the fingers and toes, occurring either as a congenital abnormality or as part of an acquired disease (such as acromegaly).

pachymeningitis (pak-i-men-in-**jy**-tis) *n.* inflammation of the dura mater (*see* meningitis).

pachymeninx (pak-i-**mee**-ninks) *n.* the dura mater, outermost of the three meninges.

pachymeter (pak-**im**-it-er) *n.* an instrument used to measure the thickness of the cornea. **—pachymetry** *n.*

pachysomia (pak-i-**soh**-miă) *n.* thickening of parts of the body, which occurs in certain diseases.

Pacinian corpuscles (pă-**sin**-iăn) *pl. n.* sensory receptors for touch in the skin, consisting of sensory nerve endings surrounded by capsules of membrane. They are especially sensitive to changes in pressure and so detect vibration particularly well. [F. Pacini (1812–83), Italian anatomist]

pack (pak) *n.* a pad of folded moistened material, such as cotton-wool, applied to the body or inserted into a cavity.

packed cell volume (PCV, haematocrit) *n.* the volume of the red cells (erythrocytes) in blood, expressed as a fraction of the total volume of the blood.

paclitaxel (pak-li-**taks**-ĕl) *n.* a cytotoxic anticancer drug (*see* taxane) administered by intravenous infusion mainly to treat ovarian cancer, breast cancer, and non-small-cell lung cancer. Trade name: **Taxol**.

PACS (picture archiving and communication system) *n.* a technology that enables the storage and transfer of digital images for display on high-resolution monitors. Images can be viewed at multiple sites simultaneously.

pad (pad) *n.* cotton-wool, foam rubber, or other material used to protect a part of the body from friction, bruising, or other unwanted contact.

Paddington alcohol test (pad-ing-tŏn) *n.* a three-question tool designed to make the connection between alcohol-related problems and A & E department attendance, enabling the potential for intervention and referral.

paed- (paedo-) *combining form denoting* children.

paediatric advanced life support (PALS) (peed-i-**at**-rik) *n.* a structured and algorithm-driven method of life support for use in severe medical emergencies in children.

paediatric early warning score (PEWS, children's early warning score, CEWS) *n.* a tool that incorporates a sliding scale for the assessment of vital signs and consciousness level to identify the degree of risk associated with the presenting physiological status of a child or young person. This enables a focused and rapid response to potentially life-threatening events.

paediatrics (peed-i-**at**-riks) *n.* the general medicine of childhood. Handling the sick child requires detailed knowledge of genetics, obstetrics, psychological development, management of handicaps at home and in school, and effects of social conditions on child health. *See also* child health clinic. —**paediatric** *adj.* —**paediatrician** (peed-i-ă-**trish**-ăn) *n.*

Paget's disease (paj-its) *n.* **1.** a chronic disease of bones, occurring in the elderly and most frequently affecting the skull, backbone, pelvis, and long bones; affected bones become thickened. There are often no symptoms, but pain, deformity, and fracture can occur. Medical name: **osteitis deformans**. **2.** a malignant condition of the nipple, resembling eczema in appearance, that is associated with underlying infiltrating cancer of the breast. [Sir J. Paget (1814–99), British surgeon]

pain (payn) *n.* an unpleasant sensation ranging from mild discomfort to agonized distress, associated with real or potential tissue damage. Pain is a subjective response to impulses from the peripheral nerves in damaged tissue, which pass to nerves in the spinal cord, where they are subjected to a gate control. This gate modifies the subsequent passage of the impulses in accordance with descending controls from the brain. Because attention is a crucial component of pain, distraction can act as a basis for pain therapy. On the other hand, anxiety and depression focus the attention and exaggerate the pain. If the nerve pathways are damaged, the brain can increase the amplification in the pathway, maintaining the sensation as a protective mechanism.

pain clinic *n.* a clinic that specializes in the management and relief of pain. Pain clinics are usually directed by anaesthetists.

paint (paynt) *n.* (in pharmacy) a liquid preparation that is applied to the skin or mucous membranes. Paints usually contain antiseptics, astringents, caustics, or analgesics.

palaeo- *combining form denoting* **1.** ancient. **2.** primitive.

palate (pal-ăt) *n.* the roof of the mouth, which separates the mouth from the nasal cavity. **hard p.** the front part of the palate. It is formed by processes of the maxillae and palatine bones and is covered by mucous membrane. **soft p.** the posterior part of the palate: a movable fold of mucous membrane that tapers at the back of the mouth to form the uvula. *See also* cleft palate.

palatine bone (pal-ă-tyn) *n.* either of a pair of approximately L-shaped bones of the face that contribute to the hard palate, the nasal cavity, and the orbits.

palato- *combining form denoting* **1.** the palate. **2.** the palatine bone.

palatoplasty (pal-a-toh-plasti) *n.* surgery to alter the shape or physical characteristics of the palate, for example to correct cleft palate or other congenital defects or to shorten and/or stiffen the palate in the treatment of snoring or obstructive sleep apnoea.

palatoplegia (pal-ă-toh-plee-jiă) *n.* paralysis of the soft palate.

palatorrhaphy (pal-ăt-o-răfi) *n. see* staphylorrhaphy.

pali- (palin-) *combining form denoting* repetition or recurrence.

palilalia (pal-i-lay-liă) *n.* a disorder of speech in which a word spoken by the individual is rapidly and involuntarily repeated.

palindromic (pal-in-drom-ik) *adj.* relapsing: describing diseases or symptoms that recur or get worse.

palliative (pal-i-ătiv) **1.** *adj.* providing relief from the symptoms of a disease but without effecting a cure. Palliative care is often used in the treatment of terminal illness. **2.** *n.* a palliative medicine.

pallidotomy (pallidectomy) (pal-i-dot-ŏmi) *n.* a neurosurgical operation to destroy or modify the effects of the globus pallidus (*see* basal ganglia) for the relief of parkinsonism and other conditions in which involuntary movements are prominent. It is now performed by stereotaxy.

pallor (pal-er) *n.* abnormal paleness of the skin, due to reduced blood flow or lack of normal pigments. Pallor may indicate shock, anaemia, cancer, or other diseases.

palmar (pal-mer) *adj.* relating to the palm of the hand. **p. arches** two arterial arches (deep and superficial) in the palm of the hand, formed by anastomosis of the ulnar and radial arteries.

palmitic acid (pal-mit-ik) *n. see* fatty acid.

palpation (pal-pay-shŏn) *n.* the process of examining part of the body by careful feeling with the hands and fingertips.

palpebral (pal-pi-brăl) *adj*. relating to the eyelid (**palpebra**).

palpitation (pal-pi-tay-shŏn) *n*. an awareness of the heartbeat. This is normal with fear, emotion, or exertion. It may also be a symptom of neurosis, arrhythmias, heart disease, and overactivity of the circulation.

PALS *n*. **1.** *see* paediatric advanced life support. **2.** *see* Patient Advice and Liaison Service.

palsy (pawl-zi) *n*. paralysis. *See* Bell's palsy, cerebral palsy.

paludism (pal-yoo-dizm) *n*. *see* malaria.

pamidronate disodium (pam-i-droh-nayt dy-soh-diŭm) *n*. *see* bisphosphonates.

pan- (pant(o)-) *combining form denoting* all; every: hence (in medicine) affecting all parts of an organ or the body; generalized.

panacea (pan-ă-see-ă) *n*. a medicine said to be a cure for all diseases and disorders. Unfortunately panaceas do not exist, despite the claims of many patent medicine manufacturers.

Panadol (pan-ă-dol) *n*. *see* paracetamol.

panarthritis (pan-arth-ry-tis) *n*. inflammation of all the structures involved in a joint. *See* arthritis.

pancarditis (pan-kar-dy-tis) *n*. an inflammatory disorder affecting the pericardium, endocardium, and heart muscle.

Pancoast syndrome (pan-kohst) *n*. pain and paralysis involving the lower branches of the brachial plexus due to infiltration by a malignant tumour of the apical region of the lung. Horner's syndrome may also be present. [H. K. Pancoast (1875–1939), US radiologist]

pancreas (pank-ri-ăs) *n*. a compound gland, about 15 cm long, that lies behind the stomach. One end lies in the curve of the duodenum; the other end touches the spleen. It is composed of clusters (acini) of cells that secrete pancreatic juice into the duodenum via the **pancreatic duct**, which unites with the common bile duct. Interspersed among the acini are the islets of Langerhans, which secrete the hormones insulin and glucagon into the bloodstream. **—pancreatic** (pank-ri-at-ik) *adj*.

pancreatectomy (pank-ri-ă-tek-tŏmi) *n*. surgical removal of the pancreas. **partial p.** removal of a portion of the gland, to remove tumours or tissue damaged by chronic or relapsing pancreatitis. **subtotal p.** removal of most of the gland. **total p.** (**Whipple's operation**) removal of the entire gland and part of the duodenum.

pancreatic juice *n*. the mixture of digestive enzymes secreted by the pancreas. Its production is stimulated by hormones secreted by the duodenum (*see* cholecystokinin, secretin).

pancreatic polypeptide *n*. a hormone released from the D cells of the islets of Langerhans of the pancreas in response to protein in the small intestine. Its actions are to inhibit pancreatic bicarbonate and protein enzyme secretion and to relax the gall bladder.

pancreatin (pank-ri-ă-tin) *n*. an extract obtained from the pancreas, containing the pancreatic enzymes. Pancreatin is administered to treat conditions in which pancreatic secretion is deficient; for example, in pancreatitis.

pancreatitis (pank-ri-ă-**ty**-tis) *n.* inflammation of the pancreas. **acute p.** a sudden illness in which the patient experiences severe abdominal pain that radiates to the back; in some cases there is rapid deterioration with shock. Treatment consists of restricting oral intake, intravenous hydration, and antibiotics if infected necrosis is present. In severe cases pancreatectomy may be required. **chronic p.** pancreatitis that may produce symptoms similar to relapsing pancreatitis or may be painless; it can lead to endocrine failure causing malabsorption and diabetes mellitus. **relapsing p.** pancreatitis in which the symptoms of acute pancreatitis are recurrent and less severe. It may be associated with gallstones or with alcoholism.

pancreatotomy (pank-ri-ă-**tot**-ŏmi) *n.* surgical incision of the duct of the pancreas in order to inspect the duct, to join the duct to the intestine, or to inject a contrast medium.

pancreozymin (pank-ri-oh-**zy**-min) *n.* the name originally given to the fraction of the hormone cholecystokinin that acts on the pancreas.

pancytopenia (pan-sy-toh-**pee**-niă) *n.* a simultaneous decrease in the numbers of red cells, white cells, and platelets in the blood. It occurs in a variety of disorders, including aplastic anaemias, hypersplenism, and tumours of the bone marrow, and may occur after chemotherapy or total body irradiation.

pandemic (pan-**dem**-ik) *n.* an epidemic so widely spread that vast numbers of people in different countries are affected. **—pandemic** *adj.*

panic disorder (**pan**-ik) *n.* a condition featuring recurrent episodes of acute distress, mental confusion, and fear. These episodes often take the form of a **panic attack** in which the core symptoms are palpitation, sweating, and tremor; overbreathing (hyperventilation) often makes the attack worse. Such attacks are especially common in people with agoraphobia.

panniculitis (pă-nik-yoo-**ly**-tis) *n.* inflammation of the panniculus adiposus, leading to multiple tender nodules in the legs and trunk.

panniculus (pă-**nik**-yoo-lŭs) *n.* a membranous sheet of tissue. **p. adiposus** the fatty layer of tissue underlying the skin.

pannus (**pan**-ŭs) *n.* vascularized granulation tissue in the superficial layers of the cornea of the eye, which grows in from the conjunctiva.

panophthalmitis (pan-off-thal-**my**-tis) *n.* inflammation involving the whole of the interior of the eye.

panosteitis (pan-osti-**I**-tis) *n.* inflammation of all the structures of a bone.

panotitis (pan-ŏ-**ty**-tis) *n.* inflammation of both the middle and the inner ears.

pant- (panto-) *combining form. see* pan-.

pantothenic acid (pan-tŏ-**theen**-ik) *n.* a B vitamin that is a constituent of coenzyme A. It plays an important role in the transfer of acetyl groups in the body.

pantropic (pan-**trop**-ik) *adj.* describing a virus that can invade and affect many different tissues of the body without showing a special affinity for any one of them.

PAP *n.* primary atypical pneumonia. *See* atypical (pneumonia).

Papanicolaou test (Pap test) (pap-ă-**nik**-ŏ-low) *n.* a test to detect cancer of the cervix or lining of the uterus. In cervical screening it is being superseded by liquid-based cytology. *See also* cervical (smear). [G. N. Papanicolaou (1883–1962), Greek physician, anatomist, and cytologist]

papaveretum (pă-pav-er-**ee**-tŭm) *n. see* papaverine.

papaverine (pă-**pav**-er-een) *n.* an alkaloid, derived from opium, that relaxes smooth muscle. It can be injected into the corpora cavernosa of the penis to treat erectile dysfunction. In combination with morphine and codeine (a mixture called **papaveretum**), it is used for the relief of postoperative pain and severe chronic pain.

papilla (pă-**pil**-ă) *n.* (*pl.* **papillae**) any small nipple-shaped protuberance. Several different kinds of papillae occur on the tongue, in association with the taste buds. **optic p.** *see* optic (disc). **—papillary** *adj.*

papillitis (pap-i-**ly**-tis) *n.* inflammation of the optic disc.

papilloedema (pap-il-ee-**dee**-mă) *n.* swelling of the optic disc, which can be a sign of raised intracranial pressure or inflammation of the optic nerve.

papilloma (pap-i-**loh**-mă) *n.* a benign tumour of nonglandular and nonsecretory epithelium producing a nipple-like growth on the surface of skin or a mucous membrane. **—papillomatous** *adj.*

papillomatosis (pap-i-loh-mă-**toh**-sis) *n.* a condition in which many papillomas grow on an area of skin or mucous membrane.

papillotomy (pap-i-**lot**-ŏmi) *n.* the operation of cutting the ampulla of Vater to widen its outlet in order to improve biliary drainage and allow the passage of stones from the common bile duct. It is usually performed using a diathermy wire through a duodenoscope during ERCP.

papovavirus (pap-**oh**-vă-vy-rŭs) *n.* one of a group of small DNA-containing viruses producing tumours in animals and humans.

Pap test (pap) *n. see* Papanicolaou test.

papule (**pap**-yool) *n.* a small raised spot on the skin. **—papular** *adj.*

papulo- *combining form denoting* a papule or pimple.

papulopustular (pap-yoo-loh-**pus**-tew-ler) *adj.* describing a rash that contains both papules and pustules.

papulosquamous (pap-yoo-loh-**skway**-mŭs) *adj.* describing a rash that is both papular and scaly.

para- *combining form denoting* **1.** beside or near. **2.** resembling. **3.** abnormal.

paracentesis (pa-ră-sen-**tee**-sis) *n.* tapping: the process of drawing off fluid from a part of the body through a hollow needle or cannula. In ophthalmology it involves an incision into the anterior chamber of the eye.

paracetamol (acetaminophen) (pa-ră-**see**-tă-mol) *n.* an analgesic drug that also reduces fever. It is taken by mouth, intravenous infusion, or as suppositories to relieve mild or moderate pain, such as headache, toothache, dysmenorrhoea, and rheumatic pain, and to treat colds and influenza. Overdosage causes liver damage. Trade names: **Calpol**, **Panadol**, **Perfalgan**, etc.

paracusis (pa-ră-**kew**-sis) *n.* any distortion of hearing.

paradoxical breathing (pa-ră-**doks**-ikăl) *n.* breathing movements in which the chest wall moves in on inspiration and out on expiration, in reverse of the normal movements. It may be seen in children with respiratory distress and patients with chronic airways obstruction. Crush injuries of the chest can lead to a severe degree of paradoxical breathing.

paraesthesia (pa-ris-**theez**-i-ă) *n.* a spontaneously occurring abnormal tingling sensation, sometimes described as **pins and needles**. *Compare* dysaesthesia.

paraffin (pa-ră-fin) *n.* one of a series of hydrocarbons derived from petroleum. **liquid p.** a mineral oil, which was formerly used as a laxative. **soft p.** a white or yellow mixture of hydrocarbons used, in combination with liquid paraffin, as an emollient, as a lubricant for treating dry eyes, and to impregnate dressings to prevent them from adhering to wounds.

paraganglioma (pa-ră-gang-li-**oh**-mă) *n.* a benign tumour arising from paraganglion cells. Such tumours can occur around the aorta, the carotid artery (carotid body tumour), and the cervical portion of the vagus nerve (*see* glomus tumour), as well as in the abdomen and the eye.

paraganglion (pa-ră-**gang**-li-ŏn) *n.* one of the small oval masses of cells in the walls of the ganglia of the sympathetic nervous system, near the spinal cord. They may secrete adrenaline.

parageusia (parageusis) (pa-ră-**gew**-siă) *n.* abnormality of the sense of taste.

paragonimiasis (endemic haemoptysis) (pa-ră-gon-i-**my**-ă-sis) *n.* a tropical disease, occurring principally in Asia, caused by the presence of the fluke *Paragonimus westermani* in the lungs or other organs. Symptoms include cough, chest pain, fatigue, and sweating.

parainfluenza viruses (pa-ră-in-floo-**en**-ză) *pl. n.* a group of large RNA-containing viruses that cause infections of the respiratory tract producing mild influenza-like symptoms. They are included in the paramyxovirus group (*see* myxovirus).

paralysis (pă-**ral**-i-sis) *n.* muscle weakness that varies in its extent, its severity, and the degree of spasticity or flaccidity according to the nature of the underlying disease and its distribution in the brain, spinal cord, peripheral nerves, or muscles. *See also* diplegia, hemiplegia, paraplegia, poliomyelitis. —**paralytic** (pa-ră-**lit**-ik) *adj.*

paramedian (pa-ră-**mee**-di-ăn) *adj.* situated close to or beside the median plane.

paramedical (pa-ră-**med**-ikăl) *adj.* describing or relating to the professions closely linked to the medical profession and working in conjunction with them. *See* allied health professional.

paramesonephric duct (pa-ră-mes-oh-**nef**-rik) *n. see* Müllerian duct.

parameter (pă-**ram**-it-er) *n.* (in medicine) a measurement of some factor, such as blood pressure, pulse rate, or haemoglobin level, that may have a bearing on the condition being investigated.

parametric test (pa-ră-**met**-rik) *n.* a test of statistical significance based on the assumption that the range of observations are distributed by chance in a normal distribution (*see* frequency distribution), where 95% of observations lie within two standard deviations of the mean (**Student's t test** to compare means). **Nonparametric tests** (**Mann–Whitney U tests**) make no assumptions about distribution patterns.

parametritis (pelvic cellulitis) (pa-ră-mi-**try**-tis) *n.* inflammation of the parametrium. The condition may be associated with puerperal infection.

parametrium (pa-ră-**mee**-triŭm) *n.* the layer of connective tissue surrounding the uterus.

paramnesia (pa-ram-**nee**-ziă) *n.* a distorted memory, such as confabulation or déjà vu.

paramyotonia congenita (pa-ră-my-ŏ-**toh**-nia kŏn-**jen**-it-ă) *n.* a rare disorder in which myotonia is precipitated by cold and exercise. It is due to a disorder of the sodium channel.

paramyxovirus (pa-ră-**miks**-oh-vy-rŭs) *n. see* myxovirus.

paranasal sinuses (pa-ră-**nay**-zăl) *pl. n.* the air-filled spaces, lined with mucous membrane, that occur in some bones of the skull and open into the nasal cavity. They comprise the **frontal sinuses** and the **maxillary sinuses** (one pair of each), the **ethmoid sinuses** (consisting of many spaces inside the ethmoid bone), and the two **sphenoid sinuses**.

paraneoplastic syndrome (pa-ră-nee-oh-**plast**-ik) *n.* signs or symptoms occurring in a patient with cancer that result from antibodies or ectopic hormones produced by the cancer and are not due directly to local effects of the cancer cells. Removal of the cancer usually leads to resolution of the problem. An example is myasthenia gravis secondary to a tumour of the thymus.

paranoia (pa-ră-**noi**-ă) *n.* **1.** a mental illness or a symptom of mental illness characterized by delusions, sometimes organized into a system. The person believes him- or herself to be a target of persecution or the victim of a conspiracy. **2.** a state of mind in which the individual has a strong belief that he or she is persecuted by others. Severe paranoia can lead to a diagnosis of personality disorder. —**paranoid** (pa-ră-noid) *adj.*

paraparesis (pa-ră-pă-ree-sis) *n.* weakness of both legs, resulting from disease of the nervous system.

paraphasia (pa-ră-**fay**-ziă) *n.* a disorder of language in which unintended syllables, words, or phrases are interpolated in the patient's speech.

paraphimosis (pa-ră-fi-**moh**-sis) *n.* retraction and constriction of the foreskin behind the glans penis. The tight foreskin cannot be drawn back over the glans and becomes painful and oedematous.

paraphrenia (pa-ră-**free**-niă) *n. see* late-onset schizophrenia.

paraplegia (pa-ră-**plee**-jiă) *n.* paralysis of both legs, usually due to disease or injury of the spinal cord. It is often accompanied by loss of sensation below the level of the injury and disturbed bladder function. —**paraplegic** *adj., n.*

parapsychology (pa-ră-sy-**kol**-ŏji) *n.* the study of mental abilities that appear to defy natural law.

Paraquat (pa-ră-kwot) *n. Trademark.* the chemical compound dimethyl dipyridilium, widely used as a weed-killer. When swallowed it exerts its most serious effects upon the lungs, the tissues of which it destroys after a few days.

parasite (pa-ră-syt) *n.* any living thing that lives in or on another living organism (*see* host). Some parasites cause irritation and interfere with bodily functions; others destroy host tissues and release toxins into the body. Human parasites include fungi, bacteria, viruses, protozoa, and worms. *See also* commensal, symbiosis. —**parasitic** (pa-ră-**sit**-ik) *adj.*

parasiticide (pa-ră-**sit**-i-syd) *n.* an agent that destroys parasites (excluding bacteria and fungi). *See also* acaricide, anthelmintic, trypanocide.

parasitology (pa-ră-sit-**ol**-ŏji) *n.* the study and science of parasites.

parastomal (pa-ră-**stoh**-măl) *adj.* relating to the area around a stoma, which often appears as a hernia or bulge. Following surgery, muscle structure is interrupted making it weaker and prone to stretching. Straining can cause intestinal contents to herniate through the weakened spot.

parasuicide (pa-ră-**soo**-i-syd) *n. see* deliberate self-harm.

parasympathetic nervous system (pa-ră-sim-pă-**thet**-ik) *n.* one of the two divisions of the autonomic nervous system, having fibres that leave the central nervous system from the brain and the lower portion of the spinal cord and are distributed to blood vessels, glands, and internal organs. It is responsible for (among other effects) slowing the heart rate and constricting the pupillary muscles. The nerve endings release acetylcholine as a neurotransmitter.

parasympatholytic (pa-ră-sim-pă-thoh-**lit**-ik) *adj.* opposing the effects of the parasympathetic nervous system. Antimuscarinic drugs have this effect.

parasympathomimetic (pa-rā-sim-pă-thoh-mi-**met**-ik) *adj.* having the effect of stimulating the parasympathetic nervous system. The actions of the parasympathomimetic drugs are **cholinergic** (resembling those of acetylcholine) and include stimulation of skeletal muscle, vasodilatation, depression of heart rate, increasing the tension of smooth muscle, increasing secretions (such as saliva), and constricting the pupil of the eye.

parathion (pa-ră-**th'**y-on) *n.* an organic phosphorus compound, used as a pesticide, that causes poisoning when inhaled, ingested, or absorbed through the skin. The symptoms are headache, sweating, salivation, lacrimation, vomiting, diarrhoea, and muscular spasms. Treatment is by administration of atropine.

parathormone (pa-ră-**thor**-mohn) *n. see* parathyroid hormone.

parathyroidectomy (pa-ră-th'y-roid-**ek**-tŏmi) *n.* surgical removal of one or more of the parathyroid glands, usually as part of the treatment of hyperparathyroidism.

parathyroid glands (pa-ră-**th'**y-roid) *pl. n.* two pairs of yellowish-brown endocrine glands that are situated behind, or sometimes embedded within, the thyroid gland. They are stimulated to produce parathyroid hormone by a decrease in the amount of calcium in the blood.

parathyroid hormone (parathormone) *n.* a hormone, synthesized and released by the parathyroid glands, that controls the distribution of calcium and phosphate in the body. A deficiency of the hormone lowers blood calcium levels, causing tetany. Recombinant parathyroid hormone (Preotact) is given by subcutaneous injection to treat menopausal osteoporosis. *Compare* calcitonin.

paratyphoid fever (pa-ră-**ty**-foid) *n.* an infectious disease caused by the bacterium *Salmonella paratyphi* A, B, or C. Symptoms include diarrhoea, mild fever, and a pink rash on the chest. Treatment with chloramphenicol is effective. The TAB vaccine provides temporary immunity against paratyphoid A and B.

paravertebral (pa-ră-**ver**-tib-răl) *adj.* close to or at the side of the backbone.

parenchyma (pă-**renk**-im-ă) *n.* the functional part of an organ, as opposed to the supporting tissue (*see* stroma).

parental responsibility (par-**rent**-ăl) *n.* the legal status that requires adults to act in the interests of a child's welfare. A birth mother always has parental responsibility unless it is removed by an adoption order, as has the father if married to the birth mother or named on the birth certificate. Same-sex parents, civil partners, both have parental responsibility. A person with parental responsibility can consent to, or refuse, treatment on behalf of a child who is too young to have capacity to make his or her own decisions about health care, providing that this person is acting in the child's best interests. *See also* Gillick competence.

parenteral (pa-**rent**-er-ăl) *adj.* administered by any way other than through the mouth: applied, for example, to the introduction of drugs into the body by injection. **p. feeding** *see* nutrition.

paresis (pă-**ree**-sis) *n.* muscular weakness caused by disease of the nervous system. It implies a lesser degree of weakness than paralysis, although the two words are often used interchangeably.

paries (**pair**-i-eez) *n.* (*pl.* **parietes**) **1.** the enveloping or surrounding part of an organ or other structure. **2.** the wall of a cavity.

parietal (pă-**ry**-ĕ-t'l) *adj.* of or relating to the inner walls of a body cavity, as opposed to the contents. **p. bone** either of a pair of bones forming the top and sides of the cranium. *See* skull. **p. cells** (**oxyntic cells**) cells of the gastric glands that secrete hydrochloric acid in the fundic region of the stomach. **p. lobe** one of the major divisions of each cerebral hemisphere (*see* cerebrum), lying beneath the crown of the skull. It contains the sensory cortex and association areas. **p. pleura** *see* pleura.

parity (**pa**-riti) *n.* a term used to indicate the number of pregnancies a woman has had that have each resulted in the birth of an infant capable of survival. *See also* grand multiparity.

parkinsonism (**par**-kin-sŏn-izm) *n.* a clinical picture characterized by tremor, rigidity, slowness of movement, and postural instability. The patient has an expressionless face, an unmodulated voice, an increasing tendency to stoop, and a shuffling walk. Parkinsonism is a disease process affecting the basal ganglia of the brain and associated with a deficiency of the neurotransmitter dopamine. Sometimes a distinction is made between **Parkinson's disease**, a degenerative disorder, and parkinsonism due to other causes, notably the long-term use of antipsychotic drugs. Relief of the symptoms may be obtained with antimuscarinic drugs, levodopa, apomorphine, and dopamine-receptor agonists (e.g. bromocriptine). [J. Parkinson (1755–1824), British physician]

SEE WEB LINKS

- Website of Parkinson's (formerly the Parkinson's Disease Society)

paronychia (whitlow) (pa-roh-**nik**-iă) *n.* an inflamed swelling of the nail folds. **acute p.** a condition that is usually caused by infection with *Staphylococcus aureus*. **chronic p.** paronychia that occurs mainly in those who habitually engage in wet work; it is associated with secondary infection with *Candida albicans*.

parosmia (pa-**roz**-miă) *n.* any disorder of the sense of smell.

parotid gland (pă-**rot**-id) *n.* one of a pair of salivary glands situated in front of each ear.

parotitis (pa-rŏ-**ty**-tis) *n.* inflammation of the parotid salivary glands. *See* mumps (infectious parotitis).

parous (**pa**-rŭs) *adj.* having given birth to one or more children.

paroxetine (pă-roks-ĕ-teen) *n.* an antidepressant drug (*see* SSRI) taken by mouth for the treatment of depression, obsessive–compulsive disorder, panic disorder, post-traumatic stress disorder, and some other anxiety disorders. Trade name: **Seroxat**.

paroxysm (pa-rŏk-sizm) *n.* **1.** a sudden violent attack, especially a spasm or convulsion. **2.** the abrupt worsening of symptoms or recurrence of disease. **—paroxysmal** (pa-rŏk-**siz**-măl) *adj.*

paroxysmal dyspnoea *n.* attacks of breathlessness occurring at night due to left ventricular heart failure.

paroxysmal tachycardia *n.* abnormally increased heart rate due to impulses generated anywhere in the heart outside the natural pacemaker (sinoatrial node), for example in the atrial muscle (**paroxysmal atrial tachycardia**, **PAT**).

parrot disease (pa-rŏt) *n. see* psittacosis.

pars (parz) *n.* a specific part of an organ or other structure, such as any of parts of the pituitary gland.

Parse's nursing theory (parz-iz) *n.* a theory that views patients as taking an active and continuous role in their development, being free to select the means of achieving a particular way of living. Nurse and patient should work together to derive the meaning of a particular situation for the patient to enable the planning of healthcare intervention. [R. Parse (20th century), nurse theorist]

parthenogenesis (par-thin-oh-**jen**-i-sis) *n.* reproduction in which an organism develops from an unfertilized ovum. It is common in plants and occurs in some lower animals (e.g. aphids).

participatory action research (par-tis-i-**pay**-tŏri) *n.* a method of improving public health by involving clients through collaboration, reflection, data collection, and actions that empower them to actively improve their own health. *See also* empowerment.

partogram (par-toh-gram) *n.* a graphic record of the course of labour, including the mother's blood pressure, heart rate, length, frequency, and strength of contractions, etc., and heart rate and amniotic fluid in the baby.

parturition (par-tewr-**ish**-ŏn) *n.* childbirth. *See* labour. **—parturient** (par-**tewr**-i-ĕnt) *adj.*

parvi- (parvo-) *combining form denoting* small size.

pascal (pas-kăl) *n.* the SI unit of pressure, equal to 1 newton per square metre. Symbol: Pa.

Paschen bodies (**pah**-skĕn) *pl. n.* particles that occur in the cells of skin rashes in patients with cowpox or smallpox; they are thought to be the virus particles. [E. Paschen (1860–1936), German pathologist]

PASI *n. see* psoriasis area severity index.

passive movement (pas-iv) *n.* movement not brought about by a patient's own efforts. Passive movements are induced by manipulation of the joints by a physiotherapist. *Compare* active movement.

passivity (pas-**iv**-iti) *n.* (in psychiatry) a symptom of schizophrenia in which the patient has the impression that his or her feelings or actions are those of another or others, usually an unknown outside power.

Pasteurella (pas-cher-**el**-ă) *n.* a genus of small rodlike Gram-negative bacteria that are parasites of animals and humans. **P. multocida** a species that usually infects animals but may be transmitted to humans through bites or scratches.

pasteurization (pas-cher-I-**zay**-shŏn) *n.* the treatment of milk by heating it to 65°C for 30 minutes, or to 72°C for 15 minutes, followed by rapid cooling, to kill such bacteria as those of tuberculosis and typhoid.

pastille (pas-t'l) *n.* a medicinal preparation containing gelatine and glycerine that is dissolved in the mouth so that the medication is applied to the mouth or throat.

PAT *n. see* paroxysmal (atrial) tachycardia.

Patau syndrome (pat-ow) *n.* a chromosome disorder in which there are three no. 13 chromosomes (instead of the usual two), causing abnormal brain development, severe learning disability, and defects in the heart, kidney, and scalp. Affected individuals rarely survive. [K. Patau (20th century), US geneticist]

patch test (pach) *n.* a test to discover which allergen is responsible for contact dermatitis in a patient. Very low concentrations of different allergens are applied under a patch on the back: a positive test will show an eczematous reaction.

patella (pă-**tel**-ă) *n.* the lens-shaped bone that forms the kneecap. It is situated in front of the knee in the tendon of the quadriceps muscle of the thigh. *See also* sesamoid bone. **—patellar** (pă-**tel**-er) *adj.*

patellar reflex (knee jerk) *n.* reflex contraction of the quadriceps (thigh) muscle, so that the leg kicks, elicited in a patient sitting with one leg crossed over the other by tapping the tendon of the muscle below the kneecap. The reflex is absent, reduced, or exaggerated when the spinal cord is damaged or diseased.

patellectomy (pat-ĕ-**lek**-tŏmi) *n.* surgical excision of the patella.

patent (**pay**-tĕnt) *adj.* open; unblocked. **p. ductus arteriosus** *see* ductus arteriosus.

path- (patho-) *combining form denoting* disease.

pathogen (**pa**-thŏ-jen) *n.* a microorganism, such as a bacterium, that parasitizes an animal (or plant) or a human and produces a disease.

pathogenesis (pa-thŏ-**jen**-i-sis) *n.* the origin and development of a disease. **—pathogenetic** (pa-thoh-ji-**net**-ik) *adj.*

pathogenic (pa-thŏ-**jen**-ik) *adj.* capable of causing disease. The term is applied to a parasitic microorganism (especially a bacterium) in relation to its host. **—pathogenicity** *n.*

pathognomonic (pa-thŏg-noh-**mon**-ik) *adj.* describing a symptom or sign that is characteristic of or unique to a particular disease.

pathological (pa-thŏ-**loj**-ikăl) *adj.* relating to or arising from disease. **p. fracture** *see* fracture.

pathology (pă-**thol**-ŏji) *n.* the study of disease processes with the aim of understanding their nature and causes. **clinical p.** the application of the knowledge of disease processes to the treatment of patients. **—pathologist** *n.*

-pathy *combining form denoting* **1.** disease. **2.** therapy.

Patient Advice and Liaison Service (PALS) (pay-shĕnt) *n.* (in England) a confidential service provided by each NHS trust to support patients, their families, and carers by giving advice and information in response to questions and concerns about local NHS services.

patient allocation (al-ŏ-**kay**-shŏn) *n.* a method of organizing nursing care in which a nurse is allocated to care holistically for all the needs of a patient on a daily basis. *Compare* task allocation.

patient-controlled analgesia (PCA) *n.* a form of pain control, used especially postoperatively, in which the patient holds a device with a button that, when pressed, administers a preset dose of an analgesic (usually morphine) into the patient's bloodstream.

patient group direction (PGD) *n.* a written instruction, signed by a doctor, that provides a legal framework for the supply and administration of medicines directly to the patient without the need for a prescription. PGDs are intended for specific groups of patients, including those requiring immunization, emergency contraception, or analgesia for minor surgery, and the medication can be given by a registered nurse.

Patient Health Questionnaire *n. see* PHQ-9.

Paul-Bunnell test (pawl-bŭ-**nel**) *n.* a haemagglutination test used in the diagnosis of glandular fever. [J. R. Paul (1893–1971) and W. W. Bunnell (1902–66), US physicians]

Paul's tube (pawlz) *n.* a glass tube with a projecting rim, used to drain the bowel after it has been brought to the surface of the abdomen and opened. [F. T. Paul (1851–1941), British surgeon]

PBC *n. see* (primary biliary) cirrhosis.

PBM *n.* peak bone mass.

p.c. (post cibum) Latin: after food, used as a direction in prescriptions.

PCA *n. see* patient-controlled analgesia.

PCO *n. see* polycystic ovary.

PCOS *n. see* polycystic ovary syndrome.

PCP *n. Pneumocystis jiroveci* (formerly *carinii*) pneumonia. *See* Pneumocystis.

PCV *n. see* packed cell volume.

PCWP *n. see* pulmonary (capillary wedge pressure).

PDA *n. see* (patent) ductus arteriosus.

PDP *n. see* personal development plan.

PE *n.* pulmonary embolus. *See* (pulmonary) embolism.

peak expiratory flow rate (PEFR) (peek eks-**pir**-ă-ter-i floh rayt) *n.* the maximum rate at which a person can forcibly expel air from the lungs at any time, usually expressed in litres per minute and used particularly to help diagnose asthma and monitor its treatment.

peau d'orange (poh daw-**rahnj**) *n.* a dimpled appearance of the skin over a breast tumour, resembling the surface of an orange. The skin is thickened and the openings of hair follicles and sweat glands are enlarged.

pecten (**pek**-tin) *n.* **1.** the middle section of the anal canal. **2.** a sharp ridge on the upper branch of the pubis (part of the hip bone). —**pectineal** (pek-**tin**-iăl) *adj.*

pectoral (**pek**-ter-ăl) *adj.* relating to the chest or breast. **p. girdle** *see* shoulder girdle. **p. muscles** the chest muscles: the pectoralis major, which draws the arm forward across the chest, and the pectoralis minor, which depresses the shoulder.

pectoriloquy (pek-ter-**il**-ŏ-kwi) *n.* abnormal transmission of the patient's voice sounds through the chest wall so that they can be clearly heard through a stethoscope.

pectus (**pek**-tŭs) *n.* the chest or breast. **p. carinatum** *see* pigeon chest. **p. excavatum** *see* funnel chest.

pedicle (**ped**-ikŭl) *n.* **1.** the narrow neck of tissue connecting some tumours to the normal tissue from which they have developed. **2.** (in plastic surgery) a narrow folded tube of skin by means of which a piece of skin used for grafting remains attached to its original site. **3.** (in anatomy) any slender stemlike process.

pediculicide (pi-**dik**-yoo-li-syd) *n.* an agent that kills lice; examples include dimeticone and permethrin.

pediculosis (pi-dik-yoo-**loh**-sis) *n.* an infestation with lice which causes intense itching. **p. capitis** infestation with **head lice**, which is quite common in schoolchildren and does not indicate poor hygiene; it may be treated with pediculicide lotions or by use of a nit comb. **p. corporis** infestation with **body lice**, which often affects the homeless and others without access to washing facilities. **Pubic** (or **crab**) **lice** (*Phthirus pubis*) are commonly sexually transmitted and respond to the same treatment as head lice.

Pediculus (pi-**dik**-yoo-lŭs) *n.* a widely distributed genus of lice. **P. humanus capitis** the head louse. **P. humanus corporis** the body louse, which in some parts of the world transmits relapsing fever and typhus. *See also* pediculosis.

peduncle (pi-**dunk**-ŭl) *n.* a narrow process or stalklike structure, serving as a connection or support. —**pedunculated** *adj.*

PEEP *n. see* positive end expiratory pressure.

PEFR *n. see* peak expiratory flow rate.

PEG *n. see* (percutaneous endoscopic) gastrostomy.

Pel-Ebstein fever (pel-**eb**-styn) *n.* a recurrent fever characteristic of patients with lymphoma or

Hodgkin's disease. [P. K. Pel (1852–1919), Dutch physician; W. Ebstein (1836–1912), German physician]

pellagra (pil-ag-ră) *n.* a nutritional disease due to a deficiency of nicotinic acid (a B vitamin). It is common in maize-eating communities. The symptoms of pellagra are scaly dermatitis on exposed surfaces, diarrhoea, and depression.

pellet (pel-it) *n.* a small pill, especially one used as an implant.

pellicle (pel-ikŭl) *n.* a thin layer of skin, membrane, or any other substance.

pelvic-floor muscle training (pel-vik) *pl. n. see* Kegel exercises.

pelvic girdle (hip girdle) *n.* the bony structure to which the bones of the lower limbs are attached. It consists of the right and left hip bones.

pelvic inflammatory disease (PID) *n.* an acute or chronic condition in which the uterus, Fallopian tubes, and ovaries are inflamed and infected. It is usually the result of chlamydial or gonorrhoeal infection ascending from the vagina and may be associated with lower abdominal pain, irregular vaginal bleeding, and vaginal discharge. Blocking of the Fallopian tubes is a common result; this can lead to ectopic pregnancy or infertility. In the chronic state, when pelvic adhesions have developed, surgical removal of the diseased tissue may be necessary.

pelvimetry (pel-vim-itri) *n.* measurement of the four internal diameters of the pelvis on an X-ray image or by CT or MR scanning. Pelvimetry has sometimes been used in determining whether it will be possible for a baby to be delivered vaginally, but this is now considered unreliable.

pelvis (pel-vis) *n.* (*pl.* **pelves**) **1.** the bony structure formed by the hip bones, sacrum, and coccyx (see illustration). The hip bones are fused at the back to the sacrum to form a rigid structure that protects the organs of the lower abdomen and provides attachment for the bones and muscles of the lower limbs. **2.** the cavity within the bony pelvis. **3.** any structure shaped like a basin. **renal p.** the expanded part of the ureter in the kidney. **—pelvic** *adj.*

pemphigoid (bullous pemphigoid) (pem-fig-oid) *n.* a chronic itchy blistering disorder most common in the elderly. The blisters most commonly occur on the limbs and may persist, unlike those of pemphigus. Pemphigoid is an autoimmune disease and responds to treatment with corticosteroids or immunosuppressant drugs. **ocular p.** a potentially blinding disease in which there is dryness, blistering, and scarring of the conjunctiva and adhesions.

pemphigus (pemphigus vulgaris) (pem-fig-ŭs) *n.* a rare but serious autoimmune skin disease marked by successive outbreaks of blisters. The blisters are superficial and do not remain intact for long; the mouth and other mucous membranes, as well as the skin, are usually affected. Systemic immunosuppressant treatment is required.

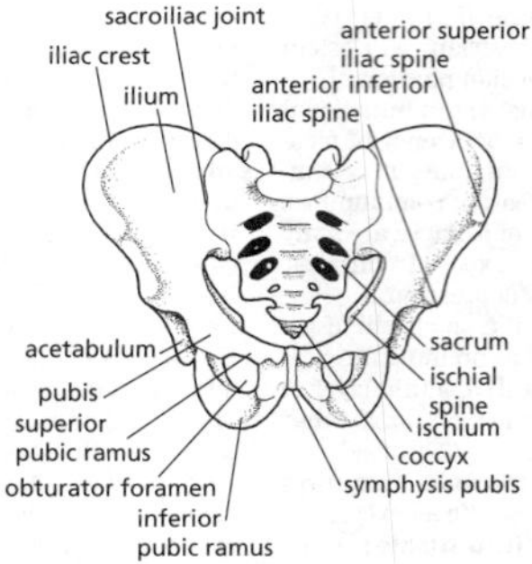

The male pelvis (ventral view)

Pendred's syndrome (pen-drids) *n.* goitre associated with congenital deafness due to deficiency of peroxidase, an enzyme that is essential for the utilization of iodine. [V. Pendred (1869–1946), British physician]

-penia *combining form denoting* lack or deficiency.

penicillamine (pen-i-**sil**-ă-meen) *n.* a drug that binds metals and therefore aids their excretion (*see* chelating agent). It is administered by mouth to treat Wilson's disease and severe rheumatoid arthritis (*see* disease-modifying antirheumatic drug). Trade name: **Distamine**.

penicillin (pen-i-**sil**-in) *n.* any one of a number of antibiotics derived from *Penicillium* moulds and used to treat infections caused by a wide variety of bacteria. Some patients are allergic to penicillin and develop such reactions as skin rashes or potentially fatal anaphylaxis. **p. G** (**benzylpenicillin**) a form of penicillin administered by injection or infusion. **p. V** (**phenoxymethylpenicillin**) an orally administered form of penicillin. **semisynthetic p.** one of a number of antibiotics derived from the penicillins, such as amoxicillin, ampicillin, and flucloxacillin.

penicillinase (pen-i-**sil**-in-ayz) *n.* an enzyme, produced by some bacteria, that is capable of antagonizing the antibacterial action of penicillin. Purified penicillinase may be used to treat reactions to penicillin.

Penicillium (pen-i-sil-iŭm) *n.* a genus of mouldlike fungi that commonly grow on decaying fruit, bread, or cheese. Some species are pathogenic to humans, causing diseases of the skin and respiratory tract. **P. rubrum** the major natural source of the antibiotic penicillin.

penile prosthesis (pee-nyl) *n. see* prosthesis.

penis (pee-nis) *n.* the male organ that carries the urethra, through which urine and semen are discharged (see illustration). Most of the organ is composed of erectile tissue (corpus cavernosum and corpus spongiosum), which becomes filled with blood under conditions of sexual excitement so that the penis is erected. *See also* glans, prepuce. —**penile** *adj.*

pent- (penta-) *combining form denoting* five.

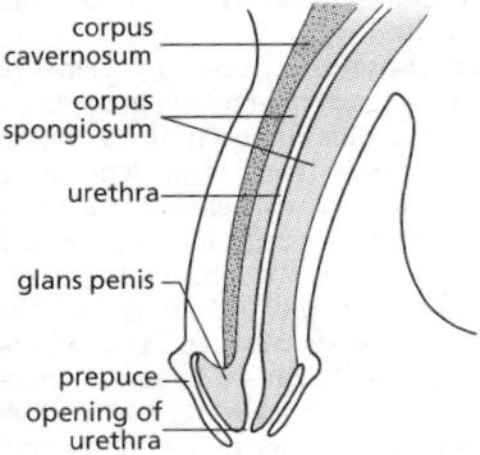

The penis (median section)

pentamidine (pen-tam-i-deen) *n.* a drug effective against protozoans and used in the treatment of *Pneumocystis* pneumonia in AIDS patients, leishmaniasis, and trypanosomiasis. It is administered by deep intramuscular injection, intravenous infusion, or inhalation. Trade name: **Pentacarinat**.

pentose (pen-tohz) *n.* a simple sugar with five carbon atoms, such as for example, ribose or xylose.

pentostatin (pen-tŏ-stat-in) *n.* a cytotoxic drug that is used in treating hairy-cell leukaemia. It is administered by intravenous injection. Trade name: **Nipent**.

pentosuria (pen-tohs-yoor-iă) *n.* an inborn defect of sugar metabolism causing abnormal excretion of pentose in the urine.

Peplau's model (pep-lowz) *n.* a model for nursing based on interpersonal relations. It emphasizes that the therapeutic nurse–patient relationship is an integral part of nursing practice and that the nurse's role evolves as a result of it. *See also* nursing models. [H. Peplau (1909–99), US nurse theorist]

peppermint (pep-er-mint) *n.* an oil extracted from a species of mint (*Mentha piperita*), used as a carminative and flavouring agent. **p. oil** an antispasmodic that relieves pain and distension in irritable bowel syndrome and diverticular disease. Trade names: **Colpermin**, **Mintec**.

pepsin (pep-sin) *n.* an enzyme in the stomach that begins the digestion of proteins by splitting them into peptones (*see* peptidase). It is produced by the action of hydrochloric acid on **pepsinogen**, which is secreted by the gastric glands.

pepsinogen (pep-**sin**-ŏ-jĕn) *n. see* pepsin.

peptic (**pep**-tik) *adj.* **1.** relating to pepsin. **2.** relating to digestion. **p. ulcer** a breach in the lining (mucosa) of the digestive tract caused by the actions of gastric acid and by pepsin. This may occur when there are abnormally high levels of pepsin or acid, or when the mucosa has been damaged by chronic *Helicobacter pylori* infection or by aspirin or NSAID use. *See* duodenal ulcer, gastric (ulcer), oesophageal ulcer.

peptidase (**pep**-tid-ayz) *n.* one of a group of digestive enzymes that split proteins in the stomach and intestine into their constituent amino acids.

peptide (**pep**-tyd) *n.* a molecule consisting of two or more amino acids linked by bonds between the amino group and the carboxyl group. *See also* polypeptide.

peptone (**pep**-tohn) *n.* a large protein fragment produced by the action of enzymes on proteins in the first stages of protein digestion.

peptonuria (pep-tohn-**yoor**-iă) *n.* the presence in the urine of peptones.

percentile (per-**sen**-tyl) *n. see* centile chart.

perception (per-**sep**-shŏn) *n.* (in psychology) the process by which information about the world, received by the senses, is analysed and made meaningful.

percussion (per-**kush**-ŏn) *n.* the technique of examining part of the body by tapping it with the fingers or an instrument (plessor) and sensing the resultant vibrations. It is used to detect the presence of fluid or abnormal solidification or enlargement in different organs.

percutaneous (per-kew-**tay**-niŭs) *adj.* through the skin: often applied to the route of administration of drugs in ointments, etc., which are absorbed through the skin. **p. coronary intervention** (**PCI**) the treatment of coronary artery disease by cardiac catheterization, usually coronary angioplasty followed by insertion of coronary stents. **Primary PCI** is the use of PCI as the first-line treatment to relieve coronary obstruction, rather than thrombolysis. **p. endoscopic gastrostomy** *see* gastrostomy. **p. nephrolithotomy** *see* nephrolithotomy. **p. transhepatic cholangiography** *see* cholangiography.

perforation (per-fer-**ay**-shŏn) *n.* the formation of a hole in a hollow organ. This may occur in the course of a disease, such as duodenal ulcer or stomach cancer. Treatment is usually by surgical repair of the perforation, but conservative treatment with antibiotics may result in spontaneous healing. Perforations may also be caused by instruments (for example a curette may perforate the uterus) or by injury (for example to the eardrum).

performance indicators (PIs) (per-**for**-mănss) *pl. n.* statistical information, based on quantitative measures of the resources and activities of the NHS, produced by health authorities and sent to the Department of Health. This enables comparisons of performance of one section with that achieved by another to be analysed and published.

performance status *n.* a scoring system used to quantify a patient's activity level and general wellbeing in order to assess suitability for chemotherapy or for taking part in a clinical trial. Commonly used systems include the WHO performance scale and the Karnofsky scale.

perfusion (per-**few**-*zhŏn*) *n.* **1.** the passage of fluid through a tissue, especially the passage of blood through the lung tissue to pick up oxygen in the alveoli and release carbon dioxide. **2.** the deliberate introduction of fluid into a tissue, usually by injection into the blood vessels supplying the tissue.

perfusion scan *n.* a technique for demonstrating an abnormal blood supply to an organ by injecting a radioactive tracer or contrast medium. Areas not being perfused show up as holes on gamma-camera images. *See also* ventilation-perfusion scanning.

pergolide (**per**-gŏ-lyd) *n.* a drug now rarely used in the treatment of Parkinson's disease. It is administered by mouth.

peri- *prefix denoting* near, around, or enclosing.

periadenitis (pe-ri-ad-in-**I**-tis) *n.* inflammation of tissues surrounding a gland.

perianal haematoma (external haemorrhoid) (pe-ri-**ay**-năl) *n.* a painful swelling composed of blood that lies next to the anus. Typically it occurs after an episode of straining to pass faeces or protracted coughing. Perianal haematomas are caused by the rupture of a small vein in the anus.

peri-arrest period (pe-ri-ă-**rest**) *n.* the recognized period, either just before or just after a full cardiac arrest, when the patient's condition is very unstable and care must be taken to prevent progression or regression into a full cardiac arrest.

periarteritis nodosa (pe-ri-ar-ter-**I**-tis) *n. see* polyarteritis nodosa.

periarthritis (pe-ri-arth-**ry**-tis) *n.* inflammation of tissues around a joint capsule, including tendons and bursae. **chronic p.** a common cause of pain and stiffness of the shoulder; it usually responds to local steroid injections or physiotherapy.

periarticular (pe-ri-ar-**tik**-yoo-ler) *adj.* around a joint, including the joint margins and surrounding area immediately adjacent to the joint capsule.

peribulbar (pe-ri-**bul**-ber) *adj.* (in ophthalmology) denoting the area around the eye.

pericard- (pericardio-) *combining form denoting* the pericardium.

pericardiectomy (pericardectomy) (pe-ri-kar-di-**ek**-tŏmi) *n.* surgical removal of the pericardium.

It is used in the treatment of chronic constrictive pericarditis and chronic pericardial effusion (*see* pericarditis).

pericardiocentesis (pe-ri-kar-di-oh-sen-**tee**-sis) *n.* removal of excess fluid from within the pericardium by means of needle aspiration.

pericardiorrhaphy (pe-ri-kar-di-**o**-răfi) *n.* the repair of wounds in the pericardium, such as those due to injury or surgery.

pericardiostomy (pe-ri-kar-di-**ost**-ŏmi) *n.* an operation in which the pericardium is opened and the fluid within drained via a tube. It is sometimes used in the treatment of septic pericarditis.

pericardiotomy (pericardotomy) (pe-ri-kar-di-**ot**-ŏmi) *n.* surgical opening or puncture of the pericardium. It is required to gain access to the heart in heart surgery and to remove excess fluid from within the pericardium.

pericarditis (pe-ri-kar-**dy**-tis) *n.* acute or chronic inflammation of the pericardium. Pericarditis may be seen alone or as part of pancarditis. It has numerous causes, including virus infections, uraemia, and cancer. **acute p.** pericarditis characterized by fever, chest pain, and a pericardial friction rub (a harsh scratching noise audible over the anterior chest wall with the aid of a stethoscope). Fluid may accumulate within the pericardial sac (**pericardial effusion**). **chronic constrictive p.** chronic thickening of the pericardium, which interferes with activity of the heart and has many features in common with heart failure.

pericardium (pe-ri-**kar**-diŭm) *n.* the membrane surrounding the heart. **fibrous p.** the outer portion of the pericardium, which completely encloses the heart and is attached to the large blood vessels emerging from the heart. **serous p.** the internal portion of the pericardium: a closed sac of serous membrane containing a very small amount of fluid, which prevents friction between the two surfaces as the heart beats. **—pericardial** *adj.*

pericardotomy (pe-ri-kar-**dot**-ŏmi) *n. see* pericardiotomy.

perichondritis (pe-ri-kon-**dry**-tis) *n.* inflammation of cartilage and surrounding soft tissues, usually due to chronic infection. A common site is the external ear.

perichondrium (pe-ri-**kon**-driŭm) *n.* the dense layer of fibrous connective tissue that covers the surface of cartilage.

pericranium (pe-ri-**kray**-niŭm) *n.* the periosteum of the skull.

pericystitis (pe-ri-sis-**ty**-tis) *n.* inflammation in the tissues around the bladder, causing pain in the pelvis, fever, and symptoms of cystitis. It usually results from infection in the Fallopian tubes or uterus.

perifolliculitis (pe-ri-fŏ-lik-yoo-**ly**-tis) *n.* inflammation around the hair follicles.

perihepatitis (pe-ri-hep-ă-**ty**-tis) *n.* inflammation of the membrane (capsule) covering the liver. It is usually associated with abnormalities of the liver or chronic peritonitis.

perilymph (pe-ri-limf) *n.* the fluid between the bony and membranous labyrinths of the ear.

perimenopause (pe-ri-men-ŏ-pawz) *n.* the period of time preceding the menopause, characterized by marked changes in the menstrual cycle and (often) hot flushes and emotional fluctuation.

perimeter (per-im-it-er) *n.* an instrument for mapping the absolute extent of the visual field and detecting any gaps or defects. —**perimetry** *n.*

perimetritis (pe-ri-mi-try-tis) *n.* inflammation of the membrane on the outer surface of the uterus. The condition may be associated with parametritis.

perimetrium (pe-ri-mee-triŭm) *n.* the peritoneum of the uterus.

perimysium (pe-ri-mis-iŭm) *n.* the fibrous sheath that surrounds each bundle of muscle fibres.

perinatal (pe-ri-nay-t'l) *adj.* relating to the period starting a few weeks before birth and including the birth and a few weeks after birth. **p. mortality rate** the number of stillbirths and deaths in the first week of life per 1000 live births and stillbirths.

perindopril (pĕ-rin-dŏ-pril) *n. see* ACE inhibitor.

perineal (pe-ri-nee-ăl) *adj.* relating to the perineum. **p. descent** abnormal bulging down of the perineum due to weakness of the pelvic floor muscles. **p. repair** *see* perineorrhaphy. **p. tear** (**p. trauma**) any injury to the perineum, which may be sustained during childbirth. First-degree tears involve only the perineal skin and vaginal mucosa. Second-degree tears involve perineal muscles but not the anal sphincter. Third-degree tears involve the external and internal anal sphincters. Fourth-degree tears involve the anal sphincters and the anal epithelium or rectal mucosa.

perineoplasty (pe-ri-nee-oh-plasti) *n.* an operation designed to enlarge the vaginal opening by incising the hymen and part of the perineum (**Fenton's operation**).

perineorrhaphy (pe-ri-ni-o-răfi) *n.* the surgical repair of a damaged perineum. The damage is usually the result of a tear in the perineum sustained during childbirth.

perinephric (pe-ri-nef-rik) *adj.* around the kidney. **p. abscess** a collection of pus around the kidney, usually secondary to pyonephrosis but also resulting from the spread of infection from other sites.

perinephritis (pe-ri-ni-fry-tis) *n.* inflammation of the tissues around the kidney, usually due to spread of infection from the kidney itself. The patient has pain in the loins, fever, and fits of shivering.

perineum (pe-ri-nee-ŭm) *n.* the region of the body between the anus and the urethral opening, including both skin and underlying muscle.

perineurium (pe-ri-newr-iŭm) *n.* the sheath of connective tissue that surrounds individual bundles of nerve fibres within a large nerve.

periocular (pe-ri-ok-yoo-ler) *adj.* adjacent to the eyeball.

periodic fever (peer-i-od-ik) *n. see* malaria.

periodontal (pe-ri-ŏ-**don**-t'l) *adj.* denoting or relating to the tissues surrounding the teeth. **p. disease** disease of the tissues that support and attach the teeth – the gums, periodontal membrane, and alveolar bone: the most common cause of tooth loss in older people. **p. membrane** (**p. ligament**) the ligament around a tooth, by which it is attached to the bone.

periodontium (pe-ri-ŏ-**don**-tiŭm) *n.* the tissues that support the teeth and attach them to the jaw: the gums (gingiva), periodontal membrane, alveolar bone, and cementum.

periodontology (pe-ri-ŏ-don-**tol**-ŏji) *n.* the branch of dentistry concerned with the tissues that support and attach the teeth and the prevention and treatment of periodontal disease.

perioperative (pe-ri-**op**-er-ă-tiv) *adj.* denoting or relating to the period that extends from the day before to the first few days after surgery.

periorbital (pe-ri-**or**-bit-ăl) *adj.* **1.** surrounding the eye socket (orbit). **2.** relating to the periosteum within the orbit.

periosteotome (pe-ri-**ost**-i-ŏ-tohm) *n.* an instrument used for cutting the periosteum and separating it from the underlying bone.

periosteum (pe-ri-**ost**-iŭm) *n.* a layer of dense connective tissue that covers the surface of a bone and provides attachment for muscles, tendons, and ligaments. The outer layer of the periosteum contains a large number of blood vessels; the inner layer contains osteoblasts and fewer blood vessels. —**periosteal** *adj.*

periostitis (pe-ri-ost-**I**-tis) *n.* inflammation of the periosteum. **acute p.** periostitis that results from direct injury to the bone and is associated with a haematoma, which may later become infected. **chronic p.** periostitis that is often due to an inflammatory disease, such as tuberculosis or syphilis, or to a chronic ulcer overlying the bone involved.

peripherally inserted central catheter *see* PICC line.

peripheral nervous system (per-**if**-er-ăl) *n.* all parts of the nervous system lying outside the central nervous system. It includes the cranial nerves and spinal nerves and their branches and the autonomic nervous system.

peripheral neuropathy *n.* *see* neuropathy.

peripheral vascular disease (PVD) *n.* any disease of the blood vessels outside the heart, especially in the extremities, most commonly due to atherosclerosis. Examples are intermittent claudication and Raynaud's disease.

periphlebitis (pe-ri-fli-**by**-tis) *n.* inflammation of the tissues around a vein: seen as an extension of phlebitis.

periproctitis (pe-ri-prok-**ty**-tis) *n.* inflammation of the tissues around the rectum and anus.

perisalpingitis (pe-ri-sal-pin-**jy**-tis) *n.* inflammation of the peritoneal membrane on the outer surface of a Fallopian tube.

perisplenitis (pe-ri-spli-**ny**-tis) *n.* inflammation of the external coverings of the spleen.

peristalsis (pe-ri-**stal**-sis) *n.* a wavelike movement that progresses along some of the hollow muscular tubes of the body, such as the intestines. It occurs involuntarily, induced by distension of the walls of the tube. Alternate contraction and relaxation of the circular and longitudinal muscles tends to push the contents of the tube forward. **—peristaltic** *adj.*

peritendinitis (pe-ri-ten-di-**ny**-tis) *n.* *see* tenosynovitis.

peritomy (per-**it**-ŏmi) *n.* an eye operation in which an incision of the conjunctiva is made in a complete circle around the cornea.

peritoneal dialysis (PD) *n.* *see* dialysis.

peritoneoscope (pe-ri-tŏn-**ee**-ŏ-skohp) *n.* *see* laparoscope.

peritoneum (pe-ri-tŏn-**ee**-ŭm) *n.* the serous membrane of the abdominal cavity (see illustration). **parietal p.** the part of the peritoneum that lines the walls of the abdomen. **visceral p.** the part of the peritoneum that covers the abdominal organs. *See also* mesentery, omentum. **—peritoneal** *adj.*

peritonitis (pe-ri-tŏn-**I**-tis) *n.* inflammation of the peritoneum. **primary p.** peritonitis caused by bacteria spread via the bloodstream. Symptoms are diffuse abdominal pain and swelling, with fever and weight loss. **secondary p.** peritonitis due to perforation or rupture of an abdominal organ, such as the vermiform appendix, allowing access of bacteria and irritant digestive juices to the peritoneum. This produces sudden severe abdominal pain and shock. Treatment is usually by surgical repair of the perforation.

peritonsillar abscess (pe-ri-**ton**-sil-er) *n.* *see* quinsy.

peritrichous (pe-ri-**try**-kŭs) *adj.* describing bacteria in which the flagella cover the entire cell surface.

perityphlitis (pe-ri-tif-**ly**-tis) *n.* *Archaic.* inflammation of the tissues around the caecum.

periureteritis (pe-ri-yoor-i-ter-**I**-tis) *n.* inflammation of the tissues around a ureter. This is usually associated with inflammation of the ureter itself (*see* ureteritis) often behind an obstruction caused by a stone or stricture.

perivascular spaces (pe-ri-**vas**-kew-ler) *pl. n.* *see* Vichow Robin spaces.

periventricular haemorrhage (PVH) (pe-ri-ven-**trik**-yoo-lă) bleeding from fragile blood vessels around the ventricles in the brain in infants born prematurely. *See also* intraventricular haemorrhage.

PERLA pupils equal, react to light and accommodation: used in hospital notes.

perle (perl) *n.* a soft capsule containing medicine.

perleche (per-**lesh**) *n.* dryness and cracking of the corners of the mouth, sometimes with infection. Perleche may be caused by persistent lip licking or by a vitamin-deficient diet.

permeability (per-mi-ă-**bil**-iti) *n.* the ability of membranes to allow

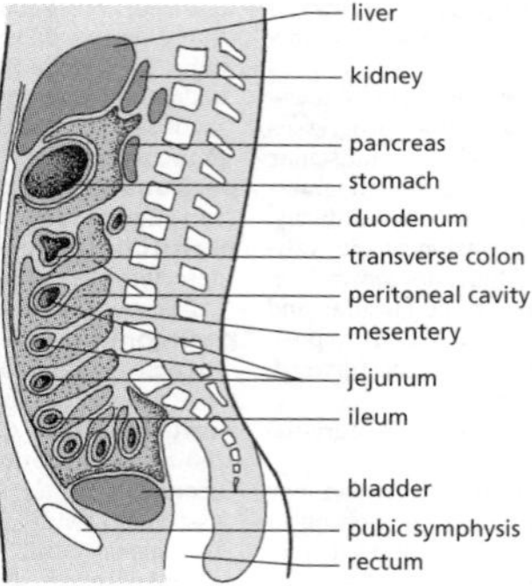

Sagittal section of the abdomen to show arrangement of the peritoneum

soluble substances to pass through them. *See also* semipermeable membrane. **—permeable** (per-mi-ăbŭl) *adj.*

permethrin (per-**meeth**-rin) *n.* a synthetic derivative of the naturally occurring insecticide pyrethrin that is applied externally as a cream to treat pubic lice and scabies. Trade name: **Lyclear**.

pernicious (per-**nish**-ŭs) *adj.* describing diseases that are highly dangerous or likely to result in death if untreated. **p. anaemia** a form of anaemia resulting from deficiency of vitamin B_{12}, due either to the body's failure to produce intrinsic factor or to dietary deficiency of the vitamin. It is characterized by defective production of red blood cells and the presence of megaloblasts in the bone marrow.

pernio (**per**-ni-oh) *n.* the medical name for a chilblain (*see* chilblains).

perniosis (per-ni-**oh**-sis) *n. see* chilblains.

pero- *combining form denoting* deformity; defect.

peromelia (pe-roh-**mee**-liă) *n.* congenital deformity of one or more limbs.

peroneal (pe-rŏ-**nee**-ăl) *adj.* relating to or supplying the outer (fibular) side of the leg.

peroneus (pe-rŏ-**nee**-ŭs) *n.* one of the muscles of the leg that arises from the fibula and helps to turn the foot outwards.

peroral (per-**or**-ăl) *adj*. through the mouth.

perphenazine (per-**fen**-ă-zeen) *n*. a phenothiazine antipsychotic drug administered by mouth to treat schizophrenia, mania, anxiety, and severe agitation and to prevent and treat severe nausea and vomiting. Trade name: **Fentazin**.

perseveration (per-sev-er-**ay**-shŏn) *n*. **1.** excessive persistence at a task that prevents the individual from turning his or her attention to new situations. It is a symptom of organic disease of the brain and sometimes of obsessive–compulsive disorder. **2.** the phenomenon in which an image continues to be perceived briefly in the absence of the object. This is a potentially serious neurological disorder.

persistent vegetative state (PVS) (per-**sist**-ĕnt) *n*. the condition that may be diagnosed after a patient has been in the vegetative state for more than four weeks and is normally regarded as permanent after twelve months. Medical treatment may be legally withdrawn from a patient in PVS but permission must first be granted by the courts. *See* vegetative state. *Compare* locked-in syndrome.

personal development plan (PDP) (**per**-sŏn-ăl) *n*. an individualized plan developed by nurses and other health-care professionals to further their commitment to continuing professional development.

personality (per-sŏn-**al**-iti) *n*. (in psychology) an enduring disposition to act and feel in particular ways that differentiate one individual from another.

personality disorder *n*. a deeply ingrained and maladaptive pattern of behaviour, which persists over many years and causes suffering, either to the patient or to other people (or both). *See* antisocial personality disorder, emotionally unstable personality disorder, hysterical.

personal protective equipment (PPE) *n*. equipment or clothing that is worn to protect the wearer from biohazards or risks that can be a part of everyday practice, such as obtaining or handling blood or sputum samples or administering medication. It can consist of gloves and eye protection. Employers have a responsibility to provide appropriate protection for staff at all times.

person-centred care (per-son-sen-tĕd) *n*. a relationship between a health-care professional and a patient that focuses on the needs of the person by negotiating and discussing care using a collaborative approach.

perspiration (per-sper-**ay**-shŏn) *n*. sweat or the process of sweating. **insensible p.** sweat that evaporates immediately from the skin and is therefore not visible. **sensible p.** sweat that is visible on the skin in the form of drops.

PERT (pancreatic enzyme replacement therapy) capsules containing the digestive enzymes lipase, amylase, and protease (**Creon**, **Pancrex**), which are given when there is insufficient endogenous production of pancreatic enzymes, for example, to patients with pancreatic cancer or cystic fibrosis. PERT treats the symptoms of steatorrhoea.

Perthes' disease (**per**-tiz) *n. see* Legg-Calvé-Perthes disease.

pertussis (per-**tus**-iss) *n. see* whooping cough.

pes (payz) *n.* (in anatomy) the foot or a part resembling a foot. **p. clavus** *see* claw-foot. **p. planus** *see* flatfoot.

pessary (**pess**-er-i) *n.* **1.** a plastic device, often ring-shaped, that fits into the vagina and keeps the uterus in position: used to treat prolapse. **2. (vaginal suppository)** a plug or cylinder of soft material containing a drug that is fitted into the vagina for the treatment of such disorders as vaginitis.

pesticide (**pest**-i-syd) *n.* a chemical agent, such as parathion, used to kill insects or other organisms harmful to crops and other cultivated plants.

PET *n. see* positron emission tomography.

petechiae (pi-**tee**-ki-ee) *pl. n.* small round flat dark-red spots caused by bleeding into the skin or beneath the mucous membrane.

pethidine (**peth**-i-deen) *n.* a potent opioid analgesic drug with mild sedative action, administered by mouth or injection to relieve moderate or severe pain of short duration (including that associated with childbirth and occurring after surgery).

petit mal (**pe**-tee mal) *n. see* epilepsy.

Petri dish (**pet**-ri) *n.* a flat shallow circular glass or plastic dish with a pillbox-like lid, used to hold solid agar or gelatin media for culturing bacteria. [J. R. Petri (1852–1921), German bacteriologist]

petrissage (pay-tri-**sahzh**) *n.* kneading: a form of massage in which the skin is lifted up, pressed down and squeezed, and pinched and rolled.

petrositis (pet-roh-**sy**-tis) *n.* inflammation of the petrous part of the temporal bone, usually due to an extension of mastoiditis.

petrous bone (**pet**-rŭs) *n. see* temporal (bone).

Peutz-Jeghers syndrome (puuts-**yeg**-erz) *n.* a hereditary disorder in which the presence of multiple polyps in the lining of the small intestine (intestinal polyposis) is associated with pigmented areas (similar to freckles) around the lips, on the inside of the mouth, and on the palms and soles. [J. L. A. Peutz (1886–1957), Dutch physician; H. J. Jeghers (1904–90), US physician]

PEWS *n. see* paediatric early warning score.

-pexy *combining form denoting* surgical fixation.

Peyer's patches (**py**-erz) *pl. n.* oval masses of lymphoid tissue on the mucous membrane lining the small intestine. [J. C. Peyer (1653–1712), Swiss anatomist]

Peyronie's disease (pay-roh-**neez**) *n.* a dense fibrous plaque in the penis. The penis curves or angulates at this point on erection and pain often results. [F. de la

Peyronie (1678–1747), French surgeon]

PGD *n.* **1.** *see* patient group direction. **2.** *see* preimplantation genetic diagnosis.

pH *n.* a measure of the concentration of hydrogen ions in a solution, and therefore of its acidity or alkalinity. A pH of 7 indicates a neutral solution, a pH below 7 indicates acidity, and a pH in excess of 7 indicates alkalinity.

phaco- (phako-) *combining form denoting* the lens of the eye.

phacoemulsification (phakoemulsification) (fakŏ-i-mul-si-fi-**kay**-shŏn) *n.* a widely used method of cataract extraction in which a high-frequency ultrasound probe is used to break up a cataract so that it can be removed through a very small incision.

phaeochromocytoma (fi-oh-kroh-moh-sy-**toh**-mă) *n.* a small vascular tumour of the medulla of the adrenal gland. Many of these tumours function by their uncontrolled and irregular secretion of the hormones adrenaline and noradrenaline. They cause attacks of raised blood pressure, increased heart rate, palpitations, and headache.

phag- (phago-) *combining form denoting* **1.** eating. **2.** phagocytes.

phage (fayj) *n. see* bacteriophage.

-phagia *combining form denoting* a condition involving eating.

phagocyte (fag-ŏ-syt) *n.* a cell that is able to engulf and digest bacteria, protozoa, cells and cell debris, and other small particles. Phagocytes include many white blood cells and macrophages, which play a major role in the body's defence mechanism. **—phagocytic** *adj.*

phagocytosis (fag-ŏ-sy-**toh**-sis) *n.* the engulfment and digestion of bacteria and other foreign particles by a phagocyte. *Compare* pinocytosis.

phakic (**fay**-kik) *adj.* denoting an eye with the natural crystalline lens still in place, as contrasted with aphakic (*see* aphakia).

phako- *combining form. see* phaco-.

phalanges (fă-**lan**-jeez) *n.* (*sing.* **phalanx**) the bones of the fingers and toes (digits). The first digit (thumb/big toe) has two phalanges. Each of the remaining digits has three phalanges. **—phalangeal** *adj.*

phalangitis (fal-ăn-**jy**-tis) *n.* inflammation of a finger or toe, caused by infection of the soft tissues, bone, or joints or by rheumatic diseases. *See also* dactylitis.

phalanx (**fal**-anks) *n. see* phalanges.

phalloplasty (**fal**-oh-plasti) *n.* surgical reconstruction or repair of the penis, performed to correct a congenital deformity or following injury to the penis.

phallus (**fal**-ŭs) *n.* the embryonic penis, before the urethral duct has reached its final state of development.

phantom limb (**fan**-tŏm) *n.* the sensation that an arm or leg, or part of an arm or leg, is still attached to the body after it has been amputated. Pain or other sensations may seem to come from the amputated part.

phantom pregnancy *n.* *see* pseudocyesis.

phantom tumour *n.* **1.** an accumulation of fluid in the lung (pleural effusion) in patients with heart failure, which resembles a tumour on radiological examination. **2.** a swelling, in the abdomen or elsewhere, caused by local muscular contraction or the accumulation of gases, that mimics a swelling caused by a tumour.

pharmaceutical (farm-ă-**sewt**-ikăl) *adj.* relating to pharmacy.

pharmacist (**farm**-ă-sist) *n.* a person who is qualified by examination and registered and authorized to dispense medicines.

pharmaco- *combining form denoting* drugs.

pharmacodynamics (farm-ă-koh-dy-**nam**-iks) *n.* the interaction of drugs with cells. It includes such factors as the binding of drugs to cells, their uptake, and intracellular metabolism.

pharmacokinetics (farm-ă-koh-ki-**net**-iks) *n.* the study of how drugs are handled within the body, including their absorption, distribution, metabolism, and excretion.

pharmacology (farm-ă-**kol**-ŏji) *n.* the science of the properties of drugs and their effects on the body. **—pharmacological** *adj.* **—pharmacologist** *n.*

pharmacopoeia (farm-ă-kŏ-**pee**-ă) *n.* a book containing a list of the drugs used in medicine, with details of their formulae, methods of preparation, dosages, standards of purity, etc.

pharmacy (**farm**-ăsi) *n.* **1.** the preparation and dispensing of drugs. **2.** premises registered to dispense medicines and sell poisons.

pharyng- (pharyngo-) *combining form denoting* the pharynx.

pharyngeal (fa-rin-**jee**-ăl) *adj.* of or relating to the pharynx. **p. pouch** (**branchial pouch**, **visceral pouch**) any of the paired segmented pouches in the side of the throat of the early embryo. They give rise to the tympanic cavity, the parathyroid glands, the thymus, and probably the thyroid gland. **p. reflex** *see* gag reflex.

pharyngectomy (fa-rin-**jek**-tŏmi) *n.* surgical removal of part of the pharynx.

pharyngitis (fa-rin-**jy**-tis) *n.* inflammation of the pharynx. It produces sore throat and may be associated with tonsillitis.

pharyngocele (fă-**ring**-oh-seel) *n.* a pouch or cyst opening off the pharynx (*see* branchial cyst).

pharyngolaryngeal (fă-ring-oh-la-rin-**jee**-ăl) *adj.* relating to both the pharynx and the larynx.

pharyngoscope (fă-**ring**-ŏ-skohp) *n.* an endoscope for the examination of the pharynx.

pharyngotympanic tube (fă-ring-oh-tim-**pan**-ik) *n.* *see* Eustachian tube.

pharynx (**fa**-rinks) *n.* a muscular tube, lined with mucous membrane, that extends from the beginning of the oesophagus (gullet) up to the base of the skull. It communicates with the posterior nares, Eustachian tube, mouth, larynx, and oesophagus. The pharynx acts as a passageway for food, as an air passage from the nasal cavity and mouth to the larynx, and as a resonating chamber for the sounds produced in the larynx. *See* hypopharynx, nasopharynx, oropharynx.

PHC *n.* primary health care. *See* primary care.

PHE *see* Public Health England.

phenelzine (fen-ĕl-zeen) *n. see* MAO inhibitor.

phenindione (fen-**in**-di-ohn) *n.* an anticoagulant drug administered by mouth to prevent or treat thrombosis in the blood vessels of the heart, lungs, or limbs. The main side-effect is bleeding (*see* warfarin).

pheniodol (fin-**I**-ŏ-dol) *n.* an iodine-containing compound that is used as a contrast medium during X-ray examination of the gall bladder (*see* cholecystography).

phenobarbital (phenobarbitone) (fee-noh-**bar**-bit-al) *n.* a barbiturate drug administered by mouth or injection as an anticonvulsant in the treatment of epilepsy and status epilepticus. It is no longer commonly prescribed.

phenol (carbolic acid) (fee-nol) *n.* a strong disinfectant, derivatives of which (**phenolics**) may be used for disinfecting the skin before surgery. **oily p.** an irritant substance administered by injection for sclerotherapy of haemorrhoids.

phenomenology (fin-om-in-**ol**-ŏji) *n.* the study of occurrences forming part of human experiences. Concerned with describing the facts of the immediate situation, rather than speculating about causes, it helps nurses and patients to understand the phenomena in question and may lead to an improved understanding of oneself and others.

phenothiazines (fee-noh-**th'**y-ă-zeenz) *pl. n.* a group of chemically related compounds with various pharmacological actions. Some (e.g. chlorpromazine) are antipsychotic drugs that are also anthelmintics.

phenotype (**fee**-noh-typ) *n.* the observable characteristics of an individual, which result from interaction between his genotype and the environment.

phenoxybenzamine (fin-oks-i-**ben**-ză-meen) *n.* a drug that dilates blood vessels (*see* alpha blocker). It is administered by mouth or intravenous infusion to reduce high blood pressure in patients with phaeochromocytoma.

phenoxymethylpenicillin (fin-oks-i-meth-il-pen-i-**sil**-in) *n. see* penicillin.

phentolamine (fen-**tol**-ă-meen) *n.* a drug that dilates blood vessels (*see* alpha blocker) and is administered by intravenous injection to reduce high blood pressure in patients with phaeochromocytoma.

phenylalanine (fee-nyl-**al**-ă-neen) *n.* an essential amino acid that is readily converted to tyrosine. Blockade of this metabolic pathway gives rise to phenylketonuria.

phenylephrine (fee-nyl-**ef**-reen) *n.* a drug that constricts blood vessels (*see* sympathomimetic) and may be given by injection or intravenous infusion to increase blood pressure in the emergency treatment of hypotension. It is also administered in eye drops to dilate the pupil for diagnosis or treatment. Trade name: **Minims Phenylephrine Hydrochloride**.

phenylketonuria (PKU) (fee-nyl-kee-tŏn-**yoor**-iă) *n.* an inherited defect of protein metabolism (*see* inborn error of metabolism) causing an excess of the amino acid phenylalanine in the blood, which damages the nervous system and leads to severe learning disability. The gene responsible for phenylketonuria is recessive, so that a child is affected only if both parents are carriers of the defective gene.

phenytoin (fen-i-**toh**-in) *n.* an anticonvulsant drug administered by mouth or intravenous injection or infusion to control tonic-clonic and partial epileptic seizures and status epilepticus. Trade name: **Epanutin**.

phial (**fy**-ăl) *n.* a small glass bottle for storing medicines or poisons.

Philadelphia chromosome (fil-ă-**del**-fiă) *n.* an abnormal chromosome (number 22), most commonly found in the marrow cells of patients with chronic myeloid leukaemia.

-philia *combining form denoting* morbid craving or attraction.

phimosis (fy-**moh**-sis) *n.* narrowing of the opening of the foreskin, which cannot therefore be drawn back over the underlying glans penis.

phleb- (phlebo-) *combining form denoting* a vein or veins.

phlebectomy (fli-**bek**-tŏmi) *n.* the surgical removal of a vein (or part of a vein), sometimes performed for the treatment of varicose veins in the legs (**varicectomy**).

phlebitis (fli-**by**-tis) *n.* inflammation of the wall of a vein, which is most commonly seen in the legs as a complication of varicose veins. A segment of vein becomes painful and tender and the surrounding skin feels hot and appears red. Thrombosis commonly develops (*see* thrombophlebitis). Treatment consists of elastic support and administration of drugs, such as NSAIDs.

phlebography (fli-**bog**-răfi) *n. see* venography.

phlebolith (**flee**-boh-lith) *n.* a stone-like structure that results from deposition of calcium in a venous blood clot.

phlebothrombosis (flee-boh-throm-**boh**-sis) *n.* obstruction of a vein by a blood clot, without preceding inflammation of its wall. It is most common within the deep veins of the calf of the leg (**deep vein thrombosis**, **DVT**). The affected leg may become swollen and tender and the clot may become detached and give rise to pulmonary embolism. Prolonged immobility, heart failure, pregnancy, injury, and surgery predispose to thrombosis by encouraging sluggish blood flow. Anticoagulant drugs (such as heparin and warfarin) are used in prevention and treatment.

phlebotomist (fli-**bot**-ŏ-mist) *n.* a specialized clinical support worker or assistant health-care scientist who collects blood from patients for examination in laboratories for diagnostic purposes.

phlebotomy (venesection) (fli-**bot**-ŏmi) *n.* the surgical opening or puncture of a vein in order to remove blood (usually for diagnostic purposes but also in the treatment of polycythaemia vera) or to infuse fluids, blood, or drugs in the treatment of many conditions. *See also* phlebotomist.

phlegm (flem) *n.* a nonmedical term for sputum.

phlycten (**flik**-tĕn) *n.* a small pinkish-yellow nodule surrounded by a zone of dilated blood vessels that occurs in the conjunctiva or in the cornea. Phlyctens are thought to be due to a type of allergy to certain bacteria.

phobia (**foh**-biă) *n.* a pathologically strong fear of a particular event or thing. Avoiding the feared situation may severely restrict one's life and cause much suffering. Treatment is with cognitive behavioural therapy, desensitization, graded self-exposure, or flooding. Antidepressants are also useful.

SEE WEB LINKS

- Information on phobias from Mind

-phobia *combining form denoting* morbid fear or dread.

phocomelia (foh-koh-**mee**-liă) *n.* congenital absence of the upper arm and/or upper leg, the hands or feet or both being attached to the trunk by a short stump.

pholcodine (**fol**-kŏ-deen) *n.* a drug that suppresses coughs and reduces irritation in the respiratory system (*see* antitussive). It is administered as a linctus for the relief of dry or painful coughs. Trade names: **Galenphol**, **Pavacol D**.

phon- (phono-) *combining form denoting* sound or voice.

phonation (foh-**nay**-shŏn) *n.* the production of vocal sounds, particularly speech.

phoniatrics (foh-ni-**at**-riks) *n.* the study of the voice and its disorders.

phonocardiogram (foh-noh-**kar**-di-ŏ-gram) *n.* *see* electrocardiophonography. **—phonocardiography** (foh-noh-kar-di-**og**-răfi) *n.*

phonophobia (foh-noh-**foh**-biă) *n.* excessive sensitivity to and fear of certain specific sounds, irrespective of the level of the sound. *See* hyperacusis, misophonia.

phonosurgery (foh-noh-**serj**-er-i) *n.* surgery performed on the larynx externally or endoscopically to improve or modify the quality of the voice.

-phoria *combining form denoting* (in ophthalmology) an abnormal deviation of the eyes or turning of the visual axis.

phosgene (**fos**-jeen) *n.* a poisonous gas developed during World War I. It is a choking agent, acting on the lungs to produce oedema, with consequent respiratory and cardiac failure.

phosphagen (**fos**-fă-jĕn) *n.* creatine phosphate (*see* creatine).

phosphataemia (fos-fă-**tee**-miă) *n.* the presence of phosphates in the blood. Sodium, calcium, potassium, and magnesium phosphates are normal constituents.

phosphatase (**fos**-fă-tayz) *n.* one of a group of enzymes capable of catalysing the hydrolysis of phosphoric acid esters. Phosphatases are important in the absorption and metabolism of carbohydrates, nucleotides, and phospholipids and are essential in the calcification of bone. **acid p.** a phosphatase present in kidney, semen, serum, and the prostate gland. **alkaline p.** a phosphatase that occurs in teeth, developing bone, plasma, kidney, and intestine.

phosphate (**fos**-fayt) *n.* any salt or ester of phosphoric acid.

phosphatidylcholine (fos-fat-i-dil-**koh**-leen) *n. see* lecithin.

phosphaturia (phosphuria) (fos-făt-**yoor**-iă) *n.* the presence of an abnormally high concentration of phosphates in the urine, making it cloudy. The condition may be associated with the formation of calculi in the kidneys or bladder.

phosphocreatine (fos-foh-**kree**-ă-teen) *n.* creatine phosphate (*see* creatine).

phospholipid (fos-foh-**lip**-id) *n.* a lipid containing a phosphate group as part of the molecule. Phospholipids are constituents of all tissues and organs, especially the brain. They are involved in many of the body's metabolic processes. Examples are cephalins, lecithins, and plasmalogens.

phosphonecrosis (fos-foh-nek-**roh**-sis) *n.* the destruction of tissues caused by excessive amounts of phosphorus in the system. The tissues likely to suffer are the liver, kidneys, muscles, bones, and the cardiovascular system.

phosphorus (**fos**-fer-us) *n.* a nonmetallic element that is toxic in its pure state. Phosphorus compounds are major constituents in the tissues of both plants and animals. In humans, phosphorus is mostly concentrated in bone. Symbol: P.

phot- (photo-) *combining form denoting* light.

photalgia (foh-**tal**-jiă) *n.* pain in the eye caused by very bright light.

photoablation (foh-toh-ăb-**lay**-shŏn) *n.* the use of light or lasers to destroy tissue.

photochemotherapy (foh-toh-kee-moh-**th'e**-ră-pi) *n. see* photodynamic therapy, PUVA.

photocoagulation (foh-toh-koh-ag-yoo-**lay**-shŏn) *n.* **1.** the destruction of tissue by heat released from the absorption of light shone on it. In eye disorders the technique is used to destroy diseased retinal tissue and to produce scarring between the retina and choroid, thus binding them together, in cases of retinal detachment. **2.** a method of arresting bleeding by causing coagulation, usually using an infrared light source.

photodermatosis (foh-toh-der-mă-**toh**-sis) *n.* any of various diseases caused by exposure to light of varying wavelength (*see* photosensitivity). The face and neck are most commonly affected. A common photodermatosis is **polymorphous light eruption**, which appears with the first sunshine of spring and abates by late summer. The photodermatoses include certain porphyrias.

photodynamic therapy (PDT, photoradiation therapy, phototherapy, photochemotherapy) (foh-toh-dy-**nam**-ik **th'**e-ră-pi) *n.* a treatment for some types of superficial cancers and for wet age-related macular degeneration. A light-sensitive agent is injected into the bloodstream, passes to the cancer cells or affected retinal blood vessels, and is activated by laser radiation, which destroys the cancer cells or seals the abnormal blood vessels.

photomicrograph (foh-toh-**my**-krŏ-grahf) *n.* *see* micrograph.

photophobia (foh-toh-**foh**-biă) *n.* discomfort caused by exposure to light. Photophobia may be associated with migraine, measles, German measles, meningitis, iritis, or corneal injury.

photophthalmia (foh-tof-**thal**-miă) *n.* inflammation of the eye due to exposure to light. It is usually caused by the damaging effect of ultraviolet light on the cornea, for example when lying under a sunbed or in snow blindness.

photoradiation (foh-toh-ray-di-**ay**-shŏn) *n.* *see* photodynamic therapy.

photorefractive keratectomy (PRK) (foh-toh-ri-**frak**-tiv) *n.* *see* keratectomy.

photoretinitis (foh-toh-ret-in-**I**-tis) *n.* damage to the retina of the eye caused by looking at the sun without adequate protection for the eyes. The central part of the visual field may be permanently lost (**sun blindness**).

photosensitivity (foh-toh-sen-si-**tiv**-iti) *n.* abnormal reaction of the skin to sunlight, which characterizes certain skin diseases (*see* photodermatosis). Drugs, such as thiazide diuretics and NSAIDs, can also cause photosensitivity. **—photosensitive** *adj.*

phototherapeutic keratectomy (foh-toh-th'e-ră-**pew**-tik) *n.* *see* keratectomy.

phototherapy (foh-toh-**th'**e-ră-pi) *n.* **1.** treatment that involves exposure to ultraviolet or infrared radiation. For example, UVB (*see* ultraviolet radiation) is used for treating severe psoriasis. **2.** *see* photodynamic therapy.

phototoxicity (foh-toh-toks-**iss**-iti) *n.* damage caused by prolonged exposure to light. **retinal p.** damage to the retina of the eye as a result of prolonged exposure to light.

photuria (foht-**yoor**-iă) *n.* the excretion of phosphorescent urine, due to the presence of certain compounds containing phosphorus.

PHQ-9 (Patient Health Questionnaire) *n.* a screening tool designed to identify people who may suffer from depression. Its nine questions are based on DSM diagnostic criteria. Each item is scored by the patient from 0 (not at all) to 3 (nearly every day). A PHQ-9 score of $\geq$10 indicates a reasonably high likelihood of major depression. It has been validated for use in primary care, in which it is commonly used not only for screening but also for monitoring the progress of treatment.

phren- (phreno-) *combining form denoting* **1.** the mind or brain.

2. the diaphragm. **3.** the phrenic nerve.

-phrenia *combining form denoting* a condition of the mind.

phrenic (**fren**-ik) *adj.* **1.** relating to the mind. **2.** relating to the diaphragm. **p. crush 1.** damage to the phrenic nerve as a result of trauma. **2.** surgical crushing of a portion of the phrenic nerve, paralysing part of the diaphragm, which is then pushed upwards and presses on the lung, partially collapsing it: formerly used in the treatment of tuberculosis. **p. nerve** the nerve that supplies the muscles of the diaphragm. On each side it arises in the neck and passes downwards between the lungs and the heart.

Phthirus (**thi**-rŭs) *n.* a widely distributed genus of lice. **P. pubis** the crab (or pubic) louse, a common parasite of humans that lives permanently attached to the body hair, particularly that of the pubic or perianal regions. *See also* pediculosis.

phthisis (**th'y**-sis) *n.* **1.** any disease resulting in wasting of tissues. **p. bulbi** a shrunken eyeball that has lost its function due to disease or damage. **2.** a former name for pulmonary tuberculosis.

phycomycosis (fy-koh-my-**koh**-sis) *n.* a disease caused by parasitic fungi of the genera *Rhizopus*, *Absidia*, and *Mucor*. The fungi grow within the blood vessels of the lungs and nervous tissue, causing blood clots that cut off the blood supply (*see* infarction). Treatment with the antibiotic amphotericin B has proved effective.

physi- (physio-) *combining form denoting* **1.** physiology. **2.** physical.

physical (**fiz**-ikăl) *adj.* (in medicine) relating to the body rather than to the mind. **p. sign** a sign that a doctor can detect when examining a patient, such as abnormal dilation of the pupils or the absence of a knee-jerk reflex.

physical medicine *n.* the medical specialty concerned with the diagnosis and management of rheumatic diseases and the rehabilitation of patients with physical disabilities. *See also* rheumatology.

physician (fiz-**ish**-ăn) *n.* a registered medical practitioner who specializes in the diagnosis and treatment of disease by other than surgical means.

physiological saline (fiz-i-ŏ-**loj**-ikăl) *n.* *see* saline.

physiological solution *n.* one of a group of solutions, including Ringer's solution, used to maintain tissues in a viable state. These solutions contain specific concentrations of substances that are vital for normal tissue function.

physiology (fiz-i-**ol**-ŏji) *n.* the science of the functioning of living organisms and of their component parts. **—physiological** *adj.* **—physiologist** *n.*

physiotherapy (fiz-i-oh-**th'e**-ră-pi) *n.* the branch of treatment that employs physical methods to promote healing, including the use of light, heat, electric current, ultrasound, massage, manipulation, hydrotherapy, and remedial exercise.

physo- *combining form denoting* air or gas.

phyt- (phyto-) *combining form denoting* plants; of plant origin.

phytomenadione (fy-toh-men-ă-**dy**-ohn) *n.* a form of vitamin K that is administered by mouth or injection as an antidote to overdosage with anticoagulant drugs and to prevent haemorrhagic disease of the newborn. It promotes the production of prothrombin, essential for the normal coagulation of blood. Trade name: **Konakion**.

phytotherapy (fy-toh-**th'e**-ră-pi) *n.* medical treatment based exclusively on plant extracts and products. Plants have provided a wide range of important drugs, but any drugs derived directly from plants should be extracted, purified, assayed, and tested before being used as medication.

pia (pia mater) (pee-ă) *n.* the innermost of the three meninges surrounding the brain and spinal cord. It contains numerous finely branching blood vessels that supply the nerve tissue within.

pian (pi-**ahn**) *n. see* yaws.

PICC line (pik) *n. p*eripherally *i*nserted *c*entral *c*atheter: a long flexible catheter usually inserted via a vein in the arm and the subclavian artery into the superior vena cava. It is used when prolonged intravenous access is required, for example, for infusional chemotherapy.

Pick's disease (piks) *n. see* frontotemporal dementia. [A. Pick (1851–1924), Czech psychiatrist]

picornavirus (pi-kor-nă-vy-rŭs) *n.* one of a group of small RNA-containing viruses. The group includes Coxsackie viruses, polioviruses, and rhinoviruses.

picric acid (trinitrophenol) (**pik**-rik) *n.* a yellow crystalline solid used as a dye and as a tissue fixative.

PICU *n.* **1.** paediatric intensive care unit: *see* intensive care. **2.** *see* psychiatric intensive care unit.

PID *n.* **1.** *see* pelvic inflammatory disease. **2.** *see* prolapsed intervertebral disc.

Pierre Robin syndrome (p'yair roh-**ban**) *n.* a congenital disease in which affected infants have a very small lower jawbone (mandible) and a cleft palate. They are susceptible to feeding and respiratory problems. [Pierre Robin (1867–1950), French dentist]

piezoelectric (peets-oh-i-**lek**-trik) *adj.* denoting or relating to an electrically generated pulse or polarity that is caused by pressure.

pigeon chest (pij-ŏn) *n.* forward protrusion of the breastbone resulting in deformity of the chest. The condition is painless and harmless. Medical name: **pectus carinatum**.

pigeon toe *n.* **(in-toe gait)** an abnormal posture in which the toes are turned inwards. It is often associated with knock-knee.

pigment (**pig**-mĕnt) *n.* a substance giving colour. Physiologically important pigments include the blood pigments (especially haemoglobin), the bile pigments, and retinal pigment (*see* rhodopsin).

pigmentation (pig-mĕn-**tay**-shŏn) *n.* coloration produced in the body by the deposition of one pigment, especially in excessive amounts. Pigmentation may be produced by natural pigments, such as melanin, or by foreign material, such as lead or arsenic in chronic poisoning.

PIH *n. see* pregnancy-induced hypertension.

piles (pylz) *pl. n. see* haemorrhoids.

pill (pil) *n.* **1.** a small ball of variable size, shape, and colour, sometimes coated with sugar, that contains one or more medicinal substances in solid form. It is taken by mouth. **2. the Pill** *see* oral contraceptive.

pillar (**pil**-er) *n.* (in anatomy) an elongated apparently supportive structure.

pilo- *combining form denoting* hair.

pilocarpine (py-loh-**kar**-peen) *n.* a parasympathomimetic drug used in the form of eye drops or gel to reduce the pressure inside the eye in angle-closure glaucoma and administered orally to treat dry mouth and dry eyes. Trade names: **Minims Pilocarpine Nitrate**, **Salagen**.

pilomotor nerves (py-loh-**moh**-ter) *pl. n.* sympathetic nerves that supply muscle fibres in the skin, around the roots of hairs. Activity of the sympathetic nervous system causes the muscles to contract, resulting in goose flesh.

pilonidal sinus (py-loh-**ny**-d'l) *n.* a short tract leading from an opening in the skin in the cleft at the top of the buttocks and containing hairs. The sinus may be recurrently infected, leading to pain and the discharge of pus.

pilosebaceous (py-loh-si-**bay**-shŭs) *adj.* relating to the hair follicles and their associated sebaceous glands.

pilosis (py-**loh**-sis) *n.* the abnormal growth of hair.

pilus (**py**-lŭs) *n.* a hair.

pimel- (pimelo-) *combining form denoting* fat; fatty.

pimozide (**pim**-oh-zyd) *n.* an antipsychotic drug administered by mouth to treat schizophrenia and some delusional disorders. Trade name: **Orap**.

pimple (**pim**-pŭl) *n.* a small inflamed swelling on the skin that contains pus. It may be the result of bacterial infection of a skin pore that has become obstructed with fatty secretions from the sebaceous glands. *See also* acne.

PIN *n. see* prostatic intraepithelial neoplasia.

Pinard's stethoscope (pee-narz) *n.* a stethoscope shaped like a listening trumpet, which is placed at a right angle over the fetus's back to hear the fetal heartbeat. [A. Pinard (1844–1934), French obstetrician]

pineal gland (pineal body) (**pin**-i-ăl) *n.* a pea-sized mass of nerve tissue attached by a stalk to the posterior wall of the third ventricle of the brain. This gland secretes the hormone melatonin. Anatomical name: **epiphysis**.

pinguecula (ping-**wek**-yoo-lă) *n.* a degenerative change in the conjunctiva of the eye, seen most commonly in the elderly. Thickened yellow triangles develop on the conjunctiva at the inner and outer margins of the cornea.

pink disease *n.* a severe illness of children of the teething age, marked by pink cold clammy hands and feet, heavy sweating, raised blood pressure, rapid pulse, and photophobia. Affected infants are very prone to secondary infection, which may be fatal. The condition may be an allergic reaction to mercury; it has virtually disappeared since all mercury-containing paediatric preparations have been banned. Medical names: **acrodynia**, **erythroedema**, **erythromelalgia**.

pink eye *n. see* conjunctivitis.

pinna (auricle) (**pin**-ă) *n.* the flap of skin and cartilage that projects from the head at the exterior opening of the external auditory meatus of the ear.

pinnaplasty (**pin**-ă-plasti) *n. see* otoplasty.

pinocytosis (pee-noh-sy-**toh**-sis) *n.* the intake of small droplets of fluid by a cell by cytoplasmic engulfment. *Compare* phagocytosis.

pins and needles (pinz) *pl. n. see* paraesthesia.

pinta (**pin**-tă) *n.* a skin disease, prevalent in tropical America, that is caused by the spirochaete *Treponema carateum*. Symptoms include thickening and eventual loss of pigment of the skin, particularly on the hands, wrists, feet, and ankles.

pinworm (**pin**-werm) *n. see* threadworm.

piriform fossae (**pi**-ri-form) *pl. n.* two pear-shaped depressions that lie on either side of the opening to the larynx.

piroxicam (py-**roks**-i-kam) *n.* a nonsteroidal anti-inflammatory drug (*see* NSAID) administered by mouth or topically to relieve pain and stiffness in osteoarthritis, rheumatoid arthritis, and ankylosing spondylitis. Trade name: **Feldene**.

PIs *pl. n. see* performance indicators.

pisiform bone (**py**-si-form) *n.* the smallest bone of the wrist (*see* carpus): a pea-shaped bone that articulates with the triquetral bone and, indirectly by cartilage, with the ulna.

pit (pit) *n.* (in anatomy) a hollow or depression.

pitting (**pit**-ing) *n.* the formation of depressed scars, as occurs on the skin following acne. **p. oedema** oedema in which fingertip pressure leaves temporary indentations in the skin.

pituitary apoplexy (pit-yoo-it-eri) *n.* acute intrapituitary haemorrhage, usually into an existing tumour, presenting as severe headache and collapse. It is a medical emergency.

pituitary gland (hypophysis) *n.* the master endocrine gland: a pea-sized body attached to the hypothalamus at the base of the skull. The anterior lobe of the gland (**adenohypophysis**) secretes thyroid-stimulating hormone, ACTH, gonadotrophins (LH and FSH), growth hormone, prolactin, lipotrophin, and melanocyte-stimulating hormone. The posterior lobe (**neurohypophysis**) secretes vasopressin and oxytocin.

pityriasis (pit-i-**ry**-ă-sis) *n.* (originally) any of a group of skin diseases typified by the development of fine branlike scales. **p. alba** a common condition in children in which pale scaly patches occur on the face. **p. capitis** *see* dandruff. **p. rosea** a common skin rash, believed to be viral in origin, that typically starts with a single patch on the trunk and is followed by an eruption of oval pink scaly macules. The rash clears completely in about eight weeks. **p. versicolor** a common chronic infection of the skin caused by the yeast *Malassezia furfur*, which produces a persistent pale or brown scaly rash on the trunk.

Pityrosporum (pit-i-**ros**-pŏ-rŭm) *n. see* Malassezia.

pivmecillinam (piv-mes-**il**-in-am) *n.* a penicillin-type antibiotic used mainly to treat urinary-tract infections caused by Gram-negative bacteria. It is administered by mouth. Trade name: **Selexid**.

pivot joint (**piv**-ŏt) *n. see* trochoid joint.

pixel (**piks**-ĕl) *n.* short for 'picture element'; the smallest individual component of an electronically produced image. *See* digital (image).

pizotifen (piz-**ot**-i-fen) *n.* an antihistamine drug used to prevent severe migraine and cluster headaches. Administered by mouth, it acts by inhibiting the effects of serotonin. Trade name: **Sanomigran**.

PKU *n. see* phenylketonuria.

placebo (plă-**see**-boh) *n.* a medicine that is ineffective but may help to relieve a condition because the patient has faith in its powers. New drugs are tested against placebos in clinical trials.

placenta (plă-**sent**-ă) *n.* an organ within the uterus by means of which the embryo is attached to the wall of the uterus. Its primary function is to provide the embryo with nourishment, eliminate its wastes, and exchange respiratory gases. It also functions as a gland, secreting chorionic gonadotrophin, progesterone, and oestrogens. *See also* afterbirth. **p. praevia** a condition in which the placenta is situated wholly or partially in the lower and noncontractile part of the uterus. When this becomes elongated and stretched during the last few weeks of pregnancy, and the cervix becomes stretched either before or during labour, placental separation and haemorrhage will occur. If the placenta is situated entirely before the presenting part of the fetus, delivery must be by Caesarean section. **—placental** (plă-**sen**-t'l) *adj.*

placental abruption *n. see* abruptio placentae.

placentography (sonoplacentography) (plas-en-**tog**-răfi) *n.* imaging of the pregnant uterus by ultrasound scanning in order to determine the position of the placenta.

plagiocephaly (play-ji-oh-**sef**-ăli) *n.* any distortion or lack of symmetry in the shape of the head, usually due to irregularity in the closure of the sutures between the bones of the skull.

plague (playg) *n.* **1.** any epidemic disease with a high death rate. **2.** an acute epidemic disease of rats and other wild rodents caused by the bacterium *Yersinia pestis*, which is transmitted to humans by rat fleas. **bubonic p.** the most common form of the disease, characterized by acute painful swellings of the lymph nodes (*see* bubo). In favourable cases the buboes burst and then heal; in other cases bleeding under the skin can lead to ulcers, which may prove fatal. **pneumonic p.** a serious form of plague in which the lungs are affected. **septicaemic p.** a serious form of plague in which bacteria enter the bloodstream.

plane (playn) *n.* a level or smooth surface, especially any of the imaginary flat surfaces used to divide the body (*see* coronal, sagittal).

planning (plan-ing) *n.* the stage of the nursing process in which an individual **care plan** is produced, stating the patient's problem(s), the objective, the goal or expected outcome, the nursing intervention, and the time or date by which the objective is expected to be achieved or by which the problem should be reviewed.

plantar (plan-ter) *adj.* relating to the sole of the foot (**planta**). **p. arch** the arch in the sole of the foot formed by anastomosing branches of the plantar arteries. **p. fasciitis** (**policeman's heel**) inflammation of the point of attachment of the fascia in the sole of the foot to the calcaneus, causing pain and tenderness of the heel. **p. reflex** a reflex obtained by drawing a bluntly pointed object along the outer border of the sole of the foot. The normal (flexor) response is a bunching and downward movement of the toes. *Compare* Babinski reflex. **p. wart** *see* wart.

plaque (plak) *n.* **1.** a layer composed of bacteria in an organic matrix that forms on the surface of a tooth, principally at its neck. It may cause caries or periodontal disease. **2.** a raised patch on the skin formed by enlarging or coalescing papules. **3.** a deposit, consisting of a fatty core covered with a fibrous cap, that develops on the inner wall of an atheromatous artery. **4.** any flattened patch or localized area of abnormality on a body surface.

-plasia *combining form denoting* formation; development.

plasm- (plasmo-) *combining form denoting* **1.** blood plasma. **2.** protoplasm or cytoplasm.

plasma (blood plasma) (plaz-mă) *n.* the straw-coloured fluid in which the blood cells are suspended. It consists of a solution of various inorganic salts of sodium, potassium, calcium, etc., with a high concentration of protein and a variety of trace substances.

plasma cells *pl. n.* antibody-producing cells found in bone-forming tissue and also in the epithelium of the lungs and gut. They develop in the bone marrow, lymph nodes, and spleen when antigens stimulate B lymphocytes to produce the precursor cells that give rise to them.

plasmacytoma (plaz-mă-sy-**toh**-mă) *n.* a malignant tumour of plasma cells, usually occurring as a single tumour in bone marrow or more rarely soft tissue (**extramedullary p.**) and often known as a 'solitary myeloma'. However, it may be multiple, in which case it is classified as a multiple myeloma.

plasmapheresis (plaz-mă-fer-ee-sis) *n.* a method of removing a quantity of plasma from the blood. Blood is withdrawn through a vein of the patient, passed through a machine (cell separator) that removes the plasma, and then returned to the patient via another vein.

plasmin (fibrinolysin) (plaz-min) *n.* an enzyme that digests the protein fibrin. Its function is the dissolution of blood clots (*see* fibrinolysis).

plasminogen (plaz-**min**-ŏ-jĕn) *n.* a substance normally present in the blood plasma that may be activated to form plasmin. *See* fibrinolysis. **p. activator** any enzyme that converts plasminogen to plasmin, of which there are two types: tissue-type plasminogen activator and urokinase-like plasminogen activator.

Plasmodium (plaz-**moh**-diŭm) *n.* a genus of protozoans that live as parasites within the red blood cells and liver cells of humans. Four species cause malaria in humans: *P. vivax*, *P. ovale*, *P. falciparum*, and *P. malariae*.

plaster (**plah**-ster) *n.* adhesive tape used in shaped pieces or as a bandage to keep a dressing in place.

plaster of Paris (POP) *n.* a preparation of gypsum (calcium sulphate) that sets hard when water is added. It is used in dentistry and orthopaedics for preparing plaster casts.

plastic lymph (plast-ik) *n.* a transparent yellowish liquid produced in a wound or other site of inflammation, in which connective tissue cells and blood vessels develop during healing.

plastic surgery *n.* a branch of surgery dealing with the reconstruction of parts of the body deformed or damaged by burns, major accidents, or cancer. It also includes the correction of congenital defects, such as cleft lip, and the replacement of parts of the body that have been lost. **aesthetic p. s.** (**cosmetic surgery**) plastic surgery performed simply to improve appearance.

SEE WEB LINKS

- Website of the British Association of Aesthetic Plastic Surgeons

plastron (**plas**-tron) *n.* the breastbone (sternum) together with the costal cartilages attached to it.

-plasty *combining form denoting* plastic surgery.

platelet (thrombocyte) (playt-lit) *n.* a disc-shaped cell structure, 1–2 μm in diameter, present in the blood. Platelets have several functions, all relating to the arrest of bleeding (*see* blood coagulation). *See also* thrombopoiesis.

platy- *combining form denoting* broad or flat.

platyhelminth (plat-i-**hel**-minth) *n. see* flatworm.

platysma (plă-**tiz**-mă) *n.* a broad thin sheet of muscle that extends from below the collar bone to the angle of the jaw. It depresses the jaw.

play (play) *n.* any spontaneous or organized activity that provides enjoyment, entertainment, amusement, or diversion. Play in childhood is essential to enable holistic development.

pledget (**plej**-it) *n.* a small wad of dressing material, such as lint, used either to cover a wound or sore or as a plug. Mounted on an instrument, it is used during operations to wipe away blood and other fluids.

-plegia *combining form denoting* paralysis.

pleio- (pleo-) *combining form denoting* **1.** multiple. **2.** excessive.

pleocytosis (plee-oh-sy-**toh**-sis) *n.* the presence of an abnormally large number of lymphocytes in the cerebrospinal fluid.

pleomorphism (plee-oh-**mor**-fizm) *n.* **1.** marked variation in the shapes of individual cells and cell nuclei, which is a feature of malignant neoplastic cells. **2.** the condition in which an individual assumes a number of different forms during its life cycle. The malarial parasite (*Plasmodium*) displays pleomorphism.

pleoptics (plee-**op**-tiks) *n.* special techniques practised by orthoptists for developing normal function of the macula, in people whose macular function has previously been disturbed because of strabismus (squint).

plessor (plexor) (**ples**-er) *n.* a small hammer used to investigate nervous reflexes and in the technique of percussion.

plethora (**pleth**-er-ă) *n.* any excess of any bodily fluid, especially blood (*see* hyperaemia). **—plethoric** (pleth-**o**-rik) *adj.*

plethysmography (pleth-iz-**mog**-răfi) *n.* the process of recording the changes in the volume of a limb caused by alterations in blood pressure. The limb is inserted into a fluid-filled watertight casing (**oncometer**) and the pressure variations in the fluid are recorded.

pleur- (pleuro-) *combining form denoting* **1.** the pleura. **2.** the side of the body.

pleura (**ploor**-ă) *n.* the covering of the lungs (**visceral p.**) and of the inner surface of the chest wall (**parietal p.**), consisting of a closed sac of serous membrane. Fluid secreted by the membrane lubricates the opposing surfaces so that they can slide painlessly over each other during breathing. See illustration. **—pleural** *adj.*

pleural cavity (**ploor**-ăl) *n.* the space between the visceral and parietal pleura, which is normally very small as the pleural membranes are in close contact.

pleurectomy (ploor-**ek**-tŏmi) *n.* surgical removal of part of the

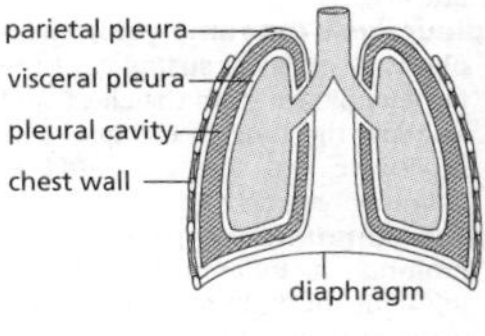

The pleura

pleura, which is sometimes done to prevent further recurrences of spontaneous pneumothorax or to remove diseased areas of pleura.

pleurisy (**ploor**-i-si) *n.* inflammation of the pleura, often due to pneumonia in the underlying lung. The pleural surfaces become slightly sticky, so that there is pain on deep breathing. Pleurisy is always associated with some other disease in the lung, chest wall, diaphragm, or abdomen.

pleurocele (**ploor**-oh-seel) *n.* herniation of the pleura.

pleurocentesis (thoracentesis, thoracocentesis) (ploor-oh-sen-**tee**-sis) *n.* the insertion of a hollow needle into the pleural cavity through the chest wall in order to withdraw fluid, blood, pus, or air.

pleurodesis (ploor-oh-**dee**-sis) *n.* a treatment for pneumothorax in which adhesions between the parietal and visceral pleura are induced by injecting a substance (e.g. silver nitrate) into the pleural cavity.

pleurodynia (ploor-oh-**din**-iă) *n.* severe paroxysmal pain arising from the muscles between the ribs. It is often thought to be of rheumatic origin.

pleurolysis (pneumolysis) (ploor-**ol**-i-sis) *n.* surgical stripping of the parietal pleura from the chest wall to allow the lung to collapse. The procedure was formerly used to help tuberculosis to heal.

pleuropneumonia (ploor-oh-new-**moh**-niă) *n.* inflammation involving both the lung and pleura. *See* pleurisy, pneumonia.

plexor (**pleks**-er) *n. see* plessor.

plexus (**pleks**-ŭs) *n.* a network of nerves or blood vessels. *See* brachial plexus.

plica (**plik**-ă) *n.* a fold of tissue. **—plicate** *adj.*

plication (pli-**kay**-shŏn) *n.* a surgical technique in which the size of a hollow organ or weakened and stretched tissue is reduced by taking tucks or folds in the walls.

ploidy (**ployd**-i) *n.* the condition of having multiple the normal number of chromosomes for the species. An increase in ploidy in the cells of a malignant tumour usually indicates greater aggressiveness and ability to invade.

plombage (plom-**bah*zh***) *n.* a surgical technique used to correct retinal detachment. A small piece of silicone plastic is sewn on the outside of the eyeball to produce an indentation over the retinal hole or tear to allow the retina to reattach.

plumbism (**plum**-bizm) *n.* lead poisoning. *See* lead.

Plummer's disease (**plum**-erz) *n.* a hyperfunctioning, usually benign, adenoma of the thyroid gland, which can be palpated and appears as a 'hot nodule' on radioactive thyroid scanning. [H. S. Plummer (1874–1937), US physician]

Plummer-Vinson syndrome (**vin**-sŏn) *n.* a disorder characterized by difficulty in swallowing associated with severe iron-deficiency anaemia. [H. S. Plummer and P. P. Vinson (1890–1959), US physicians]

pluri- *combining form denoting* more than one; several.

PMB *n. see* postmenopausal bleeding.

PMS *n. see* premenstrual syndrome.

pneo- *combining form denoting* breathing; respiration.

pneum- (pneumo-) *combining form denoting* **1.** the presence of air or gas. **2.** the lung(s). **3.** respiration.

pneumat- (pneumato-) *combining form denoting* **1.** the presence of air or gas. **2.** respiration.

pneumatocele (new-**mat**-oh-seel) *n.* herniation of lung tissue.

pneumatosis (new-mă-**toh**-sis) *n.* the occurrence of gas cysts in abnormal sites in the body. **p. cystoides intestinalis** the occurrence of multiple gas-containing cysts in the intestinal wall.

pneumaturia (new-măt-**yoor**-iă) *n.* the presence in the urine of bubbles of air or other gas, due to the formation of gas by bacteria infecting the urinary tract or to a fistula between the urinary tract and bowel.

pneumocephalus (pneumocele) (new-moh-**sef**-ă-lŭs) *n.* the presence of air within the skull, usually resulting from a fracture passing through one of the air sinuses.

pneumococcal vaccine *n.* a vaccine that protects against pneumococcal infections, including pneumonia, septicaemia, and meningitis. The pneumococcal vaccine is part of the childhood immunization programme. See Appendix 8: Immunization schedules.

pneumococcus (new-moh-**kok**-ŭs) *n.* (*pl.* **pneumococci**) the bacterium *Streptococcus pneumoniae*, which is associated with pneumonia, pneumococcal meningitis, and septicaemia and is a common bacterial cause of ear infections. —**pneumococcal** *adj.*

pneumoconiosis (new-moh-koh-ni-**oh**-sis) *n.* a group of lung diseases caused by inhaling dust. In practice industrial exposure to coal dust (*see* coal-worker's pneumoconiosis), silica (*see* silicosis), and asbestos (*see* asbestosis) produces most of the cases of pneumoconiosis.

Pneumocystis (new-moh-**sis**-tis) *n.* a genus of protozoans. **P. jiroveci** (formerly **carinii**) the cause of pneumonia in immunosuppressed patients, usually following intensive chemotherapy or in patients with AIDS. *See also* opportunistic.

pneumocyte (**new**-moh-syt) *n.* a type of cell that lines the walls separating the air sacs (*see* alveolus) in the lungs.

pneumoencephalography (new-moh-en-sef-ă-**log**-răfi) *n.* a technique used in the X-ray diagnosis of disease within the skull. Air is introduced into the ventricles of the brain to displace the cerebrospinal fluid, thus acting as a contrast medium. X-ray photographs show the size and disposition of the ventricles and the subarachnoid spaces. The technique has largely been superseded by CT and MRI scanning.

pneumogastric (new-moh-**gas**-trik) *adj.* relating to the lungs and stomach. **p. nerve** the vagus nerve.

pneumograph (**new**-moh-grahf) *n.* an instrument used to record the movements made during respiration.

pneumolysis (new-**mol**-i-sis) *n. see* pleurolysis.

pneumomycosis (new-moh-my-**koh**-sis) *n.* any infection of the lungs caused by fungi, such as aspergillosis.

pneumon- (pneumono-) *combining form denoting* the lung(s).

pneumonectomy (new-mŏ-**nek**-tŏmi) *n.* surgical removal of a lung, usually for cancer.

pneumonia (new-**moh**-niă) *n.* inflammation of the lung caused by bacteria, in which the alveoli become filled with inflammatory cells and the lung becomes solid (*see* consolidation). The symptoms include fever, malaise, cough, and chest pain, and there are shadows on the chest X-ray. Treatment with antibiotics is usually effective. **bronchopneumonia** pneumonia that starts in the small bronchi and spreads into the alveoli. **hypostatic p.** pneumonia that develops in dependant parts of the lung in people who are otherwise ill, chilled, or immobilized. **lobar p.** pneumonia that affects whole lobes of either or both lungs. *See also* atypical (pneumonia), viral pneumonia. *Compare* pneumonitis.

pneumonitis (new-mŏ-**ny**-tis) *n.* inflammation of the lung that is confined to the walls of the alveoli and often caused by viruses or unknown agents. It may be acute and transient or chronic, leading to increasing respiratory disability. It does not respond to antibiotics but corticosteroids may be helpful. *Compare* pneumonia.

pneumoperitoneum (new-moh-pe-ri-tŏn-**ee**-ŭm) *n.* air or gas in the peritoneal or abdominal cavity, usually due to a perforation of the stomach or bowel. It may be induced for diagnostic purposes (*see* laparoscopy).

pneumoretinopexy (new-moh-**ret**-in-oh-peks-i) *n.* a surgical technique in which an inert gas bubble is injected into the eye to press and seal breaks in the retina. When the retina is flat, a laser beam or cryoretinopexy is applied to cause scarring and permanently seal the tear.

pneumothorax (new-moh-**thor**-aks) *n.* air in the pleural cavity, which results from breach of the lung surface or chest wall and causes the lung to collapse. **artificial p.** the deliberate injection of air into the pleural cavity to collapse the lung: a former treatment for pulmonary tuberculosis. **spontaneous p.** pneumothorax that occurs without any apparent cause, in otherwise healthy people. **tension p.** pneumothorax in which a breach in the lung surface acts as a valve, admitting air into the pleural cavity when the patient breathes in but preventing its escape when breathing out. **traumatic p.** pneumothorax that results from injuries to the chest.

pneumotonometer (noncontact tonometer) (new-moh-toh-**nom**-it-er) *n.* an instrument that blows a puff of air at the cornea to cause flattening and hence measure intraocular pressure. It is commonly used by optometrists in tests for glaucoma.

-pnoea *combining form denoting* a condition of breathing.

POAG *n.* primary open-angle glaucoma. *See* glaucoma.

pock (pok) *n.* a small pus-filled eruption on the skin characteristic of chickenpox and smallpox rashes. *See also* pustule.

pocket resuscitation mask (**pok**-it) *n.* a compressible and easily carried mask, which can be expanded and fitted over the mouth and nose of a nonbreathing patient in order to perform mouth-to-mouth resuscitation through a small valve without contact between the mouth of the rescuer and that of the patient.

pod- *combining form denoting* the foot.

podagra (pŏ-**dag**-ră) *n.* gout of the foot, especially the big toe.

podalic version (internal podalic version) (pŏ-**dal**-ik) *n.* a procedure in which the position of a fetus in the uterus (usually a second twin that is presenting transversely or obliquely) is altered so that its feet will emerge first at birth. *See also* version.

podiatry (chiropody) (pŏ-**dy**-ă-tri) *n.* the study and care of the foot, including its normal structure, its diseases, and their treatment. The main role of a **podiatrist** (**chiropodist**) is to assess, diagnose, and treat abnormalities and diseases of the foot and to give advice on proper care of the foot and the prevention of foot problems.

SEE WEB LINKS

- Website of the Society of Chiropodists and Podiatrists

podopompholyx (poh-doh-**pom**-foh-liks) *n. see* pompholyx.

-poiesis *combining form denoting* formation; production.

poikilo- *combining form denoting* variation; irregularity.

poikilocyte (**poi**-kil-oh-syt) *n.* an abnormally shaped erythrocyte. *See also* poikilocytosis.

poikilocytosis (poi-kil-oh-sy-**toh**-sis) *n.* the presence of poikilocytes in the blood. Poikilocytosis is particularly marked in myelofibrosis but can occur to some extent in almost any blood disease.

poikilothermic (poi-kil-oh-**therm**-ik) *adj.* cold-blooded: being unable to regulate the body temperature, which fluctuates according to that of the surroundings. *Compare* homoiothermic. **—poikilothermy** *n.*

poison (**poi**-zŏn) *n.* any substance that irritates, damages, or impairs the activity of the body's tissues. The term is usually reserved for substances, such as arsenic, cyanide, and strychnine, that are harmful in relatively small amounts.

polar body (**poh**-ler) *n.* one of the small cells produced by division of an oocyte that does not develop into a functional egg cell. *See* oogenesis.

pole (pohl) *n.* (in anatomy) the extremity of the axis of the body, an organ, or a cell.

poli- (polio-) *combining form denoting* the grey matter of the nervous system.

policeman's heel (pŏ-lees-mănz) *n. see* plantar (fasciitis).

polioencephalitis (poh-li-oh-en-sef-ă-**ly**-tis) *n.* a virus infection of the brain, causing particular damage to the grey matter of the cerebral hemispheres and the brainstem. The term is now usually restricted to infections of the brain by the poliomyelitis virus.

polioencephalomyelitis (poh-li-oh-en-sef-ă-loh-my-ĕ-**ly**-tis) *n.* any virus infection of the central nervous system affecting the grey matter of the brain and spinal cord. Rabies is the outstanding example.

poliomyelitis (infantile paralysis, polio) (poh-li-oh-my-ĕ-**ly**-tis) *n.* an infectious virus disease affecting the central nervous system. Immunization, using the Sabin vaccine or the Salk vaccine, is highly effective. **abortive p.** poliomyelitis in which only the throat and intestines are infected and the symptoms are those of a stomach upset or influenza. **bulbar p.** paralytic poliomyelitis in which the muscles of the respiratory system are affected. **nonparalytic p.** a form of the disease in which the symptoms of abortive poliomyelitis are accompanied by muscle stiffness. **paralytic p.** a less common form of polio in which the symptoms of the milder forms of the disease are followed by weakness and eventual paralysis of the muscles. *See also* post-polio syndrome.

poliovirus (**poh**-li-oh-vy-rŭs) *n.* one of a small group of RNA-containing viruses causing poliomyelitis. They are included within the picornavirus group.

Politzer's bag (**pol**-it-zerz) *n.* a flexible rubber bag for inflating the middle ear through the Eustachian tube. [A. Politzer (1835–1920), Austrian otologist]

pollex (**pol**-eks) *n.* (*pl.* **pollices**) the thumb.

pollinosis (poli-**noh**-sis) *n.* a more precise term than hay fever for an allergy due to the pollen of grasses, trees, or shrubs.

poly- *combining form denoting* **1.** many; multiple. **2.** excessive. **3.** generalized; affecting many parts.

polyarteritis nodosa (periarteritis nodosa) (poli-ar-ter-**I**-tis noh-**doh**-să) *n.* a disease of unknown cause in which there is necrotizing inflammation of the walls of small and medium-sized arteries. Common manifestations include weight loss, skin rashes, testicular pain, myalgia, hypertension, neuritis, and renal disease.

polyarthritis (poli-arth-**ry**-tis) *n.* disease involving several joints, either together or in sequence, causing pain, stiffness, swelling, tenderness, and loss of function. Rheumatoid arthritis is the most common cause.

polyclinic (**pol**-i-klin-ik) *n. see* health centre.

polycystic kidney disease (poli-**sis**-tik) *n.* either of two inherited disorders characterized by cysts in the kidneys. **autosomal dominant p. k. d.** one of the most common hereditary diseases. Symptoms, including haematuria, urinary tract infection, and hypertension, are associated with progressive kidney failure. **autosomal recessive p. k. d.** a rare condition with a poor prognosis; symptoms include hypertension, excessive thirst, and underdeveloped lungs. Affected babies resemble those with Potter syndrome.

polycystic ovary (PCO) *n.* the presence of more than twelve follicles in each ovary (2–9 mm in diameter), or increased ovarian volume (>10 ml), or both. The presence of enlarged ovaries with multiple small cysts and androgen-secreting connective tissue are associated with signs of androgen excess (*see* polycystic ovary syndrome).

polycystic ovary syndrome (PCOS, Stein-Leventhal syndrome) *n.* a disorder characterized by hyperandrogenism and ovarian dysfunction (with enlarged ovaries containing multiple small cysts), which results in absent or infrequent menstrual periods and subfertility. It is associated with obesity and insulin resistance.

polycythaemia (poli-sy-**theem**-iă) *n.* an increase in the packed cell volume (haematocrit) in the blood. This may be due either to a decrease in the total volume of the plasma (**relative p.**) or to an increase in the total volume of the red cells (**absolute p.**). The latter may occur as a primary disease or as a secondary condition in association with various respiratory or circulatory disorders and with certain tumours. **p. vera** (**p. rubra vera**, **Vaquez-Osler disease**) a disease in which absolute polycythaemia is often accompanied by an increase in the numbers of white blood cells and platelets. Symptoms include headache, thromboses, cyanosis, plethora, and itching.

polydactylism (poli-**dak**-til-izm) *n. see* hyperdactylism.

polydipsia (poli-**dip**-siă) *n.* abnormally intense thirst: a symptom of diabetes mellitus and diabetes insipidus. **psychogenic p.** polydipsia in the absence of any metabolic abnormality.

polyhydramnios (hydramnios) (poli-hy-**dram**-ni-ŏs) *n.* an increase in the amount of amniotic fluid surrounding the fetus, which usually occurs in the third trimester and may be associated with maternal diabetes, multiple pregnancy, any fetal anomaly causing impaired swallowing, or placental abnormality.

polymer (**pol**-im-er) *n.* a substance formed by the linkage of a large number of smaller molecules known as **monomers**. An example of a monomer is glucose, whose molecules link together to form glycogen, a polymer.

polymorph (polymorphonuclear leucocyte) (**pol**-i-morf) *n.* a type of white blood cell with a lobed nucleus and granular cytoplasm. *See* basophil, eosinophil, neutrophil.

polymorphous light eruption (poli-**mor**-fik) *n. see* photodermatosis.

polymyalgia rheumatica (poli-my-**al**-jiă roo-**mat**-ikă) *n.* a rheumatic disease causing aching and progressive stiffness of the muscles of the shoulders and hips after inactivity. It is typically associated with loss of appetite, fatigue, night sweats, and a raised ESR. The condition is most common in the elderly and is often associated with temporal arteritis. The symptoms respond rapidly and effectively to corticosteroid treatment.

polymyositis (poli-my-oh-**sy**-tis) *n.* an autoimmune disease of the muscles that may be acute or chronic. It particularly affects the muscles of the shoulder and hip girdles, which are weak and tender to the touch. Treatment is with corticosteroids and other immunosuppressant drugs. *See also* dermatomyositis.

polymyxin B (poli-**miks**-in) *n.* an antibiotic used to treat severe infections caused by Gram-negative bacteria. Formulated with other drugs, it is administered as a solution or ointment for ear, eye, and skin infections.

polyneuritis (poli-newr-**I**-tis) *n. see* (peripheral) neuropathy.

polyneuropathy (poli-newr-**op**-ă-thi) *n. see* (peripheral) neuropathy.

polyopia (poli-**oh**-piă) *n.* the sensation of multiple images of one object. It is sometimes experienced by people with early cataract. *See also* diplopia.

polyp (polypus) (**pol**-ip) *n.* a growth, usually benign, protruding from a mucous membrane. Polyps are commonly found in the nose and sinuses, giving rise to obstruction, chronic infection, and discharge. Other sites include the ear, the stomach, and the colon; adenomatous colonic polyps may eventually become malignant. Polyps are usually removed endoscopically (*see* polypectomy). **juvenile p.** a polyp that occurs in the intestine (usually colon or rectum) of infants or young people; sometimes they are multiple (*see* polyposis). Most juvenile polyps are benign. *See also* Peutz-Jeghers syndrome.

polypectomy (poli-**pek**-tŏmi) *n.* the endoscopic or surgical removal of a polyp. The technique used depends upon the site and size of the polyp; endoscopic techniques include using a wire loop (snare) to cut through the base of the polyp (**snare p.**); this is performed with or without diathermy current (**hot snare** vs **cold snare**).

polypeptide (poli-**pep**-tyd) *n.* a molecule consisting of three or more amino acids linked together by peptide bonds. Protein molecules are polypeptides.

polyphagia (poli-**fay**-jiă) *n.* excessive eating.

polypharmacy (poli-**farm**-ă-si) *n.* treatment of a patient with more than one type of medicine.

polyploid (**pol**-i-ploid) *adj.* describing cells, tissues, or individuals in which there are three or more complete sets of chromosomes. *Compare* diploid, haploid. **—polyploidy** *n.*

polypoid (**pol**-i-poid) *adj.* having the appearance of a polyp.

polyposis (poli-**poh**-sis) *n.* a condition in which numerous polyps form in an organ or tissue. **familial adenomatous p.** (**p. coli**) a hereditary disease in which multiple adenomas develop in the gastrointestinal tract, usually the colon or rectum, at an early age. As these polyps almost invariably become malignant, patients are usually advised to undergo total removal of the affected bowel. *See also* Peutz-Jeghers syndrome. *Compare* pseudopolyposis.

polypus (**pol**-i-pŭs) *n. see* polyp.

polyradiculitis (polyradiculopathy) (poli-ră-dik-yoo-**ly**-tis) *n.* any disorder of the peripheral nerves (*see* neuropathy) in which the brunt of the disease falls on the nerve roots where they emerge from the spinal cord.

polysaccharide (poli-**sak**-eryd) *n.* a carbohydrate formed from many monosaccharides joined together in long linear or branched chains. Examples are glycogen and cellulose.

polyserositis (poli-seer-oh-**sy**-tis) *n.* inflammation of the membranes that line the chest, abdomen, and joints, with accumulation of fluid in the cavities.

polysomnograph (poli-**som**-noh-graf) *n.* a record of measurements of various bodily parameters during sleep. It is used in the diagnosis of sleep disorders, such as obstructive sleep apnoea.

polyspermia (poli-**sper**-miă) *n.* **1.** excessive formation of semen. **2.** *see* polyspermy.

polyspermy (polyspermia) (poli-**sper**-mi) *n.* fertilization of a single ovum by more than one spermatozoon: the development is abnormal and the embryo dies.

polyuria (poli-**yoor**-iă) *n.* the production of large volumes of dilute urine. The phenomenon may be due simply to excessive liquid intake or to disease, particularly diabetes mellitus, diabetes insipidus, and kidney disorders.

POM *n. see* prescription only medicine.

pompholyx (**pom**-foh-liks) *n.* eczema of the palms (**cheiropompholyx**) and soles (**podopompholyx**). Because the horny layer of the skin in these parts is so thick the vesicles typical of eczema cannot rupture. There is intense itching until the skin eventually peels. Pompholyx is commonest in early adulthood.

pons (ponz) *n.* **1. (p. Varolii)** the part of the brainstem that links the medulla oblongata and the thalamus. It contains numerous nerve tracts between the cerebral cortex and the spinal cord. [C. Varolius (1543–75), Italian anatomist] **2.** any portion of tissue that joins two parts of an organ. **—pontine** (**pon**-teen) *adj.*

POP *n. see* plaster of Paris.

popliteus (pop-**lit**-iŭs) *n.* a flat triangular muscle at the back of the knee joint, between the femur and tibia, that helps to flex the knee. **—popliteal** *adj.*

population (pop-yoo-**lay**-shŏn) *n.* **1.** the total number of people living in a defined geographical area. **2.** (in statistics) a group of people, objects, or events from which a sample is drawn for the purpose of a survey, clinical trial, or other study.

pore (por) *n.* a small opening. **sweat p.** the opening of a sweat gland on the surface of the skin.

porencephaly (por-en-sef-ăli) *n.* an abnormal communication between the lateral ventricle and the surface of the brain. This is usually a consequence of brain injury or cerebrovascular disease.

porphin (por-fin) *n.* a complex nitrogen-containing ring structure and parent compound of the porphyrins.

porphyria (por-fi-riă) *n.* one of a group of rare inborn errors of metabolism in which there are deficiencies in the enzymes involved in the biosynthesis of haem. The accumulation of the enzyme's substrate gives rise to the features of the disorder, which include the excretion of porphyrins and their derivatives in the urine, which may change colour on standing. **acute intermittent p.** a hereditary hepatic porphyria marked by recurrent attacks of acute abdominal pain, constipation, and psychotic behaviour. **erythropoietic p.** any porphyria in which the defect is primarily in the bone marrow. **hepatic p.** any porphyria in which the defect is primarily in the liver. **p. cutanea tarda** a hereditary or acquired hepatic porphyria in which light-exposed areas of the skin become blistered and fragile (*see* photodermatosis).

porphyrin (por-fi-rin) *n.* one of a number of pigments derived from porphin, which are widely distributed in living things. All porphyrins form chelates with iron, magnesium, zinc, nickel, copper, and cobalt. These chelates are constituents of haemoglobin, myoglobin, the cytochromes, and chlorophyll. *See also* protoporphyrin IX.

porphyrinuria (por-fi-rin-**yoor**-iă) *n.* the presence in the urine of porphyrins, sometimes causing discoloration. *See* porphyria.

porta (por-tă) *n.* the aperture in an organ through which its associated vessels pass. Such an opening occurs in the liver (**p. hepatis**). —**portal** *adj.*

portable (por-tă-bŭl) *adj.* (in radiography) denoting light weight equipment (and the images it produces) for use away from the radiography department, when patients cannot easily be moved (for example, on intensive therapy units).

portacaval anastomosis (portacaval shunt) (por-tă-**kay**-văl) *n.* **1.** a surgical technique in which the hepatic portal vein is joined to the inferior vena cava, thus bypassing the liver. It is no longer widely used in the treatment of portal hypertension. **2.** any of the natural communications between the branches of the hepatic portal vein in the liver and the inferior vena cava.

portal hypertension (por-t'l) *n.* a state in which the pressure within the hepatic portal vein is increased, causing enlargement of the spleen, development of oesophageal varices, and accumulation of fluid in the ascites. The commonest cause is liver cirrhosis. Treatment includes diuretic drugs, bond ligation or beta blockers for varices, or implanting a stent within the liver to join portal and hepatic veins.

portal system *n.* a vein or group of veins that terminates at both ends in a capillary bed. **hepatic p. s.** the best known portal system, consisting of the portal vein and its tributaries.

portal vein *n.* a vein that conveys blood from the stomach, intestines, spleen, and pancreas to the liver.

port-wine stain (port-wyn) *n. see* naevus.

position (pŏ-**zish**-ŏn) *n.* a posture or attitude assumed by a patient in order to facilitate nursing, diagnostic, or surgical procedures (see illustration).

positive end expiratory pressure (PEEP) (**poz**-it-iv) *n.* a technique used with the mechanical ventilation of patients with respiratory failure. The pressure at the end of expiration is kept sufficiently high to maintain the partial inflation of the lungs to prevent alveolar collapse.

positive-pressure ventilation (PPV) *n.* the forcible passage of air into the lungs to stimulate breathing movements. *See also* noninvasive ventilation, ventilator.

positive symptom *n.* (in psychiatry) a symptom of schizophrenia characterized by a distortion in some aspect of functioning, such as delusions, hallucinations, or disordered speech. *Compare* negative symptom.

positron (**poz**-i-tron) *n.* an electrically charged particle, released in some radioactive decays, that has the same mass as an electron but opposite charge. It has a very short lifetime as it quickly reacts with an electron to produce gamma rays.

positron emission tomography (PET) *n.* a cross-sectional imaging technique of nuclear medicine that enables assessment and localization of metabolic activity in tissues of the brain, chest, and abdomen by measuring their uptake of injected radioisotopes (e.g. fluorodeoxyglucose, labelled with fluorine-18, to examine glucose metabolism). As the radioisotope is metabolized, it emits positrons, which are annihilated with the production of gamma rays; these are detected by the PET scanner and used to construct images.

posology (pŏ-**sol**-ŏji) *n.* the science of the dosage of medicines.

posseting (**poss**-it-ing) *n.* the regurgitation of a small amount of milk, usually with some wind, by a baby after feeding.

Possum (**poss**-ŭm) *n.* a device that enables severely paralysed patients to use typewriters, telephones, and other machines. Modern Possums are operated by micro-switches that require only the slightest movement in any limb. The name derives from **Patient-Operated Selector Mechanism (POSM)**.

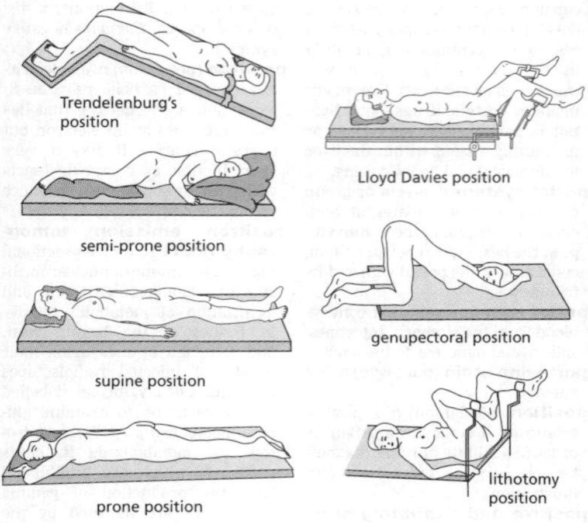

Types of position

POSSUM scoring (po-sŭm) *n.* *p*hysiological and *o*perative *s*everity *s*core for the en*um*eration of morbidity and mortality: a tool used by anaesthetists to determine the risks associated with surgery in an individual patient. This can be used to guide such decisions as the appropriateness of surgery and the requirement for intensive care postoperatively.

post- *prefix denoting* **1.** following; after. **2.** (in anatomy) behind.

postcibal (pohst-sy-băl) *adj.* occurring after eating.

postcoital (pohst-**koh**-i-t'l) *adj.* occurring after sexual intercourse. **p. bleeding** genital-tract bleeding occurring after sexual intercourse. It may be caused by sexually transmitted infections, vaginal candidiasis, atrophic vaginitis, cervical ectropion, cervical polyps, or cervical cancer. **p. contraception** (**emergency contraception**) prevention of pregnancy after intercourse has taken place. This can be achieved by an oral dose of levonorgestrel (Levonelle) or **ulipristal** (ellaOne) taken within 72 hours or 120 hours, respectively, of unprotected intercourse; or by the insertion of an IUCD within five days of unprotected intercourse. **p. test** a test used in the investigation of infertility. A specimen of cervical mucus, taken 6–24 hours after coitus in the postovulatory phase of the menstrual cycle, is examined under a microscope for the presence of motile spermatozoa.

postconcussional syndrome (pohst-kŏn-**kush**-ŏn-ăl) *n.* persistent headaches, giddiness, and lack of concentration that may follow a head injury.

postepileptic (pohst-epi-**lep**-tik) *adj.* occurring after an epileptic fit.

posterior (poss-**teer**-i-er) *adj.* situated at or near the back of the body or an organ. **p. chamber** the rear section of the eye, behind the lens, which is filled with vitreous humour.

postero- *combining form denoting* posterior.

postganglionic (pohst-gang-li-**on**-ik) *adj.* describing a neuron in a nerve pathway that starts at a ganglion and ends at the muscle or gland that it supplies. *Compare* preganglionic.

postgastrectomy syndrome (pohst-gas-**trek**-tŏmi) *n. see* dumping syndrome.

posthitis (poss-**th'y**-tis) *n.* inflammation of the foreskin. This usually occurs in association with balanitis (*see* balanoposthitis).

posthumous birth (**poss**-tew-mŭs) *n.* **1.** delivery of a child by Caesarean section after the mother's death. **2.** birth of a child after the father's death.

postmature (pohst-mă-**tewr**) *adj.* describing a baby born after 42 weeks of gestation (calculated from the first day of the last menstrual period). —**postmaturity** *n.*

postmenopausal bleeding (PMB) *n.* bleeding from the female genital tract occurring more than twelve months after the last menstrual period. Atrophic vaginitis is a common cause. Endometrial cancer occurs in up to 10% of cases.

postmenopause (pohst-**men**-ŏ-pawz) *n.* the period of a woman's life after the menopause, i.e. the following twelve months after her last menstrual period. —**postmenopausal** (pohst-men-ŏ-**pawz**-ăl) *adj.*

postmicturition dribble (pohst-mik-tewr-**ish**-ŏn **drib**-ĕl) *n.* a lower urinary tract symptom in which a dribble occurs after voiding has been completed, often after leaving the toilet. It is quite common in men but is not caused by benign prostatic hyperplasia. *Compare* terminal dribble.

post mortem (pohst **mor**-tĕm) Latin: after death. *See* autopsy.

postnasal space (pohst-**nay**-zăl) *n. see* nasopharynx.

postnatal (pohst-**nay**-t'l) *adj.* following childbirth. **p. depression** depression that affects women after childbirth, which can impair bonding between mother and child and in most cases resolves within 6 months of delivery. *Compare* postpartum (blues), puerperal (psychosis).

postoperative (pohst-**op**-er-ă-tiv) *adj.* following surgery: referring to the condition of a patient or to the treatment given at this time.

postpartum (pohst-**par**-tŭm) *adj.* relating to the period of a few days immediately after birth. **p. blues** (**baby blues**) brief episodes of tearfulness, emotional instability, poor sleep, and irritability that affect about half of all women during the first week after delivery. *Compare* postnatal (depression), puerperal (psychosis). **p. haemorrhage** (**PPH**) excessive bleeding (>500 ml) from the genital tract within 24 hours of delivery (primary PPH) or after 24 hours (secondary PPH). **p. sepsis** *see* sepsis.

post-polio syndrome (pohst-**poh**-li-oh) *n.* insidious numbness in muscles, together with fatigue and pain, that develops 15–20 years after an attack of poliomyelitis. It may be caused by loss of nerve cells that have been under greater strain than normal; there is no evidence of reactivation of the poliovirus.

postprandial (pohst-**pran**-di-ăl) *adj.* occurring after eating.

post-traumatic stress disorder (PTSD) (pohst-traw-**mat**-ik) *n.* an anxiety disorder caused by a major physical or emotional trauma, such as exposure to violence, warfare, or a disaster involving many casualties. At least one month after the event, the patient experiences the persistent recurrence of images or memories of the event, together with nightmares, insomnia, a sense of isolation, guilt, irritability, and loss of concentration. The level of anxiety may not be in direct proportion to the actual experience.

postural hypotension (poss-tewr-ăl) *n. see* hypotension.

postviral fatigue syndrome (pohst-**vy**-răl) *n. see* CFS/ME/PVF.

potassium (pŏ-**tas**-iŭm) *n.* a mineral element and an important constituent of the human body. It is the main base ion of intracellular fluid. High concentrations occur particularly in kidney failure and may lead to arrhythmia and finally to cardiac arrest. Low values result from fluid loss, e.g. due to vomiting or diarrhoea, and this may lead to general muscle paralysis. Symbol: K.

potassium-channel activator *n.* a drug that enhances the movement of potassium ions through the protein channels in cell membranes, reducing the sensitivity of smooth muscle cells in the walls of arteries to the normal stimuli to contract. The result is widening of the arteries. Potassium-channel activators, such as **nicorandil** (Ikorel), are used for improving the blood supply to the heart muscle in angina pectoris.

potassium chloride *n.* a salt of potassium administered by mouth to prevent and treat potassium deficiency, especially during treatment with digoxin or antiarrhythmic drugs. Trade names: **Kay-Cee-L**, **Sando-K**, **Slow-K**.

potassium permanganate (per-mang-ă-nayt) *n.* a salt of potassium, a solution of which has antiseptic and astringent properties and is applied to the skin as a solution to treat weeping eczema. It irritates mucous membranes and is poisonous if taken into the body. Trade name: **Permitabs**.

Potter syndrome (pot-er) *n.* a congenital condition characterized by absence of kidneys, resulting in decreased amniotic fluid (*see* oligohydramnios) and compression of the fetus. Affected babies have poorly developed lungs, a characteristic wrinkled and flattened facial appearance, and leg deformities and do not usually survive. [E. L. Potter (20th century), US pathologist]

Pott's disease (pots) *n.* tuberculosis of the backbone. Untreated, it can lead to a hunchback deformity. [P. Pott (1714–88), British surgeon]

Pott's fracture *n. see* fracture.

pouch (powch) *n.* **1.** (in anatomy) a small sac-like structure, especially occurring as an outgrowth of a larger structure. **p. of Douglas** a pouch of peritoneum occupying the space between the rectum and uterus. [J. Douglas (1675–1742), British anatomist] **2.** (in surgery) a sac created from a loop of intestine and used to replace a section of rectum that has been surgically removed, for example for ulcerative colitis. *See also* ileal pouch.

poultice (fomentation) (pohl-tis) *n.* a preparation of hot moist material applied to any part of the body to increase local circulation, alleviate pain, or soften the skin.

Poupart's ligament (poo-**parz**) *n. see* inguinal (ligament). [F. Poupart (1661–1708), French anatomist]

poverty of speech (**pov**-er-ti) *n.* brief hesitant speech using few words (often monosyllables) and lacking spontaneity. It occurs in patients with schizophrenia, dementia, and depression.

powder (**pow**-der) *n.* (in pharmacy) a medicinal preparation consisting of a mixture of two or more drugs in the form of fine particles.

power of attorney (pow-er ă-**tern**-i) *n.* authority given by an individual to another person (a proxy) to take decisions on their behalf; this may take effect immediately, after they lose mental capacity in relation to their financial affairs, or only after they lose capacity in relation to their personal welfare and health care. In the UK the proxy has responsibility for representing the patient's best interests, but he or she can refuse life-sustaining treatment for the patient only if express written provision for such a decision was made by the patient in advance (*see* advance decision, directive, or statement). The only circumstance in which the wishes of the proxy need not be followed is where clinicians believe that he or she is not acting in the patient's best interests.

SEE WEB LINKS

- An overview of power of attorney

pox (poks) *n.* **1.** an infectious disease causing a skin rash. **2.** a rash of pimples that become pus-filled, as in chickenpox and smallpox.

poxvirus (poks-vy-rŭs) *n.* one of a group of large DNA-containing viruses including those that cause smallpox (variola) and cowpox (vaccinia).

PPE *n. see* personal protective equipment.

PPH *n. see* postpartum (haemorrhage).

PPS *n.* plasma protein solution.

PPV *n. see* positive-pressure ventilation.

PQRST complex *n.* the pattern of electrical activity of the heart during one cardiac cycle as recorded by electrocardiography. *See* electrocardiogram, P–R interval, QRS complex, Q–T interval, S–T segment.

PR per rectum, i.e. via the rectum.

practice development (prak-tis) *n.* the process of sharing good practice from different areas, using interprofessional collaboration and evidence-based care, to improve patient experience.

practice nurse *n.* a trained nurse caring for the patients of one or more general practitioners in the consulting room and on domiciliary consultations. In Britain practice nurses are usually employed by GPs but may also be employed by primary care trusts as practice nurses or district nurses.

Prader orchidometer (prah-der) *n. see* orchidometer.

Prader-Willi syndrome (Prader-Willi-Labhart syndrome) (vil-i lab-hart) *n.* an inherited (autosomal dominant) condition due to an abnormality of paternal chromosome 15. It is characterized by pathological overeating and resulting obesity (children often subsequently develop type 2 diabetes), learning disabilities, and underactivity of the testes or ovaries due to lack of pituitary gonadotrophins. [A. Prader, H. Willi, and A. Labhart (20th century), Swiss paediatricians]

pravastatin (pră-vas-tă-tin) *n.* a drug taken by mouth to reduce abnormally high levels of cholesterol and other lipids in the blood (*see* statin). Trade name: **Lipostat**.

praziquantel (praz-i-kwon-tel) *n.* an anthelmintic drug used to eliminate tapeworms and schistosomes. Praziquantel is administered by mouth. Trade name: **Cysticide**.

prazosin (praz-oh-sin) *n.* a drug used in the treatment of high blood pressure (hypertension) and also to relieve urinary retention due to benign enlargement of the prostate (*see* alpha blocker). It is administered by mouth. Trade name: **Hypovase**.

pre- *prefix denoting* **1.** before; preceding. **2.** (in anatomy) in front of; anterior to.

prebiotics (pree-bI-o-tiks) *pl. n.* nondigestible constituents of food, such as inulin, which stimulate the growth of 'good' bacteria in the colon.

precancerous (pree-kan-ser-ŭs) *adj.* describing a nonmalignant condition that is known to become malignant if left untreated.

precipitin (pri-sip-it-in) *n.* any antibody that combines with its antigen to form a complex that is seen as a precipitate. The precipitin reaction is a useful means of confirming the identity of an unknown antigen or establishing that a serum contains antibodies to a known disease. *See also* agglutination.

precocious puberty (pri-koh-shŭs) *n.* the development in girls of breasts or pubic hair before the age of six or menstruation before the age of eight, and in boys the development of pubic hair or other adult sexual features below the age of nine. In girls 90% of cases have no underlying abnormalities, but in boys approximately half have a serious underlying cause, of which malignant testicular or adrenal tumours are the most common.

precordium (pree-**kor**-dium) *n.* the region of the thorax immediately over the heart. —**precordial** *adj.*

precursor (pri-**ker**-ser) *n.* a substance from which another, usually more biologically active, substance is formed. For example, trypsinogen is the precursor of the enzyme trypsin.

prediabetes (pree-dy-ă-**bee**-teez) *n. see* glucose tolerance test.

predigestion (pree-dy-**jes**-chŏn) *n.* the partial digestion of foods by artificial means before they are taken into the body.

predisposition (pree-dis-pŏ-**zish**-ŏn) *n.* a tendency to be affected by a particular disease or kind of disease. *See also* diathesis.

prednisolone (pred-**nis**-ŏ-lohn) *n.* a synthetic corticosteroid used to treat rheumatic diseases, inflammatory and allergic conditions, and some cancers. It is administered by mouth or rectally, injected into joints or muscles or applied in drops to treat eye or ear conditions. Trade names: **Deltacortril Enteric**, **Deltastab**, **Minims Prednisolone Sodium Phosphate**, **Predsol**.

pre-eclampsia (pree-i-**klamp**-siă) *n.* the combination of high blood pressure (*see* pregnancy-induced hypertension) and the presence of protein in the urine (>0.3 g in 24 hours) in a pregnant woman, with or without oedema. *See also* eclampsia.

prefrontal leucotomy (pree-**frun**-t'l) *n. see* leucotomy.

prefrontal lobe *n.* the region of the brain at the very front of each cerebral hemisphere. The functions of the lobe are concerned with emotions, memory, learning, and social behaviour.

preganglionic (pree-gang-li-**on**-ik) *adj.* describing fibres in a nerve pathway that end in a ganglion, where they form synapses with postganglionic fibres.

pre-gangrene (pree-**gang**-reen) *n.* the penultimate stage of vascular insufficiency before gangrene sets in; the term is usually applied to ischaemia of the lower limb.

pregnancy (**preg**-năn-si) *n.* the period during which a woman carries a developing fetus, normally in the uterus (*compare* ectopic pregnancy). Pregnancy lasts for approximately 266 days, from conception until the baby is born, or 280 days from the first day of the last menstrual period (*see* Naegele rule). *See also* pseudocyesis (phantom pregnancy). **p. test** any of several methods used to demonstrate whether or not a woman is pregnant. Most pregnancy tests are based on the detection, by immunological methods, of a hormone, human chorionic gonadotrophin, in the urine or in the serum. **—pregnant** *adj.*

SEE WEB LINKS

- A guide to pregnancy from the NHS Choices website

pregnancy-induced hypertension (PIH) *n.* raised blood pressure (>140/90 mmHg) developing in a woman during the second half of pregnancy. *See also* pre-eclampsia.

pregnanediol (preg-nayn-**dy**-ol) *n.* a steroid that is formed during the metabolism of the female sex hormone progesterone. It occurs in the urine during pregnancy and certain phases of the menstrual cycle.

pregnenolone (preg-**neen**-ŏ-lohn) *n.* a steroid synthesized in the adrenal glands, ovaries, and testes. Pregnenolone is an important intermediate product in steroid hormone synthesis.

preimplantation genetic diagnosis (PGD) (pree-im-plahn-**tay**-shŏn) *n.* prenatal genetic diagnosis extended to the earliest stages of embryonic development, before implantation occurs.

prelabour rupture of membranes (PROM) *n.* spontaneous rupture of the fetal membranes prior to the onset of labour. When this occurs before 37 weeks gestation in the absence of contractions, it is referred to as **preterm prelabour rupture of membranes (PPROM)**.

premature beat (**prem**-ă-tewr) *n. see* ectopic beat.

premature birth *n. see* preterm birth.

premedication (pree-med-i-**kay**-shŏn) *n.* drugs administered to a patient before an operation. Premedication usually comprises injection of a sedative (e.g. a benzodiazepine) together with a drug, such as hyoscine, to dry up the secretions of the lungs (which might otherwise be inhaled during anaesthesia).

premenstrual syndrome (PMS) (pree-**men**-stroo-ăl) *n.* a group of symptoms experienced in varying degrees by women of reproductive age up to two weeks before menstruation. These include altered mental stability, fatigue, bloating, breast tenderness, and headaches. Treatment for mild cases includes support, reassurance, dietary guidance, and stress management. More severe cases may require hormone therapy (progestogens, oral contraceptives, and gonadorelin analogues), diuretics, and SSRIs.

SEE WEB LINKS

- Website of the National Association for Premenstrual Syndrome

premolar (pree-**moh**-ler) *n.* either of the two teeth on each side of each jaw behind the canines and in front of the molars in the adult dentition.

prenatal diagnosis (antenatal diagnosis) (pree-**nay**-t'l) *n.*

diagnostic procedures carried out on pregnant women in order to detect the presence of genetic or other abnormalities in the developing fetus. Ultrasound scanning (*see* ultrasonography) remains the cornerstone of prenatal diagnosis. Other tests include chromosome and enzyme analysis of fetal cells obtained by amniocentesis or, at an earlier stage of pregnancy, by chorionic villus sampling. **Noninvasive prenatal diagnosis** involves a blood test to analyse cell-free fetal DNA in maternal blood. *See also* preimplantation genetic diagnosis.

prenatal screening *n.* screening tests carried out to estimate the risk of chromosomal or other abnormalities being present in a developing fetus. They include blood tests to measure levels of **human chorionic gonadotrophin** (**hCG**), **alpha-fetoprotein** (**AFP**), and other markers (*see also* triple test) and also scanning for the presence of ultrasound markers (*see also* nuchal translucency scanning).

preoperative (pree-**op**-er-ă-tiv) *adj.* before operation: referring to the condition of a patient or to treatment, such as sedation, given at this time.

prepatellar bursitis (pree-pă-**tel**-er) *n. see* housemaid's knee.

prepubertal (pree-**pew**-ber-t'l) *adj.* relating to or occurring in the period before puberty.

prepuce (foreskin) (**pree**-pewss) *n.* the fold of skin that grows over the glans penis. On its inner surface modified sebaceous glands (**preputial glands**) secrete a lubricating fluid over the glans. **—preputial** (pree-**pew**-shăl) *adj.*

presby- (presbyo-) *combining form denoting* old age.

presbyacusis (prezbi-ă-**kew**-sis) *n.* the progressive sensorineural deafness that occurs with age.

presbyopia (prezbi-**oh**-piă) *n.* difficulty in reading at the usual distance and in performing other close work, due to the decline with age in the ability of the eye to focus on close objects.

prescribed disease (pri-**skrybd**) *n.* one of a number of occupational diseases for which benefits are payable. Such diseases arise as a result of employment requiring close contact with a hazardous substance or circumstance and include decompression sickness in divers and infections such as anthrax in those handling wool.

prescription (pri-**skrip**-shŏn) *n.* a written direction from a registered medical practitioner to a pharmacist for preparing and dispensing a drug.

prescription only medicine (POM) *n.* a legal category of drugs that can only be dispensed with a prescription.

presenility (pree-sin-**il**-iti) *n.* premature ageing of the mind and body, so that a person shows the reduction in mental and physical abilities normally found only in old age. *See also* dementia, progeria. **—presenile** (pree-**see**-nyl) *adj.*

present (pri-**zent**) *vb.* **1.** (of a patient) to come forward for examination and treatment because of experiencing specific symptoms (**presenting symptoms**). **2.** (in obstetrics) *see* presentation.

presentation (prez-ĕn-**tay**-shŏn) *n.* the part of the fetus that is closest to the birth canal and can be felt on inserting the finger into the vagina. Normally the crown of the head presents. However, the buttocks may present (*see* breech presentation), or, if the fetus lies transversely across the uterus, the shoulder or arm may present (*see* malpresentation).

pressor (**pres**-er) *n.* an agent that raises blood pressure. *See* vasoconstrictor.

pressure area (**presh**-er) *n.* any of the areas of the body where a bone is close to the skin surface, so that pressure on that area (e.g. by lying in bed) deprives the overlying tissues of their blood supply (*see* pressure sore).

pressure index (PI) (**in**-deks) *n.* the ratio of the pressure in the posterior tibial artery to that in the brachial artery, which reflects the degree of arterial obstruction in the artery of the lower limb.

pressure point *n.* a point at which an artery lies over a bone on which it may be compressed by finger pressure, to arrest haemorrhage beyond.

pressure sore (bedsore, decubitus ulcer) *n.* an ulcerated area of skin caused by continuous pressure on part of the body in a bedridden patient. Careful nursing is necessary to prevent local gangrene. The patient's position should be changed frequently, and the buttocks, heels, elbows, and other regions at risk kept dry and clean.

SEE WEB LINKS

- Introduction to pressure sores from the NHS Choices website

pressure support ventilation (PSV) *n.* the form of mechanical ventilation used to assist patients with respiratory failure who are able to provide some breathing. It is adjusted to supplement the patient's inadequate efforts.

presystole (pree-sis-tŏ-li) *n.* the period in the cardiac cycle just preceding systole.

preterm birth (premature birth) (**pree**-term) *n.* birth of a baby before 37 weeks (259 days) of gestation (calculated from the first day of the mother's last menstrual period); a birth at less than 23 weeks is at present incompatible with life. Conditions affecting preterm babies may include respiratory distress syndrome, feeding difficulties, inability to maintain normal body temperature, apnoea, infection, necrotizing enterocolitis, and brain haemorrhages. Supportive treatment is provided in an incubator in a neonatal unit.

prevalence (**prev**-ă-lĕns) *n.* a measure of morbidity based on current levels of disease in a population, estimated either at a particular time (**point p.**) or over a stated period (**period p.**). It can be expressed either in terms of affected people (persons) or episodes of sickness per

1000 individuals at risk. *Compare* incidence rate.

preventive medicine (pri-ven-tiv) *n.* the branch of medicine whose main aim is the prevention of disease. *See also* primary prevention, secondary prevention, tertiary prevention.

priapism (pry-ă-pizm) *n.* a prolonged (greater than 4 hours) and usually painful erection of the penis. **Ischaemic priapism** is associated with blood disorders (such as sickle-cell disease) or haemodialysis; alternatively it may result from the administration of drugs used to treat erectile dysfunction, such as papaverine or alprostadil. It requires urgent decompression.

prickle cells (prik-ŭl) *pl. n.* cells with cytoplasmic processes that form intercellular bridges. The germinative layer of the epidermis is sometimes called the **prickle cell layer**.

prickly heat (prik-li) *n.* an itchy rash of small raised red spots. It occurs usually on the face, neck, back, chest, and thighs in hot moist weather. Treatment is removal of the patient to a cool (air-conditioned) place. Medical name: **miliaria rubra**.

prilocaine (pril-oh-kayn) *n.* a local anaesthetic used for nerve block, intrathecal anaesthesia, and in dentistry. It is administered by injection. Trade names: **Citanest 1%**, **Prilotekal**.

prima facie (pry-mă fay-shi) *n.* a principle that, at first sight, must be conformed with unless it conflicts with an equally important principle.

primaquine (pry-mă-kween) *n.* a drug used to treat benign malaria. It is administered by mouth after treatment with chloroquine.

primary care (pry-mer-i) *n.* health care provided by general practitioners or other health professionals to whom patients seeking medical treatment have direct access and to whom they can usually self-refer. Primary care services provided by the NHS include general practices and general dental and ophthalmic services, together with NHS walk-in centres and other community services outside the hospital service. Some primary care services are also available in the private sector. *Compare* secondary care, tertiary care.

primary care trust (PCT) *n.* formerly, one of a group of free-standing statutory bodies within the National Health Service in England that had responsibility for the health-care needs of their own geographical area. Many of their actions were determined by strategic health authorities. They were disbanded in 2013 and developed into clinical commissioning groups.

primary nursing *n.* a method of organizing nursing care in which one nurse (the **primary nurse**) is responsible for assessing the patient, planning appropriate care, and evaluating the progress of that patient throughout his or her stay in hospital and on discharge.

primary prevention *n.* avoidance of the onset of disease by behaviour modification (e.g. limiting alcohol intake) or treatment (e.g. routine childhood immunization). *See also* preventive medicine.

primary teeth *pl. n. see* dentition.

prime (prym) *vb.* (in chemotherapy) to administer small doses of a cytotoxic drug to a patient prior to high-dose chemotherapy and/or radiotherapy. This causes proliferation of the primitive bone marrow cells and aids subsequent regeneration of the bone marrow.

prime mover *n. see* agonist.

primidone (**pry**-mid-ohn) *n.* an anticonvulsant drug administered by mouth to treat tonic-clonic seizures, partial epilepsy, and essential tremor.

primigravida (pry-mi-**grav**-id-ă) *n.* a woman experiencing her first pregnancy.

primipara (pry-**mip**-er-ă) *n.* a woman who has given birth to one infant capable of survival.

primordial (pry-**mor**-di-ăl) *adj.* (in embryology) describing cells or tissues that are formed in the early stages of embryonic development.

P–R interval *n.* the interval on an electrocardiogram between the onset of atrial activity and ventricular activity.

prion (**pree**-on) *n.* a constituent protein of brain cells that, in an abnormal form, accumulates in and destroys brain tissue. This form is very stable and resistant to radiation and sterilization; it is thought to interact with normal prion protein in such a way as to convert it to abnormal prion. Prions are now widely accepted as being the causal agents of Creutzfeldt-Jakob disease and other spongiform encephalopathies.

PRK *n. see* (photorefractive) keratectomy.

p.r.n. (pro re nata) Latin: as required, used as a direction in prescriptions.

pro- *prefix denoting* **1.** before; preceding. **2.** a precursor. **3.** in front of.

probability (prob-ă-**bil**-iti) *n.* (in statistics) *see* significance.

probang (**proh**-bang) *n.* a long flexible rod with a small sponge, ball, or tuft at the end, used to remove obstructions from the larynx or oesophagus.

probe (prohb) *n.* a thin rod of pliable metal with a blunt end. The instrument is used for exploring cavities, wounds, fistulae, or sinus channels. **ultrasound p.** *see* transducer, ultrasonography. *See also* heater-probe.

probenecid (proh-**ben**-ĕ-sid) *n.* a drug that reduces the level of uric acid in the blood (*see* uricosuric drug), administered by mouth to prevent the toxic effects of cidofovir, an antiviral drug used to treat severe cytomegalovirus eye infection in AIDS patients.

problem-solving approach (**prob**-lĕm-sol-ving) *n.* a method of planning work involving assessment, problem identification, planning, implementation, and evaluation. *See* nursing process.

procarbazine (proh-**kar**-bă-zeen) *n.* a drug that inhibits growth of cancer cells by preventing cell division and is administered by mouth, principally to treat Hodgkin's disease.

process (**proh**-ses) *n.* (in anatomy) a thin prominence or protuberance.

prochlorperazine (proh-klor-per-ă-zeen) *n.* a phenothiazine antipsychotic drug used to treat schizophrenia and other psychoses, severe anxiety, and severe vertigo, nausea, and vomiting. It is administered by mouth or deep intramuscular injection. Trade names: **Buccastem**, **Stemetil**.

procidentia (pros-i-**den**-shiă) *n.* the complete prolapse of an organ, especially the uterus, which protrudes from the vaginal opening.

proct- (procto-) *combining form denoting* the anus and/or rectum.

proctalgia (proctodynia) (prok-**tal**-jiă) *n.* pain in the rectum or anus. **p. fugax** sudden severe pain that affects the rectum and may last for seconds to minutes. There is no structural disease and the pain is probably due to muscle spasm.

proctatresia (prok-tă-**tree**-ziă) *n.* *see* imperforate (anus).

proctectasia (prok-tek-**tay**-ziă) *n.* enlargement or widening of the rectum, usually due to long-standing constipation.

proctectomy (prok-**tek**-tŏmi) *n.* surgical removal of the rectum. It is usually performed for cancer of the rectum and may require the placement of a stoma (*see* colostomy).

proctitis (prok-**ty**-tis) *n.* inflammation of the rectum. Symptoms are ineffective straining to empty the bowels (tenesmus), urgency, rectal pain, diarrhoea, and the discharge of blood or mucus. Proctitis is invariably present in ulcerative colitis and sometimes in Crohn's disease.

proctocele (**prok**-toh-seel) *n.* *see* rectocele.

proctocolectomy (prok-toh-kŏ-**lek**-tŏmi) *n.* a surgical operation in which the rectum and colon are removed. Removal of the entire rectum and colon (**panproctocolectomy**) requires either a permanent opening of the ileum (*see* ileostomy) or the construction of an ileal pouch.

proctocolitis (prok-toh-kŏ-**ly**-tis) *n.* inflammation of the rectum and colon, usually due to ulcerative colitis. *See also* proctitis.

proctodynia (prok-toh-**din**-iă) *n.* *see* proctalgia.

proctogram (**prok**-tŏ-gram) *n.* an X-ray of the rectum taken after contrast material has been infused into it using a catheter. **defecating p.** a series of X-ray or MR images captured during defecation to highlight any abnormalities.

proctology (prok-**tol**-ŏji) *n.* the study of disorders of the rectum and anus.

proctorrhaphy (prokt-o-răfi) *n.* a surgical operation to stitch tears or lacerations of the rectum or anus.

proctoscope (**prok**-tŏ-skohp) *n.* an illuminated instrument that allows inspection of the distal rectum and the anus. **—proctoscopy** *n.*

proctosigmoiditis (prok-toh-sig-moid-I-tis) *n.* inflammation of the rectum and the sigmoid colon. *See also* proctocolitis.

proctotomy (prok-**tot**-ŏmi) *n.* incision into the rectum or anus to correct stricture of the canal or to open an imperforate anus.

procyclidine (proh-sy-kli-deen) *n.* an antimuscarinic drug administered by mouth or injection to reduce muscle tremor and rigidity in parkinsonism. Trade names: **Arpicolin**, **Kemadrin**.

prodromal (proh-**droh**-măl) *adj.* relating to the period of time between the appearance of the first symptoms of an infectious disease and the development of a rash or fever. **p. rash** a rash that precedes the full rash of an infectious disease.

prodrome (**proh**-drohm) *n.* a symptom indicating the onset of a disease.

proenzyme (zymogen) (proh-**en**-zym) *n.* the inactive form in which certain enzymes (e.g. digestive enzymes) are originally produced and secreted.

professionalism (prŏ-fe-shŏn-ĕ-lizăm) *n.* possession of a high level of intellectual and technical expertise, together with a commitment to public service and the ability to practise autonomously within the regulations of the discipline. It calls for a special set of values and behaviours, including honesty, integrity, reliability, responsibility, and compassion – but also self-awareness and a knowledge of limits.

proflavine (proh-**flay**-vin) *n.* a dye used as an antiseptic in the form of a cream for minor burns and abrasions.

profunda (proh-**fun**-dă) *adj.* describing blood vessels that are deeply embedded in the tissues they supply.

profundaplasty (proh-**fun**-dă-plasti) *n.* surgical enlargement of the junction of the femoral artery and its deep branch, a common operation to relieve narrowing by atherosclerosis at this point.

progeria (proh-**jeer**-iă) *n.* a very rare condition in which all the signs of old age appear and progress in a child, so that 'senility' is reached before puberty.

progesterone (proh-**jest**-er-ohn) *n.* a steroid hormone secreted by the corpus luteum of the ovary, the placenta, and also (in small amounts) by the adrenal cortex and testes. It is responsible for preparing the endometrium of the uterus for pregnancy.

progestogen (proh-**jest**-oh-jĕn) *n.* one of a group of naturally occurring or synthetic steroid hormones, including progesterone, that maintain the normal course of pregnancy. Progestogens are used to treat premenstrual tension, amenorrhoea, and abnormal bleeding from the uterus. Because they prevent ovulation, progestogens are a major constituent of oral contraceptives and other forms of hormonal contraception.

proglottis (proh-**glot**-iss) *n.* (*pl.* **proglottids** or **proglottides**) one of the segments of a tapeworm. Mature segments, situated at the posterior end of the worm, each consist mainly of a branched uterus packed with eggs.

prognathism (prog-nă-thizm) *n.* abnormal protrusion of one or both jaws. **—prognathic** (prog-**nath**-ik) *adj.*

prognosis (prog-**noh**-sis) *n.* an assessment of the future course and outcome of a patient's disease.

progressive (prŏ-**gres**-iv) *adj.* (of a disease) increasing in severity or extent; expected to get worse.

progressive supranuclear palsy (Steele-Richardson-Olszewski syndrome) *n.* a progressive neurological disorder resulting from degeneration of the motor neurons, basal ganglia, and brainstem. Starting in late middle age, it is characterized by a staring facial expression due to impaired ability to move the eyes up and down, progressing to difficulties in swallowing, speech, balance, and movement and general spasticity.

proguanil (proh-**gwan**-il) *n.* a drug that kills malaria parasites and is administered by mouth in combination with atovaquone (as **Malarone**) for the prevention and treatment of falciparum malaria. Alone or in combination with chloroquine (as **Paludrine/Avloclor**) it may be used for the prevention of malaria. Trade name: **Paludrine**.

proinsulin (proh-**ins**-yoo-lin) *n.* a substance produced in the pancreas from which the hormone insulin is derived.

projection (prŏ-**jek**-shŏn) *n.* (in psychology) the attribution of one's own qualities to other people. In psychoanalysis, this is considered to be one of the defence mechanisms; people who cannot tolerate their own feelings may cope by imagining that other people have those feelings.

prolactin (lactogenic hormone, luteotrophic hormone, luteotrophin) (proh-**lak**-tin) *n.* a hormone, synthesized and stored in the anterior pituitary gland, that stimulates milk production after childbirth and also stimulates production of progesterone by the corpus luteum in the ovary.

prolactinoma (proh-lak-tin-**oh**-mă) *n.* a benign tumour (an adenoma) of the pituitary gland that secretes excessive amounts of prolactin (*see* hyperprolactinaemia). If the tumour is large enough it may compress and damage adjacent structures.

prolapse (**proh**-laps) *n.* downward displacement of an organ or tissue from its normal position. **p. of the rectum** descent of the rectum to lie outside the anus. **p. of the uterus** descent of the cervix, or the whole of the uterus, into the vagina. The cervix may be visible at the vaginal opening or the uterus may be completely outside the vagina. It is often caused by stretching and tearing of the supporting tissues during childbirth.

prolapsed intervertebral disc (PID) *n.* a 'slipped disc': protrusion of the pulpy inner material of an intervertebral disc through a tear in the fibrous outer coat, causing pressure on adjoining nerve roots, ligaments, etc. Treatment is by rest, traction, and analgesics; if these fail, surgery may be necessary (*see* discectomy, laminectomy, microdiscectomy).

proliferate (prŏ-**lif**-er-ayt) *vb.* to grow rapidly by cell division:

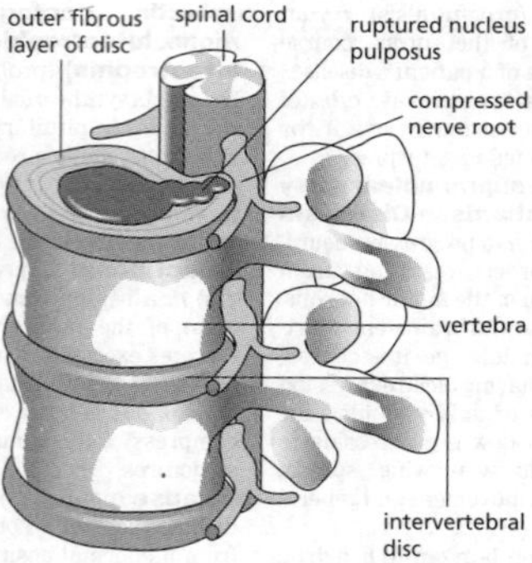

Prolapsed intervertebral disc

applied particularly to malignant tumours. **—proliferation** *n.*

proline (proh-leen) *n.* an amino acid found in many proteins.

promazine (proh-mă-zeen) *n.* a phenothiazine antipsychotic drug administered by mouth to relieve agitation, confusion, and restlessness.

promethazine (proh-meth-ă-zeen) *n.* a powerful antihistamine drug administered by mouth or injection to treat allergic conditions and insomnia. It is also used as an antiemetic. Trade names: **Avomine**, **Phenergan**.

promontory (prom-ŏn-ter-i) *n.* (in anatomy) a projecting part of an organ or other structure.

pronation (proh-nay-shŏn) *n.* the act of turning the hand so that the palm faces downwards. In this position the radius and ulna are crossed. *Compare* supination.

pronator (proh-nay-ter) *n.* any muscle that causes pronation of the forearm and hand.

prone (prohn) *adj.* **1.** lying with the face downwards. **2.** (of the forearm) in the position in which the palm of the hand faces downwards. *Compare* supine.

propantheline (proh-panth-ĕ-leen) *n.* an antimuscarinic drug that decreases activity of smooth muscle (*see* antispasmodic) and is administered by mouth to treat disorders of the digestive system. Trade name: **Pro-Banthine**.

properdin (proh-per-din) *n.* a group of substances in blood plasma that, in combination with complement and magnesium ions, is capable of destroying certain bacteria and viruses.

prophase (proh-fayz) *n.* the first stage of mitosis and of each division of meiosis, in which the chromosomes become visible under the microscope.

prophylactic (pro-fil-**ak**-tik) *n.* an agent that prevents the development of a condition or disease.

prophylaxis (pro-fil-**aks**-iss) *n.* any means taken to prevent disease, such as immunization. **—prophylactic** *adj.*

propranolol (proh-**pran**-ŏ-lol) *n.* a drug (*see* beta blocker) administered by mouth or injection to treat abnormal heart rhythm, angina, and high blood pressure. It is also used to relieve the symptoms of thyrotoxicosis and anxiety associated with palpitation or tremor and to prevent migraine headaches. Trade names: **Half-Inderal LA**, **Inderal LA**.

proprietary name (prŏ-**pry**-ĕt-er-i) *n.* (in pharmacy) the trade name of a drug: the name assigned to it by the firm that manufactured it.

proprioception (proh-pri-ŏ-**sep**-shŏn) *n.* the ability to use the senses in a coordinated way, by means of the action of proprioceptors, that enables a person to identify where parts of their body are located even when they are physiologically separate.

proprioceptor (proh-pri-ŏ-**sep**-ter) *n.* a specialized sensory nerve ending (*see* receptor) that monitors internal changes in the body brought about by movement and muscular activity. Proprioceptors in muscles and tendons assist in coordinating muscular activity.

proptosis (prop-**toh**-sis) *n.* forward displacement of an organ, especially the eye (*see* exophthalmos).

propylthiouracil (proh-pil-th'y-oh-**yoor**-ă-sil) *n.* a drug that reduces thyroid activity and is administered by mouth to treat thyrotoxicosis and to prepare patients for surgical removal of the thyroid gland.

Proscar (**pros**-kar) *n. see* finasteride.

prosop- (prosopo-) *combining form denoting* the face.

prosopagnosia (proz-oh-pag-**noh**-ziă) *n.* inability to recognize faces, either in person or in photographs, due to damage in the right occipito-temporal area of the brain. Causes include stroke and brain tumours.

prospective study (prŏ-**spek**-tiv) *n.* a systematic study of a group of individuals for a defined period or until the occurrence of a specified event (e.g. onset of illness, death) in order to observe patterns of disease and/or cause of death. *Compare* retrospective study.

prostaglandin (pros-tă-**gland**-in) *n.* one of a group of hormone-like substances present in a wide variety of tissues and body fluids. Prostaglandins have many actions; for example, they cause contraction of smooth muscle (including that of the uterus) and dilatation of blood vessels, they are mediators in the process of inflammation, and they are involved in the production of mucus in the stomach. Synthetic prostaglandins are used to induce labour or produce abortion and to treat peptic ulcers, glaucoma, and (in newborn babies) congenital heart disease.

prostate cancer (pros-tayt) *n.* a malignant tumour (carcinoma) of the prostate gland, a common form of cancer in elderly men. In most men it progresses slowly over many years and gives symptoms similar to those of benign enlargement of the prostate (*see* prostate gland).

prostatectomy (pros-tă-**tek**-tŏmi) *n.* surgical removal of some or all of the prostate gland. The operation is necessary to relieve retention of urine due to enlargement of the prostate or to reduce lower urinary tract symptoms thought to be due to benign prostatic hyperplasia. It can be performed through the bladder (**transvesical p.**), through the surrounding capsule of the prostate (**retropubic p.**), or through the urethra (**transurethral p.**). **radical** (or **total**) **p.** removal of the prostate with its capsule and the seminal vesicles, performed for the treatment of prostate cancer confined to the gland. *See also* resection.

prostate gland *n.* a male accessory sex gland that opens into the urethra just below the bladder and vas deferens. During ejaculation it secretes an alkaline fluid that forms part of the semen. The prostate may become enlarged in elderly men (**benign prostatic hyperplasia**, **BPH**). This may result in obstruction of the neck of the bladder and is treated by surgery (*see* prostatectomy, resection) or by means of drugs. See illustration.

SEE WEB LINKS

- Information about the prostate gland and PSA testing from Macmillan Cancer Support

prostate specific antigen (PSA) *n.* a protease enzyme produced by the glandular epithelium of the prostate. Its effect is to liquefy the semen within the ejaculate. Increased quantities are secreted when the gland becomes enlarged or inflamed and levels of PSA in the blood are significantly elevated in cancer of the prostate.

prostatic intraepithelial neoplasia (PIN) (pros-tat-ik) *n.* abnormal cells in the prostate that are not cancer, but may be associated with cancer within the

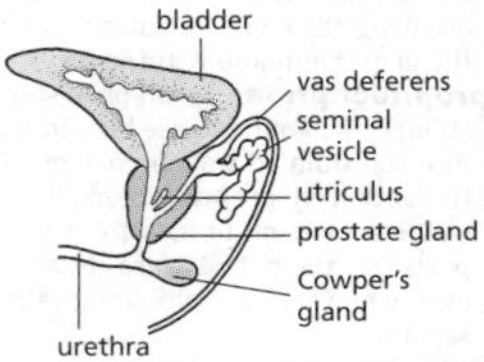

The prostate gland and associated structures (median view)

prostate. Typically, PIN will be found in prostate biopsies taken because levels of prostate specific antigen are elevated.

prostatitis (pros-tă-**ty**-tis) *n.* inflammation of the prostate gland. This may be due to bacterial infection and can be either acute or chronic.

prostatocystitis (pros-tă-toh-sis-**ty**-tis) *n.* inflammation of the prostate gland associated with inflammation of the urinary bladder.

prostatorrhoea (pros-tă-tŏ-**ree**-ă) *n.* an abnormal discharge of thin watery fluid from the prostate gland. This occurs in some patients with acute prostatitis.

prosthesis (pros-**th'ee**-sis) *n.* (*pl.* **prostheses**) any artificial device that is attached to the body as a substitute for a missing or nonfunctional part. Prostheses include artificial limbs, hearing aids and cochlear implants, dentures, and implanted pacemakers. *See also* implant. **penile p.** a malleable, semirigid, or inflatable rod inserted into the corpora cavernosa of the penis to produce rigidity sufficient for vaginal penetration in men with erectile dysfunction. **—prosthetic** (pros-**thet**-ik) *adj.*

prosthodontics (prosthetic dentistry) (pros-thoh-**don**-tiks) *n.* the branch of dentistry concerned with the provision of dentures, bridges, and implant-retained prostheses.

prostration (pros-**tray**-shŏn) *n.* extreme exhaustion.

protamine (**proh**-tă-meen) *n.* one of a group of simple proteins that can be conjugated with nucleic acids to form nucleoproteins. **p. sulphate** an antidote to heparin overdosage in oral anticoagulant therapy, given by intravenous injection or infusion. **p. zinc insulin** (Hypurin) a combination of protamine, insulin, and zinc that is absorbed much more slowly than ordinary insulin and thus reduces the frequency of injections.

protanopia (proh-tă-**noh**-piă) *n.* *see* Daltonism.

protease (**proh**-ti-ayz) *n.* any enzyme that catalyses the splitting of a protein.

protease inhibitor *n.* one of a class of antiretroviral drugs used in the treatment of HIV infection and AIDS. They inhibit the action of protease produced by HIV, required by viral growth and replication. Protease inhibitors include **atazanavir** (Reyataz), **indinavir** (Crixivan), **lopinavir** (Kaletra), and **tipranavir** (Aptivus).

protein (**proh**-teen) *n.* one of a group of organic compounds made up of one or more chains of amino acids. Proteins are essential constituents of the body; they form the structural material of muscles, tissues, organs, etc., and are equally important as regulators of function, as enzymes and hormones. Proteins are synthesized in the body from their constituent amino acids, which are obtained from the digestion of protein in the diet.

proteinuria (proh-tin-**yoor**-iă) *n.* *see* albuminuria.

proteolysis (proh-ti-**ol**-i-sis) *n.* the process whereby protein molecules are broken down by proteolytic enzymes into their constituent amino acids, which are then absorbed into the bloodstream. —**proteolytic** (proh-ti-ŏ-**lit**-ik) *adj.*

proteolytic enzyme *n.* a digestive enzyme that causes the breakdown of protein.

proteose (**proh**-ti-ohz) *n.* a product of the hydrolytic decomposition of protein.

Proteus (**proh**-ti-ŭs) *n.* a genus of rodlike Gram-negative flagellate highly motile bacteria common in the intestines and in decaying organic material. **P. vulgaris** a species that can cause urinary tract infections.

prothrombin (PT) (proh-**throm**-bin) *n.* a substance, present in blood plasma, that is the inactive precursor from which the enzyme thrombin is derived during the process of blood coagulation. *See also* coagulation factors. **p. time** (**PT**) the time taken for blood clotting to occur in a sample of blood to which calcium and thromboplastin have been added; a prolonged PT indicates a deficiency of coagulation factors. Measurement of PT is used to control anticoagulant therapy (e.g. with warfarin).

proto- *combining form denoting* **1.** first. **2.** primitive; early. **3.** a precursor.

proton-pump inhibitor (proh-ton-pump) *n.* a drug that reduces gastric acid secretion by blocking an enzyme (the **proton pump**) within the oxyntic (parietal) cells of the gastric glands. Proton-pump inhibitors include omeprazole, lansoprazole, **pantoprazole**, and rabeprazole; they are used for treating gastro-oesophageal reflux, peptic ulcer, and acid hypersecretion associated with gastrinoma.

protopathic (proh-tŏ-**path**-ik) *adj.* describing the ability to perceive only strong stimuli of pain, heat, etc. *Compare* epicritic.

protoplasm (**proh**-tŏ-plazm) *n.* the material of which living cells are made, which includes the cytoplasm and nucleus. —**protoplasmic** *adj.*

protoporphyrin IX (proh-toh-**por**-fi-rin) *n.* the most common type of porphyrin found in nature. It is a constituent of haemoglobin, myoglobin, and the commoner chlorophylls.

protozoa (proh-tŏ-**zoh**-ă) *pl. n.* a group of microscopic single-celled organisms. Most protozoa are free-living but some, such as Plasmodium and Leishmania, are important disease-causing parasites of humans. *See also* amoeba. —**protozoan** *adj.*, *n.*

protuberance (prŏ-**tew**-ber-ăns) *n.* (in anatomy) a rounded projecting part.

proud flesh (prowd) *n.* a large amount of soft granulation tissue that may develop during the healing of a wound of large surface area.

provitamin (proh-**vit**-ă-min) *n.* a substance that is not itself a vitamin but can be converted to a vitamin in the body. An example is β-carotene, which can be converted into vitamin A.

proximal (**proks**-i-măl) *adj.* (in anatomy) situated close to the origin or point of attachment or close to the median line of the body. *Compare* distal.

Prozac (proh-zak) *n. see* fluoxetine.

prune belly syndrome (Eagle-Barrett syndrome) (proon) *n.* a hereditary condition, occurring exclusively in males, characterized by a deficiency of abdominal muscles, complex malformation of the urinary tract, and bilateral undescended testes. The lungs may be underdeveloped. The name derives from the typically wrinkled appearance of the skin over the abdomen.

prurigo (proor-I-goh) *n.* an intensely itchy eruption. **Besnier's p.** chronic lichenified atopic eczema. **nodular p.** a condition of unknown cause, usually found in atopic individuals (*see* atopy), in which severely itching nodules mostly occur on the distal limbs. **p. of pregnancy** prurigo occurring in the middle trimester of pregnancy, affecting mainly the abdomen and the extensor surfaces of the limbs. It may recur in later pregnancies.

pruritus (proor-I-tŭs) *n.* itching; the predominant symptom of atopic eczema, lichen planus, and many other skin diseases. It also occurs in the elderly and may be a manifestation of psychological illness. Perineal itching is common: itching of the vulva in women is termed **p. vulvae**, whereas itching of the perianal region (**p. ani**), is most common in men. Causes of perineal itching include poor hygiene, candidiasis, threadworms, and itchy skin diseases (such as eczema). **p. gravidarum** generalized itching during pregnancy that starts in the first trimester and is associated with obstetric cholestasis.

prussic acid (prus-ik) *n. see* hydrocyanic acid.

PSA *n. see* prostate specific antigen.

psammoma (sam-**oh**-mă) *n.* a tumour containing gritty sandlike particles (**p. bodies**). It is typical of cancer of the ovary but may also be found in the meninges.

pseud- (pseudo-) *combining form denoting* superficial resemblance to; false.

pseudarthrosis (nearthrosis) (s'yood-arth-**roh**-sis) *n.* a 'false' joint, which can be a childhood condition (**congenital p.**) or occur in adults when a fracture fails to unite and the bone ends are separated by fibrous tissue.

pseudoangina (s'yoo-doh-an-**jy**-nă) *n.* pain in the centre of the chest in the absence of heart disease. It is associated with anxiety and may be part of the effort syndrome.

pseudocholinesterase (s'yoo-doh-koh-lin-**est**-er-ayz) *n.* an enzyme found in the blood and other tissues that breaks down acetylcholine, but much more slowly than cholinesterase.

pseudocoxalgia (s'yoo-doh-koks-**al**-jiă) *n. see* Legg-Calvé-Perthes disease.

pseudocrisis (s'yoo-doh-**kry**-sis) *n.* a false crisis: a sudden but temporary change in a condition, such as a fall of temperature in a patient with fever.

pseudocyesis (phantom pregnancy) (s'yoo-doh-sy-**ee**-sis) *n.* a condition in which a nonpregnant woman exhibits symptoms of pregnancy, e.g. enlarged abdomen, morning sickness, and absence of menstruation. The condition usually has an emotional basis.

pseudocyst (**s'yoo**-doh-sist) *n.* a fluid-filled space within an organ that is not enclosed by an epithelial lining. **pancreatic p.** a pseudocyst that may develop in cases of chronic pancreatitis or as a complication of acute pancreatitis. It may cause abdominal pain accompanied by a rise in the level of pancreatic enzymes in the blood. Treatment is by endoscopic or radiological drainage, or by surgery (*see* marsupialization).

pseudodementia (s'yoo-doh-di-**men**-shă) *n.* a condition in which symptoms of dementia, including memory disorders, are caused by depression rather than organic brain disease. It is most commonly seen in elderly depressed individuals.

pseudohermaphroditism (s'yoo-doh-her-**maf**-rŏ-dyt-izm) *n.* the condition of an individual who is genetically male (XY) or female (XX) and has normal internal sex organs but whose external genitalia resemble those of the opposite sex.

pseudohypertrophy (s'yoo-doh-hy-**per**-trŏ-fi) *n.* increase in the size of an organ or structure caused by excessive growth of cells that have a packing or supporting role. The result is usually a decline in the efficiency of the organ. **—pseudohypertrophic** (s'yoo-doh-hy-per-**trof**-ik) *adj.*

pseudohypoparathyroidism (s'yoo-doh-hy-poh-pa-ră-**th'y**-roid-izm) *n.* a syndrome of learning disability, restricted growth, and bony abnormalities due to a genetic defect that causes lack of response to parathyroid hormone. *See also* Albright's hereditary osteodystrophy.

pseudomembranous colitis (s'yoo-doh-**mem**-brăn-ŭs) *n. see* colitis.

Pseudomonas (s'yoo-doh-**moh**-năs) *n.* a genus of rodlike motile pigmented Gram-negative bacteria. Most live in soil and decomposing organic matter. **P. aeruginosa** a species that occurs in pus from wounds; it is associated with urinary tract infections. **P. pseudomallei** the causative agent of melioidosis.

pseudomyxoma (s'yoo-doh-miks-**oh**-mă) *n.* a mucoid tumour of the peritoneum, often seen in association with myxomas of the ovary.

pseudo-obstruction (acute colonic pseudo-obstruction, Ogilvie's syndrome) (s'yoo-doh-ŏb-**struk**-shŏn) *n.* functional impairment of intestinal peristalsis without evidence of an obstructing lesion. It commonly occurs in hospitalized patients with serious illness; vomiting, constipation, and abdominal distension are usually present.

pseudopodium (s'yoo-doh-**poh**-diŭm) *n.* (*pl.* **pseudopodia**) a temporary and constantly changing extension of the body of an amoeba or an amoeboid cell. Pseudopodia engulf bacteria and other particles as food and are responsible for the movements of the cell.

pseudopolyposis (s'yoo-doh-pol-i-**poh**-sis) *n.* a condition in which the bowel lining (mucosa) is covered by elevated or protuberant plaques (**pseudopolyps**) that are not true polyps but abnormal growth of inflamed mucosa. It is usually found in patients with long-standing ulcerative colitis.

pseudoxanthoma elasticum (s'yoo-doh-zanth-**oh**-mă i-**lass**-tik-ŭm) *n.* a hereditary disease in which elastic fibres (*see* elastic tissue) become calcified. The skin becomes lax and yellowish nodules develop in affected areas; this is accompanied by degenerative changes in the blood vessels.

psilosis (sy-**loh**-sis) *n. see* sprue.

psittacosis (parrot disease, ornithosis) (sit-ă-**koh**-sis) *n.* an endemic infection of birds, especially parrots, budgerigars, canaries, finches, pigeons, and poultry, caused by the bacterium *Chlamydia psittaci*. The infection is transmitted to humans by inhalation from handling the birds or by contact with feathers, faeces, or cage dust, but person-to-person transmission also occurs. The symptoms include fever, dry cough, severe muscle pain, and headache; occasionally a severe generalized systemic illness results. The condition responds to tetracycline or erythromycin.

psoas (psoas major) (soh-ăs) *n.* a muscle in the groin that acts jointly with the iliacus muscle to flex the hip joint. A smaller muscle (**p. minor**) has the same action but is often absent.

psoas sign *n.* an indicator of acute appendicitis. The appendix lies close to the iliopsoas muscle: if it is inflamed, any movement that involves the right psoas muscle (such as extension of the right thigh) will be painful in the right lower quadrant.

psoralen (sor-**ah**-lĕn) *n. see* puva.

psoriasis (sŏ-**ry**-ă-sis) *n.* a chronic disease in which scaly pink patches form on the elbows, knees, scalp, and other parts of the body. Psoriasis is one of the commonest skin diseases in Britain. It may occur in association with arthritis (**psoriatic arthritis**). The disease may be very severe, affecting much of the skin and causing considerable disability in the patient. **p. area severity index (PASI)** a semiobjective severity score for psoriasis, including measurement of surface area affected and the degree of erythema, induration, and scale. Commonly used in clinical trials and to ration expensive treatments, it is often interpreted with the dermatology life quality index (DLQI) score. **—psoriatic** (sor-i-**at**-ik) *adj.*

PSV *n. see* pressure support ventilation.

psych- (psycho-) *combining form denoting* **1.** the mind; psyche. **2.** psychology.

psyche (sy-ki) *n.* the mind or the soul; the mental (as opposed to the physical) functioning of the individual.

psychedelic (sy-ki-**del**-ik) *adj.* describing drugs, such as cannabis and LSD, that can induce changes in the level of consciousness of the mind.

psychiatric intensive care unit (PICU) *n.* a unit especially designed for nursing the most acutely and severely mentally ill, often a locked ward with increased staffing levels on which patients stay for the shortest possible period before being transferred to an open psychiatric ward.

psychiatrist (si-**ky**-ă-trist) *n.* a medically qualified physician who specializes in the study and treatment of mental disorders.

psychiatry (si-**ky**-ă-tri) *n.* the study of mental disorders and their diagnosis, management, and prevention. —**psychiatric** (sy-ki-**at**-rik) *adj.*

psychic (sy-kik) *adj.* **1.** of or relating to the psyche. **2.** relating to parapsychological phenomena.

psychoanalysis (sy-koh-ă-**nal**-i-sis) *n.* a school of psychology and a method of treating mental disorders based upon the teachings of Sigmund Freud (1856–1939). Psychoanalysis employs the technique of free association in the course of intensive psychotherapy in order to bring repressed fears and conflicts to the conscious mind, where they can be dealt with (*see* repression). —**psychoanalyst** (sy-koh-**an**-ă-list) *n.* —**psychoanalytic** (sy-koh-an-ă-**lit**-ik) *adj.*

psychodrama (sy-koh-drah-mă) *n.* a form of group psychotherapy in which individuals acquire insight into themselves by acting out situations from their past with other group members. *See* group therapy.

psychodynamics (sy-koh-dy-**nam**-iks) *n.* the study of the mind in action. —**psychodynamic** *adj.*

psychogenic (sy-koh-**jen**-ik) *adj.* having an origin in the mind rather than in the body. The term is applied particularly to symptoms and illnesses.

psychogeriatrics (sy-koh-je-ri-**at**-riks) *n.* the branch of psychiatry that deals with the mental disorders of older people. —**psychogeriatric** *adj.*

psychologist (sy-**kol**-ŏ-jist) *n.* a person who is engaged in the scientific study of the mind. **clinical p.** a psychologist trained in aspects of the assessment and treatment of the ill and handicapped. He or she usually works in a hospital. **educational p.** a psychologist trained in aspects of the cognitive and emotional development of children. He or she usually works in close association with schools.

psychology (sy-**kol**-ŏji) *n.* the science concerned with the study of behaviour and its related mental processes. The different schools of psychology include behaviourism, cognitive psychology, psychoanalysis, and gestaltism. —**psychological** (sy-kŏ-**loj**-ikăl) *adj.*

psychometrics (sy-koh-**met**-riks) *n.* the measurement of individual differences in psychological functions (such as intelligence and personality) by means of standardized tests. **—psychometric** *adj.*

psychomotor (sy-koh-**moh**-ter) *adj.* relating to muscular and mental activity. The term is applied to disorders in which muscular activities are affected by cerebral disturbance.

psychoneuroimmunology (sy-koh-newr-oh-im-yoo-**nol**-ŏji) *n.* the study of the effects of the mind on the functioning of the immune system, especially in relation to the influence of the mind on susceptibility to disease and the progression of a disease.

psychopath (sy-koh-path) *n.* a person who behaves in an antisocial way and shows little or no guilt for antisocial acts and little capacity for forming emotional relationships with others. *See also* antisocial personality disorder. **—psychopathic** *adj.* **—psychopathy** (sy-**kop**-ă-thi) *n.*

psychopathology (sy-koh-pă-**thol**-ŏji) *n.* **1.** the study of mental disorders, with the aim of explaining and describing aberrant behaviour. *Compare* psychiatry. **2.** the symptoms, collectively, of a mental disorder. **—psychopathological** *adj.*

psychopharmacology (sy-koh-farm-ă-**kol**-ŏji) *n.* the study of the effects of drugs on mental processes and behaviour, particularly psychotropic drugs.

psychophysiology (sy-koh-fiz-i-**ol**-ŏji) *n.* the branch of psychology that records physiological measurements, such as heart rate and size of the pupil, and relates them to psychological events. **—psychophysiological** *adj.*

psychosexual development (sy-koh-**seks**-yoo-ăl) *n.* the process by which an individual becomes more mature in his sexual feelings and behaviour. Gender identity, sex-role behaviour, and choice of sexual partner are the three major areas of development.

psychosis (sy-**koh**-sis) *n.* one of a group of mental illnesses that feature loss of contact with reality. The psychoses include schizophrenia, major disorders of affect (*see* bipolar affective disorder), major paranoid states, and organic mental disorders. Psychotic disorders may feature delusions, hallucinations, severe thought disturbances, abnormal alteration of mood, poverty of thought, and grossly abnormal behaviour. Many cases of psychotic illness respond well to antipsychotic drugs. **—psychotic** (sy-**kot**-ik) *adj.*

psychosocial (sy-koh-**soh**-shăl) *adj.* involving or relating to both the social and psychological aspects of a patient's life. **p. assessment** an interviewing technique that combines psychiatric history taking with elements of problem solving in psychotherapy, often used in patients who have presented with deliberate self-harm.

psychosomatic (sy-koh-sŏ-**mat**-ik) *adj.* relating to or involving both the mind and body: usually applied to illnesses, such as asthma and peptic ulcer, that are caused by the interaction of mental and physical factors.

SEE WEB LINKS

- Website of the journal *Psychosomatic Medicine*

psychosurgery (sy-koh-**ser**-jer-i) *n.* surgery on the brain to relieve psychological symptoms, such as severe chronic anxiety, obsessive–compulsive disorder, depression, and untreatable pain. —**psychosurgical** *adj.*

psychotherapy (sy-koh-**th'e**-răpi) *n.* psychological (as opposed to physical) methods for the treatment of mental disorders and psychological problems. There are many different approaches to psychotherapy, including psychoanalysis, client-centred therapy, group therapy, and family therapy. *See also* behaviour therapy, cognitive behavioural therapy, counselling. —**psychotherapeutic** (sy-koh-th'e-ră-**pew**-tik) *adj.* —**psychotherapist** *n.*

psychoticism (sy-**kot**-i-sizm) *n.* a dimension of personality characterized by aggression, emotional coldness, and manipulativeness.

psychotropic (sy-koh-**trop**-ik) *adj.* describing drugs that affect mood. Antidepressants, sedatives, CNS stimulants, and antipsychotics are psychotropic.

PT *n. see* prothrombin.

PTC *n. see* (percutaneous transhepatic) cholangiography.

pterion (**teer**-i-ŏn) *n.* the point on the side of the skull at which the sutures between the parietal, temporal, and sphenoid bones meet.

pteroylglutamic acid (te-roh-il-gloo-**tam**-ik) *n. see* folate.

pterygium (tĕ-**rij**-iŭm) *n.* **1.** a triangular overgrowth of the cornea, usually the inner side, by thickened and degenerative conjunctiva. **2.** a triangular overgrowth of nail-fold skin extending onto the nail bed.

pterygo- *combining form denoting* the pterygoid process.

pterygoid process (te-ri-goid) *n.* either of two large processes of the sphenoid bone.

ptomaine (**toh**-mayn) *n.* any of various substances, such as putrescine, cadaverine, and neurine, produced in decaying foodstuffs and responsible for the unpleasant taste and smell of such foods. Ptomaines themselves are harmless, but they are often associated with toxic bacteria.

ptosis (blepharoptosis) (**toh**-sis) *n.* drooping of the upper eyelid. This may be due to a disorder of the oculomotor nerve, a disease of the eye muscles, or myasthenia gravis; it may also occur as part of Horner's syndrome or as an isolated congenital feature. It is also associated with the pain of a cluster headache.

-ptosis *combining form denoting* a lowered position of an organ or part; prolapse.

PTSD *n. see* post-traumatic stress disorder.

PTTK *n.* partial thromboplastin time with kaolin, also known as **activated partial thromboplastin time** (**APTT**): a method for estimating the degree of anticoagulation induced by heparin therapy for venous thrombosis.

ptyal- (ptyalo-) *combining form denoting* saliva.

ptyalin (ty-ă-lin) *n.* an enzyme (an amylase) found in saliva.

ptyalism (sialorrhoea)˙ (ty-ă-lizm) *n.* the excessive production of saliva: a symptom of certain nervous disorders, poisoning, or infection (rabies). *Compare* dry mouth.

ptyalith (ty-ă-lith) *n.* a stone (calculus) in a salivary gland or duct.

ptyalography (ty-ă-**log**-răfi) *n. see* sialography.

puberty (**pew**-ber-ti) *n.* the time at which the onset of sexual maturity occurs and the reproductive organs become functional (*see* gonadarche). It is manifested in both sexes by the appearance of secondary sexual characteristics and in girls by the start of menstruation. *See also* precocious puberty. —**pubertal** *adj.*

pubes (**pew**-beez) *n.* **1.** the body surface that overlies the pubis, at the front of the pelvis. **2.** *see* pubis. —**pubic** *adj.*

pubiotomy (pew-bi-**ot**-ŏmi) *n.* an operation to divide the pubic bone near the symphysis, now only rarely performed during childbirth to increase the size of an abnormally small pelvis or to facilitate access to the base of the bladder and the urethra during complex urological procedures.

pubis (**pew**-bis) *n.* (*pl.* **pubes**) a bone forming the lower and anterior part of each side of the hip bone (*see also* pelvis). The two pubes meet at the front of the pelvis at the **pubic symphysis**. *See also* pubes.

Public Health England (PHE) (**pub**-lik) *n.* an executive agency of the Department of Health with responsibility for providing national leadership on health protection, health improvement, and public health knowledge. In addition to the national team, there are four regional offices and fifteen local centres providing support to clinical commissioning groups, local authorities, and health-care providers. PHE also hosts a network of specialist and reference microbiology laboratories

SEE WEB LINKS

- Public Health England website

public health medicine *n.* the speciality concerned with preventing disease in populations as distinct from individuals. Formerly known as **community** or **social medicine**, it includes epidemiology, health promotion, health service planning, health protection, and evaluation.

public health nurse *n. see* health visitor.

pudendal (pew-**den**-d'l) *adj.* relating to the pudendum. **p. block** anaesthesia of the pudendum and surrounding areas by injecting a local anaesthetic into the nerves that supply them. It is performed to relieve the pain of the expulsive stage of labour. *See also* nerve block. **p. nerve** the nerve that supplies the lowest muscles of the pelvic floor and the anal sphincter. It is often damaged in childbirth, causing incontinence.

pudendum (pew-**den**-dŭm) *n.* (*pl.* **pudenda**) the external genital organs, especially those of the female (*see* vulva).

puerperal (pew-er-per-ăl) *adj.* relating to childbirth or the period that immediately follows it. **p. infection** infection of the female genital tract arising as a complication of childbirth. **p. psychosis** a severe psychiatric disturbance, which may be depressive, manic, or schizophrenic, that is triggered by childbirth and usually arises in the first two weeks after delivery. The patient needs to be hospitalized for treatment and to prevent harm to the baby. *Compare* postnatal (depression), postpartum (blues). **p. pyrexia** a temperature of 38°C occurring on any two days within 14 days of childbirth or miscarriage. It is an indicator of postpartum sepsis.

puerperium (pew-er-peer-iŭm) *n.* the period of up to about six weeks after childbirth, during which the mother's body returns to its pre-pregnant state and her uterus returns to its normal size.

Pulex (pew-leks) *n.* a genus of widely distributed fleas. **P. irritans** the human flea: a common parasite whose bite may give rise to intense irritation and bacterial infection.

pulmo- (pulmon(o)-) *combining form denoting* the lung(s).

pulmonary (pul-mŏn-er-i) *adj.* relating to, associated with, or affecting the lungs. **p. artery** the artery that conveys deoxygenated blood from the heart to the lungs for oxygenation. **p. capillary wedge pressure** (**PCWP**) an indirect measurement of the pressure of blood in the left atrium of the heart, which indicates the adequacy of left heart function. It is measured using a catheter wedged in the most distal segment of the pulmonary artery. **p. circulation** *see* circulation. **p. embolism** *see* embolism. **p. hypertension** raised blood pressure within the blood vessels supplying the lungs. Pulmonary hypertension may complicate pulmonary embolism, septal defects, heart failure, diseases of the mitral valve, and chronic lung diseases. **p. stenosis** congenital narrowing of the outlet of the right ventricle of the heart. Severe pulmonary stenosis may produce angina pectoris, faintness, and heart failure. The defect is corrected by surgery. **p. surfactant** *see* surfactant. **p. tuberculosis** *see* tuberculosis. **p. valve** a semilunar valve in the heart, between the right ventricle and the pulmonary artery, that prevents the backflow of blood from this artery to the right ventricle. **p. vein** a vein carrying oxygenated blood from the lung to the left atrium.

pulp (pulp) *n.* **1.** a soft mass of tissue (for example, of the spleen). **2.** the mass of connective tissue containing blood vessels and nerve fibres at the centre of a tooth (**p. cavity**). **3.** the fleshy cushion on the flexor surface of the fingertip.

pulsatile (puls-ă-tyl) *adj.* characterized by regular rhythmical beating.

pulsation (pul-say-shŏn) *n.* a rhythmical throbbing or beating, as of the heart or arteries.

pulse (puls) *n.* a series of pressure waves within an artery caused by contractions of the left ventricle and corresponding with the heart rate. It is easily detected over certain superficial arteries (**p. points** – see illustration). The average adult pulse rate at rest is 60–80 per minute, but exercise, injury, illness, and emotion may produce much faster rates.

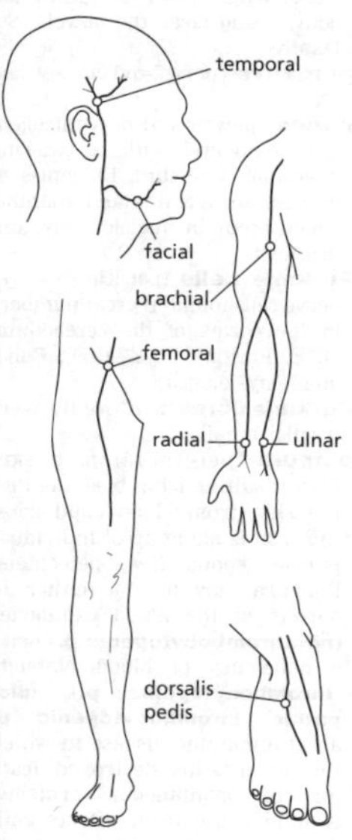

The pulse points

pulseless disease (puls-lis) *n.* *see* Takayasu's disease.

pulseless electrical activity (electromechanical dissociation) *n.* the appearance of normal-looking complexes on the electrocardiogram that are, however, associated with a state of cardiac arrest. It is usually caused by large pulmonary emboli, cardiac tamponade, tension pneumothorax, severe disturbance of body salt levels, severe haemorrhage, or hypothermia causing severe lack of oxygen to the heart muscle.

pulse oximetry (oks-im-it-ri) *n.* a technique for measuring the percentage of haemoglobin in arterial blood that is saturated with oxygen. Utilizing the fact that haemoglobin is photosensitive, it enables changes in oxygen levels to be rapidly detected. The equipment used (a **pulse oximeter**) incorporates a light-emitting sensor and photodetector placed on a finger, foot, or ear lobe; sites should be changed every 4 hours to prevent pressure necrosis. Saturation levels of less than 90% are a cause for concern.

pulse rhythm *n.* the regularity of the pulse: one of the aspects assessed when palpating a pulse. An irregular rhythm could indicate cardiac anomalies (*see* arrhythmia).

pulsus alternans (pul-sus awl-ter-nanz) *n.* a pulse in which there is a regular alternation of strong and weak beats without changes in the length of the cycle.

pulsus paradoxus (pa-ră-**doks**-ŭs) *n.* an exaggerated fall in systolic blood pressure and pulse volume when the patient breathes in. It is seen in constrictive pericarditis, pericardial effusion, and asthma.

pulvis (**pul**-vis) *n.* (in pharmaceutics) a powder.

punch-drunk syndrome *n.* a group of symptoms consisting of progressive dementia, tremor of the hands, epilepsy, and parkinsonism. It is a consequence of repeated blows to the head that have been severe enough to cause concussion.

punctate (**punk**-tayt) *adj.* spotted or dotted.

punctum (**punk**-tŭm) *n.* (*pl.* **puncta**) (in anatomy) a point or small area. **puncta lacrimalia** the two openings of the tear ducts in the inner corners of the upper and lower eyelids. *See* lacrimal (apparatus).

puncture (**punk**-cher) **1.** *n.* a wound made accidentally or deliberately by a sharp object or instrument. **needle p.** a puncture using a hollow needle to withdraw a sample of tissue (especially from the liver, bone marrow, or breast) for examination for diagnostic purposes. *See also* lumbar (puncture). **2.** *vb.* to pierce a tissue with a sharp instrument.

PUO *n.* pyrexia of unknown origin. *See* fever.

pupil (**pew**-pil) *n.* the circular opening in the centre of the iris, through which light passes into the lens of the eye. **—pupillary** (**pew**-pil-er-i) *adj.*

pupillary reflex (light reflex) *n.* the reflex change in the size of the pupil according to the amount of light entering the eye.

pupilloplasty (pew-**pil**-oh-plasti) *n.* a surgical procedure to alter the shape or function of the pupil. It is usually performed to repair a pupil damaged after trauma.

purgation (per-**gay**-shŏn) *n.* the use of drugs to stimulate intestinal activity and clear the bowels. *See* laxative.

purgative (**per**-gă-tiv) *n.* *see* laxative.

purine (**pewr**-reen) *n.* a nitrogenous compound with a two-ring molecular structure. Examples of purines are adenine and guanine, which occur in nucleic acids, and uric acid.

Purkinje cells (per-**kin**-ji) *pl. n.* nerve cells found in great numbers in the cortex of the cerebellum. [J. E. Purkinje (1787–1869), Bohemian physiologist]

Purkinje fibres *pl. n.* *see* atrioventricular bundle.

purpura (**per**-pew-ră) *n.* a skin rash resulting from bleeding into the skin from blood capillaries; the rash is made up of individual purple spots (*see* petechiae). Purpura may be due either to defects in the blood capillaries (**nonthrombocytopenic p.**) or to a deficiency of blood platelets (**thrombocytopenic p.**). **idiopathic thrombocytopenic p.** an autoimmune disease in which the platelets are destroyed, leading to spontaneous bruising. A mild acute form affects children; a more serious chronic form typically affects adults.

See also Henoch-Schönlein purpura, thrombocytopenia.

purulent (pewr-uu-lĕnt) *adj.* forming, consisting of, or containing pus.

pus (pus) *n.* a thick yellowish or greenish liquid formed at the site of an established infection. Pus contains dead white blood cells, both living and dead bacteria, and fragments of dead tissue. *See also* mucopus, seropus.

push-bang technique (puush-**bang**) *n.* a technique for removing a stone from the ureter. It consists of 'pushing' the stone back into the renal pelvis, where it can be destroyed by lithotripsy ('bang').

pustule (**pus**-tewl) *n.* a small blister on the skin that contains pus.

putamen (pew-**tay**-men) *n.* a part of the lenticular nucleus (*see* basal ganglia).

putrefaction (pew-tri-**fak**-shŏn) *n.* the process whereby proteins are decomposed by bacteria. This is accompanied by the formation of amines (such as putrescine and cadaverine) having a strong and very unpleasant smell.

PUVA (photochemotherapy) *n.* psoralen + ultraviolet A: the combination of a psoralen (a light-sensitive drug) and exposure to long-wave (315–400 nm) ultraviolet light (UVA). It is principally used for treating psoriasis.

PV per vaginam, i.e. via the vagina.

P value *n. see* significance.

PVD *n. see* peripheral vascular disease.

PVF *n. see* CFS/ME/PVF.

PVS *n. see* persistent vegetative state.

py- (pyo-) *combining form denoting* pus; a purulent condition.

pyaemia (py-**ee**-miă) *n.* blood poisoning by pus-forming bacteria released from an abscess. Widespread formation of abscesses may develop, with fatal results. *Compare* sapraemia, septicaemia, toxaemia.

pyarthrosis (py-arth-**roh**-sis) *n.* an infected joint filled with pus. *See* septic (arthritis).

pyel- (pyelo-) *combining form denoting* the pelvis of the kidney.

pyelitis (py-ĕ-**ly**-tis) *n.* inflammation of the pelvis of the kidney, usually caused by a bacterial infection. The patient experiences pain in the loins, shivering, and a high temperature. Treatment is by the administration of a suitable antibiotic, together with analgesics and a high fluid intake.

pyelocystitis (py-ĕ-loh-sis-**ty**-tis) *n.* inflammation of the renal pelvis and urinary bladder (*see* cystitis, pyelitis).

pyelogram (**py**-ĕ-loh-gram) *n.* an X-ray picture obtained by pyelography.

pyelography (py-ĕ-**log**-răfi) *n.* X-ray examination of the pelvis of the kidney using radiopaque contrast material. **anterograde p.** pyelography in which contrast material is injected directly into the renal pelvis through the skin. **intravenous p.** pyelography in which contrast material is introduced through a vein: usually part of intravenous urography. **retrograde p.** pyelography in which contrast material is injected directly into the renal pelvis through a tube inserted through the bladder and up the ureter at cystoscopy. *See also* urography.

pyelolithotomy (py-ĕ-loh-lith-**ot**-ŏmi) *n.* surgical removal of a stone from the kidney through an incision made in the pelvis of the kidney.

pyelonephritis (py-ĕ-loh-ni-**fry**-tis) *n.* bacterial infection of the kidney substance. **acute p.** pyelonephritis in which the patient has pain in the loins, a high temperature, and shivering fits. Treatment is by the administration of an appropriate antibiotic. **chronic p.** pyelonephritis in which the kidneys become small and scarred and kidney failure ensues. Vesicoureteric reflux in childhood is one of the causes.

pyeloplasty (**py**-ĕ-loh-plasti) *n.* an operation to relieve obstruction at the junction of the pelvis of the kidney and the ureter. The procedure is often perfomed laparoscopically. *See* Dietl's crisis, hydronephrosis.

pyelotomy (py-ĕ-**lot**-ŏmi) *n.* surgical incision into the pelvis of the kidney. This operation is usually undertaken to remove a stone (*see* pyelolithotomy).

pyg- (pygo-) *combining form denoting* the buttocks.

pykno- *combining form denoting* thickness or density.

pyl- (pyle-) *combining form denoting* the portal vein.

pylephlebitis (portal pyaemia) (py-li-fli-**by**-tis) *n.* septic inflammation and thrombosis of the hepatic portal vein, resulting from the spread of infection within the abdomen. The condition causes fever, liver abscesses, and ascites. Treatment is by antibiotic drugs and surgical drainage of abscesses.

pylethrombosis (py-li-throm-**boh**-sis) *n.* obstruction of the portal vein by a blood clot (*see* thrombosis), resulting from such conditions as pylephlebitis and cirrhosis of the liver. Portal hypertension is a frequent result.

PYLL *see* years of life lost.

pylor- (pyloro-) *combining form denoting* the pylorus.

pylorectomy (py-lor-**ek**-tŏmi) *n.* a surgical operation that involves the removal of the distal part of the stomach (pylorus). *See* antrectomy, pyloroplasty.

pyloric stenosis (py-**lor**-ik) *n.* narrowing of the outlet of the stomach (pylorus). This causes delay in the passage of stomach contents into the duodenum, leading to repeated vomiting, abdominal distention, dehydration, and weight loss. Pyloric stenosis in adults is caused by a peptic ulcer close to the pylorus or by a tumour invading it. **congenital hypertrophic p. s.** pyloric stenosis that occurs in babies about 3–5 weeks old (particularly boys) in which the thickened pyloric muscle can be felt as a nodule. Treatment is by pyloromyotomy.

pyloromyotomy (Ramstedt's operation) (py-lor-oh-my-**ot**-ŏmi) *n.* a surgical operation in which the muscle around the pylorus is divided down to the lining (mucosa) in order to relieve congenital pyloric stenosis.

pyloroplasty (py-**lor**-oh-plasti) *n.* a surgical operation in which the pylorus is widened by a form of reconstruction. It is done to allow the contents of the stomach to pass more easily into the duodenum.

pylorospasm (py-**lor**-oh-spazm) *n.* constriction of the pylorus due to muscle spasm, leading to delayed gastric emptying. It is usually associated with duodenal or pyloric ulcers.

pylorus (py-**lor**-ŭs) *n.* the lower end of the stomach, which leads to the duodenum. It terminates at a ring of muscle (**pyloric sphincter**), which contracts to close the opening by which the stomach communicates with the duodenum. **—pyloric** *adj.*

pyo- *combining form. see* py-.

pyocele (**py**-oh-seel) *n.* a swelling caused by an accumulation of pus in a part of the body.

pyocolpos (py-oh-**kol**-pos) *n.* the presence of pus in the vagina.

pyocyanin (py-oh-**sy**-ă-nin) *n.* an antibiotic substance produced by the bacterium *Pseudomonas aeruginosa*. It is used in medicine principally to attack Gram-positive bacteria.

pyoderma gangrenosum (py-oh-**der**-mă gang-ri-**noh**-sŭm) *n.* an acute destructive ulcerating process of the skin, especially the legs. It may be associated with ulcerative colitis or Crohn's disease or with rheumatoid arthritis or other forms of arthritis affecting many joints.

pyogenic (py-oh-**jen**-ik) *adj.* causing the formation of pus. **p. arthritis** *see* septic (arthritis). **p. granuloma** a common rapidly growing nodule on the surface of the skin. Resembling a redcurrant or (if large) a raspberry, it is composed of small blood vessels and therefore bleeds readily after the slightest injury.

pyometra (py-oh-**mee**-tră) *n.* the presence of pus in the uterus.

pyomyositis (py-oh-my-oh-**sy**-tis) *n.* bacterial or fungal infection of a muscle resulting in painful inflammation.

pyonephrosis (py-oh-ni-**froh**-sis) *n.* obstruction and infection of the kidney resulting in pus formation. A kidney stone is the usual cause of the obstruction, and the kidney becomes distended by pus and destroyed by the inflammation. Treatment is urgent nephrectomy under antibiotic cover.

pyopericarditis (py-oh-pe-ri-kar-**dy**-tis) *n.* inflammation of the pericardium, with the formation of pus.

pyopneumothorax (py-oh-new-moh-**thor**-aks) *n.* pus and gas or air in the pleural cavity. The condition can arise if air is introduced during attempts to drain the pus from an empyema. Alternatively a hydropneumothorax may become infected.

pyorrhoea (py-ŏ-**ree**-ă) *n.* a former name for periodontal disease.

pyosalpinx (py-oh-**sal**-pinks) *n.* the accumulation of pus in a Fallopian tube.

pyosis (py-**oh**-sis) *n.* the formation and discharge of pus.

pyothorax (py-oh-**thor**-aks) *n. see* empyema.

pyr- (pyro-) *combining form denoting* **1.** fire. **2.** a burning sensation. **3.** fever.

pyramid (pi-ră-mid) *n.* **1.** one of the conical masses that make up the medulla of the kidney. **2.** one of the elongated bulging areas on the anterior surface of the medulla oblongata in the brain. **—pyramidal** (pi-**ram**-i-d'l) *adj.*

pyramidal cell *n.* a type of neuron found in the cerebral cortex, with a pyramid-shaped cell body.

pyramidal system *n.* a collection of nerve fibres in the central nervous system that extend from the motor cortex in the brain to the spinal cord and are responsible for initiating movement. They form a pyramid in the medulla oblongata.

pyrazinamide (py-ră-**zin**-ă-myd) *n.* a drug administered by mouth, in conjunction with other drugs, to treat tuberculosis, particularly tuberculous meningitis. Trade name: **Zinamide**.

pyret- (pyreto-) *combining form denoting* fever.

pyrexia (py-**reks**-iă) *n. see* fever.

pyridostigmine (pi-ri-doh-**stig**-meen) *n.* a drug that inhibits the enzyme cholinesterase and is used to treat myasthenia gravis. It has a more prolonged action and is less toxic than neostigmine. Trade name: **Mestinon**.

pyridoxal phosphate (pi-ri-**doks**-ăl) *n.* a derivative of vitamin B_6 that is an important coenzyme in certain reactions of amino-acid metabolism. *See* transamination.

pyridoxine (vitamin B_6) (pi-ri-**doks**-een) *n. see* vitamin B.

pyrimethamine (pi-ri-**meth**-ă-meen) *n.* a drug administered by mouth in combination with the sulphonamide sulfadoxine (as **Fansidar**) for the treatment of falciparum malaria. It is also used, in combination with sulfadiazine, in the treatment of toxoplasmosis. Trade name: **Daraprim**.

pyrimidine (pi-**rim**-i-deen) *n.* a nitrogen-containing compound with a ring molecular structure. The commonest pyrimidines are cytosine, thymine, and uracil, which form the nucleotides of nucleic acids.

pyrogen (py-roh-jen) *n.* any substance or agent producing fever. **—pyrogenic** *adj.*

pyrosis (py-**roh**-sis) *n.* another name (chiefly US) for heartburn.

pyruvic acid (pyruvate) (py-**roo**-vik) *n.* a compound, derived from carbohydrates, that may be oxidized in the Krebs cycle to yield carbon dioxide and energy in the form of ATP.

pyuria (py-**yoor**-iă) *n.* the presence of pus in the urine, making it cloudy. This is a sign of bacterial infection in the urinary tract.

Qq

QALYs *pl. n.* *see* quality-adjusted life years.

q.d.s. (quater die sumendus) Latin: to be taken four times a day, used as a direction in prescriptions.

Q fever *n.* an acute infectious disease of many animals, including cattle, sheep, goats, deer, and dogs, that is caused by a rickettsia, *Coxiella burnetii*. It is transmitted to humans primarily through inhalation of infected particles or consumption of contaminated unpasteurized milk, but also via ticks acting as vectors. A severe influenza-like illness develops, sometimes with pneumonia, after an incubation period of up to three weeks. Treatment with tetracyclines or chloramphenicol is effective. *See also* typhus.

QOL *n.* *see* quality of life.

QRISK2 *n.* a computer algorithm that estimates the risk of a heart attack or stroke in a person over the next ten years. It uses a range of risk factors, including age, systolic blood pressure, smoking status, body mass index, and family history. Someone with a QRISK2 score of 20% (or more) is regarded as high-risk.

QRS complex *n.* the element of an electrocardiogram that precedes the S–T segment and indicates electrical activation of the ventricles.

Q–T interval *n.* the interval on an electrocardiogram between the beginning of ventricular depolarization (Q wave) and the beginning of repolarization (T wave). *See also* long QT syndrome.

quadratus (kwod-ray-tŭs) *n.* any of various four-sided muscles. **q. femoris** a flat muscle at the head of the femur, responsible for lateral rotation of the thigh.

quadri- *combining form denoting* four.

quadriceps (**kwod**-ri-seps) *n.* one of the great extensor muscles of the legs. It is situated in the thigh and is subdivided into four distinct portions: the **rectus femoris**, **vastus lateralis**, **vastus medialis**, and **vastus intermedius**.

quadriplegia (tetraplegia) (kwod-ri-**plee**-jiă) *n.* paralysis affecting all four limbs. **—quadriplegic** *adj., n.*

SEE WEB LINKS

- Peer support for people with spinal injury from a US website

qualitative research (**kwol**-it-ă-tiv) *n.* research that seeks to provide understanding of human experience, perceptions, motivations, intentions, and behaviours based on description and observation and utilizing a naturalistic interpretative approach to a subject and its contextual setting. *Compare* quantitative research.

quality-adjusted life years (QALYs) (**kwol**-iti-ă-just-id) *pl. n.* a quantitative measure, in terms of years of good-quality life, of the value of a medical procedure or service to a group of patients with similar medical conditions.

quality assurance (ă-shor-ăns) *n.* the process in which services are periodically reviewed and health-care provision assessed against benchmarks and other local or national reference points. *See* nursing audit, performance indicators. **q. a. tool** an assessment tool used by health-care practitioners to measure the quality of care provision. It can involve observation, interview, and review of written care plans and nursing orders and uses a scoring system (such as **Qualpacs** or **Monitor**).

quality circle *n.* a strategy utilized to develop and maintain nursing standards. It relies heavily on enthusiastic representatives from all disciplines participating in the process of standard development, in order to foster a personal commitment to a quality service.

quality of life (QOL) *n.* a measure of a person's physical and psychological wellbeing, especially when this is affected by disease or disability. It is usually assessed by means of patient questionnaires. It can be used to identify future management of a patient's care and to help determine who will benefit most from a treatment and who should receive priority where resources are scarce. *See* quality-adjusted life years.

Qualpacs (kwol-paks) *n.* *see* quality assurance (tool).

quantitative digital radiography (kwon-ti-tă-tiv dij-i-t'l) *n.* a method of detecting osteoporosis. A narrow X-ray beam is directed at the area of interest (usually the spine and hip), which enables a measurement to be made of its calcium content (density).

quantitative research *n.* research based on traditional scientific methods, which generates numerical data and usually seeks to establish causal relationships between two or more variables, using statistical methods to test the strength and significance of the relationships. *Compare* qualitative research.

quarantine (kwo-răn-teen) *n.* the period for which a person (or animal) is kept in isolation to prevent the spread of a contagious disease. Different diseases have different quarantine periods.

quartan (kwor-t'n) *adj.* occurring every three days, as in the case of some intermittent fevers.

quartile (kwor-tIl) *n.* one of four equal parts into which a rank-ordered data set is divided. The **interquartile** range is the difference between the upper quartile and the lower quartile and gives a clear indication of the central 50% of the values.

Queckenstedt test (kwek-ĕn-stet) *n.* a part of the routine lumbar puncture procedure. It is used to determine whether or not the flow of cerebrospinal fluid is blocked in the spinal cord. [H. H. G. Queckenstedt (1876–1918), German physician]

quickening (kwik-ĕn-ing) *n.* the first movement of a fetus in the uterus that is felt by the mother, usually after about 16 weeks of pregnancy.

quiescent (kwi-es-ĕnt) *adj.* describing a disease that is in an inactive or undetectable phase.

quinine (kwin-**een**) *n.* a drug used in the treatment of malaria due to *Plasmodium falciparum* (malignant malaria). Small doses of quinine are used to treat nocturnal leg cramps. It is administered by mouth or intravenous infusion; large doses can cause severe poisoning (*see* cinchonism).

quinism (**kwin**-izm) *n.* the symptoms of overdosage or prolonged treatment with quinine. *See* cinchonism.

quinolone (**kwin**-ŏ-lohn) *n.* one of a group of chemically related synthetic antibiotics that includes ciprofloxacin, nalidixic acid, and ofloxacin. These drugs are often useful for treating infections with organisms that have become resistant to other antibiotics.

quinsy (**kwin**-zi) *n.* pus in the space between the tonsil and the wall of the pharynx. The patient has severe pain with difficulty in opening the mouth (trismus) and swallowing. Treatment is with antibiotics; surgical incision of the abscess may be necessary. Medical name: **peritonsillar abscess**.

quotidian (kwoh-**tid**-iăn) *adj.* occurring daily, as in the case of some intermittent fevers.

quotient (**kwoh**-shĕnt) *n.* *see* intelligence quotient, respiratory quotient.

Q wave *n.* the downward deflection on an electrocardiogram that indicates the beginning of ventricular depolarization.

Rr

rabbit fever (rab-it) *n. see* tularaemia.

rabies (hydrophobia) (ray-beez) *n.* an acute virus disease of the central nervous system that may be transmitted to humans by a bite from an infected dog. Symptoms include malaise, fever, difficulty in breathing, salivation, and painful muscle spasms of the throat induced by swallowing. In the later stages of the disease the mere sight of water induces convulsions and paralysis; death occurs within 4–5 days. Injections of rabies vaccine and antiserum may prevent the disease from developing in a person bitten by an infected animal. **—rabid** (rab-id) *adj.*

racemose (ras-i-mohs) *adj.* resembling a bunch of grapes. The term is applied particularly to a compound gland the secretory part of which consists of a number of small sacs.

rachi- (rachio-) *combining form denoting* the spine.

rachis (ray-kis) *n. see* backbone.

rachischisis (ray-kis-ki-sis) *n. see* spina bifida.

rachitic (ră-kit-ik) *adj.* affected with rickets.

rad (rad) *n.* a former unit of absorbed dose of ionizing radiation. It has been replaced by the gray.

radial (ray-di-ăl) *adj.* relating to or associated with the radius. **r. artery** a branch of the brachial artery, beginning at the elbow and passing down the forearm, around the wrist, and into the palm of the hand. **r. nerve** an important mixed sensory and motor nerve of the arm, forming the largest branch of the brachial plexus. **r. reflex** flexion of the forearm (and sometimes also of the fingers) that occurs when the lower end of the radius is tapped.

radiation (ray-di-ay-shŏn) *n.* energy in the form of waves or particles, such as gamma rays, X-rays, ultraviolet rays, visible light, and infrared rays (radiant heat). **r. sickness** an acute illness caused by extreme exposure to rays emitted by radioactive substances, e.g. X-rays or gamma rays. Very high doses cause death within hours. Lower doses cause nausea, vomiting, and diarrhoea followed by damage to the bone marrow, loss of hair, and bloody diarrhoea; some of the milder symptoms can occur after therapeutic doses of radiotherapy.

radical treatment (rad-ikăl) *n.* vigorous treatment that aims at the complete cure of a disease rather than the mere relief of symptoms. *Compare* conservative treatment.

radicle (rad-ikŭl) *n.* (in anatomy) **1.** a small root. **2.** the initial fibre of a nerve or the origin of a vein. **—radicular** (ră-dik-yoo-ler) *adj.*

radiculitis (rǎ-dik-yoo-**ly**-tis) *n.* inflammation of the root of a nerve. *See* polyradiculitis.

radio- *combining form denoting* **1.** radiation. **2.** radioactive substances.

radioactivity (ray-di-oh-ak-**tiv**-iti) *n.* disintegration of the nuclei of certain elements, with the emission of energy in the form of alpha, beta, or gamma rays. Naturally occurring radioactive elements include radium and uranium. *See also* radioisotope. **—radioactive** *adj.*

radioallergosorbent test (RAST) (ray-di-oh-al-er-joh-**sor**-běnt) *n.* a blood test that identifies allergen-specific immunoglobulin E (IgE).

radioautography (ray-di-oh-aw-**tog**-rǎfi) *n. see* autoradiography.

radiobiology (ray-di-oh-by-**ol**-ǒji) *n.* the study of the effects of radiation on living tissues. **—radiobiologist** *n.*

radiodermatitis (ray-di-oh-der-mǎ-**ty**-tis) *n.* inflammation of the skin after exposure to ionizing radiation. The skin becomes dry, hairless, and atrophied, losing its colouring.

radiofrequency ablation (ray-di-oh-**free**-kwěn-si) *n. see* ablation.

radiographer (ray-di-**og**-rǎ-fer) *n.* a person who is trained in the technique either of taking X-ray images of parts of the body (**diagnostic r.**) or of treatment by radiotherapy (**therapeutic r.**).

radiography (ray-di-**og**-rǎfi) *n.* diagnostic radiology: traditionally, the technique of examining the body by directing X-rays through it to produce images (**radiographs**) on photographic film or a fluoroscope. It now also includes the production of images by computerized tomography, magnetic resonance imaging, and nuclear medicine. Radiography is used to produce images of disease in all parts of the body, to be interpreted by radiologists for physicians and surgeons. **computerized r.** radiography in which photographic film is replaced by a charged plate, from which charge is knocked off by exposure to X-rays. The resultant image is read by a laser beam, then stored digitally or printed out. **digital r.** (**DR**) radiography in which X-ray images are acquired in digital format, allowing the storage of images and their subsequent retrieval and interpretation using computers.

radioimmunoassay (ray-di-oh-im-yoo-noh-**ass**-ay) *n.* the technique of using radioactive antibodies as tracers to estimate the levels of natural substances, especially hormones, in the blood, which act as antigens. The amount of radioactivity trapped is a measure of the amount of the antigen present.

radioimmunolocalization (ray-di-oh-im-yoo-noh-loh-kǎl-I-**zay**-shǒn) *n.* a method of identifying the site of a tumour (e.g. colorectal cancer) that relies on its uptake of radioactive isotopes attached to an appropriate anticancer immune cell.

radioiodine ablation (ray-dee-oh-**I**-oh-dIn ǎ-**blay**-shǒn) *n.* the use of radioactive iodine (iodine-131) to destroy any residual thyroid tissue after thyroidectomy for cancer. Subsequent radioiodine treatment may be necessary to treat residual thyroid cancer cells.

radioisotope (ray-di-oh-**I**-sŏ-tohp) *n.* an isotope of an element that emits alpha, beta, or gamma radiation during its decay into another element. Artificial radioisotopes, such as iodine-131 and cobalt-60, are produced by bombarding elements with beams of neutrons. They are widely used in medicine as tracers and as sources of radiation for the different techniques of radiotherapy.

radiologist (ray-di-**ol**-ŏ-jist) *n.* a physician specializing in the interpretation of X-rays and other scanning techniques for the diagnosis of disease. **interventional r.** a specialist in the use of imaging to guide interventional radiology techniques.

radiology (ray-di-**ol**-ŏji) *n.* the branch of medicine involving the study of radiographs or other imaging technologies (such as ultrasound and magnetic resonance imaging) to diagnose or treat disease. **diagnostic r.** *see* radiography. **interventional r.** a branch of radiology in which complex procedures are performed using imaging guidance, which avoids patients having to undergo invasive surgery to achieve the same results. Guidance is commonly by X-ray fluoroscopy, ultrasound, computerized tomography, or magnetic resonance imaging. **therapeutic r.** *see* radiotherapy.

radiolucent (ray-di-oh-**loo**-sĕnt) *adj.* having the property of being transparent to X-rays. Gases are relatively radiolucent to X-rays and can be used as a negative contrast medium in X-ray examinations.

radionuclide (ray-di-oh-**new**-klyd) *n.* a substance containing a radioactive atomic nucleus, which can be used as a tracer for diagnosis in nuclear medicine.

radiopaque (ray-di-oh-oh-**payk**) *adj.* having the property of absorbing, and therefore being opaque to, X-rays. Radiopaque materials, such as those containing iodine or barium, are used as contrast media in radiography.

radiosensitive (ray-di-oh-**sen**-sit-iv) *adj.* describing certain forms of cancer cell that are particularly susceptible to radiation and are likely to be dealt with successfully by radiotherapy.

radiosensitizer (ray-di-oh-**sen**-sit-I-zer) *n.* a substance that increases the sensitivity of cells to radiation. The presence of oxygen and other compounds with a high affinity for electrons will increase radiosensitivity, as will chemotherapy drugs, such as fluorouracil or cisplatin, used concurrently with radiotherapy.

radiotherapist (ray-di-oh-**th'e**-ră-pist) *n.* a doctor who specializes in treatment with radiotherapy.

radiotherapy (ray-di-oh-**th'e**-răpi) *n.* therapeutic radiology: the treatment of disease with penetrating radiation, such as X-rays, beta rays, or gamma rays. Beams of radiation may be directed at a diseased part from a distance (*see* teletherapy), or radioactive material, in the form of needles, wires, or pellets, may be implanted in the body. *See also* brachytherapy.

SEE WEB LINKS

- Explanation of radiotherapy from Cancer Research UK

radium (ray-dĭŭm) *n.* a radioactive metallic element that emits alpha and gamma rays during its decay into other elements. The gamma radiation was formerly employed in radiotherapy for the treatment of cancer. Symbol: Ra.

radius (ray-di-ŭs) *n.* the outer and shorter bone of the forearm (*compare* ulna). It partially revolves about the ulna, permitting pronation and supination of the hand. —**radial** *adj.*

radix (ray-diks) *n.* *see* root.

radon (ray-don) *n.* a radioactive gaseous element that is produced during the decay of radium. It emits alpha and gamma radiation. Symbol: Rn. **r. seeds** sealed capsules containing radon, used in radiotherapy for the treatment of cancer but now largely replaced by newer agents and techniques.

RAI *n.* *see* Relatives Assessment Interview.

RAISSE *n.* Relatives Assessment Interview for Schizophrenia in a Secure Environment (*see* Relatives Assessment Interview).

rale (rahl) *n.* *see* crepitation.

raloxifene (ral-**oks**-i-feen) *n.* a drug administered orally to prevent and treat osteoporosis that develops after the menopause. It mimics the protective action of oestrogen in the bones without risk of the adverse effects (e.g. on the breast and uterus) associated with hormone replacement therapy (*see* selective (o)estrogen receptor modulator). However, it does not relieve menopausal symptoms; side-effects include hot flushes. Trade name: **Evista**.

ramipril (ram-i-pril) *n.* *see* ACE inhibitor.

Ramstedt's operation (rahm-stets) *n.* *see* pyloromyotomy. [W. C. Ramstedt (1867–1963), German surgeon]

ramus (ray-mŭs) *n.* (*pl.* **rami**) **1.** a branch, especially of a nerve fibre or blood vessel. **2.** a thin process projecting from a bone.

randomized controlled trial (ran-dŏm-yzd) *n.* *see* controlled trial.

random sample (ran-dŏm) *n.* *see* sample.

range of movement (ROM) (raynj) *n.* an observational measure of joint flexibility.

ranitidine (ra-**nit**-i-deen) *n.* an H_2-receptor antagonist (*see* antihistamine) that is used in the treatment of peptic ulcers and gastro-oesophageal reflux disease. It may be administered by mouth, intravenously, or (rarely) intramuscularly. Trade name: **Zantac**.

RANKL inhibitor *n.* *r*eceptor *a*ctivator of *n*uclear factor *k*appa B *l*igand inhibitor: an agent that works by inhibiting the development of osteoclasts and bone resorption, thus minimizing bone loss and the potential for fractures in those with postmenopausal osteoporosis and bone metastases.

ranula (ran-yoo-lă) *n.* a cyst found under the tongue, formed when the duct leading from a salivary or mucous gland is obstructed and distended.

raphe (ray-fi) *n.* a line, ridge, seam, or crease in a tissue or organ; for example, the furrow that passes down the centre of the dorsal surface of the tongue.

rarefaction (rair-i-fak-shŏn) *n.* thinning of bony tissue sufficient to cause decreased density of bone to X-rays, as in osteoporosis.

rash (rash) *n.* a temporary eruption on the skin, usually typified by discrete red spots or generalized reddening that may be accompanied by itching. A rash may be a local skin reaction or the outward sign of a systemic disorder.

Rasmussen's encephalitis (ras-muus-ĕnz) *n.* a focal encephalitis, found most commonly in children, that results in continual focal seizures (*see* epilepsy). The underlying cause is unknown but it may be due to a viral infection or an autoimmune process. [G. L. Rasmussen (20th century), US anatomist]

raspatory (rah-spă-ter-i) *n.* a file-like surgical instrument used for scraping the surface of bone. See illustration.

raspberry tumour (rahz-be-ri) *n.* an adenoma of the umbilicus.

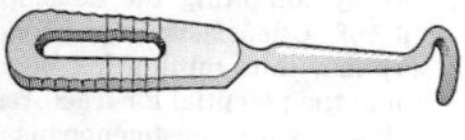

A rib raspatory

RAST *n. see* radioallergosorbent test.

Rastafarian (ras-tă-fair-iăn) *n.* an adherent of a religious and philosophical movement, originating in Jamaica in the 1920s, that accepts the Ethiopian emperor Haile Selassie (Ras Tafari Makonnen; 1892–1975) as its religious leader and god, who will return the members of the Black community who are living in exile to Africa. Many Rastafarians believe the chosen few will continue to live forever in their current bodies. See Appendix 12: Religion and nursing practice.

rat-bite fever (sodokosis) (rat-byt) *n.* a disease, contracted from the bite of a rat, due to infection by either the bacterium *Spirillum minus*, which causes ulceration of the skin and recurrent fever, or by the fungus *Streptobacillus moniliformis*, which causes inflammation of the skin, muscular pains, and vomiting. Both infections respond well to penicillin.

ratio data (ray-shi-oh) *pl. n.* data on a scale of measurement (e.g. age in years) in which differences between data can be quantified and proportions can be specified (e.g. 15 years is three times as old as 5 years).

rationalization (rash-ŏn-ă-ly-zay-shŏn) *n.* (in psychology) the explanation of events or behaviour in terms that avoid giving the true reasons.

Raynaud's disease (ray-nohz) *n.* a condition of unknown cause in which the arteries of the fingers are unduly reactive and enter spasm when the hands are cold. This produces attacks of pallor, numbness, and discomfort in the fingers. Gangrene or ulceration of the fingertips may result. Warm gloves and peripheral vasodilators may relieve the condition. **R. phenomenon** a similar condition resulting from atherosclerosis, ingestion of ergot derivatives, or use of vibrating tools. [M. Raynaud (1834–81), French physician]

RBC *n.* red blood cell (*see* erythrocyte).

RCA *n. see* root cause analysis.

RCC *n.* red cell concentrate.

RDA *n.* recommended daily allowance (of a nutrient).

reaction (ri-**ak**-shŏn) *n.* **1.** the response to a stimulus. **2.** the interaction of two or more substances that results in chemical changes in them. **3.** the effect produced by an allergen (*see* allergy).

reactive (ri-**ak**-tiv) *adj.* (in psychiatry) describing mental illnesses thought to be precipitated by events in the psychological environment. **r. hypoglycaemia** *see* hypoglycaemia.

reactive arthritis an inflammatory arthritis that develops after a gastrointestinal or a genitourinary (especially a chlamydia) infection; formerly called **Reiter's syndrome**. In a third of patients the triad of nongonococcal inflammation of the urethra, conjunctivitis, and polyarthritis occurs.

reagent (ree-**ay**-jĕnt) *n.* a compound that reacts with another, especially one used to detect the presence of the other compound.

reagin (**ree**-ă-jin) *n.* a type of antibody, formed against an allergen, that remains fixed in various tissues. Subsequent contact with the allergen causes damage to the tissue and the release of histamine and serotonin, which are responsible for the allergic reaction (*see* anaphylaxis).

reality orientation (ree-**al**-iti) *n.* therapy that aims to improve cognitive functioning and behaviour in elderly people with dementia by using repetition and a range of resources to help the memory. It involves regularly reminding the person of such information as the time, date, where he or she is, and planned events for that day, such as a visit to see a friend. The information is given verbally by a carer or written on boards placed in prominent positions in the person's home.

real-time imaging (**reel**-tym) *n.* the rapid acquisition and manipulation of ultrasound information from a scanning probe by electronic circuits to enable images to be produced on TV screens almost instantaneously. Using similar techniques, the instantaneous display of other imaging modalities, such as CT scanning and magnetic resonance imaging, can now be achieved.

reboxetine (reb-**oks**-i-teen) *n.* an antidepressant drug that acts by inhibiting reabsorption of the neurotransmitter noradrenaline, thus prolonging its action in the brain. It is administered by mouth to treat major depression. Trade name: **Edronax**.

recall (ri-kawl) **1.** *n.* the process of eliciting a representation (especially an image) of a past experience. **2.** *vb.* to elicit such a representation.

receptaculum (ree-sep-**tak**-yoo-lŭm) *n.* the dilated portion of a tubular anatomical part. **r.** (or **cisterna**) **chyli** the dilated end of the thoracic duct, into which lymph vessels from the lower limbs and intestines drain.

receptive aphasia (ri-**sep**-tiv) *n. see* aphasia.

receptor (ri-**sep**-ter) *n.* **1.** a cell or group of cells specialized to detect changes in the environment and trigger impulses in the sensory nervous system. All sensory nerve endings act as receptors. *See* exteroceptor, interoceptor, proprioceptor. **2.** a specialized area of cell membrane that can bind with a specific hormone (e.g. **oestrogen r.**), neurotransmitter (e.g. **adrenergic r.**), drug, or other chemical, thereby initiating a change within the cell.

recess (ri-**ses**) *n.* (in anatomy) a hollow chamber or a depression in an organ or other part.

recessive (ri-**ses**-iv) *adj.* describing a gene (or its corresponding characteristic) whose effect is shown in the individual only when its allele is the same, i.e. when two such alleles are present (the **double recessive** condition). *Compare* dominant. *See also* autosomal. **—recessive** *n.*

recipient (ri-**sip**-iĕnt) *n.* a person who receives something from a donor, such as a blood transfusion or a kidney transplant.

recombinant DNA (ri-**kom**-bin-ănt) *n.* DNA that contains genes from different sources that have been combined by the techniques of genetic engineering. Genetic engineering is therefore also known as **recombinant DNA technology**.

recovery position (ri-**kuv**-eri) *n.* a first-aid position into which an unconscious but breathing patient can be laid to afford maximum protection to the airway. It involves laying the patient on his or her side, with the uppermost leg bent at the knee and hip and the lower arm behind the back to prevent rolling into a position in which the patient could smother or choke.

recrudescence (ree-kroo-**des**-ĕns) *n.* a fresh outbreak of a disorder in a patient after a period during which its signs and symptoms had died down.

rect- (recto-) *combining form denoting* the rectum.

rectocele (proctocele) (**rek**-toh-seel) *n.* bulging or pouching of the rectum, usually a forward protrusion of the rectum into the posterior wall of the vagina, often in association with prolapse of the uterus.

rectopexy (**rek**-toh-peks-i) *n.* the surgical fixation of a prolapsed rectum.

rectosigmoid (rek-toh-**sig**-moid) *n.* the region of the large intestine around the junction of the sigmoid colon and the rectum.

rectovesical (rek-toh-**ves**-ikăl) *adj.* relating to the rectum and the urinary bladder.

rectum (rek-tŭm) *n.* the terminal part of the large intestine, which runs from the sigmoid colon to the anal canal. Faeces are stored in the rectum before defecation. **—rectal** (rek-t'l) *adj.*

rectus (rek-tŭs) *n.* any of several straight muscles. **r. abdominis** a long flat muscle that extends bilaterally along the entire length of the front of the abdomen. **r. femoris** *see* quadriceps. **r. muscles of the orbit** some of the extrinsic eye muscles.

recumbent (ri-kum-bĕnt) *adj.* lying down. **—recumbency** *n.*

recurrent (ri-ku-rĕnt) *adj.* **1.** (in anatomy) describing a structure, such as a nerve or blood vessel, that turns back on its course, forming a loop. **2.** occurring repeatedly. **r. miscarriage** *see* miscarriage.

red blood cell (RBC) *n. see* erythrocyte.

reduction (ri-duk-shŏn) *n.* (in surgery) the restoration of a displaced part of the body, such as a hernia or a dislocated joint, to its normal position by manipulation or operation.

reduction division *n.* the first division of meiosis, in which the chromosome number is halved.

referred pain (synalgia) (ri-ferd) *n.* pain felt in a part of the body other than where it might be expected. An abscess beneath the diaphragm, for example, may cause a referred pain in the shoulder area. The confusion arises because sensory nerves from different parts of the body share common pathways when they reach the spinal cord.

reflection (ri-flek-shŏn) *n.* the careful consideration of one's own professional practice, including the ability to review, analyse, and evaluate situations during or after events (possibly using a recognized model). It is an essential part of the learning process that will result in new methods of approaching and understanding nursing practice.

reflex (ree-fleks) *n.* an automatic or involuntary response to a stimulus, which is brought about by relatively simple nervous circuits without consciousness being necessarily involved. *See* conditioned reflex, Moro reflex, patellar reflex, plantar (reflex), pupillary reflex, rooting reflex. **r. arc** the nervous circuit involved in a reflex, being at its simplest a sensory nerve with a receptor, linked at a synapse in the brain or spinal cord with a motor nerve, which supplies a muscle or gland. See illustration.

reflexology (ree-fleks-ol-ŏji) *n.* a complementary therapy based on the theory that reflex points on the feet correspond with all body parts. Firm pressure is applied to the relevant reflex points using the thumb or fingers. Reflexology is said to be able to help with specific illnesses and may also restore the body's natural balance and harmony.

reflux (ree-fluks) *n.* a backflow of liquid, against its normal direction of movement. *See* gastro-oesophageal reflux, (reflux) oesophagitis, vesicoureteric reflux.

refraction (ri-frak-shŏn) *n.* the change in direction of light rays when they pass obliquely from one

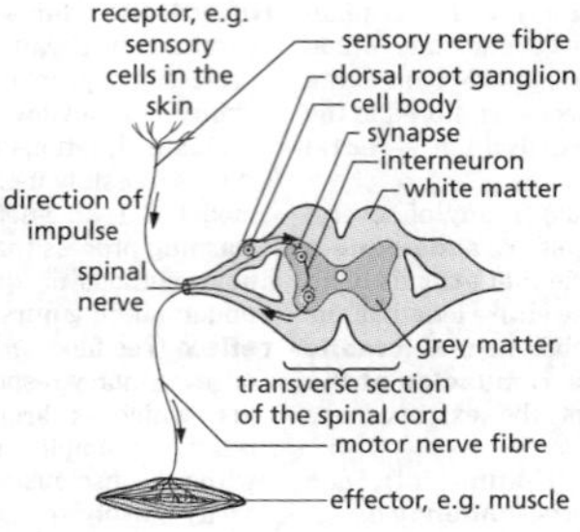

The reflex arc

transparent medium to another, of a different density. Refraction occurs as light enters the eye and passes through the cornea, lens, etc., to come to a focus on the retina. **error of r.** (**refractive error**) an abnormality of the eye, such as astigmatism or long- or short-sightedness, in which a blurred image forms on the retina due to abnormal focusing. **—refractive** (ri-**frak**-tiv) *adj.*

refractive surgery *n.* any surgical procedure that has as its primary objective the correction of any refractive error. It includes such procedures as lens extraction, LASIK, LASEK, and photorefractive keratectomy.

refractometer (ree-frak-**tom**-it-er) *n. see* optometer.

refractory (ri-**frakt**-er-i) *adj.* unresponsive: applied to a condition that fails to respond satisfactorily to a given treatment.

refractory period *n.* (in neurology) the time of recovery needed for a nerve cell that has just transmitted a nerve impulse or for a muscle fibre that has just contracted. During the refractory period a normal stimulus will not bring about excitation of the cell.

regeneration (ri-jen-er-**ay**-shŏn) *n.* the natural regrowth of a tissue or other part lost through injury.

regimen (**rej**-i-men) *n.* (in therapeutics) a prescribed systematic form of treatment, such as a diet or a course of drugs, for curing disease or improving health.

registered nurse (**rej**-is-terd) *n. see* nurse.

registrar (rej-i-**strar**) *n. see* specialist registrar.

regression (ri-**gresh**-ŏn) *n.* (in psychiatry) reversion to a more immature level of functioning.

regurgitation (ri-ger-ji-tay-shŏn) *n.* **1.** the bringing up of undigested material from the stomach to the mouth (*see* vomiting). **2.** the flowing back of a liquid in a direction opposite to the normal one. *See* aortic regurgitation, mitral regurgitation.

rehabilitation (ree-ă-bil-i-tay-shŏn) *n.* **1.** (in physical medicine) the treatment of an ill, injured, or disabled patient with the aim of restoring normal health and function. **2.** any means for restoring the independence of a patient after disease or injury.

reiki (ray-ki) *n.* a complementary therapy based on an ancient healing system rediscovered in the 20th century by a Buddhist monk. It involves the therapist putting his or her hands on or very close to the patient to boost the patient's natural invisible energy fields. It is often used as an adjunct to other therapies and is said to be helpful for many conditions.

Reiter's syndrome (ry-terz) *n.* *see* reactive arthritis [H. Reiter (1881–1969), German physician]

rejection (ri-jek-shŏn) *n.* (in transplantation) the destruction by immune mechanisms of a tissue grafted from another individual. Antibodies, complement, clotting factors, and platelets are involved in the failure of the graft to survive. Allograft rejection is a vigorous response that can be modified by drugs (such as ciclosporin and corticosteroids) and antibodies against T cells; xenograft rejection is an acute response that is at present beyond therapeutic control.

relapse (ri-laps) *n.* a return of disease symptoms after recovery had apparently been achieved or the worsening of an apparently recovering patient's condition.

relapsing fever (ri-laps-ing) *n.* an infectious disease caused by bacteria of the genus *Borrelia*, which is transmitted by ticks or lice and results in recurrent fever. The first episode of fever is accompanied by severe headache and aching muscles and joints. Subsequent attacks are milder and occur at intervals of 3–10 days.

relative density (rel-ă-tiv) *n.* the ratio of the density of a substance at a specified temperature to the density of a reference substance (for liquids, this is water at 4°C). It was formerly known as **specific gravity**.

Relatives Assessment Interview (RAI) *n.* an assessment tool designed to identify the perceptions and coping skills of relatives of patients with mental health problems. The **Relatives Assessment Interview for Schizophrenia in a Secure Environment** (**RAISSE**) is a form of the RAI adapted to examine the effects of a secure environment on the course of schizophrenia.

relaxant (ri-laks-ănt) *n.* an agent that reduces tension and strain, particularly in muscles (*see* muscle relaxant).

relaxation (ree-laks-ay-shŏn) *n.* (in physiology) the diminution of tension in a muscle, which occurs when it ceases to contract. **r. therapy** treatment by teaching patients to decrease their anxiety by reducing the tone in their muscles.

relaxin (ri-**laks**-in) *n.* a hormone, secreted by the placenta in the terminal stages of pregnancy, that causes the cervix of the uterus to dilate and prepares the uterus for the action of oxytocin during labour.

Relenza (ri-**lenz**-ă) *n. see* zanamivir.

rem (rem) *n.* a former unit dose of ionizing radiation; it was replaced by the sievert.

REM *n.* rapid eye movement: the stage of sleep during which the muscles of the eyeballs are in constant motion behind the eyelids. REM usually coincides with dreaming.

remission (ri-**mish**-ŏn) *n.* **1.** a lessening in the severity of symptoms or their temporary disappearance during the course of an illness. **2.** a reduction in the size of a cancer and the symptoms it is causing.

remittent fever (ri-**mit**-ĕnt) *n. see* fever.

renal (**ree**-năl) *adj.* relating to or affecting the kidneys. **r. artery** either of two large arteries arising from the abdominal aorta and supplying the kidneys. **r. function tests** tests for assessing the function of the kidneys, which include measurements of the specific gravity of urine, creatinine clearance time, and blood urea levels, as well as intravenous urography and renal angiography. **r. tubule** (**uriniferous tubule**) the fine tubular part of a nephron, through which water and certain dissolved substances are reabsorbed back into the blood.

renal cell carcinoma (Grawitz tumour, hypernephroma) a malignant tumour of kidney cells. It may be present for some years before giving rise to symptoms, which include fever, loin pain, and blood in the urine. Treatment is by surgery but tumours are apt to recur locally or spread via the bloodstream. Secondary tumours may be treated with Sunitinib and Sorafenib.

reni- (reno-) *combining form denoting* the kidney.

renin (**ree**-nin) *n.* an enzyme released into the blood by the kidney in response to stress. It produces angiotensin, which causes constriction of blood vessels and thus an increase in blood pressure. Excessive production of renin results in renovascular hypertension.

rennin (**ren**-in) *n.* an enzyme produced in the stomach that coagulates milk. It converts caseinogen (milk protein) into insoluble casein in the presence of calcium ions. This ensures that the milk remains in the stomach, exposed to protein-digesting enzymes, for as long as possible.

renography (isotope renography) (ri-**nog**-răfi) *n.* the radiological study of the kidneys by a gamma camera following the intravenous injection of a radioactive tracer, which is concentrated and excreted by the kidneys. A graph of the radioactivity in each kidney gives information on its function and rate of drainage.

reovirus (ree-oh-**vy**-rŭs) *n.* one of a group of small RNA-containing viruses that infect both respiratory and intestinal tracts without producing specific or serious diseases (and were therefore termed *r*espiratory *e*nteric *o*rphan viruses). *Compare* echovirus.

repetitive strain injury (RSI) (ri-**pet**-it-iv) *n.* pain in an upper limb associated with frequent repetition of a particular movement, usually related to keyboard usage. Symptoms often occur in the absence of clear signs, such as tenosynovitis or tendovaginitis.

replantation (ree-plahn-**tay**-shŏn) *n.* **1.** the reattachment of severed limbs (or parts of limbs) and other body parts (e.g. the nose) using microsurgery to rejoin nerves and vessels. **2.** (reimplantation) (in dentistry) the reinsertion of a tooth into its socket after its accidental or deliberate removal. **—replant** *vb.*

replication (rep-li-**kay**-shŏn) *n.* the process by which DNA makes copies of itself when the cell divides. The two strands of the DNA molecule unwind and each strand directs the synthesis of a new strand complementary to itself.

repolarization (ri-poh-ler-I-**zay**-shŏn) *n.* the process in which the membrane of a nerve cell returns to its normal electrically charged state after a nerve impulse has passed.

repositor (ri-**poz**-it-er) *n.* an instrument used to return a displaced part of the body to its normal position.

repression (ri-**presh**-ŏn) *n.* (in psychoanalysis) the process of excluding an unacceptable wish or an idea from conscious mental life. The repressed material may give rise to symptoms.

reproductive system (ree-prŏ-**duk**-tiv) *n.* the combination of organs and tissues associated with the process of reproduction. In males it includes the testes, vasa deferentia, prostate gland, seminal vesicles, urethra, and penis; in females it includes the ovaries, Fallopian tubes, uterus, vagina, and vulva.

research ethics committee (ri-**serch**) *n. see* ethics committee.

resection (ri-**sek**-shŏn) *n.* surgical removal of a portion of any part of the body. **submucous r.** removal of part of the cartilage septum of the nose that has become deviated, usually by injury. **transurethral r. of the prostate** (**TURP**) an operation performed when the prostate gland becomes enlarged. It involves removal of portions of the gland through the urethra using an instrument called a **resectoscope**.

resectoscope (ri-**sek**-tŏ-skohp) *n. see* (transurethral) resection.

reserve volume (ri-**zerv**) *n.* the extra volume of air that an individual could inhale (**inspiratory r. v., IRV**) or exhale (**expiratory r. v., ERV**) if not breathing to the limit of his or her capacity.

residual urine (ri-**zid**-yoo-ăl) *n.* urine remaining in the bladder after micturition.

residual volume (RV) *n.* the volume of air that remains in the lungs after the individual has breathed

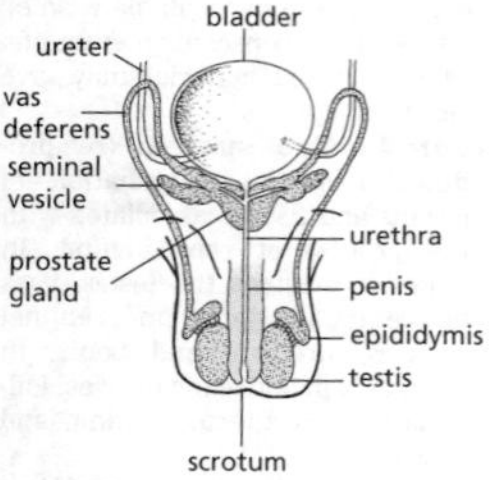

Male reproductive system

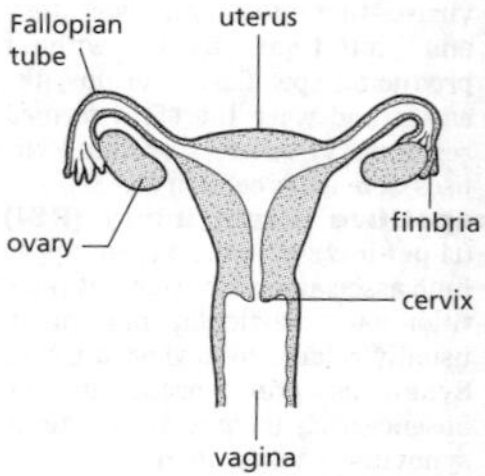

Female reproductive system

out as much as he or she can. This volume is increased in emphysema.

resistance (ri-zist-ăns) *n.* **1.** the degree of immunity that the body possesses. **2.** the degree to which a disease or disease-causing organism remains unaffected by antibiotics or other drugs.

resolution (rez-ŏ-**loo**-shŏn) *n.* **1.** the stage during which inflammation gradually disappears. **2.** the degree to which individual details can be distinguished by the eye, as through a microscope.

resonance (rez-ŏn-ăns) *n.* the sound produced by percussion of a part of the body during a physical examination. *See also* vocal resonance.

resorption (ri-sorp-shŏn) *n.* loss of substance through physiological or pathological means. In dentistry **internal resorption** occurs from within the pulp cavity; **apical resorption** occurs at the root end.

respiration (res-per-**ay**-shŏn) *n.* the process of gaseous exchange between an organism and its environment. **external r.** breathing: the stage of respiration in which oxygen is taken up by the capillaries of the lung alveoli and carbon dioxide is released from the blood. **internal r.** the stage of respiration in which oxygen is released to the tissues and carbon dioxide absorbed by the blood. *See also* lung. —**respiratory** (rĕs-**pir**-ă-ter-i) *adj.*

respirator (res-per-ayt-er) *n.* **1.** a face mask for administering oxygen or other gas or for filtering harmful fumes, dust, etc. **2.** *see* ventilator.

respiratory arrest *n.* cessation of breathing, which, without treatment, will very quickly be followed by cardiac arrest. It may result from airway obstruction, brain, spinal, or lung injury, overdose of certain medications (e.g. opioids), disease of the muscles and/or nerves necessary for breathing, or severe lung disease. Treatment includes clearance of any airway blockage and ventilatory support.

respiratory distress *n.* severe difficulty in achieving adequate oxygenation in spite of significant efforts to breathe. It is usually associated with increased breathing rate and the use of accessory muscles in the chest wall.

respiratory distress syndrome (hyaline membrane disease) *n.* the condition of a newborn infant in which the lungs are imperfectly expanded. Breathing is rapid, laboured, and shallow. The condition is most common and serious among preterm infants. It is treated by careful nursing, intravenous fluids, and oxygen, with or without positive-pressure ventilation. Surfactant administered at birth has produced encouraging results. *See also* adult respiratory distress syndrome.

respiratory quotient (RQ) *n.* the ratio of the volume of carbon dioxide transferred from the blood into the alveoli to the volume of oxygen absorbed into the alveoli. The RQ is usually about 0.8.

respiratory shock *n.* the state resulting when the respiratory process fails (due to illness or an obstruction) and the body is deprived of oxygen. *See also* respiratory arrest.

respiratory syncytial virus (RSV) *n.* a paramyxovirus (*see* myxovirus) that causes infections of the nose and throat. It is a major cause of bronchiolitis and pneumonia in young children.

SEE WEB LINKS

- Facts about RSV from the US Centers for Disease Control

respiratory system *n.* the combination of organs and tissues associated with breathing. It includes the nasal cavity, pharynx, larynx, trachea, bronchi, and lungs.

response (ri-**spons**) *n.* the way in which the body or part of the body reacts to a stimulus.

responsibility (rĕ-**spon**-si-bi-liti) *n.* the state of being accountable for one's actions. In health care, responsibility may be delegated to a less experienced clinician, but remains ultimately with the senior. At the same time responsibility for personal health is with the individual. Best health care in practice acknowledges this mutuality: the physician is an expert in medicine, the patients in themselves. *See also* accountability, professionalism.

restenosis (ree-sti-**noh**-sis) *n.* recurrent stenosis, usually in a blood vessel after such procedures as angioplasty or insertion of a stent.

restless legs syndrome (Ekbom's syndrome) (**rest**-lis) *n.* a condition in which a sense of uneasiness, restlessness, and itching, often accompanied by twitching and pain, is felt in the calves of the legs when sitting or lying down, especially in bed at night. The cause is unknown: it may be inadequate circulation, peripheral neuropathy, deficiency of iron, vitamin B_{12}, or folate, or a reaction to antipsychotic or antidepressant drugs.

rest pain (rest) *n.* pain without prior exertion, usually experienced in the feet or chest (angina pectoris), that indicates an extreme degree of ischaemia.

resuscitation (ri-sus-i-tay-shŏn) *n.* the process of reviving someone who appears to be dead by the restoration of cardiac and respiratory function. See Appendix 10: Guidelines for resuscitation **r. mannikin** a life-size model of a person for practising all aspects of basic and advanced life support.

retardation (ree-tar-**day**-shŏn) *n.* the slowing up of a process. **psychomotor r.** a marked slowing down of activity and speech. It is a symptom of severe depression. *See also* mental retardation.

retching (**rech**-ing) *n.* repeated unavailing attempts to vomit.

rete (**ree**-ti) *n.* a network of blood vessels, nerve fibres, or other strands of interlacing tissue in the structure of an organ.

retention (ri-**ten**-shŏn) *n.* inability to pass urine, which is retained in the bladder. The condition may be acute and painful or chronic and painless. The commonest cause of spontaneous **acute urinary r.** (**AUR**) is enlargement of the prostate gland in men.

retention cyst *n.* a cyst that arises when the outlet of the duct of a gland is blocked.

retention defect *n.* (in psychology) a memory defect in which items that have been registered in the memory are lost from storage. It is a feature of dementia.

reticular (ri-**tik**-yoo-ler) *adj.* (of tissues) resembling a network; branching. **r. fibres** branching fibres of connective tissue that form a delicate supportive meshwork around blood vessels, muscle fibres, glands, nerves, etc. **r. formation** a network of nerve pathways and nuclei throughout the brainstem, connecting motor and sensory nerves to and from the spinal cord, the cerebellum and the cerebrum, and the cranial nerves.

reticulocyte (ri-**tik**-yoo-loh-syt) *n.* an immature red blood cell (erythrocyte). Reticulocytes normally comprise about 1% of the total red cells.

reticulocytosis (ri-tik-yoo-loh-sy-**toh**-sis) *n.* an increase in the proportion of reticulocytes in the bloodstream: a sign of increased output of new red cells from the bone marrow.

reticuloendothelial system (RES) (ri-tik-yoo-loh-en-doh-**theel**-iăl) *n.* a community of phagocytes that is spread throughout the body. The RES is concerned with defence against microbial infection and with the removal of worn-out blood cells from the bloodstream. *See also* spleen.

reticulosis (ri-tik-yoo-**loh**-sis) *n.* abnormal overgrowth, usually malignant, of any of the cells of the lymphatic glands or the immune system. *See* Burkitt's lymphoma, Hodgkin's disease, lymphoma, mycosis fungoides.

reticulum (ri-**tik**-yoo-lŭm) *n.* a network of tubules or blood vessels. *See* endoplasmic reticulum.

retin- (retino-) *combining form denoting* the retina.

retina (**ret**-in-ă) *n.* the light-sensitive layer that lines the interior of the eye. The inner part of the retina, next to the cavity of the eyeball, contains rods and cones (light-sensitive cells) and their associated nerve fibres. The outer part (**retinal pigment epithelium**, **RPE**) is pigmented to prevent the passage of light. **—retinal** (**ret**-in-ăl) *adj.*

retinaculum (ret-in-**ak**-yoo-lŭm) *n.* (*pl.* **retinacula**) a thickened band of tissue that serves to hold various tissues in place.

retinal (**ret**-in-al) *n.* **1. (retinene)** the aldehyde of retinol (vitamin A). *See also* rhodopsin. **2.** *adj. see* retina.

retinal artery occlusion *n.* blockage of arterial blood supply to the retina, usually as a result of thrombosis or embolism. **branch r. a. o.** blockage of one of the branches of the central retinal artery, which results in visual field loss in the area of the retina supplied by the occluded vessel. **central r. a. o.** blockage of the central retinal artery, which enters the eye at the optic disc, usually resulting in sudden painless loss of vision.

retinal detachment (detached retina) *n.* separation of the inner nervous layer of the retina from the outer pigmented layer (retinal pigment epithelium), causing loss of vision in the affected part of the retina. The retina can be reattached by surgery, for example plombage, vitrectomy, or by creating patches of scar tissue between the retina and the choroid (*see* cryosurgery, photocoagulation).

retinal vein occlusion *n.* blockage of a vein carrying blood from the retina. **branch r. v. o.** blockage of one of the small branches of the central retinal vein, resulting in painless reduction of vision in the affected area. **central r. v. o.** blockage of the central retinal vein, which leaves the eye at the optic disc, usually resulting in sudden painless reduction of vision.

retinene (**ret**-in-een) *n. see* retinal.

retinitis (ret-i-**ny**-tis) *n.* inflammation of the retina, caused mainly by viral infection (e.g. cytomegalovirus, HIV). **r. pigmentosa** a non-inflammatory hereditary condition that is characterized by progressive degeneration of the retina due to malfunctioning of the retinal pigment epithelium. Night blindness and limited peripheral vision starting in childhood may progress to complete loss of vision.

retinoblastoma (ret-in-oh-blas-**toh**-mă) *n.* a rare malignant tumour of the retina, occurring mainly in children (usually under the age of 2 years).

retinoid (**ret**-in-oid) *n.* any one of a group of drugs derived from vitamin A that act on the skin to cause drying and peeling and a reduction in oil (sebum) production. Retinoids include isotretinoin, tretinoin, and alitretinoin (Toctino); they are used in the treatment of severe eczema, acne, psoriasis, ichthyosis, and other skin disorders. Possible side-effects, which may be serious, include severe fetal abnormalities (if taken by pregnant women), toxic effects on babies (if taken by breast-feeding mothers), and liver and kidney damage.

retinol (ret-in-ol) *n. see* vitamin A.

retinopathy (ret-in-**op**-ă-thi) *n.* any of various disorders of the retina resulting in impairment or loss of vision. **AIDS r.** retinopathy that occurs as a complication of AIDS. **diabetic r.** retinopathy resulting from diabetes, in which haemorrhaging or exudation may occur, either from damaged vessels into the retina or from new abnormal vessels into the vitreous humour (*see* neovascularization). **r. of prematurity** (**ROP**) abnormal growth of developing retinal vessels in premature infants, linked to high levels of oxygen therapy given to enhance their respiratory status.

retinopexy (ret-in-oh-peks-i) *n.* any surgical procedure used to repair a retinal detachment. *See* cryoretinopexy, pneumoretinopexy.

retinoschisis (ret-in-**osk**-i-sis) *n.* splitting of the layers of the neurosensory retina with accumulation of fluid between the layers. This is usually static or progresses very slowly compared to other types of retinal detachment.

retinoscope (**ret**-in-oh-skohp) *n.* an instrument used to determine the power of spectacle lenses required to correct errors of refraction of the eye. **—retinoscopy** (ret-in-**os**-kŏ-pi) *n.*

retinotomy (ret-in-**ot**-ŏmi) *n.* a surgical incision into the retina.

retraction (ri-**trak**-shŏn) *n.* **1.** (in obstetrics) the state of uterine muscle fibres remaining shortened after contracting during labour. This results in a gradual progression of the fetus downward through the pelvis. **r. ring** a depression in the uterine wall marking the junction between the actively contracting muscle fibres of the upper segment and the muscle fibres of the lower segment of the uterus. This depression is not always visible and is normal. *Compare* Bandl's ring. **2.** (in dentistry) the drawing back of one or more teeth into a better position by an orthodontic appliance.

retractor (ri-**trak**-ter) *n.* a surgical instrument used to expose the operation site by drawing aside the cut edges of skin, muscle, or other tissues. See illustration.

retro- *prefix denoting* at the back or behind.

retrobulbar neuritis (optic neuritis) (ret-roh-**bulb**-er) *n.* inflammation of the optic nerve behind the eye, causing increasingly blurred vision. Retrobulbar neuritis is one of the symptoms of multiple sclerosis but it can also occur as an isolated lesion.

retroflexion (ret-roh-**flek**-shŏn) *n.* the bending backward of an organ or part of an organ, especially the abnormal bending backwards of the upper part of the uterus.

retrograde (**ret**-roh-grayd) *adj.* going backwards, or moving in the opposite direction to the

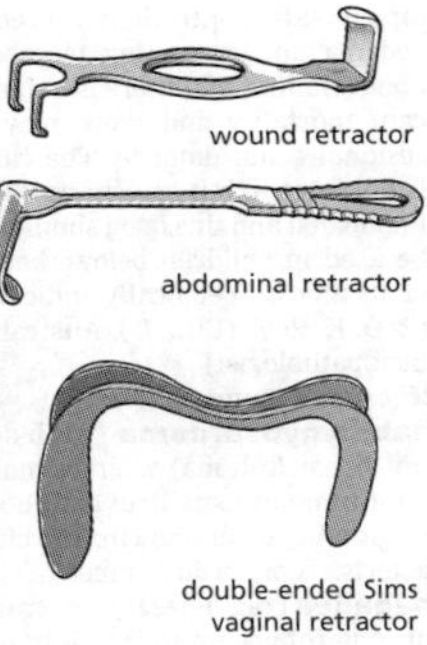

Retractors

normal. *See also* (retrograde) amnesia, (retrograde) pyelography. *Compare* antegrade.

retrogression (ret-roh-**gresh**-ŏn) *n.* return to a less complex state or condition; regression.

retrolental fibroplasia (ret-roh-**len**-t'l) *n.* *see* retinopathy (of prematurity).

retro-ocular (ret-roh-**ok**-yoo-ler) *adj.* behind the eye.

retroperitoneal fibrosis (RPF) (ret-roh-pe-ri-tŏn-**ee**-ăl) *n.* a condition in which a dense plaque of fibrous tissue develops behind the peritoneum adjacent to the abdominal aorta. The ureters become encased and hence obstructed, causing acute anuria and renal failure. The obstruction can be relieved by nephrostomy or the insertion of double J stents. In the acute phase steroid administration may help, but in established RPF ureterolysis is required.

retroperitoneal space *n.* the region between the posterior parietal peritoneum and the front of the lumbar vertebrae. This space contains important structures, including the kidneys, adrenal glands, pancreas, lumbar spinal nerve roots, sympathetic ganglia and nerves, and the abdominal aorta and its major branches.

retropharyngeal (ret-roh-fă-**rin**-ji-ăl) *adj.* behind the pharynx. **r. abscess** a collection of pus in the tissues behind the pharynx, resulting in difficulty in swallowing, pain, and fever.

retropubic (ret-roh-**pew**-bik) *adj.* behind the pubis. **r. prostatectomy** *see* prostatectomy.

retropulsion (ret-roh-**pul**-shŏn) *n.* a compulsive tendency to walk backwards. It is a symptom of parkinsonism.

retrospection (ret-roh-**spek**-shŏn) *n.* (in psychology) the systematic reviewing of past experiences.

retrospective study (ret-roh-**spek**-tiv) *n.* a review of the characteristics of a group of individuals, some of whom have a specific disease or condition, to investigate possible causes by comparing affected and unaffected individuals in terms of past experience. *Compare* prospective study.

retroversion (ret-roh-**ver**-shŏn) *n.* an abnormal position of the uterus in which it is tilted backwards, with the base lying in the pouch of Douglas, against the rectum, instead of on the bladder. *Compare* anteversion.

retrovirus (ret-roh-vy-rŭs) *n.* an RNA-containing virus that can convert its genetic material into DNA, which enables it to become integrated into the DNA of its host's cells. Retroviruses include HIV and viruses implicated in the development of some cancers.

Rett's syndrome (rets) *n.* a disorder affecting young girls, in which stereotyped movements and social withdrawal appear during early childhood. Intellectual development is often impaired and special educational help is needed. The condition is inherited as an X-linked dominant characteristic. [A. Rett (1924–97), Austrian paediatrician]

revascularization (ri-vas-kew-ler-I-zay-shŏn) *n.* **1.** the regrowth of blood vessels following disease or injury so that normal blood supply to an organ, tissue, or part is restored. **2.** the restoration of blood flow to an organ by angioplasty and stenting or by surgical bypass grafting. **coronary r.** re-establishing blood flow to ischaemic heart muscle by coronary angioplasty and insertion of stents or by means of a coronary artery bypass graft.

Reye's syndrome (rayz) *n.* a rare disorder occurring in childhood. It is characterized by the symptoms of encephalitis combined with evidence of liver failure. Treatment is aimed at controlling cerebral oedema and correcting metabolic abnormalities, but there is a significant mortality and there may be residual brain damage. The cause is not known, but aspirin has been implicated and this drug should not be used in children below the age of 16 unless specifically indicated. [R. D. K. Reye (1912–77), Australian histopathologist]

RF *n. see* rheumatic fever.

rhabdomyosarcoma (rab-doh-my-oh-sar-**koh**-mă) *n.* a rare malignant tumour, usually of childhood, originating in, or showing the characteristics of, striated muscle.

rhagades (rag-ă-deez) *pl. n.* cracks or long thin scars in the skin, particularly around the mouth. The fissures around the mouth and nose of babies with congenital syphilis eventually heal to form rhagades.

rhegmatogenous (reg-mă-**toj**-i-nŭs) *adj.* resulting from a break or tear. **r. retinal detachment** retinal detachment as a consequence of a tear in the retina.

rheo- *combining form denoting* **1.** a flow of liquid. **2.** an electric current.

rhesus factor (Rh factor) (ree-sŭs) *n.* a group of antigens that may or may not be present on the surface of the red blood cells; it forms the basis of the rhesus blood group system. Most people have the rhesus factor, i.e. they are **Rh-positive**. People who lack the factor are termed **Rh-negative**. Incompatibility between Rh-positive and Rh-negative blood is an important cause of blood transfusion reactions and of haemolytic disease of the newborn. *See also* blood group.

rheumatic fever (RF, acute rheumatism) (roo-**mat**-ik) *n.* a disease affecting mainly children and young adults that arises as a delayed complication of infection of the upper respiratory tract with haemolytic streptococci. The main features are fever, arthritis, Sydenham's chorea, and inflammation of the heart muscle, its valves, and the membrane surrounding the heart. The infection is treated with antibiotics (e.g. penicillin) and bed rest. **chronic rheumatic heart disease** a complication of rheumatic fever, in which there is scarring and chronic inflammation of the heart and its valves leading to heart failure, murmurs, and damage to the valves.

rheumatism (**room**-ă-tizm) *n.* any disorder in which aches and pains affect the muscles and joints. *See* gout, osteoarthritis, rheumatic fever, rheumatoid arthritis.

rheumatoid arthritis (**room**-ă-toid) *n.* a form of arthritis that is a disease of the synovial lining of joints. It involves the joints of the fingers, wrists, feet, and ankles, with later involvement of the hips, knees, shoulders, and neck. Diagnosis is supported by a blood test and by X-rays revealing typical changes around the affected joints. Treatment is with a variety of drugs, including anti-inflammatory analgesics, corticosteroids, and disease-modifying antirheumatic drugs; some diseased joints can be replaced by prosthetic surgery (*see* arthroplasty).

SEE WEB LINKS

- Explanation of rheumatoid arthritis from Arthritis Care

rheumatology (room-ă-**tol**-ŏji) *n.* the medical specialty concerned with the diagnosis and management of disease involving joints, tendons, muscles, ligaments, and associated structures. *See also* physical medicine. —**rheumatologist** *n.*

Rh factor *n. see* rhesus factor.

rhin- (rhino-) *combining form denoting* the nose.

rhinitis (ry-**ny**-tis) *n.* inflammation of the mucous membrane of the nose. **acute r.** *see* (common) cold. **allergic r.** *see* hay fever. **atrophic r.** rhinitis in which the mucous membrane becomes thinned and fragile. **perennial r. (vasomotor r.)** rhinitis in which there is overgrowth of, and increased secretion by, the membrane.

rhinology (ry-**nol**-ŏji) *n.* the branch of medicine concerned with disorders of the nose and nasal passages.

rhinomycosis (ry-noh-my-**koh**-sis) *n.* fungal infection of the lining of the nose.

rhinophyma (ry-noh-**fy**-mă) *n.* a bulbous craggy swelling of the nose, usually in men. It is a complication of rosacea and in no way related to alcohol intake.

rhinoplasty (**ry**-noh-plasti) *n.* surgery to alter the shape of the nose.

rhinorrhoea (ry-nŏ-**ree**-ă) *n.* a persistent watery mucous discharge from the nose, as in the common cold.

rhinoscopy (ry-**nosk**-ŏ-pi) *n.* examination of the interior of the nose using a speculum or endoscope.

rhinosinusitis (ry-noh-sy-**nūs**-I-tis) *n.* inflammation of the lining of the nose and paranasal sinuses, caused by allergies, infection, immune deficiencies, mucociliary transport abnormalities, trauma, drugs, or tumours. *See* rhinitis, sinusitis.

rhinosporidiosis (ry-noh-sper-id-i-**oh**-sis) *n.* a fungal infection of the mucous membranes of the nose, larynx, eyes, and genitals that is characterized by the formation of polyps.

rhinovirus (**ry**-noh-vy-rŭs) *n.* any one of a group of RNA-containing viruses that cause respiratory infections resembling the common cold. They are included in the picornavirus group.

rhiz- (rhizo-) *combining form denoting* a root.

rhizotomy (ry-**zot**-ŏmi) *n.* a surgical procedure in which selected nerve roots are cut at the point where they emerge from the spinal cord. The posterior (sensory) nerve roots are cut for the relief of intractable pain; the anterior (motor) nerve roots are sometimes cut for the relief of severe muscle spasm or dystonia.

rhodopsin (visual purple) (roh-**dop**-sin) *n.* a pigment in the retina of the eye consisting of retinal and a protein. The presence of rhodopsin is essential for vision in dim light. *See* rod.

rhombencephalon (rom-ben-**sef**-ă-lon) *n.* *see* hindbrain.

rhomboid (**rom**-boid) *n.* either of two muscles situated in the upper part of the back, between the backbone and shoulder blade. They help to move the shoulder blade backwards and upwards.

rhonchus (**ronk**-ŭs) *n.* (*pl.* **rhonchi**) an abnormal musical noise produced by air passing through narrowed bronchi. It is heard through a stethoscope, usually when the patient breathes out.

rhythm method (**rith**-ĕm) *n.* a contraceptive method in which sexual intercourse is restricted to the days at the beginning and end of the menstrual cycle when conception is least likely to occur (**safe period**). The method depends for its reliability on the woman having uniform regular periods and its failure rate is higher than with mechanical methods.

rib (rib) *n.* a curved strip of bone forming part of the skeleton of the thorax. There are 12 pairs of ribs. The head of each rib articulates with one of the 12 thoracic vertebrae of the backbone; the other end is attached to a costal cartilage. **false r.** any of the three pairs of ribs below the true ribs. Each is connected by its cartilage to the rib above it. **floating r.** any of the last two pairs of ribs, which end freely in the muscles of the body wall. **true r.** any of the first seven pairs of ribs, which are connected directly to the sternum by their costal cartilages. Anatomical name: **costa**.

ribavirin (ry-bă-**vy**-rin) *n.* an antiviral drug effective against a range of DNA and RNA viruses, including respiratory syncytial virus and hepatitis C. It is administered by a small-particle aerosol inhaler or by mouth. Trade names: **Copegus**, **Rebetol**, **Virazole**.

riboflavin (vitamin B_2) (ry-boh-flay-vin) *n. see* vitamin B.

ribonuclease (ry-boh-new-kli-ayz) *n.* an enzyme, located in the lysosomes of cells, that splits RNA at specific places in the molecule.

ribonucleic acid (ry-boh-new-klee-ik) *n. see* RNA.

ribose (ry-bohz) *n.* a pentose sugar that is a component of RNA and several coenzymes. Ribose is also involved in intracellular metabolism.

ribosome (ry-bŏ-sohm) *n.* a particle, consisting of RNA and protein, that occurs in cells and is the site of protein synthesis in the cell (*see* translation). **—ribosomal** *adj.*

ricewater stools (rys-waw-ter) *pl. n. see* cholera.

ricin (ry-sin) *n.* a highly toxic albumin obtained from castor-oil seeds (*Ricinus communis*) that inhibits protein synthesis and becomes attached to the surface of cells, resulting in gastroenteritis, hepatic congestion and jaundice, and cardiovascular collapse. *See also* immunotoxin.

rickets (rik-its) *n.* a disease of childhood in which the bones do not harden due to a deficiency of vitamin D (dietary or resulting from lack of exposure to sunlight). *See also* osteomalacia. **renal r.** a type of rickets that is due to impaired kidney function causing bone-forming minerals to be excreted in the urine, which results in softening of the bones.

rickettsiae (ri-ket-si-ee) *pl. n.* (*sing.* **rickettsia**) a group of very small nonmotile spherical or rod-like parasitic bacteria that cannot reproduce outside the bodies of their hosts. They cause such illnesses as rickettsial pox, Rocky Mountain spotted fever, and typhus. Rickettsiae infect arthropods (ticks, mites, etc.), through which they can be transmitted to humans. **—rickettsial** (ri-ket-si-ăl) *adj.*

rickettsial pox *n.* a disease of mice caused by the bacterium *Rickettsia akari* and transmitted to humans by mites: it produces chills, fever, muscular pain, and a rash similar to that of chickenpox. *See also* typhus.

ridge (rij) *n.* **1.** (in anatomy) a crest or a long narrow protuberance, e.g. on a bone. **2.** (in dental anatomy) the crest of the jawbone following tooth loss.

Riedel's struma (reed-ĕlz) *n.* a rare fibrosing destructive disorder of the thyroid gland that may spread to adjacent tissues and obstruct the airway. It is sometimes associated with fibrosis in other parts of the body, such as the bile duct or retroperitoneal fibrosis. [B. M. C. L. Riedel (1846–1916), German surgeon]

rifampicin (rif-am-pi-sin) *n.* an antibiotic administered by mouth or intravenous infusion to treat various infections, particularly tuberculosis and leprosy. Trade names: **Rifadin**, **Rimactane**.

rigidity (ri-**jid**-iti) *n.* (in neurology) resistance to the passive movement of a limb that persists throughout its range. It is a symptom of parkinsonism. *Compare* spasticity. **clasp-knife r.** *see* spasticity.

rigor (**ry**-ger) *n.* an abrupt attack of shivering and a sensation of coldness, accompanied by a rapid rise in body temperature. This often marks the onset of a fever and may be followed by a feeling of heat, with copious sweating. **r. mortis** the stiffening of a body that occurs within some eight hours of death in temperate climates, due to chemical changes in muscle tissue. It usually starts to disappear after about 24 hours.

riluzole (**ril**-yoo-zohl) *n.* a drug used to prolong the lives of patients with amyotrophic lateral sclerosis. It is administered by mouth. Trade name: **Rilutek**.

rima (**ry**-mă) *n.* (in anatomy) a cleft. **r. glottidis** the space between the vocal folds.

ring (ring) *n.* (in anatomy) *see* annulus.

ring block *n.* a circumferential ring of local anaesthetic solution used to block the nerves of a digit for purposes of minor surgery (*see* nerve block). Precautions are necessary to avoid vascular damage leading to gangrene.

Ringer's solution (Ringer's mixture) (**ring**-erz) *n.* a clear colourless physiological solution of sodium chloride, potassium chloride, and calcium chloride prepared with recently boiled pure water. [S. Ringer (1835–1910), British physiologist]

ringworm (**ring**-werm) *n.* *see* tinea.

Rinne's test (**rin**-iz) *n.* a test to determine whether deafness is conductive or sensorineural. A vibrating tuning fork is held first in the air, close to the ear, and then with its base placed on the mastoid process. If the sound conducted by air is heard louder than the sound conducted by bone the test is positive and the deafness sensorineural; a negative result indicates conductive deafness. [H. A. Rinne (1819–68), German otologist]

RIP *n.* raised intracranial pressure. *See* intracranial (pressure).

risk assessment (risk) *n.* (in psychiatry) an assessment of the risk that a patient may pose at a given time, which is based primarily on past behaviour and certain aspects of current behaviour. It is usually divided into risk to the patient him- or herself, risk to others, and risk of neglect.

risk factor *n.* an attribute, such as a habit (e.g. cigarette smoking) or exposure to some environmental hazard, that leads the individual concerned to have a greater likelihood of developing an illness. The relationship is one of probability and as such can be distinguished from a causal agent.

risk management *n.* an element of clinical governance in which principles are applied to aspects of health care to increase patient safety by identifying potential hazards, assessing the degree of risk, and reducing the risk or determining an acceptable balance between risk and benefit. It should include systems for learning from untoward, significant, or critical incidents and near misses.

risk register *n.* **1.** a list of infants who have experienced some event in their obstetric and/or perinatal history known to be correlated with a higher-than-average likelihood of serious abnormality. Problems associated with risk registers include limiting the designation of predisposing conditions, so to contain the number on the register within reasonable proportions, and ensuring that children not on the register receive adequate surveillance. **2.** (**at-risk register**) *see* child protection register.

risperidone (ris-pe-ri-dohn) *n.* a second-generation antipsychotic drug given by mouth or depot injection in the treatment of schizophrenia, mania, and other psychoses. Side-effects include nausea, headache, and sedation. Trade names: **Risperdal**, **Risperdal Consta**.

risus sardonicus (ry-sŭs sar-**don**-ik-ŭs) *n.* an abnormal grinning expression resulting from involuntary prolonged contraction of facial muscles, as seen in tetanus.

Ritter's disease (rit-erz) *n. see* staphylococcal scalded skin syndrome. [G. Ritter von Rittershain (1820–83), German physician]

rituximab (rit-**uks**-i-mab) *n.* a monoclonal antibody administered by intravenous infusion to treat many lymphomas and leukaemias and also severe rheumatoid arthritis and vasculitis.

rivastigmine (ry-vă-**stig**-meen) *n. see* acetylcholinesterase inhibitor.

river blindness *n. see* onchocerciasis.

RN *n.* registered nurse. *See also* nurse.

RNA (ribonucleic acid) *n.* a nucleic acid, occurring in the nucleus and cytoplasm of cells, that is concerned with synthesis of proteins (*see* messenger RNA, ribosome, transfer RNA, translation). In some viruses RNA is the genetic material.

RNLD *n.* registered nurse, learning disabilities. *See also* nurse.

RNMH *n.* registered nurse, mental health. *See also* nurse.

robotic surgery *n.* a type of laparoscopic surgery in which the operating surgeon controls the instruments via a robot. The surgeon sits at a console away from the patient and controls the robot's operating arms.

Rocky Mountain spotted fever (spotted fever, tick fever) *n.* a disease of rodents and other small mammals in North America caused by the bacterium *Rickettsia rickettsii* and transmitted to humans by ticks. Symptoms include fever, muscle pains, and a profuse reddish rash like that of measles. Treatment with tetracycline or chloramphenicol is effective. *See also* typhus.

rod (rod) *n.* one of the two types of light-sensitive cells in the retina of the eye (*compare* cone). Rods are necessary for seeing in dim light. They contain the pigment rhodopsin, which is bleached in the light and regenerated in the dark. When all the pigment is bleached (i.e. in bright light) the rods no longer function. *See also* dark adaptation, light adaptation.

rodent ulcer (roh-dĕnt) *n. see* basal cell carcinoma.

roentgen (**ront**-gĕn) *n.* a unit of exposure dose of X- or gamma-radiation.

role playing (**rohl**-play-ing) *n.* acting out another person's expected behaviour, usually in a contrived situation, in order to understand that person better. It is used in family psychotherapy, in teaching social skills to patients, and also in the training of psychiatric (and other) staff.

ROM *n. see* range of movement.

Romanowsky stains (roh-mă-**nof**-ski) *pl. n.* a group of stains used for microscopical examination of blood cells, consisting of variable mixtures of thiazine dyes with eosin. [D. L. Romanowsky (1861–1921), Russian physician]

Romberg's sign (**rom**-bergz) *n.* a finding on examination suggesting a sensory disorder affecting those nerves that transmit information to the brain about the position of the limbs and joints and the tension in the muscles. The patient is unable to maintain an upright posture with the eyes closed. [M. Romberg (1795–1873), German neurologist]

rongeur (rawn-*zh*er) *n.* powerful biting forceps for cutting tissue, particularly bone.

R on T phenomenon *n.* (in electrocardiography) the superimposition of an R wave (ventricular depolarization) on the T wave (ventricular repolarization) of the preceding heartbeat. It may trigger ventricular fibrillation. *See* QRS complex, Q–T interval, S–T segment.

root (root) *n.* **1.** (in neurology) a bundle of nerve fibres at its emergence from the spinal cord. **2.** (in dentistry) the part of a tooth that is not covered by enamel and is normally attached to the alveolar bone by periodontal fibres. **r. canal treatment** the procedure of removing the remnants of the pulp of a tooth, cleaning and shaping the canal inside the tooth, and filling the root canal. **3.** the origin of any structure, i.e. the point at which it diverges from another structure. Anatomical name: **radix**.

root cause analysis (RCA) *n.* a tool that enables the systematic investigation of a situation or an incident through the gathering of information, identification and analysis of the situation, the generation of potential recommendations, and implementation of a solution. It focuses on the origins of the situation to enable effective exploration of cause and effect and avoidance of recurrence.

root end resection *n. see* apicectomy.

rooting reflex (**root**-ing) *n.* a primitive reflex present in newborn babies: if the cheek is stroked near the mouth, the infant will turn its head to the same side to suckle.

Roper, Logan, and Tierney model (**roh**-per **loh**-găn **teer**-ni) *n.* a model for nursing that emphasizes the importance of the patient's ability to perform activities of daily living. Individuals are seen as being engaged in various activities of living throughout their lifespan; during their lives they will fluctuate between total independence and total dependence, according to age, circumstance, and health status. Nursing should provide assistance with these activities when needed. *See also* nursing models. [N. Roper, W. Logan, and A. Tierney (20th century), British nurse theorists]

ropinirole (roh-**pin**-i-rohl) *n.* a dopamine receptor agonist used to treat Parkinson's disease (either alone or in conjunction with levodopa) and restless legs syndrome. It is administered by mouth. Trade names: **Adartrel**, **Requip**.

Rorschach test (ror-shahk) *n.* a test to measure aspects of personality, consisting of ten inkblots in colour and black and white. The responses to the different inkblots are used to derive hypotheses about the subject. [H. Rorschach (1884–1922), Swiss psychiatrist]

rosacea (roh-**zay**-shiă) *n.* a chronic inflammatory disease of the face in which the skin becomes abnormally flushed. The disease occurs in both sexes and at all ages but is most common in women in their thirties.

roseola (roseola infantum, exanthem subitum) (roh-**zee**-ŏ-lă) *n.* a condition of young children in which a fever lasting for three or four days is followed by a rose-coloured rash that fades after two days. It is caused by human herpesvirus 6.

rostrum (ros-trŭm) *n.* (*pl.* **rostra**) (in anatomy) a beaklike projection, such as that on the sphenoid bone. —**rostral** *adj.*

rotator (roh-**tay**-ter) *n.* a muscle that brings about rotation of a part.

rotavirus (**roh**-tă-vy-rus) *n.* any member of a genus of viruses that occur in birds and mammals and cause diarrhoea (often severe) in children. The viruses are excreted in the faeces of infected individuals and are usually transmitted in food prepared with unwashed hands.

Rothera's test (ro*th*-er-ăz) *n.* a method of testing urine for the presence of acetone or acetoacetic acid – a sign of diabetes mellitus. [A. C. H. Rothera (1880–1915), Australian biochemist]

Roth spot (roht) *n.* a pale area surrounded by haemorrhage sometimes seen in the retina of those who have bacterial endocarditis, septicaemia, or leukaemia. [M. Roth (1839–1915), Swiss physician]

roughage (**ruf**-ij) *n.* *see* dietary fibre.

rouleau (roo-loh) *n.* (*pl.* **rouleaux**) a cylindrical structure in the blood formed from several red blood cells piled one upon the other and adhering by their rims.

round ligaments (rownd) *pl. n.* the fibromuscular bands that pass from the uterus along the broad ligaments to terminate in the labia majora.

round window *n.* *see* fenestra (rotunda).

roundworm (**rownd**-werm) *n.* *see* nematode.

Rovsing's sign (**rov**-singz) *n.* pain in the right iliac fossa induced by pressure on the left iliac fossa: a sign of acute appendicitis. [N. T. Rovsing (1868–1927), Danish surgeon]

Roy's model (roiz) *n.* a model for nursing based on the assumption that individuals are constantly adapting to changes in their environment. Adaptive responses to environmental stimuli are by means of innate or acquired mechanisms and work within the modes of physiological function, the concept of 'self', role function, and interdependence. Nursing should aim to promote and support these adaptive responses. *See also* nursing models. [C. Roy (1939–), US nurse theorist]

RPE *n.* retinal pigment epithelium. *See* retina.

-rrhagia (-rrhage) *combining form denoting* excessive or abnormal flow or discharge from an organ or part.

-rrhaphy *combining form denoting* surgical sewing; suturing.

-rrhexis *combining form denoting* splitting or rupture of a part.

-rrhoea *combining form denoting* a flow or discharge from an organ or part.

RSI *n. see* repetitive strain injury.

RSV *n. see* respiratory syncytial virus.

RSVP *n. r*eason, *s*tory, *v*ital signs, *p*lan: a communication tool that aims to enhance safe practice and ensure that essential information is communicated in a structured format.

RTA *n.* road-traffic accident.

rubefacient (roo-bi-**fay**-shĕnt) *n.* an agent that causes reddening and warming of the skin. Rubefacients are often used as counterirritants for the relief of muscular pain.

rubella (roo-**bel**-ă) *n. see* German measles.

rubeola (roo-**bee**-ŏ-lă) *n. see* measles.

rubidium-81 (roo-**bid**-iŭm) *n.* an artificial radioactive isotope, with a half-life of about four hours, that decays into krypton-81m, emitting radiations. It is used in ventilation-perfusion scanning.

rubor (**roo**-ber) *n.* redness: one of the four classical signs of inflammation in a tissue. *See also* calor, dolor, tumor.

ruga (**roo**-gă) *n.* (*pl.* **rugae**) a fold or crease, especially one of the folds of mucous membrane that line the stomach.

rule of nines (rool nynz) *n.* a method for quickly assessing the area of the body covered by burns in order to assist calculation of the amount of intravenous fluid to be given. The body is divided into areas of skin comprising approximately 9% each of the total body surface. These are as follows: each arm=9%, the head=9%, each leg=18%, the back of the torso=18%, the front of the torso=18%, with the external genitalia making up the final 1%. The rule is not applicable to children, whose body proportions change with age (in younger children the head represents a greater proportion of the total body surface area).

rumination (roo-mi-**nay**-shŏn) *n.* (in psychiatry) an obsessional type of thinking in which the same thoughts or themes are experienced repetitively. Rumination is a feature of obsessive–compulsive disorder and depression.

rupture (rup-cher) **1.** *n. see* hernia. **2.** *n.* the bursting apart or open of an organ or tissue; for example, the splitting of the membranes enclosing an infant during childbirth. **3.** *vb.* (of tissues, etc.) to burst apart or open.

Russell-Silver syndrome (Silver-Russell syndrome) (rus-ĕl sil-ver) *n.* a congenital condition characterized by short stature, a triangular face with a small mandible (lower jaw), and asymmetry of the body. [A. Russell (1914–2003), British pathologist; H. K. Silver (1918–91), US paediatrician]

Russell traction *n.* a form of traction used to align a fractured femur. The lower leg is supported in a sling just below the knee and pulling forces are exerted upwards and longitudinally by means of pulleys and weights. [R. H. Russell (1860–1933), Australian surgeon]

RV *n. see* residual volume.

RVF *n.* right ventricular failure. *See* heart failure.

Ryle's tube (rylz) *n.* a flexible tube that is inserted into the stomach through the nose of a patient and is used for aspiration of gastric secretions and evacuation of intestinal gas. [J. A. Ryle (1889–1950), British physician]

Ss

SA *n. see* (sinus) arrhythmia.

Sabin vaccine (say-bin) *n.* an oral vaccine against poliomyelitis. [A. B. Sabin (1906–93), US bacteriologist]

sac (sak) *n.* a pouch or baglike structure. Sacs can enclose natural cavities in the body, e.g. in the lungs (*see* alveolus), or they can be pathological, as in a hernia.

saccade (sa-**kahd**) *n.* a rapid movement of the eye, voluntary or occurring as a reflex, used to shift the gaze from one object to another.

sacchar- (saccharo-) *combining form denoting* sugar.

saccharide (**sak**-eryd) *n.* a carbohydrate. *See also* disaccharide, monosaccharide, polysaccharide.

saccharine (**sak**-er-een) *n.* a sweetening agent. Saccharine is 300 times as sweet as sugar and has no energy content. It is very useful as a sweetener in diabetic and low-calorie foods.

Saccharomyces (sak-er-oh-**my**-seez) *n. see* yeast.

sacculated (**sak**-yoo-layt-id) *adj.* pursed out with small pouches or sacs.

saccule (sacculus) (**sak**-yool) *n.* the smaller of the two membranous sacs within the vestibule of the ear. It contains a macula, which responds to gravity and relays information to the brain about the position of the head.

sacralization (say-krǎ-ly-**zay**-shŏn) *n.* abnormal fusion of the fifth lumbar vertebra with the sacrum.

sacral nerves (**say**-krǎl) *pl. n.* the five pairs of spinal nerves that emerge from the spinal column in the sacrum. The nerves carry sensory and motor fibres from the upper and lower leg and from the anal and genital regions.

sacral vertebrae *pl. n. see* sacrum.

sacro- *prefix denoting* the sacrum.

sacrococcygeal (say-kroh-kok-**sij**-iǎl) *adj.* relating to or between the sacrum and the coccyx.

sacroiliac (say-kroh-**il**-i-ak) *adj.* relating to the sacrum and the ilium.

sacroiliitis (say-kroh-il-i-**I**-tis) *n.* inflammation of the sacroiliac joint. Involvement of both joints is a common feature of ankylosing spondylitis and associated rheumatic diseases. The resultant low back pain and stiffness may be alleviated by rest, anti-inflammatory analgesics, or biological disease-modifying antirheumatic drugs.

sacroplasty (say-kroh-plas-ti) *n.* surgery using minimally invasive techniques and liquid cement to stabilize fragile sacral fractures, which previously would have been treated with rest and analgesia.

sacrum (**say**-krŭm) *n.* (*pl.* **sacra**) a curved triangular element of the backbone consisting of five fused vertebrae (**sacral vertebrae**). It articulates with the last lumbar vertebra above, the coccyx below, and the hip bones laterally. *See also* vertebra. **—sacral** *adj.*

SAD (seasonal affective disorder) (sad) *n.* a disorder marked by changes of mood at particular times of the year. Typically, with the onset of winter, there is depression, general slowing of mind and body, excessive sleeping, and overeating. These symptoms resolve with the coming of spring and are also relieved by phototherapy. There is evidence that mood is related to light, which suppresses the release of the hormone melatonin from the pineal gland, but the exact mechanism by which light acts as an antidepressant is unclear.

saddle-nose (sa-d'l-nohz) *n.* flattening of the bridge of the nose, such as may occur in congenital syphilis.

safe period (sayf) *n. see* rhythm method.

sagittal (saj-it'l) *adj.* describing a dorsoventral plane that extends down the long axis of the body, parallel to the median plane, dividing it into right and left parts. **s. suture** the immovable joint between the two parietal bones of the skull.

SAH *n. see* subarachnoid haemorrhage.

St Anthony's fire (sănt ant-ŏ-niz fyr) *n.* an old colloquial name for the inflammation of the skin associated with ergot poisoning. *See* ergotism.

St Thomas's Risk Assessment in Falling Elderly In-patients (STRATIFY) *n.* a validated but generic risk assessment tool that predicts the risk of falls in adult in-patients. It assesses a patient's mental status, visual acuity, mobility, and level of continence on admission and allocates a score that could be indicative of risk. It needs to be repeated during the in-patient stay. It is not disease-specific, which can increase the risk of falling.

St Vitus' dance (sănt vy-tŭs dahns) *n.* an archaic name for Sydenham's chorea.

salaam attacks (să-lahm) *pl. n. see* infantile (spasms).

salbutamol (sal-bew-tă-mol) *n.* a drug that stimulates beta-adrenergic receptors (*see* sympathomimetic). It is administered by mouth, injection, infusion, or inhalation as a short-acting bronchodilator to relieve asthma and other reversible obstructive airways diseases and to inhibit premature labour. Trade names: **Airomir**, **Asmasal Clickhaler**, **Salbulin Novolizer**, **Ventolin**, etc.

salicylate (să-lis-i-layt) *n.* a salt of salicylic acid. *See* methyl salicylate.

salicylic acid (sal-i-sil-ik) *n.* a drug that causes the skin to peel and destroys bacteria and fungi. It is applied to the skin, alone or in combination with other agents, to treat warts, corns, callus, acne, dandruff, psoriasis, and fungal nail infections. Trade names: **Cuplex**, **Duofilm**, **Salactol**, **Verrugon**, etc.

salicylism (sal-i-sil-izm) *n.* poisoning due to an overdose of aspirin or other salicylate-containing compounds. The main symptoms are headache, dizziness, tinnitus, disturbances of vision, and vomiting.

saline (normal saline, physiological saline) (say-lyn) *n.* a 0.9% solution of sodium chloride in distilled water. Saline may be used clinically for irrigating wounds, treating sodium depletion (by intravenous infusion), as a diluent for drugs, and as an ingredient of plasma substitute.

saliva (să-ly-vă) *n.* the alkaline liquid secreted by the salivary glands and the mucous membrane of the mouth. Its principal constituents are water and mucus, which keep the mouth moist and lubricate food, and enzymes (e.g. amylase) that begin the digestion of starch. *See also* dry mouth. **—salivary** (să-ly-ver-i) *adj.*

salivary gland *n.* a gland that produces saliva. There are three pairs of salivary glands: the parotid glands, sublingual glands, and submandibular glands (see illustration).

salivary stone *n. see* sialolith.

salivation (sal-i-vay-shŏn) *n.* the secretion of saliva by the salivary glands of the mouth, increased in response to the chewing action of the jaws or to the thought, taste, smell, or sight of food. *See also* ptyalism.

Salk vaccine (sawlk) *n.* a vaccine against poliomyelitis. It is administered by injection. [J. E. Salk (1914–95), US bacteriologist]

salmeterol (sal-mee-ter-ol) *n.* a drug that stimulates beta-adrenergic receptors (*see* sympathomimetic) and is used as a long-acting bronchodilator. It is administered by inhaler

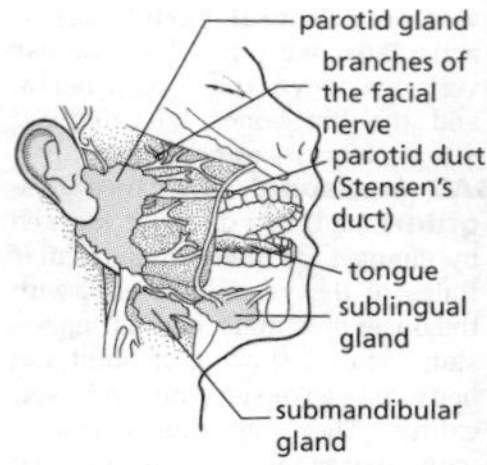

Salivary glands

to control chronic asthma and chronic obstructive pulmonary disease. Trade name: **Serevent**.

Salmonella (sal-mŏ-nel-ă) *n.* a genus of Gram-negative motile rodlike bacteria that inhabit the intestines of animals and humans. Certain species cause such diseases as food poisoning, gastroenteritis, and septicaemia. **S. paratyphi** a species that causes paratyphoid fever. **S. typhi** a species that causes typhoid fever.

salmonellosis (sal-mŏ-nel-**oh**-sis) *n.* an infestation of the digestive system by bacteria of the genus *Salmonella*. *See also* food poisoning.

salping- (salpingo-) *combining form denoting* **1.** the Fallopian tube. **2.** the auditory canal (meatus).

salpingectomy (sal-pin-**jek**-tŏmi) *n.* the surgical removal of a Fallopian tube, most commonly carried out for removal of a tubal pregnancy (*see* ectopic pregnancy). The operation involving both tubes is a permanent and completely effective method of sterilization.

salpingitis (sal-pin-**jy**-tis) *n.* inflammation of a tube, most commonly of one or both of the Fallopian tubes caused by bacterial infection spreading from the vagina or uterus or carried in the blood. **acute s.** salpingitis in which there is sharp pain in the lower abdomen. The infection may spread to the peritoneum (*see* peritonitis); in severe cases the tubes may become blocked with scar tissue.

salpingography (sal-ping-**og**-răfi) *n.* radiography of one or both Fallopian tubes after a radiopaque substance has been introduced into them via an injection into the uterus. **standardized selective s.** salpingography combined with tubal catheterization, which enables occluded tubes to be restored to patency.

salpingolysis (sal-ping-**ol**-i-sis) *n.* a surgical operation carried out to restore patency to blocked Fallopian tubes; it involves the division and removal of adhesions around the ovarian ends of the tubes.

salpingo-oophorectomy (sal-ping-oh-oh-ŏ-fŏ-**rek**-tŏmi) *n.* surgical removal of a Fallopian tube and the ovary associated with it.

salpingo-oophoritis (sal-ping-oh-oh-ŏ-fŏ-**ry**-tis) *n.* inflammation of a Fallopian tube and an ovary.

salpingostomy (sal-ping-**ost**-ŏmi) *n.* the surgical creation of an artificial opening in a blocked Fallopian tube in order to restore its patency.

salpinx (**sal**-pinks) *n.* (in anatomy) a tube, especially a Fallopian tube or the external auditory meatus.

salt (sawlt) *n.* (in chemistry) a compound formed when the hydrogen in an acid is replaced by a metal. An acid and a base react together to form a salt and water. **common s.** *see* sodium chloride. **s. depletion** excessive loss of sodium chloride from the body. This may result from sweating, persistent vomiting or diarrhoea, or loss of fluid in wounds. The main symptoms are muscular weakness and cramps.

salvage procedure (**sal**-vij) *n.* surgical measures to palliate the worst effects of a tumour but with no aim to effect a cure.

sample (**sahm**-pŭl) *n.* a subgroup of a population that is selected for study because it is regarded as representative of the population as a whole. **random s.** a sample selected by a random process ensuring that each member of the population has an equal chance of being included in it.

sanatorium (san-ă-**tor**-iŭm) *n.* **1.** a hospital or institution for the rehabilitation and convalescence of patients of any kind. **2.** an institution for patients who have suffered from pulmonary tuberculosis.

sandfly fever (**sand**-fly) *n.* a viral influenza-like disease transmitted to humans by the bite of the sandfly *Phlebotomus papatasii*. Sandfly fever occurs principally in countries surrounding the Persian Gulf and the tropical Mediterranean.

sandwich therapy (**sand**-wich) *n.* a combination of treatments in which one type of therapy (e.g. a surgical operation) is 'sandwiched' between exposures to another treatment (e.g. pre- and postoperative chemotherapy). *See also* combined therapy.

sangui- (sanguino-) *combining form denoting* blood.

sanguineous (sang-**win**-iŭs) *adj.* **1.** containing, stained, or covered with blood. **2.** (of tissues) containing more than the normal quantity of blood.

sanies (**say**-ni-eez) *n.* a foul-smelling watery discharge from a wound or ulcer, containing serum, blood, and pus.

SANS *n. see* Schedule for Assessment of Negative Symptoms.

saphena (să-**fee**-nă) *n. see* saphenous vein.

saphena varix *n.* an abnormal dilatation of the terminal section of the long saphenous vein in the groin.

saphenous nerve (să-**fee**-nŭs) *n.* a large branch of the femoral nerve that supplies the skin from the knee to below the ankle with sensory nerves.

saphenous vein (saphena) *n.* either of two superficial veins of the leg, draining blood from the foot. **long s. v.** the longest vein in the body, running from the foot to the groin. **short s. v.** the vein that runs up the back of the calf.

saponify (să-**pon**-i-fy) *vb.* (in chemistry) to hydrolyse an ester with a hydroxide, especially a fat with a hydroxide to form a soap. **—saponification** *n.*

sapr- (sapro-) *combining form denoting* **1.** putrefaction. **2.** decaying matter.

sapraemia (sap-**ree**-miă) *n.* blood poisoning by toxins of saprophytic bacteria. *Compare* pyaemia, septicaemia, toxaemia.

saprophyte (**sap**-roh-fyt) *n.* any free-living organism that lives and feeds on the dead and putrefying tissues of animals or plants. *Compare* parasite. **—saprophytic** (sap-roh-**fit**-ik) *adj.*

sarc- (sarco-) *combining form denoting* **1.** flesh or fleshy tissue. **2.** muscle.

sarcoid (**sar**-koid) **1.** *adj.* fleshy. **2.** *n.* a fleshy tumour.

sarcoidosis (Boeck's disease) (sar-koid-**oh**-sis) *n.* a chronic disorder of unknown cause in which the lymph nodes in many parts of the body are enlarged and granulomas develop in the lungs, liver, and spleen. The skin, nervous system, eyes, and salivary glands are also commonly affected, and the condition has features similar to tuberculosis.

sarcolemma (sar-koh-**lem**-ă) *n.* the cell membrane that encloses a muscle cell (muscle fibre).

sarcoma (sar-**koh**-mă) *n.* any cancer of connective tissue. These tumours may occur in any part of the body; they arise in fibrous tissue, muscle, fat, bone, cartilage, synovium, blood and lymphatic vessels, and various other tissues. *See also* chondrosarcoma, fibrosarcoma, leiomyosarcoma, liposarcoma, lymphangiosarcoma, osteosarcoma, rhabdomyosarcoma. **—sarcomatous** *adj.*

sarcoplasm (myoplasm) (**sar**-koh-plazm) *n.* the cytoplasm of muscle cells.

Sarcoptes (sar-**kop**-teez) *n.* a genus of small oval mites. **S. scabiei** the scabies mite. The female tunnels into the skin, where it lays its eggs. The presence of the mites causes severe irritation, which eventually leads to scabies.

SARS (severe acquired respiratory syndrome) *n.* an atypical pneumonia caused by a virus, SARS coronavirus (SARS CoV), that first appeared in November 2002 in China and subsequently spread to more than 20 countries in Asia, Europe, and North and South America before being contained (in June 2003). A total of 8098 people worldwide contracted SARS during the 2003 outbreak; 774 of these died. The disease itself was declared eradicated by the WHO in May 2005.

SEE WEB LINKS

- Information about SARS from the Health and Safety Executive

sartorius (sar-**tor**-iŭs) *n.* a narrow ribbon-like muscle at the front of the thigh. The longest muscle in the body, the sartorius flexes the leg on the thigh and the thigh on the abdomen.

SAS *n.* sleep apnoea syndrome (*see* (obstructive) sleep apnoea).

saucerization (saw-ser-I-**zay**-shŏn) *n.* **1.** an operation in which tissue is cut away from a wound to form a saucer-like depression. It is carried out to facilitate healing of injuries or disorders in which bone is infected. **2.** the concave appearance of the upper surface of a vertebra that has been fractured by compression.

Sayre's jacket (**say**-erz) *n.* a plaster of Paris cast used to support the backbone when the vertebrae have been severely damaged by disease, such as tuberculosis. [L. A. Sayre (1820–1900), US surgeon]

SBAR *n. see* situation, background, assessment, recommendation.

SBE *n. see* subacute bacterial endocarditis.

SBS *n. see* short bowel syndrome.

scab (skab) *n.* a hard crust of dried blood, serum, or pus that develops over a sore, cut, or scratch.

scabicide (**skay**-bi-syd) *n.* a drug that kills the mites causing scabies.

scabies (**skay**-beez) *n.* a skin infection caused by the mite *Sarcoptes scabiei*. Scabies is typified by severe itching, red papules, and often secondary infection. The mites pass from person to person by prolonged close contact. Commonly infected areas are the penis, nipples, and the finger webs. Treatment is by application of a scabicide, usually permethrin or malathion, to all areas of the body from the neck down; benzyl benzoate may be used but is more irritant.

scala (**skay**-lă) *n.* one of the spiral canals of the cochlea.

scald (skawld) *n.* a burn produced by a hot liquid or vapour, such as boiling water or steam.

scale (skayl) **1.** *n.* any of the flakes of dead epidermal cells shed from the skin. **2.** *vb.* to scrape deposits of calculus from the teeth (*see* scaler).

scalenus (skay-**leen**-ŭs) *n.* one of four paired muscles of the neck (**s. anterior**, **medius**, **minimus**, and **posterior**). They are responsible for raising the first and second ribs in inspiration and for bending the neck forward and to either side.

scalenus syndrome (thoracic outlet syndrome) *n.* the group of symptoms caused by compression of the subclavian artery and the lower roots of the brachial plexus against the outlet of the upper thoracic vertebrae. Loss of sensation and wasting may be found in the affected arm, which may also be painful.

scaler (skayl-er) *n.* an instrument for removing calculus from the teeth. It may be a hand instrument or one energized by rapid ultrasonic vibrations.

scalp (skalp) *n.* the skin that covers the cranium and is itself covered with hair.

scalpel (skal-pěl) *n.* a small pointed surgical knife with a straight handle and usually detachable disposable blades of various shapes.

scan (skan) **1.** *n.* examination of the body or a part of the body using ultrasonography, **computerized tomography** (**CT**), **magnetic resonance imaging** (**MRI**), or scintigraphy. **2.** *n.* the image obtained from such an examination. **3.** *vb.* to examine the body using any of these techniques.

scanning speech (skan-ing) *n.* a disorder of articulation in which the syllables are inappropriately separated and equally stressed. It is caused by cerebellar disease.

scaphocephaly (skaf-oh-sef-ăli) *n.* an abnormally long and narrow skull due to premature closure of the sagittal suture. **—scaphocephalic** (skaf-oh-si-fal-ik) *adj.*

scaphoid bone (skay-foid) *n.* a boat-shaped bone of the wrist (*see* carpus). It articulates with the trapezium and trapezoid bones in front, with the radius behind, and with the capitate and lunate medially. It is commonly injured by falls; for example, a **scaphoid fracture** is usually caused by a fall onto the outstretched hand.

scapul- (scapulo-) *combining form denoting* the scapula.

scapula (skap-yoo-lă) *n.* (*pl.* **scapulas** or **scapulae**) the shoulder blade: a triangular bone, a pair of which form the back part of the shoulder girdle. **—scapular** *adj.*

scar *n.* a permanent mark left after wound healing. **hypertrophic s.** an abnormal raised scar that tends to settle after a year or so, as distinct from a keloid, which is not only permanent but tends to extend beyond the original wound.

scarification (ska-rifi-kay-shŏn) *n.* the process of making a series of shallow cuts or scratches in the skin to allow a substance, such as a droplet of smallpox vaccine, to penetrate the body.

scarlatina (skar-lă-tee-nă) *n. see* scarlet fever.

scarlet fever (skar-lit) *n.* a highly contagious disease caused by toxin-producing bacteria of the genus *Streptococcus*. The symptoms include fever, tonsillitis, and a widespread scarlet rash; the tongue is also affected, becoming bright red. Treatment with antibiotics reduces the risk of secondary complications, such as ear and kidney inflammation. Medical name: **scarlatina**. *Compare* German measles.

Scarpa's triangle (skar-păz) *n. see* femoral (triangle). [A. Scarpa (1747–1832), Italian anatomist and surgeon]

scat- (scato-) *combining form denoting* faeces.

SCBU *n. see* special care baby unit.

SCC *n. see* squamous cell carcinoma.

Schedule for Assessment of Negative Symptoms (SANS) (**shed**-yool) *n.* an assessment tool designed to identify 20 negative symptoms of schizophrenia (apathy, social withdrawal, lack of spontaneity, etc.), which are numerically graded on a scale from 0 to 5.

Scheuermann's disease (adolescent kyphosis) (**shoi**-er-manz) *n.* a disorder of spinal growth, arising in adolescence, in which three or more vertebrae, usually in the thoracic spine, become wedge-shaped, resulting in backache and exaggerated outward curvature of the spine (kyphosis). [H. W. Scheuermann (1877–1960), Danish surgeon]

Schilling test (**shil**-ing) *n.* a test used to assess a patient's capacity to absorb vitamin B_{12} from the bowel. Radioactive vitamin B_{12} is given by mouth and urine collected. A patient with pernicious anaemia will excrete less than 5% of the original dose over a period of 24 hours. [R. F. Schilling (1919–2014), US physician]

schindylesis (skin-di-**lee**-sis) *n.* a form of synarthrosis (immovable joint) in which a crest of one bone fits into a groove of another.

-schisis *combining form denoting* a cleft or split.

schisto- *combining form denoting* a fissure; split.

Schistosoma (Bilharzia) (shist-ŏ-**soh**-mă) *n.* a genus of blood flukes, three species of which are important parasites of humans causing the tropical disease schistosomiasis.

schistosomiasis (bilharziasis) (shist-ŏ-soh-**my**-ă-sis) *n.* a tropical disease caused by blood flukes of the genus *Schistosoma*. The disease is contracted when larvae penetrate the skin of anyone bathing in infected water. Adult flukes eventually settle in the blood vessels of the intestine (*S. mansoni* and *S. japonicum*) or bladder (*S. haematobium*); the release of their spiked eggs causes anaemia, inflammation, and the formation of scar tissue. Additional symptoms include diarrhoea, dysentery, cirrhosis of the liver, haematuria, and cystitis. The disease is treated with praziquantel.

schiz- (schizo-) *combining form denoting* a split or division.

schizoid personality (**skits**-oid) *n.* a personality characterized by solitariness, emotional coldness to others, inability to experience pleasure, lack of response to praise and criticism, withdrawal into a fantasy world, excessive introspection, and eccentricity of behaviour. *See* personality disorder.

schizophrenia (skits-ŏ-**freen**-iă) *n.* a severe mental illness characterized by a disintegration of the process of thinking, of contact with reality, and of emotional responsiveness. Delusions and hallucinations (positive symptoms), especially of voices, are common; negative symptoms include social withdrawal and loss of energy or initiative. Treatment is with antipsychotic drugs and with vigorous psychological and social management and rehabilitation. **—schizophrenic** (skits-ŏ-fren-ik) *adj.*

Schizophrenia Nursing Assessment Protocol (SNAP) *n.* a tool used by mental health nurses to assess major issues for patients with mental health problems and their families and to plan suitable interventions.

Schlatter's disease (shlat-erz) *n. see* Osgood-Schlatter disease.

Schlemm's canal (shlemz) *n.* a channel in the eye, at the junction of the cornea and the sclera, through which the aqueous humour drains. [F. Schlemm (1795–1858), German anatomist]

Schmidt's syndrome (sh'mitz) *n.* the autoimmune destruction of the thyroid, the adrenals, and the beta cells of the islets of Langerhans, causing type 1 diabetes mellitus. It is often associated with failure of the ovaries (causing an early menopause), the parathyroids, and the parietal cells of the gastric glands (causing pernicious anaemia). [M. B. Schmidt (1863–1949), German physician]

Schmorl's nodes (shmorlz) *pl. n.* protrusions of the pulpy inner material of an intervertebral disc into the vertebral body, generally found in the thoracic and lumbar spine. Often asymptomatic and an incidental finding, they can cause back pain. [C. G. Schmorl (1861–1932), German pathologist]

Schönlein-Henoch purpura *n. see* Henoch-Schönlein purpura.

school health service (skool) *n.* (in Britain) a service concerned with promotion of health and well being in schoolchildren, the early detection of health and social problems, and their subsequent treatment and surveillance.

school nurse *n.* a registered nurse who has undertaken a course in the health care of school-age children. A member of the school health service, a school nurse is responsible for health improvement activities (including health education and promotion), developmental screening, and vaccinations.

Schwann cells (shwon) *pl. n.* the cells that lay down the myelin sheath around the axon of a medullated nerve fibre. [T. Schwann (1810–82), German anatomist and physiologist]

schwannoma (shwon-**oh**-mă) *n.* a benign tumour arising from Schwann cells, which is similar to a neurofibroma but is enclosed in a capsule. **vestibular s.** (**acoustic neuroma**) a slow-growing benign tumour of the sheath of the vestibular nerve. It progresses to cause tinnitus and hearing loss.

Schwartze's operation (shvarts-ĕz) *n.* an operation to open and drain the air cells in the mastoid in severe cases of mastoiditis. [H. H. R. Schwartze (1837–1910), German otologist]

sciatica (sy-**at**-ik-ă) *n.* pain felt down the back and outer side of the thigh, leg, and foot. It is usually caused by degeneration or tearing of an intervertebral disc, which protrudes laterally to compress a spinal nerve root. The onset may be sudden, brought on by an awkward lifting or twisting movement.

sciatic nerve (sy-**at**-ik) *n.* the major nerve of the leg and the nerve with the largest diameter. It runs down behind the thigh from the lower end of the spine.

SCID *n.* *see* severe combined immune deficiency.

scintigram (**sin**-ti-gram) *n.* a diagram showing the distribution of radioactive tracer in a part of the body, produced by recording the flashes of light given off by a scintillator as it is struck by radiation of different intensities. This technique is called **scintigraphy**. By scanning the body, section by section, a 'map' of the radioactivity in various regions is built up, aiding the diagnosis of cancer or other disorders. Such a record is known as a **scintiscan**.

scintillator (**sin**-ti-lay-ter) *n.* a substance that produces a fluorescent flash when struck by high-energy radiation, such as beta or gamma rays. A scintillator forms the basis of a gamma camera. *See also* scintigram.

scintiscan (**sin**-ti-skan) *n.* *see* scintigram.

scirrhous (**si**-rŭs) *adj.* describing carcinomas that are stony-hard to the touch, for example, carcinoma of the breast.

scissor leg (**siz**-er) *n.* a disability in which one leg becomes permanently crossed over the other as a result of spasticity of its adductor muscles or deformity of the hip. The condition occurs in children with brain damage and in adults after strokes.

scissura (scissure) (si-*zh*or-ă) *n.* a cleft or splitting, such as the splitting open of tissues when a hernia forms.

scler- (sclero-) *combining form denoting* **1.** hardening or thickening. **2.** the sclera. **3.** sclerosis.

sclera (sclerotic coat) (**skleer**-ă) *n.* the white fibrous outer layer of the eyeball. At the front of the eye it becomes the cornea. *See* eye. —**scleral** *adj.*

scleritis (skleer-**I**-tis) *n.* inflammation of the sclera.

scleroderma (skleer-oh-**der**-mă) *n.* thickening of the skin, either localized (*see* morphoea) or generalized, resulting in waxy ivory-coloured areas. Scleroderma is thought to be an autoimmune disease. Systemic sclerosis is a related multisystem disorder.

scleromalacia (skleer-oh-mă-**lay**-shiă) *n.* thinning of the sclera (white of the eye) as a result of inflammation.

sclerosis (skleer-**oh**-sis) *n.* hardening of tissue, usually due to scarring (fibrosis) after inflammation or to ageing. It can affect the lateral columns of the spinal cord and the medulla of the brain (**amyotrophic lateral s.** (**ALS**) or **Lou Gehrig's disease**), causing progressive muscular paralysis (*see* motor neuron disease). *See also* arteriosclerosis, atherosclerosis, multiple sclerosis, systemic (sclerosis), tuberous (sclerosis).

sclerotherapy (skleer-oh-**th'**e-ră-pi) *n.* treatment of varicose veins by the injection of an irritant solution. This causes thrombophlebitis, which encourages obliteration of the varicose vein by thrombosis and subsequent scarring. Sclerotherapy is also used for treating haemorrhoids and oesophageal varices.

sclerotic (skleer-**ot**-ik) **1. (sclerotic coat)** *n. see* sclera. **2.** *adj.* affected with sclerosis.

sclerotome (**skleer**-ŏ-tohm) *n.* a surgical knife used in the operation of sclerotomy.

sclerotomy (skleer-**ot**-ŏmi) *n.* an operation in which an incision is made in the sclera.

scolex (**skoh**-leks) *n.* (*pl.* **scolices**) the head of a tapeworm. Suckers and/or hooks on the scolex enable the worm to attach itself to the wall of its host's gut.

scoliosis (skoh-li-**oh**-sis) *n.* lateral (sideways) deviation of the backbone, caused by congenital or acquired abnormalities of the vertebrae, muscles, and nerves. *See also* kyphoscoliosis, kyphosis.

-scope *combining form denoting* an instrument for observing or examining.

scopolamine (skŏ-**pol**-ă-meen) *n. see* hyoscine.

scorbutic (skor-**bew**-tik) *adj.* affected with scurvy.

scoring system (**skor**-ing) *n.* any of various methods in which the application of an agreed numerical scale is used as a means of estimating the degree of a clinical situation, e.g. the severity of an injury, the degree of patient recovery, or the extent of malignancy. *See* Glasgow Coma Scale, Gleason grade, injury scoring system.

scoto- *combining form denoting* darkness.

scotoma (skoh-**toh**-mă) *n.* (*pl.* **scotomata**) an area of abnormally less sensitive or absent vision in the visual field, surrounded by normal sight. It is due to abnormalities of the visual pathway.

scotometer (skoh-**tom**-it-er) *n.* an instrument used for mapping defects in the visual field. *See also* perimeter.

scotopic (skoh-**top**-ik) *adj.* relating to or describing conditions of poor illumination. **s. vision** vision in dim light in which the rods of the retina are involved (*see* dark adaptation).

screening test (**skreen**-ing) *n.* a test carried out on a large number of apparently healthy people to separate those who may have a specified disease and would benefit from further testing from those who probably do not. Examples include newborn bloodspot screening, cervical screening, and breast screening. *See also* genetic screening.

SEE WEB LINKS

- National Screening Committee website: contains detailed notes on all screening programmes the committee has considered and the rationale for the decisions the committee has made.

scrofula (skrof-yoo-lă) *n.* tuberculosis of lymph nodes, usually those in the neck, causing the formation of abscesses. Treatment with antituberculous drugs is effective. The disease, which is now rare in the developed world, most commonly affects young children. **—scrofulous** *adj.*

scrofuloderma (skrof-yoo-loh-der-mă) *n.* tuberculosis of the skin in which the skin breaks down over suppurating tuberculous glands, with the formation of irregular-shaped ulcers with blue-tinged edges. Treatment is with antituberculous drugs.

scrototomy (skroh-tot-ŏmi) *n.* an operation in which the scrotum is surgically explored, usually undertaken to investigate patients with probable obstructive azoospermia.

scrotum (skroh-tŭm) *n.* the paired sac that holds the testes and epididymides outside the abdominal cavity. Its function is to allow the production and storage of spermatozoa to occur at a lower temperature than that of the abdomen. **—scrotal** *adj.*

scrub typhus (tsutsugamushi disease) (skrub) *n.* a disease, widely distributed in SE Asia, caused by the parasitic bacterium *Rickettsia tsutsugamushi* and transmitted to humans through the bite of mites. Symptoms include headache, chills, high temperature, a red rash, a cough, and delirium. A small ulcer forms at the site of the bite. Scrub typhus is treated with tetracycline antibiotics. *See also* rickettsiae, typhus.

scrum-pox (skrum-poks) *n.* a form of herpes simplex found in rugby players and wrestlers. It is caused by abrasive contact.

scurvy (sker-vi) *n.* a disease that is caused by a deficiency of vitamin C. It results from a lack of fresh fruit and vegetables in the diet (humans cannot synthesize vitamin C and must obtain it from their diet). The first sign of scurvy is swollen bleeding gums, and a rash of tiny bleeding spots around the hair follicles is characteristic; this may be followed by subcutaneous bleeding. Treatment is by administering vitamin C.

SDB *n. see* sleep-disordered breathing.

SDH *n. see* (subdural) haematoma.

seasickness (see-sik-nis) *n. see* motion sickness.

seasonal affective disorder (see-zŏ-năl) *n. see* SAD.

seat-belt syndrome (seet-belt) *n.* thoracic injuries that arise from violent contact with a restraining seat belt in motor vehicle accidents occurring at high speeds.

sebaceous cyst (si-bay-shŭs) *n.* **1. (epidermoid cyst, wen)** a pale or flesh-coloured dome-shaped cyst that commonly occurs in adults, especially on the face, neck, or trunk. It is firm, with a central dot, and contains keratin. It is usually removed surgically. **2.** a cyst of the sebaceous glands occurring in multiple form in a rare inherited condition, **steatocystoma multiplex**.

sebaceous gland *n.* any of the simple or branched glands in the skin that secrete an oily substance, sebum. They open into hair follicles and their secretion is produced by the disintegration of their cells.

seborrhoea (seb-ŏ-ree-ă) *n.* excessive secretion of sebum by the sebaceous glands. The glands are enlarged, especially on the nose and central face. The condition predisposes to acne and is common at puberty. Seborrhoea is sometimes associated with a kind of eczema (seborrhoeic eczema). **—seborrhoeic** *adj.*

sebum (see-bŭm) *n.* the oily substance secreted by the sebaceous glands. Sebum provides a thin film of fat over the skin, which slows the evaporation of water; it also has an antibacterial effect.

secondary care (sek-ŏnd-er-i) *n.* health care provided by hospital clinicians for a patient whose primary care was provided by the general practitioner or other health professional who first diagnosed or treated the patient. Secondary care cannot be accessed directly by patients. For example, a general practitioner who assesses a patient with an unusual skin condition may refer the patient to a dermatologist, who then becomes the source of secondary care. *Compare* tertiary care.

secondary prevention *n.* the avoidance or alleviation of the serious consequences of disease by early detection and appropriate management. *See also* preventive medicine.

secondary sexual characteristics *pl. n.* the physical characteristics that develop after puberty. In boys they include the growth of facial and pubic hair and the breaking of the voice. In girls they include the growth of pubic hair and the development of the breasts.

second-level nurse (sek-ŏnd lev-ĕl) *n.* a registered nurse (on Part 1 of the NMC register) who, having completed a two-year nursing course, provides nursing care under the direction of a first-level nurse. Second-level courses are no longer delivered. *See* enrolled nurse.

second messenger *n.* an organic molecule that acts within a cell to initiate the response to a signal carried by a chemical messenger (e.g. a hormone) that does not itself enter the cell. Examples of second messengers are inositol triphosphate and cyclic AMP.

secretin (si-**kree**-tin) *n.* a hormone secreted from the duodenum when acidified food leaves the stomach. Secretin stimulates the secretion of relatively enzyme-free alkaline juice by the pancreas and of bile by the liver.

secretion (si-kree-shŏn) *n.* **1.** the process by which a gland isolates constituents of the blood or tissue fluid and chemically alters them to produce a substance that it discharges for use by the body or excretes. **2.** the substance that is produced by a gland.

section (sek-shŏn) **1.** *n.* (in surgery) the act of cutting (the cut or division made is also called a section). **2.** *n.* (in imaging) a three-dimensional reconstruction of a body scan obtained by computerized tomography or magnetic resonance imaging. **3.** *n.* (in microscopy) a thin slice of the specimen to be examined under a microscope. **4.** *vb.* to issue an order for the compulsory admission of a patient to a psychiatric hospital for assessment and/or treatment under the appropriate section of the Mental Health Act 1983 (as amended by the Mental Health Act 2007).

section 47 removal *n.* a section of the National Assistance Act 1948 that enables a local authority to arrange for the compulsory removal to a place of care of a person who is unwilling to go voluntarily from his or her own home. It can be applied to individuals who are suffering from a grave chronic disease, or are physically incapacitated, or are living in insanitary conditions because of old age or infirmity.

secular beliefs (sek-yoo-ler) *pl. n.* nonreligious beliefs that reflect an emphasis on living in the here and now. Secularists use scepticism and rationalism to question traditional religious beliefs; they may be humanists, atheists, deists (believing in a creative force, or first cause), or agnostics.

sedation (si-day-shŏn) *n.* the production of a restful state of mind, particularly by the use of drugs (*see* sedative).

sedative (sed-ă-tiv) *n.* a drug that has a calming effect, relieving anxiety and tension. *See also* anxiolytic.

sedimentation rate (sed-i-men-tay-shŏn) *n.* the rate at which solid particles sink in a liquid under the influence of gravity. *See also* ESR (erythrocyte sedimentation rate).

segment (seg-mĕnt) *n.* (in anatomy) a portion of a tissue or an organ (e.g. the uterus or the eye), usually distinguishable from other portions by lines of demarcation.

Seidlitz powder (sed-lits) *n.* a mixture of sodium bicarbonate, sodium potassium tartrate, and tartaric acid, taken as a laxative when dissolved in water.

selective (o)estrogen receptor modulator (SERM) (si-lek-tiv) *n.* a drug that has oestrogen-like activity in some tissues and an anti-oestrogenic effect in others, depending on the manner of its binding with the oestrogen receptors. SERMs include tamoxifen, used in the treatment of breast cancer for its activity as an anti-oestrogen; and raloxifene, used in the treatment of osteoporosis for its oestrogenic effects on bone density.

selective serotonin and noradrenaline reuptake inhibitor *n. see* SNRI.

selective serotonin reuptake inhibitor *n. see* SSRI.

selegiline (sel-ej-i-leen) *n.* an MAOB inhibitor used in the treatment of Parkinson's disease. It is administered by mouth. Trade names: **Eldepryl**, **Zelapar**.

selenium (si-lee-niŭm) *n.* a trace element that has important antioxidant properties. Deficiency, which may result from prolonged parenteral feeding, can be treated by a selenium supplement (Selenase), given by mouth or injection. Vegetarians and vegans can also be at risk of deficiency. Symbol: Se.

selenium sulphide (sul-fyd) *n.* a selenium compound with antifungal properties, used to treat dandruff and scalp infections. It is administered in a shampoo. Trade name: **Selsun**.

self-actualization (self-ak-tew-ă-ly-zay-shŏn) *n.* the tendency to realize and fulfil one's maximum potential. *See* Maslow's hierarchy of human needs.

self-care (self-kair) *n.* the practice of activities that are necessary to sustain life and health, normally initiated and carried out by the individual for him- or herself.

self-catheterization (self-kath-it-er-I-zay-shŏn) *n. see* intermittent self-catheterization.

self-inflating bag (self-in-flayt-ing) *n.* a device for delivering emergency artificial ventilation by means of a tight-fitting face mask, a laryngeal mask, or an endotracheal tube. It consists of a stiff plastic bag, which is squeezed to deliver its gas contents into the patient's airway; when the pressure is released, it is reinflated from the atmosphere or an attached oxygen supply.

self-limiting (self-lim-it-ing) *adj.* describing a condition that runs a predicted course and is unaffected by any treatment.

sella turcica (sel-ă ter-sik-ă) *n.* a depression in the body of the sphenoid bone that encloses the pituitary gland.

semeiology (see-mi-ol-ŏji) *n. see* symptomatology.

semen (seminal fluid) (see-men) *n.* the fluid ejaculated from the penis at sexual climax. Each ejaculate may contain 300–500 million sperms suspended in a fluid secreted by the prostate gland and seminal vesicles with a small contribution from Cowper's glands. —**seminal** (sem-in-ăl) *adj.*

semi- *prefix denoting* half.

semicircular canals (sem-i-ser-kew-ler) *pl. n.* three tubes that form part of the membranous labyrinth of the ear. They are concerned with balance and each canal registers movement in a different plane.

semilunar cartilage (sem-i-loo-ner) *n.* one of a pair of crescent-shaped cartilages in the knee joint situated between the femur and tibia.

semilunar valve *n.* either of the two valves in the heart, each consisting of three flaps (cusps), that maintain the flow of blood in one direction. *See* aortic valve, pulmonary (valve).

seminal analysis *n.* analysis of a specimen of semen, which should be obtained after five days of abstinence from coitus, in order to assess male fertility. It includes determinations of the concentration and motility of the sperm and detection of the presence of abnormal forms of sperm. *See also* sperm count.

seminal vesicle *n.* either of a pair of male accessory sex glands that open into the vas deferens. The seminal vesicles secrete most of the liquid component of semen.

seminiferous tubule (sem-in-**if**-er-ŭs) *n.* any of the long convoluted tubules that make up the bulk of the testis.

seminoma (sem-in-**oh**-mă) *n.* a malignant tumour of the testis, appearing as a swelling, often painless, in the scrotum. The best treatment for localized disease is orchidectomy. A similar tumour occurs in the ovary (*see* dysgerminoma).

semipermeable membrane (sem-i-**per**-mi-ăbŭl) *n.* a membrane that allows the passage of some molecules but not others. Semipermeable membranes are used clinically in haemodialysis.

semiprone (sem-i-**prohn**) *adj.* describing the position of a patient lying face downwards, but with one or both knees flexed to one side. *Compare* prone, supine.

SEN *n. see* special educational needs.

senescence (si-**nes**-ĕns) *n.* the process of ageing, which is often marked by a decrease in physical and mental abilities. **—senescent** *adj.*

Sengstaken tube (sengz-tay-kĕn) *n.* a tube containing a triple lumen and inflatable balloons that is passed down the oesophagus to the stomach to compress bleeding oesophageal varicose veins. [R. W. Sengstaken (1923–78), US neurosurgeon]

senile dementia (**see**-nyl) *n. see* dementia.

senility (sin-**il**-iti) *n.* the state of physical and mental deterioration that is associated with the ageing process. **—senile** *adj.*

senna (**sen**-ă) *n.* any of various preparations of the dried fruits of certain shrubs of the genus *Cassia*, administered by mouth as a stimulant laxative to relieve constipation. Trade name: **Senokot**.

sensation (sen-**say**-shŏn) *n.* a feeling: the result of messages from the body's sensory receptors registering in the brain as information about the environment.

sense (sens) *n.* one of the faculties by which the qualities of the external environment are appreciated – sight, hearing, smell, taste, or touch. **s. organ** a collection of specialized cells (receptors), connected to the nervous system, that is capable of responding to a particular stimulus from either outside or inside the body.

sensibility (sen-si-**bil**-iti) *n.* the ability to be affected by, and respond to, changes in the surroundings. Sensibility is a characteristic of cells of the nervous system.

sensible (**sen**-sibŭl) *adj.* **1.** perceptible to the senses. **2.** capable of sensibility.

sensitive (**sen**-sit-iv) *adj.* possessing the ability to respond to a stimulus.

sensitivity (sen-sit-**iv**-iti) *n.* **1.** the degree to which a disease-causing organism responds to treatment by antibiotics or other drugs. **2.** a measure of the reliability of a screening test based on the proportion of people with a specific disease who react positively to the test: the higher the sensitivity, the fewer the false negatives. *Compare* specificity.

sensitization (sen-si-ty-**zay**-shŏn) *n.* **1.** alteration of the responsiveness of the body to the presence of foreign substances. In the development of an allergy, an individual becomes sensitized to a particular allergen. The phenomena of sensitization are due to the production of antibodies. **2.** (in behaviour therapy) a form of aversion therapy in which anxiety-producing stimuli are associated with the unwanted behaviour.

sensory (**sen**-ser-i) *adj.* relating to the input division of the nervous system, which carries information from receptors throughout the body towards the brain and spinal cord. **s. cortex** the region of the cerebral cortex responsible for receiving incoming information relayed by sensory nerve pathways from all parts of the body. **s. deprivation** a condition resulting from partial or complete absence of sensory stimuli, leading to disorientation, hallucinations, and bizarre thought patterns. **s. nerve** *see* nerve.

sentinel lymph node (**sent**-i-nĕl) *n.* the first lymph node to show evidence of metastasis of a malignant tumour (e.g. breast cancer) via the lymphatic system. Absence of cancer cells in the sentinel node indicates that more distal lymph nodes will also be free of metastasis.

sepsis (**sep**-sis) *n.* the putrefactive destruction of tissues by disease-causing bacteria or their toxins. **postpartum** (or **puerperal**) **s.** sepsis characterized by puerperal pyrexia and other signs of serious infection that occurs within six weeks of childbirth.

sept- (septi-) *combining form denoting* **1.** seven. **2.** (septo-) a septum, especially the nasal septum. **3.** sepsis.

septal defect (**sep**-t'l) *n.* a hole in the partition (septum) between the left and right halves of the heart. This congenital condition is due to an abnormality of heart development in the fetus. It may be found between the two atria (**atrial s. d.**, **ASD**) or between the ventricles (**ventricular s. d.**, **VSD**). A septal defect permits abnormal circulation of blood from the left side of the heart to the right, which results in excessive blood flow through the lungs. Pulmonary hypertension develops and heart failure may occur. Large defects are closed surgically or using percutaneous catheter techniques but small defects do not require treatment.

septic (**sep**-tik) *adj.* relating to or affected with sepsis. **s. arthritis** infection in a joint, which becomes swollen, hot, and tender; movement is very painful. The infecting organism (usually *Staphylococcus aureus*) enters the joint via the bloodstream, through a penetrating injury, or by direct spread from an area of osteomyelitis. **s. shock** a life-threatening condition that occurs when the number of bacteria in the blood multiplies uncontrollably and results in hypotension caused by septicaemia (*see* shock). Clinical manifestations include fever, rapid breathing, diarrhoea, and confusion; multi-organ failure and diffuse intravascular coagulation are associated with the condition.

septicaemia (septi-**seem**-iă) *n.* widespread destruction of tissues due to absorption of disease-causing bacteria or their toxins from the bloodstream. **meningococcal s.** *see* meningitis. *Compare* pyaemia, sapraemia, toxaemia. **—septicaemic** *adj.*

Septrin (**sep**-trin) *n.* *see* co-trimoxazole.

septum (**sep**-tŭm) *n.* (*pl.* **septa**) a partition or dividing wall within an anatomical structure. **—septal** *adj.* **—septate** (**sep**-tayt) *adj.*

sequela (si-**kwee**-lă) *n.* (*pl.* **sequelae**) any disorder or pathological condition that results from a preceding disease or accident.

sequestration (see-kwes-**tray**-shŏn) *n.* **1.** the formation of a sequestrum and its separation from the surrounding tissue. **2.** a separated part of an organ occurring as a developmental anomaly.

sequestrectomy (see-kwes-**trek**-tŏmi) *n.* surgical removal of a sequestrum.

sequestrum (si-**kwes**-trŭm) *n.* (*pl.* **sequestra**) a portion of dead bone formed in an infected bone in chronic osteomyelitis. It can cause irritation and the formation of pus, which may discharge through a sinus, and is usually surgically removed.

ser- (sero-) *combining form denoting* **1.** serum. **2.** serous membrane.

serine (**se**-reen) *n.* *see* amino acid.

SERM *n.* *see* selective (o)estrogen receptor modulator.

seroconvert (seer-oh-kŏn-**vert**) *vb.* to produce specific antibodies in response to the presence of an antigen (e.g. a vaccine or a virus). In HIV-positive patients seroconversion is accompanied by a sore throat, swollen lymph nodes, fever, and aches and pains. **—seroconversion** *n.*

serology (si-**rol**-ŏji) *n.* the study of blood serum and its constituents, particularly their contribution to the protection of the body against disease. **—serological** *adj.*

seropus (seer-oh-**pus**) *n.* a mixture of serum and pus, which forms, for example, in infected blisters.

serosa (si-**roh**-să) *n.* *see* serous membrane.

serosanguineous (seer-oh-sang-**win**-iŭs) *adj.* denoting an exudate or discharge composed of or containing serum and blood.

serositis (seer-oh-**sy**-tis) *n.* inflammation of a serous membrane. *See* polyserositis.

serotherapy (seer-oh-**th'e**-ră-pi) *n.* the use of serum containing known antibodies (*see* antiserum) to treat a patient with an infection or to confer temporary passive immunity upon a person at special risk.

serotonin (5-hydroxytryptamine, 5HT) (se-rŏ-**toh**-nin) *n.* a compound widely distributed in the tissues, particularly in the blood platelets, intestinal wall, and central nervous system. It is thought to play a role in inflammation similar to that of histamine and it is involved in the genesis of a migrainous headache. Serotonin also acts as a neurotransmitter, and its levels in the brain are believed to have an important effect on mood. *See also* $5HT_1$ agonist, SSRI.

serotype (seer-oh-typ) *n.* a category into which material is placed based on its serological activity, particularly in terms of the antigens it contains or the antibodies that may be produced against it.

serous (seer-ŭs) *adj.* **1.** relating to or containing serum. **2.** resembling serum or producing a fluid resembling serum.

serous membrane (serosa) *n.* a smooth transparent membrane lining certain large cavities of the body, such as the abdomen (*see* peritoneum) and chest (*see* pleura). The **parietal** portion of the membrane lines the walls of the cavity, and the **visceral** portion covers the organs concerned. The two form a closed sac, the inner surface of which is moistened by a thin fluid derived from blood serum, allowing frictionless movement of organs within their cavities. *Compare* mucous membrane.

serpiginous (ser-**pij**-in-ŭs) *adj.* describing a creeping or extending skin lesion, especially one with a wavy edge.

serrated (ser-**ayt**-id) *adj.* having a saw-toothed edge. —**serration** *n.*

sertraline (ser-tră-leen) *n.* an antidepressant drug (*see* SSRI) taken by mouth for the treatment of depression, panic disorder, and obsessive–compulsive disorder. Trade name: **Lustral**.

serum (blood serum) (seer-ŭm) *n.* the fluid that separates from clotted blood or blood plasma that is allowed to stand. Serum is essentially similar in composition to plasma but lacks fibrinogen and other substances that are used in the coagulation process. **s. sickness** a reaction that sometimes occurs 7–12 days after injection of a quantity of foreign antigen. Large immune complexes are deposited in the arteries, kidneys, and joints, causing vasculitis, nephritis, and arthritis.

sesamoid bone (ses-ă-moid) *n.* an oval nodule of bone that lies within a tendon and slides over another bony surface. The patella (kneecap) is a sesamoid bone.

sessile (se-syl) *adj.* (of a tumour) attached directly by its base without a stalk.

severe combined immune deficiency (SCID) (sĕ-veer kŏm-**bynd**) *n.* a rare disorder that usually manifests itself within the first three months of life by severe bacterial, fungal, and viral infection and failure to thrive. It is due to reduced numbers of T and B lymphocytes.

Sever's disease (see-verz) *n.* apophysitis caused by pulling at the point of insertion of the Achilles tendon into the calcaneus (heel bone), causing heel pain. [J. W. Sever (20th century), US orthopaedic surgeon]

sexarche (seks-ar-ki) *n.* the age when a person first engages in sexual intercourse.

sex chromatin (seks) *n.* chromatin found only in female cells and believed to represent a single X chromosome in a nondividing cell. It can be used to discover the sex of a baby before birth by examination of cells obtained by amniocentesis or chorionic villus sampling.

sex chromosome *n.* a chromosome that is involved in the determination of the sex of the individual. Women have two X chromosomes; men have one X chromosome and one Y chromosome. *Compare* autosome.

sex hormone *n.* any steroid hormone, produced mainly by the ovaries or testes, that is responsible for controlling sexual development and reproductive function. Oestrogens and progesterone are the female sex hormones; androgens are the male sex hormones.

sex-linked (seks-linkt) *adj.* describing genes (or the characteristics controlled by them) that are carried on the sex chromosomes. The genes for certain disorders, e.g. haemophilia, are carried on the X chromosome; these genes are disorders and described as **X-linked**.

sexology (seks-ol-ŏji) *n.* the study of sexual matters, including anatomy, physiology, behaviour, and techniques.

sexual deviation (seks-yoo-ăl) *n.* any sexual behaviour regarded as abnormal by society. The deviation may relate to the sexual object (as in fetishism) or the activity engaged in (for example, paedophilia or exhibitionism).

sexual intercourse (in-ter-kors) *n. see* coitus.

sexually transmitted disease (STD) *n.* any disease transmitted by sexual intercourse, formerly known as **venereal disease**. STDs include AIDS, syphilis, gonorrhoea, genital herpes, *Chlamydia* infection, and soft sore. The medical specialty concerned with STDs is **genitourinary medicine**.

SEE WEB LINKS

- Explanation of STDs from Public Health England

SFS *n. see* Social Functioning Scale.

SGA *adj. see* small for gestational age.

SGOT *n.* serum glutamic oxaloacetic transaminase. *See* aspartate aminotransferase.

SGPT *n.* serum glutamic pyruvic transaminase. *See* alanine aminotransferase.

shearing force (sheer-ing) *n.* the force between two parallel planes that occurs when one plane slides over the other. In the body the force operates when the skin moves over underlying tissues, usually when a bed-bound patient is being moved, and results in soft-tissue damage and ischaemic changes.

sheath (sheeth) *n.* (in anatomy) the layer of connective tissue that envelops structures such as nerves, arteries, tendons, and muscles.

Sheehan's syndrome (shee-ănz) *n.* subnormal activity of the pituitary gland, causing amenorrhoea and infertility, resulting from a reduction in its blood supply, due to a major haemorrhage in pregnancy. [H. L. Sheehan (20th century), British pathologist]

Shigella (shig-el-ă) *n.* a genus of nonmotile rodlike Gram-negative bacteria normally present in the intestinal tract. Some species are pathogenic. **S. dysenteriae** a species associated with bacillary dysentery.

shigellosis (shig-el-**oh**-sis) *n.* an infestation of the digestive system by bacteria of the genus *Shigella*, causing bacillary dysentery.

shin bone (shin) *n.* *see* tibia.

shingles (**shing**-ŭlz) *n.* *see* herpes (zoster).

Shirodkar's operation (shi-**rod**-karz) *n.* an operation in which the neck (cervix) of the uterus is closed by means of a purse-string suture in order to prevent miscarriage. [N. V. Shirodkar (1900–71), Indian obstetrician]

shock (shok) *n.* the condition associated with circulatory collapse, when the arterial blood pressure is too low to maintain an adequate supply of blood to the tissues. The patient has a cold sweaty pallid skin, a weak rapid pulse, irregular breathing, dry mouth, dilated pupils, a decreased level of consciousness, and a reduced flow of urine. Shock may be due to a decrease in the volume of blood (**hypovolaemic s.**), as occurs after haemorrhage, dehydration, burns, etc., or it may be caused by reduced activity of the heart (**cardiogenic s.**), as in coronary thrombosis. It may also be due to widespread dilation of the blood vessels so that there is insufficient blood to fill them. This may be caused by the presence of bacteria in the bloodstream (**septic s.**: *see* septic); a severe allergic reaction (**anaphylactic s.**: *see* anaphylaxis), drug overdosage, e.g. overdosage of insulin produces severe hypoglycaemia (**insulin s.**); or emotional shock (**neurogenic s.**). *See also* spinal shock.

short bowel syndrome (SBS) (short) *n.* intestinal failure that occurs when the small bowel is shortened by surgery or trauma, resulting in reduced absorption of nutrients. Some adaptation does occur, but if under 200 cm of small bowel remain, it is likely patients will need long-term total parenteral nutrition.

short circuit (ser-kit) *n.* *see* anastomosis.

short-sightedness (short-**syt**-id-nis) *n.* *see* myopia.

short-stretch bandage *n.* a bandage that exerts low resting pressure. It is inelastic but can stretch by up to 60% of its original length and is used in the treatment of lymphoedema and venous leg ulcers.

shoulder (**shohl**-der) *n.* the ball-and-socket joint (*see* enarthrosis) between the glenoid cavity of the scapula and the upper end (head) of the humerus. The joint is surrounded by a capsule closely associated with many tendons.

shoulder dystocia *n.* *see* dystocia.

shoulder girdle (pectoral girdle) *n.* the bony structure to which the bones of the upper limbs are attached. It consists of the right and left scapulas and clavicles.

show (shoh) *n. Informal.* a discharge of blood-stained mucus from the vagina that occurs at the start of labour.

shunt (shunt) *n.* a passage connecting two anatomical channels or sites and diverting blood or other fluid (e.g. cerebrospinal fluid) from one to the other. It may occur as a congenital abnormality (as in septal defects of the heart) or be surgically created. *See also* anastomosis.

SIADH *n. see* syndrome of inappropriate secretion of antidiuretic hormone.

sial- (sialo-) *combining form denoting* **1.** saliva. **2.** a salivary gland.

sialadenitis (sy-ăl-ad-i-**ny**-tis) *n.* inflammation of a salivary gland.

sialagogue (sy-**al**-ŏ-gog) *n.* a drug that promotes the secretion of saliva. Parasympathomimetic drugs have this action.

sialography (ptyalography) (sy-ă-**log**-răfi) *n.* X-ray examination of the salivary glands, after introducing, via a cannula, a quantity of radiopaque material into the ducts of the parotid and submandibular glands in the mouth.

sialolith (sy-**al**-oh-lith) *n.* a stone (calculus) in a salivary gland or duct. The flow of saliva is obstructed, causing swelling and intense pain.

sialorrhoea (sy-ă-lŏ-**ree**-ă) *n. see* ptyalism.

sib (sib) *n. see* sibling.

SIB *n.* self-injurious behaviour. *See* deliberate self-harm.

sibilant (**sib**-i-lănt) *adj.* whistling or hissing. The term is applied to certain high-pitched abnormal sounds heard through a stethoscope.

sibling (sib) (**sib**-ling) *n.* one of a number of children of the same parents, i.e. a brother or sister.

sickle-cell disease (drepanocytosis) (**sik**-ŭl-sel) *n.* a hereditary blood disease that mainly affects people of African ancestry. It occurs when the sickle-cell gene has been inherited from both parents and is characterized by the production of an abnormal type of haemoglobin, which precipitates in the red blood cells when the blood is deprived of oxygen. The affected cells are distorted into the characteristic sickle shape, which may block small blood vessels producing severe pain (**sickle-cell crisis**). The cells are rapidly removed from the circulation, leading to anaemia.

sickle-cell trait *n.* the carrier condition of sickle-cell disease, in which the defective gene is inherited from only one parent. It generally causes no symptoms.

side-effect (**syd**-i-fekt) *n.* an effect produced by a drug in addition to its desired therapeutic effects. Side-effects may be harmful (adverse drug reactions).

sidero- *combining form denoting* iron.

sideropenia (sid-er-oh-**pee**-niă) *n.* iron deficiency. This may result from dietary inadequacy; increased requirement of iron by the body, as in pregnancy or childhood; or increased loss of iron from the body, usually due to chronic bleeding.

siderosis (sid-er-**oh**-sis) *n.* the deposition of iron oxide dust in the lungs, occurring in silver finishers, arc welders, and haematite miners. Pulmonary fibrosis may develop if fibrogenic dusts such as silica are also inhaled.

SIDS *n. see* sudden infant death syndrome.

sievert (**see**-vŭt) *n.* the SI unit of dose equivalent, being the dose equivalent when the absorbed dose of ionizing radiation multiplied by the stipulated dimensionless factors is 1 J kg^{-1}. The sievert has replaced the rem. Symbol: Sv.

sigmoid- *combining form denoting* the sigmoid colon.

sigmoidcolectomy (sigmoidectomy) (sig-moid-col-**ek**-tŏmi) *n.* surgical removal of the sigmoid colon using either an open approach (*see* laparotomy) or laparoscopy. It is performed for tumours, severe diverticular disease, or sigmoid volvulus.

sigmoid colon (sigmoid flexure) (sig-moid) *n.* the S-shaped terminal part of the descending colon, which leads to the rectum.

sigmoidoscope (sig-**moid**-ŏ-skohp) *n.* an instrument inserted through the anus in order to inspect the interior of the rectum and sigmoid colon.

sigmoidoscopy (sig-moid-**osk**-ŏpi) *n.* examination of the rectum and sigmoid colon with a flexible or rigid sigmoidoscope. It can be used to identify the causes of diarrhoea or rectal bleeding, such as colitis or cancer.

sigmoidostomy (sig-moid-**ost**-ŏmi) *n.* an operation in which the sigmoid colon is brought through the abdominal wall and opened. *See* colostomy.

sign (syn) *n.* an indication of a particular disorder that is detected by a physician when examining a patient but is not apparent to the patient. *Compare* symptom.

significance (sig-**nif**-i-kăns) *n.* (in statistics) a relationship between two groups of observations indicating that the difference between them is unlikely to have occurred by chance alone. An assumption is made that there is no difference between the two populations from which the two groups come (the **null hypothesis**). This is tested, and a calculation indicating that there is a **probability** of less than 5% (**P value** <0.05) that the observed difference or a larger one could have arisen by chance is regarded as being **statistically significant** and the null hypothesis is rejected.

sign language (signed language) *n.* a form of communication that uses movements of the hands and other parts of the body together with facial expressions instead of sound. There are many different forms of sign language throughout the world.

sign-off mentor (syn-off) *n. see* mentor.

sildenafil (sil-**den**-ă-fil) *n.* a drug administered orally for the treatment of erectile dysfunction and by mouth or intravenous injection to treat pulmonary hypertension. During sexual stimulation, it causes smooth muscle relaxation and increased blood flow to the corpus cavernosum of the penis, which results in erection. Sildenafil is contraindicated for patients taking nitrate-based drugs. **Tadalafil** (Cialis) and **vardenafil** (Levitra) are drugs with similar effects and uses. Trade names: **Nipatra Revatio**, **Viagra**.

silicone (sil-i-kohn) *n.* any of a group of synthetic organic compounds of silicon that are water-repellent and are used in medicine in prostheses and as lubricants and adhesives.

silicosis (sil-i-**koh**-sis) *n.* a lung disease – a form of pneumoconiosis – produced by inhaling silica dust particles. It affects workers in hard-rock mining and tunnelling, quarrying, stone dressing, and boiler scaling. Silica stimulates fibrosis of lung tissue, which produces progressive breathlessness and considerably increased susceptibility to tuberculosis.

silver nitrate (**sil**-ver **ny**-trayt) *n.* a salt of silver with caustic, astringent, and disinfectant properties. It is used in the form of a stick to destroy warts and granulomas. Trade name: **AVOCA**.

Silver-Russell syndrome *n. see* Russell-Silver syndrome.

simeticone (activated dimeticone) (si-**met**-i-kohn) *n.* a silicone-based material with antifoaming properties, used in the treatment of infantile colic and often incorporated into antacid remedies. Trade names: **Dentinox**, **Infacol**.

Simmonds disease (sim-ŏnz) *n.* loss of sexual function, loss of weight, and other features of hypopituitarism caused by trauma or tumours or occurring in women after childbirth complicated by bleeding (postpartum haemorrhage). [M. Simmonds (1855–1925), German physician]

Sims's position (simz-iz) *n.* the left-sided knees-up position commonly assumed by patients undergoing examinations of the anus and rectum or vagina. [J. M. Sims (1813–83), US gynaecologist]

simultanagnosia (sim-ŭl-tan-ag-**noh**-siă) *n.* impairment of the ability to perceive or focus on more than one element of a complex visual stimulus at a time, resulting in inability to understand the overall meaning of a situation or scene. This may result from trauma or a stroke at the junction of the occipital and parietal lobes.

SIMV *n. see* (synchronized) intermittent mandatory ventilation.

simvastatin (sim-vas-tă-tin) *n.* a drug administered by mouth to reduce abnormally high levels of cholesterol in the blood (*see* statin). Trade name: **Zocor**.

Sinemet (**sin**-i-met) *n. see* levodopa.

sinew (**sin**-yoo) *n.* a tendon.

singer's nodule (**sing**-erz) *n.* a pearly white nodule that may develop on the vocal folds of people who use their voice excessively or in those with poor vocal technique.

singultus (sing-gul-tŭs) *n. see* hiccup.

sinistr- (sinistro-) *combining form denoting* left or the left side.

sino- (sinu-) *combining form denoting* **1.** a sinus. **2.** the sinus venosus.

sinoatrial node (SA node) (sy-noh-ay-tri-ăl) *n.* the pacemaker of the heart: a microscopic area of specialized cardiac muscle located in the upper wall of the right atrium near the entry of the vena cava. Fibres of the SA node contract at around 70 times per minute. Following each contraction, the impulse spreads along connecting fibres to the atrioventricular node. Impulses arriving at the SA node accelerate or decrease the heart rate.

sinogram (sy-noh-gram) *n.* an X-ray photograph of a sinus that has been injected with a radiopaque substance. **—sinography** (sy-nog-răfi) *n.*

sinus (sy-nŭs) *n.* **1.** an air cavity within a bone, especially any of the cavities within the bones of the face or skull (*see* paranasal sinuses). **2.** any wide channel containing blood, usually venous blood. **s. arrhythmia** *see* arrhythmia. **s. rhythm** a normal heart rhythm, usually as recorded on an electrocardiogram. **s. venosus** a chamber in the embryonic heart that becomes part of the right atrium after birth. **3.** a pocket or bulge in a tubular organ, especially a blood vessel. **4.** (sinus tract) an infected blind-ending tract leading from a focus of infection to the surface of the skin or a hollow organ. *See* pilonidal sinus.

sinusitis (sy-nŭs-I-tis) *n.* inflammation of one or more of the paranasal sinuses. It is often associated with rhinitis and may be acute or chronic. Symptoms may include pain, purulent discharge from the nose, nasal obstruction, and disturbances of the sense of smell. Persistent cases require treatment with antibiotics, decongestants, or steroid nose drops; surgery, such as sinus washouts or antrostomy, is occasionally required.

sinusoid (sy-new-soid) *n.* a small blood vessel found in certain organs, such as the adrenal gland and liver.

sinus rhythm *n. see* sinus.

siphonage (sy-fŏn-ij) *n.* the transfer of liquid from one container to another by means of a bent tube. The procedure is used in gastric lavage.

Sipple's syndrome (sip-ĕlz) *n. see* MENS. [J. H. Sipple (1930–), US physician]

situation, background, assessment, recommendation (SBAR) (sit-yoo-ay-shŏn) *n.* a memory prompt to enhance the communication of essential information that requires immediate attention and action. It can be used in a number of situations to enhance patient safety and aims to simplify and clarify the sharing of critical information.

sitz bath (sits) *n.* a hip bath of water or saline solution to treat conditions such as haemorrhoids and anal fissures.

SI units (Système International d'Unités) *pl. n.* the

internationally agreed system of units, based on the metre-kilogram-second system, now in use for all scientific purposes. See Appendix 15: SI units.

six-category intervention analysis *n.* a framework for exploring how care is delivered, based on the idea that there are six main styles of interaction (prescriptive, informative, confronting, cathartic, catalytic, and supportive). The analysis is widely used to help health-care professionals develop an understanding of interpersonal relationships, reflect on their own practice, and enhance their interactions.

Sjögren's syndrome (sher-grenz) *n.* an autoimmune condition affecting the salivary and lacrimal glands, resulting in a dry mouth and dryness of the eyes. In the systemic form of the disease other glands may be affected, causing dryness of the airways, vagina, or skin. The syndrome may occur secondarily to other conditions, such as rheumatoid arthritis. [H. S. C. Sjögren (1899–1986), Swedish ophthalmologist]

skatole (methyl indole) (skat-ohl) *n.* a derivative of the amino acid tryptophan, excreted in the urine and faeces.

skeletal muscle (skel-i-t'l) *n. see* striated muscle.

skeleton (skel-i-tŏn) *n.* the rigid framework of connected bones that gives form to the body, protects and supports its soft organs and tissues, and provides attachments for muscles and a system of levers essential for locomotion. **appendicular s.** the bones of the limbs. **axial s.** the bones of the head and trunk. See illustration. **—skeletal** *adj.*

skier's thumb (gamekeeper's thumb) (skee-erz) *n.* an injury to the ulnar collateral ligament of the thumb caused by forced abduction across the metacarpophalangeal joint, at the base of the thumb.

skill mix (skil miks) *n.* the various skill levels of health-service staff required, either within a particular discipline or for the total staff within a health authority, to provide effective care.

skin (skin) *n.* the outer covering of the body, consisting of an outer layer, the epidermis, and an inner layer, the dermis (see illustration). The epidermis protects the body from injury and from invasion by parasites. It also helps to prevent the body from becoming dehydrated. The combination of erectile hairs, sweat glands, and blood capillaries in the skin form part of the temperature-regulating mechanism of the body. The skin also acts as an organ of excretion (by the secretion of sweat) and as a sense organ (it contains receptors that are sensitive to heat, cold, touch, and pain). Anatomical name: **cutis**. **s. graft** a portion of healthy skin cut from one area of the body and used to cover a part that has lost its skin, usually as a result of injury, burns, or operation. *See also* split-skin graft.

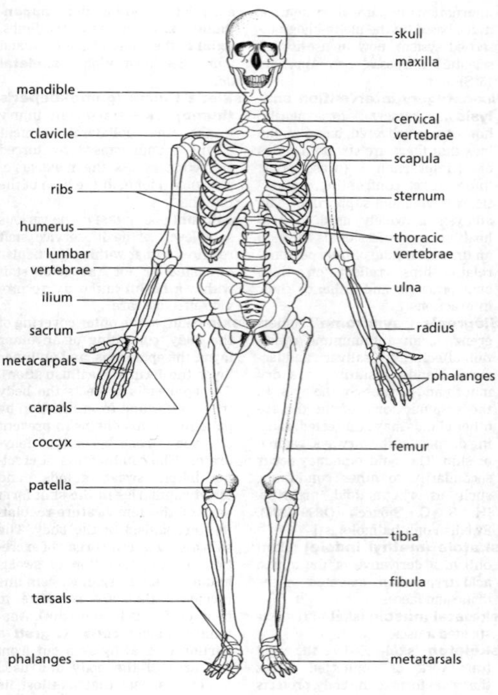

The skeleton

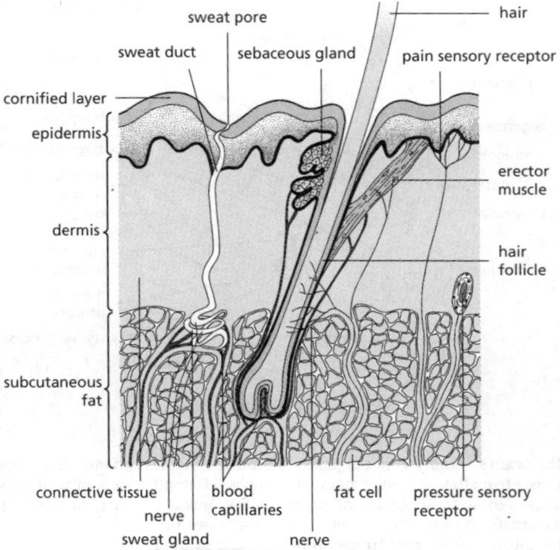

Section through the skin

ski-stick injury (skee-stik) *n.* a penetrating injury by a ski stick.

skull (skul) *n.* the skeleton of the head and face, which is made up of 22 bones. It can be divided into the cranium, which encloses the brain, and the face, including the lower jaw (mandible). (See illustration.) All the bones of the skull except the mandible are connected to each other by immovable joints (*see* suture). The skull contains cavities for the eyes and nose and a large opening at its base (foramen magnum) through which the spinal cord passes.

slapped cheek syndrome (slapt) *n. see* erythema (infectiosum).

SLE *n.* systemic lupus erythematosus: *see* lupus (erythematosus).

sleep (sleep) *n.* a state of natural unconsciousness, during which

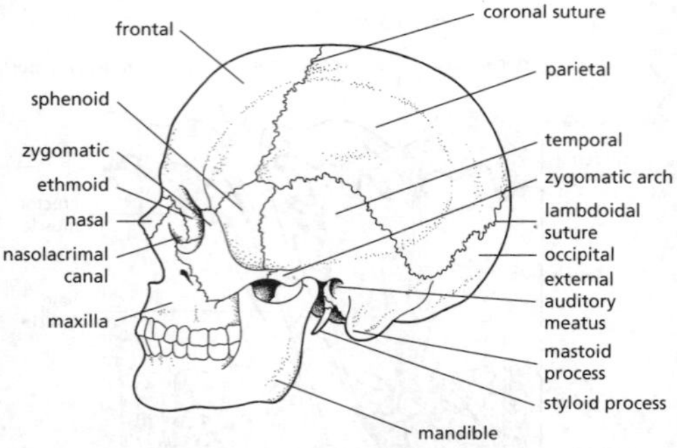

Side view of the skull bones

the brain's activity is not apparent (apart from the continued maintenance of basic bodily functions, such as breathing) but can be detected by means of an **electroencephalogram** (**EEG**). *See also* REM.

sleep apnoea *n.* cessation of breathing during sleep. **central s. a.** sleep apnoea in which there is no evidence of any voluntary efforts to breathe. **obstructive s. a. (syndrome)** (**OSA(S)**, **s. a. syndrome**, **SAS**) sleep apnoea in which airflow from the nose and mouth is restricted, resulting in more than five episodes of apnoea per hour of sleep associated with significant daytime sleepiness; snoring is a feature, but not universal. In children it is usually caused by enlarged tonsils; adult patients are often obese. Complications of prolonged OSA include heart failure and hypertension.

SEE WEB LINKS

- Website of the British Snoring and Sleep Apnoea Association

sleep-disordered breathing (SDB) *n.* abnormal patterns of respiration during sleep. Obstructive sleep apnoea is the most common SDB; other types include central sleep apnoea, such as Cheyne–Stokes respiration.

sleeping sickness (African trypanosomiasis) (sleep-ing) *n.* a disease of tropical Africa caused by the presence in the blood of the parasitic protozoans *Trypanosoma* *gambiense* or *T. rhodesiense*, which are transmitted through the bite of tsetse flies. Initial symptoms include fever, headache, and chills, followed later by enlargement of the lymph nodes, anaemia, and pains in the limbs and joints. The parasites eventually invade the minute blood vessels supplying the central nervous system, causing drowsiness and lethargy.

sleep paralysis *n.* a terrifying inability to move or speak while remaining fully alert. It occurs in up to 60% of patients with narcolepsy and may occur in other conditions, such as severe anxiety.

sleep-walking (sleep-wawk-ing) *n. see* somnambulism.

sling (sling) *n.* a bandage arranged to support and rest an injured limb so that healing is not hindered by activity. The most common sling is a triangular bandage tied behind the neck to support the weight of a broken arm.

sling procedure *n.* any of a group of surgical procedures for treating stress incontinence in women. *See* colposuspension, tension-free vaginal tape.

slipped disc (slipt) *n. see* prolapsed intervertebral disc.

slit lamp (slit) *n.* a device for providing a narrow beam of light, used in conjunction with a special microscope. It can be used to examine minutely the structures within the eye, one layer at a time.

slough (sluf) *n.* dead tissue, such as skin, that separates from healthy tissue after inflammation or infection.

slow virus (sloh) *n.* one of a group of infective disease agents now more commonly known as prions.

SMA *n. see* spinal muscular atrophy.

small bowel (smawl) *n.* the small intestine (*see* intestine). **s.-b. enema** (**enteroclysis**) a radiological technique for examining the jejunum and ileum in which barium sulphate is injected through a tube passing through the nose into the small bowel and a series of real-time images are taken. **s.-b. meal** (**barium follow-through**) a technique for examining the small bowel in which the patient swallows dilute barium sulphate suspension and then a series of abdominal radiographs are taken.

small-cell lung cancer (oat-cell carcinoma) *n.* carcinoma of the bronchus associated with the presence of oat cells (small cells with darkly staining nuclei). Small-cell lung cancer is usually related to smoking and accounts for about one-quarter of bronchial carcinomas. It carries a poor prognosis due to early distant spread.

small for gestational age (SGA) *adj.* describing a fetus or baby that has failed to reach the size or birth weight expected for its gestational age, either due to intrauterine growth restriction or because the baby is constitutionally small.

smallpox (smawl-poks) *n.* an acute infectious virus disease causing high fever and a rash that scars the skin. The rash consists of red spots (macules) that appear on the face, spread to the trunk and extremities, and gradually develop into pustules. Most patients recover but serious complications, such as nephritis or pneumonia, may develop. Treatment with thiosemicarbazone is effective. Immunization against smallpox has now totally eradicated the disease. Medical name: **variola**. *See also* alastrim, cowpox.

smear (smeer) *n.* a specimen of tissue or other material taken from part of the body and smeared on a microscope slide for examination. *See* cervical (smear).

smegma (smeg-mă) *n.* the secretion of the glands of the foreskin (prepuce), which accumulates under the foreskin and has a white cheesy appearance.

Smith-Petersen nail (smith-pee-ter-sĕn) *n.* a stainless steel nail used to fix fragments of bone when the neck of the femur is fractured. [M. N. Smith-Petersen (1886–1953), US orthopaedic surgeon]

Smith's fracture *n. see* fracture. [R. W. Smith (1807–73), Irish surgeon]

smooth muscle (involuntary muscle) (smooth) *n.* muscle that produces slow long-term contractions of which the individual is unaware. Smooth muscle occurs in hollow organs, such as the stomach, intestine, blood vessels, and bladder. *Compare* striated muscle.

SNAP *n. see* Schizophrenia Nursing Assessment Protocol.

snare (snair) *n.* an instrument consisting of a wire loop designed to remove polyps, tumours, and other projections of tissue. *See also* diathermy. See illustration.

sneeze (sneez) **1.** *n.* an involuntary violent reflex expulsion of air through the nose and mouth provoked by irritation of the mucous membrane lining the nasal cavity. **2.** *vb.* to produce a sneeze.

Snellen chart (snel-ĕn) *n.* the commonest chart used for testing sharpness of distant vision (*see* visual acuity). It consists of rows of capital letters, called **test types** (or **opto types**), the letters of each row becoming smaller down the chart. [H. Snellen (1834–1908), Dutch ophthalmologist]

snoring (snor-ing) *n.* noisy breathing while asleep due to vibration of the soft palate, uvula, pharyngeal walls, or epiglottis.

snow blindness (snoh) *n.* a painful disorder of the cornea of the eye

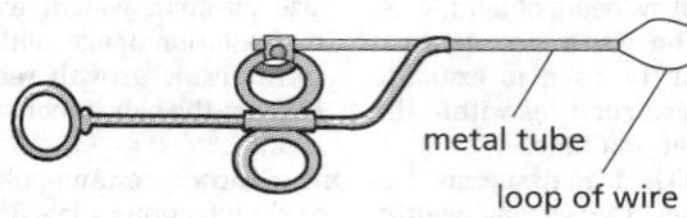

A nasal snare

due to excessive exposure to ultraviolet light reflected from the snow.

SNRI (selective serotonin and noradrenaline reuptake inhibitor) *n.* any one of a class of antidepressant drugs that increase the availability of serotonin and noradrenaline by blocking the reabsorption of these neurotransmitters by nerve endings in the brain. The group includes **venlafaxine** (Efexor XL; also licensed for the treatment of generalized anxiety disorder) and **duloxetine** (Cymbalta, Yentreve; also licensed for treating generalized anxiety disorder, diabetic neuropathy, and stress incontinence in women).

snuffles (snuf-ĕlz) *n.* **1.** partial obstruction of breathing in infants, caused by the common cold. **2.** (formerly) discharge through the nostrils associated with necrosis of the nasal bones: seen in infants with congenital syphilis.

social cleanliness (soh-shăl klen-li-nes) *n.* the first level of infection control, which includes washing with a soap substance or alcohol and maintaining high standards of personal hygiene. Further measures to avoid the spread of infection include decontamination and sterilization.

Social Functioning Scale (SFS) *n.* a scale to assess the ability of those with mental-health problems to engage in social interactions, interpersonal relationships, and activities of independent living.

socket (sok-it) *n.* (in anatomy) a hollow or depression into which another part fits.

sodium (soh-diŭm) *n.* a mineral element and an important constituent of the human body. The amount of sodium in the body is controlled by the kidneys. An excess of sodium leads to the condition of hypernatraemia, which often results in oedema. Sodium is also implicated in hypertension: a high-sodium diet is thought to increase the risk of hypertension in later life. Symbol: Na.

sodium bicarbonate (by-kar-bŏn-ayt) *n.* a salt of sodium that neutralizes acid and is administered by mouth or intravenous injection or infusion to treat metabolic acidosis (particularly renal tabular acidosis) and mild urinary-tract infections. It is also an ingredient of many antacid preparations and is used in the form of drops to soften earwax.

sodium chloride (klor-ryd) *n.* common salt: a salt of sodium that is an important constituent of the body. It is used intravenously to replace lost fluids and electrolytes, as eye drops to irrigate the eye (e.g. for eye surgery), in a mouthwash to treat minor infections, and (being instilled) to treat infections of the bladder. *See also* oral rehydration therapy, saline. Formula: NaCl.

sodium citrate (sit-rayt) *n.* a salt of sodium administered orally in the treatment of cystitis, by enema to relieve constipation (in combination with other ingredients), and by irrigation to dissolve blood clots in the bladder. It is also an ingredient of oral rehydration therapy.

sodium fusidate (few-si-dayt) *n.* an antibiotic used to treat penicillin-resistant infections caused by *Staphylococcus*, including osteomyelitis. It is administered by mouth. Trade name: **Fucidin**.

sodium nitrite (ny-tryt) *n.* a sodium salt administered by intravenous injection, with **sodium thiosulphate**, to treat cyanide poisoning.

sodium valproate (val-proh-ayt) *n.* an anticonvulsant drug administered orally or intravenously to treat all types of epilepsy and manic episodes in bipolar disorder. Trade names: **Epilim**, **Episenta**, **Epival**.

sodokosis (soh-doh-**koh**-sis) *n. see* rat-bite fever.

soft sore (chancroid) (soft) *n.* a sexually transmitted disease that is caused by the bacterium *Haemophilus ducreyi*, resulting in enlargement and ulceration of lymph nodes in the groin. Treatment with sulphonamides is effective.

solarium (sŏ-**lair**-iŭm) *n.* a room in which patients are exposed to either sunlight or artificial sunlight (a blend of visible light and infrared and ultraviolet radiation).

solar plexus (coeliac plexus) (**soh**-ler **pleks**-ŭs) *n.* a network of sympathetic nerves and ganglia high in the back of the abdomen.

soleus (**soh**-li-ŭs) *n.* a broad flat muscle in the calf of the leg. The soleus flexes the foot, so that the toes point downwards.

solution (sŏ-**loo**-shŏn) *n.* a homogeneous mixture of two or more dissimilar substances, usually of a liquid (the **solvent**) in which a solid (the **solute**) is dissolved.

solvent (**sol**-vĕnt) *n. see* solution.

soma (**soh**-mă) *n.* **1.** the entire body excluding the germ cells. **2.** the body as distinct from the mind.

somat- *combining form denoting* **1.** the body. **2.** somatic.

somatic (sŏ-**mat**-ik) *adj.* **1.** relating to the nonreproductive parts of the body. **2.** relating to the body wall (i.e. excluding the viscera). *Compare* splanchnic. **3.** relating to the body rather than the mind.

somatic symptom disorder *n.* a psychiatric disorder that is characterized by one or more chronic somatic symptoms about which patients are excessively concerned, preoccupied, or fearful. It was formerly called **somatization disorder**.

somatoform disorders (sŏ-**mat**-oh-form) *pl. n.* a group of disorders in which there is a history of repeated physical complaints with no physical basis. They include somatic symptom disorder and hypochondriacal disorder.

somatostatin (growth-hormone inhibiting hormone, GHIH) (soh-mă-toh-**stay**-tin) *n.* a hormone, produced by the hypothalamus and some extraneural tissues, including the gastrointestinal tract and the pancreas (*see* D cells), that inhibits the secretion of many hormones, including growth hormone (somatotrophin), insulin, and glucagon. **s. analogue** a drug, such as lanreotide or octreotide, used to treat symptoms caused by neuroendocrine tumours, including carcinoid syndrome and acromegaly.

somatotrophin (soh-mă-toh-**troh**-fin) *n. see* growth hormone.

somnambulism (som-**nam**-bew-lizm) *n.* sleep-walking: walking about and performing other actions in a semiautomatic way during sleep without later memory of doing so. It is common during childhood and can also arise as the result of stress or hypnosis. **—somnambulistic** *adj.*

somnolism (**som**-noh-lizm) *n.* a hypnotic trance. *See* hypnosis.

Somogyi effect (som-ŏ-gy-i) *n. see* dawn phenomenon. [M. Somogyi (1883–1971), US biochemist]

Sonne dysentery (**sonn**-i) *n.* bacillary dysentery caused by the species *Shigella sonnei.* [C. Sonne (1882–1948), Danish bacteriologist]

sonography (sonn-**og**-răfi) *n. see* ultrasonography.

sonoplacentography (soh-noh-plas-en-**tog**-răfi) *n. see* placentography.

soporific (sop-er-**if**-ik) *n. see* hypnotic.

sorbitol (**sor**-bit-ol) *n.* a carbohydrate with a sweet taste, used as a substitute for cane sugar in foods suitable for diabetics since it is absorbed slowly from the intestine.

sordes (**sor**-deez) *pl. n.* the brownish encrustations that form around the mouth and teeth of patients suffering from fevers.

sore (sor) *n.* a lay term for any ulcer or other open wound of the skin or mucous membranes. *See also* pressure sore, soft sore.

sore throat *n.* pain at the back of the mouth, commonly due to tonsillitis or pharyngitis. If infection persists the lymph nodes in the neck may become tender and enlarged (cervical adenitis).

sotalol (**soh**-tă-lol) *n.* a drug (*see* beta blocker) administered by mouth to prevent and treat abnormal heart rhythms. Trade names: **Beta-Cardone**, **Sotacor**.

souffle (soo-fĕl) *n.* a soft blowing sound heard through the stethoscope, usually produced by blood flowing in vessels.

sound (sownd) (in surgery) **1.** *n.* a long rodlike instrument, often with a curved end, used to explore body cavities or to dilate strictures in the urethra or other canals. **2.** *vb.* to explore a cavity using a sound.

Southey's tubes (**su*th***-iz) *pl. n.* fine-calibre tubes for insertion into subcutaneous tissue to drain excess fluid. They are rarely used in practice today. [R. Southey (1835–99), British physician]

spacer (**spay**-ser) *n.* a plastic container with a mouthpiece at one end and a hole for an aerosol inhaler at the other. The dose from the inhaler is sprayed into the spacer, from which it can be inhaled without needing to coordinate breathing. Spacers help to deliver a greater proportion of the dose to the airways while reducing the proportion absorbed into the body (which is the usual cause of unwanted side-effects).

Spanish fly (**span**-ish) *n.* the blister beetle, *Lytta vesicatoria*: source of the irritant and toxic chemical compound cantharidin.

spansule (**span**-sewl) *n.* a drug in the form of a capsule prepared in such a way that, when taken orally, its contents are released slowly.

spasm (spazm) *n.* a sustained involuntary muscular contraction, which may occur either as part of a generalized disorder or as a local response to an otherwise unconnected painful condition. **carpopedal s.** a spasm that affects the muscles of the hands and feet and is caused by a reduction in the blood calcium level (often transitory), as in hyperventilation.

spasmo- *combining form denoting* spasm.

spasmodic (spaz-**mod**-ik) *adj.* occurring in spasms or resembling a spasm.

spasmolytic (spaz-moh-**lit**-ik) *n.* a drug that relieves spasm of smooth muscle. *See also* antispasmodic.

spasmus nutans (spaz-mŭs **new**-tanz) *n.* a combination of symptoms including a slow nodding movement of the head, nystagmus, and spasm of the neck muscles. It affects infants and it normally disappears within a year or two.

spastic (**spast**-ik) *adj.* characterized by spasms. **s. paralysis** weakness of a limb or limbs associated with increased reflex activity. This results in spasticity and is caused by disease affecting the nerve fibres of the pyramidal system. *See also* cerebral palsy.

spasticity (clasp-knife rigidity) (spas-**tis**-iti) *n.* resistance to the passive movement of a limb that is maximal at the beginning of the movement and gives way as more pressure is applied. It is a symptom of damage to the corticospinal (pyramidal) tracts in the brain or spinal cord. *Compare* rigidity.

spatula (**spat**-yoo-lă) *n.* an instrument with a blunt blade used to spread ointments or plasters and, particularly in dentistry, to mix materials. A flat spatula is used to depress the tongue during examination of the oropharynx.

special care baby unit (SCBU) (**spesh**-ăl) *n.* a unit in a hospital that provides special care for premature, small, and sick babies. Its specialist staff is not equipped to provide intensive care.

special educational needs (SEN) *pl. n.* the requirements of children who have difficulties in learning or in accessing education. Children with SEN can be supported via mainstream schools or may attend a special school. Children identified as having SEN that cannot be met by a mainstream school should be assessed by their local authority (*see* statementing).

special hospital (secure hospital) *n.* a hospital for the care of mentally ill patients who pose a substantial risk to the community and must therefore be kept securely.

specialist community public health nurse (**spesh**-ăl-ist) *n. see* health visitor.

specialist nurse *n.* a nurse who has detailed knowledge and experience of specific conditions and takes a leading role in the care of clients in a hospital or the community. The specialist nurse works as an autonomous member of the multidisciplinary team to educate and support colleagues, patients, relatives, and carers in the provision of seamless care.

special school *n.* (in Britain) an education establishment for children with special educational needs.

specialty registrar *n.* (in a hospital) a registered doctor who undergoes a training programme in a chosen specialty in order to obtain a Certificate of Completion of Specialist Training and be eligible to apply for a consultant post. The post of specialty registrar replaced those of **registrar** and **senior registrar**.

species (spee-shiz) *n.* the smallest unit used in the classification of living organisms. Members of the same species are able to interbreed and to produce fertile offspring. Similar species are grouped together within one genus.

specific (spi-**sif**-ik) **1.** *n.* a medicine that has properties especially useful for the treatment of a particular disease. **2.** *adj.* (of a disease) caused by a particular microorganism that causes no other disease. **3.** *adj.* of or relating to a species.

specific gravity (grav-iti) *n. see* relative density.

specificity (spes-i-**fis**-iti) *n.* a measure of the reliability of a screening test based on the proportion of people free from disease who react negatively to the test: the higher the specificity, the fewer the false positives. *Compare* sensitivity.

spectroscope (**spek**-trŏ-skohp) *n.* an instrument that is used to split up light or other radiation into components of different wavelengths. The simplest spectroscope uses a prism, which splits white light into the rainbow colours of the visible spectrum.

spectrum (**spek**-trŭm) *n.* (in pharmacology) the range of effectiveness of an antibiotic. **broad s.** effectiveness against a wide range of microoganisms.

SPECT scanning (single photon emission computing tomography) (spekt) *n.* (in nuclear medicine) a cross-sectional imaging technique for observing an organ or part of the body using a gamma camera; images are produced after injecting a radioactive tracer. It is used particularly in cardiac nuclear medicine imaging (*see* MUGA scan).

speculum (**spek**-yoo-lŭm) *n.* (*pl.* **specula**) a metal instrument for inserting into and holding open a cavity of the body, such as the vagina, rectum, or nasal orifice, in order that the interior may be examined. See illustration.

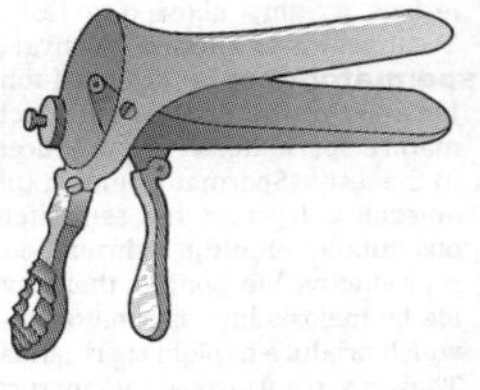

Vaginal speculum (Cusco's)

speech and language therapy (speech) *n.* the treatment of patients who have problems with communication because of congenital causes, accidents, or illness. Speech and language therapists are allied health professionals who have special training in this field.

sperm (sperm) *n.* *see* spermatozoon.

sperm- (spermi(o)- spermo-) *combining form denoting* sperm or semen.

spermat- (spermato-) *combining form denoting* **1.** sperm. **2.** organs or ducts associated with sperm.

spermatic artery (sper-**mat**-ik) *n.* either of two arteries that originate from the abdominal aorta and travel downwards to supply the testes.

spermatic cord *n.* the cord, consisting of the vas deferens, nerves, and blood vessels, that runs from the abdominal cavity to the testicle in the scrotum.

spermatocele (**sperm**-ă-toh-seel) *n.* a cystic swelling in the scrotum containing sperm. The cyst arises from the epididymis and can be felt as a lump above the testis. Treatment is by surgical removal.

spermatogenesis (sperm-ă-toh-**jen**-i-sis) *n.* the process by which mature spermatozoa are produced in the testis. Spermatogonia, in the outermost layer of the seminiferous tubules, multiply throughout reproductive life. Some of them divide by meiosis into spermatocytes, which produce haploid spermatids. These are transformed into mature spermatozoa by the process of

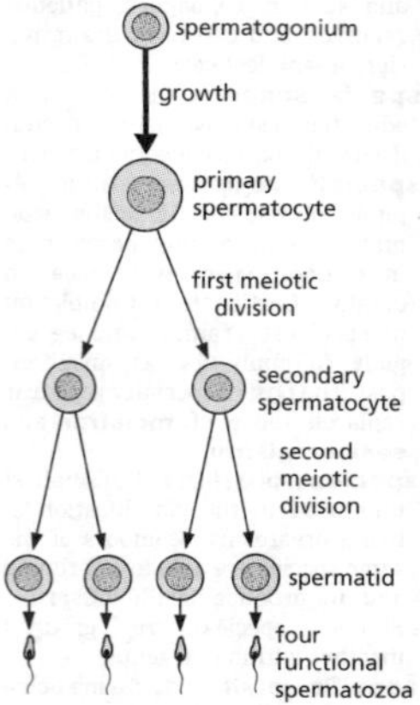

Spermatogenesis

spermiogenesis. The whole process takes 70–80 days. See illustration.

spermatorrhoea (sperm-ă-tŏ-**ree**-ă) *n.* the involuntary discharge of semen without orgasm.

spermatozoon (sperm) (sperm-ă-toh-**zoh**-ŏn) *n.* (*pl.* **spermatozoa**) a mature male sex cell (*see* gamete). The tail of a sperm enables it to swim, which is important as a means for reaching and fertilizing the ovum. (See illustration.) *See also* acrosome, fertilization.

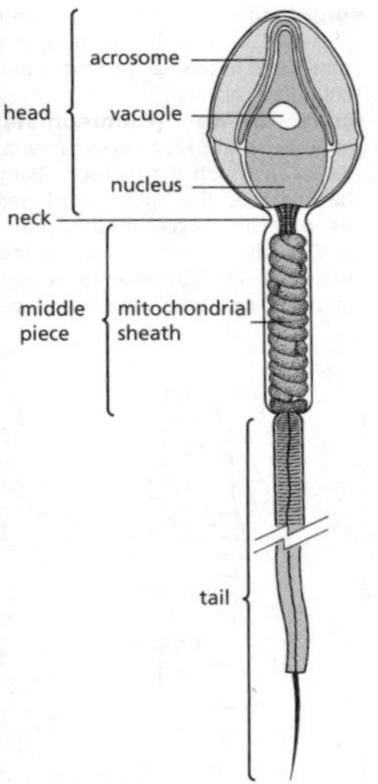

A spermatozoon

spermaturia (sperm-ăt-**yoor**-iă) *n.* the presence of spermatozoa in the urine. Abnormal ejaculation into the bladder on orgasm (retrograde ejaculation) may occur after prostatectomy or other surgical procedures or in certain neurological conditions.

sperm count *n.* an estimate of the total number of spermatozoa in a specimen of ejaculated semen, which is used as a measure of male fertility. Normal values for sperm concentration are 20–200 million spermatozoa per ml ejaculate. *See also* seminal analysis.

spermicide (**sperm**-i-syd) *n.* an agent that kills spermatozoa. Contraceptive creams and jellies contain chemical spermicides. —**spermicidal** *adj.*

spermiogenesis (sperm-i-oh-**jen**-i-sis) *n. see* spermatogenesis.

spheno- *combining form denoting* the sphenoid bone.

sphenoid bone (**sfee**-noid) *n.* a bone forming the base of the cranium behind the eyes. *See* skull.

spherocyte (**sfeer**-oh-syt) *n.* an abnormal form of red blood cell (erythrocyte) that is spherical rather than disc-shaped. They are characteristic of some forms of haemolytic anaemia. Spherocytes tend to be removed from the blood as they pass through the spleen. *See also* spherocytosis.

spherocytosis (sfeer-oh-sy-**toh**-sis) *n.* the presence in the blood of spherocytes. Spherocytosis may occur as a hereditary disorder (**hereditary s.**) or in certain haemolytic anaemias.

sphincter (**sfink**-ter) *n.* a specialized ring of muscle that surrounds an orifice. Contractions of the sphincter partly or completely close the orifice. Sphincters are found, for example, around the anus (**anal s.**) and at the openings between the stomach and the oesophagus (**lower oesophageal s.**) and the duodenum (**pyloric s.**).

sphincter- *combining form denoting* a sphincter.

sphincterectomy (sfink-ter-**ek**-tŏmi) *n.* the surgical division, usually partial, of any sphincter muscle.

sphincterotomy (sfink-ter-**ot**-ŏmi) *n.* **1.** surgical division of any sphincter muscle. **2.** surgical incision of part of the iris in the eye at the border of the pupil.

sphygmo- *combining form denoting* the pulse.

sphygmocardiograph (sfig-moh-**kar**-di-ŏ-grahf) *n.* an apparatus for producing a continuous record of both the heartbeat and the subsequent pulse in one of the blood vessels. The recording can be shown on a moving tape or on an electronic screen.

sphygmograph (**sfig**-moh-grahf) *n.* an apparatus for producing a continuous record of the pulse in one of the blood vessels, showing the strength and rate of the beats.

sphygmomanometer (sfig-moh-mă-**nom**-it-er) *n.* an instrument for measuring blood pressure in the arteries. It consists of an inflatable cuff connected to a graduated scale gauge calibrated in millimetres of mercury (mmHg).

spica (**spy**-kă) *n.* a bandage wound repeatedly in a figure-of-eight around an injured limb, forming a series of V-shapes. See illustration.

spicule (**spik**-yool) *n.* a small splinter of bone.

spider naevus (**spy**-der) *n.* *see* naevus.

spigot (**spig**-ŏt) *n.* a glass or plastic peg used to close the opening of a tube, used in nasogastric tubes and catheters.

spina bifida (rachischisis) (**spy**-nă **bif**-id-ă) *n.* a developmental defect in which the newborn baby has part of the spinal cord and its coverings exposed through a gap in the backbone (*see* neural tube defects). The symptoms may include paralysis of the legs,

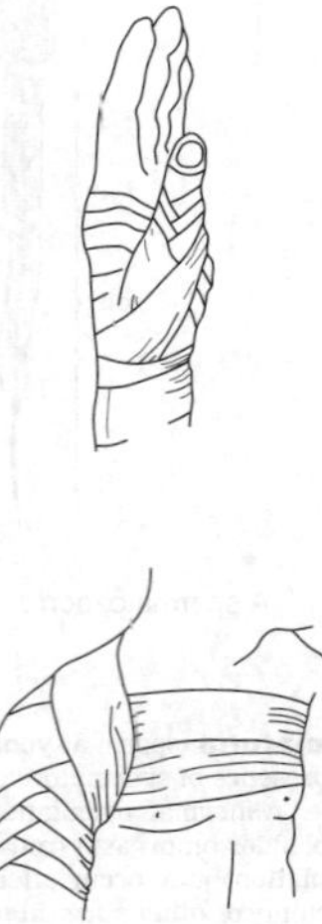

Types of spica

incontinence, and learning disabilities from the commonly associated brain defect, hydrocephalus. Spina bifida can be diagnosed at about the 16th week of pregnancy by a maternal blood test and confirmed by amniocentesis and ultrasound. **s. b. occulta** a defect in the bony arch of the spine that (unlike spina bifida) has a normal skin covering; there may be an overlying hairy patch. It is not associated with neurological involvement.

SEE WEB LINKS

- Website of Shine, the charity for people living with spina bifida and hydrocephalus

spinal accessory nerve (spy-năl) *n. see* accessory nerve.

spinal anaesthesia *n.* **1.** suppression of sensation, usually in the lower part of the body, by the injection of a local anaesthetic into the subarachnoid space, most commonly in the lumbar region of the vertebral column. Spinal anaesthesia is useful in patients whose condition makes them unsuitable for a general anaesthetic, to reduce the requirements for general anaesthetic drugs, or in circumstances where a skilled anaesthetist is not available. *See also* epidural (anaesthesia). **2.** loss of sensation in part of the body as a result of injury or disease to the spinal cord.

spinal column *n. see* backbone.

spinal cord *n.* the portion of the central nervous system enclosed in the vertebral column, consisting of nerve cells and bundles of nerves connecting all parts of the body with the brain. It extends from the medulla oblongata in the skull to the level of the second lumbar vertebra.

spinal muscular atrophy (SMA) *n.* a hereditary condition in which cells of the spinal cord die and the muscles in the arms and legs become progressively weaker. Eventually the respiratory muscles are affected and death usually results from respiratory infection. There are three types of SMA (types 1, 2, and 3), based on the severity of symptoms and age of onset; type 1, which is evident soon after birth, is the most acute and aggressive form (*see* Werdnig-Hoffmann disease).

spinal nerves *pl. n.* the 31 pairs of nerves that leave the spinal cord and are distributed to the body, passing out from the vertebral canal through the spaces between the arches of the vertebrae.

spinal shock *n.* a state of shock accompanied by temporary paralysis of the lower extremities that results from injury to the spine and is often associated with ileus. If the spinal cord is transected, permanent motor paralysis persists below the level of spinal-cord division.

spindle (spin-d'l) *n.* a collection of fibres seen in a cell when it is dividing. It plays an important part in chromosome movement in mitosis and meiosis and is also involved in division of the cytoplasm.

spine (spyn) *n.* **1.** a sharp process on a bone. **2.** the vertebral column (*see* backbone). **—spinal** *adj.*

spino- *combining form denoting* **1.** the spine. **2.** the spinal cord.

spiral bandage (spyr-ăl) *n.* a bandage wound round a part of the body, overlapping the previous section at each turn.

spiral organ *n.* *see* organ (of Corti).

Spirillum (spy-**ril**-ŭm) *n.* a genus of highly motile rigid spiral-shaped bacteria usually found in fresh and salt water containing organic matter. **S. minus** a species that causes rat-bite fever.

spiro- *combining form denoting* **1.** spiral. **2.** respiration.

spirochaetaemia (spy-roh-ki-**tee**-miă) *n.* the presence of spirochaetes in the bloodstream, occurring in the later stages of syphilis.

spirochaete (**spy**-roh-keet) *n.* any one of a group of spiral-shaped bacteria that lack a rigid cell wall and move by means of muscular flexions of the cell. The group includes *Borrelia*, *Leptospira*, and *Treponema*.

spirograph (**spy**-roh-grahf) *n.* an instrument for recording breathing movements. The record obtained is called a **spirogram**. **—spirography** *n.*

spirometer (spy-**rom**-it-er) *n.* an instrument for measuring the volume of air inhaled and exhaled. It is used in tests of ventilation. **—spirometry** *n.*

spironolactone (spy-rŏ-noh-**lak**-tohn) *n.* a synthetic corticosteroid that inhibits the activity of the hormone aldosterone and is administered by mouth as a potassium-sparing diuretic to treat fluid retention (oedema) in cirrhosis, ascites, and severe heart failure. It is also used in treating aldosteronism. Trade name: **Aldactone**.

Spitz-Holter valve (spits-**hohl**-ter) *n.* a valve used in the treatment of hydrocephalus to drain cerebrospinal fluid from the ventricles of the brain into either the right atrium or the peritoneum.

splanch- (splanchno-) *combining form denoting* the viscera.

splanchnic (**splank**-nik) *adj.* relating to the viscera. *Compare* somatic. **s. nerves** the series of nerves in the sympathetic system that are distributed to the blood vessels and viscera.

splanchnology (splank-**nol**-ŏji) *n.* the study of the viscera.

spleen (spleen) *n.* a large dark-red ovoid organ situated on the left side of the body below and behind the stomach. The spongy interior (**pulp**) of the spleen consists of lymphoid tissue within a meshwork of reticular fibres. The spleen is a major component of the reticuloendothelial system, producing lymphocytes in the newborn and containing phagocytes, which remove worn-out red blood cells and other foreign bodies from the bloodstream. Anatomical name: **lien**. **—splenic** (**splen**-ik) *adj.*

splen- (spleno-) *combining form denoting* the spleen.

splenectomy (spli-**nek**-tŏmi) *n.* surgical removal of the spleen. This is sometimes necessary in the emergency treatment of bleeding from a ruptured spleen.

splenic anaemia *n.* anaemia associated with portal hypertension and increased destruction of red blood cells by an overactive spleen.

splenitis (spli-ny-tis) *n.* inflammation of the spleen. *See also* perisplenitis.

splenomegaly (splee-noh-**meg**-ăli) *n.* enlargement of the spleen. It commonly occurs in malaria, blood disorders, leukaemia, and Hodgkin's disease. *See also* hypersplenism.

splenorenal anastomosis (splee-noh-ree-năl) *n.* a method of treating portal hypertension by joining the splenic vein to the left renal vein. *Compare* portacaval anastomosis.

splenovenography (splee-noh-vi-**nog**-răfi) *n.* X-ray examination of the spleen and veins associated with it following injection of a radiopaque dye.

splint (splint) *n.* a rigid appliance (orthosis) used to support or hold a limb or digit in position until healing of a fracture, dislocation, or soft-tissue injury has occurred.

splinter haemorrhage (splint-er) *n.* a linear haemorrhage below the nails, usually the result of trauma but also occurring in such conditions as subacute bacterial endocarditis or severe rheumatoid arthritis.

split-skin graft (SSG, Thiersch's graft) (split-skin) *n.* a type of skin graft in which thin partial thicknesses of skin are used to cover and heal a wound. They are removed from one site on the body, cut in narrow strips or sheets, and placed onto the wound area to be healed.

spondyl- (spondylo-) *combining form denoting* a vertebra or the spine.

spondylitis (spon-di-**ly**-tis) *n.* inflammation of the synovial joints of the backbone. **ankylosing s.** a type of arthritis that predominantly affects young males. The inflammation affects the joint capsules and their attached ligaments and tendons, principally the intervertebral joints and sacroiliac joints (*see* sacroiliitis). The resultant pain and stiffness are treated by analgesics (including NSAIDs), physiotherapy, and biological disease-modifying antirheumatic drugs. The disorder can lead to severe deformities of the spine (*see* ankylosis, kyphosis).

spondylolisthesis (spon-di-loh-**lis**-thi-sis) *n.* a forward shift of one vertebra upon another, due to a defect in the bone or in the joints that normally bind them together. This may be congenital or develop after injury.

spondylosis (spon-di-**loh**-sis) *n.* a spinal condition resulting from degeneration and flattening of the intervertebral discs in the cervical, thoracic, or lumbar regions. Symptoms include pain and restriction of movement. Treatment includes analgesics, NSAIDs, and physiotherapy; painful movements are prevented by wearing a neck orthosis (when the neck region is affected) or a lumbosacral corset (for the lower spine). Very severe cases sometimes require surgical fusion.

spondylosyndesis (spon-di-loh-**sin**-di-sis) *n.* surgical fusion of the intervertebral joints of the backbone.

spongiform encephalopathy (**spun**ji-form) *n.* any one of a group of rapidly progressive degenerative neurological diseases that include scrapie in sheep, **bovine spongiform encephalopathy** (**BSE**) in cattle, and Creutzfeldt-Jakob disease in humans. Human spongiform encephalopathies are characterized by rapidly progressive dementia associated with myoclonic jerks (*see* myoclonus). The diseases are thought to be caused by abnormal transmissible proteins (*see* prion).

spontaneous (spon-**tay**-niŭs) *adj.* arising without apparent cause or outside aid. The term is applied in medicine to certain conditions, such as pathological fractures, that arise in the absence of outside injury.

sporadic (sper-**ad**-ik) *adj.* describing a disease that occurs only occasionally or in a few isolated places. *Compare* endemic, epidemic.

spore (spor) *n.* a small reproductive body produced by plants and microorganisms. Some kinds of spores function as dormant stages of the life cycle, enabling the organism to survive adverse conditions. Other spores are the means by which the organism can spread vegetatively. *See also* endospore.

sporicide (**spor**-i-syd) *n.* an agent that kills spores (e.g. bacterial spores). Most germicides are ineffective since spores are very resistant to chemical action. —**sporicidal** *adj.*

sporotrichosis (spor-oh-trik-**oh**-sis) *n.* a chronic infection of the skin and superficial lymph nodes that is caused by the fungus *Sporothrix schenckii* and results in the formation of abscesses and ulcers. It occurs mainly in the tropics.

sports injury (sports) *n.* any injury related to the practice of a sport, often resulting from the overuse and stretching of muscles, tendons, and ligaments.

sports medicine *n.* a specialty concerned with the treatment of sports injuries and measures designed to prevent or minimize them.

spotted fever (**spot**-id) *n. see* Rocky Mountain spotted fever, typhus.

sprain (sprayn) *n.* injury to a ligament, caused by sudden overstretching. Sprains should be treated by cold compresses (ice-packs) at the time of injury, and later by restriction of activity.

Sprengel's deformity (**spreng**-ĕlz) *n.* a congenital abnormality of the scapula, which is small and positioned high in the shoulder. [O. G. K. Sprengel (1852–1915), German surgeon]

sprue (psilosis) (sproo) *n.* impaired absorption of food due to disease of the small intestine. **tropical s.** sprue that is characterized by diarrhoea (usually steatorrhoea), glossitis, anaemia, and weight loss; the lining of the small intestine becomes inflamed and atrophied, leading to vitamin and micronutrient deficiencies. Treatment with antibiotics and folic acid is usually effective. *See also* coeliac disease, malabsorption.

spud (spud) *n.* a blunt needle used for removing foreign bodies embedded in the cornea of the eye.

spur (sper) *n.* a sharp projection, especially one of bone.

sputum (spew-tŭm) *n.* material coughed up from the respiratory tract. Its colour, consistency, and other characteristics often provide important information affecting the diagnosis and the management of respiratory disease. Pathological examination of sputum for micro-organisms and abnormal cells may add further information.

squama (skway-mă) *n.* (*pl.* **squamae**) **1.** a thin plate of bone. **2.** a scale, such as any of the scales from the cornified layer of the epidermis. —**squamous** *adj.*

squamo- *combining form denoting* **1.** the squamous portion of the temporal bone. **2.** squamous epithelium.

squamous bone (skway-mŭs) *n.* *see* temporal (bone).

squamous cell carcinoma (SCC) *n.* any cancer of squamous epithelium. SCC is the second commonest form of skin cancer (after basal cell carcinoma), occurring usually in late-middle and old age. Cumulative exposure to the sun is the commonest cause: SCC is mainly found on areas exposed to light and is more common in men than in women. It spreads locally at first but later may spread to sites distant from its origin (*see* metastasis). Treatment is usually by surgical excision or radiotherapy.

squamous epithelium *n.* *see* epithelium.

squint (skwint) *n.* *see* strabismus.

SSG *n.* *see* split-skin graft.

SSPE *n.* *see* subacute sclerosing panencephalitis.

SSRI (selective serotonin reuptake inhibitor) *n.* any one of a group of antidepressant drugs that exert their action by blocking the reabsorption of the neurotransmitter serotonin by the nerve endings in the brain. Their effect is to prolong the action of serotonin in the brain. The group includes citalopram, fluoxetine, fluvoxamine, paroxetine, sertraline, and **escitalopram** (Cipralex). The most common side-effects are nausea, indigestion, abdominal pain, and other gastrointestinal upsets.

staccato speech (stă-kah-toh) *n.* abnormal speech in which there are pauses between words, sometimes associated with multiple sclerosis.

Stacke's operation (stak-ĕz) *n.* an operation in which the bone between the mastoid cells and the middle ear is removed to create a single cavity. It is performed when there is chronic infection of this area. [L. Stacke (1859–1918), German otologist]

stadium (stay-diŭm) *n.* (*pl.* **stadia**) a stage in the course of a disease. **s. invasionis** the period between exposure to infection and the onset of symptoms.

stage (stayj) *vb.* (in oncology) to classify a primary tumour by its size and the presence and site of metastases. In addition to clinical examination, a variety of imaging and surgical techniques provide a more accurate assessment. Staging tumours is important in prognosis and defining appropriate treatment.

staghorn calculus (stag-horn) *n.* a branched stone forming a cast of the collecting system of the kidney and therefore filling and obstructing the calyces and pelvis. It is usually associated with infection and can cause pyonephrosis and, if neglected, a perinephric abscess.

stagnant loop syndrome (stag-nănt) *n. see* blind loop syndrome.

stain (stayn) **1.** *n.* a dye used to colour tissues and other specimens for microscopical examination. **2.** *vb.* to treat a specimen for microscopical study with a stain.

stammering (stuttering) (stam-er-ing) *n.* halting articulation with interruptions to the normal flow of speech and repetition of the initial consonants of words or syllables. The symptoms are most severe when the stammerer is under any psychological stress. **—stammerer** *n.*

STAMP (Screening Tool for the Assessment of Malnutrition in Paediatrics) *n.* a validated nutritional assessment tool used in the care of children in hospital between the ages of 2 and 16. It can be administered by a nurse with assistance from the interprofessional team and allocates a score to original diagnosis or illness, nutritional intake, and weight and height to identify risk factors and the need for intervention.

standard deviation (stand-erd) *n.* (in statistics) a measure of the scatter of observations about their arithmetic mean (*see* frequency distribution), which is calculated from the square root of the **variance** of the readings in the series. The arithmetic sum of the amounts by which each observation varies from the mean must be zero, but if these variations are squared before being summated, a positive value is obtained: the mean of this value is the variance. In practice a more reliable estimate of variance is obtained by dividing the sum of the squared deviations by one *less* than the total number of observations.

stapedectomy (stay-pi-**dek**-tŏmi) *n.* surgical removal of the stapes, enabling it to be replaced with a prosthetic bone in the treatment of otosclerosis.

stapediolysis (stă-pee-di-**ol**-i-sis) *n.* an operation to restore hearing in cases of otosclerosis, in which the stapes is freed from the fenestra ovalis.

stapes (**stay**-peez) *n.* a stirrup-shaped bone in the middle ear that articulates with the incus and is attached to the membrane of the fenestra ovalis. *See* ossicle.

staphylectomy (staf-i-**lek**-tŏmi) *n. see* uvulectomy.

staphylococcal scalded skin syndrome (Ritter's disease) (staf-i-loh-**kok**-k'l **skawl**-did) *n.* a potentially serious condition of young infants in which the skin becomes reddened and then peels off. The underlying cause is a staphylococcal infection.

Staphylococcus (staf-i-loh-kok-ŭs) *n.* a genus of Gram-positive nonmotile spherical bacteria occurring in grapelike clusters. Some species are saprophytes; others parasites. Many species produce exotoxins. More serious infections that are caused by staphylococci include pneumonia, bacteraemia, osteomyelitis, and enterocolitis. **S. aureus** a species that causes boils and internal abscesses. *See also* MRSA. **—staphylococcal** *adj.*

staphyloma (staf-i-loh-mă) *n.* abnormal bulging of the cornea or sclera (white) of the eye.

staphylorrhaphy (palatorrhaphy) (staf-il-o-răfi) *n.* surgical suture of a cleft palate.

staple (stay-pŭl) *n.* (in surgery) a piece of metal used to join up pieces of tissue. Staples can be used as an alternative to sutures for an anastomosis or to bring together the skin edges of an incision; stapling machines have been produced for this purpose. *See also* endostapler.

starch (starch) *n.* the form in which carbohydrates are stored in many plants and a major constituent of the diet. Starch consists of linked glucose units and occurs in two forms, **α-amylose** and **amylopectin.** Starch is digested by means of the enzyme amylase. *See also* dextrin.

Starling's law (star-lingz) *n.* a law stating that, within certain limits, a muscle (including the heart muscle) responds to increased stretching at rest by an increased force of contraction when stimulated. [E. H. Starling (1866–1927), British physiologist]

startle reflex (star-t'l) *n. see* Moro reflex.

starvation (star-vay-shŏn) *n. see* malnutrition.

stasis (stay-sis) *n.* stagnation or cessation of flow; for example, of blood or lymph whose flow is obstructed or of the intestinal contents when peristalsis is hindered.

-stasis *combining form denoting* stoppage of a flow of liquid; stagnation.

stat (statim) Latin: at once, used as a direction in prescriptions.

statementing (stayt-mĕnt-ing) *n.* the provision by a local authority of a **statement of special educational needs** for children attending school who have mental or physical disabilities severe enough to require extra help at school. *See* special educational needs.

statin (stat-in) *n.* a drug that inhibits the action of an enzyme involved in the liver's production of cholesterol. Statins can lower the levels of **low-density lipoproteins (LDLs)** by 25–45%; they are used mainly to treat hypercholesterolaemia but also to reduce the risk of coronary heart disease in susceptible patients. *See* atorvastatin, fluvastatin, pravastatin, simvastatin.

statistical significance (stă-tist-i-kăl) *n. see* significance.

status asthmaticus (stay-tŭs ass-mat-ik-ŭs) *n.* a severe attack of asthma. Patients are very breathless and may die from respiratory failure if not treated with inhaled oxygen, bronchodilators, and corticosteroid therapy; sedatives are absolutely contraindicated.

status epilepticus (epi-**lep**-tik-ŭs) *n.* the occurrence of repeated epileptic seizures without any recovery of consciousness between them. Prolonged status epilepticus may lead to the patient's death or long-term disability.

status lymphaticus (lim-**fat**-ik-ŭs) *n.* enlargement of the thymus gland and other parts of the lymphatic system, formerly believed to be a predisposing cause to sudden death in infancy and childhood.

STD *n. see* sexually transmitted disease.

steapsin (sti-**ap**-sin) *n. see* lipase.

stearic acid (sti-**a**-rik) *n. see* fatty acid.

steat- (steato-) *combining form denoting* fat; fatty tissue.

steatoma (sti-ă-**toh**-mă) *n.* any cyst or tumour of a sebaceous gland.

steatopygia (sti-ă-toh-**pij**-iă) *n.* the accumulation of large quantities of fat in the buttocks.

steatorrhoea (sti-ă-tŏ-**ree**-ă) *n.* the passage of excess fat in the faeces due to reduced absorption of fat by the intestine (*see* malabsorption). The faeces are pale, malodorous, and may look greasy.

steatosis (sti-ă-**toh**-sis) *n.* infiltration of hepatocytes with fat. This may occur in alcoholism, obesity, metabolic syndrome, pregnancy, malnutrition, or viral hepatitis, or with some drugs.

Steele-Richardson-Olszewski syndrome (steel **rich**-ăd-sŏn ol-**zev**-ski) *n. see* progressive supranuclear palsy. [J. C. Steele and J. C. Richardson (20th century), Canadian neurologists; J. Olszewski (1913–64), Polish-born Canadian neuropathologist]

Stein-Leventhal syndrome (styn-**lev**-ĕn-thal) *n. see* polycystic ovary syndrome. [I. F. Stein (20th century) and M. L. Leventhal (1901–71), US gynaecologists]

Steinmann's pin (**styn**-manz) *n.* a fine metal nail inserted through a fractured bone through which extension is applied to the distal bone fragment. [F. Steinmann (1872–1932), Swiss surgeon]

stellate (**stel**-ayt) *adj.* star-shaped. **s. fracture** a star-shaped fracture of the kneecap caused by a direct blow. **s. ganglion** a star-shaped collection of sympathetic nerve cell bodies in the root of the neck.

Stellwag's sign (**stel**-vagz) *n.* apparent widening of the distance between the upper and lower eyelids due to retraction of the upper lid and protrusion of the eyeball. It is a sign of exophthalmic goitre. [C. Stellwag von Carion (1823–1904), Austrian ophthalmologist]

stem cell (stem) *n.* an undifferentiated cell that is able to renew itself and produce all the specialized cells within an organ. **embryonic s. c.** a cell of the blastocyst that can differentiate into almost any cell type. **haemopoietic s. c.** a cell of the bone marrow from which all blood cells are derived.

steno- *combining form denoting* **1.** narrow. **2.** constricted.

stenosis (sti-**noh**-sis) *n.* the abnormal narrowing of a passage or opening, such as a blood vessel or heart valve. *See* aortic stenosis, carotid-artery stenosis, mitral stenosis, pulmonary (stenosis), pyloric stenosis.

stenostomia (stenostomy) (sten-ŏ-**stoh**-miă) *n.* the abnormal narrowing of an opening, such as the opening of the bile duct.

Stensen's duct (**sten**-sĕnz) *n.* the long secretory duct of the parotid salivary gland. [N. Stensen (1638–86), Danish physician]

stent (stent) *n.* a tube placed inside a duct or canal to reopen it or keep it open. Stents may be used at operation to aid healing of an anastomosis, for example of a ureter, or they can be placed across an obstruction to maintain an open lumen, for example in obstruction due to tumour in the oesophagus, stomach, bile ducts, colon, or ureter. In an artery after angioplasty stents help to prevent restenosis and are increasingly used in coronary artery disease in place of coronary artery bypass grafting. **drug-eluting s.** a coronary stent coated with a drug that reduces the risk of stenosis.

stepping reflex (**step**-ing) *n.* a primitive reflex in newborn babies that should disappear by the age of two months. If the baby is held in a 'walking' position with the feet touching the ground, the feet move in a 'stepping' manner. Persistence of this reflex beyond two months is suggestive of cerebral palsy.

sterco- *combining form denoting* faeces.

stercobilin (ster-koh-**by**-lin) *n.* a brownish-red pigment formed during the metabolism of the bile pigments biliverdin and bilirubin and subsequently excreted in the urine or faeces.

stercolith (**ster**-koh-lith) *n.* a solid mass of dried compressed faeces.

stereognosis (ste-ri-og-**noh**-sis) *n.* the ability to recognize the three-dimensional shape of an object by touch alone. This is a function of the association areas of the parietal lobe of the brain. *See also* agnosia.

stereopsis (ste-ri-**op**-sis) *n. see* stereoscopic vision.

stereoscopic vision (stereopsis) (ste-ri-ŏ-**skop**-ik) *n.* perception of the shape, depth, and distance of an object as a result of having binocular vision.

stereotactic (ste-ri-ŏ-**tak**-tik) *adj.* of or relating to the accurate localization of structures within the body by using three-dimensional measurements. Stereotactic localization enables the accurate positioning within the body of radiotherapy beams or sources for the treatment of tumours and of localizing wires for the biopsy of small tumours. **s. surgery** *see* stereotaxy.

stereotaxy (stereotactic surgery) (ste-ri-ŏ-**taks**-i) *n.* a surgical procedure in which a deep-seated area in the brain is operated upon after its position has been accurately established by three-dimensional measurements using CT or MRI. The operation may be performed using an electrical current or by heat, cold, or mechanical techniques. *See also* leucotomy.

stereotypy (ste-ri-ŏ-ty-pi) *n.* the constant repetition of a complex action, which is carried out in the same way each time. It is seen in catatonia and autism; sometimes it is an isolated symptom in people with learning disability.

sterile (ste-ryl) *adj.* **1.** (of a living organism) barren; unable to reproduce its kind (*see* sterility). **2.** (of inanimate objects) completely free from microorganisms that could cause infection.

sterility (ster-**il**-iti) *n.* inability to have children, either due to infertility or (in someone who has been fertile) deliberately induced by surgical procedures as a means of contraception (*see* sterilization).

sterilization (ste-ri-ly-**zay**-shŏn) *n.* **1.** a surgical operation or any other process that induces sterility in men or women. In women this is now usually achieved by **tubal occlusion**: the permanent closure of the inner (lower) half of the Fallopian tubes through a laparoscope by means of a clip (Hulka-Clemens or Filshie clips) or a small plastic ring (Falope ring) or by introducing a rapid-setting plastic into the tubes through a hysteroscope. Men are usually sterilized by vasectomy. **2.** the process by which all types of microorganisms (including spores) are destroyed. This is achieved by the use of heat, radiation, chemicals, or filtration. *See also* autoclave.

stern- (sterno-) *combining form denoting* the sternum.

sternocleidomastoid muscle (ster-noh-kly-doh-**mas**-toid) *n. see* sternomastoid muscle.

sternohyoid (ster-noh-**hy**-oid) *n.* a muscle in the neck, arising from the sternum and inserted into the hyoid bone. It depresses the hyoid bone.

sternomastoid muscle (sternocleidomastoid muscle) (ster-noh-**mas**-toid) *n.* a long muscle in the neck, extending from the mastoid process to the sternum and clavicle. It serves to rotate the neck and flex the head.

sternomastoid tumour *n.* a small painless nonmalignant swelling in the lower half of the sternomastoid muscle, appearing a few days after birth. It is most common after breech births. The tumour may cause a slight tilt of the head, which can be corrected by physiotherapy.

sternotomy (ster-**not**-ŏmi) *n.* surgical division of the sternum, performed to allow access to the heart and its major vessels.

sternum (ster-nŭm) *n.* (*pl.* **sterna**) the breastbone: a flat bone extending from the base of the neck to just below the diaphragm and forming the front part of the skeleton of the thorax. The sternum articulates with the collar bones (*see* clavicle) and the costal cartilages of the first seven pairs of ribs. **—sternal** *adj.*

steroid (**steer**-oid) *n.* one of a group of organic compounds that include the male and female sex hormones (androgens and oestrogens), the hormones of the adrenal cortex (*see* corticosteroid), progesterone, bile salts, and sterols. Synthetic steroids have been produced for therapeutic purposes.

steroid card *n.* a card that must be carried by patients taking long-term corticosteroid medication, particularly if high doses are used. The card states that in an emergency treatment with steroids must not be suddenly stopped since this may precipitate an Addisonian crisis.

sterol (steer-ol) *n.* one of a group of steroid alcohols. The most important sterols are cholesterol and ergosterol.

stertor (ster-ter) *n.* a snoring type of noisy breathing heard in deeply unconscious patients.

steth- (stetho-) *combining form denoting* the chest.

stethoscope (steth-ŏ-skohp) *n.* an instrument used for listening to sounds within the body (*see* auscultation). A simple stethoscope usually consists of a diaphragm or an open bell-shaped structure (which is applied to the body) connected by rubber or plastic tubes to shaped earpieces for the examiner.

Stevens-Johnson syndrome (stee-vĕnz jon-sŏn) *n.* an inflammatory condition characterized by fever, large blisters on the skin, and ulceration of the mucous membranes. It may be a severe allergic reaction to certain drugs or it may follow certain infections. [A. M. Stevens (1884–1945) and F. C. Johnson (1894–1934), US paediatricians]

sthenia (sthee-niă) *n.* a state of normal or greater than normal strength. *Compare* asthenia. **—sthenic** (sthen-ik) *adj.*

stigma (stig-mă) *n.* (*pl.* **stigmata**) **1.** a mark that characterizes a particular disease, such as the café au lait spots characteristic of neurofibromatosis. **2.** any spot or lesion on the skin.

stilet (stylet, stylus) (sty-lit) *n.* **1.** a slender probe. **2.** a wire placed in the lumen of a catheter to give it rigidity while the instrument is passed along a body canal.

stillbirth (stil-berth) **(intrauterine fetal death)** *n.* birth of a fetus that shows no evidence of life (heartbeat, respiration, or independent movement) at any time later than 24 weeks after conception. A fetus born dead before this time is known as a miscarriage or abortion.

SEE WEB LINKS

- Website of the Stillbirth and Neonatal Death Society

Still's disease (stilz) *n.* **1.** *see* juvenile idiopathic arthritis. **2.** (**adult-onset Still's disease**) a systematic inflammatory disease characterized by a spiking fever, joint pain, and a pink rash that comes and goes. Treatment is by NSAIDS, corticosteroids, or disease-modifying antirheumatic drugs. [Sir G. F. Still (1868–1941), British physician]

stimulant (stim-yoo-lănt) *n.* an agent that promotes the activity of a body system or function. Amphetamines, methylphenidate, and caffeine are stimulants of the central nervous system; doxapram is a respiratory stimulant.

stimulator (stim-yoo-lay-ter) *n.* any apparatus designed to stimulate nerves and muscles for a variety of purposes. It can be used to stimulate particular areas of the brain or to block pain (as in **transcutaneous electrical nerve stimulation**, **TENS**).

stimulus (stim-yoo-lŭs) *n.* (*pl.* **stimuli**) any agent that provokes a response, or particular form of activity, in a cell, tissue, or other structure.

stirrup (sti-rŭp) *n.* (in anatomy) *see* stapes.

stitch (stich) *n.* **1.** a sharp localized pain, commonly in the abdomen, associated with strenuous physical activity. It is a form of cramp. **2.** *see* suture.

STM *n.* short-term memory.

stock culture (stok) *n. see* culture.

Stokes-Adams syndrome (stohks-ad-ămz) *n.* attacks of temporary loss of consciousness that occur when blood flow ceases due to extreme slowing of the heart rate. This syndrome may complicate heart block. [W. Stokes (1804–78) and R. Adams (1791–1875), Irish physicians]

stoma (stoh-mă) *n.* (*pl.* **stomata**) **1.** (in anatomy) the mouth or any mouthlike part. **2.** (in surgery) the artificial opening of a hollow organ that has been brought to the abdominal surface (*see* colostomy, ileostomy). **s. therapist** a nurse specially trained in the care of these openings and the appliances used with them. **—stomal** *adj.*

stomach (stum-ăk) *n.* a distensible saclike organ that forms part of the alimentary canal between the oesophagus and the duodenum. The stomach lies just below the diaphragm, to the right of the spleen. Its function is to continue the process of digestion that begins in the mouth. Gastric juice, secreted by gastric glands in the mucosa, together with the churning action of the muscular layers of the stomach, reduces the food to a semiliquid partly digested mass that passes on to the duodenum. See illustration.

stomach stapling (gastric stapling, vertical banded

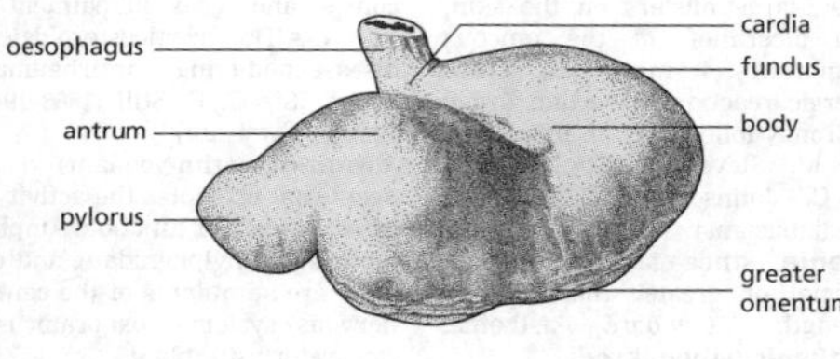

Regions of the stomach seen from the front

gastroplasty) *n.* bariatric surgery in which staples are inserted into the wall of the stomach to form a small pouch, which restricts the amount of food that can be eaten, and a gastric band is applied to limit the size of the opening between the pouch and the rest of the stomach.

stomat- (stomato-) *combining form denoting* the mouth.

stomatitis (stoh-mă-ty-tis) *n.* inflammation of the mucous lining of the mouth.

stomatology (stoh-mă-**tol**-ŏji) *n.* the branch of medicine concerned with diseases of the mouth.

-stomy (-ostomy) *combining form denoting* a surgical opening into an organ or part.

stone (stohn) *n. see* calculus.

stool (stool) *n.* faeces discharged from the anus.

stop needle (stop) *n.* a surgical needle with a shank that has a protruding collar to stop it when the needle has been pushed a prescribed distance into the tissue.

strabismus (heterotropia) (stră-**biz**-mŭs) *n.* squint: abnormal alignment of the two eyes. The strabismus is most commonly horizontal (*see* esotropia, exotropia) but it may be vertical (*see* hypertropia, hypotropia). *See also* heterophoria.

strain (strayn) **1.** *n.* excessive stretching or working of a muscle, resulting in pain and swelling. *Compare* sprain. **2.** *n.* a group of organisms obtained from a particular source or having special properties distinguishing them from other members of the same species. **3.** *vb.* to damage a muscle by overstretching.

strangulated (**strang**-yoo-layt-id) *adj.* describing a part of the body whose blood supply has been interrupted by compression of a blood vessel. **s. hernia** *see* hernia.

strangulation (strang-yoo-**lay**-shŏn) *n.* the closure of a passage, such as the main airway to the lungs (resulting in the cessation of breathing), a blood vessel, or the gastrointestinal tract.

strangury (**strang**-yoor-i) *n.* severe pain in the urethra associated with an intense desire to pass urine, resulting from irritation of the base of the bladder. It may also occur in such conditions as cancer of the base of the bladder, cystitis, or prostatitis, when it is accompanied by the painful passage of a few drops of urine.

strategic health authority (SHA) (stră-**tee**-jik) *n.* formerly, a statutory organization that was responsible for strategic leadership, building capacity, organizational development, and performance management in the local National Health Service. SHAs were established in 2002 and disbanded in 2013, when their responsibilities passed to NHS England, clinical commissioning groups, and Public Health England.

stratified (**strat**-i-fyd) *adj.* describing tissue consisting of several layers of cells. *See* epithelium.

STRATIFY *n. see* St Thomas's Risk Assessment in Falling Elderly Inpatients.

stratum (**strah**-tŭm) *n.* a layer of tissue or cells, such as any of the layers of the epidermis. **s. corneum** the outermost layer of the epidermis.

strawberry mark (strawberry naevus) (straw-bĕ-ri) *n.* *see* naevus.

streak (streek) *n.* (in anatomy) a line, furrow, or narrow band.

Streptobacillus (strep-toh-bă-**sil**-ŭs) *n.* a genus of Gram-negative aerobic nonmotile rodlike bacteria that tend to form filaments. **S. moniliformis** the cause of rat-bite fever.

streptococcal toxic shock syndrome (strep-tŏ-**kok**-k'l) *n.* *see* toxic shock syndrome.

Streptococcus (strep-toh-**kok**-ŭs) *n.* a genus of Gram-positive nonmotile spherical bacteria occurring in chains. Most species are saprophytes, but some are pathogenic. **Haemolytic streptococci** destroy red blood cells in blood agar and are the cause of many infections, including bacterial endocarditis (α-haemolytic strains) and scarlet fever (β-haemolytic strains). **S. pneumoniae** *see* pneumococcus. *See also* Lancefield classification, streptokinase. **—streptococcal** *adj.*

streptodornase (strep-toh-**dor**-nayz) *n.* an enzyme produced by some haemolytic bacteria of the genus *Streptococcus* that is capable of liquefying pus. *See also* streptokinase.

streptokinase (strep-toh-**ky**-nayz) *n.* an enzyme produced by some haemolytic bacteria of the genus *Streptococcus* that is capable of liquefying blood clots (*see* fibrinolytic). It is given by intravenous infusion to treat blockage of blood vessels, as occurs in myocardial infarction, deep vein thrombosis, and pulmonary embolism (*see* thrombolysis). Trade name: **Streptase**.

streptolysin (strep-**tol**-i-sin) *n.* an exotoxin that is produced by strains of *Streptococcus* bacteria and destroys red blood cells.

Streptomyces (strep-toh-**my**-seez) *n.* a genus of aerobic mould-like bacteria. They are important medically as a source of such antibiotics as streptomycin, dactinomycin, chloramphenicol, and neomycin.

streptomycin (strep-toh-**my**-sin) *n.* an aminoglycoside antibiotic, derived from the bacterium *Streptomyces griseus*, that is used in combination with other drugs for treating tuberculosis and brucellosis. It is administered by intramuscular injection.

stress (stres) *n.* any factor that threatens the health of the body or has an adverse effect on its functioning, such as injury, disease, overwork, or worry. Constant stress brings about changes in the balance of hormones in the body. **s. fracture** *see* fracture. **s. incontinence** *see* incontinence. **s. test** an investigation to seek evidence of cardiac ischaemia. The heart is stressed by exercise or by the administration of an intravenous drug that increases heart rate. Ischaemia may then be detected by electrocardiography, echocardiography, myocardial perfusion scan, or cardiac MRI. **s. ulcers** gastric or duodenal ulcers associated with physiological stress from severe head injury (**Cushing's ulcers**) or major burns (**Curling's ulcers**).

stretch reflex (myotatic reflex) (strech) *n.* the reflex contraction of a muscle in response to its being stretched.

stria (stry-ă) *n.* (*pl.* **striae**) (in anatomy) a streak, line, or thin band. **striae gravidarum** stretch marks: the lines that appear on the skin of the abdomen of pregnant women, due to excessive stretching of the elastic fibres. Red or purple during pregnancy, they become white after delivery.

striated muscle (stry-ayt-id) *n.* a tissue that comprises the bulk of the body's musculature. It is also known as **skeletal muscle**, because it is attached to the skeleton and is responsible for the movement of bones, and **voluntary muscle**, because it is under voluntary control.

stricture (strik-cher) *n.* a narrowing of any tubular structure in the body. A stricture may result from inflammation, muscular spasm, growth of a tumour within the affected part, or from pressure on it by neighbouring organs. **urethral s.** a fibrous narrowing of the urethra, usually resulting from injury or inflammation. The patient has increasing difficulty in passing urine and may develop urinary retention.

stricturoplasty (strik-cher-oh-plasti) *n.* an operation in which a stricture (usually in the small intestine) is widened by cutting it longitudinally and suturing transversely.

stridor (stry-dor) *n.* the noise heard on breathing in when the trachea or larynx is obstructed. It tends to be louder and harsher than wheeze.

stroke (apoplexy) (strohk) *n.* a sudden attack of weakness usually affecting one side of the body, resulting from an interruption to the flow of blood to the brain. The flow of blood may be prevented by thrombosis or embolism (**ischaemic s.**) or by haemorrhage (**haemorrhagic s.**). Prolonged reduction of blood pressure may result in more diffuse brain damage, as after a cardiorespiratory arrest. A stroke can vary in severity from a passing weakness or tingling in a limb (*see* transient ischaemic attack) to a profound paralysis, coma, and death. *See also* cerebral haemorrhage.

stroke volume *n.* the amount of blood ejected from each ventricle on each contraction, which can be affected by medication, exercise, decreases in the volume of circulating blood, or heart anomalies. In a healthy adult, stroke volume is estimated at 70 ml.

stroma (stroh-mă) *n.* the connective-tissue basis of an organ, as opposed to the functional tissue (parenchyma). For example, the stroma of the erythrocytes is the spongy framework of protein strands within a red blood cell in which the blood pigment haemoglobin is packed; the stroma of the cornea is the transparent fibrous tissue making up the main body of the cornea.

strongyloidiasis (strongyloidosis) (stron-ji-loi-**dy**-ă-sis) *n.* an infestation of the small intestine with the parasitic nematode worm *Strongyloides stercoralis*. Larvae enter the body through the skin and migrate to the lungs, where they cause tissue destruction and bleeding. Adult worms burrow into the intestinal wall and may cause ulceration, diarrhoea, abdominal pain, nausea, anaemia, and weakness. Treatment involves use of albendazole, ivermectin, or tiabendazole.

strontium (**stron**-tiŭm) *n.* a yellow metallic element, absorption of which causes bone damage when its atoms displace calcium in bone. Symbol: Sr. **strontium-89** a radioactive isotope used in the treatment of metastatic carcinoma for the relief of pain due to bone metastases. **strontium-90** a radioactive isotope used in radiotherapy for the contact therapy of skin and eye tumours and in radioimmunotherapy in combination with monoclonal antibodies.

struma (**stroo**-mă) *n.* (*pl.* **strumae**) a swelling of the thyroid gland (*see* goitre). **s. ovarii** a teratoma of the ovary containing thyroid tissue that becomes active and causes thyrotoxicosis. *See also* Riedel's struma.

strychnine (**strik**-neen) *n.* a poisonous alkaloid produced in the seeds of the East Indian tree *Strychnos nux-vomica*. Poisoning causes painful muscular spasms similar to those of tetanus; death is likely to occur from spasm in the respiratory muscles.

S–T segment *n.* the segment on an electrocardiogram that represents the interval between the end of ventricular depolarization (QRS complex) and the beginning of ventricular repolarization (T wave).

Student's t test (**stew**-dĕnts) *n.* *see* parametric test. [Pseudonym of W. S. Gosset (1876–1937), British statistician]

stupe (stewp) *n.* any piece of material, such as a wad of cottonwool, soaked in hot water (with or without medication) and used to apply a poultice.

stupor (**stew**-per) *n.* a condition of near unconsciousness, with apparent mental inactivity and reduced ability to respond to stimulation.

Sturge-Weber syndrome (sterj-**web**-er) *n.* angioma of the blood vessels overlying the brain associated with a port-wine stain on the face (*see* naevus). [W. A. Sturge (1850–1919) and F. P. Weber (1863–1962), British physicians]

stuttering (**stut**-er-ing) *n.* *see* stammering.

stye (sty) *n.* acute inflammation of a gland at the base of an eyelash, caused by bacterial infection. The gland becomes hard and tender and a pus-filled cyst develops at its centre. Medical name: **hordeolum**.

stylet (**sty**-lit) *n.* *see* stilet.

stylo- *combining form denoting* the styloid process of the temporal bone.

styloid process (**sty**-loid) *n.* **1.** a long slender downward-pointing spine projecting from the lower surface of the temporal bone of the skull. It provides attachment for muscles and ligaments of the tongue and hyoid bone. **2.** any of various other spiny projections.

stylus (sty-lŭs) *n.* **1.** a pencil-shaped instrument, commonly used for applying external medication. **2.** *see* stilet.

styptic (stip-tik) *n. see* haemostatic.

sub- *prefix denoting* **1.** below; underlying. **2.** partial or slight.

subacute (sub-ă-**kewt**) *adj.* describing a disease that progresses more rapidly than a chronic condition but does not become acute.

subacute bacterial endocarditis (SBE) *n.* a form of endocarditis characterized by a slow onset and protracted course. It is usually caused by species of *Streptococcus* or *Staphylococcus*.

subacute combined degeneration of the cord *n.* the neurological disorder complicating a deficiency of vitamin B_{12} or folate and often combined with pernicious anaemia. There is selective damage to the motor and sensory nerve fibres in the spinal cord, resulting in spasticity of the limbs and a sensory ataxia.

subacute sclerosing panencephalitis (SSPE) (skleer-**ohz**-ing pan-en-sef-ă-**ly**-tis) *n.* a rare and late complication of measles characterized by a slow progressive neurological deterioration that is usually fatal. It can occur four to ten years after the initial infection.

subarachnoid haemorrhage (SAH) (sub-ă-**rak**-noid) *n.* sudden bleeding into the subarachnoid space, which causes severe headache with stiffness of the neck. The usual source of such a haemorrhage is a cerebral aneurysm that has burst.

subarachnoid space *n.* the space between the arachnoid and pia meninges of the brain and spinal cord, containing circulating cerebrospinal fluid and large blood vessels.

subclavian artery (sub-**klay**-vi-ăn) *n.* either of two arteries supplying blood to the neck and arms. The right subclavian artery branches from the innominate artery; the left subclavian arises directly from the aortic arch.

subclavian steal syndrome (steel) *n.* a syndrome produced by proximal narrowing of the subclavian artery, in which blood is diverted to the main artery supplying the arm from smaller branches to the brain when the arm is exercised. This causes loss of consciousness (syncope).

subclinical (sub-**klin**-ikăl) *adj.* describing a disease that is suspected but is not sufficiently developed to produce definite signs and symptoms in the patient.

subconscious (sub-**kon**-shŭs) *adj.* (in psychoanalysis) denoting the part of the mind that includes memories, motives, and intentions that are momentarily not present in consciousness but can more or less readily be recalled to awareness. *Compare* unconscious.

subcutaneous (sub-kew-**tay**-niŭs) *adj.* beneath the skin. *See also* injection. **s. tissue** loose connective tissue, often fatty, situated under the dermis.

subdural (sub-**dewr**-ăl) *adj.* below the dura mater; relating to the space between the dura mater and arachnoid. **s. haematoma** *see* haematoma.

subglottis (sub-**glot**-iss) *n.* that part of the larynx that lies below the vocal folds.

subinvolution (sub-in-vŏ-**loo**-shŏn) *n.* failure of the uterus to revert to its normal size during the six weeks following childbirth.

subjective (sub-**jek**-tiv) *adj.* apparent to the affected individual but not to others: applied particularly to symptoms.

sublimation (sub-li-**may**-shŏn) *n.* the replacement of socially undesirable means of gratifying motives or desires by means that are socially acceptable. *See also* defence mechanism, repression.

subliminal (sub-**lim**-inăl) *adj.* subconscious: beneath the threshold of conscious perception.

sublingual (sub-**ling**-wăl) *adj.* beneath the tongue. **s. gland** one of a pair of salivary glands situated in the lower part of the mouth, one on either side of the tongue.

subluxation (sub-luks-**ay**-shŏn) *n.* partial dislocation of a joint, so that the bone ends are misaligned but still in contact.

submandibular gland (submaxillary gland) (sub-man-**dib**-yoo-ler) *n.* one of a pair of salivary glands situated below the parotid glands.

submaxillary gland (sub-**maks**-il-er-i) *n. see* submandibular gland.

submucosa (sub-mew-**koh**-sa) *n.* the layer of loose connective (areolar) tissue underlying a mucous membrane. **—submucosal** *adj.*

submucous (sub-**mew**-kŭs) *adj.* beneath a mucous membrane. **s. resection** *see* resection.

subphrenic abscess (sub-**fren**-ik) *n.* a collection of pus below the diaphragm, usually affecting the right side. Causes include postoperative infection and perforation of an organ.

substitution (sub-sti-**tew**-shŏn) *n.* (in psychoanalysis) the replacement of one idea by another: a form of defence mechanism.

substitution therapy *n.* treatment by providing a less harmful alternative to a drug or remedy that a patient has been receiving.

substrate (**sub**-strayt) *n.* the specific substance or substances on which a given enzyme acts.

subsultus (sub-**sul**-tus) *n.* abnormal twitching or tremor of muscles, such as may occur in feverish conditions.

subtertian fever (sub-**ter**-shăn) *n.* a form of malaria resulting from repeated infection by *Plasmodium falciparum* and characterized by continuous fever.

subtotal (sub-**toh**-t'l) *adj.* almost complete or partial: applied, for example, to surgical procedures (e.g. subtotal thyroidectomy) or to occlusion (usually of an artery).

succus (**suk**-ŭs) *n.* any juice or secretion of animal or plant origin. **s. entericus (intestinal juice)** the clear alkaline fluid secreted by the glands of the small intestine.

It contains mucus and digestive enzymes.

succussion (suk-**ush**-ŏn) *n.* a splashing noise heard when a patient who has a large quantity of fluid in a body cavity, such as the pleural cavity, moves suddenly or is deliberately shaken.

sucralfate (sewk-răl-fayt) *n.* an aluminium-containing drug that forms a protective coating over the stomach or duodenal lining. Administered by mouth, sucralfate is used in the treatment and prevention of peptic ulcer. Trade name: **Antepsin**.

sucrose (**sewk**-rohz) *n.* a carbohydrate consisting of glucose and fructose. It is the principal constituent of cane sugar and sugar beet. The increasing consumption of sucrose in the last 50 years has coincided with an increase in the incidence of dental caries, diabetes, coronary heart disease, and obesity.

suction (**suk**-shŏn) *n.* the use of reduced pressure to remove unwanted fluids or other material through a tube for disposal. During surgery, suction tubes are used to remove blood from the area of operation and to decompress the stomach (**nasogastric s.**) and the pleural space of air and blood (**chest s.**).

sudden infant death syndrome (SIDS, cot death) *n.* the sudden unexpected death of an infant less than two years old (peak occurrence between two and six months) from an unidentifiable cause. There appear to be many factors involved, the most important of which is the position in which the baby is laid to sleep: babies who sleep on their fronts (the prone position) have an increased risk.

SEE WEB LINKS

- Website of the Lullaby Trust (formerly the Foundation for the Study of Infant Death)

sudden unexpected death in epilepsy *n.* the sudden unexpected nontraumatic death of a person with epilepsy, with or without evidence of a seizure and with no obvious cause found at post mortem.

Sudek's atrophy (soo-deks) *n. see* chronic regional pain syndrome. [P. H. M. Sudek (1866–1938), German surgeon]

sudor (**s'yoo**-dor) *n. see* sweat.

sudorific (s'yoo-der-**if**-ik) *n. see* diaphoretic.

suffocation (suf-ŏ-**kay**-shŏn) *n.* cessation of breathing as a result of drowning, smothering, etc., leading to unconsciousness or death (*see* asphyxia).

suffusion (sŭ-**few**-*zh*ŏn) *n.* the spreading of a flush across the skin surface, caused by changes in the local blood supply.

sugar (**shuug**-er) *n.* any carbohydrate that dissolves in water, is usually crystalline, and has a sweet taste. Sugars are classified chemically as monosaccharides or disaccharides. Table sugar is virtually 100% pure sucrose. *See also* fructose, glucose, lactose.

suggestibility (sŭ-jes-ti-**bil**-iti) *n.* the state of readily accepting suggestions from others. —**suggestible** *adj.*

suggestion (sŭ-jes-chŏn) *n.* (in psychology) **1.** the process of changing people's beliefs, attitudes, or emotions by telling them that they will change. **2.** a thought or idea imparted to someone in a hypnotic state.

suicide (soo-i-syd) *n.* deliberately causing one's own death. **assisted s.** the act of helping a person to commit suicide by giving him or her the means (e.g. drugs) to do so, which is a criminal offence in England and Wales. Guidance on whether a person who assists a terminally ill patient to end his or her life is likely to be prosecuted in the circumstances is provided by the Director of Public Prosecutions. **attempted s.** an attempt at self-destruction in which death is averted although the person concerned intended to kill himself or herself. *Compare* deliberate self-harm.

sulcus (sul-kŭs) *n.* (*pl.* **sulci**) **1.** one of the many clefts or infoldings of the surface of the brain. **2.** any of the infoldings of soft tissue in the mouth.

sulfadiazine (sulphadiazine) (sul-fă-**dy**-ă-zeen) *n.* a drug (*see* sulphonamide) administered by mouth to prevent the recurrence of rheumatic fever and (in combination with pyrimethamine) to treat toxoplasmosis. It is applied as a cream (in the form of **silver sulfadiazine**, Flamazine) to treat infected burns, leg ulcers, and pressure sores.

sulfamethoxazole (sulphamethoxazole) (sul-fă-meth-**oks**-ă-zohl) *n. see* co-trimoxazole, sulphonamide.

sulfasalazine (sulphasalazine) (sul-fă-**sal**-ă-zeen) *n.* a drug – a combination of aminosalicylic acid and sulfapyridine (a sulphonamide) – used in the treatment of ulcerative colitis, Crohn's disease, and rheumatoid arthritis. It is given by mouth or in the form of suppositories. Trade name: **Salazopyrin**.

sulfinpyrazone (sulphinpyrazone) (sul-fin-**py**-ră-zohn) *n.* a uricosuric drug given by mouth for the control of chronic gout. It should not be taken by patients with impaired kidney function.

sulpha drug (**sul**-fă) *n. see* sulphonamide.

sulphonamide (sulpha drug) (sul-**fon**-ă-myd) *n.* one of a group of drugs, derived from sulphanilamide (a red dye), that prevent the growth of bacteria. Sulphonamides are effective against a variety of infections and were formerly widely used, particularly in treating urinary-tract infections because many of them are rapidly excreted and very soluble in the urine. However, because of their toxic side-effects, the clinical use of sulphonamides has now declined. *See* co-trimoxazole, sulfadiazine, sulfasalazine.

sulphone (**sul**-fohn) *n.* one of a group of drugs closely related to the sulphonamides. Sulphones possess powerful activity against the bacteria that cause leprosy and tuberculosis. The best known sulphone is dapsone.

sulphonylurea (sul-fŏ-nil-**yoor**-iă) *n.* one of a group of oral hypoglycaemic drugs, derived from a sulphonamide, that stimulate the beta cells in the islets of Langerhans to produce insulin and are used in the treatment of type 2 diabetes mellitus. They include glibenclamide, **gliclazide** (Diamicron), and tolbutamide.

sulphur (**sul**-fer) *n.* a nonmetallic element that is active against fungi and parasites. It is a constituent of ointments and other preparations used in the treatment of skin disorders. Symbol: S.

sulphuric acid (sul-**fewr**-ik) *n.* a powerful corrosive acid, widely used in industry. Swallowing the acid causes severe burning of the mouth and throat. The patient should drink large quantities of milk or water or white of egg; gastric lavage should not be delayed. Formula: H_2SO_4.

sumatriptan (soo-mă-**trip**-tan) *n.* *see* $5HT_1$ agonist.

sunburn (**sun**-bern) *n.* damage to the skin by excessive exposure to the sun's rays, principally UVB (*see* ultraviolet radiation). Sunburn may vary from reddening of the skin to the development of large painful fluid-filled blisters (*see* burn).

sunstroke (**sun**-strohk) *n.* *see* heatstroke.

super- *prefix denoting* **1.** above; overlying. **2.** extreme or excessive.

superciliary (soo-per-**sil**-i-er-i) *adj.* of or relating to the eyebrows (**supercilia**).

superego (soo-per-**ee**-goh) *n.* (in psychoanalysis) the part of the mind that functions as a moral conscience or judge. The superego is the result of the incorporation of parental injunctions into the child's mind.

superfecundation (soo-per-fee-kŭn-**day**-shŏn) *n.* the fertilization of two or more ova of the same age by spermatozoa from different males. *See* superfetation.

superfetation (soo-per-fee-**tay**-shŏn) *n.* the fertilization of a second ovum some time after the start of pregnancy, resulting in two fetuses of different maturity in the same uterus.

superficial (soo-per-**fish**-ăl) *adj.* (in anatomy) situated at or close to a surface. Superficial blood vessels are those close to the surface of the skin.

superinfection (soo-per-in-**fek**-shŏn) *n.* an infection arising during the course of another infection and caused by a different microorganism, which is usually resistant to the drugs used to treat the primary infection. *See also* MRSA.

superior (soo-**peer**-i-er) *adj.* (in anatomy) situated uppermost in the body in relation to another structure or surface.

superovulation (controlled ovarian stimulation) (soo-per-ov-yoo-**lay**-shŏn) *n.* stimulation of the ovary to produce more follicles with oocytes. Usually induced by gonadotrophin preparations, it is performed in in vitro fertilization and other procedures of assisted conception in order to improve the pregnancy rates. *See also* ovarian hyperstimulation syndrome.

supervisor (**soo**-per-vy-zer) *n.* an appropriately registered nurse who is accountable for a student's standard of care in a clinical area. The supervisor oversees the student's practice and learning experience during a clinical episode.

supination (soo-pi-**nay**-shŏn) *n.* the act of turning the hand so that the palm is uppermost. *Compare* pronation.

supinator (**soo**-pi-nay-ter) *n.* a muscle of the forearm that extends from the elbow to the shaft of the radius. It supinates the forearm and hand.

supine (**soo**-pyn) *adj.* **1.** lying on the back or with the face upwards. **2.** (of the forearm) in the position in which the palm of the hand faces upwards. *Compare* prone.

supportive (sŭ-**port**-iv) *adj.* (of treatment) aimed at reinforcing the patient's own defence mechanisms in overcoming a disease or disorder.

support worker (sŭ-**port**) *n.* (in the health service) a nursing auxiliary or assistant, physiotherapy helper, occupational therapy helper, speech and language therapy assistant, foot-care assistant, or ward clerk. Support workers in nursing care work under the supervision of registered practitioners (*see* health-care assistant).

suppository (sŭ-**poz**-it-er-i) *n.* a medicinal preparation in solid form suitable for insertion into a body cavity. **rectal s.** a suppository that is inserted into the rectum. It may contain drugs that act locally in the rectum or anus, drugs that are absorbed and act at other sites, or a simple lubricant. **urethral s.** a suppository that is inserted into the urethra; it may contain antibiotics, local anaesthetics (prior to procedure), or medication used in the treatment of erectile dysfunction. **vaginal s.** *see* pessary.

suppression (sŭ-**presh**-ŏn) *n.* **1.** the cessation or complete inhibition of any physiological activity. **2.** (in psychology) a defence mechanism by which a person consciously and deliberately ignores an idea that is subjectively unpleasant.

suppuration (sup-yoor-**ay**-shŏn) *n.* the formation of pus.

supra- *prefix denoting* above; over.

supraglottis (soo-pră-**glot**-iss) *n.* that part of the larynx that lies above the vocal folds and includes the epiglottis.

supraorbital (soo-pră-**or**-bit'l) *adj.* of or relating to the area above the eye orbit. **s. reflex** the closing of the eyelids when the supraorbital nerve is struck, due to contraction of the muscle surrounding the orbit.

suprapubic (soo-pră-**pew**-bik) *adj.* above the pubic bone. **s. cystotomy** *see* cystotomy.

suprarenal glands (soo-pră-**ree**-năl) *pl. n. see* adrenal glands.

supraventricular tachycardia (SVT) (soo-pră-ven-**trik**-yoo-ler) *n. see* tachycardia.

surfactant (surface-active agent) (ser-**fak**-tănt) *n.* a wetting agent. **pulmonary s.** a complex mixture of compounds, secreted by pneumocytes, that prevents the alveoli of the lungs from collapsing by reducing surface tension.

surgeon (serj-ŏn) *n.* a qualified medical practitioner who specializes in surgery.

surgery (serj-er-i) *n.* **1.** the branch of medicine that treats injuries, deformities, or disease by operation or manipulation. *See also* cryosurgery, microsurgery. **2.** the building in or from which a general practitioner or a primary care team works. **—surgical** *adj.*

surgical emphysema (serj-ikăl) *n. see* emphysema.

surgical navigation *see* computer-assisted surgery.

surgical neck *n.* the constriction of the shaft of the humerus, below the head. It is frequently the point at which fracture of the humerus occurs.

surgical spirit *n.* methylated spirit, usually with small amounts of castor oil and oil of wintergreen: used to sterilize the skin, particularly before injections.

surrogate mother a woman who becomes pregnant (by artificial insemination or embryo insertion) following an arrangement made with another party (usually a couple unable themselves to have children) in which she agrees to give the child she carries to that party when it is born.

survey (ser-vay) *n.* a study that involves the systematic collection of data from a population sample by means of questionnaires or interviews and/or through observation.

susceptibility (sŭ-sep-ti-**bil**-iti) *n.* vulnerability to disease. It is partly a reflection of general health and health-related behaviour, but is also influenced by vaccination or other methods of increasing resistance to specific diseases.

suspensory bandage (su-**spen**-ser-i) *n.* a bandage arranged to support a hanging part of the body, such as the scrotum.

suspensory ligament *n.* a ligament that serves to support or suspend an organ, such as the lens of the eye, in position.

sustentaculum (sus-ten-**tak**-yoo-lŭm) *n.* any anatomical structure that supports another structure. **—sustentacular** *adj.*

suture (soo-cher) **1.** *n.*(in anatomy) a type of immovable joint, found particularly in the skull, characterized by a minimal amount of connective tissue between the two bones. **2.** *n.*(in surgery) the closure of a wound or incision with any of various materials to facilitate the healing process. *See also* delayed suture. **3.** *n.* the material – silk, nylon, a polymer, or wire – used to sew up a wound. **4.** *vb.* to close a wound by suture. See illustration.

suxamethonium (suks-ă-měth-**oh**-niŭm) *n.* a drug that relaxes voluntary muscle (*see* muscle relaxant). It is administered by intravenous injection to produce rapid muscle relaxation for a brief period. Trade name: **Anectine**.

SVT *n. see* (supraventricular) tachycardia.

swab (swob) *n.* a pad of absorbent material (such as cotton),

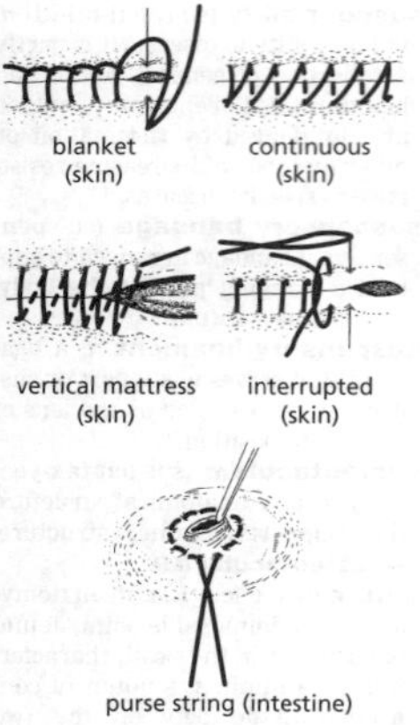

Types of surgical suturing

sometimes attached to a stick or wire, that is used for cleaning out or applying medication to wounds, operation sites, or body cavities.

swallowing (deglutition) (swol-oh-ing) *n.* the process by which food is transferred from the mouth to the oesophagus. Voluntary raising of the tongue forces food backwards towards the pharynx. This stimulates reflex actions in which the larynx and the nasal passages are closed so that food does not enter the trachea.

Swan-Ganz catheter (swon-ganz) *n.* a catheter with an inflatable balloon at its tip, which can be inserted into the pulmonary artery via the right chambers of the heart. Inflation of the balloon enables indirect measurement of pressure in the left atrium. [H. J. C. Swan (1922–2005), US cardiologist; W. Ganz (20th century), US engineer]

sweat (swet) *n.* the watery fluid secreted by the sweat glands. Its principal constituents in solution are sodium chloride and urea. The secretion of sweat is a means of excreting nitrogenous waste; it also has a cooling effect as the sweat evaporates from the surface of the skin. Anatomical name: **sudor**. **s. gland** a simple coiled tubular exocrine gland that lies in the dermis of the skin. Sweat glands occur over most of the surface of the body; they are particularly abundant in the armpits, on the soles of the feet and palms of the hands, and on the forehead.

swine influenza (swyn) *n. see* influenza.

sycosis (sy-**koh**-sis) *n.* inflammation of the hair follicles caused by infection with *Staphylococcus aureus*. It commonly affects the beard area (**s. barbae**) of men in their thirties or forties.

Sydenham's chorea (sid-ĕn-ămz) *n. see* chorea. [T. Sydenham (1624–89), English physician]

Symbicort (**sim**-bi-kort) *n. see* budesonide.

symbiosis (sim-by-**oh**-sis) *n.* an intimate and obligatory association between two different species of organism (**symbionts**) in which there is mutual aid and benefit. *Compare* commensal, parasite.

symblepharon (sim-**blef**-er-on) *n.* a condition in which the eyelid adheres to the eyeball. It is usually the result of chemical (especially alkali) burns to the conjunctiva.

symbolism (**sim**-bŏl-izm) *n.* (in psychology) the process of representing an object or an idea by something else. Psychoanalytic theorists hold that conscious ideas frequently act as symbols for unconscious thoughts and that this is particularly evident in dreaming, in free association, and in the formation of psychological symptoms. **—symbolic** (sim-**bol**-ik) *adj.*

Syme's amputation (symz) *n.* amputation of the foot just above the ankle joint. [J. Syme (1799–1870), British surgeon]

symmetry (**sim**-it-ri) *n.* (in anatomy) correspondence of form on either side of a plane or axis.

sympathectomy (sim-pă-**thek**-tŏmi) *n.* the surgical division of sympathetic nerve fibres. It is done to minimize the effects of normal or excessive sympathetic activity.

sympathetic nervous system (sim-pă-**thet**-ik) *n.* one of the two divisions of the autonomic nervous system, having fibres that leave the central nervous system in the thoracic and lumbar regions and are distributed to the blood vessels, sweat glands, salivary glands, heart, lungs, intestines, and other abdominal organs. It is responsible for increasing the heart rate and dilating the pupil, among other effects.

sympathin (**sim**-pă-thin) *n.* the name given by early physiologists to the substances released from sympathetic nerve endings, now known to be a mixture of adrenaline and noradrenaline.

sympatholytic (sim-pă-thoh-**lit**-ik) *adj.* opposing the effects of the sympathetic nervous system. Sympatholytic drugs include guanethidine, alpha blockers, and beta blockers.

sympathomimetic (sim-pă-thoh-mi-**met**-ik) *adj.* having the effect of stimulating the sympathetic nervous system by acting at alpha or beta receptors (*see* adrenergic (receptor)). Sympathomimetic drugs include **alpha-adrenergic stimulants** (**alpha agonists**), such as ephedrine, phenylephrine, metaraminol, apraclonidine, and brimonidine; and **beta-adrenergic stimulants** (**beta agonists**), such as dobutamine, salbutamol, salmeterol, and terbutaline.

sympathy (**sim**-pă-thi) *n.* (in physiology) a reciprocal influence exercised by different parts of the body on one another.

symphysiotomy (sim-fizi-**ot**-ŏmi) *n.* the operation of cutting through the front of the pelvis at the pubic symphysis in order to enlarge the diameter of the pelvis and aid delivery of a fetus whose head is too large to pass through the pelvic opening. This procedure is now rarely employed.

symphysis (**sim**-fi-sis) *n.* **1.** a joint in which the bones are separated by fibrocartilage, which minimizes movement and makes the bony structure rigid. Examples are the **symphysis pubis** (*see* pubis) and the joints of the backbone, which are separated by intervertebral discs. **s.-fundal height** *see* fundal height. **2.** the line that marks the fusion of two bones that were separate at an early stage of development. **—symphysial** or **symphyseal** *adj.*

symptom (**simp**-tŏm) *n.* an indication of a disease or disorder noticed by the patient him- or herself. *Compare* sign.

symptomatology (semeiology) (simp-tŏm-ă-**tol**-ŏji) *n.* **1.** the branch of medicine concerned with the study of symptoms of disease. **2.** the symptoms of a disease, collectively.

syn- (sym-) *prefix denoting* union or fusion.

Synacthen tests (sin-ak-thĕn) *pl. n.* tests used to assess the ability of the adrenal cortex to produce cortisol. Serum cortisol is measured before and then 30 minutes (or 5 hours) after an intramuscular injection of 250 μg (or 1 mg) tetracosactide (Synacthen), an analogue of ACTH.

synaesthesia (sin-is-**theez**-iă) *n.* a condition in which a secondary subjective sensation (often colour) is experienced at the same time as the sensory response normally evoked by the stimulus. For example, the sound of the word 'cat' might evoke the colour purple.

synalgia (sin-**al**-jiă) *n. see* referred pain.

synapse (sy-naps) *n.* the minute gap across which nerve impulses pass from one neuron to the next, at the end of a nerve fibre. Reaching a synapse, an impulse causes the release of a neurotransmitter, which diffuses across the gap and triggers an electrical impulse in the next neuron. *See also* neuromuscular junction.

synarthrosis (sin-arth-**roh**-sis) *n.* an immovable joint in which the bones are united by fibrous tissue. Examples are the cranial sutures. *See also* gomphosis, schindylesis.

synchondrosis (sin-kon-**droh**-sis) *n.* a slightly movable joint (*see* amphiarthrosis) in which the surfaces of the bones are separated by hyaline cartilage, as occurs between the ribs and sternum.

synchronized intermittent mandatory ventilation (SIMV) (**sin**-krŏ-nyzd) *n. see* intermittent mandatory ventilation.

synchysis (**sink**-i-sis) *n.* softening of the vitreous humour of the eye. **s. scintillans** (**asteroid hyalosis**) tiny refractile crystals of cholesterol suspended in the vitreous humour. They usually cause no symptoms.

syncope (fainting) (**sink**-ŏ-pi) *n.* loss of consciousness due to a sudden drop in blood pressure, resulting in a temporarily insufficient flow of blood to the brain. It commonly occurs in otherwise healthy people and may be caused by an emotional shock, by standing for prolonged periods, or by injury and profuse bleeding.

syncytium (sin-**sit**-iŭm) *n.* (*pl.* **syncytia**) a mass of protoplasm containing several nuclei. Muscle fibres are syncytia. **—syncytial** *adj.*

syndactyly (dactylion) (sin-**dak**-tili) *n.* congenital webbing of the fingers, which are joined along part or all of their length. Adjacent fingers may be joined only by skin, or the bones of the fingers may be joined.

syndesm- (syndesmo-) *combining form denoting* connective tissue, particularly ligaments.

syndesmology (sin-des-**mol**-ŏji) *n.* the branch of anatomy dealing with joints and their components.

syndesmosis (sin-des-**moh**-sis) *n.* an immovable joint in which the bones are separated by connective tissue. An example is the articulation between the bases of the tibia and fibula.

syndrome (**sin**-drohm) *n.* a combination of signs and/or symptoms that forms a distinct clinical picture indicative of a particular disorder.

syndrome of inappropriate secretion of antidiuretic hormone (SIADH) *n.* a condition of inappropriately high plasma levels of ADH (*see* vasopressin) with associated water retention, dilutional hyponatraemia, and the production of highly concentrated urine. Renal, adrenal, thyroid, and hepatic function are normal, as is the volume of circulating blood (euvolaemia). It is caused by a variety of pathological conditions and also by a number of drugs.

syndrome X *n.* *see* metabolic syndrome.

synechia (sin-**ek**-iă) *n. (pl.* **synechiae***)* **1.** an adhesion between the iris and another part of the eye. **2.** a small adhesion that forms in the nose after surgery. **anterior s.** synechia between the iris and the cornea. **posterior s.** synechia between the iris and the lens.

syneresis (sin-**eer**-i-sis) *n.* **1.** contraction of a blood clot to produce a firm mass that seals the damaged blood vessels. **2.** the degenerative shrinkage of the vitreous humour due to ageing.

synergist (**sin**-er-jist) *n.* **1.** a drug that interacts with another to produce increased activity, which is greater than the sum of the effects of the two drugs given separately. **2.** a muscle that acts with a prime mover (agonist) in making a particular movement. **—synergism, synergy** *n.* **—synergistic** (sin-er-**jist**-ik) *adj.*

synergistic gangrene *n.* gangrene of tissues produced by different bacteria acting together, usually a mixture of aerobic and anaerobic organisms. Synergistic gangrene has a pronounced tendency to spread along fascial planes, causing necrotizing fasciitis.

syngeneic (sin-jĕn-**ay**-ik) *adj.* describing grafted tissue that is genetically identical to the recipient's tissue, as when the donor and recipient are identical twins.

synoptophore (sin-**op**-toh-for) *n.* *see* amblyoscope.

synostosis (sin-os-**toh**-sis) *n.* the joining by ossification of two adjacent bones. It occurs, for example, at the cranial sutures.

synovectomy (sy-noh-**vek**-tŏmi) *n.* surgical removal of the synovium of a joint. This is performed in cases of chronic synovitis (such as rheumatoid arthritis), when other measures have been ineffective.

synovia (synovial fluid) (sy-**noh**-vi-ă) *n.* the thick colourless lubricating fluid that surrounds a joint or a bursa and fills a tendon sheath. It is secreted by the synovial membrane.

synovial joint (sy-**noh**-vi-ăl) *n. see* diarthrosis.

synovial membrane (synovium) *n.* the membrane that forms the sac enclosing a freely movable joint (*see* diarthrosis). It secretes the lubricating synovial fluid.

synovioma (sy-noh-vi-**oh**-mă) *n.* a benign or malignant tumour of the synovial membrane.

synovitis (sy-noh-**vy**-tis) *n.* inflammation of the synovial membrane, resulting in pain and swelling (arthritis). It is caused by injury, infection, or rheumatic disease.

synovium (sy-**noh**-vi-ŭm) *n. see* synovial membrane.

synthesis (**sin**-thi-sis) *n.* the formation of complex substances from simple constituents. **—synthesize** *vb.* **—synthetic** (sin-**thet**-ik) *adj.*

syphilide (syphilid) (**sif**-i-lyd) *n.* the skin rash that appears in the second stage of syphilis. Syphilides occur in crops that may last from a few days to several months. They denote a highly infectious stage of the disease.

syphilis (**sif**-i-lis) *n.* a sexually transmitted disease caused by the bacterium *Treponema pallidum*. Bacteria usually enter the body during sexual intercourse; they may also pass from an infected pregnant woman across the placenta to the developing fetus, resulting in the disease being present at birth (**congenital s.**). The primary symptom is a hard painless ulcer (chancre) at the site of infection. Secondary stage symptoms include fever, malaise, general enlargement of lymph nodes, and a faint red rash on the chest. After months, or even years, the disease enters its tertiary stage with widespread formation of tumour-like masses (gummas). Tertiary syphilis may cause serious damage to the heart and blood vessels (**cardiovascular s.**) or to the brain and spinal cord (**neurosyphilis**), resulting in tabes dorsalis, blindness, and general paralysis of the insane. *See also* bejel. **—syphilitic** (sif-i-**lit**-ik) *adj.*

syring- (syringo-) *combining form denoting* a tube or long cavity, especially the central canal of the spinal cord.

syringe (si-**rinj**) *n.* an instrument consisting of a piston in a tight-fitting tube that is attached to a hollow needle or thin tube. A syringe is used to give injections, remove material from a part of the body, or to wash out a cavity.

syringobulbia (si-ring-oh-**bulb**-iă) *n. see* syringomyelia.

syringoma (si-ring-**oh**-mă) *n.* multiple benign tumours of the sweat glands, which show as small hard swellings usually on the face, neck, or chest.

syringomyelia (si-ring-oh-my-**ee**-liă) *n.* a disease of the spinal cord in which longitudinal cavities form within the cord, usually in the cervical (neck) region. Characteristically there is weakness and wasting of the muscles in the hands with a loss of awareness of pain and temperature. An extension of the cavitation into the lower brainstem is called **syringobulbia**. Cerebellar ataxia, a partial loss of pain sensation in the face, and weakness of the tongue and palate may occur.

syringomyelocele (si-ring-oh-**my**-ĕl-oh-seel) *n.* protrusion of the spinal cord through a defect in the spine together with a fluid-filled sac continuous with the central canal of the cord.

system (**sis**-tĕm) *n.* (in anatomy) a group of organs and tissues associated with a particular physiological function, such as the nervous system or respiratory system.

systematic review (sis-tĕm-**at**-ik) *n.* a structured method of critical appraisal of all available literature relevant to a specific research topic, using a rigorous statistical approach. It is undertaken to provide information about the phenomenon of interest across a wide range of settings and empirical methods, to examine the extent to which empirical evidence supports or contradicts a hypothesis, or to generate a new hypothesis.

systemic (sis-**tem**-ik) *adj.* relating to or affecting the body as a whole, rather than individual parts and organs. **s. circulation** *see* circulation. **s. sclerosis** a rare multisystem connective-tissue disease. In the diffuse form of the disorder scleroderma may be associated with pulmonary fibrosis, renal failure, and gastrointestinal and myocardial disease. Genetic and autoimmune factors may be implicated. *See also* CREST syndrome.

systole (**sis**-tŏ-li) *n.* the period of the cardiac cycle during which the heart contracts. **—systolic** (sis-**tol**-ik) *adj.*

systolic pressure *n.* *see* blood pressure.

Tt

T_3 *n.* triiodothyronine (*see* thyroid hormone).

T_4 *n.* thyroxine (*see* thyroid hormone).

tabes dorsalis (locomotor ataxia) (tay-beez dor-**sah**-lis) *n.* a form of neurosyphilis occurring 5–20 years after the original sexually transmitted infection. The infecting organisms progressively destroy the sensory nerves. Severe stabbing pains in the legs and trunk, an unsteady gait, and loss of bladder control are common. *See also* general paralysis of the insane, syphilis.

tablet (**tab**-lit) *n.* (in pharmacy) a small disc containing one or more drugs, made by compressing a powdered form of the drug(s). It is usually taken by mouth.

tabo-paresis (tay-boh-pă-**ree**-sis) *n.* a late effect of syphilitic infection of the nervous system in which the patient shows features of tabes dorsalis and general paralysis of the insane.

TAB vaccine *n.* a combined vaccine used to produce immunity against the diseases typhoid, paratyphoid A, and paratyphoid B.

tachy- *combining form denoting* fast; rapid.

tachyarrhythmia (tak-i-ă-**ri***th*-miă) *n.* any deviation from the normal sinus rhythm of the heart that involves an increase in heart rate.

tachycardia (tak-i-**kar**-diă) *n.* an increase in the heart rate above normal. **sinus t.** tachycardia that may occur normally with exercise or excitement. It may also be due to illness, such as fever. **supraventricular t.** (**SVT**) tachycardia usually due to an accessory conduction pathway between the atria and ventricles (*see* Wolff-Parkinson-White syndrome) but sometimes stemming from an abnormal area in the atria. **ventricular t.** (**VT**) tachycardia stemming from an abnormal focus of electrical activity in the ventricles, which can result in a sudden drop in blood pressure or cardiac arrest. *See also* paroxysmal tachycardia.

tachypnoea (tak-ip-**nee**-ă) *n.* rapid breathing.

tacrolimus (tak-rŏ-**ly**-mŭs) *n.* a powerful immunosuppressant drug administered orally or by intravenous infusion to prevent rejection of transplanted organs. It is also used, in the form of an ointment, to treat atopic eczema. Side-effects may include impairment of the liver, kidneys, and heart, tremor, headache, and gastrointestinal upsets. Trade names: **Adoport**, **Advagraf**, **Capexion**, **Modigraf**, **Prograf**, **Protopic**, **Tacni**, **Vivadex**.

tactile (**tak**-tyl) *adj.* relating to or affecting the sense of touch.

taenia (tee-niă) *n.* (*pl.* **taeniae**) a flat ribbon-like anatomical structure. **taeniae coli** the longitudinal ribbon-like muscles of the colon.

Taenia *n.* a genus of large tapeworms, some of which are parasites of the human intestine. **T. saginata** the beef tapeworm: the most common tapeworm parasite of humans. *See* taeniasis. **T. solium** the pork tapeworm. Its larval stage may develop in humans, in whom it may cause cysticercosis.

taeniacide (taenicide) (tee-niă-syd) *n.* an agent that kills tapeworms.

taeniafuge (tee-niă-fewj) *n.* an agent, such as niclosamide, that eliminates tapeworms from the body of their host.

taeniasis (tee-ny-ă-sis) *n.* an infestation with tapeworms of the genus *Taenia*, resulting from ingestion of raw or undercooked meat containing the larval stage of the parasite. Symptoms include increased appetite, hunger pains, weakness, and weight loss. *See also* cysticercosis.

Tagamet (tag-a-met) *n.* *see* cimetidine.

Takayasu's disease (pulseless disease) (tak-ă-yas-ooz) *n.* progressive occlusion of the arteries arising from the arch of the aorta (including those to the arms and neck), resulting in the absence of pulses in the arms and neck. Symptoms include attacks of unconsciousness (syncope), paralysis of facial muscles, and transient blindness, due to an inadequate supply of blood to the head. [M. Takayasu (1860–1938), Japanese ophthalmologist]

tal- (talo-) *combining form denoting* the ankle bone (talus).

talc (tal'k) *n.* a soft white powder consisting of magnesium silicate, used as a dusting powder.

talipes (tal-i-peez) *n.* club-foot: a congenital deformity of one or both feet in which the patient cannot stand with the sole of the foot flat on the ground. **t. equinovarus** the most common variety of talipes, in which the foot points downwards, the heel is inverted, and the forefoot twisted. **t. valgus** talipes in which the hind foot is twisted outwards. **t. varus** talipes in which the hind foot is turned inwards.

talus (astragalus) (tay-lŭs) *n.* the ankle bone. It forms part of the tarsus, articulating with the tibia above, the fibula to the side, and the calcaneus below.

Tamiflu (tam-i-floo) *n.* *see* oseltamivir.

tamoxifen (tam-**oks**-i-fen) *n.* a drug administered orally in the treatment of breast cancer: it binds with hormone receptors in the tumour to inhibit the effect of oestrogens (*see* anti-oestrogen, selective (o)estrogen receptor modulator). It is also used to induce ovulation in the treatment of female infertility.

tampon (tam-pon) *n.* a pack of gauze, cotton wool, or other absorbent material used to plug a cavity or canal in order to absorb blood or secretions.

tamponade (tam-pon-**ayd**) *n.* **1.** the insertion of a tampon. **2.** abnormal pressure on a part of the body. **3.** the use of air, gas, or a heavy liquid injected into the vitreous humour to exert pressure on the retina during eye surgery. *See* pneumoretinopexy. **cardiac t.** a build-up of fluid around the heart within the pericardium, causing compression of the heart. This results in heart failure, a drop in blood pressure, or cardiac arrest and requires drainage of the fluid.

tamsulosin (tam-**soo**-lŏ-sin) *n.* a highly selective alpha blocker taken by mouth to treat lower urinary tract symptoms thought to be due to benign prostatic hyperplasia (*see* prostate gland). Trade name: **Flomaxtra XL**.

tantalum (**tant**-ă-lŭm) *n.* a rare heavy metal used in surgery. Tantalum sutures and plates are used for repair of defects in the bones of the skull. Symbol: Ta.

tapeworm (cestode) (**tayp**-werm) *n.* any of a group of flatworms that have a long thin ribbon-like body and live as parasites in the intestines of humans and other vertebrates. The body of a tapeworm consists of a head (*see* scolex), a short neck, and a chain of separate segments (*see* proglottis). Humans are the primary hosts for some tapeworms (*see* Taenia). However, other genera are also medically important (*see* Echinococcus).

tapotement (ta-**poht**-**mahn**) *n.* a technique used in massage in which a part of the body is struck rapidly and repeatedly with the hands.

tapping (**tap**-ing) *n. see* paracentesis.

tar (tar) *n.* a blackish viscous liquid produced by the destructive distillation of pine wood (**pine t.**) or coal (**coal t.**), used in skin preparations to treat eczema and psoriasis. As a constituent of cigarettes, tar is known to have carcinogenic properties.

tardive dyskinesia (**tard**-iv) *n. see* dyskinesia.

tars- (tarso-) *combining form denoting* **1.** the ankle; tarsal bones. **2.** the edge of the eyelid.

tarsal (**tar**-săl) **1.** *adj.* relating to the bones of the ankle and foot (tarsus). **2.** *adj.* relating to the eyelid, especially to its supporting tissue (tarsus). **t. glands** *see* meibomian glands. **3.** *n.* any of the bones forming the tarsus.

tarsalgia (tar-**sal**-jiă) *n.* aching pain arising from the tarsus in the foot.

tarsectomy (tar-**sek**-tŏmi) *n.* **1.** surgical excision of the tarsal bones of the foot. **2.** surgical removal of a section of the tarsus of the eyelid.

tarsitis (tar-**sy**-tis) *n.* inflammation of the eyelid.

tarsorrhaphy (tars-**o**-răfi) *n.* an operation in which the upper and lower eyelids are joined together. It is performed to protect the cornea or to allow a corneal injury to heal.

tarsus (**tar**-sŭs) *n.* (*pl.* **tarsi**) **1.** the seven bones of the ankle and proximal part of the foot (see illustration).

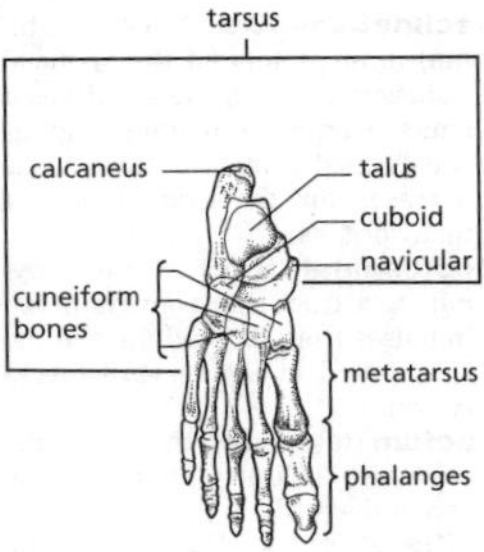

Bones of the right ankle and foot

The tarsus articulates with the metatarsals distally and with the tibia and fibula proximally. **2.** the firm fibrous connective tissue that forms the basis of each eyelid.

tartar (tar-ter) *n.* an obsolete name for calculus, the hard deposit that forms on the teeth.

task allocation (tahsk al-ŏ-kay-shŏn) *n.* an obsolete method of organizing nursing care in which patient care was divided into a number of tasks and a series of nurses was allocated to perform these tasks. The patient thus received fragmented care in which the emphasis was on the tasks (rather than the patient). *Compare* patient allocation.

taste (tayst) *n.* the sense for the appreciation of the flavour of substances in the mouth. There are four basic taste sensations – sweet, bitter, sour, and salt. **t. buds** the sensory receptors concerned with the sense of taste. They are located in the epithelium that covers the surface of the tongue and in the soft palate, the epiglottis, and parts of the pharynx. When a taste cell is stimulated by the presence of a dissolved substance impulses are sent via nerve fibres to the brain.

taurine (**tor**-een) *n.* an amino acid that is a constituent of the bile salt sodium taurocholate and also functions as a neurotransmitter in the central nervous system.

taurocholic acid (tor-oh-**koh**-lik) *n. see* bile acids.

taxane (**taks**-ayn) *n.* a cytotoxic drug that interferes with a protein involved in cell division and is used to control the growth of certain cancers. Side-effects include bone marrow suppression and hair loss. *See* docetaxel, paclitaxel.

taxis (**tak**-sis) *n.* (in surgery) the returning to a normal position of displaced bones, organs, or other parts by manipulation only.

Taxol (**taks**-ol) *n. see* paclitaxel.

Taxotere (**taks**-ŏ-teer) *n. see* docetaxel.

Tay-Sachs disease (amaurotic familial idiocy) (tay-saks) *n.* an inherited disorder of lipid metabolism (*see* lipidosis) in which abnormal accumulation of lipid in the brain leads to blindness, learning disability, and death in infancy. [W. Tay (1843–1927), British physician; B. Sachs (1858–1944), US neurologist]

TB *n. see* tuberculosis.

T bandage *n.* a T-shaped bandage used for the perineum and sometimes the head.

TBI *n.* **1.** *see* traumatic brain injury. **2.** *see* total body irradiation.

TBW *n.* total body water.

TCA *n.* *see* (tricyclic) antidepressant.

T cell *n.* a type of lymphocyte that matures in the thymus and is primarily responsible for cell-mediated immunity. **cytotoxic T c.** a T cell that destroys cancerous cells, virus-infected cells, and allografts. **helper T c.** a T cell that stimulates the production of cytotoxic T cells. **suppressor T c.** a T cell that prevents an immune response by other T cells or B cells to an antigen.

TCP *n.* **1.** *Trade name.* a solution of halogenated phenols: an effective antiseptic for minor skin injuries and irritations. It may also be used as a gargle for colds and sore throats. **2.** *see* thrombocytopenia.

Td/IPV *n.* a booster vaccine given to children between the ages of 13 and 18 years to top up immunity against tetanus, diphtheria, and polio. See Appendix 8: Immunization schedules.

t.d.s. (ter die sumendus) Latin: to be taken three times a day, used as a direction in prescriptions.

team nursing (teem) *n.* a method of organizing nursing care in which a team of nurses is responsible for the assessment, planning, implementation, and evaluation of a patient's hospital stay and subsequent discharge from the hospital.

tears (teerz) *pl. n.* the fluid secreted by the lacrimal glands to keep the front of the eyeballs moist and clean. Tears contain lysozyme, an enzyme that destroys bacteria.

technetium-99m (tek-**nee**-shi-ŭm) *n.* an isotope of the artificial radioactive element technetium. It emits gamma radiation and is widely used in nuclear medicine as a tracer for the examination of many organs.

tectospinal tract (tek-toh-**spy**-năl) *n.* a tract that conveys nerve impulses from the midbrain to the spinal cord in the cervical (neck) region.

tectum (**tek**-tŭm) *n.* the roof of the midbrain, behind and above the cerebral aqueduct.

TEDs *pl. n.* *see* thromboembolic deterrents.

teeth (teeth) *pl. n.* *see* tooth.

tegmen (**teg**-mĕn) *n.* (*pl.* **tegmina**) a structure that covers an organ or part of an organ.

tegmentum (teg-**men**-tŭm) *n.* the region of the midbrain below and in front of the cerebral aqueduct.

tel- (tele-, telo-) *combining form denoting* **1.** end or ending. **2.** distance.

tela (**tee**-lă) *n.* any thin weblike tissue. **t. choroidea** a folded double layer of pia mater containing numerous small blood vessels that extends into several of the ventricles of the brain.

telangiectasis (til-an-ji-**ek**-tă-sis) *n.* (*pl.* **telangiectases**) a localized collection of distended blood capillary vessels. It is recognized as a red spot, sometimes spidery in appearance, that blanches on pressure. Telangiectases may be found in the skin or the lining of the mouth or in the gastrointestinal, respiratory, or urinary tracts. The occurrence of multiple telangiectases is called **telangiectasia**.

teleceptor (tel-i-sep-ter) *n.* a sensory receptor that is capable of responding to distant stimuli.

telemedicine (tel-i-med-sin) *n.* the use of information technology in the diagnosis and treatment of patients. It includes telephone conversations and tele- or videoconferencing between physicians or among members of the patient's health-care team.

telencephalon (tel-en-**sef**-ă-lon) *n. see* cerebrum.

teleradiology (tel-i-ray-di-**ol**-ŏji) *n.* the process of transmitting and receiving medical images, to and from distant sites, using the telephone (or cable or satellite) network. This requires a dedicated broad-band link, such as an ISDN line, that has greater capacity for data transfer than standard telephone lines.

teletherapy (tel-i-**th'e**-ră-pi) *n.* a form of radiotherapy in which penetrating radiation is directed at a patient from a distance.

telmisartan (tel-**miss**-ar-tan) *n. see* angiotensin II antagonist.

telogen (**tel**-oh-jĕn) *n. see* anagen.

temazepam (te-**maz**-ĕ-pam) *n.* a benzodiazepine given by mouth for the short-term treatment of insomnia and in premedication before minor surgery.

template (**tem**-plăt) *n.* a design, plan, or model that enables information to be presented in a standardized and easily recognized format. A template can be applied to any aspect of nursing care to ensure that there is consistency of approach and continuity of care.

temple (**tem**-pŭl) *n.* the region of the head in front of and above each ear.

temporal (**temp**-er-ăl) *adj.* of or relating to the temple. **t. arteritis** *see* arteritis. **t. artery** a branch of the external carotid artery that supplies blood mainly to the temple and scalp. **t. bone** either of a pair of bones of the cranium. The **squamous** portion forms part of the side of the cranium. The **petrous** part contributes to the base of the skull and contains the middle and inner ears. *See also* skull. **t. lobe** one of the main divisions of the cerebral cortex in each hemisphere of the brain, lying at the side within the temple. Areas of the cortex in this lobe are concerned with the appreciation of sound and spoken language. **t. lobe epilepsy** *see* epilepsy.

temporalis (tem-per-**ay**-lis) *n.* a fan-shaped muscle at the side of the head, extending from the temporal fossa to the mandible. This muscle lifts the lower jaw.

temporo- *combining form denoting* **1.** the temple. **2.** the temporal lobe of the brain.

temporomandibular joint (TMJ) (tem-per-oh-man-**dib**-yoo-ler) *n.* the articulation between the mandible and the temporal bone. **t. j. syndrome** a condition in which the patient has painful temporomandibular joints, tenderness in the muscles that move the jaw, clicking of the joints, and limitation of jaw movement.

tenaculum (tin-**ak**-yoo-lŭm) *n.* **1.** a sharp wire hook with a handle, used in surgical operations to pick up pieces of tissue or the cut end of an artery. **2.** a band of fibrous tissue that holds a part of the body in place.

tendinitis (ten-di-**ny**-tis) *n.* inflammation of a tendon. It occurs most commonly after excessive overuse but is sometimes due to bacterial infection (e.g. gonorrhoea) or a generalized rheumatic disease (e.g. rheumatoid arthritis, ankylosing spondylitis). *See also* jumper's knee, tennis elbow. *Compare* tenosynovitis.

tendon (**ten**-dŏn) *n.* a tough whitish cord, consisting of numerous parallel bundles of collagen fibres, that serves to attach a muscle to a bone. Tendons assist in concentrating the pull of the muscle on a small area of bone. **t. sheath** a tubular sac, lined with synovial membrane and containing synovial fluid, that surrounds some tendons. *See also* aponeurosis. **t. transfer** plastic surgery in which the tendon from an unimportant muscle is used to replace the damaged tendon of an important muscle. **—tendinous** (**ten**-din-ŭs) *adj.*

tendovaginitis (tenovaginitis) (ten-doh-vaj-i-**ny**-tis) *n.* inflammatory thickening of the fibrous sheath containing one or more tendons, usually caused by repeated minor injury. It usually occurs at the back of the thumb (**de Quervain's t.**) and results in pain on using the wrists.

tenesmus (tin-**ez**-mŭs) *n.* a sensation of the desire to defecate or urinate, associated with straining and the passage of minimal volumes of faeces or urine or none at all. Rectal tenesmus may be due to proctitis, prolapse of the rectum, rectal tumour, or irritable bowel syndrome.

tennis elbow (**ten**-iss) *n.* a painful condition causing degeneration of the origin of the common extensor tendon on the lateral epicondyle of the humerus, due to overuse of the forearm muscles. *See also* tendinitis. *Compare* golfer's elbow.

teno- *combining form denoting* a tendon.

tenonectomy (ten-ŏn-**ek**-tŏmi) *n.* surgical removal of a portion of Tenon's capsule.

tenonotomy (ten-ŏn-**ot**-ŏmi) *n.* a surgical incision made into Tenon's capsule. It is most often performed to instil local anaesthetic before performing cataract surgery.

Tenon's capsule (tĕ-**nonz**) *n.* the fibrous tissue that lines the orbit and surrounds the eyeball. [J. R. Tenon (1724–1816), French surgeon]

tenoplasty (**ten**-oh-plasti) *n.* surgical repair of a ruptured or severed tendon.

tenorrhaphy (tĕn-**o**-răfi) *n.* the surgical operation of uniting the ends of divided tendons by suture.

tenosynovitis (peritendinitis) (ten-oh-sy-noh-**vy**-tis) *n.* inflammation of a tendon sheath, producing pain, swelling, and an audible creaking on movement. It may result from a bacterial infection or occur as part of a rheumatic disease.

tenotomy (tĕ-**not**-ŏmi) *n.* surgical division of a tendon. This may be necessary to correct a joint deformity caused by tendon shortening.

tenovaginitis (ten-oh-vaj-i-**ny**-tis) *n. see* tendovaginitis.

TENS *n.* transcutaneous electrical nerve stimulation: *see* stimulator.

tension-free vaginal tape (transvaginal tape, TVT) (ten-shŏn-free) *n.* a surgical sling procedure for treating stress incontinence in women in which a tape of polypropylene mesh is inserted under the mid-urethra, passing through the retropubic space on either side, and fixed to the abdominal wall just internal to the pubic symphysis. The **transobturator tape** (**TOT**) procedure is similar, but in this technique a tunnel is created out to the obturator foramen on either side, lessening the risk of vascular and bladder injuries.

tensor (**ten**-ser) *n.* any muscle that causes stretching or tensing of a part of the body.

tent (tent) *n.* **1.** an enclosure of material (usually transparent plastic) around a patient in bed, into which a gas or vapour can be passed as part of treatment. **oxygen t.** a tent into which oxygen is passed. **2.** a piece of dried vegetable material, usually a seaweed stem, shaped to fit into an orifice, such as the cervical canal. As it absorbs moisture it expands, dilating the orifice.

tentorium (ten-**tor**-iŭm) *n.* a curved infolded sheet of dura mater that separates the cerebellum below from the occipital lobes of the cerebral hemispheres above.

terat- (terato-) *combining form denoting* a monster or congenital abnormality.

teratogen (te-ră-toh-jen) *n.* any substance, agent, or process that induces the formation of developmental abnormalities in a fetus. Known teratogens include the drug thalidomide, German measles, and irradiation with X-rays. **—teratogenic** *adj.*

teratogenesis (te-ră-toh-**jen**-i-sis) *n.* the process leading to developmental abnormalities in the fetus.

teratology (te-ră-**tol**-ŏji) *n.* the study of developmental abnormalities and their causes.

teratoma (te-ră-**toh**-mă) *n.* a tumour composed of a number of tissues that are not usually found at that site and are derived from all three germ layers. Teratomas most frequently occur in the testis and ovary (*see* dermoid cyst), possibly derived from remnants of embryonic cells, and are often malignant. **malignant t. of the testis** a teratoma occurring in young men, frequently as a painless swelling of one testis. Treatment is by orchidectomy.

teratospermia (te-ră-toh-**sper**-miă) *n.* the presence in the semen of many bizarre or immature forms of spermatozoa, revealed by seminal analysis.

terbinafine (ter-**bin**-ă-feen) *n.* an antifungal drug used to treat nail infections and ringworm (*see* tinea). It is administered by mouth or topically. Trade name: **Lamisil**.

terbutaline (ter-**bew**-tă-leen) *n.* a short-acting drug that relaxes bronchial and uterine smooth muscle (*see* sympathomimetic); it is administered by mouth, injection, infusion, or inhalation in the treatment of asthma and other conditions of reversible airways obstruction, and to inhibit premature labour. Trade name: **Bricanyl**.

teres (te-reez) *n.* either of two muscles of the shoulder, extending from the scapula to the humerus. **t. major** the muscle that rotates the arm inwards. **t. minor** the muscle that rotates the arm outwards.

terlipressin (ter-li-pres-in) *n.* a drug that releases vasopressin over a period of hours. It is administered by intravenous injection to control bleeding from oesophageal varices. Trade names: **Glypressin**, **Variquel**.

terminal dribble (term-in-ăl drib-ĕl) *n.* a lower urinary tract symptom in which the flow of urine does not end quickly, but dribbles slowly towards an end. *Compare* postmicturition dribble.

tertian (ter-shăn) *adj.* occurring every two days, as in the case of some intermittent fevers.

tertiary care (ter-sher-i) *n.* the specialized services provided by centres equipped with diagnostic and treatment facilities not available at general hospitals. *Compare* primary care, secondary care.

tertiary prevention *n.* reducing the impact of complications and progression of established disease; for example, by cardiac rehabilitation following myocardial infarction. *See also* preventive medicine.

test (test) *n.* a laboratory examination or chemical analysis to determine the presence of a specific substance, microorganism, disease, etc. (See individual entries for named tests.)

testicle (test-ikŭl) *n.* the testis and its system of ducts (the vasa efferentia and epididymis) within the scrotum.

testis (tes-tis) *n.* (*pl.* **testes**) either of the pair of male sex organs that produce spermatozoa and secrete male sex hormones (*see* androgen) under the control of gonadotrophins from the pituitary gland. The testes are contained within the scrotum (*see* reproductive system). *See also* spermatogenesis.

test meal *n.* a standard meal given to stimulate secretion of digestive juices, which can then be withdrawn by tube and measured as a test of digestive function.

testosterone (test-ost-er-ohn) *n.* the principal male sex hormone (*see* androgen), formed in the testis from **androstenedione** and converted in target cells to dihydrotestosterone, which mediates most of its actions. Preparations of testosterone are used for replacement therapy in males with testosterone deficiency.

tetan- (tetano-) *combining form denoting* **1.** tetanus. **2.** tetany.

tetanus (lockjaw) (tet-ăn-ŭs) *n.* an acute infectious disease, affecting the nervous system, caused by the bacterium *Clostridium tetani*. Infection occurs by contamination of wounds by bacterial spores. Symptoms consist of muscle stiffness, spasm, and subsequent rigidity, first in the jaw and neck then in the back, chest, abdomen, and limbs; in severe cases the spasm may affect the whole body, which is arched backwards (*see* opisthotonos). Prompt treatment with penicillin and antitoxin is effective; immunization against tetanus is effective but temporary. **—tetanic** (tĕ-**tan**-ik) *adj.*

tetanus toxoid (TT) *n.* a vaccine used in active immunization against tetanus. *See* DTaP/IPV, DTaP/IPV/Hib.

tetany (**tet**-ăn-i) *n.* spasm and twitching of the muscles, particularly those of the face, hands, and feet. Tetany is usually caused by a reduction in the blood calcium level, which may be due to underactive parathyroid glands, rickets, or alkalosis.

tetra- *combining form denoting* four.

tetracaine (amethocaine) (**tet**-ră-kayn) *n.* a potent local anaesthetic applied as a gel to the skin before intravenous injections or the insertion of a cannula. It is also applied as eye drops before eye operations. Trade names: **Ametop**, **Minims Tetracaine Hydrochloride**.

tetracosactide (tetracosactin) (tet-ră-kohz-**ak**-tyd) *n. see* Synacthen tests.

tetracyclines (tet-ră-**sy**-kleenz) *pl. n.* a group of antibiotic compounds derived from cultures of *Streptomyces* bacteria. These drugs, including doxycycline, oxytetracycline, and tetracycline, are effective against a wide range of bacterial infections, including *Chlamydia*, respiratory tract infections, and acne. They are usually given by mouth.

tetradactyly (tet-ră-**dak**-tili) *n.* a congenital abnormality in which there are only four digits on a hand or foot. **—tetradactylous** *adj.*

tetralogy of Fallot (te-**tral**-ŏji ŏv fa-**loh**) *n.* a form of congenital heart disease in which there is pulmonary stenosis, enlargement of the right ventricle, and a ventricular septal defect over which the origin of the aorta lies. The affected child is blue (cyanosed). [E. L. A. Fallot (1850–1911), French physician]

tetraplegia (tet-ră-**plee**-jiă) *n. see* quadriplegia.

thalam- (thalamo-) *prefix denoting* the thalamus.

thalamencephalon (thal-ăm-en-**sef**-ă-lon) *n.* the structures, collectively, at the anterior end of the brainstem, comprising the epithalamus, thalamus, hypothalamus, and subthalamus.

thalamic syndrome (thă-**lam**-ik) *n.* a condition resulting from damage to the thalamus, often by a stroke, that is characterized by severe intractable pain and hypersensitivity in the area of the body served by the damaged brain region.

thalamotomy (thal-ă-**mot**-ŏmi) *n.* an operation on the brain in which a lesion is made in a precise part of the thalamus. It has been used to control psychiatric symptoms of severe anxiety and distress. *See also* psychosurgery.

thalamus (thal-ă-mŭs) *n.* (*pl.* **thalami**) one of two egg-shaped masses of grey matter that lie deep in the cerebral hemispheres in each side of the forebrain. The thalami are relay stations for all the sensory messages that enter the brain, before they are transmitted to the cortex.

thalassaemia (Cooley's anaemia) (thal-ă-see-miă) *n.* a hereditary blood disease, widespread in the Mediterranean countries, Asia, and Africa, in which there is an abnormality in the protein part of the haemoglobin molecule. Symptoms include anaemia, enlargement of the spleen, and abnormalities of the bone marrow. Individuals inheriting the disease from both parents are severely affected (**t. major**), but those inheriting it from only one parent are usually symptom-free.

SEE WEB LINKS

- Website of the Thalassaemia Society

thalidomide (thă-lid-ŏ-myd) *n.* a drug that was formerly used as a sedative but withdrawn because it was found to cause fetal abnormalities involving limb malformation if taken during the first three months of pregnancy. Recently it has been found to be effective in treating myeloma. It is taken by mouth. It should not be taken by women who are pregnant or capable of becoming pregnant. Trade name: **Thalidomide Celgene**.

thallium scan (thal-iŭm) *n. see* myocardial perfusion scan.

theca (th'ee-kă) *n.* a sheathlike surrounding tissue.

theine (th'ee-een) *n.* the active volatile principle found in tea (*see* caffeine).

thelarche (th'ee-lar-ki) *n.* the process of breast development, which occurs as a normal part of puberty. Isolated premature breast development in girls is not uncommon and is almost always benign.

thenar (th'ee-nar) *n.* **1.** the palm of the hand. **2.** the fleshy prominent part of the hand at the base of the thumb. *Compare* hypothenar. —**thenar** *adj.*

theobromine (thi-ŏ-broh-meen) *n.* an alkaloid, occurring in cocoa, coffee, and tea, that has a weak diuretic action and dilates coronary and other arteries.

theophylline (thi-off-i-leen) *n.* an alkaloid, occurring in the leaves of the tea plant, that has a diuretic effect and relaxes smooth muscles. Theophylline is administered by injection (as aminophylline) or by mouth and used mainly as a bronchodilator to treat severe asthma attacks. Trade names: **Nuelin SA**, **Slo-Phyllin**, **Uniphyllin Continus**.

therapeutic index (th'e-ră-pew-tik) *n.* the ratio of a dose of a therapeutic agent that produces damage to normal cells to the dose necessary to have a defined level of anticancer activity. It indicates the relative efficacy of a treatment against tumours.

therapeutics (th'e-ră-pew-tiks) *n.* the branch of medicine that deals with different methods of treatment and healing (**therapy**), particularly the use of drugs in the cure of disease.

therm (therm) *n.* a unit of heat equal to 100,000 British thermal units. 1 therm = 1.055×10^8 joules.

therm- (thermo-) *combining form denoting* **1.** heat. **2.** temperature.

thermoanaesthesia (therm-oh-anis-**theez**-iă) *n.* absence of the ability to recognize the sensations of heat and coldness. It may indicate damage to the spinothalamic tract in the spinal cord.

thermocautery (therm-oh-**kaw**-ter-i) *n.* the destruction of unwanted tissues by heat (*see* cauterize).

thermocoagulation (therm-oh-koh-ag-yoo-**lay**-shŏn) *n.* the coagulation and destruction of tissues by cautery.

thermography (ther-**mog**-răfi) *n.* a technique for measuring and recording the heat produced by different parts of the body by using photographic film sensitive to infrared radiation. The picture produced is called a **thermogram**. A tumour with an abnormally increased blood supply may be revealed on the thermogram as a 'hot spot'.

thermolysis (ther-**mol**-i-sis) *n.* (in physiology) the dissipation of body heat by such processes as the evaporation of sweat from the skin surface.

thermometer (ther-**mom**-i-ter) *n.* a device for registering temperature. **clinical t.** a sealed narrow-bore glass tube containing mercury, which expands when heated and rises up the tube. The tube is designed to register body temperatures between 35°C (95°F) and 43.5°C (110°F).

thermophilic (therm-oh-**fil**-ik) *adj.* describing organisms, especially bacteria, that grow best at temperatures of 48–85°C.

thermoreceptor (therm-oh-ri-**sep**-ter) *n.* a sensory nerve ending that responds to heat or to cold.

thermotaxis (therm-moh-**tak**-sis) *n.* the physiological process of regulating or adjusting body temperature.

thermotherapy (therm-oh-**th'e**-ră-pi) *n.* the use of heat to alleviate pain and stiffness in joints and muscles and to promote an increase in circulation.

thiabendazole (th'y-ă-**ben**-dă-zohl) *n. see* tiabendazole.

thiamine (vitamin B_1) (**th'y**-ă-min) *n. see* vitamin B.

thiazide diuretic (**th'y**-ă-zyd) *n. see* diuretic.

Thiersch's graft (**teer**-shĕz) *n. see* split-skin graft. [K. Thiersch (1822–95), German surgeon]

thigh (th'y) *n.* the upper part of the lower limb, between the hip and the knee. **t. bone** *see* femur.

thioguanine (th'y-oh-**gwah**-neen) *n. see* tioguanine.

thiopental (thiopentone) (th'y-oh-**pen**-tal) *n.* a short-acting barbiturate. It is given by intravenous injection to induce general anaesthesia. Possible complications can include respiratory depression.

Thomas's splint (**tom**-ă-siz) *n.* a metal splint used for immobilizing a fractured lower limb, especially the femur. There is a ring at the hip, a cross-piece at the foot, and side-pieces for the attachment of material to support the leg.

[H. O. Thomas (1834–1931), British orthopaedic surgeon]

thorac- (thoraco-) *combining form denoting* the thorax or chest.

thoracentesis (thor-ă-sen-**tee**-sis) *n. see* pleurocentesis.

thoracic cavity (thor-**ass**-ik) *n.* the chest cavity. *See* thorax.

thoracic duct *n.* one of the two main trunks of the lymphatic system. It receives lymph from both legs, the lower abdomen, left thorax, left side of the head, and left arm and drains into the left innominate vein.

thoracic vertebrae *pl. n.* the 12 bones of the backbone to which the ribs are attached. *See also* vertebra.

thoracocentesis (thor-ă-koh-sen-**tee**-sis) *n. see* pleurocentesis.

thoracoplasty (**thor**-ă-koh-plasti) *n.* a former treatment for pulmonary tuberculosis involving surgical removal of parts of the ribs, thus allowing the chest wall to fall in and collapse the affected lung.

thoracoscope (**thor**-ă-koh-skohp) *n.* an instrument used to inspect the pleural cavity. **—thoracoscopy** (thor-ă-**kosk**-ŏpi)*n.*

thoracotomy (thor-ă-**kot**-ŏmi) *n.* surgical opening of the chest cavity to inspect or operate on the heart, lungs, or other structures within.

thorax (**thor**-aks) *n.* the chest: the part of the body cavity between the neck and the diaphragm. The skeleton of the thorax is formed by the sternum, costal cartilages, ribs, and thoracic vertebrae. It encloses the lungs, heart, oesophagus, and associated structures. *Compare* abdomen. **—thoracic** *adj.*

thought alienation (thawt) *n.* a symptom of psychosis, especially schizophrenia, in which patients feel that their own thoughts are in some way no longer within their control by being, for example, removed or replaced by an outside force or agency.

threadworm (pinworm) (**thred**-werm) *n.* a parasitic nematode worm of the genus *Enterobius* (*Oxyuris*), which lives in the upper part of the human large intestine. Threadworms cause enterobiasis, a disease common in children throughout the world.

threonine (**three**-ŏ-neen) *n.* an essential amino acid. *See also* amino acid.

threshold (**thresh**-ohld) *n.* (in neurology) the point at which a stimulus begins to evoke a response, and therefore a measure of the sensitivity of a system under particular conditions.

thrill (thril) *n.* a vibration felt on placing the hand on the body.

-thrix *combining form denoting* a hair or hairlike structure.

thromb- (thrombo-) *combining form denoting* **1.** a blood clot (thrombus). **2.** thrombosis. **3.** blood platelets.

thrombectomy (throm-**bek**-tŏmi) *n.* a surgical procedure in which a blood clot (thrombus) is removed from an artery or a vein (*see* endarterectomy, phlebothrombosis).

thrombin (**throm**-bin) *n.* a substance (coagulation factor) that acts as an enzyme, converting the soluble protein fibrinogen to the insoluble protein fibrin in the final stage of blood coagulation. Thrombin is derived from the inactive substance prothrombin.

thromboangiitis obliterans (throm-boh-an-ji-**I**-tis ŏ-**blit**-er-anz) *n. see* Buerger's disease.

thromboarteritis (throm-boh-ar-ter-**I**-tis) *n.* inflammation of an artery (*see* arteritis) associated with thrombosis.

thrombocyte (**throm**-boh-syt) *n. see* platelet.

thrombocythaemia (throm-boh-si-**th'ee**-miă) *n.* a disease in which there is an abnormal proliferation of megakaryocytes, leading to an increased number of platelets in the blood.

thrombocytopenia (TCP) (throm-boh-sy-toh-**pee**-niă) *n.* a reduction in the number of platelets in the blood. This results in bleeding into the skin (*see* purpura), spontaneous bruising, and prolonged bleeding after injury. **—thrombocytopenic** *adj.*

thrombocytosis (throm-boh-sy-**toh**-sis) *n.* an increase in the number of platelets in the blood. It may occur in a variety of diseases, including cancers and certain blood diseases, and is likely to cause an increased tendency to thrombosis.

thromboembolic deterrents (TEDs) (throm-boh-em-**bol**-ik) *pl. n.* stockings worn to reduce the risk of deep vein thrombosis, especially after surgery.

thromboembolism (throm-boh-**em**-bŏ-lizm) *n.* the condition in which a blood clot (thrombus), formed at one point in the circulation, becomes detached and lodges at another point.

thromboendarterectomy (throm-boh-end-ar-ter-**ek**-tŏmi) *n. see* endarterectomy.

thromboendarteritis (throm-boh-end-ar-ter-**I**-tis) *n.* thrombosis complicating endarteritis, seen in temporal arteritis, polyarteritis nodosa, and syphilis.

thrombokinase (throm-boh-**ky**-nayz) *n. see* thromboplastin.

thrombolysis (throm-**bol**-i-sis) *n.* the dissolution of a blood clot (thrombus) by the infusion of a fibrinolytic agent into the blood.

thrombolytic (throm-boh-**lit**-ik) *adj.* describing an agent that breaks up blood clots (thrombi). Thrombolytic drugs are used to unblock arteries in the treatment of myocardial infarction. *See* fibrinolytic, tissue-type plasminogen activator.

thrombophilia (throm-boh-**fil**-iă) *n.* an inherited or acquired condition that predisposes individuals to thrombosis. **—thormbophilic** *adj.*

thrombophlebitis (throm-boh-fli-**by**-tis) *n.* inflammation of the wall of a vein (*see* phlebitis) with secondary thrombosis occurring within the affected segment of vein. Pregnant women are more prone to thrombophlebitis because of physiological changes in the blood and the effects of pressure within the abdomen. It may involve superficial or deep veins of the legs (the latter being less common in pregnancy than the former).

thromboplastin (Factor III, thrombokinase) (throm-boh-**plast**-in) *n.* a substance formed during the earlier stages of blood coagulation. It acts as an enzyme, converting the inactive substance prothrombin to the enzyme thrombin.

thrombopoiesis (throm-boh-poi-ee-sis) *n.* the process of blood platelet production. Platelets are formed as fragments of cytoplasm shed from giant cells (megakaryocytes) in the bone marrow by a budding process.

thromboprophylaxis (throm-boh-pro-fi-**lak**-sis) *n.* measures taken to reduce the risk of venous thrombosis and therefore avoid thromboembolism during hospitalization. Techniques include tight support stockings to minimize venous stasis and subcutaneous injections of a low-molecular-weight heparin to thin the blood.

thrombosis (throm-**boh**-sis) *n.* a condition in which the blood changes from a liquid to a solid state in the cardiovascular system and produces a mass of coagulated blood (**thrombus**). Thrombosis in an artery obstructs the blood flow to the tissue it supplies (*see* coronary thrombosis, stroke). Thrombosis can also occur in a vein (**deep vein t.**; *see* phlebothrombosis), and it may be associated with inflammation (*see* thrombophlebitis).

thrombus (**throm**-bŭs) *n.* a blood clot (*see* thrombosis).

thrush (thrush) *n.* *see* candidiasis.

thumb (thum) *n.* the first digit on the radial side of the hand. It can oppose the other four fingers of the hand.

thym- (thymo-) *combining form denoting* the thymus.

thymectomy (th'y-**mek**-tŏmi) *n.* surgical removal of the thymus.

-thymia *combining form denoting* a condition of the mind.

thymine (**th'y**-meen) *n.* one of the nitrogen-containing bases (*see* pyrimidine) occurring in the nucleic acid DNA.

thymitis (th'y-**my**-tis) *n.* inflammation of the thymus.

thymocyte (**th'y**-moh-syt) *n.* a lymphocyte within the thymus.

thymol (**th'y**-mol) *n.* an antiseptic active against bacteria and fungi, used in mouthwashes, gargles, and skin preparations.

thymoma (th'y-**moh**-mă) *n.* a benign or malignant tumour of the thymus. It is sometimes associated with myasthenia gravis.

thymus (**th'y**-mŭs) *n.* a bilobed organ in the root of the neck, above and in front of the heart. In relation to body size the thymus is largest at birth. It doubles in size by puberty, after which it gradually shrinks, its functional tissue being replaced by fatty tissue. In infancy the thymus controls the development of lymphoid tissue and immune response to microbes and foreign proteins. **—thymic** *adj.*

thyro- *combining form denoting* the thyroid gland.

thyrocalcitonin (th'y-roh-kal-si-**toh**-nin) *n.* *see* calcitonin.

thyrocele (**th'y**-roh-seel) *n.* a swelling of the thyroid gland. *See* goitre.

thyroglobulin (th'y-roh-**glob**-yoo-lin) *n.* a protein in the thyroid gland from which the thyroid hormones are synthesized.

thyroglossal (th'y-roh-**glos**-ăl) *adj*. relating to the thyroid gland and the tongue. **t. duct** a duct in the embryo between the thyroid and the back of the tongue.

thyroid cartilage (th'y-roid) *n*. the main cartilage of the larynx, consisting of two broad plates that join at the front. *See also* Adam's apple.

thyroid crisis (thyroid storm) *n*. a life-threatening condition due to an acute and severe exacerbation of previously undiagnosed or inadequately treated thyrotoxicosis. It often follows infections, childbirth, nonthyroid surgery, or trauma and presents as fever, severe agitation, nausea and vomiting, diarrhoea, abdominal pains, an accelerated heart rate, and irregularity of the heart rhythm.

thyroidectomy (th'y-roid-**ek**-tŏmi) *n*. surgical removal of the thyroid gland. **partial t.** thyroidectomy in which only the diseased part of the gland is removed. **subtotal t.** a method of treating thyrotoxicosis due to Graves' disease, in which the surgeon removes 90% of the gland.

thyroid gland *n*. a large endocrine gland situated in the base of the neck (see illustration). It consists of two lobes, one on either side of the trachea, that are joined by an isthmus. The thyroid gland is concerned with regulation of the metabolic rate by the secretion of thyroid hormone. The C cells of the thyroid gland secrete calcitonin.

thyroid hormone *n*. an iodine-containing substance, synthesized and secreted by the thyroid gland, that acts to increase the basal metabolic rate, being essential for normal mental and physical development. The principal thyroid hormone, **thyroxine** (**tetraiodothyronine**, **T_4**), is mostly converted to the metabolically more active form, **triiodothyronine** (**T_3**), within the peripheral tissues. Lack of these hormones gives rise to cretinism in infants and myxoedema in adults. Excessive production of thyroid hormones gives rise to thyrotoxicosis.

thyroiditis (th'y-roid-**I**-tis) *n*. inflammation of the thyroid gland. **acute t.** thyroiditis due to bacterial infection. **chronic t.** thyroiditis that is commonly caused by an abnormal immune response (*see* autoimmunity) in which lymphocytes invade the tissues of the gland. **subacute t.** (**de Quervain's t.**) thyroiditis caused by a viral infection. *See also* Hashimoto's disease.

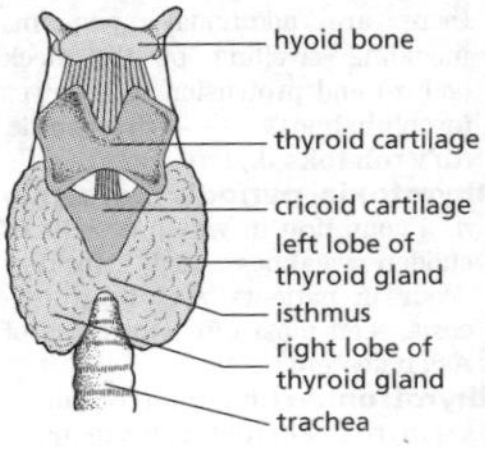

Position of the thyroid gland

thyroid-stimulating hormone (TSH, thyrotrophin) *n.* a hormone, synthesized and secreted by the anterior pituitary gland under the control of thyrotrophin-releasing hormone, that stimulates activity of the thyroid gland.

thyroid storm *n. see* thyroid crisis.

thyroplasty (**th'y**-roh-plasti) *n.* a surgical procedure performed on the thyroid cartilage of the larynx to alter the characteristics of the voice.

thyrotomy (th'y-**rot**-ŏmi) *n.* surgical incision of either the thyroid cartilage or the thyroid gland itself.

thyrotoxicosis (th'y-roh-toks-i-**koh**-sis) *n.* the syndrome due to excessive amounts of thyroid hormones in the bloodstream, causing a rapid heartbeat, sweating, tremor, anxiety, increased appetite, loss of weight, and intolerance of heat. Causes include simple overactivity of the gland, a hormone-secreting tumour, and **Graves' disease** (**exophthalmic goitre**), in which there are additional symptoms including swelling of the neck (goitre) and protrusion of the eyes (exophthalmos). **—thyrotoxic** (th'y-roh-**toks**-ik) *adj.*

thyrotoxic periodic paralysis *n.* a condition in which attacks of sudden weakness and flaccidity occur in patients with thyrotoxicosis, seen most often in males of Asian descent.

thyrotrophin (th'y-roh-**troh**-fin) *n. see* thyroid-stimulating hormone.

thyrotrophin-releasing hormone (TRH) *n.* a hormone that is secreted from the hypothalamus (in the brain) and acts on the anterior pituitary gland to stimulate the release of thyroid-stimulating hormone.

thyroxine (T_4) (th'y-**roks**-een) *n. see* thyroid hormone.

TIA *n. see* transient ischaemic attack.

tiabendazole (thiabendazole) (ty-ă-**ben**-dă-zohl) *n.* an anthelmintic administered orally to treat creeping eruption.

TIBC *n.* total iron-binding capacity (of blood serum).

tibia (**tib**-iă) *n.* the shin bone: the inner and larger bone of the lower leg. It articulates with the femur above, with the talus below, and with the fibula to the side. **—tibial** (**tib**-iăl) *adj.*

tibialis (tib-i-**ay**-lis) *n.* either of two muscles in the leg, extending from the tibia to the metatarsal bones of the foot. **t. anterior** the muscle that turns the foot inwards and flexes the toes backwards. **t. posterior** the muscle that extends the toes and inverts the foot.

tibial torsion *n.* a normal variation in posture in which there is an in-toe gait due to mild internal rotation of the tibia. The condition is often apparent in infancy when the child starts walking and resolves spontaneously with time.

tibio- *combining form denoting* the tibia.

tic (tik) *n.* a repeated and largely involuntary movement (**motor t.**) or utterance (**vocal t.**) varying in complexity from a muscle twitch or grunt to elaborate well-coordinated actions and repeated words or phrases. Simple tics occur in about a quarter of children and usually disappear within a year. *See also* Tourette's syndrome. **t. douloureux** *see* neuralgia.

ticarcillin (tik-ar-**sil**-in) *n.* a penicillin-type antibiotic administered in combination with clavulanic acid (as **Timentin**) by intravenous infusion to treat serious infections caused by *Pseudomonas* and *Proteus* bacteria.

tick (tik) *n.* a bloodsucking parasite belonging to the order of arthropods (Acarina) that also includes the mites. Tick bites can cause serious skin lesions and occasionally paralysis, and certain tick species transmit typhus, Lyme disease, and relapsing fever. Diethyltoluamide (DEET) is used as a tick repellent. **t. fever** any infectious disease transmitted by ticks, especially Rocky Mountain spotted fever.

tidal model (ty-d'l) *n.* an interprofessional mental-health model whose focus of mental-health discovery enables clients to reclaim their personal stories to start the recovery process. It encourages clients, from an early point in their illness, to actively engage with their feelings of distress in order to learn to manage and ultimately recover control of these for themselves.

tidal volume (TV) *n.* the volume of air that is taken into the lungs and exhaled in normal quiet breathing.

TILE *n.* an acronym for *t*ask, *i*ndividual (and capabilities), *l*oad, and *e*nvironment (and equipment), which enables risk assessment for any situation that requires moving and handling. It is intended to act as a prompt for effective assessment.

tilting-disc valve (tilt-ing-**disk**) *n.* the form of mechanical prosthesis most commonly used for replacing damaged heart valves.

timalation (tim-ă-**lay**-shŏn) *n.* the stimulation of the senses of touch, hearing, sight, sound, and smell. It is used in the care of patients with dementia, enabling them to experience the world in a pleasurable way.

timolol (**tim**-ŏ-lol) *n.* a beta blocker used in the treatment of hypertension, angina, and glaucoma and for long-term prophylaxis after an acute myocardial infarction. It is administered by mouth or as eye drops or gel. Trade names: **Betim**, **Timoptol**, **Tiopex**.

tincture (**tink**-cher) *n.* an alcoholic extract of a drug derived from a plant.

tinea (ringworm) (**tin**-iă) *n.* a fungal infection of the skin, scalp, or nails. It is caused by the dermatophyte fungi – *Microsporum*, *Trichophyton*, and *Epidermophyton* – and can be spread by direct contact or via infected materials. The lesions of ringworm may form partial or complete rings and may cause intense itching. The disease is treated with antifungal agents taken by mouth (such as itraconazole or terbinafine) or applied locally. **t. barbae** ringworm of the skin under a beard. **t. capitis** ringworm of the scalp. **t. cruris** ringworm of the groin and thighs. **t. pedis** *see* athlete's foot.

Tinel's sign (ti-**nelz**) *n.* a method for checking the regeneration of a nerve, usually in patients with carpal tunnel syndrome. Direct tapping over the sheath of the nerve elicits a distal tingling sensation (*see* paraesthesia), which indicates the beginning of regeneration. [J. Tinel (1879–1952), French neurologist]

tinnitus (ti-**ny**-tŭs) *n.* the sensation of sounds in the ears, head, or around the head in the absence of an external sound source. It can occur with any form of hearing loss or with normal hearing and is thought to be due to a misinterpretation of signals in the central auditory pathways in the brain. t. retraining therapy (TRT) a unified method of treating tinnitus, including explanation, counselling, cognitive behavioural therapy, mindfulness meditation, relaxation techniques, and sound therapy (*see* white noise instrument).

tintometer (tin-**tom**-it-er) *n.* an instrument for measuring the depth of colour in a liquid. The colour can then be compared with those on standard charts so that the concentration of a particular compound in solution can be estimated.

tioguanine (thioguamine) (ty-oh-**gwah**-neen) *n.* a drug that prevents the growth of cancer cells (*see* antimetabolite) and is administered by mouth in the treatment of leukaemias. Trade name: **Lanvis**.

tissue (**tis**-yoo) *n.* a collection of cells specialized to perform a particular function. Aggregations of tissues constitute organs. **t. culture** the culture of living tissues, removed from the body, in a suitable medium supplied with nutrients and oxygen. **t. typing** determination of the HLA profiles of tissues (*see* HLA system) to assess their compatibility. It is the most important predictor of success or failure of a transplant operation.

tissue-type plasminogen activator (tPA, TPA) *n.* a natural protein, found in the body and able to be manufactured by genetic engineering, that can break up a thrombus (*see* thrombolysis). It requires the presence of fibrin as a cofactor and is able to activate plasminogen on the fibrin surface, which distinguishes it from the other plasminogen activators, streptokinase and urokinase. tPAs include alteplase, **reteplase** (**Rapilysin**), and **tenecteplase** (**Metalyse**).

titration (ty-**tray**-shŏn) *n.* a method of determining the concentration of a substance in solution. A measured volume of a reagent of known concentration is added to a known volume of the test solution until the end point of the reaction has occurred.

titre (**ty**-ter) *n.* (in immunology) the extent to which a sample of blood serum containing antibody can be diluted before losing its ability to cause agglutination of the relevant antigen. It is used as a measure of the amount of antibody in the serum.

TLC *n. see* total lung capacity.

T lymphocyte *n. see* lymphocyte, T cell.

TMJ *n.* *see* temporomandibular joint.

TNF *n.* *see* tumour necrosis factor.

TNM classification *n.* a classification defined by the UICC (Union International Contre le Cancer) for the extent of spread of a cancer. T refers to the size of the tumour, N the presence and extent of lymph node involvement, and M the presence of distant spread (metastasis).

tobacco (tŏ-**bak**-oh) *n.* the dried leaves of the plant *Nicotiana tabacum* or related species, used in smoking and as snuff. Tobacco contains the stimulant but poisonous alkaloid nicotine, which enters the bloodstream during smoking. The volatile tarry material released during smoking contains carcinogenic chemicals.

tobramycin (toh-bră-**my**-sin) *n.* an aminoglycoside antibiotic used to treat septicaemia, lung infection in patients with cystic fibrosis, and urinary, skin, abdominal, central nervous system, and eye infections. It is administered by intravenous or intramuscular injection, infusion, or by inhalation, or as eye drops. Trade names: **Bramitob**, **Tobi**, **Tobravisc**.

toco- (toko-) *combining form denoting* childbirth or labour.

tocography (tok-**og**-răfi) *n.* the measuring and recording of the force and frequency of uterine contractions during labour using an instrument called a **tocodynamometer**.

tocopherol (tok-**off**-er-ol) *n.* *see* vitamin E.

tocophobia *n.* *see* tokophobia.

toddler's diarrhoea (tod-lerz) *n.* a disorder of young children characterized by the passage of frequent loose, offensive, and bulky stools in which partially digested or undigested food may be visible (the 'peas and carrot' stool). It resolves by school age.

Todd's paralysis (Todd's palsy) (todz) *n.* transient paralysis of a part of the body that has previously been involved in a focal epileptic seizure (*see* epilepsy). [R. B. Todd (1809–60), British physician]

toko- *combining form. see* toco-.

tokophobia (tocophobia) (tok-ŏ-**foh**-bia) *n.* a profound fear of childbirth. **primary t.** tokophobia that develops in adolescence and causes many women to avoid childbirth altogether. **secondary t.** tokophobia that occurs after a traumatic delivery and can stop a woman having another child.

tolbutamide (tol-**bew**-tă-myd) *n.* a short-acting drug taken by mouth in the treatment of type 2 diabetes mellitus. It is now rarely prescribed in the UK, having been superseded by other drugs. *See also* sulphonylurea.

tolerance (**tol**-er-ăns) *n.* the reduction or loss of the normal response to a substance that usually provokes a reaction in the body. **drug t.** tolerance that may develop after taking a particular drug over a long period of time. In such cases increased doses are necessary to produce the desired effect. *See also* glucose tolerance test, immunological tolerance.

tolnaftate (tol-**naf**-tayt) *n.* an antifungal drug applied topically as a cream, powder, or solution in the treatment of ringworm, especially athelete's foot. Trade name: **Mycil**.

tolterodine (tol-te-rŏ-deen) *n.* an antimuscarinic drug taken by mouth to treat detrusor overactivity giving rise to the lower urinary tract symptoms of frequency, urgency, or urge incontinence, and bedwetting in children. Trade name: **Detrusitol**.

-tome *combining form denoting* a cutting instrument.

tomo- *combining form denoting* **1.** section or sections. **2.** surgical operation.

tomography (tŏ-**mog**-răfi) *n.* the technique of rotating a radiation detector around the patient so that the image obtained gives additional three-dimensional information. In plain film tomography this produces an image of structures at a particular depth within the body, bringing them into sharp focus, while deliberately blurring structures above and below them. The visual record of this technique is called a **tomogram**. *See also* computerized tomography, positron emission tomography, SPECT scanning.

-tomy (-otomy) *combining form denoting* a surgical incision into an organ or part.

tone (tohn) *n. see* tonus.

tongue (tung) *n.* a muscular organ attached to the floor of the mouth. It is covered by mucous membrane and its surface is raised in minute projections (papillae), which give it a furred appearance. Taste buds are arranged in grooves around the papillae. The tongue helps in manipulating food during mastication and swallowing; it is the main organ of taste; and it plays an important role in the production of articulate speech. Anatomical name: **glossa**.

tongue-tie (**tung**-ty) *n.* a disorder of young children in which the tongue is anchored in the floor of the mouth more firmly than usual. No treatment is required unless the condition is extreme and associated with forking of the tongue, in which case surgery may be necessary.

tonic (**ton**-ik) **1.** *adj.* **a.** relating to normal muscle tone. **b.** marked by continuous tension (contraction), e.g. a tonic muscle spasm. **t. pupil** (**Adie's pupil**) a pupil that is dilated as a result of damage to the nerves supplying the ciliary muscle and iris. **2.** *n.* a medicinal substance purporting to increase vigour and liveliness and produce a feeling of wellbeing: beneficial effects of tonics are probably due to their placebo action.

tonicity (toh-**nis**-iti) *n.* **1.** the normal state of slight contraction, or readiness to contract, of healthy muscle fibres. **2.** the effective osmotic pressure of a solution. *See* hypertonic, hypotonic, osmosis.

tono- *combining form denoting* **1.** tone or tension. **2.** pressure.

tonography (toh-**nog**-răfi) *n.* measurement of the pressure within the eyeball while the eyeball is subjected to pressure over a period of several minutes.

tonometer (toh-**nom**-it-er) *n.* **1.** **(ophthalmotonometer)** an instrument for measuring pressure inside the eye. **Goldman applanation t.** a tonometer that measures the force required to flatten an area of cornea 3 mm^2. A greater force is required when the pressure inside the eye is increased. **2.** an instrument for measuring pressure in any other part of the body. **—tonometry** *n.*

tonsillectomy (ton-sil-**ek**-tŏmi) *n.* surgical removal of the tonsils.

tonsillitis (ton-sil-**I**-tis) *n.* inflammation of the tonsils due to bacterial or viral infection, causing a sore throat, fever, and difficulty in swallowing.

tonsillotome (ton-**sil**-ŏ-tohm) *n.* a surgical knife used for cutting into or removing a tonsil.

tonsils (**ton**-silz) *pl. n.* masses of lymphoid tissue around the pharynx, usually referring to the masses on either side of the oropharynx (**palatine t.**). *See also* adenoids (nasopharyngeal tonsil).

tonus (tone) (**toh**-nŭs) *n.* the normal state of partial contraction of a resting muscle.

tooth (tooth) *n.* (*pl.* **teeth**) one of the hard structures in the mouth used for cutting and chewing food. Each tooth is embedded in a socket in the jawbone, to which it is

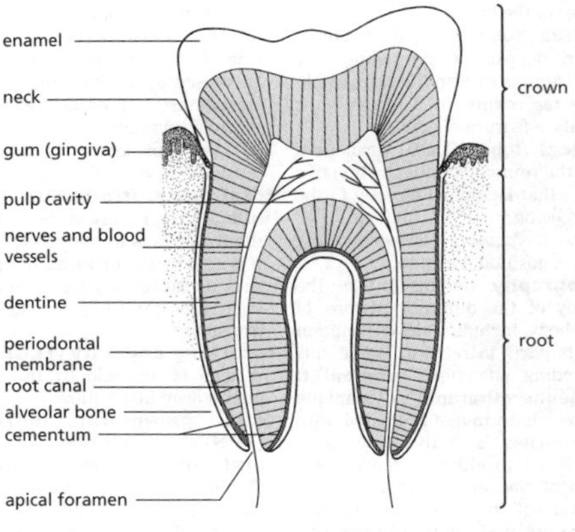

Section of a molar tooth

attached by the periodontal membrane. The exposed part of the tooth (**crown**) is covered with enamel and the part within the bone (**root**) is coated with cementum; the bulk of the tooth consists of dentine enclosing the pulp. There are four different types of teeth (*see* canine, incisor, molar, premolar). See illustration. *See also* dentition.

toothpaste (**tooth**-payst) *n. see* dentifrice.

TOP *n.* termination of pregnancy. *See* abortion.

topagnosis (top-ag-**noh**-sis) *n.* inability to identify a part of the body that has been touched. It is a symptom of disease in the parietal lobes of the brain.

tophus (**toh**-fŭs) *n.* (*pl.* **tophi**) a hard deposit of crystalline uric acid and its salts in the skin, cartilage (especially of the ears), or joints: a feature of gout.

topical (**top**-ikăl) *adj.* local: used for the route of administration of a drug that is applied directly to the part being treated.

topo- *combining form denoting* place; position; location.

topography (tŏ-**pog**-răfi) *n.* the study of the different regions of the body, including the description of its parts in relation to the surrounding structures. **corneal t.** (**videokeratography**) a technique in which an image projected onto the cornea is analysed by computer to produce a representation of the shape and refractive power of the corneal surface. **—topographical** (top-ŏ-**graf**-ikăl) *adj.*

topotecan (top-oh-**tee**-kăn) *n.* a cytotoxic drug administered orally or by intravenous infusion for treating advanced ovarian cancer, small-cell lung cancer, and recurrent cervical cancer. Trade name: **Hycamtin**.

torpor (**tor**-per) *n.* a state of sluggishness and diminished responsiveness: a characteristic of certain mental disorders and a symptom of certain forms of poisoning or metabolic disorder.

torsion (**tor**-shŏn) *n.* twisting. *See also* tibial torsion.

torticollis (wryneck) (tor-ti-**kol**-iss) *n.* an irresistible turning movement of the head that becomes more persistent, so that eventually the head is held continually to one side. A form of dystonia, it may be caused by a birth injury to the sternomastoid muscle (*see* sternomastoid tumour).

TOT *n.* transobturator tape. *See* tension-free vaginal tape.

total body irradiation (TBI) (**toh**-t'l) *n.* exposure of the whole of the patient's body to radiotherapy. It is used in certain forms of cancer, such as cancers of the blood-forming tissues, prior to a bone marrow transplant.

total lung capacity (TLC) *n.* the volume of air held by the lungs after a deep inspiration.

total parenteral nutrition (TPN) *n. see* nutrition.

total quality management (TQM) *n.* an approach to management that aims to ensure quality, effectiveness, and flexibility throughout an organization, with all individuals in the organization contributing to achieve this.

Tourette's syndrome (Gilles de la Tourette syndrome) (toor-ets) *n.* a condition characterized by multiple tics, both motor tics (e.g. eye rolling, arm movements) and vocal tics (e.g. grunts and, in a minority of patients, involuntary obscene speech), for at least one year. The condition usually starts in childhood and commonly improves with age. [G. Gilles de la Tourette (1857–1904), French neurologist]

tourniquet (toor-ni-kay) *n.* a device to compress an artery or vein to prevent flow of blood through it, usually a cord, rubber tube, or tight bandage. Tourniquets are no longer recommended as a first-aid measure to stop bleeding from a wound; direct pressure on the wound itself is considered less harmful.

tow (toh) *n.* the teased-out short fibres of flax, hemp, or jute, used in swabs, stupes, and for a variety of other purposes.

tox- (toxi-, toxo-, toxic(o)-) *combining form denoting* **1.** poisonous; toxic. **2.** toxins or poisoning.

toxaemia (toks-eem-iă) *n.* blood poisoning that is caused by toxins formed by bacteria growing in a local site of infection. *Compare* pyaemia, sapraemia, septicaemia.

toxic (toks-ik) *adj.* having a poisonous effect; potentially lethal.

toxicity (toks-iss-iti) *n.* the degree to which a substance is poisonous.

toxicology (toks-i-kol-ŏji) *n.* the study of poisonous materials and their effects upon living organisms. —**toxicologist** *n.*

toxicosis (toks-i-koh-sis) *n.* the deleterious effects of a toxin; poisoning.

toxic shock syndrome (TSS) *n.* a state of acute shock due to septicaemia. The commonest cause is a retained foreign body (e.g. a tampon or IUCD) combined with the presence of staphylococci. The condition can be life-threatening if not treated aggressively with appropriate antibiotics and supportive care (including fluid and electrolyte replacement). **streptococcal t. s. s.** a similar condition caused by Type A streptococci. *See also* necrotizing fasciitis.

toxin (toks-in) *n.* a poison produced by a living organism, especially by a bacterium (*see* endotoxin, exotoxin). In the body toxins act as antigens (*see* antitoxin).

toxocariasis (visceral larva migrans) (toks-oh-kair-I-ă-sis) *n.* an infestation with the larvae of the dog and cat roundworms, *Toxocara canis* and *T. cati*. It is characterized by enlargement of the liver, pneumonitis, fever, joint and muscle pains, vomiting, an irritating rash, and convulsions.

toxoid (toks-oid) *n.* a poisonous material (toxin) that has been rendered harmless by chemical treatment while retaining its antigenic activity. Toxoids are used in vaccines.

toxoid-antitoxin *n.* a mixture of a toxoid and its antitoxin used as a vaccine to produce active immunity.

toxoplasmosis (toks-oh-plaz-**moh**-sis) *n.* a disease of mammals and birds due to the protozoan *Toxoplasma gondii*, which may be transmitted to humans (usually by eating undercooked infected meat or food or drink contaminated with the faeces of infected cats). Generally symptoms are mild (swollen lymph nodes and an influenza-like illness), but the disease can be serious in immunocompromised patients. **congenital t.** toxoplasmosis transmitted by a woman infected during pregnancy to her fetus. It may produce severe malformations of the skull and eyes or active liver infection in the newborn.

tPA (TPA) *n. see* tissue-type plasminogen activator.

TPN *n. see* (total parenteral) nutrition.

TPR temperature, pulse, respiration.

TQM *n. see* total quality management.

trabecula (tră-**bek**-yoo-lă) *n.* (*pl.* **trabeculae**) **1.** any of the bands of tissue that pass from the outer part of an organ to its interior, dividing it into separate chambers. **2.** any of the thin bars of bony tissue in spongy bone. **—trabecular** *adj.*

trabeculectomy (tră-bek-yoo-**lek**-tŏmi) *n.* an operation for glaucoma in which a part of the **trabecular meshwork** is removed. This tissue, located at the angle between the cornea and iris, consists of tiny canals through which aqueous fluid drains into Schlemm's canal. Trabeculectomy allows aqueous fluid to filter out of the eye under the conjunctiva, thus reducing the pressure inside the eye.

trabeculoplasty (tră-**bek**-yoo-loh-plasti) *n.* a method used to selectively destroy parts of the trabecular meshwork (*see* trabeculectomy) and hence reduce intraocular pressure in the treatment of glaucoma. This may be achieved by means of a laser (**argon laser t.** or **selective laser t.**).

trace element (trayss) *n.* an element required in minute amounts for the normal functioning of the body. Examples are copper, cobalt, and manganese.

tracer (**tray**-ser) *n.* a substance that is introduced into the body and whose progress can subsequently be followed so that information is gained about metabolic processes. Radioactive tracers, which are substances labelled with radionuclides, are used for a variety of purposes in nuclear medicine.

trache- (tracheo-) *combining form denoting* the trachea.

trachea (tray-**ki**ă) *n.* the windpipe: the part of the air passage between the larynx and the main bronchi. **—tracheal** (tray-ki-ăl) *adj.*

tracheal tugging *n.* a sign indicative of an aneurysm of the aortic arch: a downward tug is felt on the windpipe when the finger is placed in the midline at the root of the neck.

tracheitis (tray-ki-I-tis) *n.* inflammation of the trachea, usually secondary to bacterial or viral infection in the nose or throat.

Tracheitis causes soreness in the chest and a painful cough and is often associated with bronchitis.

trachelorrhaphy (tray-kĕl-**o**-răfi) *n.* an operation for suturing tears in the cervix of the uterus.

tracheobronchitis (tray-ki-oh-brong-**ky**-tis) *n.* inflammation of the trachea and bronchi.

tracheostomy (tracheotomy) (tray-ki-**ost**-ŏmi) *n.* a surgical operation in which a hole is made into the trachea through the neck to relieve obstruction to breathing, as in diphtheria. A curved metal, plastic, or rubber tube is usually inserted through the hole and held in position by tapes tied round the neck. *See also* minitracheostomy.

SEE WEB LINKS

- Explanation of tracheostomy from the NHS Choices website

tracheotomy (tray-ki-**ot**-ŏmi) *n. see* tracheostomy.

trachoma (tră-**koh**-mă) *n.* a chronic contagious eye disease – a severe form of conjunctivitis caused by the bacterium *Chlamydia trachomatis* – that is common in some hot countries. If untreated, the conjunctiva becomes scarred and shrinks, causing trichiasis; blindness can be a late complication. Treatment with tetracyclines is effective in the early stages of the disease.

tract (trakt) *n.* **1.** a group of nerve fibres passing from one part of the brain or spinal cord to another, forming a distinct pathway. **2.** an organ or collection of organs providing for the passage of something, e.g. the digestive tract.

traction (**trak**-shŏn) *n.* the application of a pulling force, especially as a means of counteracting the natural tension in the tissues surrounding a broken bone, to produce correct alignment of the fragments. Considerable force, exerted with weights, ropes, and pulleys, may be necessary to ensure that a broken femur is kept correctly positioned during the early stages of healing. Traction is also used by physiotherapists for the treatment of back pain.

tractotomy (trak-**tot**-ŏmi) *n.* a neurosurgical operation for the relief of intractable pain, in which the nerve fibres that carry painful sensation to consciousness are severed within the medulla oblongata. *See also* cordotomy.

tragus (**tray**-gŭs) *n.* the projection of cartilage in the pinna of the outer ear that extends back over the opening of the external auditory meatus. It is used as a reference point in orthodontic measurements.

tramadol (**tram**-ă-dol) *n.* an opioid analgesic (*see* opiate) used for the relief of moderate or severe pain. It is administered by mouth or injection and causes less marked side-effects than other opioids. Trade names: **Maxitram SR**, **Zamadol**, **Zydol**, etc.

TRAM flap (tram) *n.* *t*ransverse *r*ectus *a*bdominis *m*yocutaneous flap: a piece of tissue (skin, muscle, and fat) dissected from the abdomen and used to reconstruct the breast after mastectomy.

trance (trahns) *n.* a state in which reaction to the environment is diminished although awareness is not impaired. It may be caused by hypnosis, meditation, catatonia, conversion disorder, or drugs.

tranexamic acid (tran-eks-**am**-ik) *n.* an antifibrinolytic drug administered by mouth or by intravenous injection or infusion as an antidote to overdosage by fibrinolytic drugs and to control severe bleeding, for example after surgery or to treat menorrhagia. Trade name: **Cyklokapron**.

tranquillizer (**trank**-wi-ly-zer) *n.* a drug that produces a calming effect, relieving anxiety and tension. **major t.** *see* antipsychotic. **minor t.** *see* anxiolytic.

trans- *prefix denoting* through or across.

transaminase (trans-**am**-in-ayz) *n.* an enzyme that is involved in the process of transamination. Examples are aspartate aminotransaminase (AST) and alanine aminotransaminase (ALT).

transamination (trans-am-i-**nay**-shŏn) *n.* a process involved in the metabolism of amino acids in which amino groups ($-NH_2$) are transferred from amino acids to certain α-keto acids, with the production of a second keto acid and amino acid. The reaction is catalysed by transaminases.

transcription (tran-**skrip**-shŏn) *n.* the process in which the information contained in the genetic code is transferred from DNA to RNA: the first step in the manufacture of proteins in cells. *See* messenger RNA, translation.

transcultural nursing (trans-**kul**-cher-ăl) *n.* a major area of nursing that focuses on the comparative study and analysis of different cultures and subcultures in the world with respect to their caring values, perceptions of health and illness, and patterns of behaviour, with the aim of developing knowledge to provide culture-specific practice. The concept of transcultural nursing was developed by US nursing theorist M. Leininger (1924–2012).

SEE WEB LINKS

- Website of the Transcultural Nursing Society

transcutaneous electrical nerve stimulation (TENS) (trans-kew-tay-niŭs) *n. see* stimulator.

transdermal (trans-**der**-măl) *adj.* through the skin: applied to the route of administration of drugs that are absorbed through the skin.

transducer (trans-**dew**-ser) *n.* a device used to convert one form of signal into another, allowing its measurement or display to be made appropriately. For example, an ultrasound probe converts reflected ultrasound waves into electronic impulses, which can be displayed on a TV monitor.

transection (tran-**sek**-shŏn) *n.* **1.** a cross section of a piece of tissue. **2.** cutting across the tissue of an organ (*see also* section).

transferase (**trans**-fer-ayz) *n.* an enzyme that catalyses the transfer of a group (other than hydrogen) between a pair of substrates.

transference (**trans**-fer-ĕns) *n.* (in psychoanalysis) the process by which a patient comes to feel and act towards the therapist as though he or she were somebody from the patient's past life, especially a powerful parent. The patient's transference feelings may be of love or of hatred.

transferrin (siderophilin) (trans-fer-in) *n.* a glycoprotein, found in the blood plasma, that acts as a carrier for iron in the bloodstream.

transfer RNA (**trans**-fer) *n.* a type of RNA whose function is to attach the correct amino acid to the protein chain being synthesized at a ribosome. *See also* translation.

transfusion (trans-few-zhŏn) *n.* **1.** the injection of a volume of blood obtained from a healthy person into the circulation of a patient whose blood is deficient in quantity or quality, through accident or disease. The blood is allowed to drip, under gravity, through a needle inserted into one of the patient's veins. Blood transfusion is routine during major surgical operations in which much blood is likely to be lost. **2.** the administration of any fluid, such as plasma or saline solution, into a patient's vein by means of a drip.

SEE WEB LINKS

- Information about giving blood from NHS Blood and Transplant

transgender (tranz-**jen**-der) *adj. see* transsexualism

transient ischaemic attack (TIA) (**tran**-zi-ĕnt isk-ee-mik) *n.* the result of temporary disruption of the circulation to part of the brain due to embolism, thrombosis to brain arteries, or spasm of the vessel walls. The most common symptoms are transient loss of vision in one eye and weakness or numbness in one limb or part of a limb.

SEE WEB LINKS

- Explanation of TIAs from the Stroke Association

transillumination (tranz-i-loo-mi-**nay**-shŏn) *n.* the technique of shining a bright light through part of the body to examine its structure. Transillumination of the paranasal sinuses is a means of detecting abnormalities.

transitional cell carcinoma (tran-**si**-*zh*ŏn-ăl) *n.* a form of cancer that affects the urothelium, which lines the urinary collecting system of the kidney, ureters, bladder, and most of the urethra. It is the most common type of bladder cancer.

transjugular (tranz-**jug**-yoo-lă) *adj.* through the jugular vein, commonly to gain access to the venous system to place lines and undertake interventions.

translation (tranz-**lay**-shŏn) *n.* (in cell biology) the manufacture of proteins in a cell, which takes place at the ribosomes. *See* messenger RNA, transfer RNA.

translational research (tranz-**lay**-shŏ-năl) *n.* scientific enquiry that focuses on developing practical applications from the findings of basic scientific research. It is sometimes divided into **T1 research** and **T2 research**. The former focuses on developing clinical treatments from laboratory-based science; the latter on embedding the findings of clinical trials into everyday practice.

translocation (tranz-loh-**kay**-shŏn) *n.* (in genetics) a type of chromosome mutation in which part of a chromosome is transferred to another part of the same chromosome or to a different chromosome. This can lead to serious genetic disorders, e.g. chronic myeloid leukaemia.

translumbar (tranz-**lum**-ber) *adj.* through the lumbar region: describing the route for injecting the aorta for aortography.

transmigration (tranz-my-**gray**-shŏn) *n.* the act of passing through or across, e.g. the passage of blood cells through the intact walls of capillaries and venules (*see* diapedesis).

transobturator tape (TOT) (tranz-**ob**-tewr-ay-ter) *n. see* tension-free vaginal tape.

transoesophageal echocardiography (tranz-ee-sof-ă-**jee**-ăl) *n. see* echocardiography.

transplacental (trans-plă-**sen**-t'l) *adj.* across the placenta: describing the transport of substances, etc., between mother and fetus.

transplantation (trans-plahn-**tay**-shŏn) *n.* the implantation of an organ or tissue from one part of the body to another, as in skin or bone grafting, or from one person to another, as in kidney or heart transplants. Transplanting organs or tissues between individuals is a difficult procedure because of the natural rejection processes in the recipient of the graft. Special treatment (e.g. with immunosuppressant drugs) is needed to prevent transplant rejection.

transposition (trans-pŏ-**zish**-ŏn) *n.* the abnormal positioning of a part of the body such that it is on the opposite side to its normal site in the body. **t. of the great vessels** a congenital abnormality of the heart in which the aorta arises from the right ventricle and the pulmonary artery from the left ventricle.

transrectal ultrasonography (TRUS) (trans-**rek**-tăl) *n. see* ultrasonography.

transsexualism (tranz-**seks**-yoo-ăl-izm) *n.* the condition of one who firmly believes that he (or she) belongs to the sex opposite to his (or her) biological gender. In adults gender reassignment surgery is sometimes justifiable, to make the externals of the body conform to the individual's view of himself (or herself). The term **transgender** is often used synonymously with transsexual, although this term also covers others who do not conform to generally recognized gender roles. *See also* gender dysphoria. —**transsexual** *adj., n.*

transudation (trans-yoo-**day**-shŏn) *n.* the passage of a liquid through a membrane, especially of blood through the wall of a capillary vessel. The liquid is called the **transudate**.

transuretero-ureterostomy (trans-yoor-ee-ter-oh-yoor-i-ter-**ost**-ŏmi) *n.* the operation of connecting one ureter to the other in the abdomen. The damaged or obstructed ureter is cut above the diseased or damaged segment and joined end-to-side to the other ureter.

transurethral (trans-yoor-**ee**-thrăl) *adj.* through the urethra. **t. resection of the prostate** *see* resection. **t. vaporization of the prostate** (**TUVP**) a technique in which the prostate is vaporized: used to treat lower urinary tract symptoms due to benign prostatic hyperplasia and urinary retention.

transvaginal (tranz-vă-**jy**-năl) *adj.* through or across the vagina. **t. tape** *see* tension-free vaginal tape. **t. ultrasonography** *see* ultrasonography.

transverse (tranz-**vers**) *adj.* (in anatomy) situated at right angles to the long axis of the body or an organ. **t. process** the long projection from the base of the neural arch of a vertebra.

transvestism (cross-dressing) (tranz-**vest**-izm) *n.* dressing in clothes normally associated with the opposite sex, which may occur in both heterosexual and homosexual people. Cross-dressing may be practised by transsexuals (*see* transsexualism), in whom it is not sexually arousing. In fetishistic transvestites (*see* fetishism) cross-dressing is sexually arousing. *See also* sexual deviation. **—transvestite** *n.*

trapezium (tră-**pee**-zium) *n.* a bone of the wrist (*see* carpus). It articulates with the scaphoid bone behind, with the first metacarpal in front, and with the trapezoid and second metatarsal on either side.

trapezius (tră-**pee**-zi-ŭs) *n.* a flat triangular muscle covering the back of the neck and shoulder. It moves the scapula and draws the head backwards to either side.

trapezoid bone (tră-**pee**-zoid) *n.* a bone of the wrist (*see* carpus). It articulates with the second metatarsal bone in front, with the scaphoid bone behind, and with the trapezium and capitate bones on either side.

trastuzumab (tras-**too**-zoo-mab) *n.* a monoclonal antibody used to treat certain types of highly malignant breast cancer and metastatic stomach cancer. It is administered by intravenous infusion. Trade name: **Herceptin**.

trauma (**traw**-mă) *n.* **1.** a physical wound or injury. **t. scores** numerical systems for assessing the severity and prognosis of serious injuries. **2.** (in psychology) an emotionally painful and harmful event. Post-traumatic stress disorder may follow from an overwhelmingly stressful event. **—traumatic** (traw-**mat**-ik) *adj.*

SEE WEB LINKS

- Website of the British Trauma Society

traumatic brain injury (TBI) *n.* injury to the brain due to external force, such as occurs following falls, traffic accidents, and violence. It is a major cause of death and disability worldwide, especially in young males.

traumatic fever *n.* a fever resulting from a serious injury.

traumatology (traw-mă-**tol**-ŏji) *n.* accident surgery: the branch of surgery that deals with wounds and disabilities arising from injuries.

travel sickness (trav-ĕl) *n. see* motion sickness.

trazodone (traz-oh-dohn) *n.* an antidepressant administered by mouth in the treatment of depression, particularly in agitated and anxious patients, and anxiety. Trade name: **Molipaxin**.

Treacher Collins syndrome (Treacher Collins deformity) (tree-cher kol-inz) *n.* a hereditary disorder of facial development. The lower jaw and zygomatic (cheek) bones are underdeveloped and the precursors of the ear fail to develop, which results in a variety of ear and facial malformations. [E. Treacher Collins (1862–1919), British ophthalmologist]

treatment field (treet-mĕnt) *n.* (in radiotherapy) an area of the body selected for treatment with radiotherapy. Radiation is administered to the field by focusing the beam of particles emitted by the radiotherapy machine and shielding the surrounding area of the body. **mantle f.** the neck, armpits, and central chest.

trematode (trem-ă-tohd) *n. see* fluke.

tremor (trem-er) *n.* a rhythmical alternating movement that may affect any part of the body. **essential t.** a slow tremor that particularly affects the hands and arms when held out. **intention t.** tremor that occurs when a patient with disease of the cerebellum tries to touch an object. **physiological t.** a feature of the normal mechanism for maintaining posture. It may be more apparent in states of fatigue or anxiety or in people with an overactive thyroid gland. **resting t.** tremor that occurs only when the patient is at rest and disappears when movement is attempted. It is a prominent symptom of parkinsonism.

trench foot (immersion foot) (trench) *n.* blackening of the toes and the skin of the foot due to death of the superficial tissues and caused by prolonged immersion in cold water or exposure to damp and cold.

Trendelenburg position (tren-del-ĕn-berg) *n.* a special operating-table posture for patients undergoing surgery of the pelvis or suffering from shock or to reduce blood loss in operations on the legs. The patient is laid on his back with the pelvis higher than the head, inclined at an angle of about 45°. *See* position. [F. Trendelenburg (1844–1924), German surgeon]

Trendelenburg's operation *n.* ligation of the long saphenous vein at the groin: performed to remove weakened portions of varicose veins.

Trendelenburg's sign *n.* a sign indicating congenital dislocation of the hip: when the patient stands on the affected leg with the other leg flexed, the pelvis is lower on the side of the flexed leg.

trephine (trif-een) *n.* a surgical instrument used to remove a circular area of tissue, usually from the cornea of the eye or from bone.

Treponema (trep-ŏ-nee-mă) *n.* a genus of anaerobic spirochaete bacteria. All species are parasitic;

some cause disease, such as *T. carateum* (pinta), *T. pallidum* (syphilis), and *T. pertenue* (yaws).

treponematosis (trep-ŏ-nee-mă-**toh**-sis) *n.* any infection caused by spirochaete bacteria of the genus *Treponema.*

trespass against the person (tres-păs) *n. see* battery.

tretinoin (tre-**tin**-oh-in) *n.* a drug (*see* retinoid) applied as a solution for the treatment of acne and sun-damaged skin and administered orally to treat acute promyelocytic leukaemia. Trade name: **Vesanoid**.

TRH *n. see* thyrotrophin-releasing hormone.

triad (**try**-ad) *n.* (in medicine) a group of three united or closely associated structures or three symptoms or effects that occur together.

triage (tree-ah*zh*) *n.* a system whereby patients are evaluated and categorized according to the seriousness of their injuries or illnesses with a view to prioritizing treatment and other resources. In emergency situations it is designed to maximize the number of survivors.

triamcinolone (try-am-**sin**-ŏ-lohn) *n.* a synthetic corticosteroid hormone that reduces inflammation but does not cause salt and water retention. Administered by intramuscular or intra-articular injection, nasal spray, or topically, it is used for treating a wide range of inflammatory and allergic conditions. Trade names: **Adcortyl**, **Aureocort**, **Kenalog**, **Nasacort**.

triamterene (try-**am**-ter-een) *n.* a potassium-sparing diuretic administered by mouth, usually in combination with a thiazide or loop diuretic, in the treatment of various forms of fluid retention (oedema).

triangle (**try**-ang-ŭl) *n.* (in anatomy) a three-sided structure or area; for example, the femoral triangle.

triangular bandage (try-**ang**-yoo-ler) *n.* a piece of material cut or folded into a triangular shape and used for making an arm sling or holding dressings in position.

triceps (**try**-seps) *n.* a muscle with three heads of origin. **t. brachii** the muscle that is situated on the back of the upper arm and contracts to extend the forearm. It is the antagonist of the brachialis.

trich- (tricho-) *combining form denoting* hair or hairlike structures.

trichiasis (trik-**I**-ă-sis) *n.* a condition in which the eyelashes rub against the eyeball, producing discomfort and sometimes ulceration of the cornea. It accompanies all forms of entropion.

trichinosis (trichiniasis) (trik-i-**noh**-sis) *n.* a disease caused by larvae of the nematode worm *Trichinella spiralis,* contracted by eating imperfectly cooked infected meat. Symptoms include diarrhoea, nausea, fever, vertigo, delirium, and pains in the limbs. The larvae eventually settle within cysts in the muscles, which may result in pain and stiffness.

trichloracetic acid (try-klor-ă-see-tik) *n.* an astringent used in solution for a variety of skin conditions. It is also applied topically to produce sloughing, especially for the removal of warts.

trichobezoar (trik-oh-**bee**-zor) *n.* hairball: a mass of swallowed hair in the stomach or gastrointestinal tract. *See* bezoar.

Trichocephalus (trik-oh-**sef**-ă-lŭs) *n. see* whipworm.

trichology (trik-**ol**-ŏji) *n.* the study of hair.

Trichomonas (trik-oh-**moh**-năs) *n.* a genus of parasitic flagellate protozoans. **T. hominis** a species that lives in the large intestine. **T. vaginalis** *see* trichomoniasis.

trichomoniasis (trik-oh-mŏ-**ny**-ă-sis) *n.* **1.** an infection of the digestive system by the protozoan *Trichomonas hominis*, causing dysentery. **2.** an infection of the vagina due to the protozoan *Trichomonas vaginalis*, causing inflammation of genital tissues with vaginal discharge. It can be transmitted to males in whom it causes urethral discharge. Treatment with metronidazole is effective.

trichomycosis (trik-oh-my-**koh**-sis) *n.* any hair disease caused by infection with a fungus.

Trichophyton (trik-oh-**fy**-tŏn) *n.* a genus of fungi, parasitic in humans, that frequently infect the skin, nails, and hair and cause tinea (ringworm). *See also* dermatophyte.

trichophytosis (trik-oh-fy-**toh**-sis) *n.* a fungal infection caused by species of *Trichophyton*.

trichromatic (try-kroh-**mat**-ik) *adj.* describing or relating to the normal state of colour vision, in which a person is sensitive to all three of the primary colours. *Compare* dichromatic.

trichuriasis (trik-yoor-**I**-ă-sis) *n.* an infestation of the large intestine by the whipworm, *Trichuris trichiura*. Symptoms, including bloody diarrhoea, anaemia, weakness, and abdominal pain, are evident only in heavy infestations. Trichuriasis can be treated with mebendazole.

Trichuris (trik-**yoor**-iss) *n. see* whipworm.

tricuspid valve (try-**kusp**-id) *n.* the valve in the heart between the right atrium and right ventricle. It consists of three cusps that channel the flow of blood from the atrium to the ventricle and prevent any backflow.

tricyclic antidepressant (try-sy-klik) *n. see* antidepressant.

tridactyly (try-**dak**-tili) *n.* a congenital abnormality in which there are only three digits on a hand or foot.

trifluoperazine (try-floo-oh-**pair**-ă-zeen) *n.* a phenothiazine antipsychotic drug taken by mouth for the treatment of schizophrenia and other psychoses, severe anxiety, and severe nausea and vomiting. Trade name: **Stelazine**.

trigeminal nerve (try-**jem**-in-ăl) *n.* the fifth and largest cranial nerve (V), which is split into the ophthalmic, maxillary, and mandibular nerves. The motor fibres are responsible for controlling the muscles involved in chewing, while the sensory fibres relay information from the front of the head and from the meninges.

trigeminal neuralgia (tic douloureux) *n. see* neuralgia.

trigeminy (try-**jem**-in-i) *n.* a condition in which the heartbeats can be subdivided into groups of three. The first beat is normal, but the second and third are premature beats (*see* ectopic beat).

trigger finger (trig-er) *n.* an impairment in the ability to extend a finger, resulting either from a nodular thickening in the flexor tendon or a narrowing of the flexor tendon sheath. On unclenching the fist, the affected finger at first remains bent then suddenly straightens.

triglyceride (try-**glis**-eryd) *n.* a lipid or neutral fat consisting of glycerol combined with three fatty-acid molecules. Triglycerides are the form in which digested fat that has been absorbed from the small intestine is transported in the bloodstream.

trigone (try-gohn) *n.* a triangular region of tissue, such as the triangular region of the wall of the bladder that lies between the openings of the two ureters and the urethra.

trigonitis (try-goh-**ny**-tis) *n.* inflammation of the trigone (base) of the urinary bladder. This can occur as part of a generalized cystitis or it can be associated with inflammation in the urethra, prostate, or neck (cervix) of the uterus.

trigonocephaly (try-gŏ-noh-**sef**-ăli) *n.* a deformity of the skull in which the vault of the skull is sharply angled just in front of the ears, giving the skull a triangular shape. **—trigonocephalic** (try-gŏ-noh-si-**fal**-ik) *adj.*

trihexyphenidyl (benzhexol) (try-hek-si-**fen**-i-dil) *n.* an antimuscarinic drug used mainly to reduce muscle tremor and rigidity in drug-induced parkinsonism. It is taken by mouth.

triiodothyronine (T_3) (try-I-oh-doh-**th'y**-rŏ-neen) *n. see* thyroid hormone.

trimeprazine (try-**mep**-ră-zeen) *n. see* alimemazine.

trimester (try-**mest**-er) *n.* (in obstetrics) any one of the three successive three-month periods into which a pregnancy may be divided.

trimethoprim (try-**meth**-oh-prim) *n.* an antibacterial drug that is active against a range of microorganisms. Administered by mouth, it is used mainly in the treatment of chronic urinary-tract infections, bronchitis, and *Pneumocystis* pneumonia. Trade name: **Trimopan**. *See also* co-trimoxazole.

trimipramine (try-**mip**-ră-meen) *n.* a tricyclic antidepressant drug that also possesses sedative properties. It is given by mouth for the treatment of depression. Trade name: **Surmontil**.

trinitrophenol (try-ny-troh-**fee**-nol) *n. see* picric acid.

triple test (**trip**-ŭl) *n.* a prenatal screening test for Down's syndrome and spina bifida; it can be performed between the 15th and 20th weeks of pregnancy but has largely been replaced by combined first-trimester PAPPA screening and nuchal translucency scanning. It measures levels of **alpha-fetoprotein (AFP)**, unconjugated oestriol (uE_3), and **human chorionic**

gonadotrophin (**hCG**) in maternal serum.

triploid (**trip**-loid) *adj.* describing cells, tissues, or individuals in which there are three complete chromosome sets. *Compare* diploid, haploid. —**triploid** *n.*

triptan (**trip**-tan) *n.* *see* $5HT_1$ agonist.

triquetrum (triquetral bone) (try-**kwee**-trŭm) *n.* a bone of the wrist (*see* carpus). It articulates with the ulna behind and with the pisiform, hamate, and lunate bones in the carpus.

trismus (**triz**-mŭs) *n.* spasm of the jaw muscles, keeping the jaws tightly closed. This is the characteristic symptom of tetanus but it also occurs as a sensitivity reaction to certain drugs and in disorders of the basal ganglia.

trisomy (**try**-soh-mi) *n.* a condition in which there is one extra chromosome present in each cell in addition to the normal (diploid) chromosome set; the cause of such disorders as Down's syndrome. —**trisomic** (try-**soh**-mik) *adj.*

tritanopia (try-tă-**noh**-piă) *n.* a rare defect of colour vision in which affected persons are insensitive to blue light and confuse blues and greens. *Compare* Daltonism, deuteranopia.

trocar (**troh**-kar) *n.* an instrument used in combination with a cannula to draw off fluids from a body cavity. It comprises a metal tube containing a removable shaft with a sharp three-cornered point.

trochanter (troh-**kant**-er) *n.* either of the two protuberances that occur below the neck of the femur.

troche (trohsh) *n.* a medicinal lozenge, taken by mouth, used to treat conditions of the mouth, throat, or alimentary canal.

trochlea (**trok**-li-ă) *n.* an anatomical part having the structure or function of a pulley; for example the fibrocartilaginous ring in the frontal bone through which the tendon of the superior oblique eye muscle passes. —**trochlear** (**trok**-li-er) *adj.*

trochlear nerve *n.* the fourth cranial nerve (IV), which supplies the superior oblique eye muscle.

trochoid joint (pivot joint) (**troh**-koid) *n.* a form of diarthrosis (freely movable joint) in which a bone moves round a central axis, allowing rotational movement.

troph- (tropho-) *combining form denoting* nourishment or nutrition.

trophic (**trof**-ik) *adj.* relating to nutrition or to the supply of nutrients, etc., to a part of the body. **t. ulcer** an ulcer due to insufficient supply of blood or nutrients to the affected part.

trophoblast (**trof**-ŏ-blast) *n.* the tissue that forms the wall of the blastocyst.

-trophy *combining form denoting* nourishment, development, or growth.

-tropic *combining form denoting* **1.** turning towards. **2.** having an affinity for; influencing.

tropical medicine (**trop**-ikăl) *n.* the study of diseases more commonly found in tropical regions than elsewhere, such as malaria, leprosy, trypanosomiasis, schistosomiasis, and leishmaniasis.

tropical ulcer (Naga sore) *n.* a skin disease prevalent in wet tropical regions. A large open sloughing sore usually develops at the site of a wound or abrasion. The ulcer is often infected with spirochaetes and bacteria and may extend deeply and cause destruction of muscles and bones.

tropicamide (trŏ-**pik**-ă-myd) *n.* an antimuscarinic drug used in the form of eye drops to dilate the pupil so that the inside of the eye can more easily be examined or operated upon. Trade name: **Mydriacyl**.

Trousseau's sign (troo-**sohz**) *n.* spasmodic contractions of muscles, especially the muscles of mastication, in response to nerve stimulation (e.g. by tapping). It is a characteristic sign of hypocalcaemia (*see* tetany). [A. Trousseau (1801–67), French physician]

TRT *n. see* tinnitus (retraining therapy).

truncus (**trunk**-ŭs) *n.* a trunk: a main vessel or other tubular organ from which subsidiary branches arise. **t. arteriosus** the main arterial trunk arising from the fetal heart. It develops into the aorta and pulmonary artery.

trunk (trunk) *n.* **1.** *see* truncus. **2.** the body excluding the head and limbs.

TRUS *n. see* (transrectal) ultrasonography.

truss (trus) *n.* a device for applying pressure to a hernia to prevent it from protruding. It usually consists of a pad attached to a belt worn under the clothing.

trust (trust) *n.* (in the NHS) a self-governing body that provides or commissions any of a range of health-care services, including hospital, community health, and mental health services. *See also* foundation trust.

trypanocide (trip-**an**-ŏ-syd) *n.* an agent that kills trypanosomes.

Trypanosoma (trip-ă-nŏ-**soh**-mă) *n. see* trypanosomiasis.

trypanosomiasis (trip-ă-nŏ-sŏ-**my**-ă-sis) *n.* any disease caused by the presence of parasitic protozoans of the genus *Trypanosoma*. The two most important diseases are Chagas' disease (**South American t.**), caused by *T. cruzi*, and sleeping sickness (**African t.**), caused by *T. rhodesiense* or *T. gambiense*.

trypsin (**trip**-sin) *n.* an enzyme that continues the digestion of proteins by breaking down peptones into smaller peptide chains (*see* peptidase). It is secreted by the pancreas in an inactive form, **trypsinogen**, which is converted in the duodenum to trypsin by the action of the enzyme enteropeptidase.

trypsinogen (trip-**sin**-ŏ-jin) *n. see* trypsin.

tryptophan (**trip**-tŏ-fan) *n.* an essential amino acid. *See also* amino acid.

T score *n.* a measure of bone mineral density used to evaluate the degree of bone thinning detected on DEXA scanning. An individual's T score is the number of standard deviations above or below the mean reference value for young healthy adults. By convention, a score above –1 is considered normal and a score below –2.5 indicates osteoporosis.

tsetse (tet-si) *n.* a large bloodsucking fly of tropical Africa belonging to the genus *Glossina*. Tsetse flies transmit the blood parasites that cause sleeping sickness, *Trypanosoma gambiense* and *T. rhodesiense*.

TSH *n. see* thyroid-stimulating hormone.

TSS *n. see* toxic shock syndrome.

tsutsugamushi disease (tsoo-tsoo-gă-**moo**-shi) *n. see* scrub typhus.

TT *n. see* tetanus toxoid.

TTTS *n. see* twin-to-twin transfusion syndrome.

T-tube *n.* a self-retaining T-shaped tube used in surgery to retain the patency of the common bile duct for postoperative drainage or to maintain an airway.

tubal occlusion (**tew**-bal) *n.* blocking of the Fallopian tubes. This is achieved by surgery as a means of sterilization; it is also a result of pelvic inflammatory disease.

tubal pregnancy (oviducal pregnancy) *n. see* ectopic pregnancy.

tube (tewb) *n.* (in anatomy) a long hollow cylindrical structure, e.g. a Fallopian tube.

tuber (**tew**-ber) *n.* (in anatomy) a thickened or swollen part.

tubercle (**tew**-ber-kŭl) *n.* **1.** (in anatomy) a small rounded protuberance on a bone. **2.** the specific nodular lesion of tuberculosis.

tubercular (tew-**ber**-kew-ler) *adj.* having small rounded swellings or nodules, not necessarily caused by tuberculosis.

tuberculide (tew-**ber**-kew-lyd) *n.* an eruption of the skin that arises in response to an internal focus of tuberculosis.

tuberculin (tew-**ber**-kew-lin) *n.* a protein extract from cultures of tubercle bacilli, used to test whether a person has suffered from or been in contact with tuberculosis (*see* Mantoux test).

tuberculoma (tew-ber-kew-**loh**-mă) *n.* a mass of cheeselike material resembling a tumour, seen in some cases of tuberculosis. Tuberculomas are found in a variety of sites, including the lung or brain.

tuberculosis (TB) (tew-ber-kew-**loh**-sis) *n.* an infectious disease caused by the bacillus *Mycobacterium tuberculosis* and characterized by the formation of nodular lesions (tubercles) in the tissues. In the most common form of the disease (**pulmonary t.**) the bacillus is inhaled into the lungs where it sets up a primary tubercle and spreads to the nearest lymph nodes (the **primary complex**). Many people become infected but show no symptoms. Others develop a chronic infection and can transmit the bacillus by coughing and sneezing. Symptoms of the active disease include fever, night sweats, weight loss, and the spitting of blood. In some cases the bacilli spread from the lungs to the bloodstream, setting up millions of tiny tubercles throughout the body (**miliary t.**). Bacilli entering by the mouth, usually in infected cows' milk, set up a primary complex in abdominal lymph nodes, leading to peritonitis, and sometimes spread to other organs, joints, and bones (*see* Pott's disease).

Tuberculosis is curable by various combinations of the antibiotics streptomycin, ethambutol, isoniazid (INH), rifampicin, and pyrazinamide. Preventive measures in the UK include the detection of cases by X-ray screening of vulnerable populations and vaccination with BCG vaccine. *See also* directly observed therapy.

SEE WEB LINKS

- Explanation of TB from Public Health England

tuberculous (tew-**ber**-kew-lŭs) *adj.* relating to or affected with tuberculosis.

tuberose (**tew**-ber-ohz) *adj. see* tuberous.

tuberosity (tew-ber-**os**-iti) *n.* a large rounded protuberance on a bone.

tuberous (tuberose) (**tew**-ber-ŭs) *adj.* knobbed; having nodules or rounded swellings. **t. sclerosis (epiloia, Bourneville's disease)** a hereditary disorder in which the brain, eyes, skin, and other organs are studded with small plaques or tumours. Symptoms include epilepsy, learning difficulties, and behavioural disorders.

tubo- *combining form denoting* a tube, especially a Fallopian tube or the Eustachian tube.

tuboabdominal (tew-boh-ab-**dom**-inăl) *adj.* relating to or occurring in a Fallopian tube and the abdomen.

tubo-ovarian (tew-boh-oh-**vair**-iăn) *adj.* relating to or occurring in a Fallopian tube and an ovary.

tubotympanal (tew-boh-**timp**-ăn-ăl) *adj.* relating to the tympanic cavity and the Eustachian tube.

tubular necrosis *n.* localized death of renal tubules. **acute t. n. (ATN)** tubular necrosis, usually as a result of ischaemia, in which urine flow is reduced and renal failure can develop.

tubule (**tew**-bewl) *n.* (in anatomy) a small cylindrical hollow structure. *See also* renal (tubule), seminiferous tubule. **—tubular** (**tew**-bew-ler) *adj.*

tularaemia (rabbit fever) (tew-lă-**ree**-miă) *n.* a disease of rodents and rabbits, caused by the bacterium *Francisella tularensis*, that may be transmitted to humans. Symptoms include an ulcer at the site of infection, inflamed and ulcerating lymph nodes, headache, aching pains, loss of weight, and a fever lasting several weeks. Treatment with chloramphenicol, streptomycin, or tetracycline is effective.

tulle gras (tewl grah) *n.* a soft dressing consisting of open-woven silk (or other material) impregnated with a waterproof soft paraffin wax.

tumefaction (tew-mi-**fak**-shŏn) *n.* the process in which a tissue becomes swollen and tense by accumulation within it of fluid under pressure.

tumescence (tew-**mes**-ĕns) *n.* a swelling, or the process of becoming swollen, usually because of an accumulation of blood or other fluid within the tissues.

tumid (tew-mid) *adj.* swollen.

tumor (tew-mer) *n.* swelling: one of the four classical signs of inflammation in a tissue. *See also* calor, dolor, rubor.

tumour (tew-mer) *n.* any abnormal swelling in or on a part of the body. The term is usually applied to an abnormal growth of tissue, which may be benign or malignant. *Compare* cyst.

tumour marker *n.* a substance produced by a tumour that can be used to aid detection of the tumour and to monitor its size and the effects of treatment. An example is alpha-fetoprotein.

tumour necrosis factor (TNF) either of two proteins, TNF-α (produced mainly by monocytes and macrophages) or TNF-β (produced by lymphoid cells), that act as mediators for immune responses. Among their many actions is destruction of tumour cells.

tunica (tew-nik-ă) *n.* a covering or layer of an organ or part; for example, a layer of the wall of a blood vessel (*see* adventitia, intima, media).

tunnel (tun-ĕl) *n.* (in anatomy) a canal or hollow groove.

tunnel vision *n.* a visual-field defect in which only the central area of the visual field remains. It occurs in advanced glaucoma.

turbinate bone (ter-bin-ayt) *n. see* nasal (concha).

turbinectomy (ter-bin-ek-tŏmi) *n.* the surgical removal (total or partial) of one of the turbinate bones, performed to treat nasal obstruction.

turgescence (ter-jes-ĕns) *n.* a swelling, or the process by which a swelling arises in tissues, usually by the accumulation of blood or other fluid under pressure.

turgid (ter-jid) *adj.* swollen and congested, especially with blood.

turgor (ter-ger) *n.* a state of being swollen or distended.

Turner syndrome (ter-ner) *n.* a genetic defect in women in which there is only one X chromosome instead of the usual two. Affected women are infertile: they have female external genitalia but their ovaries fail to develop normally, resulting in absence of menstrual periods. Characteristically they are short and have variable developmental defects. [H. H. Turner (1892–1970), US endocrinologist]

TURP *n.* transurethral resection of the prostate: *see* resection.

turricephaly (tu-ri-sef-ăli) *n. see* oxycephaly.

tussis (tus-iss) *n. see* coughing.

TUVP *n. see* transurethral (vaporization of the prostate).

TV *n. see* tidal volume.

TVT *n. see* tension-free vaginal tape.

twins (twinz) *pl. n.* two individuals who are born at the same time and of the same parents. **dizygotic** (or **fraternal**) **t.** twins resulting from the simultaneous fertilization of two egg cells; they may be of different sexes and are no more alike than ordinary siblings. **monozygotic** (or **identical**) **t.** twins resulting from the fertilization of a single egg cell that subsequently divides to give two separate fetuses. They are of the same sex and otherwise genetically identical. *See also* conjoined twins.

twin-to-twin transfusion syndrome (TTTS) *n.* a condition in which communicating vessels in the shared placenta of identical twins that share a chorion divert blood to one fetus (the recipient) from the other (the donor), resulting in one fetus with increased blood volume and one anaemic fetus.

tylosis (ty-**loh**-sis) *n.* focal keratosis occurring especially on the palms and soles. It occurs early in life and is inherited as an autosomal dominant.

tympan- (tympano-) *combining form denoting* **1.** the eardrum. **2.** the middle ear.

tympanic cavity (tim-**pan**-ik) *n. see* middle ear.

tympanic membrane (eardrum) *n.* the membrane at the inner end of the external auditory meatus, separating the outer and middle ears. When sound waves reach the ear the tympanum vibrates, transmitting these vibrations to the malleus.

tympanites (meteorism) (timp-ă-**ny**-teez) *n.* distension of the abdomen with air or gas: the abdomen is resonant on percussion. Causes include intestinal obstruction, functional bowel disorder, and aerophagy.

tympanoplasty (**timp**-ă-noh-plasti) *n.* surgical repair of defects of the eardrum and middle ear ossicles. *See* myringoplasty.

tympanotomy (timp-ă-**not**-ŏmi) *n.* a surgical operation to expose the middle ear and allow access to the ossicles.

tympanum (**timp**-ă-nŭm) *n.* the middle ear (tympanic cavity) and/or the eardrum (tympanic membrane).

typho- *combining form denoting* **1.** typhoid fever. **2.** typhus.

typhoid fever (**ty**-foid) *n.* an infection of the digestive system by the bacterium *Salmonella typhi*, causing general weakness, headache, high fever, a rash (rose spots) on the chest and abdomen, chills, and sweating; in serious cases inflammation of the spleen and bones, delirium, and intestinal haemorrhage may occur. It is transmitted through contaminated food or drinking water. Treatment is usually with antibiotics, such as ciprofloxacin or cefotaxime. Vaccines providing temporary immunity are available. *Compare* paratyphoid fever.

typhus (spotted fever) (**ty**-fŭs) *n.* any one of a group of infections caused by rickettsiae and characterized by severe headache, a widespread rash, prolonged high fever, and delirium. They all respond to treatment with chloramphenicol or tetracyclines. The rickettsiae may be transmitted by lice (**epidemic**, **classical**, or **louse-borne t.**); rat fleas (**endemic**, **murine**, or **flea-borne t.**); ticks (*see* Rocky Mountain spotted fever); or mites (*see* rickettsial pox, scrub typhus).

tyramine (ty-ră-meen) *n.* an amine naturally occurring in cheese. It has a similar effect in the body to that of adrenaline. This effect can be dangerous in patients taking MAO inhibitors (antidepressants), in whom blood pressure may become very high.

tyrosine (ty-roh-seen) *n.* *see* amino acid.

tyrosinosis (ty-roh-si-**noh**-sis) *n.* an inborn defect of metabolism of the amino acid tyrosine causing excess excretion of parahydroxyphenylpyruvic acid in the urine.

Uu

UC *n.* *see* (ulcerative) colitis.

ulcer (**ul**-ser) *n.* a break in the skin or in the mucous membrane lining the alimentary tract that fails to heal and is often accompanied by inflammation. **arterial u.** a skin ulcer due to inadequate arterial blood supply, usually seen on the feet of patients with severe atheromatous narrowing of the arteries in the legs. **decubitus u.** *see* pressure sore. **rodent u.** *see* basal cell carcinoma. **venous** (or **hypostatic** or **varicose**) **u.** the most common type of skin ulcer, occurring on the legs and caused by increased venous pressure. It most commonly affects older women. *See also* aphthous ulcer, dendritic ulcer, duodenal ulcer, gastric (ulcer), peptic (ulcer), stress (ulcer).

ulcerative colitis (**ul**-ser-ay-tiv) *n.* *see* colitis.

ulcerative gingivitis (Vincent's angina) *n.* acute painful inflammation and ulceration of the gums associated with infection by the microorganisms *Fusobacterium* and *Bacteroides*.

ule- (ulo-) *combining form denoting* **1.** scars; scar tissue. **2.** the gums.

ulna (**ul**-nă) *n.* the inner and longer bone of the forearm. It articulates with the humerus and radius above and with the radius and indirectly with the wrist bones below. **—ulnar** (**ul**-ner) *adj.*

ulnar artery *n.* a branch of the brachial artery arising at the elbow and running deep within the muscles of the medial side of the forearm to the palm of the hand.

ulnar nerve *n.* one of the major nerves of the arm. It originates in the neck and runs down the inner side of the upper arm to behind the elbow. It supplies the muscles of the forearm and the skin of the palm and fourth and fifth fingers.

ultra- *prefix denoting* **1.** beyond. **2.** an extreme degree (e.g. of large or small size).

ultradian (ul-**tray**-diăn) *adj.* denoting a biological rhythm or cycle that occurs more frequently than once in 24 hours.

ultrafiltration (ultră-fil-**tray**-shŏn) *n.* filtration under pressure. In the kidney, blood is subjected to ultrafiltration to remove the waste material that goes to make up urine.

ultramicroscopic (ultră-my-krŏ-**skop**-ik) *adj.* too small to be seen by means of an ordinary light microscope.

ultrasonics (ultră-**sonn**-iks) *n.* the study of the uses and properties of ultrasound. **—ultrasonic** *adj.*

ultrasonography (sonography) (ultră-sonn-**og**-răfi) *n.* the use of ultrasound to produce images of structures in the human body. The ultrasound probe sends out a short pulse of high-frequency sound and detects the reflected waves (echoes) occurring at interfaces within the organs. The direction of the pulse can then be moved across the area of interest with each pulse to build up a complete image. As far as is known, there are no significant adverse effects from the use of ultrasound at diagnostic energies. Ultrasonography is used extensively in obstetrics and also to examine the abdominal organs, urinary tract, blood vessels, muscles, and tendons. **transrectal u.** (**TRUS**) ultrasonography for examination of the prostate gland and seminal vesicle, in which the ultrasound probe is placed through the anus to lie directly behind these structures. **transvaginal u.** ultrasonography using a vaginal probe, which provides a detailed anatomy of the female pelvis and early accurate identification of fetal structures. *See also* Doppler ultrasound.

SEE WEB LINKS

- Further explanation of the procedure from CancerHelp UK

ultrasound (ultrasonic waves) (ul-tră-sownd) *n.* sound waves of high frequency (above 20 kHz), inaudible to the human ear. Ultrasound in the range 2–20 MHz can be used to produce images of the interior of the body as the waves reflect off structures back to the probe (*see* ultrasonography). The vibratory effect of ultrasound can also be used to break up stones (*see* lithotripsy) and cataracts (*see* phacoemulsification), to remove calculus from the teeth, to destroy tumours (**high-intensity focused u.**; **HIFU**), and in the treatment of rheumatic conditions.

ultrasound marker (mark-er) *n.* the appearance, on ultrasonography of a pregnant uterus, of a feature suggesting a structural or chromosomal abnormality in the fetus. An example is increased nuchal translucency (*see* nuchal (translucency scanning)).

ultraviolet radiation (UV) (ultră-vy-ŏ-lit) *n.* invisible short-wavelength radiation beyond the violet end of the visible spectrum, which is emitted by the sun. **UVA** UV radiation in the range 310–400 nm, which is not filtered by the atmosphere and penetrates deeply into the skin, causing age-related wrinkling and drug-induced photosensitivity reactions and contributing to the development of skin cancer. **UVB** UV radiation in the range 280–310 nm, which is largely filtered by the atmosphere. Depending on its strength, it causes suntan and sunburn and contributes to the development of skin cancer.

umbilical cord (um-**bil**-ikăl) *n.* the strand of tissue connecting the fetus to the placenta. It contains two arteries that carry blood to the placenta and one vein that returns it to the fetus.

umbilicated (um-**bil**-i-kayt-id) *adj.* having a navel-like depression.

umbilicus (omphalus) (um-**bil**-ikŭs) *n.* the navel: a circular depression in the centre of the abdomen marking the site of attachment of the umbilical cord in the fetus. **—umbilical** *adj.*

umbo (**um**-boh) *n.* a projecting centre of a round surface, especially the projection of the inner surface of the eardrum to which the malleus is attached.

unciform bone (**un**-si-form) *n. see* hamate bone.

uncinate fits (**un**-sin-ayt) *pl. n.* a form of temporal lobe epilepsy in which hallucinations of taste and smell and inappropriate chewing movements are prominent features.

unconscious (un-**kon**-shŭs) *adj.* **1.** in a state of unconsciousness. **2.** (in psychoanalysis) denoting the part of the mind that includes memories, motives, and intentions that are not accessible to awareness and cannot be made conscious without overcoming resistances. *Compare* subconscious.

unconsciousness (un-**kon**-shŭs-nis) *n.* a condition of being unaware of one's surroundings, as in sleep, or of being unresponsive to stimulation. An unnatural state of unconsciousness may be caused by factors that produce reduced brain activity, such as lack of oxygen or head injuries, or it may be brought about deliberately during general anaesthesia. *See also* coma.

uncus (**unk**-ŭs) *n.* any hook-shaped structure, especially a projection of the lower surface of the cerebral hemisphere.

undecenoates (un-des-i-**noh**-ayts) *pl. n.* antifungal agents (undecenoic acid and zinc undecenoate), applied to the skin in the form of powder, cream, or aerosol spray for the treatment of athlete's foot. Trade name: **Mycota**.

undine (**un**-deen) *n.* a small rounded container, usually made of glass, for solutions used to wash out the eye. It has a small neck for filling and a long tapering spout with a narrow outlet.

undulant fever (**un**-dew-lănt) *n. see* brucellosis.

ungual (**ung**-wăl) *adj.* relating to the fingernails or toenails (ungues).

unguentum (ung-**wen**-tŭm) *n.* (in pharmacy) an ointment.

unguis (**ung**-wis) *n.* a fingernail or toenail. *See* nail.

uni- *combining form denoting* one.

unicellular (yoo-ni-**sel**-yoo-ler) *adj.* describing organisms or tissues that consist of a single cell.

unilateral (yoo-ni-**lat**-erăl) *adj.* (in anatomy) relating to or affecting one side of the body or one side of an organ or other part.

union (**yoon**-yŏn) *n.* (in a fractured bone) the successful result of healing of a fracture, in which the bone ends have become firmly united by newly formed bone. *Compare* malunion.

uniovular (yoo-ni-**ov**-yoo-ler) *adj.* derived from a single ovum, as are identical twins. *Compare* binovular.

unipolar (yoo-ni-**poh**-ler) *adj.* (in neurology) describing a neuron that has one main process extending from the cell body. *Compare* bipolar.

Unna's paste (**oo**-năz) *n.* a dressing for varicose ulcers consisting of a mixture of zinc oxide, gelatin, and glycerine, applied between layers of a spiral bandage. [P. G. Unna (1850–1929), German dermatologist]

UPPP *n.* *see* uvulopalatopharyngoplasty.

urachus (yoor-ă-kŭs) *n.* the remains of the cavity of the allantois. It usually disappears during embryonic development, leaving a solid fibrous cord connecting the bladder with the umbilicus. —**urachal** *adj.*

uracil (yoor-ă-sil) *n.* one of the nitrogen-containing bases (*see* pyrimidine) occurring in the nucleic acid RNA.

uraemia (yoor-ee-miă) *n.* the presence of excessive amounts of urea and other nitrogenous waste compounds in the blood. This occurs in kidney failure and results in nausea, vomiting, lethargy, drowsiness, and eventually (if untreated) death. Treatment may require dialysis or transplantation. —**uraemic** *adj.*

uran- (urano-) *combining form denoting* the palate.

urataemia (yoor-ă-tee-miă) *n.* the presence in the blood of sodium urate and other urates, formed by the reaction of uric acid with bases. *See also* gout.

urate (yoor-ayt) *n.* a salt of uric acid, normally present in the urine. Excess amounts occur in the joints in gout.

uraturia (yoor-ăt-yoor-iă) *n.* the presence in the urine of urates. Abnormally high concentrations of urates in urine occur in gout.

urea (yoor-ee-ă) *n.* the main breakdown product of protein metabolism. It is the chemical form in which unrequired nitrogen is excreted by the body in the urine. Urea is formed in the liver from ammonia and carbon dioxide.

urease (yoor-i-ayz) *n.* an enzyme that catalyses the hydrolysis of urea to ammonia and carbon dioxide.

urecchysis (yoor-ek-i-sis) *n.* the escape of uric acid from the blood into spaces in the connective tissue.

uresis (yoor-ee-sis) *n.* *see* urination.

ureter (yoor-ee-ter) *n.* either of a pair of tubes, 25–30 cm long, that conduct urine from the pelvis of kidneys to the bladder. —**ureteral, ureteric** (yoor-i-te-rik) *adj.*

ureter- (uretero-) *combining form denoting* the ureter(s).

ureterectomy (yoor-i-ter-ek-tŏmi) *n.* surgical removal of a ureter. This usually includes removal of the associated kidney as well (*see* nephroureterectomy).

ureteritis (yoor-i-ter-I-tis) *n.* inflammation of the ureter. This usually occurs in association with cystitis, particularly if caused by vesicoureteric reflux.

ureterocele (yoor-ee-ter-oh-seel) *n.* a cystic swelling of the wall of the ureter at the point where it passes into the bladder. It may be associated with stenosis of the opening of the ureter and it may cause impaired drainage of the kidney with dilatation of the ureter and hydronephrosis.

ureteroenterostomy (yoor-ee-ter-oh-en-ter-ost-ŏmi) *n.* an artificial communication that is surgically created between the ureter and the bowel. *See also* ureterosigmoidostomy.

ureterolith (yoor-**ee**-ter-oh-lith) *n.* a stone in the ureter. *See* calculus, ureterolithotomy.

ureterolithotomy (yoor-ee-ter-oh-lith-**ot**-ŏmi) *n.* the surgical removal of a stone (calculus) from the ureter. If the stone occupies the lower portion of the ureter, it may be extracted by cystoscopy, thus avoiding open surgery.

ureterolysis (yoor-i-ter-**ol**-i-sis) *n.* an operation to free one or both ureters from surrounding abnormal adhesions or fibrous tissue.

ureteroneocystostomy (yoor-ee-ter-oh-nee-oh-sist-**ost**-ŏmi) *n.* the surgical reimplantation of a ureter into the bladder. This is most commonly performed to cure vesicoureteric reflux.

ureteronephrectomy (yoor-ee-ter-oh-ni-**frek**-tŏmi) *n. see* nephroureterectomy.

ureteroplasty (yoor-**ee**-ter-oh-plasti) *n.* surgical reconstruction of the ureter using a segment of bowel or a tube of bladder.

ureteropyelonephritis (yoor-ee-ter-oh-py-ĕ-loh-ni-**fry**-tis) *n.* inflammation involving both the ureter and the renal pelvis (*see* pyelitis, ureteritis).

ureteroscope (yoor-**ee**-ter-ŏ-skohp) *n.* a rigid or flexible instrument that can be passed into the ureter and up into the pelvis of the kidney. It is most commonly used to visualize a stone in the ureter and remove it safely under direct vision with a stone basket or forceps. Larger stones need to be fragmented before removal with an ultrasound probe, lithoclast, or lasers.

ureteroscopy (yoor-i-ter-**ŏs**-kŏ-pi) *n.* inspection of the lumen of the ureter with a ureteroscope.

ureterosigmoidostomy (yoor-ee-ter-oh-sig-moid-**ost**-ŏmi) *n.* the operation of implanting the ureters into the sigmoid colon. This method of permanent urinary diversion may be used after cystectomy or to bypass a diseased or damaged bladder. The urine is passed together with the faeces, avoiding the need for an external opening and appliance to collect the urine.

ureterostomy (yoor-i-ter-**ost**-ŏmi) *n.* the surgical creation of an external opening from the ureter. This usually involves bringing the ureter to the skin surface via a stent through the abdominal wall, so that the urine can drain into a suitable appliance (**cutaneous u.**).

ureterotomy (yoor-i-ter-**ot**-ŏmi) *n.* surgical incision into the ureter, most commonly performed in ureterolithotomy.

ureterovaginal (yoor-ee-ter-oh-vă-**jy**-năl) *adj.* relating to or between the ureter and vagina.

urethr- (urethro-) *combining form denoting* the urethra.

urethra (yoor-**ee**-thră) *n.* the tube that conducts urine from the bladder to the exterior. The female urethra is quite short (about 3.5 cm) and opens just within the vulva, between the clitoris and vagina. The male urethra is longer (about 20 cm) and runs through the penis. It also serves as the ejaculatory duct. —**urethral** *adj.*

urethritis (yoor-i-**thry**-tis) *n.* inflammation of the urethra, due either to infection or to the presence of a catheter in the urethra. The symptoms are those of urethral discharge with painful or difficult urination (dysuria). **nongonococcal** (or **nonspecific**) **u.** (**NGU**, **NSU**) urethritis due to a sexually transmitted infection other than gonorrhoea, often infection with *Chlamydia trachomatis*. **specific u.** urethritis due to gonorrhoea.

urethrocele (yoor-**ee**-throh-seel) *n.* prolapse of the urethra into the vaginal wall, which may be small and without symptoms or may cause a bulbous swelling to appear in the vagina, particularly on straining. The condition is associated with previous childbirth. Treatment, which is not usually required for small urethroceles, involves surgical repair of the lax tissues.

urethrography (yoor-i-**throg**-răfi) *n.* X-ray examination of the urethra, after introduction of a contrast medium, so that its outline and any narrowing or other abnormalities may be observed in X-ray images (**urethrograms**).

urethroplasty (yoor-**ee**-throh-plasti) *n.* surgical repair of the urethra, especially a urethral stricture. **Anastomotic urethroplasty** is used for a short stricture; the area of narrowing is excised and the two adjacent ends are joined directly to each other. A **substitution urethroplasty** entails the insertion of a flap or patch of skin from the scrotum or perineum into the urethra at the site of the stricture, which is laid widely open. **transpubic u.** surgical repair of a ruptured posterior urethra following a fractured pelvis. Access to the damaged urethra is achieved by partial removal of the pubic bone.

urethrorrhaphy (yoor-i-**thro**-răfi) *n.* surgical restoration of the continuity of the urethra. This may be required following laceration of the urethra.

urethrorrhoea (yoor-ee-thrŏ-**ree**-ă) *n.* a discharge from the urethra. This is a symptom of urethritis.

urethroscope (yoor-**ee**-thrŏ-skohp) *n.* an endoscope, consisting of a fine tube fitted with a light and lenses, for examination of the interior of the male urethra. —**urethroscopy** (yoor-i-**throsk**-ŏpi) *n.*

urethrostenosis (yoor-ee-throh-sti-**noh**-sis) *n.* a stricture of the urethra.

urethrostomy (yoor-i-**throst**-ŏmi) *n.* the operation of creating an opening of the urethra in the perineum in men. This can be permanent, to bypass a severe stricture of the urethra in the penis, or it can form the first stage of a urethroplasty.

urethrotomy (yoor-i-**throt**-ŏmi) *n.* the operation of cutting a short stricture in the urethra. It is performed under direct vision with a **urethrotome**: a type of endoscope that consists of a sheath down which is passed a fine knife.

urge incontinence (erj) *n.* *see* incontinence.

urgency (**er**-jĕn-si) *n.* (in urology) a compelling desire to pass urine immediately; this may be associated with infection or incontinence (urge incontinence). *See* lower urinary tract symptoms.

-uria *combining form denoting* **1.** a condition of urine or urination. **2.** the presence of a specified substance in the urine.

uric acid (**yoor**-ik) *n.* a nitrogenous organic acid that is the end-product of nucleic acid metabolism and is a component of the urine. Excess uric acid is present in the blood of people suffering from gout.

uricosuric drug (yoor-i-koh-**sewr**-ik) *n.* a drug, such as probenecid or sulfinpyrazone, that increases the amount of uric acid excreted in the urine.

uridrosis (yoor-i-**droh**-sis) *n.* the presence of excessive amounts of urea in the sweat; when the sweat dries, a white flaky deposit of urea may remain on the skin. The phenomenon occurs in uraemia.

urin- (urino-, uro-) *combining form denoting* urine or the urinary system.

urinalysis (yoor-in-**al**-i-sis) *n.* the analysis of urine, using physical, chemical and microscopical tests, to determine the proportions of its normal constituents and to detect alcohol, drugs, sugar, blood, protein, or other abnormal constituents.

urinary bladder (**yoor**-in-er-i) *n. see* bladder.

urinary diversion (dy-**ver**-shŏn) *n.* any of various techniques for the collection and diversion of urine away from its usual excretory channels, after the bladder has been removed (*see* cystectomy) or bypassed. These techniques include ureterosigmoidostomy and the construction of an ileal conduit. *See also* continent diversion.

urinary tract *n.* the entire system of ducts and channels that conduct urine from the kidneys to the exterior. It includes the ureters, the bladder, and the urethra.

urination (micturition) (yoor-in-**ay**-shŏn) *n.* the periodic discharge of urine from the bladder through the urethra.

urine (**yoor**-in) *n.* the fluid excreted by the kidneys, which contains many of the body's waste products. It is the major route by which the end-products of nitrogen metabolism – urea, uric acid, and creatinine – are excreted. The other major constituent is sodium chloride. Biochemical analysis of urine (*see* urinalysis) is commonly used in the diagnosis of diseases; immunological analysis of urine is the basis of most pregnancy tests.

uriniferous tubule (yoor-in-**if**-er-ŭs) *n. see* renal (tubule).

urinogenital (urogenital) (yoor-in-oh-**jen**-it'l) *adj.* of or relating to the organs and tissues concerned with excretion and reproduction.

urinometer (yoor-in-**om**-it-er) *n.* a hydrometer for measuring the specific gravity of urine.

urobilin (yoor-oh-**by**-lin) *n. see* urobilinogen.

urobilinogen (yoor-oh-by-**lin**-ŏ-jin) *n.* a colourless product of the reduction of the bile pigment bilirubin. Urobilinogen is formed from bilirubin in the intestine by bacterial action. Part of it is reabsorbed and returned to the liver; part of it is excreted. When exposed to air, urobilinogen is oxidized to a brown pigment, **urobilin**.

urocele (**yoor**-oh-seel) *n.* a cystic swelling in the scrotum, containing urine that has escaped from the urethra. This may arise following urethral injury.

urochesia (yoor-oh-**kee**-ziă) *n.* the passage of urine through the rectum. This may follow a penetrating injury involving both the lower urinary tract and the bowel.

urochrome (**yoor**-oh-krohm) *n.* the pigment responsible for the colour of urine.

urodynamics (yoor-oh-dy-**nam**-iks) *n.* the investigation of the function of the lower urinary tract. It involves the recording of pressures within the bladder during filling and voiding by the use of special equipment that can also record urethral sphincter pressures. It is an essential investigation in the study of urinary incontinence.

urogenital (yoor-oh-**jen**-it'l) *adj. see* urinogenital.

urogram (**yoor**-oh-gram) *n.* an X-ray of the urinary tract or any part of it. It is usually obtained after the intravenous injection of a radiopaque substance (*see* (intravenous) urography) but the contrast medium can also be introduced percutaneously or, in the case of the bladder, transurethrally (for a **cystogram**; *see* cystography).

urography (yoor-**og**-răfi) *n.* radiological examination of the urinary tract. **CT u.** urography that involves a CT scan (*see* computerized tomography). CT urography without the injection of a contrast medium is now the preferred method of demonstrating the presence of stones in the urinary tract. CT urography with contrast is used to investigate haematuria, with the aim of excluding tumours of the renal pelvis, ureter, or bladder. **intravenous u.** (**IVU**) urography following the injection into a vein of a contrast medium, which is concentrated and excreted by the kidneys. **MR u.** urography using magnetic resonance imaging. An MR contrast medium is injected into a vein and passes to the kidneys and ureters, enabling images of thin sections to be obtained. *See also* cystography, pyelography, urethrography.

urokinase (yoor-oh-**ky**-nayz) *n.* an enzyme, produced by the kidney and also present in blood and urine, that activates the system involved in dissolving blood clots. It is administered by intravenous infusion to treat deep vein thrombosis, peripheral arterial disease, and pulmonary embolism. *See* plasminogen (activator). Trade name: **Syner-KINASE**.

urolith (**yoor**-oh-lith) *n.* a stone in the urinary tract. *See* calculus.

urology (yoor-**ol**-ŏji) *n.* the branch of medicine concerned with the study and treatment of diseases of the urinary tract. **—urological** (yoor-ŏ-**loj**-ikăl) *adj.* **—urologist** *n.*

ursodeoxycholic acid (er-soh-dee-oks-i-**koh**-lik) *n.* a drug (a bile acid) used to dissolve cholesterol gallstones and to treat primary biliary cirrhosis. It is administered by mouth. Trade names: **Destolit**, **Ursofalk**.

URT *n.* upper respiratory tract.

URTI *n.* upper respiratory tract infection.

urticaria (nettle rash, hives) (er-ti-**kair**-iă) *n.* an itchy rash resulting partly from the release of histamine by mast cells. Itchy weals appear rapidly and resolve spontaneously within hours. **Angio-oedema** occurs when the weals involve the deeper levels of the skin, resulting in swelling of the lips, eyes, or tongue, which may constitute a medical emergency. **acute u.** a common and immediate response to such allergens as seafood or nuts. **cholinergic u.** a condition in which very small weals are brought on by heat, exercise, or emotion. **chronic u.** a condition that is not allergic and may persist for years.

US *n.* ultrasound scan. *See* ultrasonography.

uter- (utero-) *combining form denoting* the uterus.

uterine (**yoo**-teryn) *adj.* of or relating to the uterus.

uterovesical (yoo-ter-oh-**ves**-ikăl) *adj.* relating to the uterus and bladder.

uterus (womb) (**yoo**-ter-ŭs) *n.* the part of the female reproductive tract that is specialized to allow the embryo to become implanted in its inner wall and to nourish the growing fetus from the maternal blood. The nonpregnant uterus is a pear-shaped organ, about 7.5 cm long, suspended in the pelvic cavity. The upper two thirds (body) is connected to the two Fallopian tubes and the narrower lower third (cervix) projects at its lower end into the vagina. **u. didelphys** double uterus: a congenital condition resulting from incomplete midline fusion of the two Müllerian ducts during early embryonic development. The usual result is a double uterus with one or two cervices and a single vagina. Complete failure of fusion results in a double uterus with double cervices and two separate vaginae.

UTI *n.* urinary tract infection.

utilization behaviour (yoo-til-I-zay-shŏn) *n.* the correct use of an object at an inappropriate time or in an inappropriate situation: indicative of frontal lobe lesions.

utilitarianism (yoo-til-i-**tair**-iăn-izm) *n.* the consequentialist theory that maximizing utility (the greatest good of the greatest number) has priority over other ethical considerations. Unadulterated utilitarian policies may sometimes threaten the rights of individuals and therefore need to be balanced by considerations of deontology. *See also* consequentialism.

utricle (utriculus) (**yoo**-trik-ŭl) *n.* **1.** the larger of the two membranous sacs within the vestibule of the ear. It contains a macula, which responds to gravity and relays information to the brain about the position of the head. **2.** a small sac (the **prostatic u.**) extending out of the urethra of the male into the substance of the prostate gland.

UVA *n.* *see* ultraviolet radiation.

UVB *n.* *see* ultraviolet radiation.

uvea (uveal tract) (yoo-vi-ă) *n.* the vascular pigmented layer of the eye, which lies beneath the outer layer (sclera). It consists of the choroid, ciliary body, and iris. —**uveal** *adj.*

uveitis (yoo-vi-**I**-tis) *n.* inflammation of any part of the uveal tract of the eye, either the iris (**iritis**), ciliary body (**cyclitis**), or choroid (**choroiditis**). All types may lead to visual impairment, and uveitis is an important cause of blindness.

uveoparotitis (uveoparotid fever) (yoo-vi-oh-pa-rŏ-**ty**-tis) *n.* inflammation of the uvea and swelling of the parotid salivary gland: one of the manifestations of the chronic disease sarcoidosis.

UVPP *n. see* uvulopalatopharyngoplasty.

uvula (yoov-yoo-lă) *n.* a small soft extension of the soft palate that hangs from the roof of the mouth above the root of the tongue. It is composed of muscle, connective tissue, and mucous membrane.

uvulectomy (staphylectomy) (yoov-yoo-**lek**-tŏmi) *n.* surgical removal of the uvula.

uvulitis (yoov-yoo-**ly**-tis) *n.* inflammation of the uvula.

uvulopalatopharyngoplasty (uvulopharyngopalatoplasty, UPPP, uvulovelopharyngoplasty, UVPP) (yoov-yoo-loh-pal-ă-toh-fă-**ring**-oh-plasti) *n.* a surgical operation to remove the uvula, part of the soft palate, and the tonsils in the treatment of snoring and obstructive sleep apnoea.

Vv

vaccination (vak-si-**nay**-shŏn) *n.* a means of producing immunity to a disease by using a vaccine. The name was applied originally only to treatment with vaccinia (cowpox) virus, which gives protection against cowpox and smallpox. However, it is now used synonymously with inoculation as a method of immunization against any disease.

vaccine (**vak**-seen) *n.* a special preparation of antigenic material that can be used to stimulate the development of antibodies and thus confer active immunity against a specific disease or number of diseases. It is usually given by injection but may be introduced into the skin through light scratches; for some diseases (e.g. polio), oral vaccines are available. Many vaccines are produced by culturing bacteria or viruses under conditions that lead to a loss of their virulence but not of their antigenic nature. Other vaccines consist of specially treated toxins (toxoids) or of dead bacteria that are still antigenic. *See* immunization.

vaccinia (vak-**sin**-iă) *n.* *see* cowpox.

vaccinotherapy (vak-sin-oh-**th'e**-ră-pi) *n.* the treatment of disease by the use of vaccines.

vacuole (**vak**-yoo-ohl) *n.* a space within the cytoplasm of a cell, formed by infolding of the cell membrane, that contains material taken in by the cell.

vacuum extractor (**vak**-yoo-ŭm) *n.* *see* ventouse.

vagal (**vay**-găl) *adj.* relating to the vagus nerve.

vagin- (vagino-) *combining form denoting* the vagina.

vagina (vă-**jy**-nă) *n.* the lower part of the female reproductive tract: a muscular tube, lined with mucous membrane, connecting the cervix of the uterus to the exterior. It receives the erect penis during coitus. **—vaginal** *adj.*

vaginismus (vaj-i-**niz**-mŭs) *n.* painful spasm of the muscles surrounding the vagina, usually in response to the vulva or vagina being touched. The condition may be associated with fear of or aversion to coitus; other causative factors include vaginal infection and postmenopausal vaginal dryness (*see* (atrophic) vaginitis).

vaginitis (vaj-i-**ny**-tis) *n.* inflammation of the vagina, which may be caused by infection (commonly with *Trichomonas vaginalis*), dietary deficiency, or poor hygiene. There is often itching (*see* pruritus), increased vaginal discharge, and pain on passing urine. **atrophic v.** postmenopausal vaginal thinning caused by a reduction in the circulating levels of oestrogens: a common cause of vaginal dryness.

vaginoplasty (colpoplasty) (vă-**jy**-noh-plasti) *n.* **1.** a tissue-grafting operation on the vagina. **2.** surgical reconstruction of the vagina.

vaginosis (bacterial vaginosis) (vaj-i-**noh**-sis) *n.* a common vaginal infection caused by overgrowth of certain bacteria that are normally present in the vagina (e.g. *Gardnerella vaginalis*).

vago- *combining form denoting* the vagus nerve.

vagotomy (vag-**ot**-ŏmi) *n.* the surgical cutting of any of the branches of the vagus nerve. This is usually performed to reduce secretion of acid and pepsin by the stomach in order to cure a peptic ulcer.

vagus nerve (vay-gŭs) *n.* the tenth cranial nerve (X), which supplies motor nerve fibres to the muscles of swallowing and parasympathetic fibres to the heart and organs of the chest cavity and abdomen. Sensory branches carry impulses from the viscera and the sensation of taste from the mouth.

valaciclovir (val-ă-**sik**-lŏ-veer) *n.* an antiviral drug, similar to aciclovir, used to treat herpes infections. It is taken by mouth. Trade name: **Valtrex**.

valgus (val-gŭs) *adj.* describing any deformity that displaces the distal end of a limb away from the midline. *See* hallux (valgus), knock-knee (genu valgum), talipes (valgus).

validity (vă-**lid**-iti) *n.* an indication of the extent to which a measure (e.g. a clinical test) is a true indicator of what it purports to measure (e.g. a disease). Reduced validity can arise if the test produces different results when conducted several times on the same person under identical conditions.

valine (vay-leen) *n.* an essential amino acid. *See also* amino acid.

Valsalva manoeuvre (val-sal-vă) *n.* an attempt by a person to exhale forcibly with a closed glottis while pinching the nose and keeping the mouth closed, so that no air exits through the mouth or nose. The resulting increased pressure transplants air through the Eustachian tube, thus equalizing the negative pressure in the middle ear. This manoeuvre can often relieve the ear pain associated with flying, which is usually associated with changes in pressure. [A. M. Valsalva (1666–1723), Italian anatomist]

valsartan (val-sar-tan) *n.* *see* angiotensin II antagonist.

valve (valv) *n.* a structure found in some tubular organs or parts that restricts the flow of fluid within them to one direction only (*see* cusp). Valves are important structures in the heart, veins (*see* vein), and lymphatic vessels. *See also* aortic valve, mitral valve, pulmonary (valve), tricuspid valve.

valvoplasty (val-voh-plasti) *n.* *see* valvuloplasty.

valvotomy (valvulotomy) (val-**vot**-ŏmi) *n.* surgical cutting through a valve. The term is usually used to describe an operation to relieve obstruction caused by stenosed valves in the heart.

valvula (val-vew-lă) *n.* (*pl.* **valvulae**) a small valve. **valvulae**

conniventes circular folds of mucous membrane in the small intestine.

valvulitis (val-vew-**ly**-tis) *n.* inflammation of one or more valves, particularly the heart valves. This is most often due to rheumatic fever (*see* endocarditis).

valvuloplasty (valvoplasty) (**val**-vew-loh-plasti) *n.* therapeutic dilatation of a narrowed heart valve using balloon catheters threaded into the heart via the venous or arterial system (**balloon v.**).

vancomycin (vank-oh-**my**-sin) *n.* an antibiotic that is effective against most Gram-positive organisms and is used for treating serious infections due to strains that are resistant to other antibiotics. It is usually administered by intravenous infusion but given by mouth for treating pseudomembranous colitis. Trade name: **Vancocin**.

van den Bergh's test (van-den-**bergz**) *n.* a test to determine whether jaundice in a patient is due to haemolysis or to disease of the liver or bile duct. [A. A. H. van den Bergh (1869–1943), Dutch physician]

vanillylmandelic acid (VMA) (van-i-lil-man-**del**-ik) *n.* a metabolite of catecholamines excreted in abnormal amounts in the urine in conditions of excess catecholamine production, such as phaeochromocytoma. Measurement of VMA levels was formerly used as a screening test for phaeochromocytoma; in the UK this has been largely superseded by the urinary metanephrine test.

vaporizer (vay-per-I-zer) *n.* a piece of equipment for producing an extremely fine mist of liquid droplets by forcing a jet of liquid through a narrow nozzle with a jet of air. *See also* aerosol.

Vaquez-Osler disease (vak-ay **ohs**-ler) *n. see* polycythaemia (vera). [L. H. Vaquez (1860–1936), French physician; Sir W. Osler (1849–1919), Canadian physician]

variable (**vair**-i-ă-bŭl) *n.* a characteristic relating to an individual or group that is subject to variation. **continuous v.** a variable found at any point on a numerical scale (e.g. weight). **dependent v.** the variable in a study or experiment that is controlled by the independent variable and measured to determine the outcome of the study. **discrete v.** a variable found only at a fixed point on a numerical scale (e.g. body weight). **independent v.** the variable in a study or experiment that is manipulated in order to define the conditions of the study. **qualitative v.** a descriptive characteristic, such as sex, race, or occupation. **quantitative v.** a variable relating to a numerical scale, which may be continuous or discrete.

variance (**vair**-i-ăns) *n.* (in statistics) *see* standard deviation.

variant Creutzfeldt-Jakob disease (vCJD) (**vair**-i-ănt) *n. see* Creutzfeldt-Jakob disease.

varicectomy (va-ri-**sek**-tŏmi) *n. see* phlebectomy.

varicella (va-ri-**sel**-ă) *n. see* chickenpox.

varices (**va**-ri-seez) *pl. n. see* varicose veins.

varicocele (va-ri-koh-seel) *n.* a collection of dilated veins in the spermatic cord. It usually produces no symptoms apart from occasional aching discomfort. In some cases varicocele is associated with testicular atrophy or oligospermia, which can be improved by surgical correction or radiological embolization of the varicocele (**varicocelectomy**).

varicose veins (va-ri-kohs) *pl. n.* veins that are distended, lengthened, and tortuous. The superficial veins of the legs are most commonly affected; other sites include the oesophagus (*see* oesophageal varices) and testes (*see* varicocele). There is an inherited tendency to varicose veins but obstruction to blood flow is responsible in some cases. Treatment includes elastic support and sclerotherapy, but stripping, excision, or laser treatment is required in some cases. Medical name: **varices**.

varicotomy (va-ri-kot-ŏmi) *n.* incision into a varicose vein (*see* phlebectomy).

variola (vă-ry-ŏ-lă) *n. see* smallpox.

varioloid (vair-i-ŏ-loid) **1.** *n.* a mild form of smallpox in people who have previously had smallpox or have been vaccinated against it. **2.** *adj.* resembling smallpox.

varix (vair-iks) *n.* (*pl.* **varices**) a single varicose vein.

varus (vair-ŭs) *adj.* describing any deformity that displaces the distal end of a limb towards the midline. *See* bow-legs (genu varum), hallux (varus), talipes (varus).

vas- (vaso-) *combining form denoting* **1.** vessels, especially blood vessels. **2.** the vas deferens.

vasa efferentia (vay-să ef-er-en-shiă) *pl. n.* (*sing.* **vas efferens**) the many small tubes that conduct spermatozoa from the testis to the epididymis.

vasa vasorum (vas-or-ŭm) *pl. n.* the tiny arteries and veins that supply the walls of blood vessels.

vascular (vas-kew-ler) *adj.* relating to or supplied with blood vessels. **v. endothelial growth factor** (**VEGF**) a growth factor that creates new blood vessels during embryonic development, following trauma, and to bypass blocked vessels, thus enhancing pre-existing blood supply. VEGF has a wide range of physiological functions, including wound healing and bone formation. **v. system** *see* cardiovascular system.

vascularization (vas-kew-ler-I-zay-shŏn) *n.* the development of blood vessels (usually capillaries) within a tissue.

vasculitis (angiitis) (vas-kew-ly-tis) *n.* a patchy inflammation of the walls of blood vessels that leads to damage and thrombosis.

vas deferens (vas def-er-ĕnz) *n.* (*pl.* **vasa deferentia**) either of a pair of ducts that conduct spermatozoa from the epididymis to the urethra on ejaculation.

vasectomy (vă-sek-tŏmi) *n.* the surgical operation of severing the vas deferens. Bilateral vasectomy results in sterility and is an increasingly popular means of birth control.

vaso- *combining form. see* vas-.

vasoactive (vay-zoh-ak-tiv) *adj.* affecting the diameter of blood vessels, especially arteries. Examples of vasoactive agents are emotion, pressure, carbon dioxide, and temperature. **v. intestinal peptide** *see* vip.

vasoconstriction (vay-zoh-kŏn-**strik**-shŏn) *n.* a decrease in the diameter of blood vessels, especially arteries.

vasoconstrictor (vay-zoh-kŏn-**strik**-ter) *n.* an agent that causes narrowing of the blood vessels and therefore a decrease in blood flow. Vasoconstrictors are alpha agonists (*see* sympathomimetic), used to raise the blood pressure in disorders of the circulation, shock, or severe bleeding and to maintain blood pressure during surgery (*see* ephedrine, metaraminol, phenylephrine). Some (e.g. ephedrine, xylometazoline) are used to treat nasal congestion.

vasodilatation (vay-zoh-dy-lă-**tay**-shŏn) *n.* an increase in the diameter of blood vessels, especially arteries.

vasodilator (vay-zoh-dy-**lay**-ter) *n.* a drug that causes widening of the blood vessels and therefore an increase in blood flow. Vasodilators are used to lower blood pressure in cases of hypertension. **coronary v.** a drug, such as glyceryl trinitrate, that increases the blood flow through the heart and is used to relieve and prevent angina. **peripheral v.** a drug, such as nifedipine, that affects blood flow to the limbs and is used to treat conditions due to poor circulation.

vaso-epididymostomy (vay-zoh-epi-did-i-**mos**-tŏmi) *n.* the operation of joining the vas deferens to the epididymis in a side-to-side manner in order to bypass an obstruction in the epididymis to the passage of sperm from the testis.

vasography (vayz-**og**-răfi) *n.* X-ray imaging of the vas deferens. A contrast medium is injected either into the exposed vas deferens at surgery, using a fine needle, or by inserting a catheter into the ejaculatory duct (which discharges semen from the vesicle into the vas deferens) via an endoscope.

vasoligation (vay-zoh-ly-**gay**-shŏn) *n.* the surgical tying of the vas deferens. This is performed to prevent infection spreading from the urinary tract causing recurrent epididymitis.

vasomotion (vay-zoh-**moh**-shŏn) *n.* an increase or decrease in the diameter of blood vessels, particularly the arteries. *See* vasoconstriction, vasodilatation.

vasomotor (vay-zoh-**moh**-ter) *adj.* controlling the muscular walls of blood vessels, especially arteries, and therefore their diameter. **v. centre** a collection of nerve cells in the medulla oblongata that brings about reflex changes in the rate of the heartbeat and in the diameter of blood vessels, so that the blood pressure can be adjusted. **v. nerve** any nerve, usually belonging to the autonomic nervous system, that controls the circulation of blood through blood vessels by its action on the muscle fibres within their walls or its action on the heartbeat. **v. symptoms** subjective sensations experienced by women around the time of the menopause, often described as explosions of heat (hot flushes), mostly followed by profuse sweating. Physiological changes include peripheral vasodilatation, tachycardia with normal blood pressure, and raised skin temperature with normal body temperature.

vasopressin (antidiuretic hormone, ADH) (vay-zoh-**press**-in) *n.* a hormone, released by the pituitary gland, that increases the reabsorption of water by the kidney and causes constriction of blood vessels. Vasopressin is administered by injection or intravenous infusion to treat diabetes insipidus and to control bleeding from oesophageal varices. Trade name: **Argipressin** (synthetic vasopressin).

vasopressor (vay-zoh-**press**-er) *adj.* stimulating the contraction of blood vessels and therefore bringing about an increase in blood pressure.

vasospasm (vay-zoh-spazm) *n. see* Raynaud's disease.

vasovagal (vay-zoh-vay-găl) *adj.* relating to the action of impulses in the vagus nerve on the circulation. The vagus reduces the rate at which the heartbeats, and so lowers its output. **v. attack** excessive activity of the vagus nerve, causing slowing of the heart and a fall in blood pressure, which leads to fainting. *See* syncope.

vasovasostomy (vay-zoh-vă-**sos**-tŏmi) *n.* the surgical operation of re-anastomosing the vas deferens after previous vasectomy: the reversal of vasectomy, undertaken to restore fertility. It is ideally performed using microsurgical techniques.

vasovesiculitis (vay-zoh-ve-sik-yoo-**ly**-tis) *n.* inflammation of the seminal vesicles and vas deferens. This usually occurs in association with prostatitis and causes pain in the perineum, groin, and scrotum and a high temperature.

vector (**vek**-ter) *n.* an animal, usually an insect or a tick, that transmits parasitic microorganisms – and therefore the diseases they cause – from person to person or from infected animals to human beings.

vegetation (vej-i-**tay**-shŏn) *n.* (in pathology) an abnormal outgrowth from a membrane. In ulcerative endocarditis, such outgrowths, consisting of fibrin with enmeshed blood cells, are found on the membrane lining the heart valves.

vegetative (**vej**-i-tă-tiv) *adj.* **1.** relating to growth and nutrition rather than to reproduction. **2.** functioning unconsciously; autonomic.

vegetative state *n.* the clinical condition of unawareness of the self or the environment. The patient breathes spontaneously and has a stable circulation and sleep/wake cycles. It results from extensive damage to the cerebral cortex and thalamus while the brainstem and hypothalamus remain intact. The commonest causes are traumatic brain injury (e.g. road-traffic accidents) and cardiopulmonary arrest. *Compare* locked-in syndrome. *See also* persistent vegetative state.

VEGF *see* vascular endothelial growth factor.

vehicle (vee-ikŭl) *n.* (in pharmacy) any substance, such as sterile water or dextrose solution, that acts as the medium in which a drug is administered.

vein (vayn) *n.* a blood vessel conveying blood towards the heart. All veins except the pulmonary vein carry deoxygenated blood from the tissues to the vena cava. Veins contain valves that assist the flow of blood back to the heart. (See illustrations.) Anatomical name: **vena**. —**venous** (vee-nŭs) *adj.*

Velcade (vel-kayd) *n.* *see* bortezomib.

vena cava (vee-nă **kay**-vă) *n.* (*pl.* **venae cavae**) either of the two main veins, conveying deoxygenated blood from the other veins to the right atrium of the heart. inferior v. c. (IVC) the vein that receives blood from parts of the body below the diaphragm. **superior v. c.** the vein that drains blood from the head, neck, thorax, and arms.

vene- (veno-) *combining form denoting* veins.

venene (ven-een) *n.* a mixture of two or more venoms: used to produce antiserum against venoms (antivenene).

venepuncture (venipuncture) (**ven**-i-punk-cher) *n.* the puncture of a vein for any therapeutic purpose; for example, to extract blood for laboratory tests. *See also* phlebotomy.

venereal disease (VD) (vin-eer-iăl) *n.* *see* sexually transmitted disease.

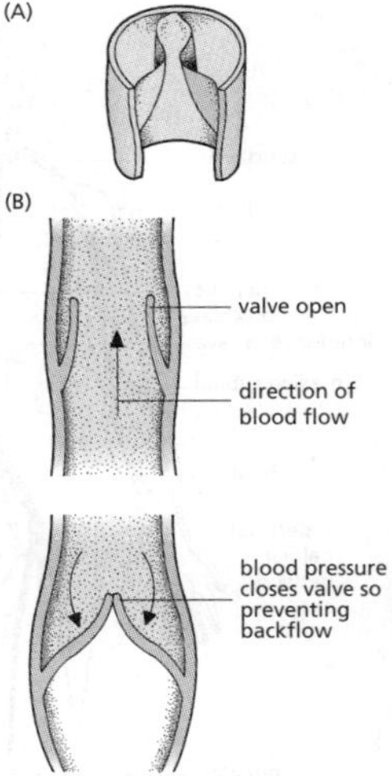

(A) cut vein showing the two cusps of a valve; (B) action of a venous valve

venesection (ven-i-**sek**-shŏn) *n.* *see* phlebotomy.

venlafaxine (ven-lă-**faks**-een) *n.* *see* SNRI.

veno- *combining form. see* vene-.

venoclysis (vi-**nok**-li-sis) *n.* the continuous infusion into a vein of saline or other solution.

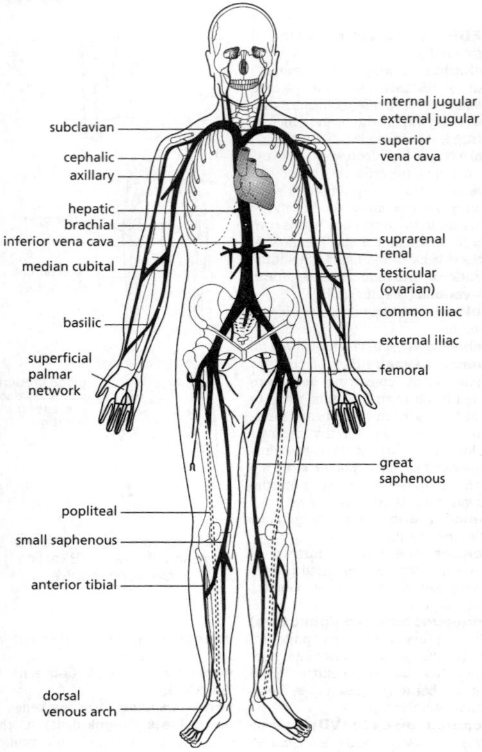

The principal veins of the body

venography (phlebography) (vi-**nog**-răfi) *n.* imaging of the anatomy of veins in a particular region of the body, commonly to demonstrate deep vein thrombosis in the legs. Traditionally, a radiopaque contrast medium is injected into a vein and X-ray photographs (**venograms**) are taken as the medium flows towards the heart. Venography can be carried out during a CT or MRI evaluation. **compression v.** an ultrasound technique to look for deep vein thrombosis. Pressing a healthy vein with the ultrasound probe usually causes it to empty and flatten, which does not occur if there is thrombus in the lumen. *See also* angiography.

venom (**ven**-ŏm) *n.* the poisonous material produced by snakes, scorpions, etc. Some venoms produce no more than local pain and swelling; others can prove lethal.

venous thromboembolism (VTE) (**vee**-nŭs) *n.* the formation of a blood clot in a vein, which may become detached and lodged elsewhere. It includes deep vein thrombosis (*see* phlebothrombosis) and pulmonary embolism. VTE is a the leading direct cause of maternal death. *See also* thromboembolism.

ventilation (ven-ti-**lay**-shŏn) *n.* **1.** the passage of air into and out of the respiratory tract. In the alveoli of the lungs gas exchange is most efficient when matched by an adequate blood flow (perfusion). Ventilation/perfusion imbalance is an important cause of anoxia and cyanosis. **2.** maintenance or support of the breathing movements of patients either by the insertion of an endotracheal tube (*see* intubation) or by noninvasive means (*see* noninvasive ventilation). *See also* ventilator.

ventilation-perfusion scanning (V/Q scanning) *n.* a nuclear medicine technique in which two different isotopes are used, one inhaled, to examine lung ventilation, and one injected, to examine lung perfusion. It is used to detect pulmonary embolism, in which the area of lung supplied by the blocked artery is not being perfused with blood but has normal ventilation.

ventilator (**ven**-ti-lay-ter) *n.* **1.** a device used to ensure a supply of fresh air. **2. (respirator)** equipment that is manually or mechanically operated to maintain a flow of air into and out of the lungs of a patient who is unable to breathe normally. **cuirass v.** a negative-pressure ventilator that encloses the chest. **Drinker v.** (**iron lung**) a negative-pressure ventilator that encloses the entire body except the head: replaced by the cuirass ventilator. **negative-pressure v.** an airtight container in which the air pressure is decreased and increased mechanically. This draws air into and out of the patient's lungs through the normal air passages. **positive-pressure v.** equipment that blows air into the patient's lungs; air is released from the lungs when the pressure from the ventilator is relaxed (*see* BiPAP, Nippy, noninvasive ventilation).

ventouse (vacuum extractor) (von-**toos**) *n.* a device to assist delivery consisting of a suction cup that is attached to the head of the fetus: traction is then applied slowly. It has now virtually replaced rotational obstetric forceps.

ventral (**ven**-trăl) *adj.* relating to or situated at or close to the front of the body or to the anterior part of an organ.

ventricle (**ven**-trik-ŭl) *n.* **1.** either of the two lower chambers of the heart. The left ventricle receives blood from the pulmonary vein and pumps it into the aorta. The right ventricle pumps blood from the venae cavae into the pulmonary artery. **2.** one of the four fluid-filled cavities within the brain. The paired first and second ventricles (lateral ventricles) communicate with the third ventricle. This leads to the fourth ventricle in the hindbrain, which is continuous with the spinal canal. Cerebrospinal fluid circulates through all the cavities.

ventricular (ven-**trik**-yoo-ler) *adj.* of or relating to one or more ventricles (of the brain or heart). **v. fibrillation** *see* fibrillation. **v. folds** *see* vocal folds. **v. septal defect** *see* septal defect. **v. tachycardia** *see* tachycardia.

ventriculitis (ven-trik-yoo-**ly**-tis) *n.* inflammation in the ventricles of the brain, usually caused by infection.

ventriculoatriostomy (ven-trik-yoo-loh-ay-tri-**ost**-ŏmi) *n.* an operation for the relief of raised pressure due to the build-up of cerebrospinal fluid that occurs in hydrocephalus.

ventriculography (ven-trik-yoo-**log**-răfi) *n.* X-ray examination of the ventricles of the brain or heart after the introduction of a contrast medium. This procedure has been largely made redundant by CT and MRI scanning.

ventriculoperitoneal shunt (ven-tri-kyoo-loh-pe-ri-tŏ-**nee**-ăl) *n.* *see* shunt.

ventriculoscopy (ven-trik-yoo-**losk**-ŏpi) *n.* observation of the ventricles of the brain through a fibre-optic instrument. *See* endoscope, fibre optics.

ventriculostomy (ven-trik-yoo-**lost**-ŏmi) *n.* an operation to introduce a hollow needle (cannula) into one of the lateral ventricles of the brain. This may be done to relieve raised intracranial pressure, to obtain cerebrospinal fluid for examination, or to introduce antibiotics or contrast material for X-ray examination.

ventro- *combining form denoting* **1.** ventral. **2.** the abdomen.

ventrosuspension (ventrofixation) (ven-troh-sus-**pen**-shŏn) *n.* surgical fixation of a displaced uterus to the anterior abdominal wall. This may be achieved by shortening the round ligaments at their attachment either to the uterus or to the abdominal wall.

venule (**ven**-yool) *n.* a minute vessel that drains blood from the capillaries.

VERA (**veer**-ră) *n.* a framework designed to improve communication between health-care professionals and patients with dementia. It consists of four stages—*v*alidation, *e*motion, *r*eassurance, and *a*ctivity—which help staff to acknowledge that their perception of reality may be different from that of their patients.

verapamil (vě-rap-ă-mil) *n.* a calcium-channel blocker administered by mouth or intravenous injection in the treatment of essential hypertension, angina, and arrhythmias. Trade names: **Cordilox**, **Securon**, **Univer**, **Verapress MR**, **Vertab SR**.

vermicide (verm-i-syd) *n.* a chemical agent used to destroy parasitic worms living in the intestine. *Compare* vermifuge.

vermiform appendix (verm-i-form) *n. see* appendix.

vermifuge (verm-i-fewj) *n.* any drug or chemical agent used to expel worms from the intestine. *See also* anthelmintic.

vermix (ver-miks) *n.* the vermiform appendix.

vernal conjunctivitis (ver-năl) *n. see* conjunctivitis.

Verner-Morrison syndrome (ver-ner mo-ri-sŏn) *n. see* VIPoma. [J. V. Verner (1927–), US physician; A. B. Morrison (1922–2008), Irish pathologist]

vernix caseosa (ver-niks kay-si-oh-să) *n.* the layer of greasy material that covers the skin of a fetus or newborn baby. It is produced by the sebaceous glands and contains skin scales and fine hairs.

verruca (plantar wart) (ver-oo-kă) *n.* (*pl.* **verrucae**) *see* wart.

verrucous carcinoma (ver-oo-kŭs) *n.* an indolent preinvasive wartlike carcinoma typically of the oral cavity, which is associated with chewing tobacco, and of the vulva.

version (ver-shŏn) *n.* a manoeuvre to alter the position of a fetus in the uterus to facilitate delivery. *See* cephalic version, podalic version.

vertebra (ver-tib-ră) *n.* (*pl.* **vertebrae**) one of the 33 bones of which the backbone is composed. Each vertebra typically consists of a **body**, from the back of which arises an arch of bone (the **vertebral** or **neural arch**) enclosing a cavity through which the spinal cord passes. Individual vertebrae are bound together by ligaments and intervertebral discs. See illustration. —**vertebral** (ver-tib-răl) *adj.*

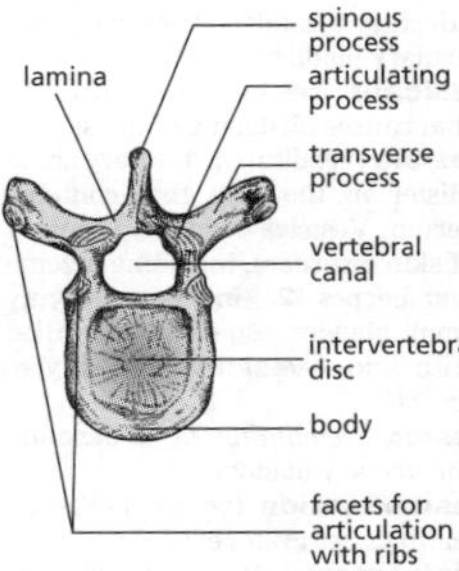

A typical thoracic vertebra (from above)

vertebral column *n.* *see* backbone.

vertex (ver-teks) *n.* the crown of the head.

vertical transmission (mother-to-child transmission) (ver-ti-kăl) *n.* transmission of an infection, such as HIV, hepatitis B, or hepatitis C, from mother to fetus via the placental circulation.

vertigo (vert-i-goh) *n.* a disabling sensation in which affected individuals feel that either they themselves or their surroundings are in a state of constant movement. It is a symptom of disease either in the labyrinth of the inner ear or in the vestibular nerve or its nuclei in the brainstem. *See also* benign paroxysmal positional vertigo.

very low-density lipoprotein (VLDL) *n.* *see* lipoprotein.

vesical (ves-ikăl) *adj.* relating to or affecting a bladder, especially the urinary bladder.

vesicant (ves-i-kănt) *n.* an agent that causes blistering of the skin.

vesicle (ves-ikŭl) *n.* **1.** a very small blister in the skin that contains serum. Vesicles occur in a variety of skin disorders, including eczema and herpes. **2.** (in anatomy) any small bladder, especially one filled with fluid. **—vesicular** (ves-ik-yoo-ler) *adj.*

vesico- *combining form denoting* the urinary bladder.

vesicofixation (ves-i-koh-fiks-ay-shŏn) *n.* *see* cystopexy.

vesicostomy (ves-i-kos-tŏmi) *n.* the surgical creation of an artificial channel between the bladder and the skin surface for the passage of urine. It is sometimes combined with closure of the urethra.

vesicoureteric reflux (VUR) (ves-i-koh-yoor-i-te-rik) *n.* the backflow of urine from the bladder into the ureters. It is classified into primary or congenital vesicoureteric reflux, which is due to defective valves, or secondary, which is due to another condition (e.g. neuropathic bladder). Infection may be conveyed to the kidneys, causing recurrent attacks of acute pyelonephritis and scarring of the kidneys in childhood.

vesicovaginal (ves-i-koh-vă-jy-năl) *adj.* relating to the bladder and vagina.

vesicular breath sounds *pl. n.* normal breath sounds, which may be increased or decreased in disease states.

vesicular mole *n.* *see* hydatidiform mole.

vesiculitis (ve-sik-yoo-ly-tis) *n.* inflammation of the seminal vesicles. *See* vasovesiculitis.

vesiculography (ve-sik-yoo-log-răfi) *n.* any technique for imaging the seminal vesicles. This is now usually performed either by injecting a contrast medium into the vas deferens during transrectal ultrasonography or by magnetic resonance imaging. Both these techniques are useful for investigation of patients with azoospermia.

vessel (ves-ĕl) *n.* a tube conveying a body fluid, especially a blood vessel or a lymphatic vessel.

vestibular glands (ves-tib-yoo-ler) *pl. n.* the two pairs of glands that open at the junction of the vagina and vulva. Their function is to lubricate the entrance to the vagina during coitus.

vestibular nerve *n.* the division of the vestibulocochlear nerve that carries impulses from the semicircular canals, utricle, and saccule of the inner ear, conveying information about posture, movement, and balance.

vestibular system *n.* those parts of the body involved in balance. The **peripheral vestibular system** (or **vestibular apparatus**) is in the inner ear. The **central vestibular system** comprises those parts of the brain that are involved in balance. It receives inputs from the ear, eyes, and proprioceptors.

vestibule (**vest**-i-bewl) *n.* (in anatomy) a cavity situated at the entrance to a hollow part. The vestibule of the ear is the cavity of the bony labyrinth that contains the saccule and utricle.

vestibulocochlear nerve (ves-tib-yoo-loh-**kok**-li-er) *n.* the eighth cranial nerve (VIII), responsible for carrying sensory impulses from the inner ear to the brain. It has two branches (*see* cochlear nerve, vestibular nerve).

vestigial (ves-**tij**-iăl) *adj.* existing only in a rudimentary form. The term is applied to organs whose structure and function have diminished during the course of evolution.

VF *n. see* (ventricular) fibrillation.

viable (**vy**-ăbŭl) *adj.* capable of living a separate existence. The legal age of viability of a fetus is 24 weeks, but some fetuses now survive birth at an even earlier gestational age due to advances in neonatal medicine.

Viagra (vy-**ag**-ră) *n. see* sildenafil.

Vibramycin (vy-bră-**my**-sin) *n. see* doxycycline.

Vibrio (**vib**-ri-oh) *n.* a genus of Gram-negative motile comma-shaped bacteria widely distributed in soil and water. **V. cholerae** the species that causes cholera.

vicarious (vik-**air**-iŭs) *adj.* describing an action or function performed by an organ not normally involved in the function. **v. menstruation** a rare disorder in which monthly bleeding occurs from places other than the vagina, such as the sweat glands, breasts, nose, or eyes.

videofluoroscopy (vid-i-oh-floo-er-**os**-kŏ-pi) *n.* the technique of viewing and recording real time X-ray investigation using a video camera (*see* real-time imaging). This enables the moving images to be reviewed at a later time, by individual frames or in slow motion.

videokeratography (vid-i-oh-ke-ră-**tog**-răfi) *n. see* (corneal) topography.

videokymography (vid-i-oh-ky-**mog**-răfi) *n.* a method of studying the vibration of the vocal folds of the larynx using high-speed digital photography. *See* laryngeal (stroboscopy).

video-otoscope (vid-i-oh-**oh**-toh-skohp) *n.* a small endoscope connected to a digital camera for examining the outer ear and eardrum.

villus (**vil**-ŭs) *n.* (*pl.* **villi**) one of many short finger-like processes that project from the surfaces of some membranes. **arachnoid v.** *see* arachnoid. **chorionic v.** any of the folds of the chorion from which the fetal part of the placenta is formed. They provide an extensive area for the exchange of oxygen, nutrients, etc., between maternal and fetal blood. *See* chorionic villus sampling. **intestinal v.** any of numerous projections that line the small intestine. Each contains a network of blood capillaries and a lacteal. Their function is to absorb the products of digestion and they greatly increase the surface area over which this can take place.

vinblastine (vin-**blas**-teen) *n. see* vinca alkaloid.

vinca alkaloid (ving-kă) *n.* one of a group of antimitotic drugs (*see* cytotoxic drug) derived from the periwinkle (*Vinca rosea*). Vinca alkaloids, usually administered intravenously, are used especially to treat leukaemias and lymphomas; they include **vinblastine** (Velbe), **vincristine** (Oncovin), and **vindesine** (Eldisine). They are highly toxic. *See also* vinorelbine.

Vincent's angina (vin-sĕnts) *n. see* ulcerative gingivitis. [H. Vincent (1862–1950), French physician]

vincristine (vin-**kris**-teen) *n. see* vinca alkaloid.

vindesine (vin-dĕ-seen) *n. see* vinca alkaloid.

vinorelbine (vin-oh-**rel**-been) *n.* a semisynthetic vinca alkaloid that is administered intravenously or orally in the treatment of advanced breast cancer and non-small-cell lung cancer. Trade name: **Navelbine**.

VIP (vasoactive intestinal peptide) *n.* a peptide hormone and neurotransmitter found widely throughout the central nervous system and intestinal tract. Its many actions include vasodilatation of blood vessels in the gut and reduction of stomach acid secretion. Large amounts cause severe diarrhoea (*see* VIPoma).

VIPoma (vy-**poh**-mă) *n.* a usually malignant tumour of islet cells of the pancreas that secrete excess VIP, causing severe diarrhoea ('pancreatic cholera' or the **Verner-Morrison syndrome**), with loss of potassium and bicarbonate and a low level of stomach acid.

viraemia (vyr-**ee**-miă) *n.* the presence in the blood of virus particles.

viral pneumonia (vy-răl) *n.* an acute infection of the lung caused by a virus, such as respiratory syncytial virus, adenovirus, influenza and parainfluenza viruses, or an enterovirus. It is characterized by headache, fever, muscle pain, and a cough that produces a thick sputum. The pneumonia often occurs with or subsequent to a systemic viral infection.

Virchow Robin spaces (perivascular spaces) (feer-koh ro-**ba**) *pl. n.* fluid-filled spaces formed around blood vessels in the pia mater as they penetrate deeper brain tissue. They may dilate, resulting in raised intracranial pressure.

virilism (vi-ril-izm) *n.* the development in a female of male secondary sexual characteristics, such as increased body hair, muscle bulk, and deepening of the voice, and male psychological characteristics.

virilization (vi-ri-ly-**zay**-shŏn) *n.* the most extreme result of excessive androgen production (hyperandrogenism) in women. It is characterized by temporal balding, a male body form, muscle bulk, deepening of the voice, enlargement of the clitoris, and hirsutism. Virilization in prepubertal boys may be caused by some tumours (*see* Leydig tumour) or the adrenogenital syndrome.

virology (vyr-**ol**-ŏji) *n.* the science of viruses. *See also* microbiology.

virulence (**vi**-rew-lĕns) *n.* the disease-producing (pathogenic) ability of a microorganism. *See also* attenuation.

virus (**vy**-rŭs) *n.* a minute particle that is capable of replication but only within living cells. Viruses are too small to be visible with a light microscope or to be trapped by filters. They infect animals, plants, and microorganisms. Viruses cause many diseases, including herpes, influenza, mumps, polio, AIDS, and rabies. Antiviral drugs are effective against some of them, and many viral diseases are controlled by means of vaccines. **—viral** *adj.*

viscera (**vis**-er-ă) *pl. n.* (*sing.* **viscus**) the organs within the body cavities, especially the organs of the abdominal cavities. **—visceral** (**vis**-er-ăl) *adj.*

visceral pouch *n. see* pharyngeal (pouch).

viscero- *combining form denoting* the viscera.

visceroptosis (vis-er-op-**toh**-sis) *n.* downward displacement of the abdominal organs.

viscid (**vis**-id) *adj.* glutinous and sticky.

viscoelastic material (vis-koh-i-**lasst**-ik) *n.* a material exhibiting both viscous and elastic properties. It is used in ophthalmic surgery (such as cataract surgery) to help maintain the shape of ocular tissues as well as lubricate and minimize trauma. Viscoelastic materials are also used in dentistry.

viscus (**vis**-kŭs) *n. see* viscera.

visual acuity (**vizh**-yoo-ăl) *n.* sharpness of vision. Acuity of distant vision is often expressed as a Snellen score (*see* Snellen chart).

visual field *n.* the area in front of the eye in any part of which an object can be seen without moving the eye.

visual purple *n. see* rhodopsin.

vital capacity (**vy**-t'l) *n.* the maximum volume of air that a person can exhale after maximum inspiration. **forced v. c. (FVC)** the maximum volume of air that the lungs can expel in a forced expiration after the deepest possible inspiration.

vital centre *n.* any of the collections of nerve cells in the brain that act as governing centres for different vital body functions, such as breathing, blood pressure, etc.

Vitallium (vy-**tal**-iŭm) *n. Trademark.* an alloy of chromium and cobalt that is used in instruments, prostheses, surgical appliances, and dentures.

vital signs *pl. n.* signs that a patient is alive, which include measurable body temperature, blood pressure, heart rate (*see* pulse), and respiratory rate.

vital statistics *pl. n.* statistics relating to the births, marriages, deaths, and incidence of disease within a population.

vitamin (vit-ă-min) *n.* any of a group of substances that are required, in very small amounts, for healthy growth and development: they cannot be synthesized by the body and are therefore essential constituents of the diet. Vitamins are divided into two groups, according to whether they are soluble in water or fat.

vitamin A (retinol) *n.* a fat-soluble vitamin that occurs preformed in foods of animal origin (especially milk products, egg yolk, and liver) and is formed in the body from the pigment β-carotene, present in some vegetable foods (for example, green leafy vegetables and carrots). Retinol is essential for growth, vision in dim light, and the maintenance of soft mucous tissue. A deficiency causes stunted growth, night blindness, xerophthalmia, keratomalacia, and eventual blindness. Recommended daily intake: 600 μg retinol equivalents for women and 700 μg for men.

vitamin B *n.* any one of a group of water-soluble vitamins that are often found together in the same kinds of food, such as liver, yeast, and eggs, and all function as coenzymes. **B_1 (thiamine, aneurine)** a vitamin deficiency of which leads to beriberi. Recommended adult intake: 0.4 mg/1000 kcal of dietary calories eaten. **B_2 (riboflavin)** a vitamin important in tissue respiration and the absorption of iron. A deficiency causes ariboflavinosis. Recommended adult intake: 1.3–1.6 mg/day. **B_6 (pyridoxine)** a vitamin from which the coenzyme pyridoxal phosphate is formed. Deficiency is very rare. Recommended adult intake: 15 μg/g dietary protein. **B_{12} (cyanocobalamin)** a vitamin that can be absorbed only in the presence of intrinsic factor, secreted in the stomach. A deficiency can lead to pernicious anaemia and degeneration of the nervous system. Recommended adult intake: 1.5 μg/day. *See also* biotin, folate, nicotinic acid, pantothenic acid.

vitamin C (ascorbic acid) *n.* a water-soluble vitamin with antioxidant properties that is essential in maintaining healthy connective tissues. A deficiency of vitamin C leads to scurvy. Recommended adult intake: 30 mg/day; rich sources are citrus fruits and vegetables.

vitamin D *n.* a fat-soluble vitamin that enhances the absorption of calcium and phosphorus from the intestine and promotes their deposition in the bone. **D_2 (ergocalciferol, calciferol)** a form obtained from the diet; good sources are fatty fish, eggs, and margarine. **D_3 (cholecalciferol)** a form manufactured in the skin in the presence of sunlight. A deficiency of vitamin D leads to rickets and osteomalacia.

vitamin E *n.* any of a group of chemically related fat-soluble compounds (**tocopherols** and **tocotrienols**) that have antioxidant properties and are thought to stabilize cell membranes. Good sources of the vitamin are vegetable oils, eggs, margarine, and wholemeal cereals. It is fairly widely distributed in the diet and a deficiency is therefore unlikely.

vitamin K *n.* a fat-soluble vitamin occurring in two main forms – **phytomenadione** and **menaquinone** – essential for the normal clotting of blood. Good dietary sources are green leafy vegetables and meat.

vitelliform degeneration (Best's disease) (vy-tel-i-form) *n.* degeneration of the macula of the eye that is inherited as a dominant characteristic and usually starts in childhood. There is widespread abnormality of retinal pigment epithelium (*see* retina) with the accumulation of a yellowish material, especially in the macular area.

vitellus (vi-tel-ŭs) *n.* the yolk of an ovum.

vitiligo (vit-i-ly-goh) *n.* a common disorder in which symmetrical white or pale macules appear on the skin (especially the face and extremities). It affects all races, but is more conspicuous in dark-skinned races. Vitiligo is an autoimmune disease and is usually progressive, although spontaneous repigmentation may occur.

vitrectomy (vi-trek-tŏmi) *n.* the removal of all or part of the vitreous humour of the eye. It is often required to repair a detached retina and to remove a vitreous haemorrhage.

vitreous detachment (vit-ri-ŭs) *n.* the separation of the vitreous humour from the underlying retina. This is a normal ageing process, but it is also more common in such conditions as diabetes and severe myopia. It can sometimes cause a tear in the retina and lead to retinal detachment.

vitreous humour (vitreous body) *n.* the transparent jelly-like material that fills the chamber behind the lens of the eye.

vitritis (vi-try-tis) *n.* inflammation within the vitreous humour of the eye.

vivisection (viv-i-sek-shŏn) *n.* a surgical operation on a living animal for experimental purposes.

VMA *n. see* vanillylmandelic acid.

vocal folds (vocal cords) (voh-kăl) *pl. n.* the two folds of tissue protruding from the sides of the larynx to form a narrow slit (glottis) across the air passage (see illustration). Their controlled interference

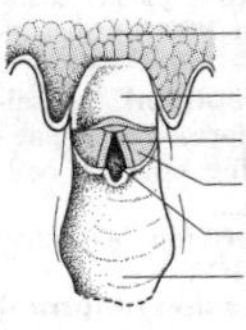

The vocal folds

with the expiratory air flow produces audible vibrations that make up speech, song, and all other vocal noises.

vocal fremitus *n. see* fremitus.

vocal resonance *n.* the sounds heard through the stethoscope when the patient speaks. These are normally just audible but they become much louder (**bronchophony**) if the lung under the stethoscope is consolidated. Vocal resonance is lost over pleural fluid except at its upper surface, when it has a bleating quality (**aegophony**). *See also* pectoriloquy.

volar (**voh**-ler) *adj.* relating to the palm of the hand or the sole of the foot (the **vola**).

volatile (**vol**-ă-tyl) *adj.* describing a liquid that evaporates at room temperature.

volition (vŏl-**ish**-ŏn) *n.* the act of or capacity for exercising the will.

Volkmann's contracture (**fohlk**-mahnz) *n.* fibrosis and shortening of muscles due to inadequate blood supply arising from arterial disease or compartment syndrome. It may be a complication of fractures, vascular surgery, or use of constricting bandages or plaster casts. [R. von Volkmann (1830–89), German surgeon]

volsellum (vulsellum) (vol-**sel**-ŭm) *n.* surgical forceps with claw-like hooks at the ends of both blades.

volt (vohlt) *n.* the SI unit of electric potential. Symbol: V.

voluntary admission (informal admission) (**vol**-ŭn-ter-i) *n.* entry of a patient into a psychiatric hospital with his (or her) agreement. *Compare* compulsory admission.

voluntary muscle *n. see* striated muscle.

volvulus (**vol**-vew-lŭs) *n.* twisting of a part of the digestive tract, usually leading to partial or complete obstruction and often reducing the blood supply, causing gangrene.

vomer (**voh**-mer) *n.* a thin plate of bone that forms part of the nasal septum.

vomica (**vom**-ik-ă) *n.* **1.** an abnormal cavity in an organ, usually a lung, sometimes containing pus. **2.** the abrupt expulsion from the mouth of a large quantity of pus or decaying matter originating in the throat or lungs.

vomit (**vom**-it) **1.** *vb.* to expel the contents of the stomach through the mouth (*see* vomiting). **2.** *n.* the contents of the stomach ejected during vomiting. Medical name: **vomitus**.

vomiting (**vom**-it-ing) *n.* the reflex action of expelling the contents of the stomach through the mouth. Vomiting is controlled by a special centre in the brain (within the medulla oblongata) that may be stimulated by certain drugs or by nerve signalling from the stomach (e.g. after ingesting toxic substances), the intestine (e.g. in intestinal obstruction), or from the inner ear (in motion sickness). Medical name: **emesis**.

von Recklinghausen's disease (von **rek**-ling-how-zĕnz) *n.* **1.** a syndrome due to hyperparathyroidism, characterized by loss of mineral from bones, which become weakened and fracture easily, and formation of kidney stones. Medical name: **osteitis fibrosa**. **2.** *see* neurofibromatosis. [F. D. von Recklinghausen (1833–1910), German pathologist]

von Willebrand's disease (von wil-i-brandz) *n.* an inherited disorder of the blood characterized by episodes of spontaneous bleeding similar to haemophilia. It is due to abnormalities in the von Willebrand factor, a glycoprotein necessary for platelet activation. [A. von Willebrand (1870–1949), Swedish physician]

voxel (voks-ĕl) *n.* short for 'volume element', the volume of tissue in a body that is represented by a pixel in a cross-sectional image.

VSD *n.* *see* (ventricular) septal defect.

VT *n.* *see* (ventricular) tachycardia.

VTE *n.* *see* venous thromboembolism.

vulsellum (vul-sel-ŭm) *n.* *see* volsellum.

vulv- (vulvo-) *combining form denoting* the vulva.

vulva (vul-vă) *n.* the female external genitalia. Two pairs of fleshy folds (*see* labium) surround the openings of the vagina and urethra and extend forward to the clitoris. *See also* vestibular glands. **—vulval** *adj.*

vulvectomy (vul-vek-tŏmi) *n.* surgical removal of the vulva. **simple v.** excision of the labia majora, labia minora, and clitoris to eradicate a nonmalignant growth. **radical v.** excision of the labia majora and minora, the clitoris, and all regional lymph nodes on both sides, together with the skin covering these areas. It is carried out for a malignant growth.

vulvitis (vul-vy-tis) *n.* inflammation of the vulva, which is often accompanied by intense itching (*see* pruritus).

vulvodynia (vul-voh-dy-niă) *n.* unexplained vulval pain, often coupled with sexual dysfunction and psychological disorder.

vulvovaginitis (vul-voh-vaj-i-ny-tis) *n.* inflammation of the vulva and vagina (*see* pruritus, vaginitis).

VUR *n.* *see* vesicoureteric reflux.

Ww

Waardenburg's syndrome (vah-den-bergz) *n.* an inherited form of deafness accompanied by a characteristic white forelock of hair and multiple colours within the irises of the eyes. It is inherited as an autosomal dominant disease, although severity is variable. [P. J. Waardenburg (1886–1979), Dutch ophthalmologist]

wafer (way-fer) *n.* a thin sheet made from moistened flour, formerly used to enclose a powdered medicine that is taken by mouth.

waist-to-hip ratio (WHR) *n.* the ratio of the circumference of the waist to that of the hips, used as a measure of obesity. It is a more reliable predictor of obesity-related mortality than body mass index alone but should be used with caution for assessment of children and young people, because of their rates of growth.

waiting list (wayt-ing) *n.* a list of the patients awaiting admission to hospital after having been assessed either as an out-patient or on a domiciliary consultation involving a specialist. In general the patients are offered places in the order in which their names were placed on the list.

Waldeyer's ring (vahl-dy-erz) *n.* the ring of lymphoid tissue formed by the tonsils. [H. W. G. von Waldeyer (1836–1921), German anatomist]

walking distance (wawk-ing) *n.* the measured distance that a patient can walk before he or she is stopped by pain in the muscles, usually the calf muscles, or breathlessness. It is a useful estimate of the degree of impairment of the blood supply. *See* claudication.

Wallerian degeneration (wol-eer-iăn) *n.* degeneration of a ruptured nerve fibre that occurs within the nerve sheath distal to the point of severance. [A. V. Waller (1816–70), British physician]

Wangensteen tube (wang-ĕn-steen) *n.* a tube with a suction apparatus that is passed into the stomach through the nose and is used to drain the contents of the stomach and duodenum to relieve abdominal distention. [O. H. Wangensteen (1898–1980), US surgeon]

ward manager (wawd man-ă-jer) *n.* a person responsible for the management of a hospital ward. The ward manager may be a non-nurse administrator with management training or the position can be (or be combined with) a nursing post.

warfarin (wor-fer-in) *n.* an anticoagulant used mainly in the prevention and treatment of deep vein thrombosis and pulmonary embolism and to prevent embolism in other patients at risk. It is given by mouth; the principal adverse effect is local bleeding. Trade name: **Marevan**.

wart (wort) *n.* a benign growth on the skin caused by infection with human papillomavirus. Treatment of warts is with over-the-counter remedies, such as lactic and salicylic acids, but cryotherapy with liquid nitrogen is also effective. **anogenital w.** a wart that is frequently associated with other genital infections (*see* condyloma). **common w.** a firm horny papule found mainly on the hands. Most will clear spontaneously within two years. **plane w.** a flat skin-coloured wart usually found on the face; it may be present in very large numbers. **plantar w.** (**verruca**) a wart occurring on the sole of the foot. Plantar warts are often tender.

Warthin's tumour (adenolymphoma) (wor-thinz) *n.* a tumour of the parotid salivary glands, containing epithelial and lymphoid tissues with cystic spaces. [A. S. Warthin (1866–1931), US pathologist]

Wassermann reaction (wass-er-măn) *n.* formerly, the most commonly used test for the diagnosis of syphilis. A sample of the patient's blood is examined for the presence of antibodies to *Treponema pallidum*. [A. P. von Wassermann (1866–1925), German bacteriologist]

water bed (waw-ter) *n.* a bed with a flexible water-containing mattress. The surface of the bed adapts itself to the patient's posture, which leads to greater comfort and reduces the potential for developing bedsores.

waterbrash (waw-ter-brash) *n.* sudden filling of the mouth with dilute saliva. This often accompanies dyspepsia, particularly if there is nausea.

water-deprivation test *n.* a test for diabetes insipidus in which fluid and food intake is withheld completely for up to 24 hours, with regular measurement of plasma and urinary osmolality and body weight. In a patient with diabetes insipidus the urine osmolality will remain low and of high volume while the patient steadily dehydrates.

water-hammer pulse *n. see* Corrigan's pulse.

Waterhouse-Friderichsen syndrome (waw-ter-howss frid-er-**ik**-sĕn) *n.* fever, cyanosis, and bleeding into the skin resulting from haemorrhage of both adrenal glands, caused by septicaemia resulting from bacterial meningitis. [R. Waterhouse (1873–1958), British physician; C. Friderichsen (20th century), Danish physician]

Waterlow score (waw-ter-loh) *n.* a pressure-ulcer risk assessment tool that identifies four levels of pressure-ulcer damage and uses body mass index, skin integrity, gender, nutritional status, continence status, and mobility to predict risk. The existence of neurological deficit, cancer, or a prolonged surgical episode are additional risk criteria. Assessment relies on the use of concomitant clinical judgment. [J. Waterlow (21st century), British nurse teacher]

Waterston's operation (waw-ter-stŏnz) *n.* the operation of joining the right pulmonary artery to the ascending aorta, performed to relieve tetralogy of Fallot. [D. Waterston (20th century), British surgeon]

watt (wot) *n.* the SI unit of power, equal to 1 joule per second. Symbol: W.

WBC *n.* white blood cell (*see* leucocyte).

weal (hive) (weel) *n.* a transient swelling, confined to a small area of the skin, that is characteristic of urticaria and occurs due to dermographism.

weaning (ween-ing) *n.* the process of gradually introducing nonmilk feeds to an infant, which is generally recommended from six months of age. This is when the gastrointestinal and renal tracts are mature enough to handle the variety of foods ingested.

Weber's test (vay-berz) *n.* a hearing test in which a vibrating tuning fork is placed at the midpoint of the forehead. If one ear is affected by conductive deafness the sound appears louder in the affected ear; if one ear has sensorineural deafness the sound appears louder in the unaffected ear. [F. E. Weber (1832–91), German otologist]

web space (web spays) *n.* the soft tissue between the bases of the fingers and toes.

Wechsler scales (weks-ler) *pl. n.* standardized scales for the measurement of **intelligence quotient** (**IQ**) in adults and children. They are administered by a psychologist. *See* intelligence test. [D. Wechsler (1896–1981), US psychologist]

Wegener's granulomatosis (vay-gĕ-nerz) *n.* *see* granulomatosis. [F. Wegener (1907–90), German pathologist]

Weil-Felix reaction (vyl fay-liks) *n.* a diagnostic test for typhus. A sample of the patient's serum is tested for the presence of antibodies against the organism *Proteus vulgaris*. [E. Weil (1880–1922), German physician; A. Felix (1887–1956), Czech bacteriologist]

Weil's disease (vylz) *n.* *see* leptospirosis. [A. Weil (1848–1916), German physician]

Welch's bacillus (welch-ŭz) *n.* *see* Clostridium. [W. H. Welch (1850–1934), US pathologist]

wen (wen) *n.* *see* sebaceous cyst.

Werdnig-Hoffmann disease (verd-nig hof-man) *n.* a hereditary disorder that is a severe form of spinal muscular atrophy affecting infants. It causes a symmetrical muscle weakness that eventually affects respiratory and facial muscles. Children usually die by the age of 20 months. [G. Werdnig (1844–1919), Austrian neurologist; J. Hoffmann (1857–1919), German neurologist]

Wermer's syndrome (werm-erz) *n.* *see* MENS. [P. Wermer, US physician]

Werner's syndrome (vair-nerz) *n.* a rare genetic disorder resulting in premature ageing that starts at adolescence. Growth may be retarded and affected individuals may suffer from a thin skin, arterial disease, leg ulcers, and diabetes. [C. W. O. Werner (1879–1936), German physician]

Wernicke's encephalopathy (ver-nik-ĕz) *n.* mental confusion or delirium occurring in combination with paralysis of the eye muscles, nystagmus, and an unsteady gait. It is caused by a deficiency of vitamin B_1 and is most commonly seen in alcoholics and in patients with persistent vomiting or an unbalanced diet. [K. Wernicke (1848–1905), German neurologist]

Wertheim's hysterectomy (ver-tymz) *n.* a radical operation performed for cervical cancer, in which the uterus, the upper vagina, broad ligaments, and parametrium are removed in conjunction with regional lymph nodes. [E. Wertheim (1864–1920), Austrian gynaecologist]

West Nile fever (west nyl) *n.* a viral disease spread by the *Culex pipiens* mosquito. It causes encephalitis, with influenza-like symptoms, enlarged lymph nodes, and a bright red rash on the chest and abdomen. In patients with a weakened immune system (such as the elderly) it can progress to convulsions, coma, and paralysis.

WETFAG *n.* a mnemonic that enables the systematic assessment of critically ill children. It consists of a series of prompts to identify elements that are essential for paediatric resuscitation: *w*eight, *e*nergy needed for defibrillation, size of required endotracheal *t*ube, *f*luid requirements, *a*drenaline requirements, and *g*lucose requirements. By knowing the weight or age of the child, each of the other elements can be calculated using a simple formula.

Wharton's duct (wor-t'nz) *n.* the secretory duct of the submandibular salivary gland. [T. Wharton (1614–73), English physician]

Wharton's jelly *n.* the mesoderm tissue of the umbilical cord, which becomes converted to a loose jelly-like mesenchyme surrounding the umbilical blood vessels.

Wheelhouse's operation (weel-howss-ŭz) *n.* an operation to relieve urethral stricture in which the incision is made through the perineum. [G. Wheelhouse (1826–1909), British surgeon]

wheeze (weez) *n.* an abnormal high-pitched (sibilant) or low-pitched sound that is heard mainly during expiration. Wheezes occur as a result of narrowing of the airways, such as results from bronchospasm or increased secretion and retention of sputum; they are commonly heard in patients with asthma or chronic bronchitis. *Compare* stridor.

whiplash injury (wip-lash) *n.* tears to the ligaments, tendons, and muscles in the neck resulting from sudden jerking back of the head and neck, usually following a rear-end motor-vehicle collision. It causes pain and stiffness in the neck; symptoms occasionally last for months or even years.

Whipple's disease (wip-ŭlz) *n.* a rare disease, usually (but not exclusively) occurring in males, in which there is malabsorption, usually accompanied by abdominal pain, skin pigmentation, and arthritis. [G. H. Whipple (1878–1976), US pathologist]

Whipple's operation *n. see* pancreatectomy. [A. O. Whipple (1881–1963), US surgeon]

Whipple's triad *n.* a combination of three clinical features that indicate the presence of an insulinoma: (1) attacks of fainting, dizziness, and sweating on fasting; (2) severe hypoglycaemia present during the attacks; (3) relief from the attacks achieved by administering glucose. [A. O. Whipple]

whipworm (wip-werm) *n.* a small parasitic whiplike nematode worm, *Trichuris trichiura* (*Trichocephalus dispar*), that lives in the large intestine. Human infection (*see* trichuriasis) results from the consumption of water or food contaminated with faecal material.

whistle-blowing (wiss-ĕl-bloh-ing) *n.* expressing concerns about patient care delivery or the professional performance of a member of staff, team, or organization. NHS organizations are required to have a whistle-blowing policy that sets out the procedures to be followed by those who wish to raise questions about an aspect of professional practice.

white blood cell (wyt) *n. see* leucocyte.

white finger *n.* the pale waxy appearance of a finger resulting from spasm of the vessels of the finger. It occurs in Raynaud's disease but can also be attributed to the long-term use of vibrating equipment (**vibrating w. f.**).

white matter *n.* nerve tissue of the central nervous system that is paler in colour than the associated grey matter because it contains more nerve fibres and thus larger amounts of myelin.

white noise instrument *n.* a device, resembling a small hearing aid, that produces sounds of many frequencies at equal intensities and is used in the treatment of tinnitus. Also known as a broad-band sound generator, wide-band sound generator, ear-level sound generator, or noiser, it was formerly known as a **tinnitus masker**.

Whitfield's ointment (wit-feeldz) *n.* an ointment containing benzoic and salicylic acids, used to treat fungal infections of the skin. [A. Whitfield (1868–1947), British dermatologist]

whitlow (wit-loh) *n. see* paronychia.

WHO *n. see* World Health Organization.

WHO checklist *n.* a process introduced by the World Health Organization to improve patient safety during surgery. There are three phases: checking before anaesthesia; checking after anaesthesia but before start of surgery (referred to as 'time out'); and checking at the end of the procedure, with identification of key concerns for the immediate postoperative period (referred to as 'sign out').

whoop (hoop) *n. see* whooping cough.

whooping cough (hoop-ing) *n.* an acute infectious disease, primarily affecting infants, due to infection of the respiratory tract by the bacterium *Bordetella pertussis*. It is characterized by a paroxysmal cough that is followed by a noisy convulsive drawing in of the breath (**whoop**) or, in the very young, by periods of apnoea. Complications include bronchopneumonia, bronchiectasis, and convulsions. Immunization, usually given in the form of the DTaP/IPV/Hib and DTaP/IPV vaccines (see Appendix 8: Immunization schedules), offers protection; an attack usually confers lifelong immunity. Medical name: **pertussis**.

WHR *n. see* waist-to-hip ratio.

Widal reaction (vi-**dahl**) *n.* an agglutination test for the presence of antibodies against the *Salmonella* organisms that cause typhoid fever. [G. F. I. Widal (1862–1929), French physician]

Williams syndrome (wil-yămz) *n.* a hereditary condition marked by a characteristic 'elfin' facial appearance, hypercalcaemia, short stature, learning disability, and aortic stenosis. Most affected children are highly sociable and have unusual conversational ability, using a rich and complex vocabulary. [J. C. P. Williams (20th century), British physician]

Wilms' tumour (vilmz) *n. see* nephroblastoma. [M. Wilms (1867–1918), German surgeon]

Wilson's disease (wil-sŏnz) *n.* an inborn defect of copper metabolism in which there is a deficiency of caeruloplasmin (which normally forms a nontoxic complex with copper). It is inherited as an autosomal recessive characteristic. The free copper may be deposited in the liver, causing jaundice and cirrhosis, or in the brain, causing learning disability and symptoms resembling parkinsonism. Medical name: **hepatolenticular degeneration**. [S. A. K. Wilson (1878–1936), British neurologist]

windpipe (**wind**-pyp) *n. see* trachea.

wisdom tooth (wiz-dŏm) *n.* the third molar tooth on each side of either jaw, which erupts normally around the age of 20 years.

witch hazel (hamamelis) (wich **hay**-zĕl) *n.* a preparation made from the leaves and bark of the tree *Hamamelis virginiana*. It is used as an astringent, especially for the treatment of sprains and bruises.

withdrawal (wi*th*-**draw**-ăl) *n.* **1. (social withdrawal)** the removal of one's interest from one's surroundings. **2.** *see* coitus (interruptus). **3.** (of treatment) the correct change to palliative care when someone is dying.

withdrawal symptoms *pl. n. see* dependence.

Wolffian body (vol-fi-ăn) *n. see* mesonephros. [K. F. Wolff (1733–94), German anatomist]

Wolffian duct *n. see* mesonephros.

Wolff-Parkinson-White syndrome (WPW syndrome) (wuulf **par**-kin-sŏn wyt) *n.* a congenital abnormality of heart conduction caused by the presence of an accessory pathway of conduction between the atria and ventricles (*see* atrioventricular bundle). It results in premature excitation of one ventricle and predisposes the patient to episodes of fast heart rate (supraventricular tachycardia). [L. Wolff (1898–1972), US cardiologist; Sir J. Parkinson (1885–1976), British physician; P. D. White (1886–1973), US cardiologist]

womb (woom) *n.* *see* uterus.

Wood's glass (wuudz) *n.* a nickel-oxide filter that holds back all but a few rays projected from an ultraviolet light source. These rays (**W. light**) cause fluorescence in hair and skin affected by some fungal and bacterial infections and are therefore useful in diagnosis. [R. W. Wood (1868–1955), US physician]

woolsorter's disease (wuul-sor-terz) *n.* *see* anthrax.

word blindness (werd) *n.* *see* alexia.

World Health Organization (WHO) (werld) *n.* an international organization working to improve global public health. Health issues are discussed and policies evolved mainly through topic-specific working groups. WHO handles information on internationally notifiable diseases and publishes the International Classification of Diseases.

SEE WEB LINKS

- The WHO website

worm (werm) *n.* any of various soft-bodied legless animals, including flatworms, nematode worms, earthworms, and leeches.

wound (woond) *n.* a break in the structure of an organ or tissue caused by an external agent; for example, a bruise, cut, or burn.

wound colonization *n.* the presence of multiplying bacteria within a wound that do not cause inflammation or clinical symptoms. This may be due to the presence of natural flora or to environmental or endogenous factors. Healing is not delayed.

WPW syndrome *n.* *see* Wolff-Parkinson-White syndrome.

wrist (rist) *n.* **1.** the joint between the forearm and hand. It consists of the proximal bones of the carpus, which articulate with the radius and ulna. **2.** the whole region of the wrist joint, including the carpus and lower parts of the radius and ulna.

wrist drop *n.* paralysis of the muscles that raise the wrist, which is caused by damage to the radial nerve.

wryneck (ry-nek) *n.* *see* torticollis.

Wuchereria (voo-ker-eer-iă) *n.* a genus of white threadlike parasitic worms (*see* filaria) that live in the lymphatic vessels. **W. bancrofti** the species that causes elephantiasis.

Xx

xanthaemia (carotenaemia) (zanth-**ee**-mia) *n.* the presence in the blood of the yellow pigment carotene, from excessive intake of carrots, tomatoes, or other vegetables containing the pigment.

xanthelasma (zanth-ĕ-**laz**-mă) *n.* yellow plaques occurring symmetrically around the eyelids.

xanthine (**zanth**-een) *n.* a nitrogenous breakdown product of the purines adenosine and guanine. Xanthine is an intermediate product of the breakdown of nucleic acids to uric acid.

xantho- *combining form denoting* yellow colour.

xanthochromia (zanth-oh-**kroh**-miă) *n.* yellow discoloration, which may affect the skin in jaundice or the cerebrospinal fluid when it contains the breakdown products of haemoglobin from red blood cells that have entered it.

xanthoma (zanth-**oh**-mă) *n.* (*pl.* **xanthomata**) a yellowish skin lesion associated with any of various disorders of lipid metabolism. **Tuberous xanthomata** are found on the knees and elbows; **tendon xanthomata** involve the extensor tendons of the hands and feet and the Achilles tendon. Crops of small yellow papules at any site are known as **eruptive xanthomata**, while larger flat lesions are called **plane xanthomata**.

xanthomatosis (zanth-oh-mă-**toh**-sis) *n.* the presence of multiple xanthomata in the skin. *See* xanthoma.

xanthopsia (zanth-**op**-siă) *n.* yellow vision: the condition in which all objects appear to have a yellowish tinge. It is sometimes experienced in digitalis poisoning.

X chromosome *n.* the sex chromosome present in both sexes. Women have two X chromosomes and men one. Genes for some important genetic disorders, including haemophilia, are carried on the X chromosomes. *See* sex-linked. *Compare* Y chromosome.

xeno- *combining form denoting* different; foreign; alien.

xenogeneic (zen-oh-ji-**nay**-ik) *adj.* describing grafted tissue derived from a donor of a different species.

xenograft (heterograft) (**zen**-oh-grahft) *n.* a living tissue graft that is made from an animal of one species to another of a different species.

xenon-133 (**zen**-on) *n.* a radioactive isotope that has a half-life of about five days and is used in ventilation scanning of the lungs in nuclear medicine (*see* ventilation-perfusion scanning). Symbol: Xe-133.

Xenopsylla (zen-op-**sil**-ă) *n.* a genus of tropical and subtropical fleas. **X. cheopis** the rat flea, which occasionally attacks humans and can transmit plague; it also transmits murine typhus and two tapeworms.

xenotransplantation (zen-oh-trans-plahn-**tay**-shŏn) *n.* the transplantation of organs from one species into another.

xero- *combining form denoting* a dry condition.

xeroderma (zeer-oh-**der**-mă) *n.* a mild form of the hereditary disorder ichthyosis, in which the skin develops slight dryness and forms branlike scales. It is common in the elderly. **x. pigmentosum** a rare genetically determined skin disorder in which there is an inherited defect in the DNA repair mechanism in the skin, which corrects damage from ultraviolet radiation. This leads to multiple skin cancers.

xerophthalmia (zeer-off-**thal**-miă) *n.* a progressive nutritional disease of the eye due to deficiency of vitamin A. The cornea and conjunctiva become dry, thickened, and wrinkled. This may progress to keratomalacia and eventual blindness.

xerosis (zeer-**oh**-sis) *n.* abnormal dryness of the conjunctiva, the skin, or the mucous membranes. In xerosis of the conjunctiva, the membrane becomes thickened and grey in the area exposed when the eyelids are open.

xerostomia (zeer-oh-**stoh**-miă) *n.* *see* dry mouth. *Compare* ptyalism.

xiphi- (xipho-) *combining form denoting* the xiphoid process of the sternum.

xiphisternum (zif-i-**ster**-nŭm) *n.* *see* xiphoid process.

xiphoid process (xiphoid cartilage) (**zif**-oid) *n.* the lowermost section of the breastbone (*see* sternum): a flat pointed cartilage that gradually ossifies until it is completely replaced by bone, a process not completed until after middle age. It does not articulate with any ribs. Also called: **ensiform process** or **cartilage**, **xiphisternum**.

X-linked disease (eks-linkt) *n.* *see* sex-linked.

X-linked lymphoproliferative syndrome (XLP syndrome, Duncan's disease) (lim-foh-prŏ-**lif**-er-ă-tiv) *n.* a hereditary disorder of the immune system caused by a defective sex-linked gene carried on an X-chromosome. There is uncontrolled proliferation of B-lymphocytes in response to infection by the Epstein–Barr virus, which can lead to fulminating hepatitis or lymphoma.

XLP syndrome *n.* *see* X-linked lymphoproliferative syndrome.

Xolair (**zŏ**-lair) *n.* *see* omalizumab.

X-rays *pl. n.* electromagnetic radiation of extremely short wavelength (beyond the ultraviolet), which passes through matter to varying degrees depending on its density. X-rays are used in diagnostic radiology (*see* nuclear medicine, radiography) and in radiotherapy. Great care is needed to avoid unnecessary exposure, because the radiation is harmful (*see* radiation (sickness)).

X-ray screening *n.* the use of an image intensifier to produce real-time imaging during an X-ray examination on a TV monitor. It is widely used in angiography and interventional radiology to guide procedures. *See* videofluoroscopy.

xylene (dimethylbenzene) (zy-leen) *n.* a liquid used for increasing the transparency of tissues prepared for microscopic examination after they have been dehydrated.

xylometazoline (zy-loh-mi-taz-oh-leen) *n.* a sympathomimetic drug that constricts blood vessels (*see* vasoconstrictor). It is applied topically (in the form of drops or a spray) as a nasal decongestant in the relief of the common cold and sinusitis. Trade names: **Otradrops**, **Otrivine**.

xylose (zy-lohz) *n.* a pentose sugar that is involved in carbohydrate interconversions within cells. It is used as a diagnostic aid for intestinal function.

Yy

YAG laser (yag) *n.* yttrium–aluminium–garnet laser: *see* laser.

yawning (yawn-ing) *n.* a reflex action in which the mouth is opened wide and air is drawn into the lungs then slowly released. It is triggered by drowsiness, fatigue, or boredom.

yaws (pian, framboesia) (yawz) *n.* a tropical infectious disease caused by the presence of the spirochaete *Treponema pertenue* in the skin and its underlying tissues. Yaws occurs chiefly in conditions of poor hygiene. It is characterized by small tumours, each covered by a yellow crust of dried serum, on the hands, face, legs, and feet. These tumours may deteriorate into deep ulcers. The disease responds well to treatment with antibiotics.

Y chromosome *n.* a sex chromosome present in men but not in women. It carries a gene (*SRY*) encoding a protein that initiates testis formation. *Compare* X chromosome.

years of life lost (YLL, years of potential life lost, YPLL, potential years of life lost, PYLL) *n.* the number of additional years a person could have expected to live, on average, had they not died prematurely. The total number of years a person might expect to live, on average, is often given in square brackets after YLL (typically YLL [75]). YLLs for different diseases can be compared across populations to give an indication of which diseases carry the greatest burden of premature mortality.

yeast (yeest) *n.* any of a group of fungi in which the body consists of individual cells, which may occur singly, in groups of two or three, or in chains. Baker's yeast (*Saccharomyces*) ferments carbohydrates to produce alcohol and carbon dioxide and is important in brewing and breadmaking. Some yeasts are a commercial source of proteins and of vitamins of the B complex; others (e.g. *Candida*, *Cryptococcus*, *Malassezia*) cause disease.

yellow fever (yel-oh) *n.* an infectious disease, caused by an arbovirus, occurring in tropical Africa and South America. It is transmitted by mosquitoes, principally *Aëdes aegypti*. The virus causes degeneration of the tissues of the liver and kidneys. Symptoms include chill, headache, pains in the back and limbs, fever, vomiting, constipation, a reduced flow of urine (which contains high levels of albumin), and jaundice. Yellow fever often proves fatal.

yellow spot *n.* *see* macula (lutea).

Yersinia (yer-sin-iă) *n.* a genus of aerobic or facultatively anaerobic Gram-negative bacteria that are parasites of animals and humans. **Y. pestis** the cause of bubonic plague. **Y. enterocolitica** a cause of intestinal infections.

YLL *see* years of life lost.

yolk sac (vitelline sac) (yohk) *n.* the membranous sac that lies ventral to the embryo. One of the extra-embryonic membranes, it probably assists in transporting nutrients to the early embryo and is one of the first sites where blood cells are formed.

Youden index (yoo-děn) *n.* a statistical test that measures the performance of a diagnostic test using the difference between the true positive rate and the false positive rate. *See* sensitivity.

YPLL *see* years of life lost.

yttrium-90 (it-riŭm) *n.* an artificial radioactive isotope of the element yttrium used in radiotherapy.

Zz

zafirlukast (zaf-eer-**loo**-kăst) *n. see* leukotriene receptor antagonist.

zanamivir (ză-**nam**-i-veer) *n.* an antiviral drug used for the treatment and prevention of influenza A and B. It is administered by inhalation. Trade name: **Relenza**.

Zantac (**zan**-tak) *n. see* ranitidine.

zein (**zee**-in) *n.* a protein found in maize.

zidovudine (AZT) (zy-**dov**-yoo-deen) *n.* an antiviral drug used, in combination with other antiretroviral drugs, in the treatment of AIDS and HIV infection. It is administered by mouth or intravenous infusion; the most common side-effects are nausea, headache, and insomnia, and it may damage the blood-forming tissues of the bone marrow. Trade name: **Retrovir**.

Zieve's syndrome (**zee**-věz) *n.* a combination of severe hyperlipidaemia, haemolytic anaemia, and jaundice seen in susceptible individuals drinking alcohol to excess. [L. Zieve (1915–2000), US physician]

ZIFT *n.* zygote intrafallopian transfer: *see* gamete intrafallopian transfer.

zinc (zink) *n.* a trace element that is a cofactor of many enzymes. It is important in the immune response and has structural properties in some proteins. Deficiency is rare with a balanced diet but may occur in alcoholics and those with kidney disease; symptoms include lesions of the skin, oesophagus, and cornea, alopecia, and (in children) retarded growth. Symbol: Zn.

zinc oxide *n.* a mild astringent used in various skin conditions, usually mixed with other substances. It is applied as a cream, ointment, dusting powder, or as a paste, often in the form of an impregnated bandage.

zinc sulphate *n.* a preparation that is used in the treatment of proven zinc deficiency. It is administered by mouth or injection. Trade name: **Solvazinc**.

zinc undecenoate (zinc undecylenate) *n. see* undecenoates.

Zollinger-Ellison syndrome (**zol**-inj-er **el**-i-sŏn) *n.* a rare disorder in which there is excessive secretion of gastric juice due to high levels of circulating gastrin, which is produced by a pancreatic tumour (*see* gastrinoma) or an enlarged pancreas. The high levels of stomach acid cause diarrhoea and peptic ulcers. [R. M. Zollinger (1903–92) and E. H. Ellison (1918–70), US physicians]

zolmitriptan (zol-mi-**trip**-tan) *n. see* $5HT_1$ agonist.

zolpidem (**zol**-pi-dem) *n. see* hypnotic.

zona pellucida (**zoh**-nă pel-**oo**-sid-a) *n.* the thick membrane that develops around the mammalian oocyte within the ovarian follicle. *See* ovum.

zonula (zon-yoo-lă) *n. see* zonule.

zonule (zonula) (zon-yool) *n.* (in anatomy) a small band or zone. **z. of Zinn** (**zonula ciliaris**) the suspensory ligament of the lens of the eye. **—zonular** *adj.*

zonulolysis (zon-yoo-**lol**-i-sis) *n.* dissolution of the zonule of Zinn, which facilitates removal of the lens in cases of cataract. This technique is not used for modern cataract surgery.

zoo- *combining form denoting* animals.

zoonosis (zoh-ŏ-**noh**-sis) *n.* any infectious disease of animals that can be transmitted to humans, such as anthrax or rabies.

zopiclone (**zop**-i-klohn) *n. see* hypnotic.

Z-track *n.* a method of injecting medication into a large muscle in which the skin and subcutaneous tissue are displaced 2.5–3.75 cm laterally during the injection and released immediately afterwards. This seals the medication deeply within the muscle and prevents leakage back into the subcutaneous tissue and skin. It is used primarily when injecting dark medications (e.g. iron solutions), which can stain the superficial tissues, and is also the method of choice for administering intramuscular medications that are highly irritant to the tissues.

zygoma (zy-**goh**-mă) *n. see* zygomatic arch, zygomatic bone.

zygomatic arch (zygoma) (zy-goh-**mat**-ik) *n.* the horizontal arch of bone on either side of the face, just below the eyes, formed by connected processes of the zygomatic and temporal bones. *See* skull.

zygomatic bone (zygoma, malar bone) *n.* either of a pair of bones that form the prominent part of the cheeks and contribute to the orbits. *See* skull.

zygote (zy-goht) *n.* the fertilized ovum before cleavage begins. **z. intrafallopian transfer** (**ZIFT**) *see* gamete intrafallopian transfer.

zym- (zymo-) *combining form denoting* **1.** an enzyme. **2.** fermentation.

zymogen (zy-moh-jen) *n. see* proenzyme.

zymosis (zy-**moh**-sis) *n.* **1.** the process of fermentation, brought about by yeast organisms. **2.** the changes in the body that occur in certain infectious diseases, once thought to be the result of a process similar to fermentation. **—zymotic** (zy-**mot**-ik) *adj.*

zymotic disease *n.* an old name for a contagious disease.

Appendix I. Biochemical reference values for blood

(B = whole blood; P = plasma; S = serum)

Table 1.1 Everyday tests

Determination	*Sample*	*Reference range*
Albumin	P	35–50 g/l
in pregnancy	P	25–38 g/l
Alcohol		
legal limit (UK)	B or P	< 17.4 mmol/l
Ammonia	B	< 40 μmol/l
α-Amylase	P	25–180 somogyi units/dl
Anion gap ($Na^+ + K^+$) – ($HCO_3^- + Cl^-$)	P	12–16 mmol/l
Bilirubin	P	3–17 μmol/l
Bicarbonate (see also Table 1.2)	P	22–28 mmol/l
Calcium		
ionized	P	1.0–1.25 mmol/l
total	P	2.12–2.65 mmol/l
total in pregnancy	P	1.95–2.35 mmol/l
Chloride	P	95–105 mmol/l
Cholesterol (see also Table 1.7)	P	3.9–7.8 mmol/l
Copper	P	12–26 μmol/l
Creatinine	P	70–150 μmol/l
in pregnancy	P	24–68 μmol/l
Digoxin		
children	P	2.0–3.0 nmol/l
adults	P	1.0–2.0 nmol/l
Glucose (fasting)	P	3.0–5.0 mmol/l
Glycated haemoglobin (HbA_{1C})	B	5–8%
Iron		
male	S	14–31 μmol/l
female	S	11–30 μmol/l
total iron-binding capacity (TIBC)	S	45–75 μmol/l

Table 1.1 *continued*

Determination	*Sample*	*Reference range*
Lactate		
venous	B	0.5–2.2 mmol/l
arterial	B	0.5–1.6 mmol/l
Magnesium	P	0.75–1.05 mmol/l
Osmolality	P	278–305 mosm/kg
Phosphate (inorganic)	P	0.8–1.45 mmol/l
Potassium	P	3.5–5.0 mmol/l
Protein (total)	P	60–80 g/l
Sodium	P	135–145 mmol/l
Urea	P	2.5–6.7 mmol/l
in pregnancy	P	2.0–4.2 mmol/l
Urea nitrogen (BUN)	P	1.16–3.12 mmol/l
Uric acid		
male	P	210–480 μmol/l
female	P	150–390 μmol/l
in pregnancy	P	100–270 μmol/l
Zinc	P	6–25 μmol/l

Table 1.2 Blood gases

Measurement	*Reference range*
Arterial CO_2 (P_aCO_2)	4.7–6.0 kPa
Mixed venous CO_2 (P_vCO_2)	5.5–6.8 kPa
Arterial oxygen (P_aO_2)	12.0–14.5 kPa
Mixed venous oxygen (P_vO_2)	4.0–6.0 kPa
Newborn arterial oxygen	5.3–8.0 kPa
H^+ ion activity	36–44 nmol/l
Arterial pH	7.35–7.45 pH units

Table 1.2 *continued*

Measurement	*Reference range*
Bicarbonate	
arterial – whole blood	19–24 mmol/l
venous – plasma	22–28 mmol/l
cord blood	14–22 mmol/l
Base excess	± 2 mmol/l
Carboxyhaemoglobin	
non-smoker	< 2%
smoker	3–15%
toxic at:	>15%
coma at:	>50%

Table 1.3 Diagnostic enzymes

Enzyme	*Sample*	*Reference range*
Acid phosphatase		
total	S	1–5 U/l
prostatic	S	0–1 U/l
Alkaline phosphatase	P	80–250 U/l
Alanine aminotransferase (ALT)	P	5–35 U/l
α-Amylase	P	25–180 somogyi units/dl
Angiotensin-converting enzyme (ACE)	S	21–54 U/l
Aspartate aminotransferase (AST)	P	15–42 U/l
Creatine kinase (CK)		
male	P	24–195 U/l
female	P	24–170 U/l
Gamma-glutamyl transferase (GGT)		
male	P	11–51 U/l
female	P	7–35 U/l
Lactate dehydrogenase (total)	P	240–525 U/l

Table 1.4 Hormones

Hormone	*Sample*	*Reference range*
ACTH	P	3.3–15.4 pmol/l
Adrenaline (epinephrine)	P	0.03–1.31 nmol/l
Aldosterone		
recumbent	P	100–450 pmol/l
midday	P	2-fold increase of recumbent level
Angiotensin II	P	5–35 pmol/l
Antidiuretic hormone (ADH)	P	0.9–4.6 pmol/l
Calcitonin		
male	P	< 100 nmol/l
female	P	< 30 nmol/l
Cortisol		
00.00 h	P	80–280 nmol/l
09.00 h	P	280–700 nmol/l
Follicle-stimulating hormone (FSH)		
follicular phase	P or S	0.5–5.0 U/l
ovulatory peak	P or S	8–15 U/l
luteal phase	P or S	2–8 U/l
postmenopause	P or S	>30 U/l
male	P or S	0.5–5.0 U/l
Gastrin		
male + female (>60 yr)	P	< 50 pmol/l
female (16–60 yr)	P	< 38 pmol/l
Glucagon	P	< 50 pmol/l
Growth hormone	P	< 20 mU/l
Human chorionic gonadotrophin	S	< 5 U/l
Insulin (fasting)	P	< 15 mU/l
Insulin C-peptide (fasting)	P	< 0.4 nmol/l (undetectable in hypoglycaemia)
Insulin-like growth factor-1 (IGF-1)	P	0.52–3.4 kU/l
Luteinizing hormone		
premenopausal	P or S	6–13 U/l
follicular phase	P or S	3–12 U/l
ovulatory peak	P or S	20–80 U/l

Table 1.4 *continued*

Hormone	*Sample*	*Reference range*
luteal phase	P or S	3–16 U/l
postmenopause	P or S	>30 U/l
male	P or S	3–8 U/l
Noradrenaline	P	0.47–4.14 mmol/l
17-β-oestradiol		
follicular phase	P	75–260 pmol/l
mid-cycle	P	370–1470 pmol/l
luteal phase	P	180–1100 pmol/l
male	P	<220 pmol/l
Pancreatic polypeptide	P	<200 pmol/l
Parathyroid hormone (intact)	P	0.9–5.4 pmol/l
Progesterone		
male	P	<5 nmol/l
female postovulation	P	15–77 nmol/l
follicular (newborn)	P	<3 nmol/l
17-Hydroxyprogesterone	P	7–16 nmol/l
Prolactin		
male	P	<450 U/l
female	P	<600 U/l
Renin activity	P	
recumbent		1.1–2.7 pmol/ml per hr
erect after 30 min		3.0–4.3 pmol/ml per hr
Somatostatin	P	30–166 pmol/l
Testosterone		
male	P or S	9–42 nmol/l
female	P or S	1–2.5 nmol/l
Thyroid-stimulating hormone	P	0.5–5.5 mU/l
Thyroid-binding globulin	P	13–28 mg/l
Tri-iodothyronine (T_3)	P	1–3 nmol/l
Free T_3	P	3.3–8.2 pmol/l
Thyroxine (T_4)	P	70–140 nmol/l
Free T_4	P	9–25 pmol/l
Vasoactive intestinal peptide (VIP)	P	<30 pmol/l

Please note that reference ranges vary from lab to lab, and it is important to check the local laboratory reference ranges rather than relying solely on those given in the above table.

Table 1.5 Proteins and immunoproteins

Protein/immunoprotein	*Sample*	*Reference range*
Albumin	P	35–50 g/l
α_1-Antitrypsin	S	107–209 mg/l
Complement		
C3		65–190 mg/dl
C4		15–50 mg/dl
Caeruloplasmin	S	16–60 mg/dl
C1 esterase inhibitor	S	15–35 mg/dl
C-reactive protein (CRP)	S	< 10 mg/l
Ferritin	S	14–200 μg/l
Fibrinogen	P	2–4 g/l
D-dimer	S	< 500 μg/l
Haptoglobins	S	0.6–2.6 g/l
Immunoglobulins		
IgG	S	6.0–13.0 g/l
IgA	S	0.8–3.0 g/l
IgM	S	0.4–2.5 g/l
IgE	S	< 120 kU/l
β_2-Microglobulin	S	< 3 mg/l
Thyroid microsomal antibodies		
male	S	< 1/400
female (< 44 yr)	S	< 1/400
female (>44 yr)	S	< 1/6400
Total protein	P	60–80 g/l
β_1-Transferrin	S	1.2–2.0 g/l

Table 1.6 Paediatric reference values

Determination	*Sample*	*Reference range*
Alkaline phosphatase	P	
< 1 year		30–250 IU/l
1–14 years		150–570 IU/l
>14 years		80–250 IU/l
Ammonia	P	
newborn		64–107 μmol/l
0–2 weeks		56–92 μmol/l
>1 month		21–50 μmol/l
Aspartate aminotransferase	P	
1–3 years		20–60 IU/l
4–6 years		15–50 IU/l
Bicarbonate	P	
infants		18–22 mmol/l
older children		20–26 mmol/l
Bilirubin	P	
first week of life		100–200 μmol/l (total)
after first week of life		2–14 μmol/l (total)
and throughout childhood		0–0.4 μmol/l (direct)
Calcium	P	
1–3 weeks		1.9–2.85 mmol/l
3 weeks and above		2.12–2.65 mmol/l
β-Carotene	S	
< 1 year (upper limit falls with age up to 3½ years)		1.3–6.3 μmol/l
3½ years onwards		1.9–2.8 μmol/l
Creatinine	P	
cord blood		57–100 μmol/l
2 weeks–6 years		33–61 μmol/l
6 years–10 years		39–70 μmol/l
>12 years		49–81 μmol/l
Creatinine clearance	P	
3–13 years		94–142 ml/min per 1.73m^2
Creatine kinase (CK)	P	
neonates		75–400 U/l

Table 1.6 *continued*

Determination	*Sample*	*Reference range*
infants 3–12 months		10–145 U/l
children 1–15 years		15–130 U/l
Gamma-glutamyl transferase (GGT)	P	
0–1 month		12–271 U/l
1–2 months		9–159 U/l
2–4 months		7–98 U/l
4–7 months		5–45 U/l
7–12 months		4–27 U/l
1–15 years		3–30 U/l
Glucose (fasting)	S	
cord		2.5–5.3 mmol/l
premature/low birth wt		1.1–3.3 mmol/l
neonates		1.67–3.3 mmol/l
1 day		2.2–3.3 mmol/l
1–7 days		2.8–4.6 mmol/l
>7 days		3.3–5.5 mmol/l
Total protein	P	
1st month		51 g/l (mean)
1st year		61 g/l (mean)
1–6 years		61–78 g/l
7–16 years		66–82 g/l
Immunoglobulins		
IgG	S	
cord		5.2–18.0 g/l
0–2 weeks		5.0–17.0 g/l
2–6 weeks		3.9–13.0 g/l
6–12 weeks		2.1–7.7 g/l
3–6 months		2.4–8.8 g/l
6–9 months		3.0–9.0 g/l
9–12 months		3.0–10.9 g/l
1–2 years		3.1–13.8 g/l
2–3 years		3.7–15.8 g/l
3–6 years		4.9–16.1 g/l

Table 1.6 *continued*

Determination	*Sample*	*Reference range*
6–9 years		5.4–16.1 g/l
9–12 years		5.4–16.1 g/l
12–15 years		5.4–16.1 g/l
IgA	S	
cord		0.00–0.02 g/l
0–2 weeks		0.01–0.08 g/l
2–6 weeks		0.02–0.15 g/l
6–12 weeks		0.05–0.4 g/l
3–6 months		0.1–0.5 g/l
6–9 months		0.15–0.7 g/l
9–12 months		0.20–0.7 g/l
1–2 years		0.3–1.2 g/l
2–3 years		0.3–1.3 g/l
3–6 years		0.4–2.0 g/l
6–9 years		0.5–2.4 g/l
9–12 years		0.8–2.8 g/l
12–15 years		0.8–2.8 g/l
IgM	S	
cord		0.02–0.2 g/l
0–2 weeks		0.05–0.2 g/l
2–6 weeks		0.08–0.4 g/l
6–12 weeks		0.15–0.7 g/l
3–6 months		0.20–1.0 g/l
6–9 months		0.40–1.6 g/l
9–12 months		0.60–2.1 g/l
1–2 years		0.50–2.2 g/l
2–3 years		0.50–2.2 g/l
3–6 years		0.50–2.0 g/l
6–9 years		0.50–1.8 g/l
9–12 years		0.50–1.9 g/l
12–15 years		0.50–1.9 g/l
Lactate	P (venous)	0.5–2.2 mmol/l
	P (arterial)	0.5–1.6 mmol/l
	B	0.5–1.7 mmol/l

Table 1.6 *continued*

Determination	*Sample*	*Reference range*
Phosphate (inorganic)	P	
newborn		1.20–2.78 mmol/l
young children		1.29–1.78 mmol/l
girls 15 years		0.9–1.38 mmol/l
boys 17 years		0.83–1.49 mmol/l
Potassium	P	
newborn		up to 6.6 mmol/l
>1 month–6 years		4.1–5.6 mmol/l
boys 7–16 years		3.3–4.7 mmol/l
girls 7–16 years		3.4–4.5 mmol/l
Sweat sodium		10–40 mmol/l
Sweat chloride		0–50 mmol/l
Thyroid-stimulating hormone (TSH) (outside neonatal period)	S	0.5–5.0 mU/l
Uric acid	P	
childhood		0.06–0.24 mmol/l
boys 16 years		0.23–0.46 mmol/l
girls 16 years		0.19–0.36 mmol/l

Table 1.7 Lipids and lipoproteins

Lipid/lipoprotein	*Sample*	*Reference range*
Cholesterol	P	3.9–7.8 mmol/l
ideal upper limit		5.2 mmol/l
acceptable upper limit		6.5 mmol/l
Triglyceride (fasting)	P	0.55–1.90 mmol/l
Nonesterified (free) fatty acids (NEFA)	S	
male		0.19–0.78 mmol/l
female		0.06–0.9 mmol/l

Table 1.7 *continued*

Lipid/lipoprotein	*Sample*	*Reference range*
Lipoproteins (as cholesterol)		
low-density (LDL)	S	1.55–4.4 mmol/l
ideal upper limit		3.4 mmol/l
acceptable upper limit		4.2 mmol/l
high density (HDL)	S	0.8–2.0 mmol/l
ideal (male)		>0.9 mmol/l
ideal (female)		>1.2 mmol/l
Total cholesterol/HDL	S	
ideal		< 5 ratio

Table 1.8 Vitamins

Vitamin	*Sample*	*Reference range*
Vitamin A		
retinol	S	
male		1.06–3.35 μmol/l
female		0.84–2.95 μmol/l
β-carotene	S	
male		0.01–6.52 μmol/l
female		0.019–2.93 μmol/l
Vitamin B		
Thiamin (B_1)	P	>40 nmol/l
Riboflavin (B_2)	S	100–630 nmol/l
Pyridoxine (B_6)	P (EDTA)	20–120 nmol/l
Vitamin B_{12}	S	138–780 nmol/l
Folate	S	12–33 μmol/l
red blood cell folate	B	500–1300 μmol/l
Vitamin D metabolites		
25-(OH) D	S	17–125 nmol/l
1,25-$(OH)_2$ D_3	S	50–120 pmol/l
Vitamin E (α-tocopherol)	S	11.5–35 μmol/l

Appendix 2. Biochemical reference values for urine

Determination	*Reference range*
Aldosterone	10–50 nmol/24 h
Albumin	< 80 mg/24 h
α-Aminolaevulinic acid	9.9– 53.4 μmol/24 h
Amylase	
secretion rate	1–17 somogyi U/h
clearance	0.01–0.04 of creatinine clearance value
Arginine	1.3–6.5 μmol/mol creat
Ascorbic acid	34–68 μmol/l
Calcium	2.5–7.5 mmol/24 h
Catecholamines	< 2.6 μmol/24 h
Chloride	110–250 mmol/24 h
Copper	0.47–0.55 μmol/l
Cortisol	60–1500 nmol/l < 280 nmol/24 h
Creatinine	
male	9.0–17.0 mmol/24 h
female	7.5–12.5 mmol/24 h
pregnancy	8.0–13.5 mmol/24 h
Glucose	0.06–0.84 mmol/l
Homovanillic acid (HVA) – adults	< 43 μmol/24 h
Hydroxyindoleacetic acid (5-HIAA)	16–73 μmol/24 h
Hydroxymethylmandelic acid (HMMA)	16– 48 μmol/24 h
Iron	< 1.8 μmol/24 h
Lead	< 0.4 μmol/l
β_2-Microglobulin	4–370 μg/l
Magnesium	3.3–4.9 mmol/24 h
Osmolality	350–1000 mosm/kg
Oxalate	< 450 μmol/24 h
Phosphate (inorganic)	15–50 mmol/24 h
Porphyrins	
coproporphyrin	50–350 nmol/24 h

Appendix 2. *continued*

Determination	*Reference range*
porphobilinogen	0.9–8.8 μmol/24 h
uroporphyrin	0–49 nmol/24 h
Potassium	20–60 mmol/l
	40–120 mmol/24 h
Protein	< 120 mg/24 h
pregnancy	< 300 mg/24 h
Sodium	50–125 mmol/l
	100–250 mmol/24 h
Urea	250–500 mmol/24 h
Uric acid	< 5.0 mmol/24 h
pregnancy (except late)	< 7.0 mmol/24 h
Urobilinogen	< 6.7 μmol/24 h
Vanillylmandelic acid (VMA)	< 35 μmol/24 h
Zinc	2.1–11.0 μmol/24 h

Appendix 3. Biochemical reference values for faeces

Determination	*Reference range*
Fat (on normal diet)	< 7 g/24 h
Nitrogen	70–140 mmol/24 h
Urobilinogen	67–473 μmol/24 h
Coproporphyrin	< 0.46 nmol/g dry weight
Protoporphyrin	< 2.67 μmol/24 h
Protoporphyrin	≤0.11 nmol/kg dry weight
Total porphyrin	
(ether soluble)	10–200 nmol/g dry weight
(ether insoluble)	0–24 nmol/g dry weight

Appendix 4. Haematological reference values

Measurement	*Reference range*
haemoglobin	(male) 13.5–18.0 g/dl
	(female) 11.5–16.0 g/dl
packed cell volume or haematocrit (PCV)	(male) 0.40–0.54 l/l
	(female) 0.37–0.47 l/l
red cell count	(male) 4.5–6.5 $\times 10^{12}$/l
	(female) 3.9–5.6 $\times 10^{12}$/l
mean cell volume (MCV)	81–100 fl
mean cell haemoglobin (MCH)	27–32 pg
mean cell haemoglobin concentration (MCHC)	32–36 g/dl
reticulocyte count	0.8–2.0 per cent
absolute count	25–100 $\times 10^{9}$/l
total blood volume	70 $\pm$ 10 ml/kg
plasma volume	45 $\pm$ 5 ml/kg
red cell volume	(male) 30 $\pm$ 5 ml/kg
	(female) 25 $\pm$ 5 ml/kg
white cell count	4.0–11.0 $\times 10^{9}$/l
neutrophils	2.0–7.5 $\times 10^{9}$/l
lymphocytes	1.3–3.5 $\times 10^{9}$/l
eosinophils	0–0.44 $\times 10^{9}$/l
basophils	0–0.10 $\times 10^{9}$/l
monocytes	0.2–0.8 $\times 10^{9}$/l
platelet count	150–400 $\times 10^{9}$/l
bleeding time	1–9 min
coagulation time	5–11 min
thrombin time	10–15 s
prothrombin time	10–14 s
activated partial thromboplastin time	35–45 s
fibrinogen concentration	1.6–4.2 g/l
fibrinogen titre	normal – up to 1/128
erythrocyte sedimentation rate	(male) 0–10 mm
	(female) 0–15 mm
cold agglutinin titre at 4°C	less than 64

Appendix 5. Body mass index (BMI)

Calculation of body mass index

BMI can be calculated using metric units (kilograms and metres) or imperial units (pounds and inches). The metric system is more widely used.

Metric calculation

Weight in kilograms is divided by height in metres squared, i.e. weight (kg)/height^2 (m)

For example:
height = 1.65 m, weight = 67 kg

Calculation:
$67 \div (1.65)^2 = 24.6$

Imperial calculation

Weight in pounds is divided by height in inches squared and multiplied by 703, i.e. [weight (kg)/height^2 (in)] × 703

For example:
weight = 144 lb, height = 60″

Calculation:
$[144 \div (60)^2] \times 703 = 28.12$

Interpretation of body mass index

The range within which a person's BMI falls will help determine whether they are of a healthy weight for their height. The ranges are as follows:

Weight status	*BMI*
Starvation	< 15
Underweight	< 18.5
Normal weight	18.5–24.9
Overweight	25–29.9
Obesity	30–40
Morbid obesity	>40

The first of the example BMIs given above, 24.6, would fall within the 'normal' range, indicating good health with no need to lose weight.

The second example BMI, 28.12, would fall within the 'overweight' range. A person with a BMI of 25 or over is probably overweight, with a greater risk of developing heart disease, osteoarthritis, diabetes, high blood pressure, stroke, some cancers, and other diseases. Steps should be taken to lose weight, which can include a healthier diet and regular exercise.

A BMI of 18.5 or under may indicate that the person is deliberately restricting their food intake in order to achieve a desired degree of thinness. This is unhealthy and may lead to such health problems as malnutrition and osteoporosis, which are associated with the eating disorders anorexia nervosa and bulimia nervosa. A BMI of 17.5 or less is one of the criteria stipulated by the World Health Organization for a diagnosis of anorexia nervosa. For someone with a BMI of 30 or over, advice from a health professional about how to lose weight may be beneficial. Caution must be exercised when using the BMI as it is a screening tool, not a diagnostic tool.

BMI and children

Weight status	*Centile range*
Underweight	Less than the 5th centile
Healthy weight	5th percentile to less than the 85th centile
At risk of overweight	85th to less than the 95th centile
Overweight	Equal to or greater than the 95th centile

Although the BMI number is calculated in the same way for children and adults, the criteria used to interpret the meaning of the BMI number for children and teenagers are different from those used for adults. For children and teens, BMI age- and sex-specific centiles are used for the following reasons:

- the amount of body fat changes with age
- the amount of body fat differs between girls and boys
- healthy weight ranges change with each month of age for each sex
- healthy weight ranges change as height increases

Appendix 6. Formulae for calculating drug dosages

Solid drugs

A whole tablet is always preferable to a broken tablet as the latter will have no definite and predictable dose. Always check with the pharmacy department whether a drug in tablet form can be broken to achieve the prescribed dose.

$$\text{dose required} = \frac{\text{strength required}}{\text{stock strength}} \times \text{volume or number of stock tablets}$$

Example:

A patient is prescribed 30 mg amitriptyline. Amitriptyline is available in 10-mg tablets.

Calculation:

$$\text{Number of tablets required} = \frac{30}{10} \times 1 = 3$$

Liquid drugs

$$\text{volume required} = \frac{\text{strength required}}{\text{stock strength}} \times \text{volume of stock solution}$$

Example:

A child is prescribed 240 mg paracetamol. Paracetamol suspension is available as a solution of 120 mg/5 ml.

Calculation:

$$\text{volume of paracetamol required} = \frac{240}{120} \times 5 = 10 \text{ ml}$$

Drugs measured in units

Some medications may be available in different strengths and it is essential that the planning of administration includes the selection of a suitable combination of strengths to provide the prescribed dose in the minimum amount of tablets or liquid.

$$\text{amount required} = \frac{\text{strength required}}{\text{stock strength}} \times \text{volume of solution}$$

Examples with calculations:

1. A patient is prescribed 100 000 units of nystatin. The stock solution or unit measurement is 100 000 units in 1 ml of solution.

$$\text{volume of solution required} = \frac{100\ 000 \text{ units}}{100\ 000 \text{ units}} = 1 \text{ ml}$$

2. A patient is prescribed 12 000 units of heparin (for subcutaneous injection). Stock ampoules contain 25 000 units in 5 ml of solution.

$$\text{volume required} = \frac{12\ 000}{25\ 000} \times 5 = \frac{60\ 000}{25\ 000} = 2.4 \text{ ml}$$

Preparation of solutions

$$\text{volume required} = \frac{\text{strength required}}{\text{stock strength}} \times \text{volume of stock solution}$$

Example with calculation:

A vial of amoxicillin (500 mg) is mixed with 4.6 ml water for injections to give a concentration of 100 mg/ml. What volume of the solution is required to give an injection of 125 mg?

$$\frac{125}{100} \times 1 = 1.25 \text{ ml}$$

Intravenous infusions

There are two main types of giving set in use and they deliver fluid at the rate of 20 or 60 drops per millilitre. Blood-giving sets deliver fluid at the rate of 15 drops per millilitre.

$$\text{time for infusion (hours)} = \frac{\text{volume (ml)}}{\text{rate (ml/hour)}}$$

Example with calculation:

If a patient is to receive 500 ml normal saline at the rate of 100 ml per hour, how long will it take to deliver the fluid?

$$\frac{500}{100} = 5 \text{ hours}$$

Rate of drops per minute

$$\text{rate} = \frac{\text{volume (ml)}}{\text{time (hours)}} \times 60$$

(a) If the giving set has a flow rate of 20 drops per millilitre:

$$\text{rate} = \frac{500 \times 20 \text{ (drops/ml)}}{5 \times 60} = 33 \text{ drops per minute}$$

(b) If the giving set has a flow rate of 60 drops per millilitre:

$$\text{rate} = \frac{500 \times 60 \text{ (drops/ml)}}{5 \times 60} = 100 \text{ drops per minute}$$

(c) For a blood-giving set (rate 15 drops per millilitre) when the patient is to receive a blood transfusion over 4 hours:

$$\text{rate} = \frac{500 \times 15 \text{ (drops/ml)}}{4 \times 60} = 31.25 \text{ drops per minute}$$

https://www.nursingtimes.net/clinical-archive/medicine-management/how-to-calculate-drug-dosage-accurately-advice-for-nurses/199884.article

This website, from the *Nursing Times*, provides a selection of more examples for nurses to practise calculating drug dosages.

Appendix 7. Alcohol: ABV and recommended intake

ABV (alcohol by volume)

The strength of an alcoholic drink is printed on the label of a bottle (or on the container) and is indicated by the initials 'ABV' (or alcohol by volume, or simply 'vol') following a number or percentage. For example, '13.5% ABV' on a bottle of wine means that the wine contains 13.5% pure alcohol (ethanol).

Table 7.1 A range of alcoholic drinks with their typical ABVs

Drink	*ABV(%)*
cider	2–8.5%
beer	2–12%
alcopops	4–17.5%
wine	9–16%
liqueur	15–55%
fortified wine	15.5–20% (18–22% in EU)
vodka	35–50%
gin	40–50%
whisky	40–55%

Recommended intake

The amount of alcohol in a drink is measured in units. One unit is 10 ml or 8 g pure alcohol; for example: 300 ml 4% beer, or 85 ml 11% red wine.

The relationship of units to ABV is given by a simple formula:

$$\frac{\text{strength (ABV)} \times \text{volume (in ml)}}{1000} = \text{no. of units}$$

For example:

half a pint of cider would contain:

$$\frac{7\ \text{(ABV)} \times 284\ \text{(ml in } \tfrac{1}{2} \text{ pint)}}{1000} = 2 \text{ units}$$

two glasses of wine would contain:

$$\frac{13\ \text{(ABV)} \times 240\ \text{(ml in 2 glasses)}}{1000} = 3 \text{ units}$$

The Department of Health recommends a maximum weekly intake of no more than 14 units for both men and women and suggests that the total intake should be spread across 3 days or more and that 'several' drink-free days should be adopted each week. Current guidelines suggest that alcohol should be avoided during pregnancy to minimize the risks of low birth weight or organ defects. Women who find that they are pregnant having drunk alcohol during the earlier part of their pregnancy should avoid further drinking but should also be aware that the risk of harm to their baby is likely to be low. However, women who consistently drink above the recommended alcohol intake risk their child being born with fetal alcohol syndrome.

Appendix 8. Immunization schedules

Routine immunizations (excluding catch-up campaigns)

Age due	*Disease protected against*	*Vaccine*	*Usual site*
8 weeks	Diphtheria, tetanus, pertussis (whooping cough), polio and *Haemophilus influenzae* type b (Hib)	DTaP/IPV/Hib	thigh
	Pneumococcal (13 serotypes)	Pneumococcal conjugate vaccine (PCV)	thigh
	Meningococcal group B (MenB)2	MenB2	left thigh
	Rotavirus gastroenteritis	Rotavirus	oral
12 weeks	Diphtheria, tetanus, pertussis (whooping cough), polio and *Haemophilus influenzae* type b (Hib)	DTaP/IPV/Hib	thigh
		MenC	thigh

Appendix 8. *continued*

Age due	*Disease protected against*	*Vaccine*	*Usual site*
	Meningococcal group C (MenC)		
	Rotavirus gastroenteritis	Rotavirus	oral
16 weeks	Diphtheria, tetanus, pertussis (whooping cough), polio and *Haemophilus influenzae* type b (Hib)	DTaP/IPV/Hib	thigh
	Meningococcal group B (MenB)2	MenB2	left thigh
	Pneumococcal (13 serotypes)	PCV	thigh
1 year	Hib and MenC	Hib/MenC booster	upper arm/thigh
	Pneumococcal (13 serotypes)	PCV booster	upper arm/thigh
	Measles, mumps, and rubella (German measles)	MMR	upper arm/thigh
	Meningococcal group B (MenB)2	MenB booster	left thigh
2 to 6 years	Influenza	Live attenuated influenza vaccine LAIV4	both nostrils
3 years, 4 months	Diphtheria, tetanus, pertussis and polio Measles, mumps, and rubella	DTaP/IPV MMR	upper arm
Girls aged 12 to 13 years	HPV types 16 and 18	HPV (two doses 6–24 months apart)	upper arm

Appendix 8. *continued*

Age due	*Disease protected against*	*Vaccine*	*Usual site*
14 years	Tetanus, diphtheria and polio Meningococcal groups A, C, W, and Y disease	Td/IPV (check MMR status) MenACWY	upper arm
65 years	Pneumococcal (23 serotypes)	Pneumococcal polysaccharide vaccine (PPV)	upper arm
65 years +	Influenza	Inactivated influenza vaccine	upper arm
70 years	Shingles	Shingles	upper arm, subcutaneous.

When babies are born prematurely, they should follow the immunization schedule according to their chronological age, not their predicted age.

Nonroutine immunizations

Vaccine	*Age*	*Groups immunized*
BCG (tuberculosis)	at birth	babies who are more likely to come into contact with tuberculosis than the general population
	adult life	at risk groups (patients or health-care professionals)
Hep B (hepatitis B)	at birth	babies whose mothers are hepatitis B positive
	adult life	at risk groups (patients or health-care professionals)
Flu Chickenpox Whooping cough	adult life	at risk groups (patients or health-care professionals)

Appendix 9. Essential skills clusters

The NMC introduced the concept of essential skills clusters (ESC) in 2007 following a review of practice-related issues around fitness to practise at the point of registration. It wished to demonstrate that newly qualified practitioners are fit for purpose and able to practise safely and effectively on the completion of the nursing programme. The underlying purposes of the cluster skills were to encourage the ongoing support of students during their practice periods, to enhance the strength of practice assessment, and to demonstrate how the cluster skills relate to the NMC outcomes and proficiencies in the preregistration nursing curriculum. These skills form the basis for practice assessment and are assessed at three key progression points in the programme. The very name 'essential skills cluster' demonstrates that safe practice is developed through the existence of a strong evidence base, which should imbue confidence in the public on what to expect from the newly registered graduate nurse.

- cluster skill 1: care, compassion, and communication
- cluster skill 2: organizational aspects of care
- cluster skill 3: infection prevention and control
- cluster skill 4: nutrition and fluid management
- cluster skill 5: medicine management

Appendix 10. Guidelines for resuscitation

The process of resuscitation should only be attempted, following practice, if the practitioner is competent and confident. Practitioners must be familiar with the position and contents of the resuscitation trolley and the emergency number in the event of a cardiac arrest. They must also attend an annual resuscitation update session.

The following information is a summary of the Resuscitation Council's most recent guidelines, which were last updated in 2015 and are current at the time of publication. The full guidelines should be studied. Ensure that you are using the current version of the guidelines (the ratios of breaths to chest compressions may change) by checking on the Council's website: https://www.resus.org.uk

The collapsed adult patient in hospital

- On discovery of the patient, shout for HELP and assess the safety of the environment for potential hazards.
- Assess the patient urgently: is he or she breathing, does he or she have a carotid or central pulse, what is his or her skin colour?

If there are no apparent signs of life:

- Call the resuscitation team and start cardiopulmonary resuscitation (CPR). Ensure that the patient is positioned so that effective CPR can begin. Start cardiac compressions, at the rate of 30 compressions to 2 forced breaths to the lungs via the mouth. Observe the movement of the chest during the procedure.
- Apply the defibrillation pads/monitor and attempt defibrillation if competent to do so, otherwise wait for the resuscitation team to arrive and take over the care.

If there are signs of life:

- Assess the patient's airway (note any obstruction), breathing (for the rate and depth of respiration), and circulation or pulse (for capillary refill time); check whether there is any evidence of disability.
- Give the patient oxygen, attach monitoring (pulse oximetry, ECG, blood pressure), record vital signs, and take blood samples.
- Call the resuscitation team if appropriate and prepare for handover.

There should be a debriefing session to review the process at a suitable time.

Paediatric basic life support

- On discovery of the child, shout for HELP and assess the safety of the environment for potential hazards.
- Assess the child urgently: is he or she breathing, does he or she have a carotid or brachial pulse, what is the skin colour?
- Ensure that the airway is open by using the head tilt/chin lift manoeuvre. If the child is not breathing normally and there is no evidence of obstruction to the airway, perform 5 rescue breaths to the lungs via the nose and mouth, depending on the size of the child. Observe the movement of the chest during the procedure.
- If the child remains unresponsive, start cardiac compressions at the rate of 2 rescue breaths to 15 chest compressions, using fingers or one hand (depending on the size of the child) at the level of the nipples and to a depth of at least one third of the diameter of the child's chest (or by 4 cm for a infant and 5 cm for a child), and then call the resuscitation team. Aim for a rate of 100–120 compressions per minute. Continue until the team arrives.

There should be a debriefing session to review the process at a suitable time.

Foreign body causing airway obstruction (children or adults)

- Carefully assess the severity of the obstruction taking care not to force the obstruction further down the upper airway.

If the child or adult has an effective cough:

- Encourage deeper coughing.
- Observe carefully for evidence of deterioration to ineffective coughing or relief of the obstruction, which will be demonstrated by a rapid change in the colour of the patient.

If the child has an ineffective cough and is unconscious:

- Perform 5 rescue breaths and start chest compressions at the rate of 15 compressions to 2 rescue breaths.

If the child has an ineffective cough and is conscious:

- Perform either 5 sharp back blows or 5 thrusts (abdominal for children aged one year or over; chest for children aged under one year); this should dislodge the obstruction.
- The child will need careful continuing observation.

If the adult has an ineffective cough and is unconscious:

- Start cardiopulmonary resuscitation.

If the adult has an ineffective cough and is conscious:

- Give up to 5 sharp back blows.
- If this fails to relieve the obstruction, give up to 5 abdominal thrusts.
- Alternate 5 back blows with 5 abdominal thrusts until the obstruction is relieved.

Appendix 11. The Human Rights Act

The introduction to the Human Rights Act 1998 (HRA) describes it as "an Act to give greater effect to rights and freedoms guaranteed under the European Convention on Human Rights" (also known as the Convention).

As health-care professionals, nurses have a duty to protect the human rights of their patients. Not only is this enshrined within the NMC Code of Professional Conduct (2008) but the Human Rights Act 1998, which came into force in October 2000, clearly identifies a range of issues that relate to nursing practice. The rights set out in the Convention and its protocols that are incorporated into British law by the HRA are those in Articles 2 to 12 and Article 14 of the Convention, plus those in the first and sixth protocols. Under the Act, NHS trusts and all health authorities will be classed as "public authorities": as such, they are obliged to act in accordance with the Convention and could be liable for breaches of the HRA.

The following articles cover rights that are relevant to nursing practice and the provision of nursing care.

Article 2 enshrines the right to life and imposes a duty on public authorities to protect someone whose life is at risk. This protection could be extended to a patient needing treatment that would save his or her life.

Article 3 prohibits torture or inhuman or degrading treatment or punishment. Many forms of conduct have been found to be capable of breaching Article 3, including serious assaults, prison conditions, rape, and corporal punishment, and degrading treatment could include subjection of a patient to multiple examinations for training purposes.

Article 5 recognizes the right to liberty and freedom from arbitrary detention. For detention to be lawful, it must be only for one of the specified purposes set out in the article; these can include the detention and treatment of patients with mental health problems. Article 5 limits the circumstances under which someone can be detained, the terms of detention being regularly reviewed on an individual basis. In such reviews the onus is on the public authority to justify continued detention rather than on the detainee to show why he or she should be released.

Article 6 guarantees the right to a fair trial in civil and criminal proceedings and sets standards for the way that proceedings are run. It may be relevant if there are accusations of bias in a Mental Health Review Tribunal or a Child Protection Conference.

Article 8 refers to the right to privacy and family life. Many rights are safeguarded under this article, including bodily integrity (which affords protection against forced treatment or physical restraint), sexuality, personal autonomy, the right to die with dignity, access of family members, privacy of correspondence and phone calls, and environmental protection (including freedom from excessive noise).

Article 9 guarantees freedom of thought and the opportunity to hold any religious belief. Individuals cannot be forced to follow a particular religion and cannot be prevented from changing their religion. It also protects the right to practise one's religion or beliefs provided that these are part of a sufficiently coherent philosophical scheme; veganism and pacifism, for example, are protected. Possible areas of relevance for nursing practice include the provision of facilities for worship, provision of culturally appropriate food, and sensitivity over the use of mixed wards for those to whom they are not acceptable for religious reasons.

Article 10 guarantees the right to hold and express opinions and ideas. It also guarantees the right to pass information to other people and to receive information from others; however, it is essential to consider the reputation or rights of others and the issues that relate to the disclosure of information received in confidence.

Article 12 relates to the right to marry and found a family. Although this does not cover issues that relate to transgender individuals and same-sex marriage, it could be applied to those with a mental illness or learning disability or those who wish to have a family by nonconventional means, such as IVF. It could also apply to those for whom sterilization is being suggested as a result of their lack of mental capacity.

Article 14 guarantees the prohibition of discrimination and clearly states that the enjoyment of the rights and freedoms covered in the other articles will be available without discrimination on any ground, such as sex, race, colour, language, religion, political or other opinion, national or social origin, association with a national minority, or other status.

This review of the HRA is not exhaustive and merely identifies elements that may have an impact on nursing practice. Further details of the Act are available on the Equality and Human Rights Commission website https://www.equalityhumanrights.com/en/human-rights/human-rights-act.

Appendix 12. Religion and nursing practice

Adherence to the particular set of beliefs, values, and practices that constitute their religion may have varying levels of importance for patients and their families. It is therefore essential that nurses should acquire at least a basic knowledge of the most common religions in order to deliver holistic care that meets their patients' needs. Religious beliefs may have implications for diet, dress, and medication, as well as procedures followed at birth and death. The sections below are outlines of the most commonly encountered religions. They focus on elements likely to have relevance to nursing practice and are by no means exhaustive, being intended only as a guide to enable appropriate care to be given. It should also be stressed that patients may not adhere rigidly to all the tenets of their religion. Nurses are urged to check the details of their patients' religious practices and not to make assumptions. They should also recognize that there is an important distinction between offering spiritual support for their patients as part of a holistic therapeutic approach and making any direct religious intervention, which may be considered unethical.

Roman Catholics recognize the pope, based in the Vatican City State within Rome, as the successor to St Peter, whom Christ appointed as the first head of his church. Like other Christians, they regard certain rituals – the sacraments – as having special significance, being visible signs of inner grace. Catholics accept seven sacraments: baptism, confirmation, reconciliation (confession and penance), the Eucharist (or Holy Communion; receiving consecrated bread and wine), marriage, holy orders (joining the priesthood), and anointing the sick (formerly known as extreme unction or the last rites). Catholics are encouraged to attend an act of worship – Mass – at least once a week, during which participants may receive the Eucharist having made confession; they are under an obligation to do this once a year (during the Easter season). Catholics are usually expected to fast for at least one hour before receiving Holy Communion, but this may be waived for those who are ill or over 60 years of age. There is no objection to taking water or any kind of medicine before Communion. Catholics may take great comfort from the support of a priest and often wish to make confession or be anointed before an operation. Fridays are traditionally regarded as 'fasting' days, on which no meat is eaten; Catholics who follow the practice may eat a vegetarian or fish diet on that day. Fasting is also practised during the season of Lent. The faith endorses organ donation. The Church believes that using artificial methods of contraception is "intrinsically evil", regardless of the consequences: Catholics are supposed to use only natural methods of birth control. Abortion is regarded as a moral evil whatever the reasons for it. Holding that human life begins at fertilization, Catholics are opposed to experimentation on human embryos and reject IVF treatment for couples who cannot conceive naturally. The Church considers it morally acceptable to refuse extraordinary and aggressive medical means to preserve life. It sees the refusal of such treatment not as euthanasia (which the Church regards as morally wrong) but as a proper acceptance of the human condition in the face of death.

Protestants are of the Christian faith; they include, among others, members of the Church of England and the other churches of the Anglican Communion, Baptists, Presbyterians, and Methodists. Their beliefs and practices vary widely. The only generally accepted sacraments are baptism and Holy Communion: patients may wish to take Communion in a similar way to Roman Catholics. Access to a chaplain may be important and some patients may wish to fast on Fridays or during Lent. Although most Protestants are opposed in principle to abortion, many accept that there are some situations in which it is indicated, as when the health of the mother would be severely compromised by continuing the pregnancy, when rape has led to the pregnancy, and when overwhelming disability has been diagnosed in the fetus. They generally regard suicide as morally wrong and do not support euthanasia.

Quakers – also known as the Religious Society of Friends – believe that there is something of God in everybody and that each human being is of unique worth. Most Quakers regard themselves as Christians; others see themselves as agnostic or prefer to avoid such labels altogether. They do not accept the sacraments, have no formal creeds or ceremonies, and refuse to take oaths. There is no clergy as Quakers feel that all believers can minister to one another; Quaker services may include readings and periods of silence. Quakers are divided as to whether animal experimentation should be allowed for medical research; they regard abortion as a matter of individual conscience.

Jehovah's Witnesses are members of a Christian-based religious movement with an evangelistic approach. They refuse blood transfusions, including autologous transfusions in which a person's own blood is stored for later use in a medical procedure. As a result of this approach, children and young people under the age of 16 years who require a blood transfusion may need protection (under the legal system). Jehovah's Witnesses refuse military service and are discouraged from voting in elections. Abortion is regarded as murder, and IVF treatment is unacceptable as it involves the destruction of some embryos. Smoking, drinking alcohol, chewing betel nut, and taking other drugs for pleasure are not acceptable. Adherents are not required to be vegetarian but many choose to eat meat only occasionally. They believe that God's intervention at the end of the world is imminent and may become upset at the prospect of dying before this event.

Christian Scientists do not rely on conventional medicine but hold that illness and injury can be healed through prayer. The Church respects the work of the medical profession and does not forbid the use of medicine by its members, but many Christian Scientists prefer to rely on prayer. Those who choose to undergo medical treatment for a specific problem normally give up Christian Science treatment for the period of treatment. This is because one treatment approaches healing from a material and the other from a spiritual perspective, and the approaches are considered to be incompatible. Christian Scientists accept the use of material aids, such as lenses for vision correction, splints for broken bones, and dental services.

Mormons are members of a sect – the Church of Jesus Christ of the Latter-Day Saints – who follow a nontraditional pattern of Christianity. They have no clergy and reject infant baptism. Mormons prefer to bury their dead rather than cremate them. They oppose abortion, the consumption of tobacco, alcohol, tea, coffee, and the use of illicit drugs. They are encouraged to fast once a month (usually on the first Sunday) by going without food and drink for two consecutive meals. Some Mormons wear a sacred undergarment, which is only removed for hygiene and medical treatments and must be treated with great respect.

Islam, whose followers are called Muslims, hold that there is one God – Allah – whose prophet is Mohammed. The most important Muslim practices are the Five Pillars of Islam, which are incumbent on all Muslims. They are:

- *shahadah* – reciting the Muslim profession of faith
- *salat* – reciting ritual prayers five times each day, facing towards Mecca
- *zakat* – paying alms to help the poor and the needy
- *sawm* – fasting during the month of Ramadan
- *hajj* – a pilgrimage to Mecca that must be made at least once in a Muslim's lifetime

A copy of the Qur'an (Koran) should be available for Muslim patients. They may use a mat to pray and will need to know the direction of east so that they can pray towards Mecca.

Certain foods are prohibited, including pork and its by-products, blood, and the flesh of animals that have died without being ritually slaughtered and fully bled. Although Muslims fast during other times of the year, Ramadan is the only time when fasting during daylight hours is obligatory for every able-bodied adult Muslim. The rules for fasting and praying may be relaxed for ill people, the elderly, pregnant or breastfeeding women, and those with certain medical conditions, such as diabetes. Insulin treatment for diabetics who wish to fast may need to be adjusted during Ramadan. Forbidden food and medicines are termed *haraam*; acceptable foods and medicines are described as *halal*. There may be issues of compliance if patients find that they have been prescribed life-saving but *haraam* medications (these may contain pork products, such as gelatine). Alcohol is forbidden.

Circumcision is not compulsory in Islam but it is an important ritual aimed at improving cleanliness. It is therefore strongly encouraged. Suicide and euthanasia are explicitly forbidden. Muslims regard abortion as wrong and forbidden but may allow it if continuing the pregnancy would put the mother's life in real danger.

Niqab refers to the piece of cloth that is worn by Muslim women to cover the face; women who wear it usually also cover their hands. Some Muslim women wear full-body garments that only expose their eyes; some cover every part of the body except their face and hands. Some believe that only their hair and/or their cleavage should be covered, while others do not observe any special dress rules. Some Muslims consider that it is not permitted to touch an adult person of the opposite sex other than one's spouse. This means that some Muslim women may refuse to be examined by a male member of the medical staff, especially if no other females are present.

Muslims treat the dead body with gentleness and respect. The body is cleaned, scented, and covered with a clean cloth for burial, which should be performed – by Muslims – as soon as possible after death. Cremation is forbidden. Wherever possible, burial should take place within 24 hours of death.

Judaism holds that there is one God, who appointed the Jews to be his chosen people in order to set an example of holiness and ethical behaviour to the world. Orthodox Jews require strictly kosher food, i.e. food prepared according to Jewish dietary laws. Some hospitals provide both a regular kosher and a strictly kosher diet. It must be served in the original container, unopened if possible, so that the patient can see the *hecksher* (seal of reliability). Pork and shellfish are forbidden, as is any food that has come into contact with prohibited food or the utensils used to cook or serve prohibited food. All meat must be killed in the approved way (*shechita*), and meat and milk must not be consumed at the same meal (meat must not be served in a cream sauce or milky drinks served after a meat meal). If Jewish patients are fasting, food needs to be available before sunrise and after sunset. The pork restriction may have implications for diabetes management: nonporcine insulin will be required. Orthodox Jewish men always wear a skullcap (a *kippah* or *yarmulke*). Every week religious Jews observe the Sabbath (or Shabbat), which lasts from sunset on Friday to sunset on Saturday, and keep its laws and customs. Male patients will need to pray. Orthodox patients are forbidden to use or touch electrical appliances (such as light switches) or to carry anything during Shabbat. When dealing with patients of the opposite sex, avoid touching or other contact unless medically necessary. Women prefer to keep their bodies and limbs completely covered.

Circumcision for male babies shortly after birth is a religious and cultural practice that is considered to be fundamental to Judaism. However, not all Jews regard circumcision as an absolute requirement. All forms of contraception are permitted in Judaism in appropriate circumstances. Jewish law does not forbid abortion but does not permit it on demand; because the mother's life takes precedence over the life of the fetus, abortion may be performed to save the life of the mother. Jewish law forbids suicide and active euthanasia. Although organ donation is allowed in order to save lives, some ultra-Orthodox Jews do not permit it.

Dying patients should not be left alone and their relatives may wish to stay. After death, the body should be touched as little as possible: it is traditionally regarded as sacred and should not be damaged in any way. Orthodox Jews do not permit post mortems unless required by law. Relatives may wish to keep vigil over the body. If death happens during the Sabbath, the body should be left and burial should take place within 24 hours if possible.

Hinduism is a religious tradition that originated in the Indian subcontinent. It is a diverse and ancient religion in which a variety of deities are worshipped in temples and the home. Of central importance is the belief in reincarnation, resulting in a profound respect for all forms of life. Most Hindus are vegetarians (those who do eat meat abstain from beef and pork) and many avoid dairy products. Onions and garlic are avoided by many Hindus, as is alcohol. Fasts take place at various prescribed times. The cow is considered to be sacred, which may have implications in the treatment of diabetics (nonbovine/non-porcine insulin should be used). Hinduism is generally opposed to abortion except when it is necessary to save the mother's life. Cleanliness and modesty are features of the religion. Decisions about organ donation and transplantation are left to individuals to make, but there are many references in Hindu scriptures that support the concept.

Sikhs believe that God is one, the ultimate and eternal guru who provides enlightenment and understanding for the disciple who sets his or her heart on finding him and serving him. Male Sikhs are distinguished by their adoption of the five *k*s:

- *kesh* (uncut hair)
- *kangha* (the comb that is used to keep hair clean)
- *kara* (a metal bangle)
- *kaccha* (knee-length underwear)
- *kirpan* (a dagger)

There are no strict dietary requirements but many Sikhs are vegetarians or avoid beef. Those who eat meat should not eat *halal* meat (meat killed according to Muslim law). Sikhs believe in reincarnation and therefore death may not be perceived as threatening or frightening. Their passing may be supported by readings from the holy texts and the attendance of family and friends. After death, religious symbols should not be removed from the body and the family should be asked about last offices.

Buddhism is based on the teachings of Gautama Siddhartha (the Buddha) in the 6th century bc and focuses on personal spiritual development. Buddhists strive for a deep insight into the true nature of life and do not worship gods or adhere to a fixed set of doctrines. Traditional Buddhists reject abortion because it involves the deliberate destruction of a life; however, they may be willing to review this belief if abortion appears to be the lesser evil in the circumstances. Some schools of Buddhism prohibit the eating of meat, because the killing of animals violates the First Moral Precept and because meat is considered an intoxicant to the body, which violates the Fifth Moral Precept. Alcohol is likewise avoided by many Buddhists.

Rastafarians accept Haile Selassie, the former emperor of Ethiopia, as the living God incarnate. Many adhere to the dietary prohibitions in the Old

Testament and will not eat pork or shellfish. Others are vegans or strict vegetarians and avoid any foods containing artificial additives. Some Rastafarians also reject synthetic or extracted drugs, insisting on purely natural remedies.

Appendix 13. Health-care websites

(excluding those that can be accessed directly via entry-specific web links)

Professional, regulatory, and government bodies, and organizations providing advice and support

Action for Sick Children www.actionforsickchildren.org
Action on Hearing Loss www.actiononhearingloss.org.uk
Age UK www.ageuk.org.uk
American Association of Critical Care Nurses www.aacn.org/
AskSARA www.asksara.dlf.org.uk
Advice about health, home, and daily activities to promote independent living
Association for Child and Adolescent Mental Health www.acamh.org.uk
Association for Continence Advice www.aca.uk.com/
Association for Perioperative Practice www.afpp.org.uk/home
Association for Professionals in Infection Control and Epidemiology www.apic.org
Association for Young People's Health www.youngpeopleshealth.org.uk
Association of Pediatric Hematology/Oncology Nurses www.aphon.org
BLISS www.bliss.org.uk
A special-care baby charity
British Anaesthetic and Recovery Nurses Association www.barna.co.uk
British Association for Sexual Health and HIV www.bashh.org
British Association of Critical Care Nurses www.baccn.org.uk/
British Deaf Association www.bda.org.uk
British National Formulary (for adults and children) www.bnf.org/products/bnf-online/
British Pharmacological Society www.bps.ac.uk/
Child Accident Prevention Trust www.capt.org.uk
Child Bereavement Trust www.childbereavementuk.org/
Child Growth Foundation www.childgrowthfoundation.org
Childline www.childline.org.uk
Choices in Recovery www.choicesinrecovery.com
Mental health information and support
College of Operating Department Practitioners www.codp.org.uk/
Contact a Family www.unison.org.uk/at-work/health-care/representing-you/unison-partnerships/codp/
For families with disabled children http://www.cafamily.org.uk/
Continence Foundation www.continence-foundation.org.uk

Down Syndrome Medical Interest Group www.dsmig.org.uk/
Foundation for People with Learning Disabilities www.learningdisabilities.org.uk
Great Ormond Street Institute of Child Health www.ucl.ac.uk/ich
Health and Care Professions Council www.hpc-uk.org
Healthcare Infection Society www.his.org.uk
Infection Prevention Society http://www.ips.uk.net/
International Council of Nurses www.icn.ch
International Society of Advance Care Planning and End of Life Care www.acpelsociety.com
International Society of Psychiatric Mental Health Nurses www.ispn-psych.org/
KidsHealth https://kidshealth.org/
Information about children's health for young people, parents, and health professionals
King's Fund www.kingsfund.org.uk
Macmillan Cancer Support www.macmillan.org.uk/
Medicines for Children www.medicinesforchildren.org.uk
A website for health-care providers and families that gives guidance and information about medication
Marie Curie Cancer Care www.mariecurie.org.uk/
Medicines and Healthcare products Regulatory Agency www.gov.uk/government/organisations/medicines-and-healthcare-products-regulatory-agency#page=DynamicListMedicines
Mencap www.mencap.org.uk/
Mental Health Foundation www.mentalhealth.org.uk
Mind www.mind.org.uk/
NAM AIDSmap www.aidsmap.com/
HIV and AIDS information
National Association of Pediatric Practitioners www.napnap.org/
National Children's Bureau www.ncb.org.uk
National Institute for Health Research www.nihr.ac.uk/
National Institute of Mental Health www.nimh.nih.gov/index.shtml
National Network for Learning Disability Nurses www.nnldn.com
National Poisons Information Service www.npis.org/
Oncology Nursing Society www.ons.org/
Pituitary Foundation www.pituitary.org.uk/
Public Health England www.gov.uk/government/organisations/public-health-england
Rethink www.rethink.org/
Royal College of Midwives www.rcm.org.uk
Royal College of Nursing www.rcn.org.uk
Royal College of Obstetricians and Gynaecologists www.rcog.org.uk/en/guidelines-research-services/

Royal College of Paediatrics and Child Health www.rcpch.ac.uk
Royal National Institute of Blind People www.rnib.org.uk/
Royal Society for the Prevention of Accidents www.rospa.com
Sexual Advice Association http://sexualadviceassociation.co.uk/
Society for Endocrinology www.endocrinology.org/
Society of Sexual Health Advisors www.ssha.info/
Spotting the Sick Child www.spottingthesickchild.com/?
A valuable resource that helps health professionals spot children with serious illness
Terrence Higgins Trust www.tht.org.uk/
Tissue Viability Society www.tvs.org.uk/
Together for Short Lives www.togetherforshortlives.org.uk/
Children's palliative care information
Women's Aid www.womensaid.org.uk/
Women's Health Concern https://www.womens-health-concern.org/
YoungMinds www.youngminds.org.uk

Sites for research and information

American Society for Pharmacology and Experimental Therapeutics www.aspet.org/knowledge/what-is-pharmacology/
Centre for the Advancement of Interprofessional Education www.caipe.org.uk/
Cochrane Library www.cochranelibrary.com
A collection of reviews of health-care interventions mainly for professionals
College of Emergency Medicine http://www.rcem.ac.uk/
eMedicine Specialties www.emedicine.medscape.com
Online specialty textbooks
Emergency Nursing World http://enw.org/TOC.htm
English Centre for Practice Development www.canterbury.ac.uk/health-and-wellbeing/england-centre-for-practice-development/england-centre-for-practice-development.aspx
Evidence in Health and Social Care www.evidence.nhs.uk/
Female Genital Mutilation
www.who.int/gender/other_health/guidelinesnursesmid.pdf
Guide to Internet Resources for Cancer www.cancerindex.org/clinks1.htm
Healthcare Improvement Scotland www.healthcareimprovementscotland.org/
Mental Health in Higher Education hub http://mhhehub.ning.com
MIDIRS www.midirs.org
An information resource on midwifery
National Audit Office www.nao.org.uk
NHS Digital http://digital.nhs.uk/
Includes statistics on health care
NICE databases www.nice.org.uk/about/what-we-do/evidence-services/journals-and-databases

OBGYN.net www.obgyn.net/
Research in women's health mainly for professionals
Paediatric Nursing Forum www.jiscmail.ac.uk/cgi-bin/webadmin?A0=paediatric-nursing-forum
Psychiatric Nursing www.psychiatricnursing.org/
UK Centre for the History of Nursing and Midwifery http://sites.nursing.manchester.ac.uk/ukchnm
UK Foundation of Nursing Studies www.fons.org/
Women's Health Information www.womens-health.co.uk/

Appendix 14. Degrees and diplomas

BA	Bachelor of Arts
BEd	Bachelor of Education
BN	Bachelor of Nursing
BSc	Bachelor of Science
CMT	Clinical Midwife Teacher
CPH	Certificate of Public Health
DCD	Diploma of Child Development
DCH	Diploma in Child Health
DipHE	Diploma in Higher Education
DipNEd	Diploma in Nursing Education
DN	Diploma in Nursing
DPH	Diploma in Public Health
DPhil	Doctor of Philosophy
DPM	Diploma in Psychological Medicine
DTM&H	Diploma in Tropical Medicine and Hygiene
EN(G)	Enrolled Nurse (General)
EN(M)	Enrolled Nurse (Mental)
EN(MH)	Enrolled Nurse (Mental Handicap)
FETC	Further Education Teaching Certificate
FRCN	Fellow of the Royal College of Nursing
FRSH	Fellow of the Royal Society of Health
HV	Health Visitor
MA	Master of Arts
MBA	Master of Business Administration
MBIM	Member of the British Institute of Management
MEd	Master of Education
MSc	Master of Science
MTD	Midwife Teachers' Diploma
NVQ	National Vocational Qualification
OHNC	Occupational Health Nursing Certificate
ONC	Orthopaedic Nurses' Certificate

OND	Ophthalmic Nursing Diploma
PhD	Doctor of Philosophy
RCNT	Registered Clinical Nurse Tutor
RGN	Registered General Nurse
RM	Registered Midwife
RMN	Registered Mental Nurse
RN	Registered Nurse
RNMH	Registered Nurse for the Mentally Handicapped
RNT	Registered Nurse Teacher
RSCN	Registered Sick Children's Nurse
SCM	State Certified Midwife
SEN	State Enrolled Nurse
SRN	State Registered Nurse

Appendix 15. SI units

Table 15.1 Base and supplementary SI units

Physical quantity	*Name of unit*	*Symbol for unit*
length	metre	m
mass	kilogram	kg
time	second	s
electric current	ampere	A
thermodynamic temperature	kelvin	K
luminous intensity	candela	cd
amount of substance	mole	mol
*plane angle	radian	rad
*solid angle	steradian	sr

*supplementary units

Table 15.2 Derived SI units with special names

Physical quantity	*Name of unit*	*Symbol for unit*
frequency	hertz	Hz
energy	joule	J
force	newton	N
power	watt	W
pressure	pascal	Pa
electric charge	coulomb	C
electric potential difference	volt	V
electric resistance	ohm	Ω
electric conductance	siemens	S
electric capacitance	farad	F
magnetic flux	weber	Wb
inductance	henry	H
magnetic flux density (magnetic induction)	tesla	T
luminous flux	lumen	lm
illuminance (illumination)	lux	lx
absorbed dose	gray	Gy
activity	becquerel	Bq
dose equivalent	sievert	Sv

Table 15.3 Decimal multiples and submultiples to be used with SI units

Submultiple	*Prefix*	*Symbol*	*Multiple*	*Prefix*	*Symbol*
10^{-1}	deci	d	10^{1}	deca	da
10^{-2}	centi	c	10^{2}	hecto	h
10^{-3}	milli	m	10^{3}	kilo	k
10^{-6}	micro	μ	10^{6}	mega	M
10^{-9}	nano	n	10^{9}	giga	G
10^{-12}	pico	p	10^{12}	tera	T
10^{-15}	femto	f	10^{15}	peta	P
10^{-16}	atto	a	10^{16}	exa	E
10^{-21}	zepto	z	10^{21}	zetta	Z
10^{-24}	yocto	y	10^{24}	yotta	Y

Table 15.4 Conversion of units to and from SI units

From	*To*	*Multiply by*
in	m	0.0254
ft	m	0.3048
sq in	m^2	0.00064516
sq ft	m^2	0.092903
cu in	m^3	0.0000164
cu ft	m^3	0.0283168
l(itre)	m^3	0.001
gal(lon)	m^3	0.0045609
gal(lon)	litres	4.5609
lb	kg	0.453592
g cm^{-3}	kg m^{-3}	1000
lb/in^3	kg m^{-3}	27679.9
mmHg	Pa	133.322
cal	J	4.1868
m	in	39.3701
cm	in	0.393701
cm^2	sq in	0.155
m^2	sq in	1550
m^2	sq ft	10.7639
m^3	cu in	61023.6
m^3	cu ft	35.3146
m^3	l(itre)	1000
m^3	gal(lon)	219.969
kg	lb	2.20462
kg m^{-3}	g cm^{-3}	0.001
kg m^{-3}	lb/in^3	0.0000363
Pa	mmHg	0.0075006
J	cal	0.238846

Temperature conversion

°C (Celsius) = 5/9(°F – 32)

°F (Fahrenheit) = (9/5 × °C) + 32

Appendix 16. Abbreviations

An asterisk (*) denotes that the subject has an entry in the Dictionary.

AA	*Alcoholics Anonymous
AAA	abdominal aortic aneurysm
A&E	accident and emergency (department)
ABPI	*ankle–brachial pressure index
ACE	angiotensin-converting enzyme
ACTH	*adrenocorticotrophic hormone
ADH	*antidiuretic hormone
ADHD	*attention-deficit/hyperactivity disorder
ADLs	*activities of daily living
ADP	*adenosine diphosphate
ADR	adverse drug reaction
AED	antiepilepsy drugs
AF	atrial fibrillation
AFB	acid-fast bacilli
AFP	*alpha-fetoprotein
AGA	appropriate for gestational age
AHF	*antihaemophilic factor
AIDS	*acquired immune deficiency syndrome
AIH	artificial insemination by husband
AKI	*acute kidney injury
ALD	*adrenoleukodystrophy
ALG	antilymphocyte globulin
ALL	acute lymphoblastic leukaemia
ALS	*advanced life support; *antilymphocyte serum; amyotrophic lateral sclerosis
ALT	*alanine aminotransferase
AMD	*age-related macular degeneration
AML	acute myeloid leukaemia
AMP	*adenosine monophosphate
ANDI	abnormal development and involution
APD	*auditory processing disorder; automated peritoneal dialysis
APEL	Accreditation of Prior Experiential Learning
APL	Accreditation of Prior Learning
APT	alum precipitated toxoid
APTT	activated partial thromboplastin time
ARC	AIDS-related complex
ARDS	*adult respiratory distress syndrome
ARF	*acute renal failure; acute respiratory failure
ARM	*artificial rupture of membranes

ARMD	*age-related macular degeneration
ARV	*antiretroviral
ASD	atrial septal defect
AST	*aspartate aminotransferase
ATLS	*advanced trauma life support
ATN	acute tubular necrosis
ATP	*adenosine triphosphate
ATT	antitetanus toxoid
AUR	acute urinary retention
AV	*atrioventricular
AVM	arteriovenous malformation
AVPU	alert, voice (responses present), pain (responses present), unresponsive
AVT	*auditory verbal therapy
BAHA	bone-anchored hearing aid
BAI	*Beck Anxiety Inventory
BAL	*bronchoalveolar lavage; British Anti-Lewisite
BBB	*bundle branch block; *blood–brain barrier
BBV	blood-borne virus
BCC	*basal cell carcinoma
BCG	*bacille Calmette-Guérin
BDI	*Beck Depression Inventory
BFHI	*baby-friendly hospital initiative
BiPAP	*bi-level positive airways pressure
BLS	*basic life support
BMI	*body mass index
BMR	*basal metabolic rate
BMT	bone-marrow transplant
BNF	*British National Formulary
BNP	brain natriuretic peptide
BOO	*bladder outlet obstruction
BOOP	*bronchiolitis obliterans organizing pneumonia
BP	*blood pressure
BPAD	*bipolar affective disorder
BPD	*bronchopulmonary dysplasia
BPH	benign prostatic hyperplasia
BPPV	*benign paroxysmal positional vertigo
BPRS	*Brief Psychiatric Rating Scale
BSA	body surface area
BSE	*bovine spongiform encephalopathy
BSER	*brainstem evoked response audiometry
BSL	*British Sign Language
BSS	*balanced salt solution; *Beck Scale for Suicide Ideation
CABG	*coronary artery bypass graft
CAF	*common assessment framework
CAH	*congenital adrenal hyperplasia

CAPD	chronic (or continuous) ambulatory peritoneal dialysis
CAPE	*Clifton Assessment Procedures for the Elderly
CAT	computerized axial tomography
CATS	*Credit Accumulation Transfer Scheme
CBF	cerebral blood flow
CBT	*cognitive behavioural therapy
CCF	*congestive cardiac failure
CCU	coronary care unit
CD	*controlled drug
CDH	congenital diaphragmatic hernia; *congenital dislocation of the hip
CDS	*Calgary Depression Scale
CEMACH	Confidential Enquiry into Maternal Deaths and Child Health
CESDI	Confidential Enquiries into Stillbirths and Deaths in Infancy
CF	*cystic fibrosis
CFS/ME/PVF	*chronic fatigue syndrome/myalgic encephalomyelitis (or encephalopathy)/postviral fatigue syndrome
CHD	*coronary heart disease
CHF	congestive heart failure
CIN	cervical intraepithelial neoplasia
CIS	*carcinoma in situ
CISC	clean intermittent self-catheterization
CIWA-Ar	Clinical Institute Withdrawal Assessment for Alcohol, revised scale
CJD	*Creutzfeldt-Jakob disease
CML	chronic myeloid leukaemia
CMV	*cytomegalovirus
CNS	central nervous system
COAD	chronic obstructive airways disease
COPD	*chronic obstructive pulmonary disease
COSHH	*control of substances hazardous to health
CPAP	*continuous positive airways pressure
CPD	*continuing professional development
CPK	creatine phosphokinase
CPN	community psychiatric nurse
CPR	*cardiopulmonary resuscitation
CQC	*Care Quality Commission
CRF	chronic renal failure
CRH	*corticotrophin-releasing hormone
CRP	*C-reactive protein
CSF	*cerebrospinal fluid
CSI	*Caregiver Strain Index
CSOM	chronic suppurative otitis media
CSSD	Central Sterile Supplies Department

CT	*computerized tomography
CVA	*cerebrovascular accident
CVAD	*central venous access device
CVP	*central venous pressure
CVS	*chorionic villus sampling
CXR	chest X-ray
D and C	*dilatation and curettage
DCIS	*ductal carcinoma in situ
DEXA	dual-energy X-ray absorptiometry
DH	*Department of Health
DHEA	*dehydroepiandrosterone
DI	donor insemination
DIC	*disseminated intravascular coagulation
DKA	*diabetic ketoacidosis
DLE	*discoid lupus erythematosus
DM	diabetes mellitus
DMARD	*disease-modifying antirheumatic drug
DMD	*Duchenne muscular dystrophy
DMSA	dimercaptosuccinic acid
DNA	*deoxyribonucleic acid
DNAR	*do not attempt resuscitation
DOT	*directly observed therapy
DR	digital radiography
DRS	*Delusions Rating Scale
DSH	*deliberate self-harm
DSM	*Diagnostic and Statistical Manual of Mental Disorders
DTaP	diphtheria, tetanus, and pertussis (vaccine)
DTPA	diethylenetriaminepentaacetic acid
DU	*duodenal ulcer
DVT	*deep vein thrombosis
EB	*epidermolysis bullosa
EBM	expressed breast milk
EBP	*evidence-based practice
EBV	*Epstein-Barr virus
ECF	extracellular fluid
ECG	*electrocardiogram
ECI	*Experience of Caregiving Inventory
ECMO	extracorporeal membrane oxygenation
ECoG	*electrocochleography
ECT	*electroconvulsive therapy
ED	emergency department
EDD	expected date of delivery
EDTA	ethylenediaminetetraacetic acid
EDV	*end-diastolic volume
EEG	*electroencephalogram
EIA	exercise-induced asthma

ELISA	*enzyme-linked immunosorbent assay
EMG	*electromyography
EMLA	eutectic mixture of local anaesthetics (cream)
ENT	ear, nose, and throat
EOG	*electrooculography
EPS	extrapyramidal side-effects
ERCP	*endoscopic retrograde cholangiopancreatography
ERG	*electroretinography
ERPC	evacuated retained products of conception
ERV	expiratory reserve volume
ESC	essential skills clusters
ESR	*erythrocyte sedimentation rate
ESRF	*end-stage renal failure
ESV	*end-systolic volume
ESWL	extracorporeal shock-wave lithotripsy
ET	*endotracheal
EUA	examination under anaesthetic
EWS	*early warning system
FAS	*fetal alcohol syndrome
FBC	full blood count
FBS	fasting blood sugar
FESS	*functional endoscopic sinus surgery
FEV	*forced expiratory volume
FFP	fresh frozen plasma
FIM	*Functional Independence Measure
FOBT	*faecal occult blood test
FQ	*Fear Questionnaire
FRAT	*Falls Risk Assessment Tool
FRC	*functional residual capacity
FSH	*follicle-stimulating hormone
FTT	*failure to thrive
FVC	*forced vital capacity
GABA	*gamma-aminobutyric acid
GAD	glutamic acid decarboxylase
GCS	*Glasgow Coma Scale
GDS	*Geriatric Depression Scale
GFR	*glomerular filtration rate
GH	*growth hormone
GHIH	growth-hormone inhibiting hormone
GHQ	*General Health Questionnaire
GI	*gastrointestinal
GIFT	*gamete intrafallopian transfer
GIST	gastrointestinal stromal tumour
GN	*glomerulonephritis
GnRH	*gonadotrophin-releasing hormone
GOLD	Global Initiative for Chronic Obstructive Lung Disease

GOR	*gastro-oesophageal reflux
GPI	*general paralysis of the insane
GRAF-PIF	General Risk Assessment for Paediatric In-patient Falls
GTN	*glyceryl trinitrate
GUM	genitourinary medicine
GUS	genitourinary system
GVHD	*graft-versus-host disease
HADS	*Hospital Anxiety and Depression Scale
HAI	*hospital-acquired infection
HAV	hepatitis A virus
Hb	*haemoglobin
HC	head circumference
hCG	*human chorionic gonadotrophin
HCV	hepatitis C virus
HD	*Huntington's disease
HDL	*high-density lipoprotein
HDU	*high-dependency unit
HEMS	*helicopter-based emergency medical services
HFEA	*Human Fertilization and Embryology Authority
HGP	*Human Genome Project
5-HIAA	*5-hydroxyindoleacetic acid
Hib	*Haemophilus influenzae* type B (vaccine)
HIFU	high-intensity focused ultrasound
HIV	*human immunodeficiency virus
HMG	*human menopausal gonadotrophin
HoNOS	*Health of the Nation Outcome Scale
HPV	*human papillomavirus
HR	heart rate
HRS	*Hallucinations Rating Scale
HRT	*hormone replacement therapy
HSDU	Hospital Sterilization and Disinfection Unit
HSE	*Health and Safety Executive
HSV	herpes simplex virus
5HT	*5-hydroxytryptamine
HTLV	human T-cell lymphocytotrophic virus
HUS	*haemolytic uraemic syndrome
HYCOSY	hysterosalpingo-contrast sonography
IBD	*inflammatory bowel disease
IBS	irritable bowel syndrome
IC	*inspiratory capacity
ICD	*International Classification of Diseases
ICP	intracranial pressure
ICSH	*interstitial-cell-stimulating hormone
ICSI	*intracytoplasmic sperm injection
ICU	intensive care unit
ID	*intradermal

IDDM	insulin-dependent diabetes mellitus
IDT	*incident decision tree
IGT	*impaired glucose tolerance
IHD	*ischaemic heart disease
IM	*intramuscular
IMV	*intermittent mandatory ventilation
INH	*isoniazid
INO	internuclear ophthalmoplegia
IOUS	intraoperative ultrasound examination
IPD	intermittent peritoneal dialysis
IPPV	intermittent positive-pressure ventilation
IPV	inactivated poliomyelitis vaccine
IQ	*intelligence quotient
IRV	inspiratory reserve volume
ISS	*injury scoring system
ITU	intensive therapy unit
IUCD	intrauterine contraceptive device
IUGR	intrauterine growth restriction
IUI	intrauterine insemination
IUS	intrauterine system
IV	*intravenous
IVC	inferior vena cava
IVF	*in vitro fertilization
IVI	intravenous infusion
IVU	intravenous urography
JCA	juvenile chronic arthritis
JVP	jugular venous pressure
LASEK	laser in situ epithelial keratomileusis
LASIK	laser in situ keratomileusis
LAUP	*laser-assisted uvulopalatoplasty
LBC	*liquid-based cytology
LDL	*low-density lipoprotein
LE	lupus erythematosus
LFTs	*liver function tests
LGA	large for gestational age
LH	*luteinizing hormone
LHRH	luteinizing hormone releasing hormone
LMP	(date of) last menstrual period
LOC	level of consciousness
LP	lumbar puncture
LRTI	lower respiratory tract infection
LSD	*lysergic acid diethylamide
LUTS	*lower urinary tract symptoms
LVF	left ventricular failure
MAO	*monoamine oxidase
MAS	*mandibular advancement splint

MBC	*maximum breathing capacity
MCU	*micturating cystourethrogram
MDT	*multidisciplinary team
ME	*myalgic encephalomyelitis
MenC	*meningitis C (vaccine)
MENS	multiple endocrine neoplasia syndromes
MET	*medical emergency team
MHRA	*Medicines and Healthcare products Regulatory Agency
MI	*myocardial infarction
MLD	minimal lethal dose
MMR	measles, mumps, rubella (vaccine)
MNAT	*Mini-Nutrition Assessment Tool
MND	*motor neuron disease
MODS	*multiple organ dysfunction syndrome
MODY	*maturity-onset diabetes of the young
MOF	*multi-organ failure
MPQ	*McGill Pain Questionnaire
MR	magnetic resonance
MRI	*magnetic resonance imaging
MRSA	meticillin- or multiple-resistant *Staphylococcus aureus*
MS	*multiple sclerosis
MSA	*multiple system atrophy
MSH	*melanocyte-stimulating hormone
MSP	*Munchausen's syndrome by proxy
MSU	*midstream specimen of urine
NAD	nicotinamide adenine dinucleotide
NAI	*nonaccidental injury
NBM	nothing (or nil) by mouth
NCVQ	*National Council for Vocational Qualifications
NVQ	National Vocational Qualification
NDU	Nursing Development Unit
NEC	*necrotizing enterocolitis
NG	*nasogastric
NGU	nongonococcal urethritis
NHL	non-Hodgkin's lymphoma
NHS	*National Health Service
NICE	*National Institute for Health and Care Excellence
NICU	*neonatal intensive care unit
NIPPV	noninvasive intermittent positive-pressure ventilation
NIV	*noninvasive ventilation
NMC	*Nursing and Midwifery Council
NMR	*nuclear magnetic resonance
NPF	*nurse prescribers' formulary
NSAID	*nonsteroidal anti-inflammatory drug
NSFs	*national service frameworks
NSU	nonspecific urethritis

OAE	*otoacoustic emissions
OCD	*obsessive–compulsive disorder
OGD	*oesophagogastroduodenoscopy
ORT	*oral rehydration therapy
OSA	*obstructive sleep apnoea
OTC	*over-the-counter (medicine)
PACS	picture archiving and communication system
PALS	*paediatric advanced life support; *Patient Advice and Liaison Service
PAP	primary atypical pneumonia
PAT	paroxysmal atrial tachycardia
PBC	primary biliary cirrhosis
PBM	peak bone mass
PCA	*patient-controlled analgesia
PCI	percutaneous coronary intervention
PCO	*polycystic ovary
PCOS	*polycystic ovary syndrome
PCP	*Pneumocystis jiroveci* (formerly *carinii*) pneumonia
PCT	*primary care trust
PCV	*packed cell volume
PCWP	pulmonary capillary wedge pressure
PDA	patent ductus arteriosus
PDP	*personal development plan
PE	pulmonary embolus
PECT	positron emission computed tomography
PEEP	*positive end expiratory pressure
PEFR	*peak expiratory flow rate
PEG	percutaneous endoscopic gastrostomy
PERLA	pupils equal, react to light and accommodation
PET	*positron emission tomography
PGD	*preimplantation genetic diagnosis
PHC	primary health care
PICC	*peripherally inserted central catheter
PICU	paediatric intensive care unit; *psychiatric intensive care unit
PID	pelvic inflammatory disease; *prolapsed intervertebral disc
PIH	*pregnancy-induced hypertension
PIN	*prostatic intraepithelial neoplasia
PIs	*performance indicators
PKU	*phenylketonuria
PMB	*postmenopausal bleeding
PMS	*premenstrual syndrome
POAG	primary open-angle glaucoma
POM	*prescription only medicine
POP	*plaster of Paris

PPE	*personal protective equipment
PPH	postpartum haemorrhage
PPS	plasma protein solution
PPV	*positive-pressure ventilation
PR	per rectum
PREP	Post-Registration Education and Practice
PRK	*photorefractive keratectomy
PSA	*prostate specific antigen
PSV	*pressure support ventilation
PT	*prothrombin
PTC	percutaneous transhepatic cholangiography
PTSD	*post-traumatic stress disorder
PTTK	partial thromboplastin time with kaolin
PUO	pyrexia of unknown origin
PUVA	photochemotherapy psoralen + ultraviolet A
PV	per vaginam
PVD	*peripheral vascular disease
PVF	*postviral fatigue syndrome
PVS	*persistent vegetative state
QALYs	*quality-adjusted life years
QOL	*quality of life
RAI	*Relatives Assessment Interview
RAISSE	Relatives Assessment Interview for Schizophrenia in a Secure Environment
RAST	*radioallergosorbent test
RBC	*red blood cell
RCA	*root cause analysis
RCC	red cell concentrate
RDA	recommended daily allowance (of a nutrient)
REM	rapid eye movement
RF	*rheumatic fever
RIP	raised intracranial pressure
RNA	*ribonucleic acid
ROM	*range of movement
RPE	retinal pigment epithelium
RSI	*repetitive strain injury
RSV	*respiratory syncytial virus
RTA	road-traffic accident
RV	*residual volume
RVF	right ventricular failure
SA	sinus arrhythmia
SAD	*seasonal affective disorder
SAH	subarachnoid haemorrhage
SANS	*Schedule for Assessment of Negative Symptoms
SARS	severe acute respiratory syndrome
SAS	sleep apnoea syndrome
SBE	*subacute bacterial endocarditis

SBS	*short bowel syndrome
SCBU	*special care baby unit
SCC	*squamous cell carcinoma
SCID	*severe combined immune deficiency
SDH	subdural haematoma
SEN	*special educational needs
SERM	*selective (o)estrogen receptor modulator
SFS	*Social Functioning Scale
SGA	*small for gestational age
SGOT	serum glutamic oxaloacetic transaminase
SGPT	serum glutamic pyruvic transaminase
SHA	*strategic health authority
SIADH	*syndrome of inappropriate secretion of antidiuretic hormone
SIB	self-injurious behaviour
SIDS	*sudden infant death syndrome
SIMV	*synchronized intermittent mandatory ventilation
SLE	systemic lupus erythematosus
SMA	*spinal muscular atrophy
SNAP	*Schizophrenia Nursing Assessment Protocol
SNRI	*selective serotonin and noradrenaline reuptake inhibitor
SPECT	single photon emission computing tomography
SSG	*split-skin graft
SSPE	*subacute sclerosing panencephalitis
SSRI	*selective serotonin reuptake inhibitor
STAMP	Screening Tool for the Assessment of Malnutrition in Paediatrics
STD	*sexually transmitted disease
STI	sexually transmitted infection
STRATIFY	*St Thomas's Risk Assessment Tool in Falling Elderly In-patients
STM	short-term memory
SVT	*supraventricular tachycardia
TB	*tuberculosis
TBI	*total body irradiation
TBW	total body water
TCA	*tricyclic antidepressant
TEDs	*thromboembolic deterrents
TENS	*transcutaneous electrical nerve stimulation
TIA	*transient ischaemic attack
TIBC	total iron-binding capacity
TLC	*total lung capacity
TMJ	*temporomandibular joint
TNF	*tumour necrosis factor
TOP	termination of pregnancy

TOT	*transobturator tape
tPA	*tissue-type plasminogen activator
TPN	*total parenteral nutrition
TPR	temperature, pulse, respiration
TQM	*total quality management
TRH	*thyrotrophin-releasing hormone
TRT	tinnitus retraining therapy
TRUS	*transrectal ultrasonography
TSH	*thyroid-stimulating hormone
TSS	*toxic shock syndrome
TT	*tetanus toxoid
TTTS	*twin-to-twin transfusion syndrome
TURP	transurethral resection of the prostate
TUVP	transurethral vaporization of the prostate
TV	*tidal volume
TVT	*tension-free vaginal tape
U+E	urea and electrolytes
UC	*ulcerative colitis
UPPP	*uvulopalatopharyngoplasty
URT	upper respiratory tract
URTI	upper respiratory tract infection
US	ultrasound scan
UTI	urinary tract infection
UVA	ultraviolet radiation A
UVB	ultraviolet radiation B
UVPP	*uvulopalatopharyngoplasty
VF	ventricular fibrillation
VIP	vasoactive intestinal peptide
VMA	*vanillylmandelic acid
VSD	ventricular septal defect
VT	ventricular tachycardia
VTE	*venous thromboembolism
VUR	*vesicoureteric reflux
WBC	*white blood cell
WHO	*World Health Organization
YAG	yttrium–aluminium–garnet (laser)
ZIFT	zygote intrafallopian transfer

Appendix 17. The NMC code of professional conduct: Standards for conduct, performance, and ethics

(Nursing and Midwifery Council, March 2015)

Prioritize people

You put the interests of people using or needing nursing or midwifery services first. You make their care and safety your main concern and make sure that their dignity is preserved and their needs are recognized, assessed, and responded to. You make sure that those receiving care are treated with respect, that their rights are upheld, and that any discriminatory attitudes and behaviours towards those receiving care are challenged.

1 **Treat people as individuals and uphold their dignity**. To achieve this, you must:
  - 1.1 treat people with kindness, respect, and compassion
  - 1.2 make sure you deliver the fundamentals of care effectively
  - 1.3 avoid making assumptions and recognize diversity and individual choice
  - 1.4 make sure that any treatment, assistance, or care for which you are responsible is delivered without undue delay, and
  - 1.5 respect and uphold people's human rights.

2 **Listen to people and respond to their preferences and concerns**. To achieve this, you must:
  - 2.1 work in partnership with people to make sure you deliver care effectively. The fundamentals of care include, but are not limited to, nutrition, hydration, bladder and bowel care, physical handling, and making sure that those receiving care are kept in clean and hygienic conditions. They also include making sure that those receiving care have adequate access to nutrition and hydration, and making sure that you provide help to those who are not able to feed themselves or drink fluid unaided.
  - 2.2 recognize and respect the contribution that people can make to their own health and wellbeing
  - 2.3 encourage and empower people to share decisions about their treatment and care
  - 2.4 respect the level to which people receiving care want to be involved in decisions about their own health, wellbeing, and care
  - 2.5 respect, support, and document a person's right to accept or refuse care and treatment, and

2.6 recognize when people are anxious or in distress and respond compassionately and politely.

3 Make sure that people's physical, social, and psychological needs are assessed and responded to. To achieve this, you must:

3.1 pay special attention to promoting wellbeing, preventing ill health, and meeting the changing health and care needs of people during all life stages

3.2 recognize and respond compassionately to the needs of those who are in the last few days and hours of life

3.3 act in partnership with those receiving care, helping them to access relevant health and social care, information, and support when they need it, and

3.4 act as an advocate for the vulnerable, challenging poor practice and discriminatory attitudes and behaviour relating to their care.

4 Act in the best interests of people at all times. To achieve this, you must:

4.1 balance the need to act in the best interests of people at all times with the requirement to respect a person's right to accept or refuse treatment

4.2 make sure that you get properly informed consent and document it before carrying out any action

4.3 keep to all relevant laws about mental capacity that apply in the country in which you are practising, and make sure that the rights and best interests of those who lack capacity are still at the centre of the decision-making process, and

4.4 tell colleagues, your manager, and the person receiving care if you have a conscientious objection to a particular procedure and arrange for a suitably qualified colleague to take over responsibility for that person's care.

5 Respect people's right to privacy and confidentiality. As a nurse or midwife, you owe a duty of confidentiality to all those who are receiving care. This includes making sure that they are informed about their care and that information about them is shared appropriately. To achieve this, you must:

5.1 respect a person's right to privacy in all aspects of their care

5.2 make sure that people are informed about how and why information is used and shared by those who will be providing care

5.3 respect that a person's right to privacy and confidentiality continues after they have died

5.4 share necessary information with other healthcare professionals and agencies only when the interests of patient safety and public protection override the need for confidentiality, and
5.5 share with people, their families, and their carers, as far as the law allows, the information they want or need to know about their health, care, and ongoing treatment sensitively and in a way they can understand.

Practise effectively

You assess need and deliver or advise on treatment, or give help (including preventative or rehabilitative care), without too much delay and to the best of your abilities, on the basis of the best evidence available and best practice. You communicate effectively, keeping clear and accurate records and sharing skills, knowledge, and experience where appropriate. You reflect and act on any feedback you receive to improve your practice.

6 **Always practise in line with the best available evidence**. To achieve this, you must:
6.1 make sure that any information or advice given is evidence-based, including information relating to using any healthcare products or services, and
6.2 maintain the knowledge and skills you need for safe and effective practice.

7 **Communicate clearly**. To achieve this, you must:
7.1 use terms that people in your care, colleagues, and the public can understand
7.2 take reasonable steps to meet people's language and communication needs, providing, wherever possible, assistance to those who need help to communicate their own or other people's needs
7.3 use a range of verbal and non-verbal communication methods, and consider cultural sensitivities, to better understand and respond to people's personal and health needs
7.4 check people's understanding from time to time to keep misunderstanding or mistakes to a minimum, and
7.5 be able to communicate clearly and effectively in English.

8 **Work cooperatively**. To achieve this, you must:
8.1 respect the skills, expertise, and contributions of your colleagues, referring matters to them when appropriate
8.2 maintain effective communication with colleagues
8.3 keep colleagues informed when you are sharing the care of individuals with other healthcare professionals and staff

8.4 work with colleagues to evaluate the quality of your work and that of the team
8.5 work with colleagues to preserve the safety of those receiving care
8.6 share information to identify and reduce risk, and
8.7 be supportive of colleagues who are encountering health or performance problems. However, this support must never compromise or be at the expense of patient or public safety.

9 Share your skills, knowledge, and experience for the benefit of people receiving care and your colleagues. To achieve this, you must:
9.1 provide honest, accurate, and constructive feedback to colleagues
9.2 gather and reflect on feedback from a variety of sources, using it to improve your practice and performance
9.3 deal with differences of professional opinion with colleagues by discussion and informed debate, respecting their views and opinions, and behaving in a professional way at all times, and
9.4 support students' and colleagues' learning to help them develop their professional competence and confidence.

10 Keep clear and accurate records relevant to your practice. This includes but is not limited to patient records. It includes all records that are relevant to your scope of practice. To achieve this, you must:
10.1 complete all records at the time or as soon as possible after an event, recording if the notes are written some time after the event
10.2 identify any risks or problems that have arisen and the steps taken to deal with them, so that colleagues who use the records have all the information they need
10.3 complete all records accurately and without any falsification, taking immediate and appropriate action if you become aware that someone has not kept to these requirements
10.4 attribute any entries you make in any paper or electronic records to yourself, making sure they are clearly written, dated and timed, and do not include unnecessary abbreviations, jargon, or speculation
10.5 take all steps to make sure that all records are kept securely, and
10.6 collect, treat, and store all data and research findings appropriately.

11 Be accountable for your decisions to delegate tasks and duties to other people. To achieve this, you must:
11.1 only delegate tasks and duties that are within the other person's scope of competence, making sure that they fully understand your instructions
11.2 make sure that everyone you delegate tasks to is adequately supervised and supported so they can provide safe and compassionate care, and
11.3 confirm that the outcome of any task you have delegated to someone else meets the required standard.

12 Have in place an indemnity arrangement which provides appropriate cover for any practice you take on as a nurse or midwife in the United Kingdom. To achieve this, you must:

12.1 make sure that you have an appropriate indemnity arrangement in place relevant to your scope of practice. You make sure that patient and public safety is protected.

Preserve safety

You work within the limits of your competence, exercising your professional 'duty of candour' and raising concerns immediately whenever you come across situations that put patients or public safety at risk. You take necessary action to deal with any concerns where appropriate.

13 Recognize and work within the limits of your competence. To achieve this, you must:

13.1 accurately assess signs of normal or worsening physical and mental health in the person receiving care

13.2 make a timely and appropriate referral to another practitioner when it is in the best interests of the individual needing any action, care, or treatment

13.3 ask for help from a suitably qualified and experienced healthcare professional to carry out any action or procedure that is beyond the limits of your competence

13.4 take account of your own personal safety as well as the safety of people in your care, and

13.5 complete the necessary training before carrying out a new role.

14 Be open and candid with all service users about all aspects of care and treatment, including when any mistakes or harm have taken place. To achieve this, you must:

14.1 act immediately to put right the situation if someone has suffered actual harm for any reason or an incident has happened which had the potential for harm

14.2 explain fully and promptly what has happened, including the likely effects, and apologize to the person affected and, where appropriate, their advocate, family, or carers, and

14.3 document all these events formally and take further action (escalate) if appropriate so they can be dealt with quickly.

15 Always offer help if an emergency arises in your practice setting or anywhere else. To achieve this, you must:

15.1 only act in an emergency within the limits of your knowledge and competence

15.2 arrange, wherever possible, for emergency care to be accessed and provided promptly, and

15.3 take account of your own safety, the safety of others, and the availability of other options for providing care.

16 Act without delay if you believe that there is a risk to patient safety or public protection. To achieve this, you must:

16.1 raise and, if necessary, escalate any concerns you may have about patient or public safety, or the level of care people are receiving in your workplace or any other healthcare setting, and use the channels available to you in line with our guidance and your local working practices

16.2 raise your concerns immediately if you are being asked to practise beyond your role, experience, and training

16.3 tell someone in authority at the first reasonable opportunity if you experience problems that may prevent you working within the Code or other national standards, taking prompt action to tackle the causes of concern if you can

16.4 acknowledge and act on all concerns raised to you, investigating, escalating, or dealing with those concerns where it is appropriate for you to do so

16.5 not obstruct, intimidate, victimize, or in any way hinder a colleague, member of staff, person you care for, or member of the public who wants to raise a concern, and

16.6 protect anyone you have management responsibility for from any harm, detriment, victimization, or unwarranted treatment after a concern is raised.

17 Raise concerns immediately if you believe a person is vulnerable or at risk and needs extra support and protection. To achieve this, you must:

17.1 take all reasonable steps to protect people who are vulnerable or at risk from harm, neglect, or abuse

17.2 share information if you believe someone may be at risk of harm, in line with the laws relating to the disclosure of information, and

17.3 have knowledge of and keep to the relevant laws and policies about protecting and caring for vulnerable people.

18 Advise on, prescribe, supply, dispense, or administer medicines within the limits of your training and competence, the law, our guidance, and other relevant policies, guidance, and regulations. To achieve this, you must:

18.1 prescribe, advise on, or provide medicines or treatment, including repeat prescriptions (only if you are suitably qualified) if you have enough knowledge of that person's health and are satisfied that the medicines or treatment serve that person's health needs

18.2 keep to appropriate guidelines when giving advice on using controlled drugs and recording the prescribing, supply, dispensing, or administration of controlled drugs

18.3 make sure that the care or treatment you advise on, prescribe, supply, dispense, or administer for each person is compatible with any other care or treatment they are receiving, including (where possible) over-the-counter medicines

18.4 take all steps to keep medicines stored securely, and

18.5 wherever possible, avoid prescribing for yourself or for anyone with whom you have a close personal relationship.

19 Be aware of, and reduce as far as possible, any potential for harm associated with your practice. To achieve this, you must:

19.1 take measures to reduce as far as possible the likelihood of mistakes, near misses, harm, and the effect of harm if it takes place

19.2 take account of current evidence, knowledge, and developments in reducing mistakes and the effect of them and the impact of human factors and system failures

19.3 keep to and promote recommended practice in relation to controlling and preventing infection, and

19.4 take all reasonable personal precautions necessary to avoid any potential health risks to colleagues, people receiving care, and the public.

Promote professionalism and trust

You uphold the reputation of your profession at all times. You should display a personal commitment to the standards of practice and behaviour set out in the Code. You should be a model of integrity and leadership for others to aspire to. This should lead to trust and confidence in the profession from patients, people receiving care, other healthcare professionals, and the public.

20 Uphold the reputation of your profession at all times. To achieve this, you must:

20.1 keep to and uphold the standards and values set out in the Code

20.2 act with honesty and integrity at all times, treating people fairly and without discrimination, bullying, or harassment

20.3 be aware at all times of how your behaviour can affect and influence the behaviour of other people

20.4 keep to the laws of the country in which you are practising

20.5 treat people in a way that does not take advantage of their vulnerability or cause them upset or distress

20.6 stay objective and have clear professional boundaries at all times with people in your care (including those who have been in your care in the past) and their families and carers

20.7 make sure you do not express your personal beliefs (including political, religious, or moral beliefs) to people in an inappropriate way

20.8 act as a role model of professional behaviour for students and newly qualified nurses and midwives to aspire to

20.9 maintain the level of health you need to carry out your professional role, and

20.10 use all forms of spoken, written, and digital communication (including social media and networking sites) responsibly, respecting the right to privacy of others at all times.

21 **Uphold your position as a registered nurse or midwife**. To achieve this, you must:

21.1 refuse all but the most trivial gifts, favours, or hospitality, as accepting them could be interpreted as an attempt to gain preferential treatment

21.2 never ask for or accept loans from anyone in your care or anyone close to them

21.3 act with honesty and integrity in any financial dealings you have with everyone you have a professional relationship with, including people in your care

21.4 make sure that any advertisements, publications, or published material you produce or have produced for your professional services are accurate, responsible, ethical, do not mislead or exploit vulnerabilities, and accurately reflect your relevant skills, experience, and qualifications

21.5 never use your professional status to promote causes that are not related to health, and

21.6 cooperate with the media only when it is appropriate to do so, and then always protecting the confidentiality and dignity of people receiving treatment or care.

22 **Fulfil all registration requirements**. To achieve this, you must:

22.1 meet any reasonable requests so we can oversee the registration process

22.2 keep to our prescribed hours of practice and carry out continuing professional development activities, and

22.3 keep your knowledge and skills up to date, taking part in appropriate and regular learning and professional development activities that aim to maintain and develop your competence and improve your performance.

23 Cooperate with all investigations and audits. This includes investigations or audits either against you or relating to others, whether individuals or organizations. It also includes cooperating with requests to act as a witness in any hearing that forms part of an investigation, even after you have left the register. To achieve this, you must:

- 23.1 cooperate with any audits of training records, registration records, or other relevant audits that we may want to carry out to make sure you are still fit to practise
- 23.2 tell both us and any employers as soon as you can about any caution or charge against you, or if you have received a conditional discharge in relation to, or have been found guilty of, a criminal offence (other than a protected caution or conviction)
- 23.3 tell any employers you work for if you have had your practice restricted or had any other conditions imposed on you by us or any other relevant body
- 23.4 tell us and your employers at the first reasonable opportunity if you are or have been disciplined by any regulatory or licensing organization, including those who operate outside of the professional healthcare environment, and
- 23.5 give your NMC Pin when any reasonable request for it is made.

24 Respond to any complaints made against you professionally. To achieve this, you must:

- 24.1 never allow someone's complaint to affect the care that is provided to them, and
- 24.2 use all complaints as a form of feedback and an opportunity for reflection and learning to improve practice.

25 Provide leadership to make sure people's wellbeing is protected and to improve their experiences of the healthcare system. To achieve this, you must:

- 25.1 identify priorities, manage time, staff, and resources effectively, and deal with risk to make sure that the quality of care or service you deliver is maintained and improved, putting the needs of those receiving care or services first, and
- 25.2 support any staff you may be responsible for to follow the Code at all times. They must have the knowledge, skills, and competence for safe practice; and understand how to raise any concerns linked to any circumstances where the Code has, or could be, broken.